TRAVEL MEDICINE

Commissioning Editor: Tom Hartman
Project Development Manager: Louise Cook
Project Manager: Jess Thompson
Illustration Manager: Mick Ruddy
Design Manager: Jayne Jones
Illustrator: Marion Tasker

TRAVEL MEDICINE

EDITED BY

JAY S. KEYSTONE MD MSC (CTM) FRCPC

Professor, Department of Medicine, University of Toronto; Staff Physican,
Center for Travel and Tropical Medicine, Toronto General Hospital, Toronto,
ON, Canada

PHYLLIS E. KOZARSKY MD

Professor of Medicine, Infectious Diseases; Chief, Travelers' Health and Tropical
Medicine Section, Emory University School of Medicine, Atlanta, GA, USA

DAVID O. FREEDMAN MD

Professor of Medicine and Epidemiology/International Health,
Division of Geographic Medicine, University of Alabama at Birmingham; Director,
University of Alabama Travelers Health Clinic, Birmingham, AL, USA

HANS D. NOTHDURFT MD

Professor, Department of Infectious Diseases and Tropical Medicine;
Head, University Travel Clinic, University of Munich, Munich, Germany

BRADLEY A. CONNOR MD

Clinical Associate Professor of Medicine, Division of Gastroenterology and
Hepatology, Weill Medical College of Cornell University; Medical Director,
The New York Center for Travel and Tropical Medicine, New York, NY, USA;
President, International Society of Travel Medicine

M Mosby

Edinburgh ■ London ■ New York ■ Oxford ■ Philadelphia ■ St Louis ■ Sydney ■ Toronto 2004

MOSBY
An imprint of Elsevier Limited

First published 2004
   Reprinted 2004, 2005, 2007

ISBN 978-0-323-02521-8

British Library Cataloguing in Publication Data
A catalogue record for this book is available from the British Library

Library of Congress Cataloging in Publication Data
A catalog record for this book is available from the Library of Congress

Notice
Medical knowledge is constantly changing. Standard safety precautions must be followed, but as new research and clinical experience broaden our knowledge, changes in treatment and drug therapy may become necessary or appropriate. Readers are advised to check the most current product information provided by the manufacturer of each drug to be administered to verify the recommended dose, the method and duration of administration, and contraindications. It is the responsibility of the practitioner, relying on experience and knowledge of the patient, to determine dosages and the best treatment for each individual patient. Neither the Publisher nor the editors/contributor assumes any liability for any injury and/or damage to persons or property arising from this publication.

The Publisher

 ELSEVIER   your source for books, journals and multimedia in the health sciences
www.elsevierhealth.com

Working together to grow
libraries in developing countries
www.elsevier.com | www.bookaid.org | www.sabre.org
ELSEVIER   BOOK AID International   Sabre Foundation

The Publisher's policy is to use **paper manufactured from sustainable forests**

Printed in Spain

CONTENTS

LIST OF CONTRIBUTORS

Rebecca Wolfe Acosta RN MPH
Executive Director, Travelers' Medical
Service of New York, NY, USA

John W. Aldis MD MPH&TM
Research Physician, Special
Immunizations Program, US Army
Medical Research Institute of Infectious
Diseases, Ft. Detrick, MD, USA

Susan A. Anderson MD MS
Travel, Tropical and Wilderness
Medicine Consultant, Clinical Assistant
Professor of Medicine, Division of
Infectious Disease and Geographic
Medicine, Stanford University School Of
Medicine, Palo Alto Medical Foundation,
CA, USA

Vernon Ansdell MD
Director, Travel and Tropical Medicine,
Hawaii Permanente Medical Group Inc.,
Honolulu, HI, USA

Howard Backer MD MPH
Acting Chief, Immunization Branch,
California Department of Health
Services, Berkeley, CA, USA

Michael Bagshaw MB MRCS FFOM
DAVMed
Head of Medical Services, British
Airways, Harmondsworth, UK

Trish L. Batchelor MBBS FRACGP MPH
(Trop Med)
Medical Officer, CIWEC Travel Medicine
Centre, Kathmandu and Medical Advisor
to The Travel Doctor New Zealand,
Kathmandu, Nepal

Carrie Beallor MD CCFP DTM&H
Clinical Consultant, Center for Travel
and Tropical Medicine, University Health
Network, University of Toronto,
Toronto, ON, Canada

Ronald H. Behrens MD FRCP
Consultant in Travel and Tropical
Medicine, Travel Clinic, Hospital for
Tropical Diseases, London, UK

Steven J. Brewster MD MPH
Chief, Preventive Medicine, Family
Physician Lieutenant Colonel US Army
Medical Corps, Department of
Preventative Medicine, Fort Drum,
NY, USA

William B. Bunn MD JD MPH
Vice President – Health, Safety, Security
and Productivity, International Truck
and Engine Corporation, Warrenville,
IL, USA

Michael V. Callahan MD DTM&H
MSPH
Assistant Professor of International
Health
Center for International Health, Boston
University School of Public Health,
Center for International Health &
Development, Boston, MA, USA

Francesco Castelli MD
Associate Professor of Infectious
Diseases, Institute for Infectious and
Tropical Diseases, University of Brescia,
Brescia, Italy

Eric Caumes MD
Professor of Medicine, Department of
Infectious and Tropical Diseases,
Hôpital Pitie – Salpetrière, Paris, France

Martin Cetron MD
Deputy Director, Division of Global
Migration and Quarantine, Centers for
Disease Control and Prevention;
Associate Professor, Division of
Infectious Diseases, Department of
Medicine, Emory University School of
Medicine, Rollins School of Public
Health, Atlanta, GA, USA

Jean Francois Chicoine MD FRCP(c)
Scientific Consultant, Travel Medisys,
Medisys Health Group Inc., Montreal,
QC, Canada

Jan C. Clerinx MD DTM
Lecturer in Tropical Medicine,
Department of Clinical Sciences, Prince
Leopold Institute of Tropical Medicine,
Antwerp, Belgium

Bradley A. Connor MD
Clinical Associate Professor of Medicine,
Division of Gastroenterology and
Hepatology, Weill Medical College of
Cornell University; Medical Director,
The New York Center for Travel and
Tropical Medicine, New York, NY,
USA; President, International Society of
Travel Medicine

Richard Dawood MD DTM&H
Specialist in Travel Medicine, Fleet Street
Clinic, London, UK

Thomas E. Dietz MD
Clinical Assistant Professor, Department
of Family Medicine, Oregon Health and
Science University, Portland, OR, USA

Yoram Epstein PhD
Professor of Physiology, Heller Institute
of Medical Research, Sheba Medical
Center; Tel Hashomer, Israel

Charles D. Ericsson MD
Professor and Clinical Director, Division
of Infectious Diseases, University of
Texas-Houston Medical School,
Houston, TX, USA

Philip R. Fischer MD DTM&H
Professor of Pediatrics, Department of
Pediatrics and Adolescent Medicine,
Mayo Medical School, Mayo Clinic,
Rochester, MN, USA

Mark S. Fradin MD
Clinical Associate Professor of
Dermatology, University of North
Carolina at Chapel Hill, Chapel Hill,
NC, USA

David O. Freedman MD
Professor of Medicine and
Epidemiology/International Health,
Division of Geographic Medicine,
University of Alabama at Birmingham;
Director, University of Alabama
Travelers Health Clinic, Birmingham,
AL, USA

Ken L. Gamble MD
Lecturer, University of Toronto, Center for Travel and Tropical Medicine, Toronto; Executive Director, Missionary Health Institute, North York, ON, Canada

Martin P. Grobusch MD MSc DTM&H
Department of Parasitology, Institute of Tropical Medicine, Eberhard Karls University, Tuebingen, Germany

Peter H. Hackett MD
President, ISMM; Associate Clinical Professor, Division of Emergency Medicine, University of Colorado Health Sciences Center, Ridgway, CO, USA

Davidson H. Hamer MD FACP
Assistant Professor of Medicine and Nutrition, Tufts University School of Medicine and Friedman School of Nutrition Science and Policy; Adjunct Assistant Professor of International Health, Boston University School of Public Health, Division of Geographic Medicine and Infectious Diseases, Tufts-New England Medical Center, Boston, MA, USA

Urban Hellgren MD
Associate Professor, Karolinske Institut, Division of Infectious Diseases, Huddinge University Hospital, Stockholm, Sweden

David R. Hill MD DTM&H
Professor of Medicine and Director of National Travel Health Network and Centre, Hospital for Tropical Diseases, London, UK

Jessica Herzstein MD MPH
Global Medical Director, Air Products and Chemicals, Inc., Allentown, PA, USA

Elaine C. Jong MD
Clinical Professor of Medicine and Director, Hall Health Primary Care Center; Medical Director, Campus Health Services; Co-Director, UW Travel and Tropical Medicine Service and Hall Health Travel Medicine Clinic, University of Washington School of Medicine, Seattle, WA, USA

Kevin C. Kain MD FRCPC
Professor of Medicine, University of Toronto, Canada Research Chair in Molecular Parasitology, Director for Travel and Tropical Medicine, Toronto General Hospital, Toronto, ON, Canada

Jay S. Keystone MD MSc (CTM) FRCPC
Professor, Department of Medicine, University of Toronto; Staff Physician, Center for Travel and Tropical Medicine, Toronto General Hospital Toronto, ON, Canada

Amy D. Klion MD
Staff Physician, Laboratory of Parasitic Disease, National Institutes of Allergy and Infectious Diseases, National Institutes of Health, Bethesda, MD, USA

Herwig Kollaritsch MD DTM
Head of Department and Associate Professor, Department of Specific Prophylaxis and Tropical Medicine, Institute of Pathophysiology, University of Vienna, Vienna, Austria

Phyllis E. Kozarsky MD
Professor of Medicine, Infectious Diseases; Chief, Travelers' Health and Tropical Medicine Section, Emory University School of Medicine, Atlanta, GA, USA

Andrea Kropf Dipl.-Psych
Psychotherapist, Berlin, Germany

Susan M. Kuhn MD MSc DTM&H FRCPC
Clinical Assistant Professor, Departments of Pediatrics and Medicine, University of Calgary; Director, Odyssey Travel and Tropical Medicine Clinic, Calgary, AB, Canada

Brian R. Landzberg MD
Clinical Assistant Professor of Medicine, Weill Medical College of Cornell University, New York, NY, USA

Edith R. Lederman MD
US Naval Medical Research Unit No. 2. Jakarta, Indonesia

Thomas Löscher MD
Professor of Internal Medicine and Tropical Medicine, Department of Infectious Diseases and Tropical Medicine, University of Munich, Munich, Germany

Deborah M. Lovell-Hawker BA PhD D Clin, Psy
Principal Clinical Psychologist, Oxford University Psychiatry Department, Warneford Hospital, Oxford, UK

Sheila M. Mackell MD
Pediatrician & Travel Medicine Consultant, Mountain View Pediatrics, Flagstaff, AZ, USA

Alan J. Magill MD FACP
Science Director, Walter Reed Army Institute of Research, Silver Spring, MD, USA

Stephan Mann MD MPH
Medical Director, Corporate Occupational Health Solutions, Corp OHS, Frederick, MD, USA

Alberto Matteelli MD
Responsible Community Medicine Unit, Institute of Infectious and Tropical Diseases, University of Brescia, Brescia, Italy

Anne E. McCarthy MD FRCPC DTM&H
Assistant Professor, Division of Infectious Diseases, University of Ottawa, Ottawa, ON, Canada

Marilynne McKay MD
Professor Emerita of Dermatology, Emory University School of Medicine, Atlanta; Chairman of Dermatology, Lovelace Health System, Albuquerque, NM, USA

Susan L.F. McLellan MD MPH
Associate Professor of Medicine, Infectious Diseases Section, School of Medicine; Clinical Assistant Professor of Tropical Medicine, Department of Tropical Medicine, SPHTM, Tulane University Health Sciences Center, New Orleans, LA, USA

Maria D. Mileno MD
Associate Professor of Medicine and Director, Travel Medicine Service, Department of Medicine, The Miriam Hospital, Providence, RI, USA

Daniel S. Moran PhD
Doctor of Physiology, Heller Institute of Medical Research, Sheba Medical Center, Tel Hashomer, Israel

Helmut Müller-Ortstein MD
Psychiatrist and Psychotherapist, Munich, Germany

Cloe Murray RN BSN COHN-S
Nurse Consultant, Hill-Rom Corporation, Batesville, IN, USA

Hans D. Nothdurft MD
Professor, Department of Infectious Diseases and Tropical Medicine, and Head, University Travel Clinic, University of Munich, Munich, Germany

Luis Ostrosky-Zeichner MD
Assistant Professor of Medicine,
Division of Infectious Diseases,
University of Texas-Houston Medical
School, Houston, TX, USA

John Piacentino MD MPH
Regional Chief Physician , Corporate
Occupational Health Solutions,
North Bethesda, MD, USA

Cecilia Pizzocolo MD
Fellow, Institute for Infectious and
Tropical Diseases, University of Brescia,
Brescia, Italy

Pamela Rendi-Wagner MD MSc
DTM&H
Assistant Professor, Department of
Specific Prophylaxis and Tropical
Medicine, Institute of Pathophysiology,
University of Vienna, Vienna, Austria

Nuccia Saleri MD
Fellow Infectious Diseases, Institute of
Infectious and Tropical Diseases,
Brescia, Italy

Patricia Schlagenhauf MD
Research Scientist, WHO Collaborating
Centre for Travelers' Health, Division of
Epidemiology and Communicable
Diseases, Institute for Social and
Preventative Medicine, University of
Zurich, Zurich, Switzerland

Eli Schwartz MD DTMH
Director, Center of Geographic Medicine
and Department of Medicine, Sheba
Medical Center, Tel Hashomer, Israel

David R. Shlim MD
Medical Director, Jackson Hole Travel
and Tropical Medicine, Kelly, WY, USA

Alan M. Spira MD, DTM&H, FRSTM
Medical Director, The Travel Medicine
Center, Beverly Hills CA, USA

Robert Steffen MD
Director; Professor of Travel Medicine,
WHO Collaborating Centre for Travelers'
Health, Division of Communicable
Disease, Institute for Social and
Preventative Medicine, University of
Zurich, Zurich, Switzerland

Kathryn N. Suh MD FRCPC
Lecturer, Department of Medicine,
Division of Infectious Diseases, Queen's
University, Kingston, ON, Canada

Frederick J. Summers MD
Regional Psychiatrist for Latin America
for Department of State, American
Embassy Peru

David N. Taylor MD
Research Professor
Department of International Health,
John Hopkins University,
Bloomberg School of Public Health,
Baltimore, MD, USA

Dominique Tessier MD CCFP FCFP
Medical Director, Medisys Travel Health
Clinic and Travelmedisys.com, Montreal,
QC, Canada

Thomas H. Valk MD MPH
President and CEO, VEI Inc., Great Falls,
VA, USA

Alfons Van Gompel MD DTM
Associate Professor of Tropical Medicine,
Institute of Tropical Medicine, Antwerp,
Belgium

Abinash Virk MD DTM&H
Assistant Professor of Medicine, Mayo
Graduate School of Medicine; Director,
Travel and Tropical Medicine Clinic,
Mayo Clinic Consultant, Division of
Infectious Diseases, Mayo Clinic,
Rochester, MN, USA

Michelle Weinberg MD MPH
Medical Epidemiologist, Division of
Global Migration and Quarantine,
US Centers for Disease Control and
Prevention, Atlanta, GA, USA

Eric A. Weiss MD FACEP
Assistant Professor of Emergency
Medicine; Associate Director of Trauma;
Chair, Disaster Committee and
Bioterrorism Task Force, Stanford
University Medical Center, Palo Alto,
CA, USA

Eric L. Weiss MD DTM&H
Assistant Professor of Emergency
Medicine & Infectious Diseases; Director,
Stanford Travel Medicine; Medical
Director, Stanford Life Flight; Division of
Emergency Medicine, Palo Alto, CA, USA

Jeffrey Wilks BA(Hons) PhD LLB
(Hons) Grad Dip Legal Practice
Professor of Tourism, Centre for
Tourism and Risk Management,
The University of Queensland, Ipswich,
QLD, Australia

Mary E. Wilson MD FACP
Associate Professor of Medicine, Harvard
Medical School, Mount Auburn Hospital,
Cambridge, MA, USA

Martin S. Wolfe MD DCMT FACP
Director, Travelers' Medical Service of
Washington; Clinical Professor of
Medicine, George Washington Medical
School, Georgetown Medical School,
Washington, DC, USA

ACKNOWLEDGEMENTS

The editors wish to acknowledge Dr. Jamie Macguire for his excellent, extensive, and very pertinent comments on the glossary in this book. A special thank you to Deborah Russell and Louise Cook from Elsevier whose vision, enthusiasm, dedication and sense of humour helped to bring this book to fruition. Above all, thank you to our families and partners for their everlasting patience and understanding.

PREFACE

Some people assert, and we would agree, that travel is necessary.

'We all live in the same neighborhood now and can perhaps better come to terms with our various beliefs and ways of life through travel' (Lyer P. *Time Magazine, Essay, page 82 May 27, 2002*).

Physical and psychological challenges do face us when we venture outside of our norms, and the optimal way of dealing with these issues is to educate ourselves in advance. The healthy traveler travels again, whereas the unhealthy traveler does not, nor do the family, friends and colleagues who are expected to listen, in great detail, about 'the vacation from Hell'.

The global village is a reality indeed. When an event affects the population in one part of our world, it inevitably will have an impact on all others.

'Virtually any destination can be reached from any other in only 36 hours of travel. This 36-hour window is well within the incubation period of most infectious diseases, thus providing ample opportunity for disease transmission to travelers and by them.' (S. Ostroff, 7th conference of the International Society of Travel Medicine, Innsbruck Austria, 2001).

The recent outbreak of SARS is a dramatic example of this concept. One traveler, an infected physician from Southern China, spread the newly described coronavirus infection to his contacts, and through them in a matter of weeks to more than 16 countries around the world. The evolution of travel medicine as a unique specialty owes its origins to the marked increase in global travel for tourism, business, education, family reunification, and migration, and to the health risks posed by these population movements.

As travel medicine is in its formative years, we have a unique opportunity to create this textbook to meet the hands-on needs of travel medicine practitioners. We have thus chosen to write this textbook with a unique purpose in mind. This book goes far beyond merely supplementing courses of instruction in school or post-graduate training, or serving as a reference book. It is a 'how to' book which can be read from beginning to end as a complete course in travel medicine.

The job of the travel medicine practitioner is to conduct an individualized risk assessment, educate the traveler about the risks, and counsel them regarding prevention of illnesses and injuries. Also, travelers may receive advice on self-treatment of a variety of ailments. Limited post-travel triage information is included in this book for those providers who care for returned travelers. The purpose of triage is to ensure that the ill-returned traveler is referred, where necessary, for immediate evaluation to avoid a potentially life threatening situation or serious public health risk that may be unrecognized by an unqualified practitioner.

This text provides a diverse approach to the presentation of material via wide-ranging and highly effective algorithms, photographs, sample tools, and other graphics. The book distinguishes itself through its high quality artwork that supplements and amplifies learning. Additionally, each chapter contains a list of 'key points' that summarize the most important issues discussed within the chapter. Therefore, it is hoped that the well-designed, practical approach taken by the authors will make this book an essential resource that the travel health provider will keep close at hand.

Jay S. Keystone
Phyllis E. Kozarsky
David O. Freedman
Hans D. Nothdurft
Bradley A. Connor
2003

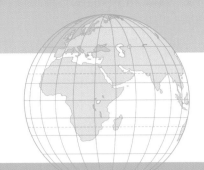

CHAPTER 1   Introduction to Travel Medicine

Phyllis E. Kozarsky and Jay S. Keystone

KEYPOINTS

- Despite the risks of emerging and re-emerging infectious diseases and the recent threat of terrorism, international tourist arrivals remain high, as does travel from industrialized to developing countries

- Travel medicine is the discipline devoted to the maintenance of the health of international travelers through health promotion and disease prevention

- The global focus and knowledge base of travel medicine distinguishes this unique specialty from most other fields of medicine and nursing

- There is a continuing need for improvement in knowledge among those giving pre-travel health advice

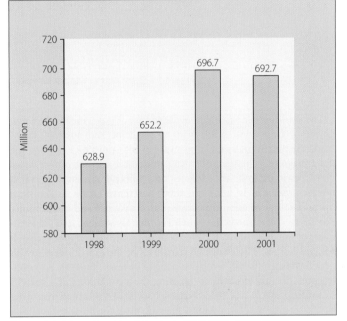

Figure 1.1 International tourist arrivals 1998–2001 (WTO, 2001).

INTRODUCTION

Travel remains one of the largest 'businesses' in the world, in spite of the global threat of emerging and re-emerging infectious diseases and the recent concerns about international terrorism. According to data released in June 2002 by the World Tourism Organization, international tourist arrivals amounted to 693 million in 2001,[1] only 4 million down from the 697 million of 2000 due to the weakening economies of major tourism markets and the impact of the terrorist attacks of September 11, 2001 (Figs 1.1 and 1.2). To keep this in perspective, the number of international tourist arrivals was only 50 million in 1950, 150 million in 1970, and 500 million in 1993.

Now, more people than ever are traveling to exotic and remote destinations; in 1999 over 75 million traveled from industrialized to developing countries. This represented a 50% increase from 1993 (Robert Steffen, personal communication 2002). In 2001, the travel health website at the Centers for Disease Control and Prevention (CDC) received 13.7 million requests for documents, a 60% increase over the previous year (Leisa Weld, CDC, personal communication 2002).

With the movement of people over centuries of exploration, documentation exists for the spread of diseases such as the plague, yellow fever, smallpox, malaria and cholera around the world (Fig. 1.3).[2] It is clear, however, that today's traveler faces not only the ailments of years gone by, but also the threat of acquiring new, emerging, and re-emerging illnesses such as HIV, leptospirosis, variant CJD, and multi-drug resistant malaria. Severe Acute Respiratory Syndrome (SARS) is the latest emerging infectious disease that was spread globally in a matter of weeks entirely by infected travelers and their contacts. Fears of contagion and global advisories from the WHO all but eliminated

tourist travel to affected countries and contributed to the bankruptcy of some of the world's major airlines.[3,4] In addition, and far more important in terms of traveler mortality, is the threat of problems such as injury (due to motor vehicle accidents) or the exacerbation of underlying illness (e.g., cardiac disease). Given these challenges, during the 1970s and 1980s, several visionary clinicians began exploring the medical requirements and recommendations that would better ensure healthy travel. This initial dabbling in the study and practice of the prevention of travel-related illness has now grown along with the escalation of travel itself, and has become a highly specialized area of medicine.

Thus travel medicine is the discipline devoted to the maintenance of the health of international travelers through health promotion and disease prevention. It is still a fledgling multidisciplinary field encompassing a wide variety of specialties and subspecialties, including infectious and tropical diseases, public health and preventive medicine, primary care, and geographic, occupational, military, and wilderness medicine. Recently, travel medicine has broadened to include migration medicine, immigrant health, and a focus on the impact of travel on receiving countries. Unlike many other health-care specialties, depending upon the country, travel medicine is often practiced by nurses and physicians alike.

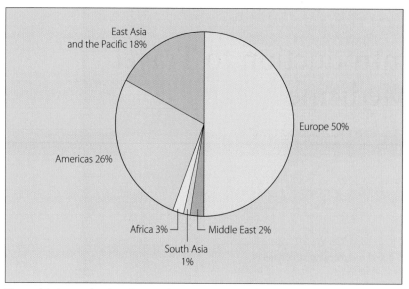

Figure 1.2 International tourism receipts: market share 2001 (WTO, 2001).

The worldwide focus and knowledge base of travel medicine distinguishes it from most other fields of medicine and nursing. Travel medicine practitioners must be aware of infectious disease risks and their magnitude, patterns of drug resistance, current outbreaks of illness, civil and military conflicts, and political barriers to travel at border crossings. In addition, they must have access to the most up-to-date information on travel-related vaccines and medications. For some travel medicine providers, the assessment and management of the ill-returned traveler is an important component of their responsibilities. The challenge remains that for practitioners in this new field, there is still a relative paucity of texts, journals, and conferences that are devoted to teaching the new aspects and reviews of information in the field. National societies in various countries have thus emerged to provide a meeting place for those with similar interests in travel health, and The International Society of Travel Medicine was started just over a decade ago with a mission to address educational needs for professionals and the public. Their conferences, journal, and newsletter have provided a central place for the gathering of this unique body of information and for travel health professionals themselves from across the world. In addition, along with the annual or biennial publication of authoritative information

from institutions such as the World Health Organization and the Centers for Disease Control and Prevention (CDC), new global surveillance systems, including GeoSentinel and TropNet Europ, have been developed to track travel-related morbidity so that all can better understand the emerging health problems related to population movements.

Though the first international conference of travel medicine practitioners took place in 1988, the beginnings of travel medicine may truly have dated back hundreds, or even thousands of years, when healers or practitioners advised explorers, missionaries and military conquerors of the extreme hazards of their occupations. Today, the focus of travel medicine is on recreational tourists, business persons, overseas volunteers, missionaries, and the military. More recently, however, the field has expanded to include migrant populations fleeing civil and military conflicts or looking for political asylum or economic opportunities. In addition, the current era of the increasing popularity of ecotourism and extreme travel has added a new dimension to the field, including the challenges faced as practitioners counsel increasing numbers of immunocompromised individuals, such as those with HIV, cancer, autoimmune disease, or organ transplants.

The complexity and variety of travel itineraries, combined with the many health issues of enthusiastic travelers of all ages, shapes and sizes, ensure that it takes much longer than appreciated to acquire the expertise necessary to provide travel medicine services. It is no longer adequate for advice to pass informally from friends, family, or travel counselors to travelers – or even from health-care specialists in other fields to their patients – warning them only about the potential hazards of tap water. Indeed, data gathered over the last decade have clearly shown that health information for travel continues to be sought by far less numbers than it should. Depending on the study of travelers to malarious areas, 50% or more seek travel health advice, but far fewer adhere to recommendations for chemoprophylaxis and insect protection.[5–7] Recent data obtained from the CDC have shown that less than one third of US travelers to areas of the world at risk for yellow fever have received the vaccine (Martin Cetron, personal communication, 2002).

The key now is to increase awareness of this field, to educate the clinician, and to promote greater use of travel medicine experts. The chapters in this textbook address the most important issues in this rapidly growing and ever-changing field, and represent an important step in the education of all travel medicine providers.

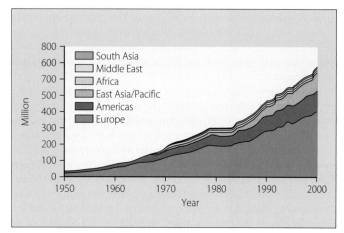

Figure 1.3 Population growth and time to circumnavigate the globe.[3]

REFERENCES

1. World Tourism Organization. *Facts and Figures.* Madrid: World Tourism Organization; 2001: www.world-tourism.org.
2. Murphy GG, Nathanson NM. New and Emerging Virus Diseases. *Seminars in Virology* 1994; **5**:87-102.
3. Lee N, Hui D, Wu A, et al. A major outbreak of Severe Acute Respiratory Syndrome in Hong Kong. *N Engl J Med.* 2003; **348**:1986–94
4. Potanen SM, Low DE, Henry B. Identification of Severe Acute Respiratory Syndrome in Canada. *N Engl J Med* 2003; **348**:1995–2005
5. Provost S, Soto JC. Predictors of pretravel consultation in tourists from Quebec (Canada). *J Travel Med* 2001; **8**(2):66–75.
6. Lobel HO, Baker MA, Gras FA, *et al.* Use of malaria prevention measures by North American and European travelers to East Africa. *J Travel Med* 2001; **8**(4):167–172.
7. dos Santos CC, Anvar A, Keystone JS, Kain KC. Survey of use of malaria prevention measures by Canadians visiting India. *CMAJ* 1999; **160**(2):195–200.

CHAPTER 2   Epidemiology: Morbidity and Mortality in Travelers

Robert Steffen

KEYPOINTS

- Travel health risks are dependent on the itinerary, season and duration of travel, purpose of travel, lifestyle, and host characteristics

- Motor vehicle injuries and drowning are the major causes of preventable deaths in travelers, while malaria remains the most frequent cause of infectious disease deaths

- Complications of cardiovascular conditions are a major cause of deaths in travelers as well. More recent concerns include the greater recognition of the risk of pulmonary embolism which occurs very rarely among long distance air travelers

- Travelers' diarrhea (TD) remains the most frequent illness among travelers; risk of TD can be divided basically into three risk categories based on destination

- According to surveys, participation in casual sex without the regular use of condom protection is practiced by up to 19% of male travelers when enroute alone

INTRODUCTION

Compared with staying home, mortality and morbidity is increased in those traveling, especially when their destination is in developing countries. Travel health risks vary greatly according to:

Where
- industrialized versus developing countries
- city or highly developed resort versus off-the-tourist-trail.

When
- season of travel, e.g., rainy versus dry

How long
- duration of stay abroad

What for (purpose of travel)
- tourism versus business versus rural work versus visiting friends or relatives (VFR)
- other (military, airline crew, adoption, etc.)

How (travel characteristics)
- hygiene standard expected: high (e.g., multistar hotels) versus low (e.g., low budget backpackers)
- special activities: high altitude trekking, diving, hunting, camping, etc.

Host characteristics
- healthy versus pre-existing condition, non-immune versus (semi)-immune.

This chapter will concentrate on the available epidemiological data associated with travel health risks in general; it will not describe the epidemiology of individual diseases. The data are often unsatisfactory because they are incomplete, old, or they were generated in studies, which may have been biased. Among the infectious health risks only those will be mentioned about which travel related incidence rates have been published. The reader should consult tropical medicine textbooks for information about less common travel-related infections, such as, trypanosomiasis.

CORNERSTONES OF TRAVEL HEALTH EPIDEMIOLOGY

As shown in Figure 2.1 health problems in travelers are frequent. Three out of four Swiss travelers to developing countries had some health impairment, defined as the use of any therapeutic medication or reporting to have been subjectively ill. At first glance, this proportion is alarming, but also 50% of short-term travelers who crossed the Northern Atlantic had health impairments, here most often constipation.[1] According to other surveys, 22–64% of Finnish, Scottish or American travelers reported some health complaint, usually dependent on the destination. Also the season may play a role as exemplified in Scottish Package tourists to eastern or southern Europe, where the illness rates in summer were 57% and 77% respectively, compared with much lower rates during other seasons (12% and 32% respectively). A larger follow-up study shows that only few of these self-reported health problems are severe. Less than 10% of travelers to developing countries consulted a doctor either abroad or after returning home, or were confined to bed due to travel related illness or an accident; less than 1% was hospitalized, usually for a few days only.[1] But it is still disturbing that more than 14% of such travelers are incapacitated. Among visitors to Paris, less than 1% attended emergency medical care.[2] The most tragic consequence of travel is death abroad, which occurs in approximately 1/100 000; in trekkers in Nepal a 15 times higher risk of dying has been documented.

A study based on medical insurance claims among World Bank staff and consultants demonstrates that business travel may also pose health risks beyond exposure to infectious diseases and that medical claims are increasing with the increasing frequency of travel[3] (Fig. 2.1).

MORTALITY

At first sight, data on the primary cause of deaths abroad appear contradictory. While some studies claim that accidents are the leading cause of death, others demonstrate the predominance of cardiovascular events.[4] These differences are primarily due to the varied examined populations and destinations. Southern Europe, Florida and parts of the Caribbean are favorite destinations of senior travelers, in whom elevated mortality rates due to a variety of natural causes are to be expected, whereas in developing destinations, the risk of fatal accidents is clearly higher. Assaults or terrorism are infrequent causes of death at present (Table 2.1).

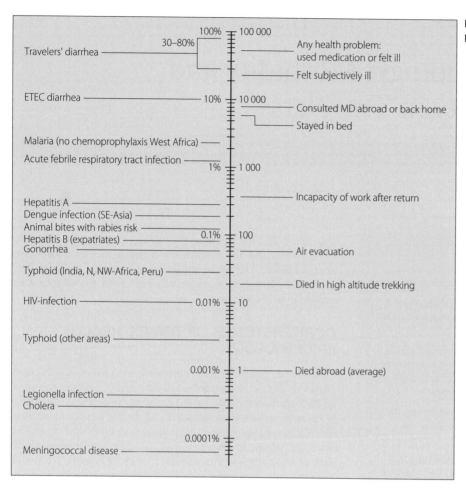

Figure 2.1 Monthly incidence rates of health problems during stays in developing countries.

Accidents

Deaths abroad due to injuries are two- to three-fold higher in 15–44-year-old travelers than in the same age group in industrialized countries.[4] Fatal accidents are mostly due to motor vehicle injury. Per 10 000 motor vehicles, 1.4 deaths per annum are reported in the UK, compared with 9–67 in Asia and 20–118 in Africa. Motorbikes are frequently implicated (partly because in many countries there is no obligation to wear a helmet); alcohol often plays a role. Tourists are reported to be several times more likely than local drivers are to have accidents.[5]

Drowning is also a major cause of death and accounted for 16% of all deaths (due to injuries) among US travelers. The reasons for these included alcohol, the presence of unrecognized currents or undertow, and being swept out to sea.

Table 2.1 Causes of death among different populations of travelers (%)

Origin of traveler Destination of traveler	USA (PCV) Developing country	USA Anywhere	Swiss Europe	Swiss Overseas	Foreign USA	Australia Overseas	Scotland Abroad
Year of travel	1962–1983	1975/1984	1987	1987	1991	1995	1991
Total number of deaths	185	2463	247	68	17,988	421	952
Cardiovascular	8.0	49.0	14.0	15.0	45.0	35.0	68.9
Infection	5.0	1.0	–	3.0	–	2.4	3.6
Other illness	8.0	?	2.0	9.0	–	–	–
Accidents							
Road accident	36.0	7.0	13.0	12.0	37.0	28.3	–
Air crash	5.0	2.0	4.0	12.0	7.0	–	–
Drowning	14.0	4.0	4.0	9.0	15.0	–	–
Other injuries	23.0	12.0	2.0	11.0	23.0	26.0	20.7
Unknown	–	25.0	58.0	29.0	–	17.0	7.0

PCV, Peace Corps Volunteers (US).

Kidnapping and killing has been increasing, but this usually is limited to employees of international and nongovernmental organizations. Fatal assaults on tourists and terrorism may occur anywhere, not only in developing countries.

Animals are a relatively uncommon cause of death among travelers. There are now some 60 confirmed shark attacks worldwide, the number is rising possibly due to neoprene wetsuits, which allow the wearer to stay longer in colder water, where the risk is greater.[6] Among safari tourists in South Africa, three foreigners were killed by wild mammals, in a 10-year period, two by lions after the tourists left their vehicle to approach them. The number of fatal snakebites is estimated to be 40 000 worldwide (mainly in Nigeria and India), but few victims are travelers.

Also a broad variety of toxins may be a risk to travelers. Ciguatoxin leading to ciguatera syndrome after the consumption of tropical reef fish is a major risk; the case fatality is 0.1–12%. 'Body-packing' of heroin, cocaine and other illicit drugs in the gastrointestinal tract or in the vagina may result in the death of travelers when the condoms or other packages break. Fatal toxic reactions and life threatening neurological symptoms after the application of highly concentrated N,N-diethyl-m-toluamide (also called N,N-diethyl-3-methylbenzamide), or DEET, in small children have rarely been observed. Lead-glazed ceramic purchased abroad may result in lead poisoning and could remain undetected for a long period of time.

Infectious diseases

Malaria is the most frequent cause of infectious death among travelers. Between 1989 and 1995, 373 fatalities due to malaria were reported in nine European countries, with 25 deaths in the United States.[7] This was almost exclusively due to *P. falciparum*, the case fatality rate ranging from 0–3.6%.

Among deaths due to infectious diseases, HIV should have a prominent place, although it does not appear in the statistics, since it is a late consequence of infection abroad. In Switzerland it is estimated that 10% of HIV infections are acquired abroad. In the UK, the risk of acquiring HIV is considered to be 300 times higher while abroad, compared with staying home.[8] Every traveler may be exposed to risk: seamen, military personnel, those visiting friends and relatives in high endemicity countries, businessmen or tourists. HIV patients while traveling have a higher risk of complications, which ultimately may be fatal.[9]

There is a multitude of other infections which may result in the death of a traveler, including the usually harmless travelers' diarrhea, and rabies, which untreated has a case fatality rate of almost 100%. Overall, however, fatal infections are quite effectively prevented in the traveler.

Non-infectious disease

Senior travelers in particular may experience a new illness, or complications of a pre-existing illness. Of particular concern are cardiovascular conditions,[4] and evidence has been generated that pulmonary embolism associated with long distance air travel may occur in five per million travelers; many of these cases are fatal. Risk factors for this have been clearly identified.[10]

AEROMEDICAL EVACUATION

Accounts on repatriation are instructive, as they are a mirror of serious health problems, many of which are not reported otherwise. Fifty percent of aeromedical evacuation is because of accidents and 50% due to illness. In the latter group, cardio- or cerebrovascular and gastrointestinal problems are the most frequent causes. Psychiatric problems have decreased as a reason for air evacuation.

MORBIDITY

Travelers' diarrhea

Classical travelers' diarrhea (TD) is defined as three or more unformed stools per 24 h, with at least one accompanying symptom, such as fecal urgency, abdominal cramps, nausea, vomiting, fever, etc. Also milder forms of TD may result in incapacitation (Fig. 2.2).[11]

There are three levels of risk for TD: (1) travelers from industrialized countries who stay for two weeks in Canada, the USA, northern and central Europe, or Australia and New Zealand have a low incidence rate of up to 8%; (2) intermediate incidence rates (8–20%) are experienced by travelers to most destinations in the Caribbean, southern Europe, Japan and South Africa, and (3) the incidence rates of TD in journeys to developing countries vary between 20% and 66% during the first 2 weeks of stay.[11] Travelers' diarrhea is still the most frequent illness among travelers who originate from industrialized countries and visit developing countries (Fig. 2.1), while those who live in areas of high endemicity have a lower risk as a result of acquired immunity. Groups at particularly high risk of illness include infants, young adults and persons with impaired gastric acid barrier. TD often has a particularly severe and long-lasting course in small children.[1]

Over the last two decades of the twentieth century, the rates of TD remained fairly stable in developing countries (Fig. 2.3). Tunisia is one of the few host countries worldwide where the ministries of health and tourism jointly tried to reduce the burden of gastrointestinal infections in their guests, initially with success. This is explained mainly by the rapid growth in the main tourist sector, while there was insufficient investment in the infrastructure, particularly in water supply and removal of wastage. In southern Europe, however, much improvement has been noted (Fig. 2.3).

The symptoms of TD in tourists frequently start on the third day of the stay abroad, with second episodes in 20% of the cases beginning about a week after arrival. Untreated, the mean duration of TD is 4 days (median 2 days), and in 1%, the symptoms may persist over a month. Twenty-two percent of patients show signs of mucosal invasive or inflammatory disease with fever and/or blood in the stools. Fecal leukocytes and hemoccult are found positive in such feces. TD is usually caused by fecal contamination of food and beverages. The pathogens responsible for TD are described elsewhere in this volume (Chapter 16).

Malaria

Annually, almost 10 000 malaria infections are imported by travelers and reported in industrialized nations.[7] In view of incomplete reporting, this is an underestimate, and as demonstrated by Swiss data, probably less than 50% of imported infections are not reported. Patients treated abroad are also typically not included in reporting data. The proportion of *P. falciparum* infection varies depending on the destination (Fig. 2.4). As shown in Figure 2.1, malaria would be a frequent diagnosis among travelers to tropical Africa if they failed to use prophylactic medication.

Using the existing surveillance data and the numbers of travelers to the respective destinations, the relative risk of malaria in travelers visiting different countries can be estimated. Such data will only indicate a risk per country, and not a precise destination. The annual entomological inoculation rate clearly demonstrates broad differences within a country. This is illustrated in Kenya, with rates

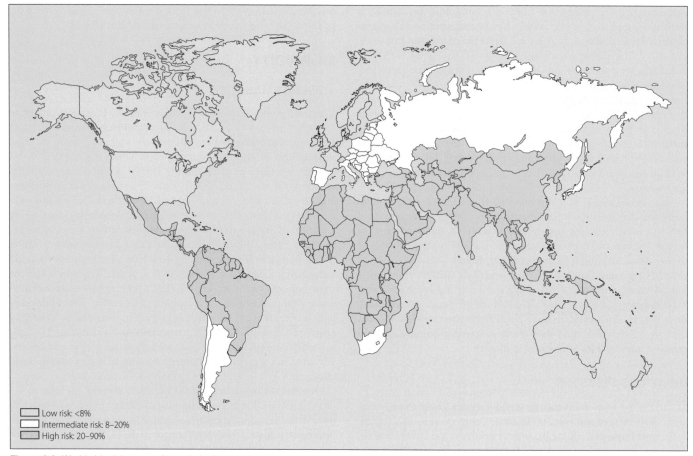

Figure 2.2 Worldwide risk areas of traveler's diarrhea.

from 0–416 (at the coast locally exceeding 200), or within a city and its suburbs, such as Kinshasa, 3–612 (equivalent to two infective bites each night).[12] Seroconversion surveys for circumsporozoite antibodies in travelers initially seemed to overestimate the infection rate (up to 49%), but the more recently published rate of 5% is closer, though still markedly higher than the incidence rate per month of 1.5% observed in travelers who had not used any chemoprophylaxis.[13] This may indicate that asymptomatic malaria infection can occur.

Risk of infection is influenced not only by destination but also by:
- number of vectors

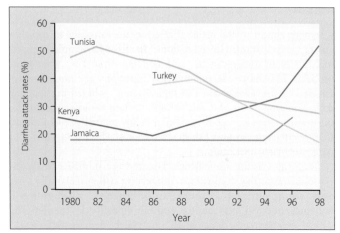

Figure 2.3 Evolution of traveler's diarrhea attack rates.

- *Anopheles* species (infected vector density)
- population density (infected population density)
- infrastructure condition (housing, water management, mosquito control)
- resistance to insecticides
- seasonality, particularly rainfall
- duration of exposure (the cumulative risk of contracting malaria is proportional to the length of stay in the transmission area)
- compliance (personal protection measures, chemoprophylaxis)
- style of travel (camping versus staying in air conditioned or well-screened urban hotel)
- host factors (such as semi-immunity, pregnancy)

These variables illustrate that it is impossible to predict the risk of malaria transmission by more than a rough order of magnitude in any specific traveler. The travel health physician and even the traveler will often ignore at least some of these parameters. Finally, old data may have become obsolete in view of global warming: in Nairobi, previously free of transmission at an elevation of 1700 m, an increasing risk of malaria is reported. Nevertheless, at least one can estimate whether a traveler will be at high or low risk (Fig. 2.4).

A more detailed account on malaria epidemiology with maps, is found in Chapter 12, where the adverse events due to prophylactic medication against malaria is discussed.

Vaccine preventable infections

For most vaccine preventable diseases, no recent morbidity and mortality data (Fig. 2.1) exist, although there are indications that the incidence rates identified in the 1970s and 1980s are decreasing. It

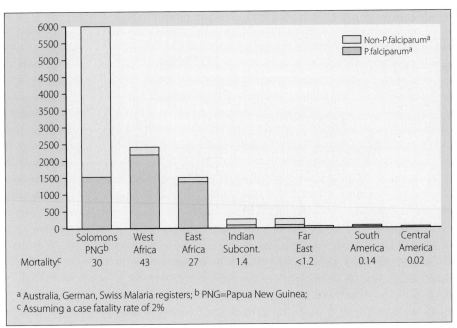

Figure 2.4 Risk of *P. falciparum* malaria infection.

	Solomons PNG[b]	West Africa	East Africa	Indian Subcont.	Far East	South America	Central America
Mortality[c]	30	43	27	1.4	<1.2	0.14	0.02

[a] Australia, German, Swiss Malaria registers; [b] PNG=Papua New Guinea;
[c] Assuming a case fatality rate of 2%

is uncertain to what degree this is due to improved hygienic conditions at the destinations – somewhat a contradiction to observations related with TD – or to immunization. It is unlikely that the current risk in travelers can be studied, as ethically it is impossible to leave cohorts unprotected just for an epidemiological assessment. Subsequently, the epidemiological data of the various infections will be grouped here (as in Chapter 10) in required, routine and recommended immunizations.

Required immunizations

Yellow fever occurs only in tropical Africa and northern South America (Fig. 2.5). Usually a few hundred cases are reported to WHO annually, but it is estimated that more than 200 000 cases occur. Yellow fever has never occurred in Asia although the vectors, *Aedes* and *Haemagogus* have been observed there. Yellow fever is extremely rare in travelers, but several cases in unvaccinated travelers have been reported in the last 10 years, despite the fact these travelers should have been immunized.[14] Four travelers recently reported with yellow fever died (Fig. 2.5).

Cholera and plague would be the other two diseases subject to the currently (February 2003) valid International Health Regulations, but since immunization is not required (exceptions being cholera for Palau and Sudan after transit through endemic areas).

Meningococcal disease has frequently been observed during or after the *hajj* or *umrah* pilgrimage to Mecca (200/100 000), but it is rare even in travelers staying in countries where the infection is highly endemic (0.04/100 000). The case fatality rate among travelers slightly exceeded 20%. Rarely, *Neisseria meningitidis* may be transmitted during air-travel of at least 8 h duration. More recently, measles vaccination has also become a requirement for those entering Panama from Venezuela or Colombia.

Routine immunizations

To the author's knowledge, no cases of tetanus have been recently reported in travelers, but such may be hidden in national surveillance data.

As demonstrated by a large epidemic in the former Soviet Union 1990 to 1997, diphtheria may flare up under specific circumstances.[15] This epidemic resulted in dozens of importations to Western Europe

and North America, some travelers died while still in Russia. Far less serious forms of cutaneous diphtheria are occasionally imported mainly from developing countries.

Poliomyelitis, although almost eradicated from most parts of the world (Fig. 2.6) may rarely still be associated with a virus imported by asymptomatic persons, as demonstrated in Bulgaria and China recently. In travelers, poliomyelitis has not been observed since the 1990s (Fig. 2.6).

Very little data exist on pertussis, *haemophilus influenzae* B, measles, mumps and rubella in travelers. In view of suboptimal compliance with vaccination, European, African and Asian travelers are responsible for outbreaks on the American continent, where vaccine uptake is far superior.

Hepatitis B – now a routine immunization in most industrialized countries – is mainly a problem for expatriates living close to the local population and for travelers breaking the most basic hygiene rules; the monthly incidence is 25/100 000 for symptomatic infections; 80–420/100 000 for all infections.[14] While minute quantities of the virus are sufficient for transmission and the exact mode of transmission may remain undetected in many individuals, clear risk factors, such as casual unprotected sex, nosocomial transmission, etc. have often been suspected. Behavioral surveys have shown that 10–15% of travelers voluntarily or involuntarily expose themselves to blood and body fluids while abroad in high-risk countries. Besides the risk factors mentioned above such persons also went to the dental hygienist, for acupuncture, cosmetic surgery, tattoos, ear piercing, scarification, etc.

Recommended immunizations

The most frequent vaccine preventable infection in non-immune travelers to developing countries is hepatitis A with an average incidence rate of 300/100 000 per month; in high-risk backpackers or foreign-aid-volunteers this rate is 2000/100 000.[14] In various studies reviewed it has been shown that luxury tourists staying at multistar resorts may be at risk of infection.

Typhoid fever is diagnosed with an incidence rate of 30/100 000 per month among travelers to the Indian subcontinent, North and West Africa (except Tunisia), and Peru; elsewhere this rate is ten-fold lower. A fair proportion of infections are imported by those visiting friends

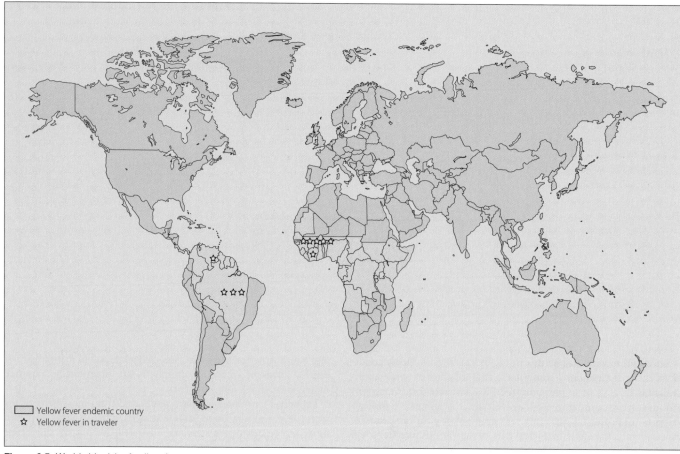

Figure 2.5 Worldwide risk of yellow fever.

and relatives, but also people originating in industrialized countries are affected. The case fatality rate is 0–1% among travelers.

The risk of rabies is particularly high in Asia, from where 90% of all human rabies deaths are reported, but there may be under-reporting in other parts of the world. Rabies free areas include Australia, New Zealand, the Pacific Islands, Scandinavia, the UK, Ireland, Iceland and Switzerland. Many among the monthly 0.2–0.4% who in developing countries experience an animal bite, are at risk of rabies. Rabies is a risk particularly in those who are in close contact with natives over a prolonged time, e.g. missionaries, those en route with bikes, and in those working with animals, or who explore caves.

Based on post-travel skin tests, the incidence rate of *M. tuberculosis* infections is 3000/100 000 person-months of travel, and 60/100 000 had active tuberculosis. The prevalence of transmissible tuberculosis among air travelers is estimated to be 5–100/100 000 passengers, depending on the route of the plane. Nevertheless, transmission in flight, also during prolonged train and bus rides has only rarely been reported and outdoor transmission can be neglected, except if there is repeated exposure, as may occur particularly among long-term, low-budget travelers or expatriates.

The risk of cholera is approximately 0.2/100 000, although asymptomatic and oligosymptomatic infections may be more frequent, as demonstrated in Japanese travelers. The case fatality rate is less than 2% among travelers.

For several potentially vaccine-preventable diseases, the risk of infection is less than 1 per million. Although a few dozen cases of Japanese encephalitis have been diagnosed in civilian travelers within the last 25 years, the attack rate in civilians is less than 1 per

million in view of the number of travelers. Exceptionally, a short-term tourist in Bali may be affected. Only two international travelers were diagnosed with plague since 1966. Very few anecdotal reports have documented tick-borne encephalitis in international travelers, although they certainly occur in persons hiking or camping in endemic areas.

To date, no data have been published on the risk of influenza in this population, but various outbreaks on cruise ships or after a flight have been described.

Other infections

Only a few select infections can be mentioned in this section. Those about which no more than anecdotal reports have been published will be omitted.

Sexually transmitted diseases

Casual sex, according to most surveys, in almost 50% without regular condom protection, is practiced by 4–19% of travelers while they are abroad.[16] This results in HIV infection and other sexually transmitted diseases (STD). The WHO estimates that 75% of all HIV infections worldwide are sexually transmitted and that the efficiency of transmission per sexual contact ranges from 0.1% to 1%. The transmission probability of HIV is greatly enhanced by the presence of other STD and genital lesions, as is often the case in female prostitutes and other infected persons in developing countries. Typically, 14–25% of cases of gonorrhea and syphilis diagnosed in Europe were imported from abroad.

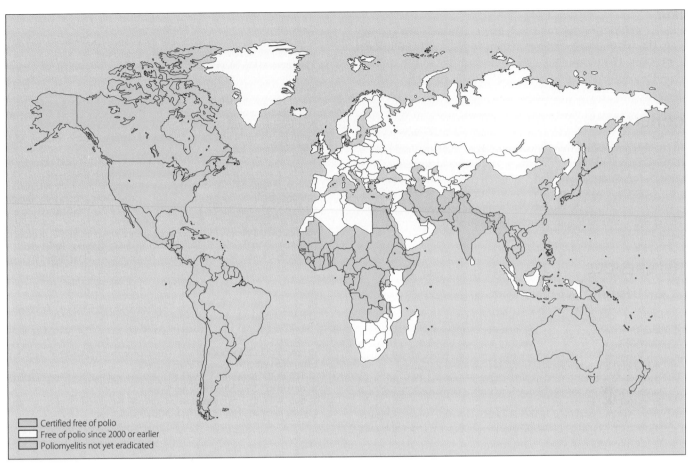

Figure 2.6 Worldwide risk of poliomyelitis (2001).

Legend on map:
Certified free of polio
Free of polio since 2000 or earlier
Poliomyelitis not yet eradicated

Common cold

This is one of the most frequent health problems, with an attack rate of 13% in short-term travelers; among them 40% are incapacitated for an average of 2.6 days. From interviews in Chinese hospitals, there is anecdotic evidence that lower respiratory tract infections occur particularly often in this country.

Dengue

In Southeast Asia, the seroconversion rate of dengue in travelers is 200/100 000,[17] but travelers may less frequently also be at risk in other endemic areas. However, there are some indications that dengue is a reemerging illness in other parts of the world as well, and surveillance systems are documenting larger numbers of returning travelers with dengue from most endemic regions.

Legionella

With easier diagnostic means, the rate of *legionella* infections reported to Eurosurveillance is continuously increasing: it reached 289 in 1999. The highest rate found among British travelers was after a stay in Turkey, 1/100 000 compared with, e.g., ten times fewer when the destination was in the USA.[18]

Leishmaniasis

This has frequently been described in travelers, but to the author's knowledge, no systematic review with data has been published.

Schistosomiasis

Using newer serological tests, there is some indication that schistosomiasis is an infection that long-term travelers, missionaries and volunteers acquire in endemic areas. However, it is currently unknown whether or not most of these exposed travelers would ever develop the typical signs and symptoms of the disease.

Trypanosomiasis

Trypanosomiasis, in its African form, has been reported in only 29 cases in the USA in the twentieth century, but the risk seems to be increasing.

Non-infectious health problems

This covers a broad variety of problems, accidents and illnesses, which can be divided into environment- or host-related.

Environmental

Travel may result in stress, particularly fear of flying – most prominent during take-off and landing – and flight delays, which are frequent causes for anxiety.[19] Motion sickness may affect up to 80% of passengers in small vessels in rough seas, but also affects passengers (though fewer) on jet flights. In-flight emergencies occur in 1/11 000 passengers, the most frequent ones being gastrointestinal, cardiac, neurological, vasovagal and respiratory.

Also changes in climate and altitude create problems. In particular, high altitude sickness (described in Chapter 38) will affect every passenger if ascent is rapid to extremely high altitudes. Health impairments related to diving are described in Chapter 39.

In addition to the accidents described in the mortality section, small bruises acquired while swimming, other marine hazards or lacerations due to sporting activities may take longer to heal in view of suprainfection. Sprained ankles and other sports injuries are frequent, particularly among senior travelers who tend to fall, e.g., in dimly lit hotels.

Host

Persons with pre-existing conditions may experience some aggravation. This is particularly common in those with chronic constipation, diarrhea or other gastrointestinal ailments, while others, such as dermatological conditions or degenerative joint pain may improve under a sunny, warm climate.[20]

CONCLUSION

In conclusion, health professionals who advise travelers need to keep the described epidemiological facts in mind when determining what preventive measures are needed. Ultimately, the decision regarding to what degree one wishes to protect future travelers is an arbitrary one – nobody should give the illusion that 'complete protection' is possible. Travel will always have some inherent additional risks compared with staying home.

REFERENCES

1. Steffen R, Lobel HO. Epidemiologic basis for the practice of travel medicine. *J Wilderness Med* 1994; **5**:56–66.
2. Prazuck T, Semaille C, Halioua B, *et al*. Health hazards in international tourists visiting Paris in August: a five-year retrospective epidemiologic survey. *J Travel Med* 1998; **5**:178–183.
3. Liese B, Mundt KA, Dell LD, *et al*. Medical insurance claims associated with international business travel. *Occup Environ Med* 1997; **54**:499–503.
4. Hargarten SW, Baker TD, Guptill K. Overseas fatalities of United States citizen travelers: an analysis of deaths related to international travel. *Ann Emerg Med* 1991; **20**:622–626.
5. Wilks J. International tourists, motor vehicles and road safety: a review of the literature leading up to the Sydney 2000 Olympics. *J Travel Med* 1999; **6**:115–121.
6. Woolgar JD, Cliff G, Nair R, *et al*. Shark Attack: Review of 86 Consecutive Cases. *J Trauma Inj, Inf, Crit Care* 2001; **50**:887–891.
7. Muentener P, Schlagenhauf P, Steffen R. Imported malaria (1985–95): trends and perspectives. *Bull WHO* 1999; **77**:560–566.
8. Thomson MM, Najera R. Travel and the introduction of human immunodeficiency virus type 1 non-B subtype genetic forms into Western countries. *Clin Infect Dis* 2001; **32**:1732–1737.
9. Furrer H, Chan P, Weber R, *et al*. Increased risk of wasting syndrome in HIV-infected travelers: prospective multicentre study. *Trans R Soc Trop Med Hyg* 2001; **95**:484–486.
10. Ansell JE. Air travel and venous thromboembolism – is the evidence in? *N Engl J Med* 2001; **345**:828–829.
11. Sonnenburg F von, Tornieporth N, Waiyake P, *et al*. Risk and aetiology of diarrhoea at various tourist destinations. *Lancet* 2000; **356**:133–134.
12. Hay SI, Rogers DJ, Toomer JF, *et al*. Annual Plasmodium falciparum entomological inoculation rates (EIR) across Africa: literature survey, internet access and review. *Trans R Soc Trop Med Hyg* 2000; **94**:113–127.
13. Nothdurft HD, Jelinek T, Blüml A, *et al*. seroconversion to circumsporozoite antigen of plasmodium falciparum demonstrates a high risk of malaria transmission in travelers to East Africa. *Clin Infect Dis* 1999; **28**:641–642.
14. Steffen R, Connor B. Prioritization of vaccines in travel medicine. *J Travel Med* 2003; in press.
15. Galazka A. The changing epidemiology of diphtheria in the vaccine era. *J Infect Dis* 2000; **181(suppl 1)**:2–9.
16. Hawkes S, Hart GJ, Johnson AM, *et al*. Risk behaviour and HIV prevalence in international travelers. *AIDS* 1994; **8**:247–252.
17. Jelinek T. Dengue fever in international travelers. *Clin Infect Dis* 2000; **31**:144–147.
18. Joseph CA. On Behalf Of EWGLI. Travel associated legionnaires' disease in Europe in 1999. *Euro Surveill* 2001; **6**:53–60.
19. McIntosh IB, Swanson V, Power KG. Anxiety and health problems related to air travel. *J Travel Med* 1998; **5**:198–204.
20. Steffen R, Linde F Van der. Intercontinental travel and its effect on pre-existing illnesses. *Aviat Space Envir Med* 1981; **52**:57–58.

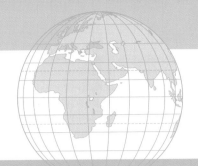

CHAPTER 3 Starting, Organizing and Marketing a Travel Clinic

David R. Hill

KEYPOINTS

■ One of the many reasons for the increase in the number of travel clinics include the need for education regarding prevention and self-treatment of travel related ailments. Travel health advisors maintain up-to-date information on these issues as well as a panel of immunizations for travelers

■ Provider knowledge and training have become critical pieces in the development of the travel medicine specialty

■ Prevention advice is dependent not only on the traveler's itinerary, but also on a variety of host variables, such as the medical history

■ Knowing the information and resources available and how to access them are the keys to the provision of excellent travel medicine advice

■ Having good policies and procedures in place, as well as a marketing strategy for the travel clinic, will enable a clinic to function well, grow, and be successful

INTRODUCTION

The growth of travel medicine as a specialty over the last 20 years has been paralleled by the growth of specialized services providing pre-travel care. These services, known as travel clinics, have become a main focus of travel medicine worldwide. It is in travel clinics that travelers can receive up-to-date advice on vaccine preventable disease, malaria, diarrhea, the care of chronic medical conditions, and receive required or recommended immunizations. Nevertheless, it is not known how many persons visit a travel clinic before departing on a trip. Some estimate that fewer than 10% consult such a service.[1] If travel medicine is to accomplish its goal of protecting all travelers who venture to areas of health risk, there needs to be an improved effort to inform both travelers and health-care providers of the benefits of pre-travel care as it is rendered in a travel clinic.

Why should the traveling public visit a travel clinic? The publication of this book as well as several others devoted entirely to the field of travel medicine[2,3] supports the premise that travel medicine has a defined area of expertise and knowledge. There are sufficient risks to the traveler – such as the frequent occurrence of traveler's diarrhea, occasional cases of life-threatening malaria, and the occurrence of vaccine preventable disease – which establish the point that all travelers should receive education and counseling prior to their trips. Indeed, the simple acts of education and provision of prophylactic medication are the least expensive and most cost-effective interventions in all of travel medicine.[4]

But why visit a travel medicine specialist and not a generalist? Some of these reasons are detailed in Table 3.1. There is a body of knowledge in travel medicine that is sufficiently different from general medicine and even infectious diseases and tropical medicine, that it is best practiced by health-care personnel who have been trained in the field, who are constantly updating their knowledge, and who have the information and resources to provide pre-travel care. This knowledge base has been recently defined[5] and now formally assessed by an examination given by the International Society of Travel Medicine (ISTM).

There is ample evidence that health-care practitioners who are not familiar with the field of emporiatrics make errors in judgment and advice, particularly about the prevention of malaria.[6–9] These errors have led to adverse outcomes for travelers, such as malaria deaths in travelers who were advised to take no or incorrect chemoprophylaxis.[10]

The practice of travel medicine requires that health-care providers maintain up-to-date information on the geography of illness, provide a full panel of immunizations against both common and uncommon vaccine-preventable disease, and have access to the recommendations of expert bodies such as the World Health Organization (WHO) and the Centers for Disease Control and Prevention (CDC). If a travel clinic can provide this level of expert care, it will distinguish itself from a generalist's office and increase the value of the service to the traveling public.

Finally, it will be made clear throughout this book, that providing only immunizations without making a complete assessment of the traveler and providing other preventive health advice is not the practice of travel medicine and is not an appropriate level of service. It is not sufficient to be certified to administer yellow fever vaccine and then not give advice on malaria chemoprophylaxis. Although there may not be specific laws that proscribe this behavior, it is prudent that all who give travel vaccines do so in the context of a travel medicine service as outlined in this chapter. This same admonition should apply to travel operators who book tours, but may fail to inform the

Table 3.1	Benefits of a travel medicine service

Comprehensive pre-travel care (see Table 3.5)

Knowledgeable and experienced providers (see Table 3.4)

Up-to-date advice (in verbal and written form) on the wide range of travel-related health risks

Access to current epidemiologic resources and expert opinion

Availability of immunizations against vaccine-preventable illness

Provision of medications/prescriptions for self-treatment of travelers' diarrhea, and chemoprophylaxis against malaria and environmental illness

Post-travel screening and referral

traveler of health risks or required immunizations. The European Community has developed guidelines describing the minimum health information that should be conveyed to travelers by a travel operator (European Directive 90/314/EEC).[11] The implementation and enforcement of these guidelines, however, has not been uniform and is subject to interpretation. Nevertheless, continued links between travel medicine practitioners and the travel industry will contribute to healthier travel.

THE PRACTICE OF TRAVEL MEDICINE

What is the current practice of travel medicine and can this help in deciding which elements are necessary for the establishment of a new travel clinic? In an effort to define how travel medicine was being practiced, the Education Committee of the ISTM surveyed its membership in 1994 and the results were published in 1996.[12] What was clear from this survey was that the practice of travel medicine in the mid-1990s was very diverse (see Table 3.2). The care of travelers was being provided by those with formal training in tropical and travel medicine who saw thousands of travelers each year, to those with generalist training who only saw a few patients. Despite these differences, a few consistent themes emerged. Nearly all clinics were from North America, Western Europe and Australia (94%), a private office was the most frequent setting for the clinics (41%), and physicians (94%) nearly always directed them. Most clinics saw only a modest number of patients: less than 20 patients per week were seen by 61% of clinics (14% saw less than 2 patients/week), and only 13% saw more than 100 patients/week. Nearly all clinics (≥97%) provided advice about malaria, insect avoidance, and the prevention and treatment of traveler's diarrhea, and most administered a wide range of vaccines. Although clinics were usually directed by physicians, advice and care were rendered nearly equally by physicians and nurses, particularly in the USA, and in many European clinics.[13] A further analysis of European travel medicine services and their funding sources and affiliations is given in Table 3.3. Finally, most physicians (63%) who were involved in travel medicine trained in infectious disease or tropical medicine. There were also marked regional differences. Physicians in Canada trained in general medicine or family practice (54%), and physicians in Europe in infectious diseases and tropical medicine (77%).

Where are these travelers going (Fig. 3.1)? Data from the World Tourism Organization indicate that for all travel during 2001, Europe was most frequently visited (58%). As expected, for those visiting a travel medicine service (1984–2002), developing regions were more common with travelers going to destinations in the Americas (31%), Africa (29%), East Asia and the Pacific (23%) with almost equal frequency.

Table 3.2 Survey of 341 travel clinics worldwide – 1994

	(%)
Location	
USA	57
Europe	20
UK & Ireland	6
Canada	6
Australia & New Zealand	5
Other	6
Affiliation	
Private	41
School of Medicine	20
Hospital	10
Corporate/Student Health	10
Public Health	8
Other	11
Number of travelers seen/year	
≤ 100	14
101–500	30
501–1000	17
1001–5000	26
> 5000	13
Providers of advice	
Nurse only	16
Physician only	41
Nurse and physician	42
Other	2
Physician training	
Family or general practice	16
Internal medicine	17
Infectious disease or tropical medicine	63
Other	4

Data from Hill DR, Behrens RH, 1996.[12]

ELEMENTS OF A TRAVEL MEDICINE PRACTICE

Provider knowledge and training

The decade of the 1990s was a period of rapid growth in travel medicine – from the initial convening of the International Society of Travel Medicine in 1991 to biennial meetings of the Society that are now attended by several thousand persons. With this marked growth, it is likely that the face of travel medicine has also changed. Nevertheless, referring to the initial survey[12] it is possible to discern those elements

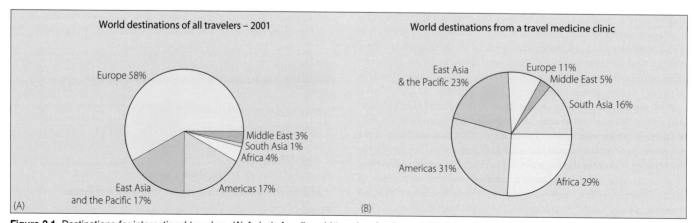

Figure 3.1 Destinations for international travelers. (A) Arrivals for all world travelers for the year 2001 (*n* = 692 700 000). Data from the World Tourism Organization (www.world-tourism.org/index.htm accessed 10/5/02). (B) Destinations for travelers receiving pre-travel care at the International Traveler's Medical Service at the University of Connecticut, USA, from January 1984 through June 2002 (*n* = 14 071 travelers).

Table 3.3 Delivery of pre-travel health services by health-care professionals in Europe

Country	Proportion of service delivery (%)			Proportion of institution delivering service (%)		
	Physician	Nurse	Main funding of pre-travel health activity[a]	Public health	Hospital/University	Primary care
Austria	100	–	Private	20	30	40
Belgium	90	10	Private	0	0	70
Denmark	90	10	Private	–	–	70
Finland	20	80	Private/Govt. funded	5	5	70
France	75	20	Private/Govt. funded	–	25	45
Germany	97	0	Private	10	10	60
Greece	20	80	Govt. funded	40	30	40
Ireland	100	under medical direction	Private	–	10	65
Italy	80	20	Private/Govt. funded	75	10	10
Luxembourg	100	0	Private	2	0	96
Netherlands	30	50	Private	50	15	25
Norway	20	80	Mostly private	85	2	5
Portugal	70	30	Mostly Govt. funded	70	30	–
Spain	30	45	Govt. funded	90	5	3
Sweden	n/a	n/a	Private	–	15	10
Switzerland	80	20	Private/Govt. funded	10	30	40
UK	75	20	Private/Govt. funded	0	7	70

[a]Simplified assessment. *Source:* Scientific Analysis of Risks Relating To Communicable Diseases Linked to Tourism and Travel. A summary of a project report funded by the Public Health Directorate of the European Commission (1999), the Scottish Centre for Infection and Environmental Health (United Kingdom) & Société de Médecine des Voyages (France).

that should be part of any travel medicine practice. These are listed in Tables 3.4 and 3.5, and have been more completely defined by the Canadian Committee to Advise on Tropical Medicine and Travel (CATMAT) in their Guidelines for the Practice of Travel Medicine published in 1999.[1] The key elements to a travel medicine practice are: provider knowledge, training, and experience in the field, the assessment of the traveler, provision of advice about prevention and management of travel-related disease (both infectious and non-infectious), the administration of vaccines, and recognition of key syndromes in returned travelers.

First, the providers, whether physician, nurse, or other licensed health-care personnel, should be trained in travel medicine. The many examples of inadequate advice rendered to travelers by those who were not knowledgeable in the field emphasize the importance of an adequate knowledge base.[6,7,9,14–16] Training includes education and experience.

There are numerous venues to study in the fields of travel and tropical medicine. These range from short-term review courses (one to several days) or the biennial ISTM meeting in travel medicine, to several-month intensive courses in traveller's health and/or tropical medicine, which may include an overseas clinical experience.[17] Even short-term education in travel medicine has been associated with improved knowledge.[18] It is not considered necessary that providers of travel medicine also have expertise in tropical medicine, but they should have enough knowledge of syndromes in returned travelers to be able to recognize and triage important post-travel conditions such as fever, rash, diarrhea, and respiratory conditions. The body of knowledge for travel medicine providers has been defined by the ISTM[5] and is outlined in Table 3.4. Both the ISTM and the American Society of Tropical Medicine and Hygiene (ASTM&H) have developed examinations that lead to a certificate of knowledge. The ISTM has emphasized travel medicine[5] and the ASTM&H has emphasized tropical medicine.[17]

Experience is the other component of being able to practice travel medicine. It is only with regular assessment of travelers of all ages who have multiple health conditions, and are planning a wide variety of travel destinations and activities, that one can gain competence in the field. Although there are only a limited number of sites worldwide where travelers can have training in travel medicine (e.g., Glasgow, Scotland, Basel, Switzerland, and Tel Hashomer, Israel), the ISTM is actively engaged in developing additional sites. Persons who are interested should contact the ISTM secretariat to locate places where they can receive this training. Some international courses also host their own exams.

The travel clinic survey indicated that 14% of clinics saw less than two patients/week.[12] This number is far too few to maintain competency. Although it is difficult to assign a minimum number of pre-travel consultations, 10 to 20 per week seems to be a reasonable number to maintain the experience needed to provide competent advice and care.

Personnel and models of care

The survey of travel clinics indicated that most practices have both physicians and nurses participating in the care of patients. Although physicians direct the majority of clinics, nurses are frequently the sole providers of advice. The specialty of travel medicine is ideally suited to the involvement of and care rendered by nurses, nurse practitioners and physician assistants. Given the variety of providers, each clinic will need to decide how to divide the responsibilities.

For clinics in which both physicians and nurses provide care there are two models (as outlined in Fig. 3.2). In the first model, the physician obtains the travel itinerary, planned activities, and the patient's

Table 3.4	Elements of a travel medicine practice: provider qualifications

Knowledge
  Geography
  Travel-associated infectious diseases: epidemiology, transmission, prevention
  Travel-related drugs and vaccines: indications, contraindications, pharmacology, drug interactions, adverse events
  Non-infectious travel risks both medical and environmental: prevention and management
  Recognition of major syndromes in returned travelers: e.g., fever, diarrhea, rash and respiratory illness
  Access to travel medicine resources: texts, articles, Internet sites

Experience
  6 months in a travel clinic with at least 10–20 pre-travel consultations/ week

Continuing education
  Short or long courses in travel medicine
  Membership in specialty society dealing with travel and tropical medicine, (e.g.,) The International Society of Travel Medicine and national societies

Table 3.5	Elements of a travel medicine practice: services

Assessing the health of the traveler[a]
  Underlying medical conditions and allergies
  Immunization history

Assessing the health risk of travel
  Itinerary
  Duration
  Reason for travel
  Planned activities

Preventive advice[b]
  Vaccine-preventable illness
  Traveler's diarrhea prevention and self-treatment
  Malaria prevention
  Other vector-borne and water-borne illness
  Personal safety and behavior
  Environmental illness – altitude, heat, cold
  Animal bites and rabies avoidance
  Travel medical kits
  Travel health and medical evacuation insurance
  Access to medical care overseas

Vaccination

Post-travel assessment

[a]Permanent records should be maintained
[b]Advice should be given both verbally and in written form

medical and immunization history. They then give the health advice and decisions are made concerning recommended and required immunizations. The care of the patient is then transferred to a nurse (or to a person who has competency to administer vaccines). The nurse reviews vaccine side-effects, obtains informed consent, and administers the vaccines. After giving the vaccines they record vaccine administration information in the medical record. The record is now complete, and can be filed or entered into a clinic database if one has been developed.

In the second model the nurse, nurse practitioner or physician assistant provides the complete pre-travel care from the medical and travel history, to preventive advice, to administration and recording of vaccines.

Some clinics which are entirely private or which are part of a larger franchise system will have nurses (or other non-physician health providers) as the sole providers of care. If this is the case, it is necessary that detailed protocols be developed, which the nursing staff can follow. These have to be clinic-specific (reflecting the standard of care within the region) and in written form with standing orders for administration of vaccines and writing of prescriptions.

In the UK this model of independent care rendered by nurses is supported by a legal framework known as Patient Group Directions (PGD). This requires a clear and detailed written protocol, agreed and signed by doctors, nurses and pharmacists. The document details the indications and situations when a nurse can select, prescribe and administer a prescription-only medication without recourse to a physician. The PGD requires that the nurse receive appropriate training, updating and audit of practice.

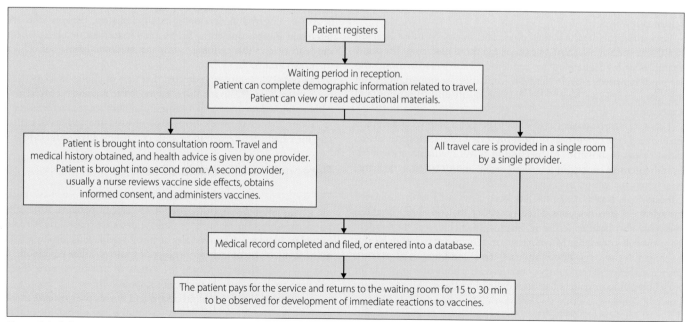

Figure 3.2 A flow chart for patient care in a travel medicine clinic. Two options are presented – two-provider or single-provider care.

Assessment of the traveler and travel health risks

The medical record

The initial phase of the pre-travel visit is the assessment of the traveler. It is necessary to determine who the traveler is (their demographics and any medical conditions which might affect travel or prophylactic measures) and what health risks they will potentially be exposed to during their trip. This assessment needs to be consistent and so a standard travel clinic form should be used. The importance of a permanent medical record for all travelers cannot be overemphasized. This record will document everything provided for the traveler. For insurance companies, it will document the level of care that has been provided. For the traveler, it is a record of the immunizations and advice they received and can be very useful if they lose their immunization card at some time in the future. For the travel clinic, it can be accessed to create a database of all travelers seen at a given site.

Some clinics have chosen to have the traveler complete demographic and travel information either before their visit by using a form that is mailed to them when their appointment is made, or in the waiting room just before they are seen. Because many travelers make appointments only a few days in advance of their clinic visit, and other clinics will see 'walk-ins', it is often logistically difficult to mail the form to the traveler. And, if they forget to bring it to their appointment, it will need to be completed by the provider in any case. We have also found in our travel medicine service, that if the traveler completes their form while they wait to be seen, the information has to be reviewed during the visit and is often corrected or amended and little time is saved. We choose, then, to obtain all information during the visit. Elements of the assessment phase of the visit, which should be recorded in the medical record, are listed in Table 3.6.

After recording the traveler's demographics, itinerary, travel activities, and medical history, an immunization history should be obtained. Because the pre-travel visit is an ideal time to update recommended childhood, adolescent, or adult vaccines, the dates or intervals of these

routinely recommended vaccines need to be recorded. Parents should be instructed to bring in their child's immunization record. Immunizations given for previous travel can often be determined by examining a traveler's International Certificate of Vaccination.[19] Finally, a telephone number should be available to contact the traveler's primary care physician to confirm dates of administration if they are not known.

The last part of the travel record documents the immunizations administered, the prophylactic and self-treatment medications prescribed, and the advice provided. There should also be space to record additional care given to the traveler or documentation of patient refusal to receive certain recommended vaccines or prophylactic measures. Because much of the information in a pre-travel visit is similar among travelers, there is frequently little need for narrative documentation, and the visit lends itself to standardization and efficient recording of data.

Figure 3.3 illustrates an immunization form that can be easily adapted for an individual clinic's requirements. Elements required by law in the USA include: vaccine type, dose, date of administration, manufacturer and lot number, site of administration, and name and title of administrator. This information should be recorded for several reasons. First, it becomes a permanent record of the traveler's immunizations. Second, if a traveler calls with a side-effect, it is easier to determine which vaccine is causing the reaction since the administration site has been documented. Third, in the event of a vaccine recall, lot numbers have been recorded and patients who need to be contacted can be readily identified. Entering patients into a computerized database will make the task of identifying patients much easier since records can be searched by vaccine type and lot number. A database will also allow rapid access to the information in a patient's chart if they call some months or years following their visit. Fourth, as stated in the National Childhood Vaccine Injury Act of 1986 in the USA,[20] all administrators of vaccines are required to report adverse events via the Vaccine Adverse Events Reporting System.

The methods and forms for reporting adverse events can be obtained by calling 1-800 822-7967 in the USA or accessing www.fda.gov/cber/vaers/vaers.htm. The Division of Immunization in Canada has a similar reporting system and can be reached by calling 1 613-957-1340 or 1 800-363-6456, or accessing http://www.hc-sc.gc.ca/hpb/lcdc/bid/di/vaae_e.html. In the UK, suspected adverse event reports are made to the Committee on Safety of Medicines through the 'Yellow Card Scheme' at http://www.mca.gov.uk/aboutagency/regframework/csm/csmhome.htm. Many other countries and regions also have their own reporting systems.

INFORMATION AND RESOURCES

For the travel medicine specialist

The advent of computerized information systems and web-based resources has provided access to constantly updated information that supplements traditional text-based resources (e.g., Health Information for International Travel, known as the yellow book) for the US provider,[21] Health Information for Overseas Travel for British providers,[22] and International Travel and Health published by the WHO.[23] This has moved the practice of travel medicine to a specialty that can respond on a daily basis to changes in the epidemiology of disease and the resistance patterns of parasitic and bacterial infections. Practicing travel medicine without use of these resources leads to a decreased level of service.

A complete listing of computerized resources is detailed by Keystone et al. (2001) in an excellent review[24] and will not be duplicated by this chapter. Nevertheless, Table 3.7 lists resources that all travel medicine specialists should find useful in their clinics. Many national

---

Table 3.6	The travel clinic record

Traveler demographics
   Name, date of birth, address, telephone number, and e-mail address
   Referring physician name, address, and telephone/fax numbers
   Referring business name and address (if applicable)
   Dates of departure and return
   Destination – countries and areas within countries, (e.g.,) rural vs. urban
   Nature of travel – business, pleasure, visiting friends and relatives, study
      or teaching, missionary or service
   Accommodation during travel

Medical history:
   Including pregnancy, immunosuppressing conditions, HIV risk factors
   Medications taken
   Medication or food allergies (particularly to eggs)
   Past history of hepatitis or jaundice

Travel history – previous travel-related illness

Country of birth and duration of residence – unusual illness

Immunization history

Advice given

Medications prescribed

Immunization form for vaccines administered

Comment section

Signature line

Immunization form

Vaccine	Dose, Route	Date	Manufact.	Lot#	Exp. Dt.	Site	Sig.
Tetanus/Diph.							
Typhoid							
Cholera							
Yellow fever							
Polio (inact.)							
Immune glob.							
Hep. A (inact.)							
Meningococcal							
Measles (M/R)							
Japan. Enceph.							
Hepatitis B							
Rabies							
Other							
PPD							

Figure 3.3 A sample immunization form containing elements for vaccine administration documentation.

societies–such as those in France, Germany, and Scotland–have developed resources that can be used by their travel medicine specialists.

There are 'listservs' that provide information and discussion about newly developing outbreaks or tropical medicine and travel related clinical cases (Table 3.7). The ASTM&H and ISTM listservs require membership in the organization. ProMedmail, a program of the Infectious Diseases Society of America, is a discussion group that posts up-to-date information on tropical medicine and infectious disease outbreaks (sometimes unverified) throughout the world.

Text-based resources should include, as a minimum, a textbook of travel medicine,[2,3,25] journals of subspecialty societies with an interest in travel and tropical medicine (see Table 3.7), and a textbook of tropical medicine.[26–28]

A world atlas is an invaluable resource. By using an atlas the exact itinerary can be defined. This itinerary can be compared with a map that details the regions of risk, and a decision can be made whether or not to provide prevention against diseases such as malaria or administer vaccines against yellow fever or meningococcal meningitis, as examples. If the epidemiology maps are computer-based or in loose-leaf form, they can be printed or copied and provided to the traveler.

Each travel clinic should decide how these resources are put into practice. It is helpful to standardize pre-travel care. The use of a travel clinic form allows standardization of the intake information, and assures that the same information is obtained on each patient. It is more difficult to standardize the advice and vaccines administered. The nature of travel medicine is that there are frequent differences of opinion whether to give a particular immunization or which anti-malarial to prescribe. However, the situation should never arise that travelers who are going on the same trip and have the same medical circumstances, but who come into the clinic at different times and are seen by different providers, receive different advice, vaccines and medications.

To avoid this situation, specific protocols for each country visited can be used. These can be developed by the personnel within the practice or obtained from one of the commercially available data-base programs (some of which are listed in Table 3.7 and also by Keystone et al.[24]). To further complicate this, there will be variation between countries as to which vaccines are available (e.g. BCG, oral polio, and tick-borne encephalitis vaccines), the indications and schedules for immunization, and the standard of malaria chemoprophylaxis. Therefore, it is important to match any protocols to the practice standard of the region, province, or country in which the travel clinic is located.

For the traveler

Education is the mainstay of travel care. It is difficult to measure acquisition of knowledge during the pre-travel visit,[29,30] and equally difficult to assess whether or not this knowledge is employed during travel.

The best information about travelers acting on pre-travel advice comes from studies of compliance with malaria chemoprophylaxis and the use of preventive measures to avoid traveler's diarrhea. Travelers frequently stray from the advice they received: only 50%–60% of travelers are completely compliant with malaria medications,[31,32] and more than 90% make errors in food and beverage choice within a short time period after arrival at their travel destination.[33,34] Nevertheless, it is still important to provide travelers with the tools to remain safe and healthy, and consistent and clear

Table 3.7 Information resources for the travel specialist[a]
World Health Organization Home page – www.who.int/home-page Weekly Epidemiologic Record – www.who.int/wer/ Emerging Infections – www.who.int/csr/don/er/
Internet resources **USA** Centers for Disease Control and Prevention – Travel Medicine Home page – www.cdc.gov/travel/index.htm Morbidity Mortality Weekly Report – www.cdc.gov/mmwr Vaccine Information Statements – www.cdc.gov/nip/publications/vis US State Department Travel Advisories – travel.state.gov Vaccine Adverse Event Reporting – www.fda.gov/cber/vaers/vaers.htm
Canada Health Canada – Travel Medicine – www.travelhealth.gc.ca Committee to Advise on Tropical Medicine and Travel – www.hc-sc.gc.ca/pphb-dgspsp/tmp-pmv/catmat-ccmtmv/index.html Canadian Society for International Health – www.csih.org/trav_inf.html Communicable Disease Report – www.hc-sc.gc.ca/pphb-dgspsp/publicat/ccdr-rmtc/ Vaccine Adverse Event Reporting – www.hc-sc.gc.ca/hpb/lcdc/bid/di/vaae_e.html
UK Department of Health – www.doh.gov.uk/traveladvice/index.htm Communicable Disease Report – www.phls.co.uk/publications/cdr/index.html Fit for Travel – Scotland – www.fitfortravel.scot.nhs.uk National Travel Health Network and Centre – www.nathnac.org
European Surveillance website – www.eurosurveillance.org
Societies with interest in international medicine American Society of Tropical Medicine and Hygiene – www.astmh.org British Travel Health Association – www.btha.org German Society of Tropical Medicine and International Health – www.dtg.mwn.de/index.htm Infectious Diseases Society of America – www.idsa.org International Society of Travel Medicine – www.istm.org Pan American Health Organization – www.paho.org Royal Society of Tropical Medicine and Hygiene (UK) – www.rstmh.org Wilderness Medical Society – www.wms.org
Commercial travel medicine databases Travax EnCompass (Shoreland, Inc., US) – www.shoreland.com Travax (Travel Medicine – Scotland) – www.travax.scot.nhs.uk MASTA (England) – www.masta.org Exodus Software Ltd (Ireland) – www.exodus.ie Edisan (Médecine des Voyages – France) – www.edisan.fr Tropimed ® (Switzerland, Germany, USA) – www.tropimed.com
Listserv Discussion Groups International Society of Travel Medicine – listserv/@yorku.ca; type: subscribe Travelmed your name in message[b] American Society of Tropical Medicine and Hygiene – listserv/@yorku.ca; type: subscribe Tropmed your name in message[b] ProMed mail – majordomo@promedmail.org; type: subscribe Promed your name in message
[a]See Keystone *et al*.[24] for a comprehensive listing. [b]Requires membership in parent society to join discussion group.

advice has been shown to lead to improved compliance with antimalarials.[35]

It is not enough to educate travelers using only verbal discussion. They may be overwhelmed in the pre-travel session and have difficulty retaining information only from memory. As an example of the challenge faced by travelers, consider the amount of information they are given just in the discussion about malaria chemoprophylaxis. They have to retain information about the mosquito vector, the time periods for risk of exposure to the vector, the geographic regions of risk, the measures to avoid exposure e.g., repellents, insecticides, clothing, use of netting, and the indications, side-effects, and schedule for administration of malaria chemoprophylactics. This advice is given when the traveler may be really worried about, and focusing on, how many injections they will be receiving. Therefore, most travel health advisors

recommend providing the traveler with written materials that summarize and highlight the information. The traveler can refer to this material and process the information when they are under less pressure. In the survey of travel medicine clinics, written advice on malaria was provided 94% of the time, information on insect avoidance 86% of the time, and information on traveler's diarrhea 91% of the time.[12] Slightly more than 20% of clinics presented videos on these topics to travelers.

Clinics may want to write their own education material. This has the advantage of reinforcing what was said in the pre-travel visit and emphasizes concepts in a consistent fashion.

There are several commercial sources of advice, such as computer-based travel advice that can be printed or hard copy material that can be copied and presented to the traveler (see Table 3.7 and Keystone *et* al.[24]). Booklets and monographs can deal with a wider range of topics and can be purchased separately by the traveler. It is important, however, that written advice on the key medical and health issues is included as part of the visit, and is not an optional, extra expense item.

Travelers can also access many of the same Internet sites used by travel medicine providers. Much of the information in these sites, particularly that of the CDC and Fit for Travel–Scotland, is easily understood by the traveling public. In addition to those listed in Table 3.7, there are others specifically oriented toward the traveler listed in Table 3.8, and discussed more completely by Keystone et al.[24] This article also lists several sites of benefit to travelers with special needs or chronic illness.

In addition to education about the main topics in travel medicine, such as avoidance of malaria and diarrhea and the indications for vaccines, travel clinics should be able to provide advice in other, less common areas. These areas include health issues for special needs traveler, such as pregnant women, diabetics, elderly persons, and those who travel with chronic cardiac or pulmonary disease. The access of safe and reliable medical care overseas is another important topic for both the short and long-term expatriate traveler. Providing brochures on travel medical insurance programs is useful. In the USA, the US State Department maintains a listing of air evacuation and medical insurance companies at travel.state.gov/medical.html. Providing these additional resources will further distinguish a travel medicine service from a generalist's office that is giving travel vaccines and enhance the level of care.

POLICIES AND PROCEDURES

All patients who receive a vaccine are required to have informed consent. The initial decision about which vaccines to receive occurs during the pre-travel counseling session when the traveler's risks for vaccine-preventable diseases are identified and discussed. However, it is still necessary to undergo a more formal process of obtaining con-

Table 3.8	Internet information resources for the traveler[a]
World Health Organization Home page – www.who.int/home-page
US Centers for Disease Control and Prevention – Travel Medicine Home page – www.cdc.gov/travel/index.htm
US State Department – Medical Information for Americans – travel.state.gov/medical.html
US CIA World Factbook – www.odci.gov/cia/publications/factbook
Divers Alert Network (DAN) – www.diversalertnetwork.org/
Expedia – www.expedia.com/daily/travnews
Travel Health On-Line (Shoreland, Inc., Milwaukee, US) – www.tripprep.com
International Association for Medical Assistance to Travelers (IAMAT) – www.iamat.org
Health Canada – Travel Medicine Program – www.hc-sc.gc.ca/pphb-dgspsp/tmp-pmv/pub_e.html
MASTA (Australia) – www.masta.edu.au/
Traveller's Medical and Vaccination Centres (Australia) – www.tmvc.com.au
MASTA (England) – www.masta.org/home.html
UK Department of Health – www.doh.gov.uk/traveladvice/index.htm
Fit for Travel – Scotland – www.fitfortravel.scot.nhs.uk/

Travel Clinic Directories
    ISTM – www.istm.org/disclinics.html
    ASTM&H – www.astmh.org/clinics/clinindex.html

[a]See Keystone et al.[24] for a comprehensive listing

sent that includes hearing and reading information about the potential benefits and side effects of each vaccine. Following the decision to receive a vaccine, the traveler will sign the consent form. The need for signed consent varies worldwide, and in some areas of Europe and Africa, after the provision of relevant information, a verbal agreement to receive vaccinations is acceptable.

In order to facilitate the presentation of consistent and accurate information about vaccines, the US Public Health Service has written a 'Vaccine Information Statement' (VIS) on each vaccine given for routine health-care in the USA. These may be downloaded from the CDC at www.cdc.gov/nip/publications/vis. A sample of the VIS for measles-mumps-rubella vaccine is seen in Figure 3.4. For vaccines that are not covered by these documents, the vaccine manufacturer may have written one that can be used; otherwise, the clinic should write their own information statements.

Infection control practices should be in place at all immunization sites. These are usually set by the hospital or medical school where a clinic is located, or by the state or regional health departments for free standing clinics. The use of gloves, and the disposal of sharps and spent vaccine vials, are all regulated items.

TRAVEL CLINIC FACILITIES, EQUIPMENT AND SUPPLIES

Facilities

The variation in settings for travel medicine practices makes it difficult to recommend a standard configuration for the clinic. Some clinics will be set within an internal medicine or a generalist practice, and may not have dedicated space for travel. Generally, these will be ones that have lower patient volumes. Nevertheless, all clinics will have a reception area where the patient registers for their appointment, and an area where they wait prior to their appointment. The waiting area can be used for patient education where travel magazines, health bulletins, and even educational videos may be made available.

For the busy travel medicine practice, dedicated space is important. This entails having both consultation rooms and vaccine administration rooms. As discussed previously, one model for care is to have a travel specialist obtain the travel and medical history, render advice, and review vaccines in a separate consultation room in which vaccines are not administered. The patient is then brought into another room where vaccines are given. In clinics that also provide pre-travel physical exams or post-travel care, this room can be used as an examination room. In another model, the same person obtains the travel history, renders advice, and administers vaccines. This can occur in a single room, or two rooms can be used as described above.

Travel clinics that are located in hospitals or within a medical school or group practice will typically have access to laboratory testing. Pre-travel testing might include serology for immunity to hepatitis A, hepatitis B, or measles, and testing for HIV as a requirement by some countries prior to obtaining an entry visa. A laboratory on site will make it easier to evaluate patients for post-travel illness. It is best if the laboratory has expertise in interpreting blood smears and in examining stools for ova and parasites.

Equipment

Ideally, each consultation room should have a computer. This allows the provider to access the travel medicine practice database if one has been created. They can immediately determine the vaccines a patient received during a previous consultation if the hard copy of their medical record is not available. The computer should also have the

MEASLES MUMPS & REBELLA VACCINES

WHAT YOU NEED TO KNOW?

1 | Why get vaccinated?

Measles, mumps, and rubella are serious diseases.

Measles
- Measles virus causes rash, cough, runny nose, eye irritation, and fever.
- It can lead to ear infection, pneumonia, seizures (jerking and staring), brain damage, and death. Ask your doctor or nurse for more information.

Mumps
- Mumps virus causes fever, headache, and swollen glands.
- It can lead to deafness, meningitis (infection of the brain and spinal cord covering), painful swelling of the testicles or ovaries, and, rarely, death.

Rubella (German Measles)

- Rubella virus causes rash, mild fever, and arthritis (mostly in women).
- If a woman gets rubella while she is pregnant, she could have a miscarriage or her baby could be born with serious birth defects.

You or your child could catch these diseases by being around someone who has them. They spread from person to person through the air.

Measles, mumps, and rubella (MMR) vaccine can prevent these diseases.

Most children who get their MMR shots will not get these diseases. Many more children would get them if we stopped vaccinating.

2 | Who should get MMR vaccine and when?

Children should get 2 doses of MMR vaccine::

The first at **12-15 months of age** and the second at **4-6 years of age.**

These are the recommended ages. But children can get the second dose at any age, as long as it is at least 28 days after the first dose.

Some **adults** should also get MMR vaccine: Generally, anyone 18 years of age or older, who was born after 1956, should get at least one dose of MMR vaccine, unless they can show that they have had either the vaccines or the diseases. MMR vaccine may be given at the same time as other vaccines.

3 | Some people should not get MMR vaccine or should wait

- People should not get MMR vaccine who have ever had a life-threatening allergic reaction to **gelatin**, the antibiotic **neomycin**, or **a previous dose of MMR vaccine**
- People who are moderately or severely ill at the time the shot is scheduled should usually wait until they recover before getting MMR vaccine.

- Pregnant women should wait to get MMR vaccine until after they have given birth. Women should not get pregnant for 4 weeks after getting MMR vaccine.

- Some people should check with their doctor about whether they should get MMR vaccine, including anyone who:
  - Has HIV/AIDS, or another disease that affects the immune system
  - Is being treated with drugs that affect the immune system, such as steroids, for 2 weeks or longer.
  - Has any kind of cancer
  - Is taking cancer treatment with x-rays or drugs
  - Has ever had a low platelet count (a blood disorder)

Figure 3.4 A Vaccine Immunization Sheet that describes the Measles-Mumps-Rubella vaccine. These sheets are available in the US from the CDC (www.cdc.gov/nip/publications/vis). They should be read and retained by the traveler prior to administration of the vaccine as part of the informed consent process. Clinics may also obtain information sheets from vaccine manufacturers or write their own if necessary.

Continued

- People who recently had a transfusion or were given other blood products should ask their doctor when they may get MMR vaccine

Ask your doctor or nurse for more information.

4 What are the risks from MMR vaccine?

A vaccine, like any medicine, is capable of causing serious problems, such as severe allergic reactions. The risk of MMR vaccine causing serious harm, or death, is extremely small.

Getting MMR vaccine is much safer than getting any of these three diseases.
Most people who get MMR vaccine do not have any problems with it.

Mild Problems
- Fever (up to 1 person out of 6)
- Mild rash (about 1 person out of 20)
- Swelling of glands in the cheeks or neck (rare)
  If these problems occur, it is usually within 7-12 days after the shot. They occur less often after the second dose.

Moderate Problems
- Seizure (jerking or staring) caused by fever (about 1 out of 3,000 doses)
- Temporary pain and stiffness in the joints, mostly in teenage or adult women (up to 1 out of 4)
- Temporary low platelet count, which can cause a bleeding disorder (about 1 out of 30000 doses)

Severe Problems (Very Rare)
- Serious allergic reaction (less than 1 out of a million doses)
- Several other severe problems have been known to occur after a child gets MMR vaccine. But this happens so rarely, experts cannot be sure whether they are caused by the vaccine or not. These include:
  - Deafness
  - Long-term seizures, coma, or lowered consciousness
  - Permanent brain damage

5 What if there is a moderate or severe reaction?

What should I look for?
Any unusual conditions, such as a serious allergic reaction, high fever or behavior changes. Signs of a serious allergic reaction include difficulty breathing, hoarseness or wheezing, hives, paleness, weakness, a fast heart beat or dizziness within a few minutes to a few hours after the shot. A high fever or seizure, if it occurs, would happen 1 or 2 weeks after the shot.

What should I do?
- Call a doctor, or get the person to a doctor right away.
- Tell your doctor what happened, the date and time it happened, and when the vaccineation was given.
- Ask your doctor, nurse, or health department to file a Vaccine Adverse Event reporting System (VAERS) form, or call VAERS yourself at 1-800-822-7967

6 The National Vaccine Inquiry Compensation Program

In the rare event that you or your child has a seriuos reaction to a vaccine, a federal program has been created to help you pay for the care of those who have been harmed.

For details about the National Vaccine Injury Compensation Program, call **1-800-338-2382** or visit the program's website at
http://www.hrsa.gov/bhpr/vicp

7 How can I learn more?

- Ask your doctor or nurse. They can give you the vaccine package insert orsuggest other sources of information.

- Call your local or state health department's immunization program.

- Contact the Centers for Disease Control and Prevention (CDC):
  - Call **1-800-232-2522** (English)
  - Call **1-800-232-0233** (Epañol)
  - Visit the National Immunization program's website at **http://www.cdc.gov/nip**

U.S. DEPARTMENT OF HEALTH & HUMAN SERVICES
Centres for disease Control and Prevention
National Immunization program

Vaccine information Statement (Interim)
MMR (6/13/02)   42 U.S.C. § 300aa-26

Figure 3.4 cont'd A Vaccine Immunization Sheet that describes the Measles-Mumps-Rubella vaccine. These sheets are available in the US from the CDC (www.cdc.gov/nip/publications/vis). They should be read and retained by the traveler prior to administration of the vaccine as part of the informed consent process. Clinics may also obtain information sheets from vaccine manufacturers or write their own if necessary

commercial, off-line database if the clinic has subscribed to one. Lastly, if the computer is connected to the Internet, web-based information services can be consulted when questions arise about such issues as the status of an outbreak or the location of travel medicine clinics in other areas of the country or world.

Each consultation room should have a telephone, and a fax machine should be available within the clinic. The latter is particularly useful in receiving vaccine records or insurance referrals from travelers' primary care physicians.

A refrigerator and freezer are required for vaccines; vaccine storage should be their sole use. If possible they should be connected to an emergency power source so that if power is lost, the cold chain will not be disrupted. It is mandatory to monitor and record the temperature and in some areas of the world (e.g., the European Union) this is a requirement for yellow fever registration. Temperature recording should be undertaken twice daily. If the refrigerator/freezer is not connected to emergency power, an alarm should be installed to indicate if the temperature deviates from the standard. Vaccines requiring refrigeration should be maintained at 2°–8°C (35°–46°F), with an optimal temperature of 5°C (40°F).[36] Vaccines that require frozen storage (e.g., yellow fever and varicella) should be maintained at –15°C (5°F) or cooler with an optimal temperature of –20°C (0°F). Because the refrigerator door will be exposed to warmer temperatures, vaccines should never be stored on the door.

Vaccines

Vaccines are generally ordered from the manufacturers. If a clinic is part of a hospital or school of medicine practice, purchasing will be through the pharmacy services. It is typical that hospital pharmacies have purchasing contracts with vaccine manufacturers with whom they have agreed price structures. This may limit a clinic's ability to independently choose between two similar products. For example, if a clinic would like to use Vaqta (Merck) for protection of its travelers against hepatitis A, but the hospital has a contract with GlaxoSmithKline, then Havrix will be the vaccine supplied in the clinic. A log of vaccine use should be maintained in order that supplies always remain sufficient to meet demand.

The ability to administer yellow fever vaccine is usually regulated by state, regional, or provincial health departments. An application is required and certain conditions have to be met before being registered to give the vaccine. These may include proof that the clinic is staffed by licensed health-care personnel, that the vaccine will be maintained at the proper storage temperatures and given promptly after reconstitution, or that the clinic can handle potential anaphylactic reactions to the vaccine. Once approved, the regulating health agency provides the clinic with a validation stamp to be recorded in the WHO 'International Certificate of Vaccination'[19] as required by international health regulations.

Supplies

Most supplies relate to the administration of vaccines: gloves, syringes of multiple sizes, needles of different lengths and gauge (for intramuscular and intradermal use with patients of different size and weight), bandages, alcohol pads, cotton gauze. Some clinics carry a topical anesthetic such as Emla cream® (Astra), which can be applied in children to the immunization site approximately half an hour prior to receipt of the injections.

Infection control safety features include having a 'sharps receptacle' readily available for the disposal of needles and syringes. The authors have mounted it on the wall adjacent to the examination table where vaccines are given. Once the injection is completed, the administrator simply turns and drops the syringe with the attached needle into the bucket.

An important safety feature is the ability to deal with an anaphylactic reaction after vaccination. Adrenaline compounds and antihistamines should be readily available. Some hospital-based clinics have the advantage of on-site emergency medical technicians and an emergency room that can take care of rare, severe adverse reactions.

OPTIONAL TRAVEL CLINIC SERVICES

In addition to the basic provision of advice, vaccines and preventive prescriptions, many travel clinics have expanded their care to other areas. These include providing telephone advice, selling travel-related items, and rendering post-travel care. Some have combined their travel clinic with a vaccination clinic. The range of potential services is defined in Table 3.9. Giving travel advice over the telephone is controversial and has been cited by travel medicine specialists as a major challenge. Most clinics are willing to provide advice to physicians, but fewer are willing to provide it to the general public. To give advice appropriately takes both time and expertise, and this effort for the public may not translate into patient visits to the clinic. In order to gain some remuneration for telephone advice to the public, 16% of clinics actually charged for this advice.[12]

With the advent of e-mail and the listing of travel clinics on the ISTM and ASTM&H web pages (as well as other sites), questions now come via e-mail. Responding to these requests requires an equal effort. It also provides the person requesting the information with a written statement of your recommendations, which, if acted upon by the patient, could make you legally responsible for the recommendations if the traveler had a deleterious side effect from a drug or vaccine.

If a clinic chooses to provide telephone or e-mail advice, it should be clear who will respond to the requests, and when the response will happen. Setting aside a certain time each day to deal with the queries will make the effort more efficient.

A clinic also needs to decide how detailed to make their advice. We have found that giving general rather than specific advice to public inquiries is best, and because you have not established a formal physician-patient relationship, it may be the safest course from a medical-legal point of view. It is not possible or practical to obtain all of the medical and itinerary information over the telephone to properly assess health risks, and therefore, any specific recommendations that you give would be based on incomplete data.

The following is a suggested way to respond to a request for medical advice for travel to Kenya for a safari:

'There are several health issues to consider when traveling to Kenya. These involve protecting yourself against insect carriers of disease, receiving vaccines against some diseases, being careful about what you eat and drink to avoid diarrhea, and exercising common sense behavior. The following immunizations can be considered depending upon your planned activities, whether or not you have any medical conditions, and which vaccines you may have previously received: tetanus-diphtheria, hepatitis A, hepatitis B, polio, typhoid, and yellow fever. Malaria is a common and very serious problem in Kenya, and you should take care to avoid the mosquitoes transmitting infection and take malaria preventive medication. There are several medications to choose from and you should discuss with your doctor which one would be best for you. You should also know how to access medical care during your trip if you need it. A visit to a travel medicine specialist can help you to determine which preventive measures are best for you and you will be able to discuss these and other issues in more detail.'

Table 3.9	Optional travel clinic services
Telephone or e-mail advice to physicians and the traveling public
Sale of travel-related items, e.g., repellents, netting, rehydration salts, first aid kits
Pre-travel physical exams
Evaluation and screening for post-travel illness
Combining travel medicine services with a vaccination clinic
Pharmacy services
Clinical laboratory testing

Some larger travel medicine practices have developed automated response lines. These are complex to develop, however, and need constant updating to remain current.

Selling travel related health items is a way to provide increased revenue, but it also benefits the patient by allowing them to immediately purchase items that may be otherwise difficult to locate. There are several companies that produce items targeted to the traveler.[24]

In some clinics (predominantly in the UK) pre-packaged antimalarial drugs, standby treatment drugs for traveler's diarrhea or malaria, and drugs to prevent acute mountain sickness can be provided to travelers during the consultation. This allows specific explanation of the medications. Malaria diagnostic kits (in countries where they are available) can also be offered to long-term travelers.

The setting, training and interests of the travel medicine providers within a clinic will determine whether or not pre-travel physical exams or post-travel evaluation and care are performed. Clinics that are part of a university student health service or an occupational medicine program with contracts with corporations might perform physical exams as part of visa or program participation requirements. Additional time would need to be allotted to render these services.

The consensus statement by Canadian travel medicine experts[1] as well as the body of knowledge developed by the ISTM,[5] does not include the requirement for extensive knowledge of tropical disease by travel medicine specialists. The Canadians recommend that 'all post-travel consultations should be managed by a physician and should include the following: recognition of any travel-related illness, and timely medical assessment, with referral if required, for the management of travel-related illnesses'.[1] Therefore, all travel medicine specialists should be able to recognize key syndromes in the returned traveler and know how to refer them for adequate care. For clinics with personnel with expertise in infectious diseases and tropical medicine, it will be appropriate to evaluate and treat ill returned travelers without referral. In these settings, it is necessary to have adequate laboratory assistance to diagnose or confirm suspected illness.

The combination of a vaccine clinic and a travel clinic is a natural association. The vaccines are available, and the expertise of the staff is immediately at hand. Vaccine clinics can immunize immigrants who need immunizations to obtain entry visas, students who need immunizations for schooling, such as meningococcal vaccine, that might not be carried by local physicians, and veterinarians and animal handlers who require rabies vaccination. The clinic can also be open to any others who require a vaccine, but do not have access to a physician who can provide it.

In some cases, such as with immigrants or veterinarians, it is necessary to use laboratory services to check serology for proof of immunity to measles or varicella, as examples, or whether the titer of rabies antibody in previously immunized persons is sufficient to preclude a booster dose of rabies vaccine.

Vaccine clinic visits are of short duration and efficient, and leads to increased productivity of the clinic. A separate vaccine clinic form should be generated that contains patient demographic data, pertinent medical, immunization and medication history, and the reason for the vaccine. The reverse side of the form can be a standard immunization form. Once completed, this can be entered into the clinic database, or filed in the chart.

FEES AND REVENUE FOR A TRAVEL MEDICINE PRACTICE

In few other areas of travel medicine is there as much controversy as that of fee structures and reimbursement. In the USA, travel clinics range from being entirely private, fee-for-service facilities in which the providers do not join any third-party carrier plans, to hospital or medical school-based clinics in which fees are set by the hospital or university practice plan and all providers participate with insurance programs. In addition, there is wide variability in the reimbursement levels for travel medicine by insurance carriers, with many carriers refusing to cover vaccines and medications prescribed for travel. In many other areas of the world, such as Canada, the travel visit and vaccine charges are usually not covered by provincial health plans.

In the USA, travel medicine specialists who are participating providers for third-party carriers are required to accept the terms of reimbursement of those carriers. The travel clinic, then, cannot request that the traveler pay more than the insurance company's level of reimbursement for a covered service. This frequently leads to underpayment for rendered services, particularly for vaccines that may cost the provider more than the amount of the insurance company payment. For uncovered services, the travel clinic can request a cash payment. A waiver that indicates that the traveler is responsible for payment for uncovered services will need to be agreed and signed before the traveler can be billed. This waiver should be obtained for all patients as they register for their appointment.

In clinics that participate with insurance plans, a physician must be physically present in the clinic when care is rendered by a nurse in order for the nurse to bill for the travel visit. In this case the nurse is billing 'incident to' the physician. Nurses can bill independently in entirely private clinics that are fee-for-service.

US Medicaid will not cover any services related to travel, so Medicaid patients have to pay cash for the advice and vaccines that they receive. Some clinics require Medicaid patients to pay before they are seen rather than sending a bill to them. Medicare will cover routinely recommended vaccines for adults: influenza, pneumococcal, tetanus, hepatitis B, and also rabies.

Finally, most patients will require a referral from their primary care physician in order for the clinic to bill the patient's insurance company. These referrals should be initiated when the appointment is booked, although with the ready availability of facsimile machines, the referral can be made when the patient arrives for their appointment and registers. However, this process will take increased time and effort on the part of office staff.

A clinic needs to determine their method for collection of charges. Should the clinic bill the insurance company, should it bill the patient and have the patient seek reimbursement from their insurance company, or should the clinic collect payment at the time of service? It is easier to collect cash or credit card payment at the time of the visit to decrease costs associated with billing. If the clinic is a participating provider with an insurance carrier and more is initially collected than the amount paid by the insurance company, however, the clinic is obligated to return the difference. This can be a cumbersome process that diminishes profitability of the travel service.

Most care in travel medicine consists of a consultation fee, vaccine fees, and vaccine administration charges. The correct billing codes should be applied to each of these services. In the USA, both a diagnostic code called an ICD-9 code (International Classification of Diseases),[37] and a procedural code called a CPT code (Current Procedural Terminology)[38] are applied for each service, including each vaccine administered. For example, yellow fever vaccine has an ICD-9 code of V04.4 and a CPT code of 90717. There is also a procedural code for the administration of the vaccine: 90471 for the administration of a single vaccine, and 90472 for the administration of each additional vaccine. The specific codes can be found in the publications referenced.[37,38]

For the travel consultation, office visit, or other outpatient visit, CPT codes are used. For new patients the codes range from 99201 (10 min) to 99205 (60 min) depending upon the complexity of the visit. For follow-up visits the codes are 99211 (5 min) through 99215 (40 min). The problem with using these codes in travel medicine is that they require a physical examination as part of the visit (except for 99211). A physical exam is not routinely part of pre-travel evaluation. Therefore, in our practice, we use preventive medicine, individual or group counseling coding. These codes are to be used when services are 'provided to individuals (or groups) at a separate encounter for the purpose of promoting health and preventing illness or injury.'[38] The codes are 99401 (15 min), to 99404 (60 min). Codes 99411 (30 min) or 99412 (60 min) are used for group counseling when there is one or more traveler. The diagnostic code for travel visits that we use is V65.8.

The preventive medicine codes seem more appropriate to describe what is taking place during the pre-travel visit. Because many insurance carriers will not cover preventive medicine services the traveler will have to pay cash for them. Travelers should be informed of this at the time of making the appointment or at registration and sign a waiver indicating that they are responsible for payment.

Items sold separately in the clinic, such as repellents, netting, and travel health books, can be charged on a cash basis.

MARKETING AND PROMOTING A TRAVEL CLINIC

Table 3.10 indicates the wide range of ways to promote a travel medicine service among travelers and referring physicians. Word of

Table 3.10	Marketing a travel medicine service
Word of mouth among travelers, referral physicians, health agencies, or travel agencies
News releases to print, radio or television media concerning travel medicine care

Direct advertising in:
   print media
   telephone directories
   regional/state medical journals

Development of a clinic brochure with mailings to:
   physicians
   retail travel agencies
   regional/state health departments

Letters to referring physicians that details vaccines administered and medications prescribed
Education sessions for physicians and lay public

mouth between travelers and referring physicians can increase awareness about a clinic and lead to referrals. The first step in this process is to make clear to the traveler the advantages of the visit to a travel clinic compared with receiving care from a primary care physician. These advantages have been described earlier: provider knowledge of disease epidemiology and prevention, availability of all vaccines necessary for travel, provision of advice and preventive strategies on uncommon diseases, and availability of written resources on disease prevention. Travelers will recognize the value of clinics that can deliver this level of service and will share their enthusiasm with family and friends. It is not uncommon in our practice for travelers to say after their visit how impressed they were with the service; they had expected to come and only get shots, not to also receive detailed information on a wide variety of travel health risks.

Physicians will refer patients to a clinic if they perceive that their patient has received excellent care in a timely fashion and are provided with information about their patient's visit. All referral physicians should be sent a letter that details which vaccines were administered and which medications were prescribed. This provides the physician with a written record that can be filed with their chart. We also include with the letter a brochure that describes the clinic and its services. Many generalist offices do not want to stock costly and infrequently used immunizations, and find it difficult to keep up with changing global patterns of disease and prevention strategies. Therefore, if they are pleased with your service they are generally more than willing to let your clinic provide the care.

More direct measures can be employed. News releases about the clinic can generate publicity in newspapers, television, and radio. These releases are timely around holiday periods, or when world events provide an opportunity to describe the advantages of pre-travel care. If one is practicing travel medicine in a private office, it may be difficult to develop publicity for the press. Hospital- and medical school-based practices can, however, take advantage of their facility's marketing departments. These departments can make public service announcements for radio, arrange radio talk show interviews, and promote items for television. Clinic health-care providers can also give lectures to lay groups on the topic of health and travel, or more for-mal educational sessions (e.g., Grand Rounds) to the medical community

Direct advertising is another way to gain recognition. All clinics should be listed in the telephone directory. Larger advertisements can be taken out in these directories, in local newspapers, or in regional medical journals.

Direct mailings with a clinic brochure can be employed. Targets for these mailings include local physician's offices, schools and universities, and local and regional businesses that have international markets. Sending brochures to travel agencies may lead to referrals when they book international tours and travel. To generate business from these sources it can be helpful to visit the sites directly and present to them what your travel service has to offer. Meeting with the directors of travel agencies, student health center staff at schools and universities, and with human resource personnel in corporations is a way to effectively inform them of the advantages of having their client, students, or employees visit your service. If the volume of patients is sufficient from a particular site (school or business), a contract can be established. Under this contract, the clinic would agree to provide certain services at a reduced price and the facility would agree to have all of their travel care administered through your clinic. If the travel clinic also has a vaccine clinic as part of its services, contracts can be established with veterinary offices to provide rabies immunizations, or state or provincial health departments to provide hepatitis B immunizations, as examples.

A clinic brochure should contain information detailing reasons to obtain pre-travel care, what care will be provided, the hours of operation, directions to the facility, contact numbers, and a web address if developed. Including statistics about the travel population served by your clinic and pictures of travel destinations can enhance the appeal of a brochure.

Most travelers have access to Internet resources, and if a clinic develops its own website, the traveler can review this. The ISTM and ASTM&H websites maintain a listing of travel clinics that are directed by members of the respective societies. Accessing these sites is particularly useful when either a provider or traveler is trying to locate a clinic in another part of the country or the world. These lists have also been incorporated into some of the commercial travel information sites.

TROUBLESHOOTING

The survey of travel clinics identified several areas of challenge to the practice of travel medicine in 1994.[12] The top ten problems cited by practitioners are listed in Table 3.11; these represent more than 80% of all of the difficulties listed by clinics. Many of these remain a challenge today, and if those who are developing a clinic pay attention to and anticipate them during the planning stages, then it is likely that the clinic will be able to deal with them more efficiently.

CONCLUSION

With the growth of travel medicine, the importance of a specialized travel medicine service has become evident. Advantages of this service include provision of care by a health professional who has training and experience in the field and has access to information and resources from expert bodies to provide care based on current recommendations. In a travel clinic, the traveler should be able to receive advice on a wide range of topics, be administered any required or recommended vaccines, and be given prescriptions for prevention or self-treatment of problems such as malaria, diarrhea and high altitude illness. Providing pre-travel care at this level of service will distinguish the travel clinic from a generalist's office, and establish it as a critical aspect in the care of international travelers.

ACKNOWLEDGMENT

The author thanks Ron H. Behrens for helpful comments and suggestions.

Table 3.11	Top ten problems encountered in travel clinics[a]
Insufficient space, time, and staff to meet demands	
Travelers presenting with a short time interval before departure	
Phone calls for advice	
Need for standardized, up-to-date advice for clinic personnel	
Conflicting and unreliable advice provided to travelers	
Patient concern about the cost of service and vaccines	
Difficulty in assessing patient compliance with and understanding of advice	
Difficulty in accessing new medications and vaccines	
Failure of insurance carriers to pay for services	
Travelers having preconceived ideas about their needs	

[a]Adapted from Hill DR, Behrens RH, 1996[12]

REFERENCES

1. Committee to Advise on Tropical Medicine and Travel (CATMAT). Guidelines for the practice of travel medicine. An Advisory Committee Statement (ACS). *Can Commun Dis Reps* 1999; **25**:1–6.
2. DuPont HL, Steffen R, eds. *Textbook of Travel Medicine and Health*. 2nd edn. Hamilton, Ontario: B.C. Decker; 2001.
3. Zuckerman JN, ed. *Principles and Practice of Travel Medicine*. New York: John Wiley & Sons; 2001.
4. Behrens RH, Roberts JA. Is travel prophylaxis worth while? Economic appraisal of prophylactic measures against malaria, hepatitis A, and typhoid in travellers. *BMJ* 1994; **309**:918–922.
5. Kozarsky PE, Keystone JS. Body of knowledge for the practice of travel medicine. *J Travel Med* 2002; **9**:112–115.
6. Demeter SJ. An evaluation of sources of information in health and travel. *Can J Public Health* 1989; **80**:20–22.
7. Keystone JS, Dismukes R, Sawyer L, et al. Inadequacies in health recommendations provided for international travelers by North American travel health advisors. *J Travel Med* 1994; **1**:72–78.
8. Blair DC. A week in the life of a travel clinic. *Clin Micro Rev* 1997; **10**:650–673.
9. Leggat PA. Sources of health advice given to travelers. *J Travel Med* 2000; **7**:85–88.
10. Kain KC, MacPherson DW, Kelton T, et al. Malaria deaths in visitors to Canada and in Canadian travellers: a case series. *Can Med Assoc J* 2001; **164**:654–659.
11. Schiff AL. Travel industry and medical professionals. In: DuPont HL, Steffen R, eds. *Textbook of Travel Medicine and Health*. 2nd edn. Hamilton, Ontario: BC Decker; 2001:11–15.
12. Hill DR, Behrens RH. A survey of travel clinics throughout the world. *J Travel Med* 1996; **3**:46–51.
13. Carroll B, Behrens RH, Crichton D. Primary health care needs for travel medicine training in Britain. *J Travel Med* 1998; **5**:3–6.
14. Grabowski P, Behrens RH. Provision of health information by British travel agents. *Trop Med Int Health* 1996; **1**:1–3.
15. Shafer RT, Correia J, Patel V, et al. Travel advice from embassies (letter). *Lancet* 1996; **348**:757–758.
16. Townend M. Sources and appropriateness of medical advice to trekkers. *J Travel Med* 1998; **5**:73–79.
17. Barry M, Maguire JH, Weller PF. The American Society of Tropical Medicine and Hygiene initiative to stimulate educational programs to enhance medical expertise in tropical diseases. *Am J Trop Med Hyg* 1999; **61**:681–688.
18. Gardner TB, Hill DR. Knowledge of travel medicine providers: analysis from a continuing education course. *J Travel Med* 1999; **6**:66–70.
19. Superintendent of Documents USPHS. *International Certificates of Vaccination (PHS-731)*. Washington, DC: Government Printing Office.
20. Centers for Disease Control. National childhood vaccine injury act: Requirements for permanent vaccination records and for reporting of selected events after vaccination. *MMWR* 1988; **37**:197–200.
21. Centers for Disease Control and Prevention. *Health Information for International Travel, 2001–2002*. Atlanta: US Department of Health and Human Services; 2001.
22. Lea G, Lesse J, eds. *Health Information for Overseas Travel*. London: The Stationery Office; 2001.
23. World Health Organization. International Travel and Health. *Vaccination Requirements and Health Advice*. Geneva, Switzerland: World Health Organization; 2002.
24. Keystone JS, Kozarsky PE, Freedman DO. Internet and computer-based resources for travel medicine practitioners. *Clin Infect Dis* 2001; **32**:757–765.
25. Keystone JS, Kozarsky PE, Nothdurft HD, et al., eds. *Travel Medicine*. London: Harcourt Publishers; 2003.
26. Guerrant RL, Walker DH, Weller PF, eds. *Tropical Infectious Diseases. Principles, Pathogens, & Practice*. Vol. 1. Philadelphia: Churchill Livingstone; 1999.
27. Strickland GT, ed. *Hunter's Tropical Medicine and Emerging Infectious Diseases*. 8th edn. Philadelphia: W.B. Saunders; 2000.
28. Cook G, Zumia A, eds. *Manson's Tropical Diseases*. 21st edn. London: W. B. Saunders; 2003.
29. Genton B, Behrens RH. Specialized travel consultation. Part II: acquiring knowledge. *J Travel Med* 1994; **1**:13–15.
30. Packman CJ. A survey of notified travel-associated infections: implications for travel health advice. *J Pub Health Med* 1995; **17**:217–222.
31. Lobel HO, Phillips-Howard PA, Brandling-Bennett AD, et al. Malaria incidence and prevention among European and North American travellers to Kenya. *Bull WHO* 1990; **68**:209–215.
32. Steffen R, Heusser R, Mächler R, et al. Malaria chemoprophylaxis among European tourists in tropical Africa: use, adverse reactions, and efficacy. *Bull WHO* 1990; **68**:313–322.

33. Kozicki M, Steffen R. Schär M. 'Boil it, cook it, peel it or forget it': does this rule prevent travellers' diarrhoea? *Int J Epidemiol* 1985; **14**:169–172.

34. Steffen R, Collard F, Tornieporth N, *et al*. Epidemiology, etiology, and impact of traveler's diarrhea in Jamaica. *JAMA* 1999; **281**:811–817.

35. Hill DR. Health problems in a large cohort of Americans traveling to developing countries. *J Travel Med* 2000; **7**:259–266.

36. Laboratory Centre for Disease Control. National guidelines for vaccine storage and transportation. *Can Commun Dis Rep* 1995; **21**:93–97.

37. American Medical Association. *International Classification of Diseases.* 9th revision. Clinical Modification. Chicago, IL: AMA Press; 2001.

38. American Medical Association. *Current Procedural Terminology.* Chicago, IL: AMA Press; 2001.

CHAPTER 4 Sources of Travel Medicine Information

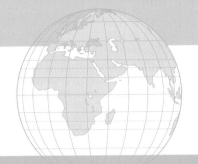

David O. Freedman

KEYPOINTS

- Authoratative bodies such as the World Health Organisation (WHO) and the Centers for Disease Control and Prevention (CDC) host websites that contain comprehensive travel health information. Numerous national bodies as well as commercial organisations also provide excellent travel health information on public or membership-only websites.

- Itinerary driven databases that generate comprehensive reports for use in travel health counseling have largely migrated from PC-based software to formats that can be accessed in real time over the Internet via a web-browser interface at the user's end

- Broad reference texts in travel medicine can be supplemented from a list of specialized texts that contain detailed discussions, factual tables, and primary references that are sometimes needed to deal with select or uncommon patients situations

- TravelMed is an important electronic discussion forum of issues related to the practice of travel medicine (see http://www.istm.org/listserv.html)

INTRODUCTION

Travel medicine is concerned with keeping international travelers alive and healthy. To an extent beyond that in most other disciplines, travel medicine providers need to keep constantly current with changing disease risk patterns in over 220 different countries. The knowledge base on which preventative and therapeutic interventions are based continues to change rapidly. An increasingly wired world allows for frequent and detailed dissemination of disease incidence patterns, information on new outbreaks, the description of new diseases affecting travelers, as well as data on new drug resistance patterns in old diseases. Travelers are finding ever more exotic and previously unvisited locales to go to. In addition, travelers are bringing ever more sophisticated and updated information with them at the time of the pre-travel medical encounter.

Electronic media are now the major source of updated information for travel medicine providers. Essentially all the most important authoritative national and international surveillance bulletins, outbreak information, and official governmental recommendations are available on the World Wide Web. For the most part, these authoritative sources still provide print output but uniformly with the delays inherent in producing print media. Printed reference sources serve for detailed reading on a particular topic. Individuals almost everywhere have open access to these medical information resources on the Internet. Travel medicine providers who are not current with

what is posted on the popular and authoritative Internet sites will be at a disadvantage when interacting with their patients.

This chapter will provide mostly in tabular form, information on key travel medicine oriented information resources targeted to travel medicine professionals. Selected consumer-targeted resources will be outlined briefly. By their nature, electronic resources change both location (web address or URL) and content more frequently than can be compensated for in a printed resource text such as this. As the Internet has matured and as certain key websites have emerged as pre-eminent a stability has emerged that was not present in the late 1990s. The electronic resources discussed below were current at press time, but some information may be outdated by the time this chapter is in the hands of the reader.

REFERENCE TEXTS

The first section of Table 4.1 lists selected core reference texts whose primary emphasis is a comprehensive approach to travel medicine and to keeping travelers alive and healthy. Any of these high quality resources is certainly sufficient to cover completely the practical aspects of caring for those to be seen in a travel medicine practice. The next sections list by category large reference texts that contain detailed discussions, factual tables, and primary references that would be helpful in dealing with select or uncommon situations. Some special groups may be more frequent in certain health-care settings and the listed publications may be worthwhile for providers who see many of a particular type of traveler. Both the WHO and CDC books are available over the Internet (see Table 4.3), but due to the frequent use that both these publications see in many settings, most providers still prefer to keep a hard-copy bound version on hand. Many very high-quality travel medicine reference booklets that are produced by national or regional societies or governmental entities are not covered here. Popular English language books targeted at consumers are listed last, so that providers can be aware of what the travelers are reading in order to be able to understand concerns and correct any misunderstandings that can arise from a lay literature of varying quality.

JOURNALS

Table 4.2 lists selected English language journals that consistently and frequently feature articles on travel medicine. Most of these journals have their complete contents available electronically in a format that is restricted to their own subscribers.

TRAVEL CLINIC SOFTWARE PROGRAMS

Since the early 1990s, electronic information systems for travel health counseling have become widely utilized and increasingly sophisti-

Table 4.1   Books

Comprehensive Travel Medicine Resources

Health Information for International Travel, 2003–2004 edn. (The 'CDC Yellow Book'). Order from the Public Health Foundation www.phf.org. Phone orders 1-877-252-1200 or 301-645-7773 outside USA.

International Travel and Health 2002. (WHO 'Green' Book (formerly yellow)). Published annually. Available from authorized WHO book agents. www.who.int/ith (not downloadable as one document – ISBN 92 4 158027 5).

Health Information for Overseas Travel, 2nd edn. Lea, G. and Leese, J. (editors). UK: The Stationery Office; 2001. www.archive.official-documents.co.uk/document/doh/hinfo/index.htm/(ISBN 0 11 322329 3).

Textbook of Travel Medicine and Health, 2nd edn. DuPont, H.L. and Steffen R. (editors). Hamilton, Ontario, Canada: B.C. Decker, Inc.; 2000. www.bcdecker.com (ISBN 1-55009-137-9).

Manual of Travel Medicine and Health, 2nd edn. Steffen R., DuPont H.L. Wilder-Smith, A. (editors). Hamilton, Ontario, Canada: B.C. Decker, Inc.; 2003. www.bcdecker.com (ISBN 1-55009-227-8).

Travel Medicine and Migrant Health Lockie, C. Walker, E. Calvert, L. Cossar, J. Raeside, F. Knill-Jones, R. (editors). UK: Churchill Livingstone; 2000 (ISBN 0443062420).

The Travel and Tropical Medicine Manual, 3rd edn. Jong, E.C., McMullen, R. UK: W.B. Saunders; 2002. www.us.elsevierhealth.com (ISBN 0-7216 7678 2)

Travel Medicine. Infectious Disease Clinics of North America Freedman D.O. (editor). Philadelphia, PA: W.B. Saunders; 1998, Vol. 12:2 (ISSN 0891-5520).

Travel Medicine. Medical Clinics of North America Jong E.C. (editor). Philadelphia, PA: W.B. Saunders; 1999, Vol. 83: 4.

Comprehensive Immunization Resources

Vaccines, 4th edn. Plotkin, S.A. and Orenstein, W.A. Philadelphia, PA: W.B. Saunders; 2004. www.us.elsevierhealth.com (ISBN 0-7216-9688-0).

Epidemiology and Prevention of Vaccine Preventable Diseases ('The Pink Book'), 7th edn. Atlanta, USA:.CDC; 2002. With 2003 update www.cdc.gov/nip/publications/pink/ (Free download available.)

Canadian Immunization Guide, 6th edn. Ottawa, Ontario, Canada: National Advisory Committee on Immunization; 2002. www.hc-sc.gc.ca/ pphb-dgspsp/publicat/cig-gci/index.html#toc (ISBN 0-660-18803-1 – Entire publication can be downloaded and printed free of charge.)

Travel and Routine Immunizations. Thompson R.F., Milwaukee, WI: Shoreland; 2003. Annual updates. http: //www.shoreland.com

Pharmacopoeias

Martindale, the Complete Drug Reference, 33rd edn. Sweetman S, (editor). London: Pharmaceutical Press; 2002, 085369 4990. www.pharmpress.com

Drug Information for the Health Care Professional. US Pharmacopeia DI, 22nd edn. Englewood, USA: Micromedex; 2002. www.micromedex.com (ISBN 156363 3310).

British National Formulary, 45th edn. Mehta, D.K. (editor). London: Pharmaceutical Press; 2003. www.bnf.org (ISBN: 0 85369 510 5).

Specialized Resource Texts (in-depth coverage of important areas)

Tropical Medicine and Emerging Infectious Diseases, 8th edn. Strickland, T. Hunter's Philadelphia: W.B. Saunders; 2000. www.elsevierhealth.com (ISBN 0-7216-6223-4).

Manson's Tropical Diseases, 21st edn. Cook, G. and Zumla, A. (editors). UK: W.B.Saunders; 2002. www.us.elsevierhealth.com. (ISBN 0-7020-2640-9).

A World Guide to Infections Wilson, ME. New York: Oxford University Press; 1991. www.oup-usa.org/medical/

Control of Communicable Disease Manual, 17th edn., Washington DC: Chin J. American Public Health Association; 2000. www.apha.org (ISBN 087553242X).

Red Book. Report of the Committee on Infectious Diseases, 26th edn. Elk Grove, IL: American Academy of Pediatrics; 2003. www.aap.org

Travelers' Malaria Schlagenhauf, P. Hamilton, Ontario, Canada: B.C. Decker; 2001. www.bcdecker.com (ISBN 1 55009 157 3).

Special Groups of Travelers

High Altitude Medicine. Hultgren, H. Stanford, CA: Hultgren Publications; 1997. www.highaltitudemedicine.com

Wilderness Medicine, 4th edn., Auerbach, P.S. St. Louis: Mosby; 2001 (ISBN 0 323 00950 6).

International Occupational and Environmental Medicine Herzstein, J.A. St. Louis, MO: Mosby; 1998. www.mosby.com

Refugee Health Medecins Sans Frontieres. London: Macmillan Education; 1997. www.msf.org

Field Guide to Wilderness Medicine Auerbach, P.S. et al. St. Louis, MO: Mosby; 1999 (ISBN 0815109261).

Consumer Oriented Books (what the travelers are reading)

International Travel Health Guide, 12th edn. Rose, S.R. Northampton, MA: Travel Medicine Inc; 2001. Downloadable in sections from http: //www.travmed.com.

Travelers Health – How to Stay Healthy Abroad, 4th Edn. Dawood R. Oxford University Press 2002.

Lonely Planet The 'Healthy Travel' Series Young, I., 2000. Separate volumes on Africa, Asia & India, Australia, New Zealand and the Pacific, Central & South America. www.lonelyplanet.com

The Travellers' Good Health Guide. Lankester, T. London: Sheldon Press; 1999. www.sheldonpress.com (ISBN 0 85969 827 0).

Bugs, Bites and Bowels, Healthy Travel, 2nd edn. Wilson-Howarth, J. Cadogan Guides; 2002. www.cadoganguides.com (ISBN 1-86011-868-2).

The Pocket Doctor: A Passport to Healthy Travel, 3rd edn. Bezruchka, Stephen. Seatle, WA: Mountaineers Books; (ISBN 0 89886 6 146).

The Rough Guide to Travel Health. Jones, N. London: Rough Guides, Inc; 2001. www.roughguides.com (ISBN 1 85828 570 4).

Travelling Well, 9th edn. Mills, D. Brisbane: Travelling Well; 2000. www.travellingwell.com.au/page1.html (ISBN 0 9577179 0 3).

Table 4.2   Journals frequently publishing papers on travel medicine

American Journal of Tropical Medicine & Hygiene
Aviation Space and Environmental Medicine
British Medical Journal
Bulletin of the World Health Organization
Clinical Infectious Diseases
Emerging Infectious Diseases Journal
Eurosurveillance Weekly
Eurosurveillance Monthly
Journal of Infectious Diseases
Journal of Occupational and Environmental Medicine
Journal of Travel Medicine
The Lancet
Military Medicine
Morbidity and Mortality Weekly Report
Pediatric Infectious Diseases Journal
Transactions of the Royal Society of Tropical Medicine & Hygiene
Tropical Medicine and International Health
Vaccine
Weekly Epidemiological Record
Wilderness and Environmental Medicine

cated. These systems allow the user to query large electronic databases containing information on disease risk, epidemiology, and vaccine recommendations across more than 220 countries in the world. These systems allow a rapid, convenient means of accessing a large body of changing information.

With the advent of active server page or ASP technology in recent years, these databases can be accessed in real time over the Internet via a web-browser interface at the user's end. All the major vendors of travel clinic software now make their products available via the web. Thus, the most widely used English language packages are all listed in Table 4.3 under the heading 'Destination Specific Database Programs for Health Care Providers'. In all cases, the software is also available on diskette or CD for providers who have no or slow Internet access. The advantage to Internet access is the availability of seamless access to real time updating. Diskettes and CDs must be shipped and loaded and updating can only occur as frequently as the vendor ships.

Most high quality systems have at least two major components: (1) displays of information including country by country information on health risks within a given country, country by country vaccine recommendations, and disease by disease fact sheets for major diseases; (2) an itinerary maker feature that, after input of a complete traveler itinerary, prints out summary recommendations for the entire itinerary in the order of travel. These printouts generally include a vaccination plan, malaria recommendations, destination risks, in-country resources, and are individualized with the name of the patient and the clinic. In addition, detailed country-by-country disease maps, especially for malaria or yellow fever, are important features to consider in evaluating a system. Printouts of these can be important in educating patients who may have indefinite or changeable itineraries. Many software packages also now include global distribution maps for a number of important tropical diseases. As described individually

in Table 4.3, a number of other important and useful features are included in many of the available packages.

The quality and timeliness of the information contained in a software package should be the premier consideration. The listed databases all contain high quality information and the recommendations generated consistently represent those of authoritative national or international bodies. In case of discrepancy between WHO, CDC and national bodies, many of the software packages highlight these differences, and allow for selection of one or the other in generating a final report.

TRAVEL MEDICINE WEBSITES

Only selected websites that have data of generally high quality and of a broader international interest to travel medicine providers are referenced in Table 4.3. Checking more than one authoritative site on a specific issue is always recommended. First, authoritative recommendations still contain some element of opinion. Thus, even major sources like the WHO and the CDC can disagree on some issues. Second, because of changing disease patterns, what was accurate yesterday may not be accurate today and some sites are more timely in updating than others. Fortunately, most sites now put an indicator at the bottom of each page stating when the last update was. Always be suspicious of information on a web page that carries no date.

The URLs listed in Table 4.3 are grouped by general categories, which are self-explanatory. The sites maintained by the WHO and the CDC contain the most comprehensive primary information. Some valuable subsidiary web pages on these sites are not specifically listed in the table, but are linked from the WHO and CDC pages that are listed in the table. Many of the vendors that provide database software (discussed above) to health-care providers provide high quality, but less comprehensive versions in lay language to the public for free. The consumer-oriented sites are widely accessed by the public as a primary source of travel health information, so that it is important for practitioners to be familiar with what the travelers are reading.

ELECTRONIC DISCUSSION FORUMS AND LISTSERVS

'Listservs' are electronic distribution lists that function using e-mail. Anyone who has joined a particular listserv group can e-mail a posting to a central server. The posting is then disseminated to all members who have subscribed to the same list. Four electronic discussion groups are recommended for travel medicine providers (Table 4.4). To join one of these listservs, an e-mail message must be sent to the server as specified in Table 4.4 or in some cases a form can be filled out on a website that automatically generates the required e-mail. Once a person is accepted as a list member, the computer will generate, by e-mail, a list of instructions on how to participate in the discussion for that group. TravelMed is an unmoderated discussion of issues related to the practice of Travel Medicine (see www.istm.org/listserv.html for further information). Pro-Med is a moderated discussion of emerging infections with ability to post only a proportion of submissions received. It presently has over 25 000 subscribers.

Some listservs are set up to provide information only and not to allow interactive discussion. For example, with MMWR-TOC subscribers receive by e-mail each Thursday evening, the table of contents of that week's CDC Morbidity and Mortality Weekly Report. Subscribers can then decide whether or not to bother downloading the whole issue from the CDC server.

Table 4.3 **Travel medicine websites**

Authoritative Travel Medicine Recommendations

US CDC Travelers' Health Home	www.cdc.gov/travel/index.htm
US CDC Online Health Information for International Travel (The Yellow Book)	www.cdc.gov/travel/yb/index.htm
WHO On-line International Travel and Health (The Green (formerly yellow) Book)	www.who.int/ith/
Health Canada Travel Medicine Program Information for Professionals	www.hc-sc.gc.ca/pphb-dgspsp/tmp-pmv/prof_e.html
Canadian Committee to Advise on Tropical Medicine and Travel (CATMAT) Guidelines	www.hc-sc.gc.ca/pphb-dgspsp/tmp-pmv/catmat-ccmtmv/index.html
Canadian Immunization Guide (Health Canada)	www.hc-sc.gc.ca/pphb-dgspsp/publicat/cig-gci/
Health Information for Overseas Travel (UK Department of Health)	www.archive.official-documents.co.uk/document/doh/hinfo/index.htm
2001 Malaria Prevention Guidelines (UK Public Health Laboratory Service)	www.phls.org.uk/publications/cdph/issues/CDPHvol4/No2/malaria_guidelinesp.pdf

Travel Warnings and Consular Information

US Department of State Travel Warnings and Consular Information	travel.state.gov/travel_warnings.html
UK Foreign and Commonwealth Office Country Advice	www.fco.gov.uk/travel (click Country Advice)
Canada Department of Foreign Affairs & International Trade Travel Reports	www.voyage.gc.ca/dest/intro-en.asp
Australia Department of Foreign Affairs and Trade Travel Advice by Country	www.dfat.gov.au/consular/advice/advices_mnu.html
US Department of State HIV Testing Requirements for Entry into Foreign Countries	www.travel.state.gov/HIVtestingreqs.html
US Department of State Foreign Entry Requirements (visas needed etc.)	www.travel.state.gov/foreignentryreqs.html
Aircraft Disinsection Requirements by Country	ostpxweb.dot.gov/policy/safety/disin.htm

Vaccine Resources

US Advisory Committee on Immunization Practices Vaccine Specific Guidelines	www.cdc.gov/nip/ACIP/
US Vaccine Information Safety (VIS) Statements for Supply to Patients	www.cdc.gov/nip/publications/VIS/default.htm
Epidemiology and Prevention of Vaccine Preventable Diseases (The CDC Pink Book)	www.cdc.gov/nip/publications/pink/
Immunize.org (IAC)	www.immunize.org/index.htm
List of Names of Vaccine Products Country by Country	www.health.state.mn.us/divs/dpc/adps/forgnvac.htm

Disease Specific Information

WHO Health Topics A-Z Links to Disease Specific Web pages	www.who.int/health_topics/en/
CDC Health Topics A to Z Links to Disease Specific Web pages	www.cdc.gov/health/
Malaria Foundation International	www.malaria.org/
Roll Back Malaria Program	mosquito.who.int/

Multisource Destination Specific Database Programs (for health-care providers)

Travax and Travax Encompass (USA)[a]	www.shoreland.com
Travax NHS UK (unrelated to US site)[a]	www.travax.scot.nhs.uk
TropiMed[a]	www.tropimed.com
Walkabout 2000[a]	www.traveldoctor.com.au/
MASTA UK (Medical Advisory Services for Travellers Abroad)[a]	www.masta.org
GIDEON (Global Infectious Diseases Epidemiology Network)[a]	www.gideononline.com

Multisource Destination Specific Database Programs (for travelers)

Shoreland's Travel Health On-line (derived from US Travax)	www.tripprep.com
Scottish Centre for Infection and Environmental Health's Fit for Travel Site (derived from UK Travax)	www.fitfortravel.scot.nhs.uk/
Fit-for-Travel from the University of Munich (unrelated to Scottish site)	www.fit-for-travel.de/en/index.html
The TravelDoctor TMVC Australia Trip Planner (derived from Walkabout2000)	www.traveldoctor.com.au/
International Association for Medical Assistance to Travelers 1) Malaria and 2) Immunization Guides	www.iamat.org
International SOS Online Country Guides[a]	www.internationalsos.com/online
Mdtravelheath.com	www.MDtravelhealth.com
Travel-Vax (Ireland)	www.travelvax.net/travelvax/whatis.html
Travel Medicine, Inc.	www.travmed.com/

Table 4.3   Travel medicine websites—cont'd

Emerging Diseases & Outbreaks

ProMedmail; The ISID Program for Monitoring Emerging Infectious Diseases	www.promedmail.org
WHO Communicable Disease Surveillance and Response (CSR) Homepage	www.who.int/csr/en/
WHO CSR Disease Outbreak News	www.who.int/csr/don/en/
Health Canada Division of Disease Surveillance Infectious Disease News Brief	www.hc-sc.gc.ca/pphb-dgspsp/bid-bmi/dsd-dsm/nb-ab/index.html

Surveillance & Epidemiological Reports

Weekly Epidemiological Record (WHO)	www.who.int/wer/
Eurosurveillance Weekly	www.eurosurveillance.org/
WHO EURO Computerized Information System for Infectious Diseases	cisid.who.dk/
Morbidity and Mortality Weekly Report (US CDC)	www.cdc.gov/mmwr
Canada Communicable Diseases Report	www.hc-sc.gc.ca/pphb-dgspsp/publicat/ccdr-rmtc/index.html
UK CDR Weekly	www.phls.co.uk/publications/cdr/index.html
Australia Communicable Diseases Intelligence (CDI)	www.health.gov.au/pubhlth/cdi/cdihtml.htm
Eurosurveillance Links Page to the National European Bulletins	www.eurosurveillance.org/links/links-02.asp
PAHO Links to the National Bulletins	www.paho.org/English/SHA/shavsp.htm
WHO Links Page the Ministries of Health and National Surveillance Institutes Around the World	www.who.int/emc/surveill/mohglobal.html
EpiNorth-Bulletin of the Network for Communicable Disease Control in Northern Europe	www.epinorth.org/
GeoSentinel Global Surveillance Network[b]	www.istm.org/geosentinel/main.html
TropNetEurop Surveillance Network[b]	www.tropnet.net

General Travel Medicine Advice for Travelers

Lonely Planet Health	www.lonelyplanet.com/health/health.htm
Health Canada Travel Medicine Program Information for Travelers	www.hc-sc.gc.ca/pphb-dgspsp/tmp-pmv/pub_e.html

Disability Resources

Access-able Page	www.access-able.com/
Mobility International	www.miusa.org
Society for Accessible Travel and Hospitality (SATH)	www.sath.org/

Overseas Assistance

International SOS[b]	www.intsos.com/
BC/BS (Blue Cross/Blue Shield) Participating Worldwide Providers	www.bluecares.com/healthtravel/worldwide_hospitals.html
US Department of State List of Doctors and Hospitals Abroad	www.travel.state.gov/acs.html
International Association for Medical Assistance to Travelers[b]	www.iamat.org/
US Department of State List of Medical Evacuation Vendors	travel.state.gov/medical.html
Highway To Health[b]	www.highwaytohealth.com/

Maps & Country Information

United Nations Map Homepage	www.un.org/Depts/Cartographic/english/htmain.htm
US Department of State Country by Country Background Notes	www.state.gov/r/pa/ei/bgn/
MapQuest Online Location Finder	www.mapquest.com/
CIA World Factbook (Country by Country)	www.odci.gov/cia/publications/factbook/index.html
Links to Map-related Websites	www.lib.utexas.edu/maps/map-sites/map-sites.html/
National Geographic Map Machine	plasma.nationalgeographic.com/mapmachine/

Safety and Security

Association for Safe International Travel Country by Country Road Safety Information	www.asirt.org/
US Department of State Overseas Security Advisory Council (OSAC)[b]	www.ds-osac.org/
iJet Travel Intelligence Travel Risk Management	www.ijet.com
Kroll Inc. Risk Consulting[a]	www.krollworldwide.com/
Control Risks Group Risk Consultancy[a]	www.crg.com/
Global Business Access, Ltd. Consulting[a]	www.globalltd.com/

General Travel Information of Frequent Interest to Patients

CDC Division of Quarantine	www.cdc.gov/ncidod/dq/index.htm
Times Around the World	times.clari.net.au/index.htm
Embassies in the USA List of Links to Web pages	www.embassy.org/embassies/index.html
Embassies in the USA US Department of State Official List	www.state.gov/s/cpr/rls/fco/index.cfm?id=4194

Table 4.3	Travel medicine websites—cont'd
Electrical Outlet Configurations Country by Country	www.teleadapt.com/
International Civil Aviation Organization (UN Agency)	www.icao.int/
International Air Transport Association (airline industry consortium)	www.iata.org/
US Federal Aviation Administration International Aviation Safety Assessment Program Country by Country List	www.faa.gov/avr/iasa/index.htm
World Tourism Organization	www.world-tourism.org/
Training in Travel Medicine	
HealthTraining.org Database of Training Opportunities	www.healthtraining.org
TropEd Europ List of Accredited Programs	www.troped.org/
TrainingFinder PHF Database of Training Opportunities	www.trainingfinder.org/
International Society of Travel Medicine Certification Process	www.istm.org/certificate_of_knowledge/cok_top_frame.html
American Society of Tropical Medicine and Hygiene Certification Process	www.astmh.org/certification.html
Short Courses and Meetings in Travel Medicine	
Swiss Tropical Institute Basel Annual Short Course in Travel Medicine	www.sti.ch/kurse.htm
London School of Hygiene & Tropical Medicine Annual Short Course	www.lshtm.ac.uk/
Royal Free Hospital University College London	r.hargreaves@rfc.ucl.ac.uk
Wilderness Medical Society	www.wms.org
International Society of Travel Medicine Congresses (odd years only)	www.istm.org
American Society of Tropical Medicine and Hygiene Annual Meetings	www.astmh.org
British Travel Health Association Annual Meetings	www.btha.org
Travel & International Medicine Course (odd years only)	www.dom.washington.edu/cme/
Asia Pacific Travel Health Society Congresses (even years only)	www.apths.com
Diploma Courses in Travel and/or Tropical Medicine	
The Gorgas Course in Clinical Tropical Medicine	info.dom.uab.edu/gorgas/
London School of Hygiene & Tropical Medicine	www.lshtm.ac.uk/
Scottish Centre for Infection and Environmental Health Travel Medicine Diploma	www.travelcourses.scieh.scot.nhs.uk scieh.htm
Swiss Tropical Institute Basel	www.sti.ch/kurse.htm
Royal Free and University College	r.hargreaves@rfc.ucl.ac.uk
Liverpool School of Tropical Medicine	www.liv.ac.uk/lstm/lstm.html
James Cook University	www.jcu.edu.au/school/sphtm/phtm/subjects/tm5512.htm
Mahidol Tropical Medicine	www.tm.mahidol.ac.th/index.htm/
Tulane School of Public Health Department of Tropical Medicine	www.tropmed.tulane.edu/
Professional Societies	
International Society of Travel Medicine	www.istm.org
American Society of Tropical Medicine and Hygiene	www.astmh.org/
Royal Society of Tropical Medicine and Hygiene	www.rstmh.org/
Wilderness Medical Society	www.wms.org/
Divers Alert Network[b]	www.diversalertnetwork.org/
American College of Occupational and Environmental Medicine[b]	www.acoem.org/
American Association of Occupation Health Nurses[b]	www.aaohn.org/
Undersea & Hyperbaric Medicine Society	www.uhms.org/
Vendors of Travel Health Products	
MASTA UK (Medical Advisory Services for Travellers Abroad)	www.masta.org/products/index.html
Chinook Medical Inc.	www.chinookmed.com
Travel Medicine, Inc.	www.travmed.com
Magellan's	www.magellans.com

[a]Access restricted to fee-paying subscribers/members or to specific professionals. Sample material usually available.
[b]Access to some sections of the website restricted to fee-paying subscribers or members. Sample material usually available.

Table 4.4	Listservs relevant to travel medicine practice
Type in the body of the message:	**Send to this address:**
Discussion groups	
subscribe TRAVELMED your name[a]	listserv@yorku.ca
subscribe TROPMED your name[b]	listserv@yorku.ca
ProMedmail (complete on-line form)	www.promedmail.org
subscribe MALARIA your name	listserv@wehi.edu.au
e-mail Table of Contents New Issues/Bulletins	
MMWR (complete on-line form)	www.cdc.gov/mmwr/ mmwrsubscribe.html
subscribe EID-TOC	listserv@cdc.gov
subscribe WER-REH	majordomo@who.ch
subscribe DOSTRAVEL your name	listserv@lists.state.gov
Eurosurveillance Weekly	www.eurosurveillance.org/ subscribe/subscribe-O2.asp
UK FCO Travel Bulletins	www.fco.gov.uk/subscribe

[a]List restricted to members of the International Society of Travel Medicine.
[b]List restricted to members of the American Society of Tropical Medicine and Hygiene.

Similar arrangements are in place for the Emerging Infectious Diseases Journal (EID), for Eurosurveillance, and for the WHO Weekly Epidemiological Record (WER). The travel advisories listserv automatically e-mails US State Department Consular Information sheets each time one is updated or changed, or when a travel advisory or warning is issued.

CHAPTER 5   The Pre-travel Consultation

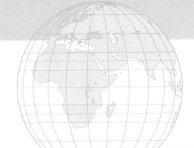

Martin S. Wolfe and Rebecca Wolfe Acosta

KEYPOINTS

■ The two key elements of the pre-travel consultation are: (1) the risk assessment, during which health risks are determined on the basis of traveler, travel, and destination factors and (2) the risk management, during which appropriate, individualized recommendations and prevention strategies are provided to the traveler on the basis of the risk assessment

■ Psychosocial variables such as risk perception and risk aversion, as well as perceived benefits and barriers to action, impact significantly on the implementation of and adherence to preventive measures

■ Optimal risk communication includes the clear and concise sharing of relevant and reputable information to help promote understanding and informed decision making

■ The major elements of risk management include appropriate travel immunizations, malaria chemoprophylaxis, insect precautions, and prevention and self-treatment of travelers' diarrhea

■ Additional travel-related health issues that must be considered include: jetlag, motion sickness, women's health, sexually transmitted diseases, environmental illness, water- and insect-borne diseases, personal safety and security, and motor vehicle accidents

INTRODUCTION

The basis of the pre-travel consultation is risk assessment and risk management. Risk assessment is the process by which the travel health provider evaluates the multitude of factors that may impact on the health of the traveler i.e., the traveler him/herself, the travel, and the destination. The traveler's health, medical history, attitudes, and likely risk behavior are evaluated, the style, mode and purpose of travel are considered, and the health and safety issues of the destination are assessed. The risk management portion of the travel medicine consult is focused on counseling the traveler on preventive measures to reduce illness and injury during travel. The extent of the counseling required by the travel medicine practitioner and the recommendations for preventive measures are dependent entirely upon the results of the risk assessment. It is this individualized approach to the travel medicine consultation that distinguishes those with expertise in travel medicine from those who use the 'cookie cutter' approach in which recommendations for preventive measures are based on a map or a table that lists countries and diseases within them. Finally, it is important to remember that in addition to an excellent risk assessment and well-developed knowledge of appropriate preventive recom-

mendations, the ultimate success or failure of the travel medicine consultation will hinge on the ability of the travel medicine advisor to communicate effectively with the traveler.

STRUCTURE AND ORGANIZATION OF THE PRE-TRAVEL CONSULTATION

Even when the travel medicine provider is proficient with the travel medicine knowledge base, the essence of travel health care is demonstrated through the well-conducted risk assessment and consultation. Conducting the effective consultation requires travel medicine providers to rely on their assimilation of the travel medicine knowledge base, experience, keen assessment/evaluation skills and effective communication.

In this section, the general elements of the pre-travel consultation process will be reviewed from the risk assessment and risk communication through vaccine administration and documentation.

The general elements of the pre-travel consultation include:

■ The risk assessment
■ Risk communication
■ The recommendations and the individualized care plan
■ Vaccine recommendations
■ Prescription medications as indicated (i.e., malaria chemoprophylaxis; travelers' diarrhea self treatment etc.)
■ Advice on preventive measures and risk reduction
■ Counseling on risk reduction and prevention advice
■ Administration of vaccinations
■ Informed consent
■ Documentation of all vaccines, prescriptions and advice given.

A sample methodology for providing the consultation is outlined in Table 5.1.

Risk assessment

The risk assessment forms the basis for the advice and care that is provided during the consultation. Risk management on the other hand is an efficient way of providing international travelers with evidence-based advice.[1] A risk is the probability of a hazard, or a set of circumstances that may have harmful consequences, occurring.[2] In order to conduct a meaningful risk assessment, and effective pre-travel consultation, the travel medicine provider must have a working understanding of the travel medicine knowledge base. This knowledge base includes the hazards (diseases and other risks) by destination/itinerary, the interventions to reduce exposure to the hazards (risk reduction) and knowledge regarding contraindications to vaccinations and medications which may be indicated. Many resources are available to assist in developing the knowledge base, remaining current,

Table 5.1 Sample counseling methodology. The following outline presents a summary of important clinical issues to be considered during a pre-travel counseling session. Specific advice and methodology may vary according to the traveler's needs and clinic/practice specific policies and procedures. Consistent counseling methods should be adopted within each clinic/practice setting and should be supported by policy and procedures specific to each topic

Risk assessment (RA) I (Travel variables)

Itinerary
    Include departure date, countries, regions, city/rural, season and length of time in each area
    Consider activities (e.g., safari, hiking, rafting, golfing etc.) and purpose of travel (e.g. business vs tourism)
Assess trip accommodations and mode of travel (e.g. cruise ship, overland)
    (e.g., high-end/luxury; moderate/tourist; budget)

Risk assessment (RA) II (Health/medical variables)

Age/gender
Vaccination history (include previous adverse reactions/fainting)
Medical/health history
    Allergies
    Medications
    Medical/health conditions – current or recurrent
    Pregnancy status

Risk assessment (RA) III (Psycho-social variables)

Assess type of traveler
    General attitudes regarding risks
    Personality (e.g., risk taker, conservative etc.)
    Reference/peer groups (e.g. VFR)

Risk management: Vaccine recommendations

Review standard and individualized recommendations
    Based on risk assessment I-III (RA I–III)
    Assist with decision making, based on facts while considering other concerns (cost, vaccine anxiety etc.)
    Review and discuss benefits/risks of all recommended vaccines
    Consult with traveler's primary/specialist physician(s) as appropriate (e.g., pregnant traveler)
    Finalize care plan with traveler

Risk management: Administration of vaccinations

Provide and review written information (i.e., Vaccine Information Statements-VIS) for all selected vaccines
Obtain verbal/written consent for any vaccines to be administered
Administer vaccination(s)
Complete related documentation including 'Yellow Card'/immunization record

Risk management: Malaria counseling (if/as indicated by RA I–II) and insect precautions

Utilize teaching tools including maps, insect precautions handout etc.
Discuss anti-malarial medication options based on RA I–III
    In addition to RA I–II factors, consider patient comfort level and other possible barriers to adherence such as cost etc. (RA–III)
Provide appropriate anti-malarial prophylaxis with verbal and written medication information sheet (MIS)
Provide risk reduction counseling on other important insect-borne diseases (i.e., dengue, trypanosomiasis etc.) and information on risk reduction measures
    (i.e. insect repellents, impregnated bednets etc.) as indicated by RA I–III

Risk management: Food and beverage precautions/travelers' diarrhea (TD) management

Review basic prevention issues for all travelers
Utilize counseling/teaching aids
Provide specific advice, based on RA I–III
    Example: Budget/rural travelers should consider taking water filter/purifier
Provide advice on travelers' diarrhea management with verbal and written instructions
    Consider providing self-therapy along with Medication Information Sheet (MIS) as appropriate

Risk management: Other advice

Provide all travelers with information on personal safety, accident prevention, rabies prevention, avoiding/minimizing contact with fresh water etc as indicated by RA I-III.
Provide 'special needs' traveler (e.g., diabetic, pregnant, pediatric traveler etc.) with advice specific to individual needs and medical issues as appropriate
    Encourage traveler to discuss specific management issues with primary physician (e.g., insulin adjustment; travelers' diarrhea management etc.)
    Coordinate/consult with primary physician as necessary
Provide all travelers with basic information on medical-evacuation/medical – assist plan and services
    Stress the importance of this for those with underlying medical conditions; rural and/or long-term travelers
Counsel all travelers on signs/symptoms that require medical care during or after travel,
    e.g. fever; persistent diarrhea/gastrointestinal problems; unusual rashes etc.

Table 5.1	Sample counseling methodology. The following outline presents a summary of important clinical issues to be considered during a pre-travel counseling session. Specific advice and methodology may vary according to the traveler's needs and clinic/practice specific policies and procedures. Consistent counseling methods should be adopted within each clinic/practice setting and should be supported by policy and procedures specific to each topic—cont'd

Risk management: Other actions

Coordinate and document follow-up plan as needed (e.g., multiple visits for vaccination series etc.)
Allow time for patient to ask questions; encourage them to call after the visit with any questions or concerns
Review 'after hours' care policy with patients.
Document all vaccines, prescriptions and advice given

Risk management: Documentation/Counseling Aides: utilize forms/materials to assist with counseling process and documentation

Patient Questionnaire
    Provides Yes/No and qualified answers to RA I–II issues
Care Plan Record or Client Encounter Form
    Encourages consistency of practice
    Provides for efficient, effective documentation of all vaccines, medications and advice given including client consent
    Acts as a 'check-list' or guide for provider during the consultation
Patient Handouts
    Vaccine Information Statements (VIS), Medication Information Sheets (MIS)
    Travel-related disease and hazard information pamphlets (rabies, altitude, travel insurance, Japanese encephalitis, dengue, food and water precautions, insect precautions, jet lag, deep vein thrombosis (DVT), HIV/STDs etc.)
Counseling aides (e.g., wall charts, maps, demonstration materials)

and assisting in the general risk assessment (see Chapters 2 and 4). A risk assessment must be conducted in order to ascertain the risks and make appropriate recommendations for each traveler. A risk assessment involves gathering as much pertinent information as possible from the traveler: their proposed itinerary (itinerary variables), health status (health/medical variables), and the type of traveler and background (psychosocial variables), so that the advice given to the traveler will be relevant to their needs.

A basic summary of the risk assessment is:

Who will be traveling (age, gender, health/medical and vaccination history)
Where (country(ies), urban/rural)
When (departure date, duration and season of travel) are they traveling?
Why are they traveling?
What will they be doing when they get there?
How will they be traveling and living while there?

A patient questionnaire is an essential tool to assist in the collection and organization of important information about travelers and their itinerary. Table 5.2 lists topics that should be included in a questionnaire. Presenting the questions related to health and medical history in a Yes/No format with space for additional explanatory information as necessary, allows for the provider to view the information in an efficient manner and focus on issues of need and concern. The questionnaire may be filled out by the traveler in advance, either at home or in the clinic waiting area. Although itinerary and health and medical variables may be easily captured in a questionnaire, psychosocial variables such as attitudes and peer or reference groups are more subtle. The travel medicine provider will need to rely on interpersonal and assessment skills during the consultation to assist in the evaluation of these important factors.

Itinerary variables (where, when, why, what and how)

The most basic level of the risk assessment relates to itinerary variables that will answer the questions of where, when, why, how is the trip

being taken and what will the traveler be doing on the journey. Where and when are they traveling? This should include: countries/regions to be visited; the amount of time in urban versus rural areas; season and length of time in each area etc. In general, a traveler who only visits an urban area for several days to a few weeks will have less exposure to diseases and other health hazards than one going for several months to rural areas. The date of departure should also be requested. This will help to assess any need for accelerated doses of

Table 5.2	Topics to include in the pre-travel health/medical questionnaire

Countries, regions, cities to be visited
Date of departure; length of total trip
Duration of stay in each location
Purpose of travel (i.e., business, vacation)   Examples of proposed activities including side excursions (e.g., hiking, golfing, safari etc.)
Types of accommodation (i.e., luxury–budget/camping)
Age

Vaccination history
    Travel vaccines
    Routine vaccines
    History of adverse reactions/vaso-vagal events

Current medical conditions (include immune-suppression)
Underlying and intermittent medical conditions
Current or underlying psychological or psychiatric conditions (include depression, anxiety, suicidal ideation)
Medications (daily and intermittent)
Allergies   Medications, foods, environmental etc.

Womens' health issues
    Current or planned pregnancy within 3 months
    Breast feeding
    History of vaginitis or urinary tract infections
    Current contraceptive measure(s)

vaccines such as hepatitis B, Japanese encephalitis and rabies should these be indicated. Why is the traveler going on the trip? What will they be doing while there? The purpose and nature of the trip reveal valuable information about potential risks. The general risks of a 'backpack' traveler visiting remote villages or a humanitarian worker, may be very different for a 'package' tourist or business traveler to the same country. However, it is also important to inquire about planned and possible activities, including excursions and side trips (e.g., safari, beaching, biking, hiking, rafting, golfing etc.) as such activities affect the risk profile. How will the traveler live and travel during the trip? It is important to have some information on major modes of transportation; type of accommodations (e.g., luxury, business, tourist or budget level) and overall budget for the trip. Although some of this information may be subjective (i.e., perception of 'luxury versus budget' and uncertainty of specific plans), it can help the provider in tailoring prevention advice such as the need for the traveler to bring along a bed-net or a water filter/purifier if 'budget' accommodations are anticipated in developing countries.

Travelers should be asked to describe their preferred traveling style and any previous travel experiences. Are they likely to seek the road less traveled, the most exotic foods, the novel experience? A self-described adventure seeker may be at higher risk of exposure to disease and injury and will require appropriate advice. The subjective variables along with psychosocial variables, such as perception of risks, may have as much influence on the risk assessment and overall adherence with recommended prevention measures as the objective variables and should be carefully considered (see later).

Health and medical variables

In order to safely recommend and prescribe vaccinations and medications and screen for fitness for travel, all pertinent health and medical variables must be reviewed. These variables include age, medical conditions, vaccination history, medications, pregnancy and allergy. The travel medicine provider must be familiar with the indications, risks, contraindications and benefits of any vaccinations and medications that may be prescribed to the traveler. Contraindications and precautions to vaccination generally dictate circumstances when vaccines will not be given.[3] However, in some situations the benefit from the vaccine may outweigh the risks and the provider will need to consider this in the risk assessment. An example of this would be the relative contraindication to vaccinating a pregnant woman against yellow fever. If a pregnant woman cannot avoid traveling to an area with current yellow fever activity (versus traveling to an endemic area without reports of current yellow fever activity), the risk of disease may be higher than the risk from the vaccine.[4] This must be taken into consideration and included in the risk-benefit discussion with the traveler.

The importance of vaccination history and previous adverse reactions to vaccines should not be overlooked. Many people have poor recall of vaccination history and official records may not exist or be easily accessible. The travel medicine provider should inquire about the possibility of previous vaccinations during routine physicals (influenza, tetanus-diphtheria, pneumococcal disease), following injury (tetanus toxoid or tetanus-diphtheria), school entrance or military service requirements, or related to previous travel. If there is doubt about the previous vaccination history and no records are available, the traveler should be offered the vaccinations as indicated.

Once the travel medicine provider has information on the health and medical history of the traveler, the needs related to fitness for travel become more evident. Individuals with underlying medical conditions may need clearance from a personal physician and more specific preparation and advice related to travel. The travel medicine

provider's understanding of the medical condition in the context of the proposed itinerary is essential to determining needs and maximizing fitness for travel. Many travelers with underlying conditions can continue with their proposed itineraries but they must understand the overall heightened risks. Including the personal or specialist physician in necessary modifications in medical and daily regimens and encouraging the traveler to have adequate travel insurance are important steps. Some travelers may be advised to modify their proposed itineraries and avoid certain activities based on underlying conditions. For example, individuals with sickle cell disease and trait are at higher risk for crises and splenic infarctions above 10 000 ft (3050 m). Frequent tourist itineraries to high elevations in South America, the Himalayan region, and Europe could pose significant risk to such travelers and they may need to consider an alteration in the itinerary to reduce the risk.

Common medications prescribed by travel medicine providers, such as antimalarial drugs and travelers' diarrhea self-treatment, have contraindications and precautions. In addition to the possibility of aggravating underlying conditions, these medications may interact with non-travel-related medications used by the traveler. One example would be the contraindication of prescribing mefloquine (Lariam®) to anyone with underlying psychiatric problems or disease including recent depression or psychosis. The travel medicine provider must be well informed on the products, and astute enough to prescribe them to the right traveler for the right reasons.

Psycho-social variables

'Who' will be traveling includes the traveler's general perception regarding risk and prevention, personality (risk taker/conservative), and reference and peer groups. These can be described as psychosocial variables. These variables are not easily qualified through a pre-travel questionnaire and may not become fully evident during the pre-travel consultation. However, during the course of consultation the travel medicine provider should remain alert to clues about these variables and recognize the importance of the influence of these variables.

Psychosocial variables become very important with regard to adherence to preventive health behaviors. Travelers may have their own perceptions about the risks of exposure to a disease or other hazards and prevention methods. The traveler will be faced with many barriers to utilizing recommended prevention methods such as the cost of vaccines and antimalarial prophylactic drugs, the fear of vaccine or medication side-effects, or simply the overriding temptation to sample exotic foods from a street vendor. The Health Belief Model (HBM) was one of the first models that adapted theory from the behavioral sciences to health problems, and it remains one of the most widely recognized conceptual frameworks of health behavior.[5] The HBM explains the likelihood of an individual's undertaking a preventive health action. The HBM is summarized in Table 5.3. The HBM emphasizes that behavioral change is affected strongly by beliefs about benefits and barriers to changing the target health behavior. According to the HBM, when people perceive a 'threat of disease,' they assess the 'benefits' of and 'barriers' to taking a recommended health action. If the perceived benefits of the action outweigh the perceived barriers, the model predicts a higher likelihood of taking and maintaining the recommended health action.[6]

Perception is a key aspect to understanding 'patient' choice.[2]

The most promising application of the HBM is in the development of messages that are likely to persuade individuals to make healthy decisions.[5] The messages can be delivered in print educational materials, in one-to-one counseling, or through mass media. Travelers have their own unique set of psychosocial variables which may influence

Table 5.3 Summary of Health Belief Model from *Theory at a Glance, A Guide for Health Promotion Practice*, National Institutes of Health, National Cancer Institute (1997)[5]

Concept	Definition	Application
Perceived susceptibility	One's opinion of chances of getting a condition	Define population(s) at risk, risk levels; personalize risk based on a person's features or behavior; heighten susceptibility if too low
Perceived severity	One's opinion of how serious a condition and its sequelae are	Specify consequences of the risk and the condition
Perceived benefits	One's opinion of the efficacy of the advised action to reduce risk or seriousness of impact	Define action to take; how, where, when; clarify the positive effects to be expected
Perceived barriers	One's opinion of the tangible and psychological costs of the advised action	Identify and reduce barriers through reassurance, incentives, assistance
Cues to action	Strategies to activate 'readiness'	Provide how-to information, promote awareness, reminders
Self-efficacy	Confidence in one's ability to take action	Provide training, guidance in performing action

their acceptance and rejection of recommended vaccinations and medications as well as adherence to behaviors for reducing risk (such as regularly taking the antimalarial medication). Quality information sharing and risk communication, including the relevance of the risks as well as background experiences and values, will influence the individual's decision making.[7]

Risk communication

Risk communication is defined as the open two-way exchange of information and opinion about risk, leading to better understanding and better decisions.[8] Effective communication is a dialogue, which is refined as it evolves. Effective communication about risk, and incorporating the relevance of the risk to the individual, can assist in informed decisions about behavior.[2] There are several fundamental aspects to maximize the effectiveness of risk communication: (1) Risk information relevant to the individual is more valuable than average population data. (2) Information must be presented clearly for people to make good use of it. (3) Care must be taken to avoid an overload of information. (4) Sources of information must be reputable, valid and accessible. (5) Decision aids such as booklets, videos and paper-based charts can help with the presentation and discussion of risk information with patients.[8]

Given the importance of risk communication, it should take place during the risk assessment process and continue into counseling and teaching about specific preventive measures. Travelers must be actively involved in treatment decisions such as vaccinations and the choice of which antimalarial medication is best for them. They should be provided with relevant information about risks, possible consequences, and how to minimize exposure to hazards during travel. For example travelers planning a rafting trip may have exposure to potentially contaminated water. Telling them to avoid contact with water makes no sense in this context. Informing them about some of the potential hazards (i.e., schistosomiasis, leptospirosis), possible consequences and some means to reduce risk, such as wearing protective clothing/ foot wear and in some cases taking prophylactic antibiotics) will allow the traveler to make informed decisions and take actions relevant to them. The goal should be to optimally (versus maximally) prepare travelers (with necessary vaccines, medications, and risk information and avoidance tools) to confidently meet and handle hazards, not to scare them into unnecessary vaccinations or overly restrictive behavior.

The recommendations and the individualized care plan

The care plan includes recommended vaccines, medications and relevant teaching and counseling based on the risk assessment. Once the travel medicine provider has reviewed the questionnaire with the traveler, the 'who, when, where, why, what, and how' should provide a meaningful context for refining recommendations and formulating an individual care plan for the traveler. Risk communication should continue throughout this process to maximize informed decisions about recommended vaccines and medications and to tailor prevention counseling to the traveler's needs. Patient handouts and informational pamphlets on all vaccines, medications and specific advice given should be reviewed and provided to the traveler to facilitate discussion, to promote and reinforce understanding, and for the traveler's future reference. Patient educational materials are available from a variety of sources, including pharmaceutical companies and other commercial resources. In some instances travel clinic staff may produce their own materials such as charts listing the risk/benefits of antimalarial medication options, medication information sheets (MIS) and disease/hazard specific information and prevention advice which may be reviewed with and then given to the patient.

Vaccine administration

The pre-travel consultation almost always involves the administration of vaccinations. In settings where vaccines are provided there must be policies and procedures regarding the entire vaccination process including inventory, storage, informed consent, administration, documentation and management of anaphylaxis (see Chapters 4 and 10).

One of the objectives of the risk assessment process and pre-travel consultation is to select the appropriate vaccines for the traveler. Considerations must include risk/benefit discussions and timing of vaccine series if indicated. Informed decision-making will evolve from effective risk communication. Informed decision-making has been institutionalized in some settings. For example in the USA, the National Childhood Vaccine Injury Act requires that adults and the parent/legal guardian for children be provided with Vaccine Information Statements (VIS) prior to immunization with routine vaccinations (e.g., DTaP, Td, MMR, varicella, polio, Hib, hepatitis B, or pneumococcal conjugate vaccine). VIS are available for other vaccines and their use is recommended, but not required by federal law. The date the VIS was given to the patient and the publication date of the VIS must be documented in the patient's chart. Signed consent is not mandated but documentation of consent is recommended or required by certain state or local authorities.[9] Regardless, signed consent should be considered as a part of good practice and may offer some protection should any legal action occur. All vaccinations administered must be documented in the traveler's medical record, including date and location of administration, manufacturer, dose, lot number, site and route. This information is essential in the event of an adverse reaction, future recall of a vaccine, and to minimize over-vaccination. If yellow fever vaccine has been provided it must be appropriately documented in the International Certificate of Vaccination ('yellow card') which must be provided to the traveler. All other vaccines given should be documented in the traveler's yellow card or on another suitable document.

Documentation and the care plan record

Regardless of laws concerning documentation, it is quality practice to document in the patient record any vaccines and medications given. A care plan record, or patient encounter form, should also include topics discussed and advice that was given to the traveler including patient information handouts/booklets. A form with blanks and space for check marks can be created to capture all of the necessary information. The form can include a section for documenting the traveler's signature/initials consenting to the vaccines and medications that were given. The clinic may wish to have a legal consultant review a consent document prior to putting it into practice. A well-organized form will reduce the time the provider needs to spend on documentation, while ensuring a complete record of all that transpired during the consultation. A complete record will also enhance patient care by allowing for continuity of care in settings with multiple providers, providing for access to the information for future patient questions/issues about the services provided; and facilitating appropriate follow-up in future visits to the clinic.

Conclusion

Those providing pre-travel health care must consider the elements that make up the structure of the pre-travel consultation, including the risk assessment. By adopting a consistent methodology based on sound knowledge and utilizing effective tools for delivering care, the travel medicine provider will enhance both the quality and efficiency of the care that is delivered. Each provider may have their own unique style for conducting the pre-travel consultation; however the goal should always be the same: travelers who are well informed and appropriately prepared for their particular journey and needs.

RISK MANAGEMENT: GENERAL ADVICE FOR TRAVELERS

Each year, over 50 million people from the developed world visit the developing world, where they are exposed to numerous infectious and non-infectious risks. In a study reported by Steffen *et al.* in 1987, 1–5% of international travelers seek medical attention; 0.01–0.1% require emergency medical evacuation; and one in 100 000 dies.[10] Cardiovascular disease and trauma from accidents are the most frequent causes of death and are much more likely than infectious diseases to cause mortality.[11] Although there is little that can be done systematically to prevent non-infectious deaths, many if not most of the infection-related deaths are preventable.[12] In recent years, the best source of specific, up-to-date advice on infectious and non-infectious diseases of travelers is the specialized travel clinic and the travel medicine specialist.

Travel clinics and travel medicine specialists, physicians and nurses, must be familiar with the geographic distribution and risk of vaccine preventable diseases, malaria, other exotic infections, environmental problems and the available preventative measures for these. As noted earlier, preventive health measures and recommendations must be individualized for each traveler, depending on the type of itinerary, style of travel, proposed activities, living conditions and meals, the traveler's pre-existing medical conditions, allergies and other variables. The major differences between lower and higher risk travel are listed in Table 5.4. All of this knowledge regarding the traveler, his or her itinerary and the destination come together as the overall risk assessment for the individual traveler. In addition, travel medicine specialists with tropical medicine expertise should be capable of recognizing, diagnosing and treating returned travelers with exotic diseases.

The principal areas involved in protecting the traveler's health include:

- Basic pre-travel preparation
- Fitness for travel
- Travel health insurance
- Locating a physician abroad
- Preparation of a travel medical kit
- Vaccines: routine, required and recommended
- Prevention of malaria and other insect-borne diseases
- Travelers' diarrhea: prophylaxis and self-treatment
- Other traveler and itinerary specific advice
- Post-travel care (where the expertise is available)

Basic pre-travel preparation

Given a basic knowledge of travel medicine on the part of the primary health care provider, and a rather straightforward uncomplicated itinerary for a healthy traveler, the needs of such a traveler may be satisfied by his or her own personal practitioner. However, if it is not feasible for a practitioner to provide the most current and up-to-date recommendations and advice, or if the travel consult is complicated, the traveler should be referred to the nearest travel clinic or travel medicine specialist for more thorough preparation. Also, some vaccines (such as yellow fever) may not be readily available to the primary care provider and may be obtained only from a specialized travel medicine advisor.

Fitness for travel

All travelers should be screened for underlying medical problems and medications that may impact upon the pre-travel advice and the care

Table 5.4	Factors influencing risk of contracting a disease or illness while traveling	
Factor	Lower risk	Higher risk
Geographical destination	Developed countries	Developing countries
Length of stay	Short term	Long-term
Location within country	Urban	Rural
Type of accommodation	Luxury	Economy
Purpose of travel	Business	Leisure
Age	Older	Younger
Type of travel	Usual tourist	Adventure

Adapted from *Travel Health Tips*, Aventis Pasteur Inc., Discovery Drive, Swiftwater, PA 18370, 2002.

that is provided. Travel medicine providers need this information in order to screen appropriately for contraindications and possible problems with the vaccinations and other preventive measures that may be indicated. In most cases, it is sufficient to elicit a medical and health care history directly from the traveler, including history of underlying medical problems/issues, medications, allergies etc. However in some instances, travelers with underlying medical issues, including pregnancy, may need clearance to travel and input from their primary care or specialist care providers (see later). In these cases, the travel medicine provider should, whenever possible, work with the traveler's personal physician or specialist to obtain the additional information necessary to develop an appropriate care plan for vaccinations and other recommendations. For example, travelers with cardiac disease should carry pertinent medical records from their cardiologist; a copy of a recent electrocardiogram and a copy of recent pertinent laboratory tests; a notice of having an implanted defibrillator or pacemaker; and a list of cardiac medications and doses. Travelers who will be carrying medications and other medical supplies (i.e., syringes for the traveler with diabetes) should carry a letter from the prescribing physician listing the medications/supplies with a statement of medical necessity. In addition, travelers with underlying medical conditions or allergies should consider obtaining engraved bracelets or health cards with a brief summary of their conditions in case of emergency. These can be obtained from a number of sources, including Medic Alert Foundation, P.O. Box 1009, Turlock, CA 15380. A suggested checklist of important documents to be carried by the traveler is listed in Table 5.5.

The travel medicine provider plays an important role in stressing the overall concept of 'fitness for travel' and helping the traveler to understand the potential impact of his or her proposed journey on an underlying health condition or ongoing medical needs. A pre-travel physical examination, preferably performed by the primary care provider, or, if necessary, by the travel clinic practitioner, is recommended for travelers with serious underlying medical problems, for those planning a long or physically demanding trip, and for those planning to reside abroad for prolonged periods. Standard age and gender-specific recommendations for physical examinations should be utilized with the addition of other tests, such as a tuberculin skin test (PPD), where indicated. A useful example is the screening procedures performed on United States Foreign Service personnel planning to live abroad, shown in Table 5.6. In a corporate or government

Table 5.6 Routine screening procedures performed periodically on US Foreign Service personnel

History and physical examination
Pulmonary function tests (as indicated and for postings above 8000 feet)
Electrocardiogram (after age 50 or as indicated)
Flexible sigmoidoscopy (offered after age 50)
Tuberculin skin test (PPD)
Chest X-ray
PAP smear and pelvic exam (after age 21)
Mammogram (required after age 50; recommended age 40 and over)
Stool Hemoccult (x 3) (age 50 or earlier when indicated)
Complete blood count
Urinalysis
Blood chemistry profile
Blood type (pre-employment only)
Glucose 6-phosphate dehydrogenase (pre-employment only)
Hepatitis B antigen, hepatitis C antibody (after age 12)
HIV I and II (after age 12)
RPR or VDRL (after age 12)
Prostate specific antigen (males 50 years or earlier when indicated)
Stool exams for ova and parasites (x 3)
Schistosomiasis serology (returnees from endemic areas)

setting, and occasionally for the unaffiliated traveler, these screening procedures may be used to determine whether an individual is cleared unconditionally for travel, or under what circumstances foreign travel may be appropriate from a health perspective. Also, long stay travelers or those traveling in remote destinations are advised to have up-to-date dental and eye examinations before departure.

Travel health insurance

Despite the best preparation and caution, illness and injury may occur during travel or residence abroad. It is essential that all travelers, particularly those with underlying medical conditions, review their health insurance to determine whether coverage applies to pre-existing medical conditions, to conditions acquired during travel, to hospitalization abroad, or to medical evacuation from foreign countries. It is also important to determine whether there is phone access for 24-hour/7-day a week medical assistance/referrals during travel. Otherwise, an appropriate policy for such coverage should be obtained from one of the many companies available to fill the various needs of travelers. It is important that travelers review the offerings carefully, read the fine print, and select the one that will best meet their needs.

Locating a physician abroad

Travelers with underlying health problems should be given names of physician specialists in the places to be visited, usually available from specialist directories. A number of resources listing recognized English-speaking physicians overseas are available, including a directory available from the International Association for Medical Assistance to Travelers (IAMAT, 417 Center St., Lewiston, NY 14092, Tel: 716 754 4883). North American travelers can contact their local Embassy or Consulate to locate a doctor. Citizens of other countries will usually

Table 5.5 Checklist of important documents to be carried

Certificate of vaccination (yellow card)
Any vaccine or other exemption letters
Passport with any necessary visas. Extra passport photos
Copies of medical records, electrocardiogram, recent chest X-ray
List of current medications with trade and generic names and doses
A list of allergies
Blood type and group
Name, address, fax and e-mail of personal physician
Name and contacts for next of kin
International driver's license
Travel insurance card
Photocopies of original documents should be left at home and also carried with the traveler in a place separate from the originals.

find a similar service at their local diplomatic representative. A number of travel insurance companies include medical assistance abroad, accessed by the company's assistance contact number. Resources available for medical care abroad and evacuation are discussed in Chapter 49.

Necessary medications and personal travel medical kit

Travelers with chronic illnesses or medical needs should carry a sufficient supply of necessary medications. Longer-term residents should assure re-supply or purchase of reputable identical drugs while abroad. In some countries, drugs may lack label warnings and preparations may not meet government standards of preparation or potency. Travelers should be cautioned that potentially dangerous drugs may be included in such preparations including chloramphenicol, sulfas, butazolidin and aminopyrine, among others. Travelers carrying syringes and needles should be provided with an official-looking statement, on letter-head stationery, explaining why they are traveling with the syringes, as a document may be requested by customs/immigration officials on arrival at their destination. In addition, travelers should be advised to bring along new or extra eyeglasses or contact lenses, hearing aids, prosthetic devices etc., prior to travel, as the necessary material and technology may not be available in developing countries.

The travel medicine provider should also provide advice on the components of a traveler's personal medical kit. The contents of the medical kit will vary according to pre-existing medical needs, length, and type of journey. For example travelers who will be visiting large cities may only need to carry their own medications along with additional supplies to manage symptoms of minor ailments such as the common cold and simple wounds. Travelers to more remote regions may need a kit with additional first aid materials and an instructional guide for their use. As a convenience to the traveler, as well as a source of revenue to the travel medicine practitioner, some travel clinics may sell basic pre-stocked kits and certain travel items, or else prescribe them. The most common items include insect repellents, antimalarial prophylactic drugs, water purification tablets or devices, oral rehydration salts, antimotility agents, and basic first aid supplies. The travel kit for emergency or routine use is covered fully in Chapter 8.

Vaccines: routine, required and recommended

Vaccinations are considered central to pre-travel medical care by the traveler and practitioner. Vaccines may be categorized as 'routine' for pediatric and adult populations, regardless of whether or not travel is planned; 'required' for those who need them to cross international borders (i.e., yellow fever and meningitis vaccines); and/or 'recommended' according to risk of infection. Vaccine recommendations will vary according to a number of factors including the traveler's immunization history, itinerary, duration and season of travel, proposed activities and purpose of travel, style of travel, and pre-existing medical history. Vaccine requirements by country are published annually by the Centers for Diseases Control (CDC); Health Information for International Travel,[13] and the World Health Organization (WHO) in International Travel and Health: Vaccination Requirements and Health Advice.[14] A number of commercial computer and on-line programs are also available for guidance on vaccine recommendations (see Chapter 4). It is important that the travel medicine provider understands the contraindications and risks as well as benefits of vaccinations, especially when providing care to special populations such as the pregnant traveler, the HIV positive traveler, and children. Live vaccines, such as measles, varicella and yellow fever, are contraindicated during pregnancy and in the immunocompromised traveler.[13] Clinics that provide care to the pediatric population should take special measures to ensure that routine immunization schedules and records are maintained, particularly if doses of certain vaccines are accelerated to ensure protection during travel.[13] Routine vaccination schedules should be coordinated with the pediatrician of record whenever possible.

The travel clinic should stock all vaccines that may be indicated for travel, including routine vaccines, and have clearly defined policies and procedures for the storage, recommendations and administration of vaccines (see Chapter 9). Yellow Fever vaccine is given only in approved travel clinics and other approved state-licensed official vaccination centers. Certain vaccines may be difficult to obtain and are more cost-effective when administered at travel clinics and certain government facilities where a large volume of travelers are seen. These include Japanese B encephalitis, quadrivalent meningococcal meningitis, plague, tick-borne encephalitis, and rabies vaccines.

Complete details on Immunizations are given in Chapters 9, 10, and 11. Chapters 25 and 26 discuss the Immunocompromised Traveler and the Traveler with HIV.

Prevention of malaria and other insect-borne diseases

The most serious potential infectious risk for travelers to the tropics is malaria. In recent years, approximately 1000 to 1500 malaria cases and four deaths have been reported in the USA, annually.[15] Invariably, these cases were in travelers who either took no recommended antimalarial drug prophylaxis or used these drugs inappropriately.[15] Incorrect advice is frequently given by physicians to travelers who are not aware of the distribution of malaria, drug resistant malaria, and the availability and proper use of antimalarial drugs and measures to protect against mosquito bites. It is imperative that travel medicine practitioners be expert in the provision of advice concerning the prevention of malaria. Particularly good maps on the distribution of malaria in affected countries, updated regularly, are available from a number of sources (see Chapter 4). Each traveler must be evaluated and counseled individually before a malaria prophylactic drug is prescribed. Factors to be considered include: specific areas to be visited; the presence of drug resistant malaria; age, health and medical history such as pregnancy; history of depression etc.; prior use of and tolerance of antimalarial drugs; the travelers comfort level with the options available, and the cost of various drugs. Personal protection measures to prevent mosquito bites from the night-biting *Anopheles* mosquito must also be discussed.[16,17] Travel information handouts on general insect protective measures and on details of specific antimalarial drugs should be given to the traveler. The traveler must be made aware that no drug or anti-mosquito measures can totally guarantee protection against illness from malaria. It is also important to stress that malaria may occur for up to 3 years (in the case of relapsing *Plasmodium vivax* and *Plasmodium ovale* malaria) after return from a malarious area. Any febrile illness 7 days after entering to 3 years from departing a malarious area must be presumed to be malaria until ruled out. Detailed discussions of malaria epidemiology, chemoprophylaxis, self-diagnosis and self-treatment, and the approach to the patient with malaria are in Chapters 12 to 15.

Malaria is not the only insect-borne infection that travelers may encounter, although it is the most important. Diseases such as dengue fever, transmitted by the *Aedes* mosquito, which bites in the early morning and late afternoon, and Lyme disease, transmitted by tick bite, may be prevented only by avoiding contact with the insect vectors. Insect Protection is discussed in more detail in Chapter 7.

Travelers' diarrhea

Travelers' diarrhea is the most frequent problem affecting travelers, particularly those traveling in the developing world. Up to half of the travelers from industrialized countries who visit the developing world develop this malady.[18] Low-grade fever, abdominal cramping, or vomiting may occur along with diarrhea. Infection is usually acquired by ingesting microbes contaminating food or water, or by coming into contact with the contaminated hands of an infected person. Although travelers' diarrhea may be caused by bacteria, viruses, or parasites, the most common cause is infection with enterotoxigenic *Escherichia coli* bacteria. Other frequently occurring bacterial pathogens that potentially cause more severe illness, include Campylobacter, Shigella, and Salmonella species. Viruses and parasites are less frequent causes of illness although the latter (particularly giardiasis) tends to be responsible for persistent bowel problems in adventurous travelers going off the usual tourist routes.[18] Recommended preventive measures are listed in Table 5.7 and are discussed in more detail in Chapter 17. Table 5.8 lists some of the inadequate preventive measures used by travelers. Most authorities agree that prophylactic antibiotics should not be routinely recommended because the potential risk may outweigh the benefit.[19] Bismuth subsalicylate (Pepto-Bismol®) in a dosage of two tablets four times a day for periods of less than 3 weeks is a safe and effective way of reducing the occurrence of travelers' diarrhea by approximately 65% in those persons at risk.[20] The most important factor in treating travelers' diarrhea is the replacement of lost fluids and electrolytes. This can be accomplished by drinking tea, broth, or carbonated beverages. Better yet are oral rehydration electrolyte mixtures that are mixed with potable water to prepare a more balanced replacement fluid. Bland, usually well-tolerated foods, such as toast, plain rice and broth should be eaten, and milk products should be avoided. For many travelers, especially those with mild diarrhea, this is the only treatment necessary because in most cases illness is self-limited and short-lived. However, self-treatment may be desirable to reduce the length and severity of illness, and to avoid care from local practitioners who may not have the resources or ability to treat the condition properly. In this case, travelers should be given a prescription for an appropriate antibiotic, such as a quinolone or azithromycin, along with detailed written instructions on their use in the event of moderate-to-severe travelers' diarrhea. It should be emphasized that diarrhea that develops one week or more after a traveler returns home is more likely to be caused by a intestinal protozoan. A written handout outlining the important aspects of prevention and self-treatment of travelers' diarrhea should be reviewed with

Table 5.7   Recommended preventive measures against travelers' diarrhea

Eat well – cooked steaming hot food (meats, fish, rice/noodles, vegetables)
Avoid cold or raw vegetable salads and fruit peeled by others
Drink bottled water (properly sealed and carbonated adds a measure or protection) and other commercially bottled beverages (soda, juice, beer, wine)
Disinfect untreated water with portable iodine resin filters or iodine tablets, or boil it for 3 mins
Avoid ice-cubes unless made with potable water
Use only pasteurized and refrigerated dairy products
Avoid custards, cream pastries and mayonnaise products, particularly if storage and handling are questionable
Avoid raw or poorly steamed shellfish

Table 5.8   Inadequate preventive measures used by travelers

Not bringing water to a boil
Large hand-held pump filters – may not remove viruses
Inadequate concentration or contact time of drinking water with chlorine or iodine
Using tap water for tooth brushing
Drinking fruit drinks using ice made with impure water
Steaming shellfish (may not inactivate hepatitis A)
Assuming that staying in luxury hotels in major cities assures safe water and food
Swimming in polluted ocean or body of fresh water
Eating fruits peeled by locals, and salads in restaurants

and given to the traveler during the consultation. Travelers' diarrhea epidemiology, prevention, clinical presentation and self-treatment are thoroughly discussed in Chapters 16 to 19. Other food-borne illnesses are covered in Chapter 47.

Women's health

Although most pre-travel health care is not gender-specific there are some particular issues important to women travelers. Some vaccinations, antimalarial drugs, and other medications are contraindicated during pregnancy (see Chapter 20). All non-pregnant women of childbearing age, should be offered vaccination against rubella, measles and varicella if they are not immune to these diseases, which pose a particular risk if contracted during pregnancy.[13]

Prior to an extended foreign trip or residence, women travelers should visit their gynecologist for an age and risk-specific gynecological examination, which could include a Pap smear, a mammography, and if indicated, advice on contraception. A discussion on the risks and benefits of various forms of contraception and their availability overseas, particularly in rural areas, should be included in the gynecological examination. Not all methods of contraception are equally problem-free during travel, and an appropriate method should be chosen carefully before departure. Although travel medicine providers usually do not provide direct gynecological care, they should alert women to some of the basic issues and encourage them to have a discussion with their gynecologist or women's health provider as necessary.

It is important for the travel medicine provider to inform women taking oral contraceptives (OC) that the presence of diarrhea can reduce absorption of the OC and lead to decreased protection. Should diarrhea develop, an additional barrier contraceptive may need to be added to maximize contraception. In addition, certain antibiotics, including tetracycline and ampicillin can reduce the absorption and effectiveness of the OC, and an alternative method should be utilized while these antibiotics are being taken and for 7 days afterwards. When crossing time zones, it is important to take the OC every 24 h, and every day at the same time. Women taking OC are at increased risk for developing deep vein thrombosis.[21] During periods of inactivity related to travel, such as long air and bus trips, preventive measures such as frequent walking and stretching should be advised.

When a contraceptive method fails or when a woman has had unprotected sex, emergency or post-coital contraception may be indicated. Women wishing to have an abortion may find this impossible in many countries and potentially dangerous in others.[21–23]

Women travelers should carry their own personal hygiene products as well as medication for menstrual cramps, urinary tract or vaginal infections, if they are prone to these problems. To reduce the risk of urinary tract infections, especially in hot climates, women should be encouraged to keep well hydrated. Finally, women travelers should be encouraged to learn about local customs in the countries they will be visiting. It may be necessary to adapt clothing, interactions, and activities, to be sensitive to local cultures and minimize unwanted attention during travel to some countries. For example, in many cultures, most women wear skirts or dresses below the knee, and blouses that cover the shoulders. Many guidebooks have sections on cultural issues and advice that is important for the safety and security of women travelers in some parts of the world, particularly for those who are traveling alone.

Sexually transmitted and blood-borne diseases

The travel medicine literature is filled with studies showing that travelers not infrequently engage in anonymous casual sex with fellow travelers, locals, or commercial sex workers. In a UK study of international travelers seen for a post-travel check-up, 19% reported a new sexual partner during their trip and only one-third reported consistent condom use. A survey of American Peace Corps Volunteers revealed that 60% reported having sex with another Peace Corps Volunteer, and 39% reported having sex with a host-country national and either inconsistent (49%) or no (19%) condom use.[24] Coupled with the high prevalence of HIV and other sexually transmitted diseases in the populations of many parts of the world, travelers displaying a less cautious approach to sexual encounters are at high risk of contracting these diseases. Although most travelers are rightfully concerned over contracting HIV, they must also be counseled on the risk of other important sexually transmitted diseases such as multi-drug-resistant *gonorrhea*, hepatitis B, syphilis, herpes type 2, chancroid, *lymphogranuloma venereum* and *granuloma inguinale*. Hepatitis B vaccine should be recommended for any traveler contemplating sexual contact with a new partner, and for those who will reside overseas.[25] The safest course for the traveler is abstinence. Short of this, men should use reliable condoms and women should use diaphragms or female condoms, with spermicides. Unfortunately, none of these methods are 100% protective. Travelers who admit to a high-risk sexual contact should be tested for HIV, syphilis, and hepatitis B and C on their return. Appropriate cultures should be taken for gonorrhea and chlamydia.

Due to the potential transmission of blood-borne pathogens, travelers should not use another person's razor, shaver, or toothbrush. Also, in areas with a high prevalence of these pathogens, intravenous drug use, body piercing, or tattooing should be avoided. Emergency blood transfusions present a difficult situation. At some embassies in developing countries, 'walking blood banks' have been established. The 'blood bank' consists of a number of expatriates who are at low risk of blood-borne pathogens, and who have been identified as potential blood donors. In some situations, a seriously ill traveler may have access to this resource. A traveler who has been sexually assaulted or who otherwise has had high-risk contact with blood or bodily fluids of another individual should receive post-exposure prophylaxis (PEP), with antiretroviral drugs.[26,27] This should be started as soon after exposure as possible and within 72 h. HIV antibody testing should be done immediately, to establish a baseline of the current HIV status at time of exposure, and repeated at 6 weeks, 3 months and 6 months.[23]

OTHER INTINERARY SPECIFIC ADVICE

Aircraft travel

At cabin pressure (~8500 ft) of jet aircraft, gas expands and therefore eating produces bloating, and the effect of alcohol is more potent.

Recommendations to decrease these problems include: wearing loose clothing; avoiding gas producing and greasy foods; eating slowly, minimal use of alcohol before and during the flight; and drinking one pint of fluid every 3 h (water or fruit juice, rather than carbonated drinks) to counteract the dryness of the cabin. Dryness of the nose or eyes can be helped by using saline nose drops or spray and artificial tear drops, respectively.[28] Walking around the cabin periodically can help avoid venous stasis and the development of blood clots in the legs, that can lead to pulmonary embolism. This is particularly important for pregnant women and those on oral contraceptives. Tight undergarments and stockings should be avoided so that the circulation to the feet is not impeded. In the presence of varicose veins or circulatory problems, elastic support hose may be useful.[29]

Jet lag

Crossing time zones in international travel causes disturbance in the sleep-wake cycle. This can lead to insomnia, sleepiness during the day, general malaise, anorexia, and difficulty concentrating – the symptoms of jet lag. Various dietary measures have been advocated, but none has been scientifically validated. Exposure to natural sunlight at specific times of day has some support by experts as a means to improve jet lag, but that regimen may not always be easy to follow. A more practical and simpler way of adapting to a new time zone is the use of a short-acting hypnotic such as zolpidem (Ambien®) at the new bed time, for the first few days after arrival, or during a long night-flight. Alcoholic beverages should be avoided with these drugs, and ideally, during the first days of adaptation to the new time zone.[30] Melatonin is not considered a drug, nor is it licensed or supervised by the US Food and Drug Administration. It is available as a dietary supplement and no toxicity has been associated with its use. Although extensive research has been conducted on melatonin use to combat jet lag, the results are mixed and sufficiently modest that melatonin cannot be definitely recommended for this purpose.[31,32]

Jet lag is discussed in more detail in Chapter 42.

Acclimatization

Gradual ascent is the cornerstone of prevention of altitude sickness. Current recommendations are to avoid abrupt ascents to altitudes higher that 3000 m and to spend 2–3 nights at 2500 to 3000 m before further ascent. Initial moderate activity and avoidance of alcoholic beverages, tobacco, and excessive food are helpful in acclimatizing to high altitude. Increased water intake is necessary at high altitudes in order to prevent dehydration, an aggravating factor for altitude sickness. Unless contraindicated, acetazolamide (Diamox®) at a dose of 125–250 mg twice a day taken 24 h before ascent and continued for the first few days at the higher altitude may be beneficial. Acetazolamide reduces the symptoms of altitude illness by speeding acclimatization and decreases susceptibility to AMS (acute mountain sickness).[33] Travelers to altitudes above 3,000m should be well informed about the symptoms of AMS, the basic prevention measures, and warned to avoid further ascent if symptoms occur until the symptoms have resolved. (See Chapter 38 for a complete discussion of Altitude illness, prevention and management).

Sun and heat disorders

Travelers should choose a broad-spectrum sunscreen that protects against UV-A and UV-B rays and has a sun protection factor (SPF), of at least 15, which offers a long period of protection. A waterproof brand should be used if the traveler will be sweating or swimming. Sunscreen should be applied about 30 min before sun exposure, so that it can be absorbed by the skin.[34] Heat disorders can be avoided by abstaining from prolonged sun exposure and overly strenuous exercise. Drinking more fluids and adding salt to food can be very helpful. Sun-associated disorders are discussed in Chapter 41 and extremes of temperature and hydration in Chapter 40.

Water-borne diseases and skin infections

Where schistosomiasis occurs, all bodies of fresh water must be considered to be infected with these parasites and contact with this water must be avoided. If travelers feel compelled to swim in endemic areas, they should try to stay in the middle of the lake or swim in fast moving rivers where contact with the infectious organisms will be low. Should contact with potentially infested water occur, exposed areas should be quickly rubbed and dried with a towel to prevent penetration of parasites. Schistosomiasis cannot be contracted in salt water or chlorinated swimming pools.[35] Caution must be observed before swimming at beaches near urban areas, which may be highly polluted. Leptospirosis, a potentially fatal zoonosis, is primarily contracted through contact with contaminated soil or surface water in tropical areas. Outbreaks and individual cases of leptospirosis have been associated with activities such as kayaking, canoeing, rafting, scuba diving, jungle trekking, and swimming in jungle rivers. Travelers planning these activities should be advised on how to minimize exposure to potentially contaminated soil and water, and in some cases, might consider the use of antibiotic prophylaxis with a tetracycline derivative. Protective clothing and footwear should be worn and submersion in and drinking of surface water should be avoided.[36] Jellyfish, corals, and other biting and stinging aquatic creatures are a hazard to bathers.[37] Walking barefoot or lying on sandy beaches can allow for infection with helminthic parasites such as hookworm and strongyloides, burrowing sand-fleas (*Tunga penetrans*), and injuries from coral, shells, glass or splinters. Many tropical beaches contain the excrement of dogs and cats infected with hookworms. Larval forms of these animal hookworms (which differ from human hookworms) can penetrate unprotected feet or other parts of the body that are in direct contact with the sand. This leads to the condition of cutaneous larva migrans, which gives a very pruritic, serpiginous, erythematous, migrating lesion under the skin.[38]

Many pre-existing skin conditions may be aggravated by humid and hot tropical climates. Skin and clothing must be kept dry and clean to avoid chafing and prickly heat. Scabies and lice are best prevented by careful washing of the body and clothes.[39] Tumbu fly-larva infection of the skin in tropical Africa occurs when the fly deposits eggs on clothing or bathing suits dried out of doors. Larvae hatch in a few days and then penetrate the skin when they come in contact with the garments, causing a tender boil-like sore. This infection can be prevented by ironing clothes dried outdoors.[40]
(A review of Skin Diseases is provided in Chapter 53).

Other travel-related risks

African trypanosomiasis, or sleeping sickness, is a potential hazard, particularly in the game parks of East, Central, and South Africa, where wild animals are the reservoir and the tsetse fly is the vector. Infection in expatriate travelers is uncommon. The risk of tsetse fly bites can be decreased by wearing long shirts and trousers, by keeping vehicle windows rolled up, and by using insect repellents.[41] South American trypanosomiasis (Chagas' disease) can be avoided by sleeping under bed nets in rural endemic areas when local accommodation consists of thatched roofed or adobe (mud-walled) huts.

Snakes are usually nocturnal and will generally bite during the day only if they are attacked or surprised. Boots with long trousers tucked

into them should be worn in areas where poisonous snakes are present. For travel to remote areas, a snake-bite kit, and under exceptional circumstances (e.g., potential occupational exposure), antivenom against local snakes or scorpions should be taken along.[42] Travelers with histories of anaphylactic reactions to bites of venomous insects should carry an anaphylactic kit (Ana-Kit®, Bayer, West Haven, CT or EpiPen® Center Laboratories, Port Washington, NY) and wear an allergy bracelet.[43]

Rabies remains a risk in much of the world. Travelers must be advised to avoid contact with potentially infected animals particularly dogs. Some travelers may benefit from receiving pre-exposure rabies vaccination. Regardless of vaccination status all travelers should be informed about the importance of post-exposure medical care. [13] Chapter 46 discusses 'Bites, Stings and Envenomation'.

Motor vehicle accidents

The leading cause of accidental deaths of travelers to developing countries is motor vehicle accidents.[11] Travelers should be advised to avoid overcrowded public transport, travel by road after dark in rural areas, and riding on mopeds and motorcycles. Whenever possible, travelers should wear a helmet when riding a bicycle (or moped, scooter, or motorcycle) and wear a seat belt in an automobile. It is important to drive defensively and be aware of the local rules of the road, which in some developing countries appear to be non-existent.

POST-TRAVEL CARE

Many travel clinic personnel have the capability to recognize, diagnose, and treat unusual infections and other conditions contracted during tropical travel. Evaluation by a physician is usually unnecessary for persons who remain healthy during and after short-term travel. Travelers who have undertaken longer term or rigorous travel, as well as expatriate residents returning from the developing world, should undergo a post-travel checkup even if they are asymptomatic. Such a checkup should include a short travel history, a physical examination, complete blood count, urinalysis, blood chemistry profile, tuberculin skin test, and stool examinations for ova and parasites. If potential exposure to an infectious agent has occurred, serologic testing should be performed for such infections as HIV, syphilis, hepatitis B and C, schistosomiasis or filariasis.[44,45] Both travelers and physicians must always consider previous travel in the evaluation of symptoms that appear months or, rarely, years after return home. Significant symptoms of concern include fever, chills, sweats, fatigue, persistent diarrhea or other gastrointestinal symptoms and weight loss.[46] Differential diagnosis, diagnostic methods, and treatment for symptomatic returnees are thoroughly described in Section 11 of this volume, 'Post-Travel Care', and in textbooks on tropical medicine.[47,48,49]

One important caveat in this new age of SARS. Travel medicine practitioners must be particularly vigilant concerning this new serious respiratory infection since health care workers appear to be at highest risk. Knowledge of epidemic areas, clinical features, and a detailed travel history from the patient will enable one to institute aerosol & contact precautions before direct contact with the patient occurs.[50] (See Chapter 56 for more information on SARS).

CONCLUSION

The art of travel medicine is distinguished by the ability to efficiently provide individualized care based on sound knowledge, keen risk assessment skills and the ability to effectively communicate with the traveler. The assessment and provision of the appropriate information, the necessary vaccinations and medications are the foundations of the travel medicine consultation. However, the traveler must remain central to the process, and the interventions must be relevant to his/her needs. The travel medicine provider's challenge is to help travelers "pack" what they need, not burden them with excess, or leave them ill-prepared once en-route. After all, once the travelers have left the travel clinic setting, they will be making the decisions and choices that will ultimately affect their health.

REFERENCES

1. Stringer C, Chiodini J, Zuckerman J. International travel and risk assessment. *Nurs Stand* 2002; **16**(39):49–54.
2. Calman KC. Cancer: science and society and the communication of risk. *BMJ* 1996; **313**:799–802.
3. CDC. *Epidemiology and Prevention of Vaccine-Preventable Diseases.* 7th edn. GA: Department of Human Services, Centers for Disease Control and Prevention, Atlanta; 2002.
4. Roche Laboratory. *Physicians Desk Reference (PDR) Product information,* 56th edn. Basel, Switzerland: Roche Laboratory; 2002:2989–2992.
5. National Institutes of Health, National Cancer Institute. *NIH Theory at a Glance: A Guide for Health Promotion Practice.* Bethesda, MD: National Institutes of Health, National Cancer Institute; 1997.
6. Becker M. *The Health Belief Model and Personal Health Behavior.* Thorofare, NJ: Slack; 1974.
7. Institute of Medicine. *Risk Communication and Vaccination.* Washington DC: National Academy Press; 1997.
8. Edwards A, Elwyn G, Mulley A. Explaining risks: turning numerical data into meaningful pictures. *BMJ* 2002; **324**:827–830.
9. CDC. General Recommendation on Immunizations, Recommendations of the Advisory Committee on Immunization Practice (ACIP) and the American Academy of Family Physicians (AAFP). *MMWR* 2002; **51**(RR-2):1–36.
10. Steffen R, Rickenbach M, Wilhelm U, *et al.* Health problems after travel to developing countries. *J Infect Dis* 1987; **156**:84–91.
11. Hargarten SW, Baker TD, Guptell K, *et al.* Overseas fatalities of United States citizen travelers: an analysis of deaths related to international travel. *Ann Emerg Med* 1991; **20**:622–626.
12. Blair DC. A week in the life of a travel clinic. *Clin Microbiol Rev* 1997; **10**:650–673.
13. CDC. *Health Information for International Travel 2001–2002.* Atlanta: Centers for Disease Control; 2001.
14. World Health Organization. *International Travel and Health: Vaccination Requirements and Health Advice.* Geneva, Switzerland: World Health Organization; 2003
15. CDC. Malaria Surveillance – United States, 1999. *MMWR* 2002; **51**(SS–01):1–18.
16. Kain KC, Shanks GD, Keystone JS. Malaria Chemoprophylaxis in the age of drug resistance. I. Currently recommended drug regimens. *Clin Infect Dis* 2001; **33**:226–234.
17. Schlagenhauf P. *Travelers' Malaria.* Hamilton: BC Decker; 2001.
18. Ericsson CD. Travelers' diarrhea: epidemiology, prevention, and self-treatment. *Infect Dis Clin North Am* 1998; **12**:285–303.
19. National Institutes of Health Consensus Conference. Travelers' diarrhea. *JAMA* 1985; **253**:2700–2704.
20. DuPont HL, Ericsson CD, Johnson PC, *et al.* Prevention of travelers' diarrhea by the tablet form of bismuth subsalicylate. *JAMA* 1987; **257**:1347–1350.
21. Hatcher RA, Trussell TJ, Stewart FH, *et al.*, eds. Contraceptive Technology. 17th ed. New York: Ardent Media; 1998.
22. Christopher E. Contraception and travel. In: Dawood R, ed. *Travelers' Health.* New York: Random House; 1994:430–439.
23. CDC. Sexually transmitted diseases treatment guidelines 2002. *MMWR* 2002; **51**(RR–6):1–79.
24. Wong CC, Celum CL. Global risk of sexually transmitted diseases. *Med Clin North Am* 1999; **83**:975–995.
25. Mast EE, Williams IT, Alter MJ, *et al.* Hepatitis B vaccination of adolescent and adult high-risk groups in the United States. *Vaccine* 1998; **16(suppl)**:S27–S29.
26. Bamberger JD, Waldo CR, Gerberding JL, *et al.* Post-exposure prophylaxis for infection following sexual assault. *Am J Med* 1999; **106**:323–326.
27. CDC. Public Health Service Guidelines for the management of health care worker exposures to HIV and recommendations for post-exposure prophylaxis. *MMWR* 1998; **47**(RR–7):1–33.
28. Harding R. Air travel. In: Dawood R, ed. *Travelers' Health.* New York: Random House; 1994:225–237.
29. Kesteven PJL, Robinson BJ. Clinical risk factors for venous thrombosis associated with air travel. *Aviat Space Environ Med* 2001; **72**:125–128.
30. Waterhouse J, Reilly T, Atkinson G. Jet-lag. *Lancet* 1997; **350**:1611–1616.
31. Brzezinski A. Melatonin in humans. *N Engl J Med* 1997; **336**:186–195.
32. Caldwell JL. The use of melatonin: an information paper. *Aviat Space Environ Med* 2000; **71**:238–244.
33. Bezruchka S. High altitude medicine. *Med Clin N Am* 1992; **76**:1481–1497.
34. Potts JF. Sunlight, sunburn and sunscreens. *Postgrad Med* 1990; **87**:52–63.
35. Corachon M. Schistosomiasis in travelers. *J Travel Med* 1995; **2**:1–3.
36. Haake DA, Dundoo M, Cader R, *et al.* Leptospirosis, water sports, and chemoprophylaxis. *Clin Infect Dis* 2002; **34**:40–43.
37. Auerbach PS, Halstead BW. Hazardous aquatic life. In: Auerbach PS, Geehr PC, eds. *Management of Wilderness and Environmental Emergencies 2nd ed.* St. Louis, MO: Mosby; 1989:953–965.
38. Wilson ME. Skin problems in travelers. *Infect Dis Clin North Am* 1998; **12**:471–488.
39. Chosidow O. Scabies and pediculosis. *Lancet* 2000; **355**:819–826.
40. Rice PL, Gleason N. Two cases of myiasis in the United States by the African Tumbu fly, *Cordylobia anthropophaga* (Diptera, Calliphoridae). *Am J Trop Med Hyg* 1972; **21**:62–65.
41. McMullen R, Hill CD. African sleeping sickness (Trypanosomiasis). In: Jong EC, McMullen R, ed. *The Travel and Tropical Medicine Manual,* 3rd ed. Philadelphia: WB Saunders; 2003:383-393.
42. Davidson TD. Approach to snakebite for international and adventure travelers. In: Bia, F, ed. *Travel Medicine Advisor.* Atlanta: The American Health Consultants Inc; 1994:1–23.
43. Frazier CA. Insect stings – a medical emergency. *JAMA* 1976; **235**:2410–2411.
44. Carroll B, Dow C, Snashall D, *et al.* Post-tropical screening: how useful is it? *BMJ* 1993; **307**:541.
45. Whitty CJ, Carroll B, Armstrong M, *et al.* Screening travelers and expatriates returning from the tropics. *Trop Med Int Health* 2000; **5**:818–823.
46. Wolfe MS. Medical evaluation of the returning traveler. In: Bia, F, ed. *Travel Medicine Advisor.* Atlanta: American Health Consultants Inc; 1991:26.1–26.15.
47. Strickland GT. *Hunter's Tropical Medicine,* 8th edn. Philadelphia: WB Saunders; 2000.
48. Guerrant RL, Walker DH, Weller PF. *Tropical Infectious Diseases.* Philadelphia: Churchill Livingstone; 1999.
49. Cook GC, Zumla A. *Manson's Tropical Diseases,* 21st edition, Philadelphia: WB Saunders; 2002.
50. Booth CM, Matukas LM, Tomlinson GA, *et al.* Clinical features and short-term outcomes of 144 patients with SARS in the Greater Toronto Area. *JAMA* 2003;**289**:1–9.

CHAPTER 6 Water Disinfection for International Travelers

Howard Backer

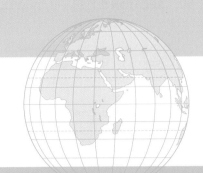

KEYPOINTS

- Risk of water-borne illness depends on the number of organisms consumed, volume of water, concentration of organisms, host factors, and the treatment system efficacy

- An understanding of the unique vocabulary of terms such as disinfection and purification is important for the travel medicine practitioner in order to be able to educate the traveler

- Methods of water treatment include heat, clarification filtration and chemical disinfection

- The use of halogens (e.g., chlorine and iodine) is popular for water disinfection, and an understanding of their toxicity, the appropriate concentrations to use as well as how to improve taste with their use is important

- Different microorganisms have varying susceptibilities to heat, filtration, and halogenation

INTRODUCTION

Safe and efficient treatment of drinking water is among the major public health advances of the twentieth century. Without it, water-borne disease would spread rapidly in most public water systems served by surface water.[1] However, worldwide, more than one billion people have no access to potable water, and 2.4 billion do not have adequate sanitation. This results in billions of cases of diarrhea every year and a reservoir of enteric pathogens for travelers to these areas. In certain tropical countries, the influence of high-density population, rampant pollution, and absence of sanitation systems means that available raw water is virtually wastewater. Contamination of tap water commonly occurs because of antiquated and inadequately monitored disposal, water treatment, and distribution systems. Travelers have no reliable resources to evaluate local water system quality. Less information is available for remote surface water sources.[2] Even in developed countries with low rates of diarrhea illness, regular water-borne disease outbreaks indicate that microbiologic quality of the water, especially surface water, is not assured.[3] As a result, travelers should take appropriate steps to ensure that the water they drink does not contain infectious agents. Look, smell, and taste are not reliable to estimate water safety.

ETIOLOGY AND RISK OF WATER-BORNE INFECTION

Infectious agents with the potential for water-borne transmission include bacteria, viruses, protozoa, and non-protozoan parasites (Table 6.1). Alhtough the primary reason for disinfecting drinking water is to destroy microorganisms from animal and human biologic wastes, water may also be contaminated with industrial chemical pollutants, organic or inorganic material from land and vegetation, biologic organisms from animals, or organisms that reside in soil and water. *E. coli* and *Vibrio cholerae* may be capable of surviving indefinitely in tropical water. Most enteric organisms, including *Shigella, S. typhi*, hepatitis A, and *Cryptosporidium* parvum, can retain viability for long periods in cold water and can even survive for weeks to months when frozen in water. In temperate water, however, enteric bacterial and viral pathogens remain viable only for several days.

Risk of water-borne illness depends on the number of organisms consumed, which is in turn determined by the volume of water, concentration of organisms, and treatment system efficiency.[4] Additional factors include virulence of the organism and defenses of the host. Microorganisms with a small infectious dose (e.g., *Giardia, Cryptosporidium, Shigella*, hepatitis A, enteric viruses, enterohemorrhagic *E. coli*) may cause illnesses even from inadvertent drinking during water-based recreational activities.[5] Because total immunity does not develop for most enteric pathogens, reinfection may occur. Most diarrhea among travelers is probably food-borne; however, the capacity for water-borne transmission must not be underestimated.

WATER TREATMENT METHODS FOR TRAVELERS

Several techniques for improving microbiologic quality of water are available to individuals and small groups who encounter questionable water supplies while traveling (Table 6.2). As with all advice in travel medicine, the specific recommendation for any traveler depends on the destination, style and purpose of travel. Most travelers should become familiar with more than one technique. Travelers may stay in hotels at night and explore remote villages or wilderness parks during the day, requiring an understanding of methods for a spectrum of water conditions. Bottled water may be a convenient and popular solution but creates ecological problems in countries that do not recycle the plastic.

The term *disinfection*, the desired result of field water treatment, is used here to indicate the removal or destruction of harmful microorganisms, which reduces the risk of illness. It is impractical to eliminate all microorganisms from drinking water; generally the goal is a 3–5 log reduction. Table 6.3 lists other important definitions.

Heat

Heat is the oldest and most reliable means of water disinfection (Table 6.4). Heat inactivation of microorganisms is exponential and follows first-order kinetics.[10] Thus, the thermal death point is reached

Table 6.1   Examples of water-borne pathogens

Bacterial	Viral	Protozoa	Other parasites[a]
Enterotoxigenic *E. coli; E. coli* O157: H7	Hepatitis A	*Giardia lamblia*	*Ascaris lumbricoides*
Shigella species	Hepatitis E	*Entamoeba histolytica*	*Ancylostoma duodenale*
Campylobacter species	Norovirus	*Cryptosporidium parvum*	*Fasciola hepatica*
Vibrio cholerae	Poliovirus	*Blastocystis hominis*	*Dracunculus medinensis*
Salmonella (primarily typhi) species	Miscellaneous enteric viruses (more than 100 types)	Isospora belli	*Strongyloides stercoralis*
Yersinia enterocolitica		*Balantidium coli*	*Trichuris trichiura*
Aeromonas species		Acanthamoeba Cyclospora	*Clonorchis sinensis* *Paragonimus westermani* *Diphyllobothrium latum* *Echinococcus granulosus*

[a]Water-borne transmission is possible but uncommon for all these parasites except *D. medinesis*.

in shorter time at higher temperatures, while lower temperatures are effective if applied for a longer time. Pasteurization uses this principle to kill enteric food pathogens and spoiling organisms at temperatures between 60°C and 70°C, well below boiling, for up to 30 mins.[11]

All common enteric pathogens are readily inactivated by heat, though microorganisms vary in heat sensitivity (Table 6.5). Bacterial spores like *Clostridium* are heat resistant (some can survive 100 °C for long periods) and ubiquitous in the natural environment, but they are not water-borne enteric pathogens. Thus, sterilization, the destruction or removal of all life forms, is not necessary for drinking water.

Since enteric pathogens are killed within seconds by boiling water and rapidly at temperatures above 60°C, the traditional advice to boil water for ten minutes to assure potable water is excessive. Because the time required to heat water from 55°C to a boil works toward disinfection, any water brought to a boil should be adequately disinfected. Boiling for 1 min, or keeping the water covered and allowing it to cool slowly after boiling will add an extra margin of safety. The boiling point decreases with increasing altitude but this is not significant compared with the time required for thermal death at these temperatures.

Although attaining boiling temperature is not necessary, boiling is the only easily recognizable endpoint without using a thermometer. Hot tap water temperature and the temperature of water perceived to be too hot to touch vary too widely to be reliable measures for pasteurization of water. Nevertheless, if no reliable method of water treat-ment is available, tap water that has been kept hot in a tank for at least 30 min and is too hot to keep a finger immersed for 5 seconds (estimated 55°–65°C; 131°–149°F) is a reasonable alternative. Travelers with access to electricity can boil water with either a small electric heating coil or a lightweight electric beverage warmer brought from home. In very austere and desperate situations with hot, sunny climate, adequate pasteurization temperature can be achieved with a solar oven or simple reflectors.[12]

Clarification

Clarification refers to techniques that reduce turbidity or cloudiness, of surface water that is caused by natural organic and inorganic material. These techniques can markedly improve the appearance and taste of water. They may reduce the number of microorganisms, but not enough to assure potable water. However, clarifying the water facilitates disinfection by filtration or chemical treatment. Cloudy water can rapidly clog microfilters. Moreover, cloudy water requires increased levels of halogens for treatment and the combined effects of the water contaminants plus the additional halogen can be quite unpleasant.

Sedimentation

Sedimentation is the separation of suspended particles like sand and silt that are large enough to settle rapidly by gravity. Microorganisms, especially protozoan cysts, also settle eventually, but this takes much longer. Sedimentation should not be considered a means of disinfection. Simply allow the water to sit undisturbed for about one hour or until sediment has formed on the bottom of the container, then decant or filter the clear water from the top.

Coagulation-flocculation

Coagulation-flocculation (C-F), a technique in use since 2000 BC, can remove smaller suspended particles and chemical complexes too small to settle by gravity (colloids). Coagulation is achieved with addition of a chemical that causes particles to stick together by electrostatic and ionic forces. Flocculation is a physical process that promotes formation of larger particles by gentle mixing. Alum (an aluminum salt), lime (alkaline chemicals principally containing calcium or magnesium with oxygen), or iron salts are commonly used coagulants. Alum is non-toxic and used in the food industry for pickling. It is readily available in any chemical supply. In an emergency, baking powder or even the fine white ash from a campfire can be used as a coagulant. Other natural substances are used in various

Table 6.2   Methods of water treatment that can be applied by travelers

Heat
Clarification
 Sedimentation
 Coagulation-flocculation
 Granular activated charcoal

Filtration
 Reverse osmosis

Halogens
 Chlorine
 Iodine
  Iodine resins

Miscellaneous
 Chlorine dioxide
 Silver
 Ultraviolet

Table 6.3   Definition of terms

Clarification	Techniques that reduce turbidity of water.
Coagulation-flocculation	Removes smaller suspended particles and chemical complexes too small to settle by gravity (colloids).
Contact time	The length of time that the halogen is in contact with microorganisms in the water.
Disinfection	The desired result of field water treatment, used here to indicate the removal or destruction of harmful microorganisms.
Enteric pathogen	Microorganisms capable of causing intestinal infection after ingested; may be transmitted through food, water, or direct fecal-oral contamination.
Halogen	Oxidant chemical that can be used for disinfection of water (e.g., chlorine, iodine).
Halogen demand	The amount of halogen reacting with impurities in the water.
Potable	Implies 'drinkable' water, but technically means that a water source, on average, over a period of time, contains a 'minimal microbial hazard,' so that the statistical likelihood of illness is acceptable.
Purification	Frequently confused with disinfection, but is more accurately used to indicate the removal of organic or inorganic chemicals and particulate matter to improve offensive color, taste and odor.
Residual halogen concentration	The amount of active halogen remaining after halogen demand of the water is met.
Reverse osmosis	A process of filtration that uses high pressure to force water through a semi-permeable membrane that filters out dissolved ions, molecules, and solids.
Turbidity	Cloudiness in water caused by natural organic and inorganic material.

part of the world. C-F removes 60–98% of microorganisms, heavy metals, and some chemicals and minerals.

The amount of alum added in the field, approximately a large pinch (one-eighth teaspoon) per gallon of water, need not be precise. Stir or shake briskly for 1 min to mix, and then agitate gently and frequently for at least 5 mins to assist flocculation. If the water is still cloudy, add more flocculent and repeat mixing. After at least 30 min for settling, pour the water through a fine-woven cloth or paper filter. Although most microorganisms are removed with the floc, a final process of filtration or halogenation should be completed to ensure disinfection.

Granular-activated carbon

Granular-activated carbon (GAC) purifies water by adsorbing organic and inorganic chemicals thereby improving odor and taste. GAC is a common component of field filters. It may trap but does not kill organisms; in fact, non-pathogenic bacteria readily colonize GAC.[13] In field water treatment, GAC is best used after chemical disinfection, to make water safer and more palatable by removing disinfection by-products and pesticides, as well as many other organic chemicals and heavy metals. It removes the taste of iodine and chlorine (see Halogens).

Filtration

Filtration is both a physical and a chemical process influenced by characteristics of filter media, water, and flow rate. The primary determinant of a microorganism's susceptibility to filtration is its size (Table 6.6). Portable filters can readily remove protozoan cysts and bacteria, but may not remove all viruses, which are much smaller than the pore size of most field filters.[14] Only the semi-permeable membranes in reverse osmosis filters are inherently capable of removing viruses (see below). However, viruses often clump together or to other larger particles or organisms, and electrochemical attraction may cause viruses to adhere to the filter surface. In general, mechanical filters such as ceramic filters, can reduce viral loads by 2–3 logs, but should not be considered adequate for complete removal of viruses. Recently, First Need filter (General Ecology, Exton, PA) was able to meet the EPA standards for water purifiers, which include 4-log removal of viruses.[15]

There are a large number of filters available commercially for individual and small groups. Their ease of use is attractive to many travelers (Table 6.7). Most of the filters sold for field water treatment are maze, or depth, filters made of various media (including ceramic, com-

Table 6.4   Heat for disinfection

Advantages	Disadvantages
Does not impart additional taste or color to water.	Does not improve the taste, smell or appearance of poor quality water.
Single-step process that inactivates all enteric pathogens.	Fuel sources may be scarce, expensive, or unavailable.
Efficacy is not compromised by contaminants or particles in the water, like halogenation and filtration.	

Relative susceptibility of microorganisms to heat: Protozoa > Bacteria > Viruses

Table 6.5 Heat inactivation of microorganisms (selected data)[6-8]

Organism	Lethal temperature/time
Giardia	70°C for 10 min
Cryptosporidium	72°C (water heated up over 1 min)[6]
Salmonella, Shigella, and Campylobacter	75°C for 3 min
V. cholerae	60°C for 10 min 100°C for 10 s
E. coli	60°C for 5 min 70°C for 1 min
Most enteric viruses	56-60°C in 20–40 min < 1 minute above 70°C (158°F).
Hepatitis A	85°C for 1 min[7]

pressed GAV, or fibers) that create long, irregular labyrinthine passages to trap the organism (Fig. 6.1). A depth filter has a large holding capacity for particles, so it lasts longer than a single-layer membrane filter before clogging. Flow can be partially restored to a clogged filter by back flushing or surface cleaning, as with ceramic filters, which removes the larger particles trapped near the surface. Most filters incorporate a pre-filter on the intake tubing to remove large particles, protecting the inner micro-filter; if lacking, a fine-mesh cloth or coffee filter can be used. See clarification techniques for cloudy water.

In pristine protected watersheds where human activity (and viral contamination) is minimal and the main concerns are bacteria and cysts, mechanical filtration alone can provide adequate disinfection. However, for developing world travel and for surface water with heavy levels of fecal or sewage contamination, mechanical filters should not be used as the sole means of disinfection. Additional treatment with heat or halogens before or after filtration guarantees effective virus removal.

Several factors influence the decision of which filter to buy: (1) how many persons are to use the filter; (2) what microbiologic demands will be put on the filter (claims); and (3) what is the preferred means of operation (function). Cost may also be an important consideration (Table 6.8).

Reverse osmosis

Reverse osmosis filtration uses high pressure (100–800 PSI) to force water through a semi-permeable membrane that filters out dissolved ions, molecules, and solids. This process can both remove microbiologic contamination and desalinate water. Although small hand pump reverse osmosis units have been developed, their high price and slow output currently prohibit use by land-based travelers. They are, however, important survival aids for ocean voyagers.

Filter testing and registration

The United States Environmental Protection Agency (EPA) developed consensus-based performance standards as a guideline for testing and evaluation of portable water treatment devices.[16] Many companies now use the standards as their testing guidelines. Testing is done or contracted by the manufacturer. Challenge water at specified temperatures, turbidity, and numbers of microorganisms is pumped through the filter at given intervals within the claimed volume capacity. Units that claim to remove, kill, or inactivate all types of disease-causing microorganisms from the water, including bacteria, viruses, and protozoan cysts, are designated as a 'microbiologic water purifier.' They must demonstrate that they meet the testing guidelines, which require a 3-log (99.9%) reduction for cysts, 4-log (99.99%) for viruses and 5–6 log reduction for bacteria. Filters can make limited claims to serve a definable environmental need, for example, removal of protozoan cysts or cysts and bacteria only. The EPA does not endorse, test, or approve mechanical filters; it merely assigns registration numbers.

Halogens

Worldwide, chemical disinfection with halogens, chiefly chlorine and iodine, is the most commonly used method for improving and maintaining microbiologic quality of drinking water and can be used by individuals and groups in the field (Table 6.9).[17] Hypochlorite, the major chlorine disinfectant, is currently the preferred means of municipal water disinfection worldwide, so extensive data support its use. Both calcium hypochlorite ($Ca[OCl]_2$) and sodium hypochlorite ($NaOCl$) readily dissociate in water. Iodine is effective in low concentrations for killing bacteria, viruses, and cysts, and in higher concentration against fungi and even bacterial spores; however, it is a poor algicide. Elemental (diatomic) iodine (I_2) and hypoiodous acid (HOI)

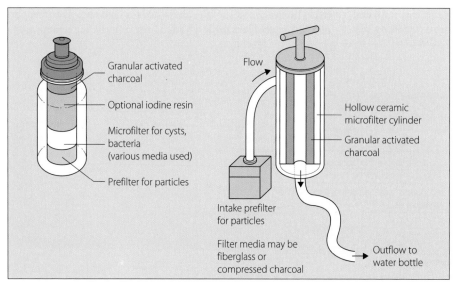

Figure 6.1 Design of typical portable 3-stage microfilter with hand pump and 4-stage water bottle insert.

Granular activated charcoal

Optional iodine resin

Microfilter for cysts, bacteria (various media used)

Prefilter for particles

Flow

Hollow ceramic microfilter cylinder

Granular activated charcoal

Intake prefilter for particles

Filter media may be fiberglass or compressed charcoal

Outflow to water bottle

Table 6.6 Microorganism susceptibility to filtration

Organism	Approximate size (µm)	Maximum recommended filter rating (µm)
Viruses	0.03	n/a.[a]
Escherichia coli	0.5 by 3–8	0.2–0.4
Campylobacter	0.2–0.4 by 1.5–3.5	0.2–0.4
V. cholerae	0.5 by 1.5–3.0	0.2–0.4
Cryptosporidium oocyst	2–6	1
Giardia cyst	6–10 by 8–15	3–5
Entamoeba histolytica cyst	5–30 (average 10)	3–5
Nematode eggs	30–40 by 50–80	20
Schistosome cercariae	50 by 100	Coffee filter or fine cloth, or double thickness closely woven cloth
Dracunculus larvae	20 by 500	

[a]Not applicable. Most portable filters, except reverse osmosis membrane filters, rely on electrostatic trapping of viruses or viral attachment to larger particles

are the major germicides in an aqueous solution. Bromine is another halogen with germicidal action that is sometimes used for treatment of swimming pool water, but has not been used for drinking water treatment in the field. The germicidal activity of halogens results from oxidation of essential cellular structures and enzymes. Disinfection effectiveness is determined by characteristics of the disinfectant, the microorganism, and environmental factors.

Given adequate concentrations and contact times, both iodine and chlorine are effective disinfectants with similar biocidal activity under most conditions. Of the halogens, iodine reacts least readily with organic compounds and is less affected by pH, indicating that low iodine residuals should be more stable and persistent than corresponding concentrations of chlorine. Taste preference is individual. Common sources and doses of iodine and chlorine are given in Table 6.10.

Vegetative bacteria (non-spore forming) are very sensitive to halogens; viruses have intermediate sensitivity, requiring higher concentrations or longer contact times. Protozoal cysts are more resistant than enteric bacteria and enteric viruses, but can be inactivated by field doses of halogens (Table 6.11).[18–29] *Cryptosporidium* oocysts, however, are much more resistant to halogens and inactivation is not practical with common doses of iodine and chlorine used in field water disinfection.[20] Little is known about *Cyclospora*, but it is assumed to be similar to *Cryptosporidium*. Certain parasitic eggs, such as *Ascaris*, are also resistant, but these are not commonly spread by water. All these resistant cysts and eggs are susceptible to heat or filtration. Relative resistance between organisms is similar for iodine and chlorine.

The disinfection reaction

Several factors influence the disinfection reaction. Understanding these allow flexibility with greater reassurance (Table 6.12). The primary factors of the first-order chemical disinfection reaction are concentration and contact time.[21,22] Their relationship is illustrated in Figure 6.2. The amount of halogen added must be enough to meet halogen demand and leave a residual halogen concentration (see definitions in Table 6.3). In field disinfection, concentrations of 1 to 16 mg/L for 10 to 60 minutes are generally effective. Even clear surface water often has at least 1 mg/L of halogen demand, so it is prudent to use 4 mg/L as a target halogen concentration for clear water.[23] Lower concentrations (e.g., 2 mg/L) can be used for back-up treatment of questionable tap water (Table 6.13). The need for prolonged contact times with low halogen concentrations are suggested by (1) data that extended contact times are required for 99.9% kill of *Giardia* in very cold water;[24,25] and (2) uncertainty of residual concentration.

Iodine resins

Iodine resins are considered demand disinfectants. The resin has low solubility, so that as water passes through, little iodine is released into

Table 6.7 Filtration

Advantages	Disadvantages
Simple to operate	Add bulk and weight to baggage
Mechanical filters require no holding time for treatment (water is treated as comes out of filter)	Most filters not reliable for removal of viruses
Large choice of commercial products	Expensive relative to halogens
Adds no unpleasant taste and often improves taste and appearance of water	Channeling of water or high pressure can force microorganisms through the filter
Rationally combined with halogens for removal or destruction of all microorganisms	Eventually clog from suspended particulate matter; may require some maintenance or repair in field

Susceptibility of microorganisms to filtration: Protozoa > Bacteria > Viruses

Table 6.8 Choice of portable field water filters and purification devices

Capacity	Microbiologic claims	Operation	Primary filter	Manufacturer brand[a]	Additional elements, stages, comments and manufacturer's website[b]	Retail price[c]
1–2 person	Protozoa only	Hand pump	Ceramic	General Ecology Microlite	Intake strainer, GAV www.generalecology.com/	US$30
			Ceramic	Katadyn Mini	www.katadyn.com (new site for Katadyn, PUR, and Exstream)	US$70
		Sport bottle	Microfilter	PentaPure Spring	GAV www.pentapure.com/	US$25
	Protozoa, bacteria	Hand pump	Ceramic	Katadyn Mini	Prefilter	US$90
				Stern's Outdoors Filter Pump	www.stearnsinc.com/	US$26
				Timberline Eagle	www.timberlinefilters.com/	US$24
			Pleated glass-fiber	Katadyn Hiker	GAV; for high quality source water, remove 'most' bacteria	US$50
			Borosilicate fiber	Cascade Designs Walkabout	GAV	US$35
		Sport bottle	Hollow fiber	Innova; ANOVA	GAV www.ipur.com	US$40
	All, including viruses	Hand pump	Iodine resin	PUR Voyager	Intake filter www.katadyn.com	US$35
		Sport bottle	Iodine resin	PentaPure Sport	Filter for protozoan cysts and GAV	US$35
				Exstream (3 models)	Filter for protozoan cysts and GAV www.exstreamwater.com	US$40–60
		Hand pump	Reverse osmosis	Katadyn Survivor 06	Desalinates, for ocean survival; very low flow rate, 1 L/h	US$550
		Battery-operated	Ultraviolet	Hydro-Photon Steri-Pen	www.hydro-photon.com	US$199
Small group	Protozoa only	Gravity drip	Ceramic filter	Stern's Outdoors High flow	Plastic collection bag	US$72
	Protozoa, bacteria	Hand pump	Ceramic	Katadyn Pocket	Prefilter	US$200
				Katadyn Combi	GAV cartridge	
					Add-on: counter-top (faucet attach)	US$150
				MSR Waterworks II	Prefilter, GAV and third stage membrane filter	US$140
				MSR Miniworks	Prefilter, GAV	US$65
			Borosilicate fiber	Cascade Designs	Prefilter, GAV, Viral Stop (chlorine solution) to kill viruses	
				Sweetwater Filter	http://www.cascadedesigns.com/	US$60
			Pleated fiberglass	Katadyn Guide	Prefilter	US$80
		Gravity siphon	Ceramic	Katadyn Siphon		US$70
				Marathon ceramics e-water siphon	GAV www.marathonceramics.com	US$30
				AquaRain siphon	www.aquarain.com	US$32
		Gravity drip bucket filter	Ceramic	Katadyn TRK Drip	3 ceramic candles, water drips between 2 buckets; optional GAV	US$160–190
				British Berkfeld LP-2	2 ceramic elements www.jamesfilter.com	US$145
				AquaRain 200	2 ceramic elements	US$189
	All, including viruses	Hand pump	Compressed GAC	First-Need Deluxe	Claims viral removal by electrostatic attraction; no chemicals used	US$70
			Reverse osmosis	Katadyn Survivor 35	Desalinates, for ocean survival; low flow rate, 1.2 gal/h	US$1425
		Hand pump	Iodine resin	PUR Explorer	Prefilter, GAV, iodine resin models currently pulled from market	US$140

Table 6.8	Choice of portable field water filters and purification devices—cont'd					
Capacity	Microbiologic claims	Operation	Primary filter	Manufacturer brand[a]	Additional elements, stages, comments and manufacturer's website[b]	Retail price[c]
				PUR Scout	Prefilter, GAV, iodine resin models currently pulled from market[d]	US$90
		Faucet attachment	Iodine resin	PentaPure Travel Tap	GAV	
		Gravity drip bucket filter	Iodine resin 'candles'	PentaPure Bucket	Filter for protozoan cysts and GAV	US$170
Large Group	Protozoa, bacteria	Gravity drip bucket filter	Ceramic	British Berkfeld Big Berkey	4 ceramic elements	US$279
				AquaRain 400	4 ceramic elements	US$239
		Large hand pump	Ceramic	Katadyn KFT Expedition		US$890
			Compressed GAC	General Ecology Base Camp	Similar element to First Need, but not tested for viral. Electric models also available.	US$500
	All, including viruses	Large hand pump	Iodine resin	PentaPure Outdoor 600	Filter for protozoan cysts and GAV	US$1475

[a]Consider additional features, such as flow rate, filter capacity, size, and filter weight.
[b]This is not a comprehensive list. Models change frequently. Manufacturer site provided if it contains product information; otherwise search manufacturer and brand with any major search engine to find large retail sites that provide detailed product information.
[c]Retail prices vary.
[d]Recent testing failed to demonstrate complete viral inactivation, so company recommends two passes through filter and 20 min contact time; see http://www.purwater.com/camping.shtml

aqueous solutions. On the other hand, when microorganisms contact the resin, iodine is transferred and binds to the microorganisms, apparently aided by electrostatic forces.[30] Bacteria and cysts are effectively exposed to high iodine concentrations, which allow reduced contact time compared with dilute iodine solutions. However, some contact time is necessary, especially for cysts. Resins have demonstrated effectiveness against bacteria, viruses, and cysts, but not against *Cryptosporidium parvum* oocysts or bacterial spores.

The concept of demand disinfectants has great potential for water disinfection in small or individual systems. Filters containing iodine resins have been designed for field use. Most incorporate a 1 μm cyst filter to remove *Cryptosporidium, Giardia,* and other halogen-resistant parasitic eggs or larva, in an attempt to avoid prolonged contact time. Carbon that removes residual dissolved iodine, preventing excessive iodine ingestion in long-term users, may not allow sufficient contact time for cyst destruction. Cloudy or sediment-laden water may clog the resin, as it would any filter, or coat the resin, inhibiting iodine transfer.

The effectiveness of the resin is highly dependent on the product design and function, and more testing is needed on specific products. Recently, two companies pulled iodine resins from the market due to repeat testing that demonstrated viral break-through, despite initial pre-marketing testing that passed the EPA protocol. The companies were not able to determine whether the failure was due to channeling of water that allowed organisms to avoid contact with the resin, lack of residual iodine concentration in effluent water, or need for greater contact time.

Improving halogen taste

Objectionable taste and smell limit the acceptance of halogens, but taste can be improved by several means. One method is to use the minimum necessary dose with a longer contact time. Several chemical means are available to reduce free iodine to iodide or chlorine to chloride that have no color, smell, or taste. These chemical species also have no disinfection action, and so these techniques should be used only after the required contact time. The best and most readily

Table 6.9	Halogenation
Advantages	Disadvantages
Inexpensive	Potential toxicity (especially iodine)
Iodine and chlorine are widely available	Corrosive, stains clothing
Very effective for bacteria, viruses and most protozoa	Not effective for *Cryptosporidium*
Taste can be removed	Impart taste and odor
Flexible dosing	Requires understanding of disinfection principles
As easily applied to large quantities as small quantities	
Relative susceptibility of microorganisms to halogens: Bacteria > Viruses > Protozoa	

Table 6.10   Dose of halogen for field water disinfection[26,28]

	Amount added to 1 L for 4 p.p.m.	Amount added to 1 L for 8 p.p.m.
Iodination methods		
Iodine tabs (tetraglycine hydroperiodide)	1/2 tab	1 tab
EDWGT (emergency drinking water germicidal tablet)		
Potable Aqua		
Globaline		
2% iodine solution (tincture)	0.2 mL; 4–5 drops[a]	0.4 mL; 8–10 drops
10% povidone-iodine solution	0.35 mL; 7–8 drops	0.70 mL; 14–16 drops
Saturated solution: iodine crystals in water	13 mL	26 mL
	Amount added to I L for 5 p.p.m.	**Amount added to 1 L for 10 p.p.m.**
Chlorination methods		
Household bleach 5%; Sodium hypochlorite	0.1 mL; 2 drops	0.2 mL; 4 drops
Chlorine tablets (Sodium dichloroisocyanurate); AquaClear		1 tab
Chlorine plus flocculating agent; AquaCure, AquaPure, Chlor-floc		8 p.p.m./tab

[a]Measure with dropper (1 drop ~ 0.05 mL)

available agent is ascorbic acid (Vitamin C), available in crystalline or powder form. A common ingredient of flavored drink mixes, it accounts for their effectiveness in covering up the taste of halogens. Other safe and effective means of chemical reduction are sodium thiosulfate, hydrogen peroxide, and zinc-copper alloys (KDF resins) that act as catalysts to reduce free iodine and chlorine through an electrochemical reaction. GAV will remove the taste of iodine and chlorine partially by adsorption and partially by chemical reduction. Finally, alternative techniques such as filtration or heat that do not affect taste can be used in many situations.

Halogen toxicity

Chlorine has no known toxicity when used for water disinfection. Sodium hypochlorite is not carcinogenic; however, reactions of chlorine with certain organic contaminants yield chlorinated hydrocarbons, chloroform, and other trihalomethanes, which are considered carcinogenic. Nevertheless, the risk of death from infectious diseases if disinfection is not used is far greater than any risk from by-products of chlorine disinfection.

There is much more concern with iodine because of its physiologic activity, potential toxicity, and allergenicity. Data recently reviewed

Table 6.11   Halogen disinfection data[21–29]

Halogen	Organism	Concentration (mg/L)[a]	Time (min)	Temperature (°C)	Disinfection constant (Ct)[b]
Iodine	Escherichia coli	1.3	1	2-5	1.3
	E. histolytica cysts	3.5	10	25	35
	E. histolytica cysts	6.0	5	25	30
	Poliovirus 1	1.25	39	25	49
	Coxsackie virus	0.5	30	5	15
	Giardia cysts	4	15	30	60[d]
	Giardia cysts	4	120	5	480[d]
Chlorine	Escherichia coli	0.1	0.16	5	0.016
	Campylobacter	0.3	0.5	25	0.15
	20 enteric viruses	0.5	60	2	30
	Hepatitis A virus	0.5	5	5	2.5[c]
	E. histolytica cysts	3.5	10	25	35
	Giardia cysts	2.5	60	5	150
	Cryptosporidium oocyst	80 / 10	90 / 720	20	7200–9600 / 1440
	Schistosome cercariae	1.0	30	28	30

[a]Residual concentration of active chlorine disinfectant compounds
[b]Most experiments use 2–3 log (99–99.9%) reduction as endpoint
[c]4-log reduction
[d]100% kill; viability tested only at 15, 30, 45, 60, and 120 min

Table 6.12   Factors affecting halogen disinfection

	Effect	Compensation
Primary factors Concentration	Measured in mg/L or the equivalent, parts per million (p.p.m.); higher concentration increases rate and proportion of microorganisms killed.	Higher concentration allows shorter contact time for equivalent results. Lower concentration requires increased contact time.
Contact time	Usually measured in minutes; longer contact time assures higher proportion of organisms killed.	Contact time is inversely related to concentration; longer time allows lower concentration
Secondary factors Temperature	Cold slows reaction time.	Some treatment protocols recommend doubling the dose (concentration) of halogen in cold water, but if time allows, exposure time can be increased instead, or the temperature
Water contaminants, cloudy water (turbidity)	Halogen reacts with organic nitrogen compounds from decomposition of organisms and their wastes to form compounds with little or no disinfecting ability, effectively decreasing the concentration of available halogen. In general, turbidity increases halogen demand	Doubling the dose of halogen for cloudy water is a crude means of compensation that often results in a strong halogen taste on top of the taste of the contaminants. A more rational approach is to first clarify water to reduce halogen demand.
pH	The optimal pH for halogen disinfection is 6.5–7.5. As water becomes more alkaline, approaching pH 8.0, much higher doses of halogens are required.	Most surface water is neutral to slightly acidic, so compensating for pH is usually not necessary. Tablet formulations of halogen have the advantage of some buffering capacity.

by Backer and Hollowell[31] suggest the following guidelines as appropriate:

■ High levels of iodine (16–32 mg/day) such as those produced by recommended doses of iodine tablets should be limited to short periods of one month or less.

■ Iodine treatments that produces a low residual ≤1–2 mg/L appear safe, even for long periods of time in people with normal thyroids.

■ Anyone planning to use iodine for prolonged periods should have their thyroid examined and thyroid function tests done to assure that they are initially euthyroid. Optimally, repeat thyroid function test and examine for iodine goiter after 3–6 months of continuous iodine ingestion and monitor occasionally for iodine-induced goiter thereafter. If this is not feasible, assure low-level iodine consumption (see above) or use a different technique.

Certain groups should not use iodine for water treatment:

■ pregnant women (due to concerns of neonatal goiter);
■ those with known hypersensitivity to iodine;
■ persons with a history of thyroid disease, even if controlled on medication;
■ persons with a strong family history of thyroid disease (thyroiditis); and
■ persons from countries with chronic iodine deficiency.

Miscellaneous disinfectants

Ozone and chlorine dioxide are both effective disinfectants that are widely used in municipal water treatment plants, but until recently, were not available in stable form for field use. These disinfectants have been demonstrated effective against *Cryptosporidia* in commonly used concentrations.[32]

A stabilized solution of chlorine dioxide has been developed and marketed under the name of Aquamira (McNett Outdoor, Bellingham, WA) and Pristine (Advanced Chemicals Ltd., Vancouver, British Columbia). US EPA registration for use as a 'water purifier' is pending, however, these products currently are approved for sale in the USA under more limited bactericidal claims.

A process has been developed that uses an electrochemical process to convert simple salt into a mixed-oxidant disinfectant containing free chlorine, chlorine dioxide and ozone. The device has been reduced to a cigar-sized unit that operates on camera batteries (Miox Corp, Albuquerque, NM).[33]

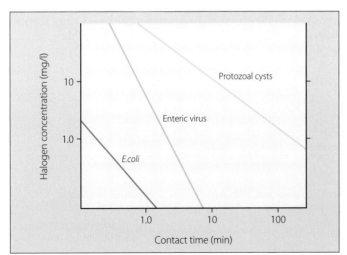

Figure 6.2 Graph of disinfection reaction for 99.9% kill, halogen concentration versus time. Note relative susceptibility of microorganisms. Slope and position of lines will vary with specific organism, disinfectant, and water temperature. Adapted from Chang SL, *WHO Bulletin* 1968; 38:401–414.

Table 6.13   Recommended contact time (min) for specified concentration of halogen and water temperature[a]

Concentration of halogen	5°C	15°C	25°C
2 p.p.m.	240	180	60
4 p.p.m.	180	60	45
8 p.p.m.	60	30	15

[a]Contact times are extended from usual recommendations to account for uncertainty of residual halogen and time necessary to kill *Giardia* cysts in very cold water.[24]

Silver

Silver ion has bactericidal effects in low doses and some attractive features, including absence of color, taste and odor. However, the concentrations are strongly affected by adsorption into the surface of any container as well as common substances in water, and scant data for disinfection of viruses and cysts indicate limited effect, even at high doses. The use of silver as a drinking water disinfectant has been much more popular in Europe, where silver tablets (MicroPur, Katadyn Corp., Wallisellen, Switzerland) are sold widely for field water disinfection. The EPA has not approved them for this purpose in the USA, but they were approved as a water preservative, to prevent bacterial growth in previously treated and stored water. Recently, the company has combined a chlorine solution with the silver (Micropur Forte) to provide water disinfection plus preservation.

Ultraviolet

Ultraviolet (UV) radiation is widely used to sterilize water used in beverages and food products and for secondary treatment of waste-water. It has not been well adapted to field use because of the requirements for power. In order to kill, the ultraviolet waves must actually strike the organism in sufficient doses of energy. The water must be free of particles that would act as a shield. The UV rays do not alter the water, but they also do not provide any residual disinfecting power. Recently a portable, battery operated unit was marketed for small quantity disinfection (Hydro-Photon Inc, Blue Hill, ME). Although previous data suggested limited ability of monochromatic UV rays to inactivate protozoan cysts, company product testing appears solid and shows effectiveness against important water-borne pathogens, including *Cryptosporidia*.

Preferred technique

Optimal water treatment technique for an individual or group will depend on the number of persons to be served, space and weight accommodations, quality of source water, personal taste preferences, and fuel availability. Since halogens do not kill *Cryptosporidia* and filtration misses some viruses, optimal protection for all situations may require a two-step process of (1) filtration or coagulation-flocculation followed by (2) halogenation (Tables 6.14 and 6.15). Heat is effective as a one-step process in all situations, but will not improve the aesthetics of the water. The iodine resins, combined with micro-filtration to remove resistant cysts, are also a viable one-step process, but questions have recently surfaced of product effectiveness under all conditions.

Table 6.14	Summary of field water disinfection techniques			
	Bacteria	Viruses	*Giardia* or amebic cysts	*Cryptosporidium*
Heat	+	+	+	+
Filtration	+	+/–[a]	+	+
Halogens	+	+	+	–

+, susceptible to removal or inactivation.
[a]Most filters make no claims for viruses. General Ecology claims virus removal by First Need Filter. Reverse osmosis filtration can remove viruses.

Where the water will be stored for a period of time, such as on a boat, motor home, or a home with rainwater collection, halogens, chlorine dioxide, or silver should be used to prevent the water from becoming contaminated. This can be supplemented by filtration before or after storage. A minimum chlorine or iodine free residual concentration of 3–5 mg/L should be maintained in the water. Iodine will work for short periods (i.e., weeks) but not for prolonged storage, since it is a poor algaecide. For prolonged storage, a tightly sealed container is best to decrease risk of contamination. Narrow mouth jars or containers with water spigots prevent contamination from repeated contact with hands or utensils.[34]

On long-distance, ocean-going boats where water must be desalinated as well as disinfected during the voyage, only reverse osmosis membrane filters are adequate.

SANITATION

As demonstrated among local communities in developing countries, both good sanitation and potable water are necessary to prevent enteric illness.[35,36] Personal hygiene, particularly hand washing, prevents spread of infection from food contamination during preparation of meals. Disinfect dishes and utensils by rinsing in water containing enough household bleach to achieve a distinct chlorine odor. The sanitation challenge for wilderness and rural travelers is proper waste disposal to prevent additional contamination of water supplies. Human waste should be buried 8 to 12 inches deep, at least 100 ft from any water, and at a location from which water runoff is not likely to wash organisms into nearby water sources. Groups of three persons

Table 6.15	Choice of method for various source water			
Source Water	'Prisitine' wilderness water with little human or domestic animal activity	Tap water in developing country	Developed or developing country	
			Clear surface water near human and animal activity[a]	Cloudy water
Primary concern	*Giardia,* enteric bacteria	Bacteria, *Giardia*, small numbers of viruses	All enteric pathogens, including *Cryptosporidium*	All enteric pathogens
Effective methods	Any single step method[b]	Any single step method[b]	Heat	CF followed by second step (heat, filtration or halogen)
			Filtration plus halogen (can be done in either order); Iodine resin filters (see text)	

CF, Coagulation-flocculation.
[a]Includes agricultural run-off with cattle grazing, or sewage treatment effluent from upstream villages or towns.
[b]Includes heat, filtration, or halogens.

or more should dig a common latrine to avoid numerous individual potholes and inadequate disposal.

CONCLUSION

Although food-borne illness probably accounts for most enteric illness that affects travelers, nearly all causes of traveler's diarrhea can also be water-borne. It is not possible for travelers to judge the microbiologic quality of surface water, and it is not prudent to assume the potability of tap water in many areas. Many simple and effective field techniques to improve microbiologic water quality are available to travelers. It is important to learn the basic principles and limitations of heat, filtration, and chemical disinfection, then become familiar with at least one technique appropriate for the destination, water source, and group composition. Detailed information about these techniques is also available in Auerbach's *Wilderness Medicine*.[37]

REFERENCES

1. WHO/UNICEF. *Global Water Supply and Sanitation Assessment 2000.* Geneva, Switzerland: WHO; 2000.
2. Geldreich E. Microbiological quality of source waters for water supply. In: McFeters G, ed. *Drinking Water Microbiology.* New York, NY: Springer; 1990:3–32.
3. CDC. Surveillance for water-borne-disease outbreaks – United States, 1997–1998. *MMWR* 2000; **49**:1–33.
4. Hurst C, Clark R, Regli S. Estimating the risk of acquiring infectious disease from ingestion of water. In: Hurst C, ed. *Modeling Disease Transmission and its Prevention by Disinfection.* Melbourne, Australia: Cambridge University Press; 1996:99–139.
5. Steiner T, Thielman N, Guerrant R. Protozoal agents: what are the dangers for the public water supply? *Annu Rev Med* 1997; **48**:329–340.
6. Thraenhart O. Measures for disinfection and control of viral hepatitis. In: Block S, ed. *Disinfection, Sterilization, and Preservation.* 4th ed. Philadelphia, PA: Lea & Febiger; 1991:445–472.
7. Fayer R. Effect of high temperature on infectivity of Cryptosporidium parvum oocysts in water. *Appl Environ Microbiol* 1994; **60**:273–275.
8. Bandres J, Mathewson J, DuPont H. Heat susceptibility of bacterial enteropathogens. *Arch Intern Med* 1988; **148**:2261–2263.
9. Groh C, MacPherson D, Groves D. Effect of heat on the sterilization of artificially contaminated water. *J Travel Med* 1996; **3**:11–13.
10. Joslyn L. Sterilization by heat. In: Block S, ed. *Disinfection, Sterilization, and Preservation.* 4th edn. Philadelphia: Lea and Febiger; 1991:495–527.
11. Frazier W, Westhoff, D. Preservation by use of high temperatures. Food Microbiology. New York, NY: McGraw-Hill; 1978.
12. McGuigan K, Joyce T, Conroy R, Gillespie J, Elmore-Meegan M. Solar disinfection of drinking water contained in transparent plastic bottles: characterizing the bacterial inactivation process. *J Appl Microbiol* 1998; **84**:1138–1148.
13. Le Chevallier M, McFeters G. Microbiology of activated carbon. In: McFeters G, ed. *Drinking Water Microbiology.* New York, NY: Springer; 1990:104–120.
14. Environmental Health Directorate Health Protection Branch. *Assessing the effectiveness of small filtration systems for point-of-use disinfection of drinking water supplies (80-EHD-54).* Ottawa: Department of National Health and Welfare; 1980.
15. Gerba C, Naranjo J. Microbiological water purification without the use of chemical disinfection. *Wilderness Environ Med* 1999; **10**:12–16.
16. US Environmental Protection Agency. Guide standard and protocol for testing microbiological water purifiers. *Report to Task Force.* Cincinnati: US Environmental Protection Agency; 1987.
17. National Academy of Sciences. The disinfection of drinking water. *Drinking Water Health* 1980; **2**:5–139. Available: http://www.nap.edu/books/0309029317/html/index.html accessed 12/15/2001.
18. Jarrol E, Hoff J, Meyer E. Resistance of cysts to disinfection agents. In: Erlandsen S, Meyer E, eds. *Giardia and Giardiasis: biology, pathogenesis and epidemiology.* New York, NY: Plenum Press; 1984:311–328.
19. Ongerth J, Johnson RL, MacDonald SC, *et al.* Backcountry water treatment to prevent giardiasis. *Am J Public Health* 1989; **79**:1633–1637.
20. Carpenter C, Fayer R, Trout J, Beach M. Chlorine disinfection of recreational water for Cryptosporidium parvum. *Emerging Infect Dis* 1999; **5**:579–584.
21. White G. *Handbook of Chlorination.* 3rd edn. New York, NY: Van Nostrand Reinhold; 1992.
22. Hoff J. *Inactivation of microbial agents by chemical disinfectants.* Cincinnati: USEPA; EPA/600/1986; **67**:2–86.
23. LeChevallier M, Evans T, Seidler R. Effect of turbidity on chlorination efficiency and bacterial persistence in drinking water. *Appl Environ Microbiol* 1981; **42**:159–167.
24. Fraker L, Gentile DA, Krivoy D, *et al.* Giardia cyst inactivation by iodine. *J Wilderness Med* 1992; **3**:351–358.
25. Hibler CP, Hancock CM, Perger LM, *et al.* Inactivation of Giardia cysts with chlorine at 0.5 °C to 5.0 °C. *American Water Works Association Research Report.* Denver: AWWA Research Foundation; 1987.
26. Powers E. *Efficacy of flocculating and other emergency water purification tablets.* United States Army Natick Research, Development and Engineering Center; Report Natick/TR-93/033. MA: Natick; 1993.
27. Rogers M, Vitaliano J. Military and small group water disinfecting systems: an assessment. *Milit Med* 1979; **7**:267–277.
28. Powers E. *Inactivation of Giardia cysts by iodine with special reference to Globaline: a review.* United States Army Natick Research, Development and Engineering Center; Technical report natick/TR-91/022. MA: Natick; 1993.
29. Gerba C, Johnson D, Hasan M. Efficacy of iodine water purification tablets against Cryptosporidium oocysts and Giardia cysts. *Wilderness Environ Med* 1997; **8**:96–100.
30. Marchin G, Fina L. Contact and demand-release disinfectants. *Crit Rev Environ Control* 1989; **19**:227–290.
31. Backer H, Hollowell J. Use of iodine for water disinfection: iodine toxicity and maximum recommended dose. *Environ Health Perspect* 2000; **108**:679–684.
32. Peeters J, Mazas E, Masschelein W, Maturana I, DeBacker E. Effect of disinfection of drinking water with ozone or chlorine dioxide on survival of Cryptosporidium. *Appl Environ Microbiol* 1989; **55**:1519–1522.
33. Venczel L, Arrowood M, Hurd M, Sobsey M. Inactivation of Cryptosporidium parvum oocysts and Clostridium perfringens spores by a mixed-oxidant disinfectant and by free chlorine. *Appl Environ Microbiol* 1997; **63**:1598–1601.
34. Sobel J, Mahon B, Mendoza C, Passaro D, Cano F, *et al.* Reduction of fecal contamination of street-vended beverages in Guatemala by a simple system for water purification and storage, handwashing, and beverage storage. *Am J Trop Med Hyg* 1998; **59**:380–387.
35. Mertens T, Frenando M, Cousens S, *et al.* Childhood diarrhoea in Sri Lanka: a case-control study of the impact of improved water sources. *Trop Med Parasit* 1990; **41**:98–104.
36. Huttly SR. The impact of inadequate sanitary conditions on health in developing countries. *World Health Stat Q* 1990; **43**:118–126.
37. Backer H. Field Water Disinfection. In: Auerbach P, ed. *Wilderness Medicine* 4th edn. St. Louis, MO: Mosby; 2001:1186–1236.

CHAPTER 7 Insect Protection

Mark S. Fradin

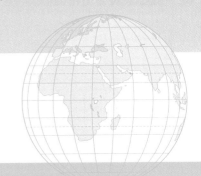

KEYPOINTS

- A number of variables play a role in the effectiveness of insect repellents. Little known examples are that N,N-diethyl-m-toluamide (also called N,N-diethyl-3-methylbenzamide), (DEET)-based repellents may work less well in women than in men, and with each 10 °C increase in ambient temperature, there can be as much as a 50% reduction in protection

- Host movement, dark clothing, carbon monoxide, skin warmth and moisture, and presence of perfumes all may lure biting insects

- Despite common beliefs, DEET toxicity is minimal, with only 16 cases of encephalopathy reported over the last half century (13 in children <8 years)

- Herbal insect repellents are less effective than DEET

- There are numerous methods to use for personal protection against insect bites, such as protective clothing and bed nets. These may be purchased through a variety of websites

INTRODUCTION

In preparation for travel to many tropical and subtropical locations, the well-informed traveler needs to be aware of the potential risks of insect and arthropod-transmitted disease. Mosquitoes, flies, ticks, midges, chiggers, and fleas are capable of transmitting multiple bacterial, viral, protozoan, parasitic and rickettsial infections to humans (Table 7.1). A multi-pronged approach is necessary to prevent becoming a victim of vector-borne disease: protection from bites is best achieved through avoiding infected habitats, wearing protective clothing, and applying repellents. This chapter will review all available techniques for preventing insect and arthropod bites, and will provide practical information to the traveler that will make it possible to distinguish between effective and ineffective methods of protection. A summary of the topics covered in this chapter is shown in Figure 7.1.

STIMULI THAT ATTRACT INSECTS

Scientists have not yet elucidated the exact mechanism by which insects and arthropods are attracted to their hosts. The stimuli that attract mosquitoes have been best studied. Mosquitoes use visual, thermal, and olfactory stimuli to locate a bloodmeal.[1,2] For mosquitoes that feed during the daytime, host movement and the wearing of dark-colored clothing may initiate orientation towards an individual. Visual stimuli appear to be important for in-flight orientation, par-

Table 7.1 Examples of diseases transmitted to humans by biting insects and arthropods

Mosquitoes

Eastern equine encephalitis
Western equine encephalitis
St. Louis encephalitis
La Cross encephalitis
West Nile virus
Japanese encephalitis
Venezuelan equine encephalitis
Malaria
Yellow fever
Dengue fever
Bancroftian filariasis
Epidemic polyarthritis (Ross River virus)
Chikungunya fever
Rift Valley Fever

Ticks

Lyme disease
Rocky mountain spotted fever
Colorado tick fever
Relapsing fever
Ehrlichiosis
Babesiosis
Tularemia
Tick paralysis
Tick typhus

Flies

Tularemia
Leishmaniasis
African trypanosomiasis (sleeping sickness)
Onchocerciasis
Bartonellosis
Loa loa

Chigger Mites

Scrub typhus (tsutsugamushi fever)
Rickettsial pox

Fleas

Plague
Murine (endemic) typhus

Lice

Epidemic typhus
Relapsing fever

Kissing bugs

American trypanosomiasis (Chagas' disease)

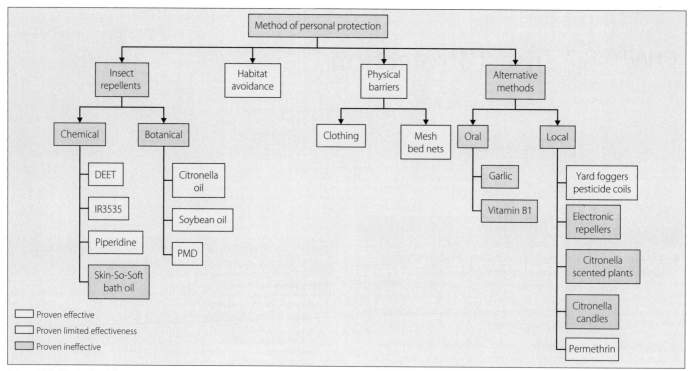

Figure 7.1 Methods of Personal Protection.

ticularly over long ranges. As a mosquito nears its host, olfactory stimuli then help guide the mosquito to its host. Carbon dioxide, released from breath and skin, serves as a long-range airborne attractant, at distances up to 36 m. Lactic acid, skin warmth, and moisture also serve as attractants. Volatile compounds, derived from sebum, eccrine and apocrine sweat, and/or the cutaneous microflora bacterial action on these secretions, may also act as chemoattractants. Different species of mosquitoes may show strong biting preferences for different parts of the body, related to local skin temperature and sweat gland activity. Floral fragrances, found in perfumes, lotions, detergents and soaps, may also lure biting insects and arthropods.

There can be significant variability in the attractiveness of different individuals to the same or different species of mosquitoes. Men tend to be bitten more readily than women, and adults are more likely to be bitten than children. Adults tend to be bitten less as they get older. Heavyset individuals tend to attract more mosquitoes, perhaps due to their greater relative heat or carbon dioxide output.

PERSONAL PROTECTION

Personal protection against bites is best achieved by avoiding infested habitats, using protective clothing and shelters, and applying repellents.[3,4]

Habitat avoidance

It is obvious that avoiding infested habitats, when feasible, will reduce the risk of being bitten. Many species of mosquitoes and other blood-sucking insects and arthropods are particularly active at dusk, making this a good time to remain indoors. If camping outdoors, to avoid common resting places, it is wise to be situated in areas that are high, dry, open, and as free from vegetation as possible. Any area with standing or stagnant water should be avoided, as these are ideal breeding grounds for mosquitoes.

Physical protection

By blocking access to the skin, physical barriers can be very effective in preventing bites. A long-sleeved shirt, socks, full-length pants, and a hat will readily protect most of the skin surface. Ticks and chigger mites usually gain access to the skin around the ankle area, so tucking pant legs into socks or boots will reduce the risk of being bitten. Loose-fitting shirts, made of tightly woven fabric, and worn over a tucked-in undershirt will effectively reduce bites to the upper body. Light-colored clothing will attract fewer mosquitoes and biting flies, and will make it easier to see any ticks that might have crawled onto the fabric. A broad-brim, preferably light-colored, hat will also help protect the head and neck and reduce the chance of being bitten by mosquitoes, deerflies, blackflies and biting midges.

Mesh garments or garments made of tightly-woven material can block ready access to the skin surface, thereby reducing the risks of being bitten. Hooded jackets, pants, mittens and head nets are available from several manufacturers in a wide range of styles for both adults and children. (Table 7.2). With a mesh size of less than 0.3 mm, these garments are woven tightly enough to exclude even biting ticks and midges. The main limitation of these garments is that, like any clothing, bending or sitting may pull the garments close enough to the skin to enable insects to bite through the fabric. Some people may also find mesh garments to be uncomfortable to wear during vigorous activity or in hot weather.

Lightweight insect nets and mesh shelters are also available to protect travelers while they sleep. (Table 7.2 and Fig. 7.2). The simplest net is a large piece of mesh fabric that is suspended above and draped over a bed or sleeping bag to protect the occupant. More complex free-standing, tent-like shelters are also available, made with flexible hoops that support the protective mesh over the occupant. The efficacy of insect nets or shelters may be greatly enhanced by spraying them with a permethrin-based contact insecticide, which can provide weeks of protection following a single application.

Table 7.2   Manufacturers of protective clothing, protective shelters, and insect nets

Protective clothing (includes hooded jackets, pants, headnets, ankle guards, gaiters, and mittens)	Protective shelters and insect nets
Bug Baffler, Inc. P.O. Box 444 Goffstown, NH 03045 (800) 662-8411 www.bugbaffler.com	Long Road Travel Supplies 111 Avenida Drive Berkeley, CA 94708 (800) 359-6040 www.longroad.com
Insect Out, Inc. P.O. Box 49643 Colorado Springs, CO 80949 (888) 488-0285 www.insectout.com	Wisconsin Pharmacal Co. 1 Repel Road Jackson, WI 53037 (800) 558-6614 www.wpcbrands.com
BugOut Outdoorwear, Inc. P.O. Box 185 901 East Stewart Centerville, Iowa 52544 (877) 928-4688 www.bug-out-outdoorwear.com	Travel Medicine, Inc. 369 Pleasant Street Northampton, MA 01060 (800) 872-8633 www.travmed.com
Skeeta P.O. Box 3422 Fayetteville, AR 72702 (501) 521-7324 www.skeeta,com	GearZone www.gearzone.co.uk
The Original Bug Shirt Company P.O. Box 127 Trout Creek, ON P0H 2L0 (888) 998-9096 www.bugshirt.com	Medical Advisory Services for Travellers Abroad, Ltd. (MASTA) www.masta.org
Shannon Outdoor Bug Tamer P.O. Box 444 Louisville, GA 30434 (800) 852-8058 www.bugtamer.com	Nomad Travellers Store www.nomadtravel.co.uk
Nomad Travellers Store www.nomadtravel.co.uk	

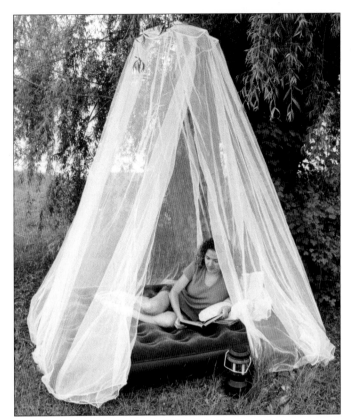

Figure 7.2A Bed net. (Courtesy of Wisconsin Pharmacal Co.).

Insect repellents

For many people, applying insect repellents may be the most effective and easiest way to protect against bites. The search for the 'perfect' insect repellent has been ongoing for decades, and has yet to be achieved. The ideal agent would repel multiple species of biting insects and arthropods, remain effective for at least 8 h, cause no irritation to skin or mucous membranes, possess no systemic toxicity, be resistant to abrasion, wash off, and be greaseless and odorless. No presently-available insect repellent meets all of these criteria. Efforts to find such a compound have been hampered by the multiplicity of variables that affect the inherent repellency of any chemical. Repellents do not all share a single mode of action, and different species of insects may react differently to the same repellent.

To be effective as an insect repellent, a chemical must be volatile enough to maintain an effective repellent vapor concentration at the skin surface, but not evaporate so rapidly that it quickly loses its effectiveness. Multiple factors play a role in effectiveness, including concentration, frequency and uniformity of application, the user's activity level and inherent attractiveness to blood-sucking insects and arthropods, and the number and species of the organisms trying to bite. Gender may also play a role in how well a repellent works – one study has shown that DEET-based repellents worked less well in women than in men.[5] The effectiveness of any repellent is reduced by abra-

sion from clothing; evaporation and absorption from the skin surface; wash off from sweat, rain, or water; and a windy environment.[2] Each 10°C increase in ambient temperature can lead to as much as 50% reduc-tion in protection time, due to greater evaporative loss of the repel-lent from the skin surface. One of the greatest limitations of insect repellents is that they do not 'cloak' the user in a chemical veil of pro-tection; any untreated exposed skin will be readily bitten by hungry insects and arthropods.

Chemical repellents
DEET
N,N-diethyl-m-toluamide (also called N,N-diethyl-3-methylbenzamide), or DEET, remains the gold standard of presently available insect repellents. In the United States, DEET has been registered for use by

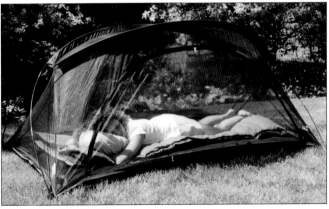

Figure 7.2B Protective shelter.

the general public since 1957. It is a broad spectrum repellent, effective against many species of crawling and flying pests, including mosquitoes, biting flies, midges, chiggers, fleas, and ticks. The United States Environmental Protection Agency estimates that about 30% of the US population uses a DEET-based product every year; worldwide use exceeds 200 million people annually.[6] More than 45 years of empirical testing of more than 20 000 other compounds has not led to a superior repellent being brought to market.[7]

DEET may be applied to skin, clothing, mesh insect nets or shelters, window screens, tents, or sleeping bags. Care should be taken to avoid inadvertent contact with plastics (such as watch crystals and glasses frames), rayon, spandex, leather, or painted and varnished surfaces, since DEET may damage these. DEET does not damage natural fibers like wool and cotton.

Choosing a deet formulation DEET is sold worldwide in concentrations of 5–100%. DEET is available in lotion, solution, towelette, gel, solid stick, and spray forms. As a general rule, higher concentrations of DEET will provide longer-lasting protection. Mathematical models of repellent effectiveness show that the protection is proportional to the logarithm of the concentration of the product. This curve tends to plateau out at higher repellent concentrations, providing relatively less additional protection for each incremental dose of DEET over 50%. Hence, for most activities, 10–35% DEET will usually provide adequate protection. The 100% DEET formulations are rarely needed. The higher strengths of DEET repellent are appropriate to use under circumstances in which the wearer will be in an environment with a very high density of insects (e.g., a rain forest), where there is a high risk of disease transmission from bites, or under circumstances where there may be rapid loss of repellent from the skin surface, such as under conditions of high temperature and humidity, or rain. Under these circumstances, re-application of the repellent will still likely be necessary to maintain its effectiveness.

At least two companies (3M, and Sawyer Products) currently manufacturer extended-release formulations of DEET that make it possible to deliver long-lasting protection without requiring the use of high concentrations of DEET. 3M's product, Ultrathon, was developed for the US military. This acrylate polymer 35% DEET formulation, when tested under multiple different environmental/climatic field conditions, was as effective as 75% DEET, providing up to 12 h of >95% protection against mosquito bites.[2] Sawyer Products' controlled-release 20% DEET lotion traps the chemical in a protein particle which slowly releases it to the skin surface, providing repellency equivalent to a standard 50% DEET preparation, lasting about 5 h. About 50% less of this encapsulated DEET is absorbed when compared with a 20% ethanol-based prepa-ration of DEET.

Deet safety and toxicity Given its use by millions of people worldwide for 45 years, DEET continues to show a remarkable safety profile. In 1980, to comply with more current standards for repellent safety, the US EPA issued an updated Registration Standard for DEET.[6] As a result, 30 new animal studies were conducted to assess acute, chronic, and subchronic toxicity; mutagenicity; oncogenicity; and developmental, reproductive, and neurological toxicity.[8] The results of these studies neither led to any product changes to comply with current EPA safety standards, nor indicated any new toxicities under normal usage. The EPA's Re-registration Eligibility Decision (RED) released in 1998 confirmed the Agency position that 'normal use of DEET does not present a health concern to the general U.S. population'.[9]

Case reports of potential DEET toxicity exist in the medical literature, and have been summarized in several medical literature reviews.[2,10] Fewer than 50 cases of significant toxicity from DEET exposure have been documented in the medical literature over the last four decades; over three-quarters of these resolved without sequelae. Many of these cases had long-term, excessive, or inappropriate use of DEET repellents; the details of exposure were frequently poorly documented, making causal relationships difficult to establish. These cases have not shown any correlation between the risk of toxicity and the concentration of the DEET product used or the age of user.

The reports of DEET toxicity that raise the greatest concern involve 16 cases of encephalopathy, 13 in children under age 8 years.[2,10] Three of these children died, one of whom had ornithine carbamoyltransferase deficiency, which might have predisposed her to DEET-induced toxicity. The other children recovered without sequelae. The EPA's analysis of these cases concluded that they 'do not support a direct link between exposure to DEET and seizure incidence'.[9] Animal studies in rats and mice show that DEET is not a selective neurotoxin.[6] According to the EPA, even if a link between DEET use and seizures does exist, the observed risk, based on DEET usage patterns, would be less than 1/100 million users.[9] Other studies have confirmed that children under 6 years old are not at greater risk for developing adverse effects from DEET when compared with older individuals.[11]

Consumers applying both a DEET-based repellent and a sunscreen should be aware that the repellent might reduce the sunscreen's effectiveness. In a study of 14 patients who sequentially applied a 33% DEET repellent and an SPF 15 sunscreen, the sunscreen SPF was decreased by a mean of 33%, although the repellent maintained its potency.[12] Combination sunscreen/DEET products are available, and will deliver the SPF as stated on the label. However, these products are generally not the best choice, as it is rare that the need for re-application of sunscreen and repellent is exactly the same. In an effort to maintain adequate sun protection, consumers applying combination products will often apply more repellent than they would otherwise have needed.

There are always special concerns about the use of insect repellents during pregnancy. Most repellents are not tested in pregnant women. One published study followed 450 Thai women who used 20% DEET daily during the second and third trimesters of pregnancy to reduce the risk of contracting malaria.[13] Four percent of these women had detectable levels of DEET in umbilical cord blood at the time of delivery. However, no differences in survival, growth, or neurological development could be detected in the infants borne to mothers who used DEET when compared with an equal number of mothers treated with a daily placebo cream during their pregnancies.

The EPA has issued guidelines to ensure safe use of DEET-based repellents (Table 7.3).[14] Careful product choice and common-sense application will greatly reduce the possibility of toxicity. In the past the American Academy of Pediatrics recommended that DEET-containing repellents used on children contained no more than 10% DEET.[2] However, more recently, it has reevaluated the situation and is recommending the same concentrations for children as for adults (except for in small infants). See chapter 21. When required, reapplication of low-strength repellent can compensate for their inherent shorter duration of protection. Individuals adverse to applying DEET directly to their skin may get long-lasting repellency by applying DEET only to their clothing. DEET-treated garments, stored in a plastic bag between wearings, will maintain their repellency for several weeks.

Questions regarding the safety of DEET may be addressed to the EPA-sponsored National Pesticide Telecommunications Network, available every day from 06:30 to 16:30. PST at (800) 858-7378 or via their website at http://npic.orst.edu.

IR3535 (ethyl-butylacetylaminoproprionate)

IR3535 (butylacetylaminopropionate) is an analogue of the amino acid β alanine, and has been used in Europe for 20 years. In the USA, this compound is classified by the EPA as a biopesticide, effective against mosquitoes, ticks, and flies. In July 1999, 7.5% IR3535 was

Table 7.3	Guidelines for safe and effective use of insect repellents (adapted from EPA guidelines)[14]

For casual use, choose a repellent with no more than 35% DEET though up to 50% DEET is acceptable. Repellents with the same percent DEET may be used in children, however not in small infants.

Use just enough repellent to lightly cover the skin; do not saturate the skin.

Repellents should be applied only to exposed skin and/or clothing – do not use under clothing.

For maximum effectiveness, apply to all exposed areas of skin.

To apply to the face, dispense into palms, rub hands together, and then apply thin layer to face.

Avoid contact with eyes and mouth – do not apply to children's hands to prevent possible subsequent contact with mucous membranes.

After applying, wipe repellent from the palmar surfaces to prevent inadvertent contact with eyes, mouth and genitals.

Never use repellents over cuts, wounds, inflamed, irritated or eczematous skin.

Do not inhale aerosol formulations or get in eyes.

Frequent reapplication is rarely necessary, unless the repellent seems to have lost its effectiveness. Reapplication may be necessary in very hot, wet environments, due to rapid loss of repellent from the skin surface.

Once inside, wash off treated areas with soap and water. Washing the repellent from the skin surface is particularly important under circumstances where a repellent is likely to be applied for several consecutive days.

brought to the US market, sold exclusively by the Avon Corporation as *Skin-So-Soft Bug Guard Plus*. Very little data are available to the public on IR3535. In the initial studies submitted to the EPA for registration of this product, IR3535 was shown to work for up to 4 hours against mosquitoes. However, a comparative laboratory study of insect repellents, using *Aedes aegypti* mosquitoes, showed that the product was effective for an average of only about 23 min.[22]

Although Avon never marketed its *Skin-So-Soft* Bath Oil as a repellent, this product received considerable media attention several years ago when it was reported by some consumers to be effective as a mosquito repellent. When tested under laboratory conditions against *Aedes aegypti* mosquitoes, *Skin-So-Soft* Bath Oil's effective half-life was found to be 0.51 h.[2] In one study, against *Aedes albopictus*, *Skin-So-Soft* oil provided 0.64 hours of protection from bites, 10 times *less* effective than 12.5% DEET.[2] *Skin-So-Soft* oil has been found to be somewhat effective against biting midges, but this effect is likely due to its trapping the insects in an oily film on the skin surface. It has been proposed that the limited mosquito repellent effect of *Skin-So-Soft* oil could be due to its fragrance, or to the other chemicals used in its formulation.

Piperidine

Piperidine-based repellents are available in Europe under the trade name of *Autan Bayrepel*, and may be purchased in lotion, spray and stick formulations. The few available published studies of this product show that it may provide repellency comparable with DEET, protecting against many species of mosquitoes and biting flies for up to 8 h, and against ticks for up to 4 h. The repellents are cosmetically pleasant and, unlike DEET, show no detrimental effects on contact with plastics. Piperidine-based repellents are not yet available for sale in the USA.

Botanical repellents

Literally thousands of plants have been tested as sources of insect repellents. Although none of the plant-derived chemicals tested to date demonstrate the broad effectiveness and duration of DEET, a few show repellent activity. Plants with essential oils that have been reported to possess repellent activity include citronella, cedar, verbena,

pennyroyal, geranium, lavender, pine, cajeput, cinnamon, rosemary, basil, thyme, allspice, garlic, and peppermint.[15,16] Unlike DEET-based repellents, botanical repellents have been relatively poorly studied. When tested, most of these essential oils tended to show short-lasting protection, lasting minutes to 2 h. A summary of readily available plant-derived insect repellents is shown in Table 7.4.

Citronella

Oil of citronella was initially registered as an insect repellent by the US EPA in 1948. It is the most common active ingredient found in 'natural' or 'herbal' insect repellents. Originally extracted from the grass plant *Cymbopogon nardus*, oil of citronella has a lemony scent.

Conflicting data exist on the efficacy of citronella-based products, varying greatly depending on the study methodology, location, and species of biting insect tested. One citronella-based repellent was found to provide no repellency when tested in the laboratory against *Aedes aegypti* mosquitoes.[17] Another study of the same product, however, conducted in the field, showed an average of 88% repellency over a 2-h exposure. The product's effectiveness was greatest within the first 40 min after application, and then decreased with time over the remainder of the test period.[17] In a recent comparative laboratory study of the efficacy of insect repellents, no tested citronella-based product (concentration range of 0.1–12%) completely repelled mosquitoes for more than 19 min.[22]

The short duration of action of citronella can be partially overcome by frequent re-application of the repellent. In 1997, after analyzing available data on the repellent effect of citronella, the EPA concluded that citronella-based insect repellents must contain the following statement on their labels: 'For maximum repellent effectiveness of this product, repeat applications at one hour intervals.'[18]

Citronella candles have been promoted as an effective way to repel mosquitoes from one's local environment. One study compared the efficacy of commercially available 3% citronella candles, 5% citronella incense, and plain candles to prevent bites by *Aedes* species mosquitoes under field conditions.[2] Subjects near the citronella candles had 42% fewer bites than controls who had no protection (a statistically significant difference). However, burning ordinary candles reduced the number of bites by 23%. There was no difference in efficacy between

Table 7.4	Botanical insect repellents		
Manufacturer	**Product name**	**Form(s)**	**Active ingredient**
Travel Medicine, Inc. Northampton, MA (800) 872-8633	FiteBite Plant-Based Insect Repellent	Lotion	Eucalyptus oil (PMD) 30%
Repel Jackson, WI (800) 558-6614	Lemon eucalyptus	Lotion	Eucalyptus oil (PMD) 30%
SC Johnson Wax Racine, WWI (800) 558-5566	OFF! Botanicals	Lotion	Eucalyptus oil (PMD) 10%
Laboratorios OTC Ibérica SA	Mosi-Guard	Lotion & pump spray	Eucalyptus oil (PMD) 50%
HOMS, Inc. www.biteblocker.com	Blocker	Lotion & pump spray	Soybean oil 2%
Quantum, Inc. Eugene, OR (800) 448-1448	Buzz Away Buzz Away, SPF 15	Towelette & pump spray Lotion	Citronella oil 5%; oils of cedarwood, peppermint, eucalyptus, lemongrass
Tender Corp. Littleton, NH (800) 258-4696	Natrapel	Lotion and pump spray	Citronella 10%
All Terrain Co. Encinitas, CA (800) 246-7328	Herbal Armor Herbal Armor SPF 15 Herbal Armor	Lotion Lotion Pump spray	Citronella oil 12%, oils of cedar, peppermint oil 2.5%, cedar oil 2% lemongrass oil 1%, geranium oil 0.05%, in a slow-release encapsulated formula
Green Ban Norway, IA (319) 446-7495	Green Ban For People: Regular Double Strength	 Oil Oil	 Citronella oil 5%, peppermint oil 1% Citronella oil 10%, peppermint oil 2%

citronella incense and plain candles. The ability of plain candles to decrease biting may be due to their serving as a 'decoy' source of warmth, moisture, and carbon dioxide.

The citrosa plant (*Pelargonium citrosum* 'Van Leenii') has been marketed as being able to repel mosquitoes through the continuous release of citronella oils. Unfortunately, when tested, these plants offer no protection against bites. Mosquitoes were found to readily land on the leaves of the plant themselves.[2]

Blocker

Although available in Europe for several years, Blocker, a 'natural' repellent, was not released to the US market until 1997. Blocker combines soybean oil, geranium oil, and coconut oil into lotion and spray forms. Studies conducted at the University of Guelph (Ontario, Canada) showed that this product was capable of providing over 97% protection against *Aedes* species mosquitoes under field conditions, even after 3.5 h of application. During the same time period, a 6.65% DEET-based spray gave 86% protection.[2] A second study showed that Blocker provided a mean of 200 ± 30 (SD) min of complete protection from mosquito bites.[2] Blocker also provided about 10 h of protection against biting black flies; in the same test, 20% DEET only gave 6.5 h of complete protection.[2]

Eucalyptus

A derivative (*p*-menthane-3,8-diol, or PMD) isolated from oil of the lemon eucalyptus plant has shown promise as an effective 'natural' repellent. This menthol-like repellent has been very popular in China

for years, and is currently available in Europe under the brand name *Mosi-guard*. PMD was registered as a biopesticide by the US EPA and licensed for sale in the USA in March 2000.[19] In the USA, it is presently available as Repel's Lemon Eucalyptus Insect Repellent, *OFF!* Botanicals, and as Travel Medicine's FiteBite Lemon Eucalyptus Repellent (see Table 7.4). In a laboratory study against Anopheles mosquitoes, 30% PMD showed efficacy comparable with 20% DEET, but required more frequent reapplication to maintain its potency.[17,20]

Efficacy of DEET versus botanical repellents

Limited data are available from studies that directly compare plant-derived repellents to DEET-based products. Available data proving the efficacy of 'natural' repellents are often sparse, and there is no uniformly-accepted standard for testing these products. As a result, different studies often yield varied results, depending on how and where the tests were conducted. In general, when compared to 'natural' products, DEET-based repellents demonstrate longer-lasting effectiveness. In a laboratory study against *Aedes aegypti* mosquitoes, two commercially-available 'natural' repellents containing citronella (and other plant-derived essential oils) demonstrated no repellent effect, even when applied at twice the concentration that would typically be expected to be used.[21] In the same study, DEET-based repellents (at various concentrations) provided at least 2 h of protection.[21]

One study has been done that compares the relative efficacy of botanical repellents to DEET-based products. To eliminate the confounding variables commonly found in outdoor field experiments tested against wild populations of mosquitoes, this study was

Figure 7.3 Protection times of insect repellents.

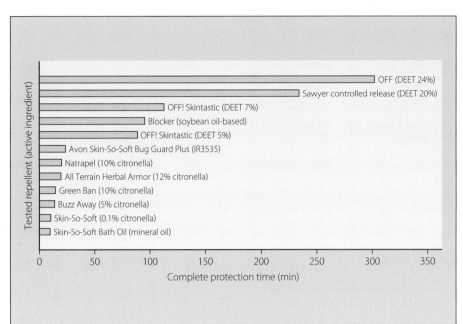

Figure 7.3 Protection times of insect repellents.

conducted in a laboratory using controlled numbers of *Aedes aegypti* mosquitoes. This study showed that only the DEET-based repellents were able to provide complete protection from mosquito bites for up to 6 h, depending on the DEET concentration of the product tested. The oil of eucalyptus (PMD)-based repellent protected for an average of 120 min, and the soybean oil-based Blocker provided a mean of about 90 min of complete protection. In contrast, all other tested botanical repellents, regardless of concentration and active ingredient, protected for an average of less than 23 min[22] (Fig. 7.3). Wristbands impregnated with either DEET or citronella offered no protection against bites.[22]

For people who choose to use 'natural' repellents, reapplication of the repellent on a frequent basis, preferably hourly, will help to compensate for the short duration of action of these repellents. Travelers in areas of the world where insect-borne disease is a real threat would be better protected by using a DEET-based repellent, which, depending on the product chosen, can provide 6–12 h of complete protection against insect bites from a single application of the repellent.

Alternative repellents

There has always been great interest in finding an oral insect repellent. Oral repellents would be convenient and would eliminate the need to apply creams to the skin or put on protective clothing. Unfortunately, no effective oral repellent has been discovered. For decades, lay literature has made the claim that Vitamin B$_1$ (thiamine) works as a systemic mosquito repellent. When subjected to scientific scrutiny, however, thiamine has unanimously been found not to have a repellent effect on mosquitoes. The United States Food and Drug Administration, prompted by misleading consumer advertising, issued the following statement in 1983: 'There is a lack of adequate data to establish the effectiveness of thiamine or any other ingredient for OTC (over the counter) internal use as an insect repellent. Labeling claims for OTC orally administered insect repellent drug products are either false, misleading, or unsupported by scientific data.'[23] Tests of over 100 ingested drugs, including other vitamins, failed to reveal any that worked well against mosquitoes.[2] Ingested garlic has also never proven to be an effective pest deterrent.

Permethrin

Pyrethrum is a powerful, rapidly-acting insecticide, originally derived from the crushed dried flowers of the daisy *Chrysanthemum cinerariifolium*. Permethrin is a man-made synthetic pyrethroid. It does not repel insects, but instead works as a contact insecticide, causing nervous system toxicity, leading to death, or 'knockdown', of the insect. The chemical is effective against mosquitoes, flies, ticks, fleas, lice, and chiggers. Permethrin has low mammalian toxicity, is poorly absorbed by the skin, and is rapidly metabolized by skin and blood esterases.[24]

Permethrin should be applied directly to clothing or to other fabrics (tent walls, mosquito nets), not to skin. Permethrins are non-staining, nearly odorless, resistant to degradation by heat or sun, and will maintain their effectiveness for at least two weeks, through several launderings.[2]

The combination of permethrin-treated clothing and skin application of a DEET-based repellent creates a formidable barrier against biting insects. In an Alaskan field trial against mosquitoes, subjects wearing permethrin-treated uniforms and a polymer-based 35% DEET product had greater than 99.9% protection (1 bite/h) over 8 h; unprotected subjects were bitten an average of 1188 bites/h.[25]

Permethrin-sprayed clothing also proved very effective against ticks. One hundred percent of *D. occidentalis* ticks (which carry Rocky Mountain Spotted Fever) died within 3 h of touching permethrin-treated cloth.[3] Permethrin-sprayed pants and jackets also provided 100% protection from all three life stages of *Ixodes dammini* ticks, the vector of Lyme disease.[3] In contrast, DEET alone (applied to the skin), provided 85% repellency at the time of application; this protection deteriorated to 55% repellency at 6 h, when tested against the lone star tick *Amblyomma americanum*.[3] *Ixodes scapularis* ticks, which may transmit Lyme disease, also seem to be less sensitive to the repellent effect of DEET.[26]

Permethrin-based insecticides available in the USA are listed in Table 7.5. To apply to clothing, spray each side of the fabric (outdoors) for 30 to 45 s, just enough to moisten. Allow to dry for 2–4 h before wearing. Permethrin solution is also available for soak-treating large items, such as mesh bed nets.

Table 7.5 **Permethrin insecticides**

Manufacturer	Product name	Form(s)	Active ingredient
Coulston Products Easton, PA (610) 253-0167	Duranon	Aerosol & pump sprays	Permethrin 0.5%
	Perma-Kill	Liquid concentrate	Permethrin 13.3%
Sawyer Products Tampa, FL (800) 940-4464	Permethrin Tick Repellent	Aerosol & pump sprays	Permethrin 0.5%
United Industries Corp. St. Louis, MO (800) 767-9927	Cutter Outdoorsman Gear Guard	Aerosol spray	Permethrin 0.5%
Wisconsin Pharmacal Co. Jackson, WI (800) 558-6614	Repel Permanone	Aerosol spray	Permethrin 0.5%
LifeSystems England www.lifesystems.co.uk		Pump spray	Permethrin 0.5%

Reducing local mosquito populations

Consumers may still find advertisements for small ultrasonic electronic devices meant to be worn or carried and claim to repel mosquitoes by emitting a noise such as that of a dragonfly (claimed to be the 'natural enemy' of the mosquito), male mosquito, or bat. Multiple studies, conducted both in the field and laboratory, show that these devices do not work.[27] Pyrethrin-containing 'yard foggers' set off prior to an outdoor event can temporarily reduce the number of biting insects and arthropods in a local environment. These products should be applied before any food is brought outside, and should be kept away from animals or fishponds. Burning coils that contain natural pyrethrins or synthetic pyrethroids (such as d-allethrin or d-transallethrin) can also temporarily reduce local populations of biting pests.[17] Some concerns have been raised about the long-term cumulative safety of use of these coils in an indoor environment.

RELIEF FROM MOSQUITO BITES

Cutaneous responses to mosquito bites range from the common localized wheal-and-flare reactions, to delayed bite papules, rare systemic Arthus-type reactions, and even anaphylaxis.[2] Bite reactions are the result of sensitization to mosquito salivary antigens, which lead to the formation of both specific IgE and IgG antibodies. Immediate-type reactions are mediated by IgE and histamine, while cell-mediated immunity is responsible for the delayed reactions.

Several strategies exist for relieving the itch of mosquito bites. Topical corticosteroids can reduce the associated erythema, itching, and induration; a short, rapidly-tapering course of oral prednisone can also be very effective in reducing extensive bite reactions. Topical diphenhydramine and ester-type topical anesthetics should be avoided, due to concerns about inducing allergic contact sensitivity. Oral antihistamines can be effective in reducing the symptoms of mosquito bites. Cetirizine was given prophylactically in a double-blind, placebo-controlled, 2-week, cross-over trial to 18 individuals who had previously experienced dramatic cutaneous reactions to mosquito bites.[28] Subjects given the active drug had a statistically-significant 40% decrease in both the size of the wheal response at 15 min, as well as in the size of the 24-h bite papule. The mean pruritus score, measured at 0.25, 1, 12, and 24 h after being bitten, was 67% less than that of the untreated controls. Similar benefits have been reported with elastine. In highly sensitized individuals, prophylactic treatment with antihistamines may safely reduce the cutaneous reactions to mosquito bites.

AfterBite, a 3.6% ammonium solution has been found to relieve type I hypersensitivity symptoms associated with mosquito bites. In a double-blind, placebo controlled trial, 64% of mosquito bitten subjects experienced complete relief of symptoms after a single application of the ammonium solution; the remaining 36% experienced partial relief, lasting 15–90 min after a single application. No subjects treated with placebo reported complete symptom relief.[29]

CONCLUSION

Comprehensive approach to personal protection

An integrated approach to personal protection is the most effective way to prevent insect and arthropod bites, regardless of where one is in the world and which species may be biting. Maximum protection is best achieved through avoiding infested habitats, and using protective clothing, topical repellents and permethrin-treated garments to prevent nocturnal bites. When appropriate, mesh bed nets or tents should be used to prevent nocturnal insect bites.

DEET-containing repellents are the most effective products presently on the market, providing broad-spectrum, long-lasting repellency against multiple species. Of the currently-available, non-DEET repellents, the most effective (in descending order of duration of protection) are piperidine, PMD (oil of eucalyptus), and the soybean oil-based Blocker. Repellents alone, however, should not be relied upon to provide complete protection. Mosquitoes, for example, can find and bite any untreated skin, and may even bite through thin clothing. Deerflies, biting midges, and some black-flies prefer to bite around the head, and will readily crawl into the hair to bite where there is no protection. Wearing protective clothing, including a hat, will reduce the chances of being bitten. Treating one's clothes and hat with permethrin will maximize their effectiveness, by causing 'knockdown' of any insect that crawls or lands on the treated clothing. To prevent chiggers or ticks from crawling up the legs, pants should also be tucked into the boots or stockings. Wearing smooth, closely woven fabrics, such as nylon, will make it more difficult for ticks to cling to the fabric. After returning indoors, the skin should be inspected for the presence of ticks. Any ticks found attached to the skin should be removed to reduce the potential risk of disease trans-mission. Most ticks require over 48 h of attachment to transmit Lyme disease.[30] The best method of tick removal is to simply grasp the tick with a forceps as close to the skin surface as possible, and pull upwards, with a steady, even force.

The US military relies on this integrated approach to protect troops deployed in areas where insects and arthropods constitute either a significant nuisance or medical risk. The Department of Defense's Insect Repel-lent System consists of DEET applied to exposed areas of skin, and permethrin-treated uniforms, worn with the pant legs tucked into boots, and the undershirt tucked into the pant's waistband. This system has been proven to dramatically reduce the likelihood of being bitten.

Travelers visiting parts of the world where vector-borne diseases are potential threats will be best able to protect themselves if they learn about indigenous pests and the diseases they might transmit. Protective clothing, mesh covered tents or bedding, repellents, and permethrin spray should be carried. Travelers would be wise to check the most-current World Health Organization (WHO) www.who.int/en or Centers for Disease Control and Prevention (CDC) www.cdc.gov/travel/index.htm recommendations about traveling to countries where immunizations (for example, against yellow fever), or chemoprophy-laxis (for example, against malaria) should be addressed prior to departure.

REFERENCES

1. Bock GR, Cardew G, ed. *Olfaction in Mosquito-Host Interactions*. New York: J Wiley; 1996.
2. Fradin MS. Mosquitoes and mosquito repellents: a clinician's guide. *Ann Int Med* 1998; **128**(11):931–940.
3. Fradin MS. Protection from blood-feeding arthropods. In: Auerbach PS, ed. *Wilderness Medicine*. 4th edn. St. Louis: Mosby; 2001:754–768.
4. Curtis CF. Personal protection methods against vectors of disease. *Rev Med Vet Entomol* 1992; **80**(10):543–553.
5. Golenda CF, Solberg VB, Burge R, Gambel JM, Wirtz RA. Gender-related efficacy difference to an extended duration formulation of topical N,N-diethyl-m-toluamide (DEET). *Am J Trop Med Hyg* 1999; **60**(4):654–657.
6. U.S. Environmental Protection Agency. Office of Pesticides and Toxic Substances. Special Pesticide Review Division. *N,N-diethyl-m-toluamide (DEET) Pesticide Registration Standard* (EPA 540/RS-81-004). Washington DC: U.S. Environmental Protection Agency; 1980.
7. King WV. Chemicals evaluated as insecticides and repellents at Orlando, Fla. *USDA Agric Handb* 1954; **69**:1–397.
8. The DEET Joint Venture Group. *Completed studies for the DEET Toxicology Data Development Program*. Washington, DC: The DEET Joint Venture Group, Chemical Specialties Manufacturers Association; 1996.
9. U.S. Environmental Protection Agency. Office of Pesticide Programs, Prevention, Pesticides and Toxic Substances Division. *Reregistration Eligibility Decision (RED): DEET* (EPA 738-F-95-010). Washington, DC: U.S. Environmental Protection Agency; 1998.
10. Osimitz TG, Grothaus RH. The present safety assessment of DEET. *J Am Mosq Control Assoc* 1995; **11**(2):274–278.
11. Veltri JC, Osimitz TG, Bradford DC, Page BC. Retrospective analysis of calls to poison control centers resulting from exposure to the insect repellent N,N-diethyl-m-toluamide (DEET) from 1985–1989. *J Toxicol Clin Toxicol* 1994; **32**(1):1–16.
12. Murphy ME, Montemarano AD, Debboun M, Gupta R. The effect of sunscreen on the efficacy of insect repellent: A clinical trial. *J Am Acad Derm* 2000; **43**:219–222.
13. McGready R, Hamilton KA, Simpson JA, *et al.* Safety of the insect repellent N, N-diethyl-m-toluamide (DEET) in pregnancy. *Am J Trop Med Hyg* 2001; **65**:285–289.
14. United States Environmental Protection Agency. Office of Pesticide Programs, United States Environmental Protection Agency (EPA-735/F-93-052R). Washington DC: United States Environmental Protection Agency; 1998.
15. Quarles W. Botanical mosquito repellents. *Common Sense Pest Control* 1996; **12**(4):12–19.
16. Duke J. USDA-Agricultural Research Service Phytochemical and Ethnobotanical Databases. http://www.ars-grin.govduke.
17. Fradin MS. Insect repellents. In: Wolverton S, ed. *Comprehensive Dermatologic Drug Therapy*. Philadelphia, PA: WB Saunders; 2001:717–734.
18. United States Environmental Protection Agency. Office of Pesticide Programs, Prevention, Pesticides and Toxic Substances Division: Reregistration eligibility decision (RED) for oil of citronella (EPA-738-F-97-002). Washington DC: United States Environmental Protection Agency; 1997.
19. United States Environmental Protection Agency. Office of Pesticide Programs. p-Menthane-3,8-diol. Washington, DC 2000. Washington, DC: United States Environmental Protection Agency. Available: www.epa.gov/pesticides/biopesticides/factsheets/fs011550e.htm.
20. Trigg JK, Hill N. Laboratory evaluation of a eucalyptus-based repellent against four biting arthropods. *Phytother Res* 1996; **10**:313–316.
21. Chou JT, Rossignol PA, Ayres JW. Evaluation of commercial insect repellents on human skin against Aedes aegypti (Diptera: Culicidae). *J Med Entomol* 1997; **34**:624–630.
22. Fradin MS, Day JF. Comparative efficacy of insect repellents. *N Engl J Med* 2002; **347**:13–18.
23. Food and Drug Administration. Drug products containing active ingredients offered over-the-counter (OTC) for oral use as insect repellents. *Fed Red* 1983; **48**.
24. Insect repellents. *Med Lett Drugs Ther* 1989; **31**:45–47.
25. Lillie TH, Schreck CE, Rahe AJ. Effectiveness of personal protection against mosquitoes in Alaska. *J Med Entomol* 1988; **25**(6):475–478.
26. Schreck CE, Fish D, McGovern TP. Activity of repellents applied to skin for protection against Amblyomma americanum and Ixodes scapularis ticks (Acari: Ixodidae). *J Am Mosq Control Assoc* 1995; **11**:136–140.
27. Coro F, Suarez S. Review and history of electronic mosquito repellers. *Wing Beats* 2000; **Summer:**6–32.
28. Reunala T, Brummer-Korvenkontio H, Karppinen A, Coulie P, Palosuo T. Treatment of mosquito bites with cetirizine. *Clin Exp Allergy* 1993; **23**:72–75.
29. Zhai H, Packman EW, Maibach HI. Effectiveness of ammonium solution in relieving type I mosquito bite symptoms: a double-blind, placebo-controlled study. *Acta Derm Venereol (Stockh)* 1998; **78**:297–298.
30. Sood SK, Salzman MB, Johnson BJ, *et al.* Duration of tick attachment as a predictor of the risk of Lyme disease in an area in which Lyme disease is endemic. *J Infect Dis* 1997; **175**(4):996–999.

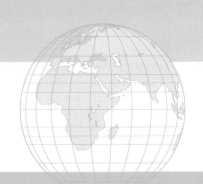

CHAPTER 8 Travel Health and Medical Kits

Eric A. Weiss

KEYPOINTS

- Travel health advisors should recommend that travelers wander through the aisles of their favorite pharmacy and purchase over the counter items that assist with minor ailments

- Medications should always be carried with the traveler and stored in carry-on baggage

- Items placed in a travel health/first aid kit are determined by a number of factors: the traveler, destination, and his/her risk factors

- Adventuresome travel requires special supplies and knowledge of how to use the supplies in order to help care for injuries that occur

- Prescription medications should be a part of the travel health kit and include extras of usual medications along with items for exposures such as malaria and altitude

INTRODUCTION

Travelers often venture to locations where comprehensive medical care is not readily available. Evidence of this trend can be seen in Nepal, where the number of travelers obtaining trekking permits annually has increased from 14 000 in 1976 to almost 75 000 in 1996.[1] Many travelers are inadequately prepared for their trips and are naive about the associated risks. Surveys of trekkers in the Khumbu region of Nepal from 1995–1997 revealed that only 18% of respondents carried a comprehensive kit.[2]

Thus, it appears that most travelers are busy checking their passports, paperwork, and reservations, and spend little, if any time preparing a travel health kit. Even if traveling near home or within one's own country, it is helpful to carry a kit containing items that include a person's usual medications and anything that could be of assistance should even a minor illness occur. It is strongly recommended that travelers take the time to walk the aisles of their local pharmacy and purchase items that they feel most comfortable using when minor health problems occur. In this way, they will not be forced to spend time finding a place to buy these items (which are often not equivalent) during travel. While many medications available only by prescription may be found over the counter in developing countries, the standards by which they are manufactured may vary, with even counterfeit medications being found in many parts of the world.

THE BASIC TRAVEL HEALTH KIT

The basic travel health kit should address the most common adverse health events that typically occur during travel (Table 8.1). In one series, 64% of travelers experienced some health complaint during travel to a developing country.[3] Duration of travel correlates strongly with risk of illness or injury, with each additional day of travel adding a 3–4% increase risk.[4] This statistic emphasizes the need for longer-term travelers to carry a more comprehensive travel medical kit. Diarrhea and respiratory tract symptoms are the most common complaints during travel to developing countries.[3,5–7] Nearly one out of every four travelers experience respiratory symptoms during their trip, which include cough, sore throat, runny nose, or ear ache.[3,5] Nearly 8% of travelers experience skin problems related to stinging or biting insects, heat or sun exposure, dermatophytes or contact allergens.[3] Nearly 5% of travelers experience trauma from accidents or injuries.[3] Most are minor, consisting of blisters, cuts, abrasions or bruises and amenable to self-treatment with components of a basic first aid kit.

Travel health advisors should help patients assemble a basic medical kit and prescribe medication that might be needed during the trip. Travelers should be reminded to carry their kits with them at all times, even during their journeys. Many times, exacerbations of chronic problems or new problems occur on board aircraft and the traveler's kit is with their checked baggage; it should always be stored in the carry-on baggage. Bearing in mind the new regulations regarding allowable items, anything sharp should remain in a checked bag.

Table 8.2 gives suggestions for the contents of a basic travel health kit, while Table 8.3 lists a dental kit. The design of a kit, however, should take into consideration the following factors:

- Medical expertise of the intended user
- The location and environmental extremes of the destination
- Endemic diseases

Table 8.1	Reported illness during travel to developing countries
Symptom	**Number (%)**
Diarrhea	358 (64)
Respiratory tract symptoms	204 (34)
Skin problem	63 (8)
High altitude illness	45 (6)
Motion sickness	37 (5)
Accidents or injuries	35 (4)
Febrile episodes (malaria most common)	21 (3)
Modified from.[3]	

Table 8.2	Suggested contents for the basic travel health kit
Usual prescription medications (including extras)	
Analgesic (aspirin or acetaminophen and/or non-steroidal anti-inflammatory)	
Throat lozenges	
Decongestant	
Antihistamine	
Cough suppressant/expectorant	
Loperamide	
Antibacterial wipes or towelettes	
Antibiotic for diarrhea	
Bismuth subsalicylate	
Sunscreen	
Antifungal cream	
Steroid cream	
Antimalarial medication	
Insect repellent	
Bandages and adhesive	
Water purification tablets	
Oral rehydration salts	
Tweezers/scissors	
Antacid	
Digital thermometer	

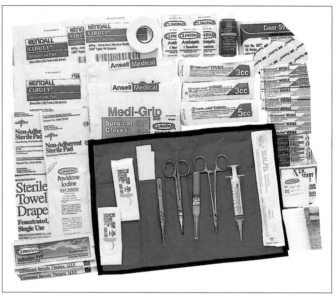

Figure 8.1 A commercial 'Suture/Syringe Kit'.

The travel medical kit should be well organized in a protective and convenient carrying case or pouch. A nylon or cordura organizer bag is both lightweight and durable (Fig. 8.2). Bags made of silicone impregnated ripstop nylon are even lighter but are not as tough.

- Duration of travel
- Distance from definitive medical care and availability of rescue
- Group size
- Pre-existing illnesses
- Weight and space limitations

Extremes of weather, terrain, and activity interact to increase the risk of illness or injury during travel, and thus need to be factored into the contents of the travel health/first aid kit. Travel to areas that are more than 1 h from definitive medical care mandates a more comprehensive kit than travel to just urban areas.

For travel to developing countries, some suggest carrying needles, syringes, and intravenous catheters, particularly for long-term remote travel. Unfortunately, in some countries, these instruments are reused under nonsterile conditions. In addition, commercial 'Suture/ Syringe Kits' are available (Fig. 8.1) that contain supplies to be given to and used by the local health care provider (Travel Medicine, Inc., Tel: 800 872 8633, www.travmed.com).

Table 8.3	Suggested items for a dental kit
Mouth mirror	
Dental floss	
Cavit® temporary filling material (Chinook Medical Gear, Inc. Tel: 1 800 766 1365; www.chinookmed.com)	
Cotton rolls/cotton pellets	
Zinc oxide: mixed with eugenol, forms a paste that can be used as a temporary filling or to repair a broken tooth (Chinook Medical Gear)	
Eugenol (oil of cloves): a dental anesthetic	

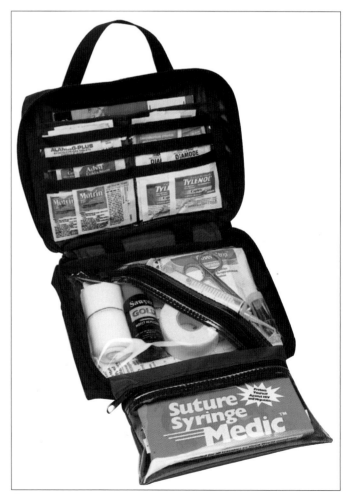

Figure 8.2 A nylon or cordura organizer bag.

Newer-generation bags with clear, vinyl compartments have proven superior to mesh covered pockets for protecting the components from the environment (Adventure Medical Kits, Tel: 800 324 3517, www.adventuremedicalkits.com). The vinyl protects the components from dirt, moisture, and insects and prevents the items from falling out when the kit is turned on its side or upside down.

For aquatic environments, the kit should be stored in a waterproof dry bag (Northwest River Supply, Tel: 800 635 5202, www.nrsweb.com) or watertight container, such as a Pelican® Box (Pelican Products, Tel: 310 326 4700, www.pelican.com). Inside, items should be sealed in resealable plastic bags since moisture will invariably make its way into any container. Aloksak® bags (Watchful Eye Designs, Tel: 800 355 1126), which feature a leakproof, waterproof and airtight seal are now available for this purpose. According to the manufacturer, they have been tested by the US Navy and are waterproof to 200 feet.

Some medicines may need to be stored outside of the main kit to ensure protection from extreme temperatures. Capsules and suppositories melt when exposed to temperatures above 37 °C, and many liquid medicines (e.g., insulin) become useless after freezing.

Another consideration is that of passing through foreign customs while carrying kits containing controlled medications (e.g., narcotics). Travelers should carry a letter written by their health care provider regarding their need for controlled items. Physicians themselves should carry a copy of their medical license and DEA certificate, and anyone carrying narcotics or injectable medication should carry copies of their prescriptions.

FIRST AID KITS

In addition to the basic travel health kit, many travelers should also consider carrying a greater number of items that would be helpful for treatment of injuries. After all, injuries remains a major cause of morbidity and mortality in travelers, and as mentioned previously, more and more travelers are venturing into more remote environments. First aid kits can be assembled at home or purchased at an outdoor retail store. It may actually be less expensive to buy a ready-made first aid kit as the manufactures buy the hard-to-find components in bulk and pass on the savings to their customers. One travel medical kit company has developed a useful algorithm in conjunction with their line of travel medical kits to assist the customer in choosing a kit that is appropriate for their destination of travel. 'How to Choose a Kit' charts identify kit components and delineate the kits according to group size, trip duration, and area of travel. Table 8.4 lists suggested items for a basic wound management kit.

An important item to consider as well is 2-octyl cyanoacrylate (Dermabond), a topical skin adhesive. In the USA, it is packaged in small single-use applicators (cost ~US$30.00). It is ideal because it precludes the need for topical anesthesia, is easy to use, reduces risk of needle stick injury, and takes up less space than a conventional suture kit. When applied to a skin surface, the material provides strong tissue support, and can be easily peeled off in 4–5 days without leaving evidence of its presence.[9] Studies in facial lacerations in children have shown that it provides a faster and less painful method of closing wounds than does suturing;[10] in addition, it yields

Table 8.4	Suggested items for basic wound management

10–20 cc wound irrigation syringe with an 18 or 19-gauge catheter.

Povidone iodine solution USP 10% Betadine® to disinfect backcountry water and to sterilize wound edges; when diluted tenfold with water, can be used for wound irrigation. May help to kill the rabies virus in wounds inflicted by animals.

One-quarter by 4-inch wound closure strips. When combined with tincture of benzoin, wound closure strips can adequately close shallow, non-gaping lacerations and have several advantages over suturing, including reduced need for anesthesia, ease of application, and decreased incidence of wound infection. hey are stronger, longer, stickier, and more porous than butterfly-type adhesive bandages.

Tincture of benzoin: a liquid adhesive that enhances the stickiness of wound closure strips, moleskin, or tape.

Polysporin or double-antibiotic ointment. Avoid Neosporin or triple-antibiotic ointment because of allergic reactions to Neosporin.

Forceps or tweezers for removing embedded objects from the skin such as splinters, cactus thorns, ticks, or stingers.

First-aid cleansing pads with lidocaine: these pads have a topical anesthetic, and a textured surface that makes them ideal for scrubbing dirt and embedded objects out of abrasions.

Antiseptic towelettes with benzalkonium chloride.

Surgical scrub brush: A sterile scrub brush for cleaning embedded objects and dirt from abrasions.

Aloe vera gel: A topical anti-inflammatory gel for treating burns, frostbite, and poison oak/ivy dermatitis.

Scalpel with No. 11 blade: for draining abscesses.

Nitrile gloves.

4 x 4 inch sterile dressings.

Non-adherent sterile dressings. Spenco 2nd Skin® (a polyethylene oxide gel laminate composed of 96% water) is an excellent alternative and provides an ideal covering for burns, blisters, and abrasions.

Gauze roller bandages or Kling® bandages.

Elastic roller bandage (Ace® wrap).

Assortment of strip and knuckle adhesive bandages.

Stockinet bandage: A net style bandage particularly useful for holding dressings in place over joints.

Molefoam or Moleskin: A padded adhesive material for preventing blisters and for protecting them once they occur.

Assorted widths of adhesive tape.

similar cosmetic results without tissue necrosis.[11] One should bear in mind, however that petroleum based ointments and salves, including antibiotic ointments, should not be used on wounds after gluing, as these substances can weaken the polymerized film and cause wound dehiscence. Table 8.5 provides the technique for gluing lacerations.

An alternative to gluing wounds is skin stapling, a technique that has evolved significantly in the last several years.[12] For travel use, a particularly handy item is the 3M Precise Disposable Skin Stapler, which contains 25 staples. See Table 8.6 for the appropriate technique for skin stapling.

As mentioned previously, the requirements and sophistication of the travel health and first aid kits will be determined by the degree of 'adventure' of the trip and its environment: the climate, the duration, and how remote from medical care and the ease in which this care can be accessed. Certainly the health care provider on an expedition will require additional equipment and this information is covered in Chapter 31. Nonetheless, some find it helpful to 'always be prepared,' and carry with them other supplies in case of need such as:

- Sam® Splint (Adventure Medical Kits, Tel: 1 800 324 3517, www.adventuremedicalkits.com): a versatile and lightweight malleable, foam padded splint that can be adapted for use on almost any part of the body.
- Hyperthermia/Hypothermia thermometer: Ideally should be able to read temperatures down to 29.4 °C (85 °F) and up to 41.6 °C (107 °F).
- CPR Microshield® (Chinook Medical Gear, Inc., Tel: 800 766 1365, www.chinookmed.com): a compact, easy-to-use, clear, flexible barrier with a one-way air valve for performing mouth-to-mouth rescue breathing. Prevents physical contact with a victim's secretions.
- Bandage scissors: Designed with a blunt tip to protect the victim while cutting through clothes, boots or bandages.
- Cotton tipped applicators: May be used to remove insects or other foreign material from the eye. Also useful to roll fluid out from beneath a blister, or to evert an eyelid to locate a foreign body.
- Plastic resealable (Zip-Lock™) bags
- Safety pins
- Accident Report Form
- Pencil

A variety of prescription and other specialized medications and supplies have been found useful for travelers based upon their medical histories, their itineraries, and their risk factors. Table 8.7 includes a variety of medications listed by category that may be carried if their use is anticipated.

In sum, thinking about the contents of an appropriate travel health kit/first aid kit provides the opportunity for the travel health advisor to carefully assess the risks of travel for any given individual. Just as travel health advice should be tailored to the person, and not just to the destination, so should the contents of a travel health kit. The trekker should be prepared for not only injury, but diarrhea, dehydration, and overexposure to the sun. At the same time, the deluxe leisure traveler will be just as uncomfortable as the unprepared trekker if he or she is suffering with a severe headache and is without an analgesic on arrival at a first class hotel. Obviously, anyone with an underlying chronic illness, or those who have special needs must be even more vigilant. Issues regarding these travelers such as diabetics (who may want to carry glucose paste), or women who are pregnant are discussed elsewhere.

Table 8.5	Technique for gluing lacerations
Irrigate the wound with copious amounts of disinfected water.	
Control any bleeding with direct pressure.	
Once hemostasis is obtained, approximate the wound edges using fingers or forceps.	
Paint the tissue glue over the opposed wound edges using a very light brushing motion of the applicator tip. Avoid excessive pressure of the applicator on the tissue as this can separate the skin edges, forcing glue into the wound. Apply multiple thin layers (at least three), allowing the glue to dry between each application (about 2 min).	
Glue can be removed from unwanted surfaces with acetone, or loosened from skin with petrolatum jelly.	

Table 8.6	Technique for stapling wounds
Squeeze the stapler partway until it clicks and resistance is felt. The two points of the staple should be protruding out from the stapler.	
Grab one edge of the laceration with one of the staples and use it as a hook to pull the wound closed. Use an index finger on the other hand to push the other wound edge in until the wound edges just meet. Hold the stapler upright at a 90° angle to the wound, and make sure that the stapler is positioned evenly over the cut so that it does not overlap one wound edge more than the other.	
Gently and evenly squeeze the stapler with a thumb to advance the staple into the tissue.	
Once the staple is seated, relax pressure on the stapler and back the stapler out to disengage.	

Table 8.7   Examples of prescription medications and other supplies that may be useful for travelers and/or medical personnel caring for travelers

Respiratory
Beta2 agonist metered-dose inhaler and spacer (for asthma and other allergic reactions): Salmeterol (Serevent®), a long-acting beta-adrenergic agonist, is recommended because it only requires twice-daily inhalation.
Prednisone

Cardiovascular
Nitroglycerin tablets or spray
Aspirin
Metoprolol (Lopressor®) 5 mg tablets

Gastrointestinal
Prochlorperazine (Compazine®) or Promethazine (Phenergan®) 25 mg suppositories
Diphenoxylate hydrochloride and atropine sulfate (Lomotil®)
Hydrocortisone acetate (Anusol-HC suppositories®)
Bisacodyl 10 mg suppositories (Dulcolax®)
Scopolamine (Transderm Scop®) patches for motion sickness

Analgesics and sedatives
Acetaminophen with oxycodone (Vicodin® or Percocet®)
Morphine sulfate for injection and naloxone (Narcan®)
Diazepam (Valium®) or midazolam (Versed®) p.o. or i.v./i.m. and flumazenil (Romazicon®)
Fentanyl oral transmucal (Actiq®)

Allergic reactions
Epinephrine 1:1000 solution, or Epi E•Z Pen® auto injector.

Antibiotics and antifungals
Azithromycin (Zithromax®) 250 mg capsules
    Indications: Tonsillitis, ear infections, bronchitis, pneumonia, sinusitis, traveler's diarrhea, skin infections, urethritis, pelvic infections.
Amoxicillin Clavulanate (Augmentin®) 500 mg tablets
    or
Cefuroxime (Ceftin®) *or* Cephalexin (Keflex®) 500 mg tablets
    Indications: Bite wounds, skin infections, pneumonia, urinary tract infections, ear infections, bronchitis, tonsillitis and sinusitis.
Ciprofloxacin (Cipro®) 500 mg tablets (or other fluoroquinolone)
    Indications: Diarrhea including travelers diarrhea, urinary tract infections, pelvic infections, bone infections.
Metronidazole (Flagyl®) 250 mg tablets
    Indications: Infections with Giardia or amoebae, intra-abdominal infections including peritonitis and appendicitis, dental infections.
Fluconazole (Diflucan®) 150 mg single dose tablets
    Indications: Vaginal candidiasis

High risk of venomous snakes
Elastic roller bandage to apply the pressure immobilization technique for venom sequestration.

High risk of altitude illness (See Chapter 38)
Oxygen
Portable hyperbaric bag (Gamow Bag®)
Acetazolamide (Diamox®) 125 mg b.i.d. for prophylaxis, and 250 mg b.i.d. for treatment of altitude illness
Dexamethasone (Decadron®) 4 mg tablets
Nifedipine (Procardia®)10–25 mg tablets

High risk of ultraviolet photokeratitis (Snowblindness)
Ophthalmic anesthetic (e.g., proparacaine or tetracaine 0.5%)
    To facilitate eye examination and to provide short-term analgesia
Fluorescein stain
Ophthalmic cycloplegic (e.g., cyclopentolate 1%)
Ophthalmic corticosteroid-antibiotic combination (e.g., Maxitrol)
Ophthalmic antibiotic drops ciprofloxacin ophthalmic solution 0.3%

High risk of heat illness
Hyperthermia thermometer
Intravenous normal saline solutions and administration supplies
Chemical ice packs
Oral rehydration salt packets

Cold climates
Hypothermia (low-reading) thermometer: should be able to read down to at least 30 °C.
Glutose® paste (an energy source to help facilitate shivering)

Table 8.7	Examples of prescription medications and other supplies that may be useful for travelers and/or medical personnel caring for travelers—cont'd

Marine environment
5% acetic acid (vinegar)
Prednisone
Scopolamine (Transderm Scop®) patches for motion sickness

Tropical or jungle environment
Clotrimazole or betamethasone dipropionate cream (Lotrisone®)
Permethrin 5% cream and 1% shampoo.
Sunscreen and insect repellent

For remote or extended expeditions
Stethoscope
Pleural decompression set with one-way Heimlich valve
Foley catheter
Airway supplies (oral or nasal airways, endotracheal and cricothyrotomy tubes)
Pre-buffered 1% Xylocaine for topical anesthesia
Intravenous catheters, solutions and tubing
Needles and syringes
Urine chemstrips
Urine pregnancy test

REFERENCES

1. His Majesty's Government of Nepal. *Nepal Tourism Statistics, 1996.* Kathmandu, Nepal: Asian Printing Press; 1996.
2. Weiss EA. *Wilderness 911 – A Step-By-Step Guide for Medical Emergencies and Improvised Care in the Backcountry.* Seattle, WA: The Mountaineers; 1998.
3. Hill DR. Health problems in a large cohort of Americans traveling to developing countries. *J Travel Med* 2000; **7**:259–266.
4. Stenbeck JL. Health hazards in Swedish field personnel in the tropics. *Travel Med Internat* 1991; **9**:51–59.
5. Kendrick MA. Study of illness among Americans returning from international travel. *J Infect Dis* 1972; **126**:684–685.
6. Scoville SL, Bryan JP, Tribble D, *et al.* Epidemiology, preventive services, and illness of international travelers. *Milit Med* 1997; **162**:172–178.
7. Steffen R, Rickenbach M, Wilhelm U, *et al.* Health problems after travel to developing countries. *J Infect Dis* 1987; **156**:84–91.
8. Reid D, Dewar RD, Fallon RJ, *et al.* Infection and Travel: the experience of package tourists and other travelers. *J Infect* 1980; **2**:365–370.
9. Toriumi DM, Raslan WF, Friedman M, *et al.* Variable histotoxicity of histoacryl when used in a subcutaneous site. *Laryngoscope* 1991; **101**:339–343.
10. Watson DP. Use of cyanoacrylate tissue adhesive for closing facial lacerations in children. *BMJ* 1989; **299**:1014.
11. Quinn JV, Drzewiecki A, Li MM, *et al.* A randomized, controlled trial comparing a tissue adhesive with suturing in the repair of pediatric facial lacerations. *Ann Emerg Med* 1993; **22**:1130–1135.
12. Dunmire SM. Staples versus sutures for wounds closure in the pediatric population. *Ann Emerg Med* 1989; **18**:448.

CHAPTER 9 Principles of Immunization

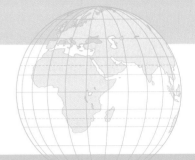

Pamela Rendi-Wagner and Herwig Kollaritsch

KEYPOINTS

- Both live attenuated and killed vaccines are in current use. Each category has advantages in terms of potential for induction of long-term memory cells, adverse effects, duration of response, and amount of antigen needed

- Intramuscular vaccinations are used for adjuvant-containing, potentially irritating antigens, subcutaneous injection is preferred for live viral vaccines, and intradermal injection can reduce the amount of antigen needed

- The oral route of administration is used for certain vaccines where the stimulation of intestinal IgA and other mucosal immune mechanisms defend against the pathogenesis of infection (e.g. oral polio vaccine, oral typhoid vaccine, oral cholera vaccine)

- Live and inactivated vaccines can be safely and effectively (in terms of seroconversion rates) administered at the same time. Vaccines can be administered at any time before or after a different vaccine with the exception of some live vaccines, if not given simultaneously, should be separated by at least 4 weeks

- Strict guidelines for body site, route of administration, and length of needle are in place for each vaccine and should be adhered to regardless of desire to maximize convenience or patient comfort. Separate recommendations are in place for children

INTRODUCTION

Recent decades have provided the indisputable insight that the control of major infectious diseases is less effective by therapeutic than preventive means of intervention, in particular by well targeted use of vaccines. The global eradication of smallpox in 1977 serves as the primary example for effective disease control through immunizations. Application of modern biotechnological tools has resulted in an array of vaccine candidates arising from various sources, creating the promise of effective prevention (and treatment) of many more diseases that are associated with high mortality and morbidity.

IMMUNOLOGY OF VACCINATION

Active immunization

Generally, active immunization represents a harmless, yet highly effective active interaction between the host's immune system and specific pathogens. The main requirement of a successful vaccine is the induction of a sufficiently high titer of protective antibody including

immunological memory, both memory T- and memory B-cells (sero-protection), enabling the organism to respond to a recurring confrontation with the same pathogen in an effective manner by enhanced and accelerated recruitment of protective antibodies (Table 9.1). Three main categories of vaccines can be defined:

- Live vaccines
- Killed vaccines
- Genetically engineered vaccines (DNA-, RNA-vaccines, transgenic plants)

Active immunization involves administration of either killed (inactivated) or live (attenuated) whole pathogens, parts of inactivated microorganisms, or modified pathogen's product (e.g. tetanus toxoid) by either oral or parenteral route. The induction of antibodies of antitoxin, anti-invasive, or neutralizing activity usually represent an indirect measure of protection (immunogenicity).[1] However, in some cases, such as pertussis vaccine, serum antibody titers are not necessarily predictive of protection (Table 9.1). If so, reliance can only be placed on quantifying the protection rate against natural infection in the field (efficacy, Table 9.2).

Live vaccines

Live vaccines contain live attenuated microorganisms, which are still capable of replicating within the host (vaccinee). The microorganisms are attenuated, meaning that they have lost most of their disease causing capacity but still need to be in possession of their immunogenic properties. In most cases, live vaccines show a significantly higher immunogenicity (Table 9.2) than inactivated vaccines since natural infection is imitated almost perfectly by eliciting a wider range of immunologic responses both humoral (B cells) as well as cellular immunity (CD8$^+$ and CD4$^+$ T cells). A single vaccine administration is usually sufficient to induce long-term sometimes even lifelong protection.

However, the main disadvantage of this vaccine category is the potential of reversion to natural virulence via back mutations of the attenuated vaccine organism and the possibility of causing a symptomatic infection similar to wild-virus infection in the recipient or in unprotected contacts (e.g. Vaccine-associated-paralytic-poliomyelitis, VAPP, after oral poliovirus vaccine, OPV).

Killed vaccines

The vaccines for some viruses and most bacteria are inactivated (killed) whole cell or subunit preparations (Table 9.2), which are incapable of replicating within the vaccinee. These types of vaccines need to contain a higher antigenic quantum than live vaccines to induce an adequate immunologic response usually including B cell and CD4$^+$ T cell response. Therefore, most of the killed pathogens or their products need immunomodulators, so called adjuvants, mostly aluminum-hydroxide or -phosphate, to improve antigen presentation and prolong

Table 9.1   Degree of correlation[a] between different immune mechanisms and clinical protection induced by vaccines

Vaccine type	Humoral immune response	Cell mediated immunity	Comments
Diphtheria	++		Protective titer ELISA >0.01 IU/mL. Serology indicated in the case of unclear vaccination status and lack of documentation.
Hib	++	+	Precise minimal protective Ab titer not known; possibly 0.15–1.0 mcg anti-PRP Ab. Test not routinely used.
Hepatitis A	++		Pre-vaccination serology might be cost-effective for persons with likely prior natural infection. (ELISA >10 mIU: protective titer).
Hepatitis B	++		Post-vaccination serology indicated in high-risk persons (protective ELISA titer >10 mIU/mL, except UK: ≥100 mIU/mL).
Influenza (inact.)	++	+	Protective anti-hemagglutinin titer: 1/40. Immunity rarely exceeds 1 year. Concomitant CTL induction? Testing recommended in the immunocompromised.
Japanese encephalitis (mouse brain)	++		No international standard for protective Ab titer established. Caveat: Cross-reactive antibodies (flavivirus).
Measles	++	+	Protective titer: NT >1: 4; induction of important cellular immune response?
Meningococcus	++		Correlation between post-vaccination ELISA titers and vaccine efficacy suggest that >2 mcg of antibody to be protective.
Mumps	++		Post-vaccination serology (ELISA) correlates with protection. Precise minimal protective Ab titer not known.
Pertussis (acellular)	+	+	Precise minimal protective Ab titer not known. Routine tests not available. Efficacy tested in controlled field trials.
Pneumococcus	++		23 subtypes, determination of Ab titer not feasible for routine use.
Polio[b]	++		IPV: protective Ab titer NT >1:8. Correlated with immunity. OPV: serum+ mucosal Ab response. NT does not necessarily correlate with immunity.
Rabies	++	+	Protective Ab titer: RFFIT: > 0.5 IU/mL or NT: 1:25.
Rubella	++		Protective Ab titer: >1:32 (hemagglutination-inhibition-test) or ELISA. Tests correlate with protection. Mucosal Ab involved in protection.
Tick-born-encephalitis	++		ELISA test (VIE/mL) give surrogate markers for immunity. Caveat: cross-reactivity of antibodies (flavivirus) – NT required!
Tetanus	++		Protective Ab titer: ELISA >0.01 IU/mL but usually >0.1 IU/mL (more reliable). See also under diphtheria.
Tuberculosis (BCG)	–	++	No easily measurable correlate of immunity to tuberculosis.
Typhoid[b]	+		Testing almost impossible. Mucosal antibodies following live typhoid vaccine (oral).
Varicella	+	+	Regular antibody testing indicated for leukemia patients.
Yellow fever	++		Caveat: cross-reactive antibodies (flavivirus). Neutralization-test only available at the CDC.

[a]–, no correlation; + low correlation; ++ high correlation.
[b]Depending on vaccine type.

the stimulatory effect by an antigen depot formation.[2] More recently various other potent adjuvant systems, such as virosomes, biodegradable microspheres or novel adjuvant substances like MF59 or MPLA are undergoing clinical evaluation.

The maintenance of long-term immunity of some vaccines, including toxoids, recombinant subunit and polysaccharide conjugate vaccines (Table 9.2) require multidose immunization courses consisting of two to three inoculations, followed by periodic administration of booster doses (Table 9.2). Doses administered at intervals less than the minimum interval can lead to a suboptimal immune response. In clinical practice, however, it is recommended that vaccine doses administered ≤4 days before the minimum interval may be counted as valid (except rabies vaccine).

Unconjugated polysaccharide vaccines, however, do not require multiple doses. In general, bacterial antigens do not induce long-term immunity irrespective of the route of vaccination. Because of immunological memory, delays of recommended booster intervals

or interruption of primary immunization courses are usually negligible and do never require reinstitution of the complete vaccination series.

However, some inactivated vaccines are incapable of eliciting immunological memory, thus being booster-incompetent. These vaccines include all preparations using capsular polysaccharides as vaccine antigens. Yet another shortcoming of carbohydrate vaccines is that capsular polysaccharides, being T-cell-independent immunogens, are poorly immunogenic in vaccinees younger than 2 years of age owing to the immature status of their immune systems. However, coupling of those antigens with protein carriers renders the polysaccharides visible to T cells, which provide help for antibody response including stimulation of B cell memory, also induced in the young (e.g. conjugated Hib and pneumococcus vaccines).

The main advantage, regardless of the type, of inactivated vaccines lies in their superior safety profile due to the inability of antigen multiplication and reversion to pathogenicity within the host.

Table 9.2   Major terms to aid perusal of clinical vaccine literature

Acellular vaccines	Purified component vaccines
ACIP	Advisory Committee on Immunization Practices
Adjuvant	Constituent particularly of killed vaccines to increase immunogenicity and prolong the stimulatory effect (e.g. aluminium salt)
Adverse reaction	Very rarely unpredictable events which may result in permanent sequelae or be life-threatening. Occurrence does not necessarily prove causality
Antigenicity	(Syn: Immunogenicity) The ability of an agent(s) to elicit systemic or local immunologic response
Booster	Repeated immunizations in defined intervals to generate further antibody secreting cells and memory B cells to provide long-term immunity
CMI	Cell mediated immunity (T-cell response)
Conjugate vaccine	Chemical linking of polysaccharide antigen to a carrier protein which converts the polysaccharide from a T-cell independent into a T-cell dependent antigen
Efficacy of vaccines	(Syn: Protective efficacy). Proportion of subjects in the placebo group of a vaccine trial who would have not become ill if they had received the vaccine
GMT	Geometric Mean Titer
Immunity	Resistance developed in response to a stimulus by an antigen (infecting agent or vaccine) and usually characterized by the presence of antibodies
Immunogenicity	The ability of an infectious agent or vaccine antigen to induce specific immunity
Immunologic memory	Ability of the immune system (B-cell and T-cell memory) to recognize antigens and response in a reinforced manner after reinfection or booster
Inactivated vaccines	Vaccines containing killed whole cell, subunit, or toxoid preparations of the pathogen which are incapable of replicating within the vaccinee
Live attenuated vaccines	Vaccines containing live attenuated micro-organisms, which are still capable of replicating within the vaccinee
Priming	Stimulation of adequate humoral immune response including immunologic memory to be accelerated by follow-up booster inoculations
Recombinant vaccine	Vaccine containing antigens (e.g. HBs Antigen) attained by expression of a gene encoding for a specific protein in a heterologous host
Seroconversion	Detectable humoral immune response after natural infection or vaccination
Seroprotection	Specific serum antibody titer predictive of protection
Side-effect	Unavoidable reactions intrinsic to the antigen or other vaccine components are mild to moderate in severity without permanent sequelae
Subunit vaccine	Active vaccines merely containing purified protective epitopes and their corresponding polypeptides
Toxoid	Active vaccines containing detoxified bacterial toxins (e.g. Tetanus, Diphtheria) as immunogenic agent
Vaccination	Procedure for immunization against infectious diseases
Vaccine	Immunobiological substance used for active immunization
Vaccine coverage	Proportion of vaccinated individuals within a group or population
Whole cell vaccine	Vaccines containing inactivated whole bacteria or whole viruses

DNA-vaccines

A recent new technology has been the injection (via gene guns) of naked DNA encoding for a specific vaccine antigen. The aim of DNA vaccines is to be uptaken by host cells in which it generates the synthesis and secretion of the vaccine antigen thus triggering a humoral or cellular immune response. Prior to clinical use of DNA-based vaccines in humans, detailed safety issues need to be investigated and there are unlikely to be any commercial products available during the lifespan of this textbook.

Passive immunization

In some circumstances, immediate protection against a specific infection proves to be necessary. Since active immunization elicits protective antibodies not until 1 to 2 weeks following inoculation, administration of specific preformed antibodies, such as hepatitis B immunoglobulin (HBIG), Rabies IG, Tetanus IG, or Varicella-Zoster IG, seems to be indicated if potential disease exposure is given in recent past or near future. These specific hyperimmunoglobulins, derived from adult donors with high titers of the desired antibodies (95% IgG, trace amounts of IgA and IgM), stimulated by immunization or recent natural infection, are not known to transmit viruses such as HIV-1, or any other infectious agent. Hyperimmunoglobulins are usually recommended for intramuscular (i.m.) administration followed by peak serum antibody levels about 48 to 72 h after administration.

Vaccine handling and administration

Personnel administering vaccines should take necessary precautions to minimize risk for spreading of disease. Hands should be washed before and after each patient contact. Gloves are not required unless the person vaccinating has a lesion on their hands, is likely to come into contact with potentially infectious body fluids, or as long as hand contact with blood or other potentially infectious materials is not reasonably anticipated. To prevent contamination, syringes and needles must be sterile and a separate needle and syringe should be used for each injection. Changing the needle between drawing the vaccine into the syringe and injecting it is not necessary. Unless specifically licensed, different vaccines should never be mixed in the same syringe.

To prevent needle stick injury, needles should never be recapped after use and should be discarded promptly in puncture-proofed, specifically labeled containers. In the USA, federal regulations require safer injection devices (needle-free injectors) to be used if such technology is commercially available and medically appropriate. Additional information concerning this regulation may be obtained at: http://www.immunize.org/genr.d/needle.htm

Anesthetic techniques

Anxiety about vaccinations is widespread. Some local anesthetic agents such as 5% lidocaine-prilocaine emulsion (EMLA® manufactured by AstraZeneca), applied 30–60 min before injection, may relieve discomfort during vaccination without interfering with the immune response. Because of the risk of methemoglobinemia, such lidocaine-prilocaine treatment should not be used in infants younger than 12 months old under treatment with methemoglobin-inducing agents. A topical refrigerant spray may be administered shortly before vaccination to reduce short-term pain. Moreover, in newborn infants, sucrose placed on the tongue immediately before injection may have a calming effect.

Techniques of vaccine administration

Route of immunization

The route of vaccination is generally determined in pre-licensure studies. Intramuscular vaccinations are used for adjuvant-containing, potentially irritating antigens (e.g. tetanus/diphtheria vaccine). Administration by subcutaneous injection is preferred for live viral vaccines, to lessen the discomfort due to local inflammation (e.g. yellow fever vaccine). Intradermal injection, such as for BCG vaccine requires careful technique to avoid inadvertent subcutaneous antigen injection and consequent diminished immunologic response. The oral route of administration is used for certain vaccines where the stimulation of intestinal IgA and other mucosal immune mechanisms defend against the pathogenesis of infection (e.g. oral polio vaccine, oral typhoid vaccine, oral cholera vaccine). Vaccines for administration by nasal, rectal and vaginal routes are under investigation.

Local pain and swelling at the site of injection are the most common side-effects of all vaccines given by injection. The severity of the symptoms and number of patients experiencing them may vary from vaccine to vaccine, depending on the components of the vaccine.

However, it is advisable to use only the administration technique and site of injection recommended by the manufacturer, unless data are available to support using alternative sites. Using unapproved alternate sites could reduce the immune response to the vaccine.

Intramuscular route

The choice of site for intramuscular administration (Table 9.3)[3] is based on the volume of injected material and the size of the muscle. For infants younger than 18 months of age the preferred site for intramuscular injections is the musculus vastus lateralis in the anterolateral aspect of the thigh (Fig. 9.1). In older children and adults the deltoid muscle provides the ideal site for i.m. injections (Fig. 9.2). The needle length used for i.m. injections in young infants (<12 months) should be 7/8 to 1 inch, for older children (<18 years) 7/8–11/4 inches, depending on the size of the muscle. For adults (>18 years), the suggested needle size is 1 to 2 inches. A 23- to 25-gauge needle is appropriate for administration of most i.m. vaccinations (Fig. 9.3).

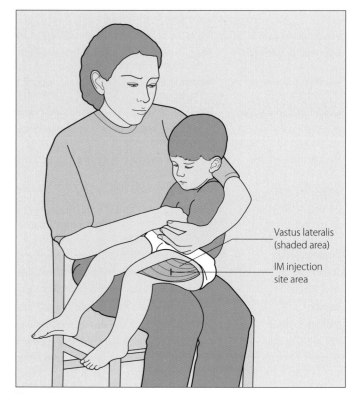

Vastus lateralis (shaded area)

IM injection site area

Figure 9.1 Intramuscular injection site for infants and toddlers (birth to 36 months of age). Insert needle at an 80–90 degree angle into vastus lateralis muscle in anterolateral aspect of middle or upper thigh.

Table 9.3	How to administer vaccines via the intramuscular route	
Patient's age	Site	Needle size[12]
Infants (birth to 12 months of age)	Vastus lateralis muscle in anterolateral aspect of middle or upper thigh	7/8 inch to 1 inch needle, 23–25 gauge
Toddlers (12 to 36 months of age)	Vastus lateralis muscle. Preferred until deltoid muscle has developed adequate mass] (~age 36 months)	7/8 inch to 1 inch needle, 23–25 gauge
Toddlers (>36 months of age), children and adults	Densest portion of deltoid muscle, above armpit and below acromion	1–2 inch needle, 23–25 gauge

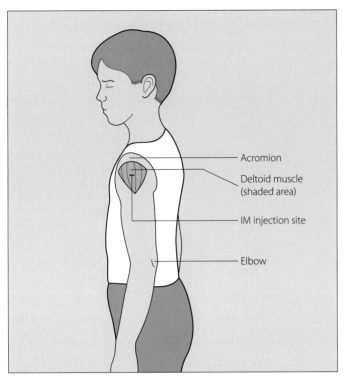

Figure 9.2 Intramuscular injection site for older toddlers, children and adults. Insert needle at an 80–90 degree angle into the densest portion of deltoid muscle – above armpit and below acromion.

- Use a needle long enough to reach deep into the muscle. Insert the needle at an 80°–90° angle to the skin with a quick thrust.

- Retain pressure on the skin around injection site with thumb and index finger while needle is inserted.

- There are no data to document the necessity of aspiration, however, if performed and blood appears after negative pressure, the needle should be withdrawn and a new site selected.

- Multiple injections given in the same extremity should be separated as far as possible (preferably 1" to $1\frac{1}{2}$" with minimum of 1" apart

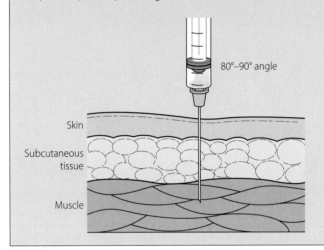

Figure 9.3 Angle of needle insertion for intramuscular injection.

Due to the thickness of overlying subcutaneous fat and the consequentially decreased immune response, moreover, because of the possibility of damaging the nearby sciatic nerve, the gluteal region should be avoided for active i.m. vaccinations. However, the gluteal site is often used for i.m. administration of large volumes of immunoglobulin preparations. At this site of injection, caution should be taken to avoid nerve injury, which is most perfectly done by injecting in the center of a triangle bordered by the anterior superior iliac spine, the tubercle of the iliac crest, and the upper border of the greater trochanter of the femur.

Many experts recommend 'aspiration' by pulling back the syringe plunger before injection, although there exists no data to document the necessity for this procedure. However, if blood appears after aspiration, the needles should be withdrawn and a new site selected.

In patients with bleeding disorders, the risk of bleeding after i.m. injection can be reduced by application of firm pressure to the site of inoculation, vaccinating shortly after application of clotting factor replacement, or using smaller needles (23-gauge or smaller). Moreover, some vaccines recommended for i.m. application may excep-

tionally be given subcutaneously to persons at risk for bleeding. If a patient with bleeding diathesis must receive an intramuscular injection, using a smaller gauge needle, placing steady pressure over the injection site for at least 2 min and limiting the movement of the extremity for a few hours may decrease the development of bleeding complications.

Subcutaneous route
Subcutaneous injections (Table 9.4)[3] can be administered in the anterolateral aspect of the thigh or the upper arm by inserting the needle at about 45-degree angle in a pinched-up skinfold. A 5/8 inch, 23–25 gauge needle is recommended (see Figs 9.4, 9.5 and 9.6).

Intradermal route
Intradermal injections are usually administered on the volar surface of the forearm or the deltoid region by inserting the needle parallel to the long axis of the arm and raising a small bleb with the injected material. A 3/8 to 3/4 inch, 25 or 27-gauge needle is optimal (Figs 9.7, 9.8).

Table 9.4	How to administer vaccines via the subcutaneous route	
Patient's age	**Site**	**Needle size[12]**
Infants (birth to 12 months of age)	Vastus lateralis muscle in anterolateral	7/8 inch to 1 inch needle, 23–25 gauge
Toddlers (12 to 36 months of age)	Fatty area of the thigh or outer aspect of upper arm	5/8 to 3/4 inch needle 23–25 gauge
Children and adults	Outer aspect of arm	5/8 inch to 3/4 inch needle 23–25 gauge

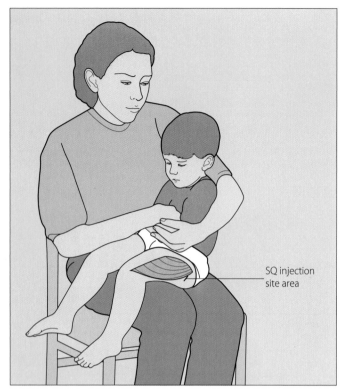

Figure 9.4 Subcutaneous injection site for infants and toddlers (birth to 36 months of age). Insert needle at a 45 degree angle into the fatty area of anterolateral thigh. Make sure subcutaneous tissue is pinched, to prevent injection into muscle.

Oral application

Vaccines given orally such as OPV or live typhoid vaccine should be swallowed and retained. The dose should be repeated if the person fails to retain the vaccine longer than 10 min following the first application.

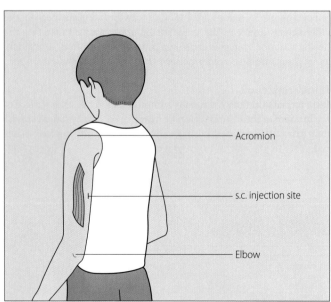

Figure 9.5 Subcutaneous injection site for injection of toddlers, children and adults. Insert needle at a 45 degree angle into the outer aspect of upper arm. Make sure subcutaneous tissue is pinched, to prevent injection into muscle.

- Insert the needle at 45° angle to the skin.

- Pinch up on s.c. tissue to prevent injection into muscle.

- There are no data to document the necessity of aspiration, however, if performed and blood appears after negative pressure, the needle should be withdrawn and a new site selected.

- Multiple injections given in the same extremity should be separated as far as possible (preferably 1" to $1\frac{1}{2}$" with minimum of 1" apart).

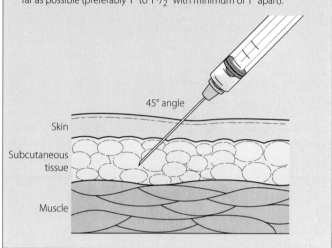

Figure 9.6 Angle of needle insertion for subcutaneous injection.

Simultaneous administration of different vaccines

Simultaneous administration of different vaccines is of particular importance when preparing for international travel. Moreover, simultaneous administration of vaccines is critical for childhood immunization programs. Since combination vaccines increase the

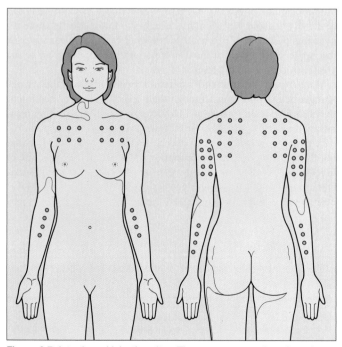

Figure 9.7 Intradermal injection sites. The most common intradermal injection site is the ventral forearm. Other sites (indicated by dotted areas) include the upper chest, upper arm, and shoulder blades. Skin in these areas is usually lightly pigmented, thinly keratinized, and relatively hairless, facilitating detection of adverse reactions.

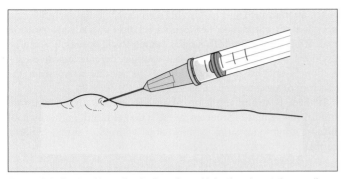

Figure 9.8 Angle of insertion for intradermal injection. Insert the needle at a 10–15 degree angle, so it punctures the skin's surface. When injected, the drug should raise a small wheal.

probability that a child will be fully immunized at the appropriate age, immunization rates are raised significantly. Usually, most widely used live and inactivated vaccines can be safely and effectively (in terms of seroconversion rates) administered at the same time[4,5] (Table 9.5).

With the exception of live vaccines administered within an interval of 4 weeks of each other, vaccines can be administered at any time before or after a different vaccine. Due to the potential immunological interference, some live vaccines, if not given simultaneously, should be separated by at least 4 weeks. No evidence, however, exists indicating that OPV and Ty21a interfere with other parenterally administered live vaccines when administered concurrently or within 4 weeks.

The administration of immunoglobulin (IG)-containing preparations shortly before or simultaneously with certain vaccines may also adversely affect the immune response of the active immunizations (e.g. measles and rubella vaccine), depending on the dose of IG. The immune response following yellow fever and oral polio vaccine seems not to be influenced by co-administration of immunoglobulin.[6] Similarly, Ty21a can be administered at anytime with respect to IG. The interference with inactivated vaccines is far less pronounced than with attenuated vaccines. For example, concurrent administration of HBIG, or Tetanus IG and the corresponding vaccine or toxoid in the course of pre- or post-exposure prophylaxis has not been demon-

strated to cause inhibition of the immune response, yet providing immediate and long-term protection. The combined administration of hepatitis A vaccine and IG has been observed to negligibly decrease serum antibody titers, but does not impair seroconversion rates.

Interchangeability of vaccine products

Although precise data concerning safety, immunogenicity, and efficacy is lacking, vaccines against the same diseases with similar antigens from different manufactures are usually considered interchangeable when used according to their licensed indication. Available data indicate, that all brands of diphtheria, tetanus toxoids, live and inactivated polio, hepatitis A, hepatitis B, and rabies vaccines can be used interchangeably within a vaccination series. Due to a lacking correlate for *Bordetella pertussis* infection, the interchangeability of acellular pertussis vaccines is difficult to assess. Therefore, whenever feasible, the same brand of DTaP should be used. Vaccination series should never be interrupted if the same brand is not available.

Special caution is indicated, when using vaccines of the same brand and vaccine name obtained in different countries, since differences in vaccine formulation might exist.

Serologic testing before and after immunizations

In any case, except BCG, vaccination may be undertaken regardless of prior knowledge of the immunity status of the vaccinee. This is particularly true for low-priced vaccines such as polio, diphtheria or tetanus vaccines. Whereas in the case of high-priced vaccines (e.g. Hepatitis A or B vaccine), it may be more cost-effective to test immunity status prior to vaccination, particularly if acquisition of immunity via natural infection in the past is very likely. Moreover, serologic testing may be reasonable in the case of unclear immunization status due to incomplete or lack of documentation of vaccination courses.

Checking post-vaccination antibody titer for healthy vaccinees is generally indicated only after hepatitis B and rubella vaccine. Unresponsiveness to the hepatitis B vaccine poses a serious problem since more than 10% of healthy immunocompetent adults fail to develop protective antibody levels after the recommended three-dose intramuscular vaccination course (non-responders).[7] In chronic dialysis populations current hepatitis B vaccination regimens result in a disappointing 50% to 75% rate of development of anti-HBs.[8] In addition, all women of child-bearing age need to be protected adequately against rubella infection. Due to similarly potential unresponsiveness to rubella vaccine, it appears most reasonable to check antibody titer post-vaccinally.

Moreover, seroconversion rates and antibody levels after vaccinations may be reduced in immunocompromised subjects who should be considered for post-vaccination serologic testing.

However, when interpreting serological results by employing specific antibody titers as surrogate markers for level of protection, we have to bear in mind, that assessed serum antibodies, such as antibodies after pertussis vaccination, are not reliably of neutralizing activity and therefore may not be necessarily predictive of protection. Thus, we may not always rely on serology as the standard means of measurement of post-vaccination clinical protection[1] (Table 9.1). Though specific methods to measure cellular immunity exist, they are unsuitable for routine application.

Vaccination in those with impaired immunity

In the case of impaired immunocompetence, including congenital immune deficiencies, HIV infection, malignant neoplasm, or recipients

Table 9.5	Recommended spacing of different vaccines
Combination of different vaccine antigens	**Minimum interval**
Killed – Killed	None
Live – Killed	None
Killed – Live	None
Live – Live	~4 weeks, if not given simultaneously (except OPV – MMR – oral typhoid vaccines: no interval required)
Killed – Immunoglobulin	None
Immunoglobulin – Killed	None; if simultaneously: at different sites
Live – Immunoglobulin	~2–3 weeks (except OPV, yellow fever, oral typhoid: no interval required)
Immunoglobulin – Live	~3–5[a] months (except OPV, yellow fever, oral typhoid: no interval required)

[a]Dose-dependent.

of immunosuppressive therapy, cautious considerations about risks and benefits of vaccinations need to be made.[9] In general, patients with uncertain or severely impaired immune status should not receive live vaccines because of the risk of disease from the vaccines strains after administration of attenuated viral or bacterial vaccines.

Since decreased immunity results in reduced immunogenicity of vaccines reflected by significantly diminished seroconversion rates and antibody levels these patients should be considered for post-vaccination serologic testing.

Detailed management of specific risk groups will be covered elsewhere (see chapters 24, 25 and 26).

MANAGEMENT OF ADVERSE REACTIONS

It is beyond doubt, that currently licensed modern vaccines are safe and effective and have to undergo extensive and strictly controlled preclinical and clinical safety trials before licensed for routine use by public health authorities. However, despite all sorts of safety precautions one can not absolutely exclude sporadic cases of undesirable vaccine-associated adverse reactions (Table 9.6). Therefore, vaccine recommendations should always be orientated on the basis of careful evaluation of vaccine benefits and safety weighed against the risk of vaccine preventable disease.

Vaccine-associated side effects (Table 9.2) are usually mild and harmless. On average, about 5% to 10% of all vaccinees complain about post-vaccination problems of mostly moderate local (redness, swelling and pain of the limb), or systemic (fever, headache) nature, occurring shortly after vaccination (6–48 h).

Although anaphylactic reaction is an extremely rare event after vaccination, immediate facilities (epinephrine and equipment for maintaining an airway) and personnel should always be available for treating such allergic emergencies.

Very rarely, unpredictable serious life-threatening adverse reactions may occur. However, occurrence does not necessarily prove causality.

Association of such an event is only considered, if there is timely and symptomatic correlation between vaccination and adverse reaction and, if other diseases with similar symptomatic appearance can be excluded. For most attenuated virus-vaccines, definite causative association is established by isolation of the vaccine strain from the vaccinee or vaccinee's contacts.

If there is strong suspicion of such a serious adverse reaction, official reporting of this event to the national health authority is of utmost importance since in the context with other similar reports, further clues about this incidence may be detected.

CONTRAINDICATIONS TO VACCINATIONS

Absolute contraindications against administration of vaccines are most uncommon. Except for severe hypersensitivity to vaccine constituents, no further contraindications exist against killed vaccines. Whereas, administration of live vaccines may be contraindicated in special situation such as pregnancy and impaired immunity.

Hypersensitivity reactions can vary in severity from mild local symptoms to severe anaphylaxis (Table 9.6). However, allergic reactions occurring immediately after vaccination are very suggestive of an anaphylactic reaction and act as a contraindication for follow-up vaccinations. However, persons with history of systemic anaphylactic-like symptoms after egg ingestion who need yellow fever vaccine may be skin tested before vaccination and desensitized. Local delayed-type hypersensitivity reactions, such as allergic response to neomycin, are not contraindications for vaccinations. If a person reports an anaphylactic reaction to latex, vaccines supplied in vials containing natural rubber should be avoided unless the benefit of the vaccination outweighs the risk of an allergic reaction.

No evidence indicates any influence on vaccine-associated reactogenicity or efficacy, if vaccine is administered during minor illness (≤38°C, ≤100°F). However, if fever (≥38°C, ≥100°F) or clinical symp-

Table 9.6	Potential hypersensitivity reactions to common vaccine components	
Vaccine component	**Contained in the vaccine against**	**Hypersensitivity reaction**
Egg protein	Yellow fever[c] Influenza[b] Measles[a] Mumps[a] Rabies[a] TBE[a]	On rare occasions, anaphylaxis or immediate hypersensitivity reaction; dose-dependent risk.
Antibiotics (gentamycin, neomycin etc.)	Measles Mumps Rubella TBE Rabies	Mostly delayed-type (cell-mediated) local contact dermatitis; no contraindication to vaccinations.
Mercury compounds (Merthiolate)	Almost eliminated from modern vaccines	Mostly delayed-type local contact dermatitis, no contraindication to vaccinations.
Phenol	Cholera (old killed vaccine) Pneumococcus	Delayed-type local contact dermatitis, no contraindication.
Gelatin	Measles Mumps Rubella Yellow fever	Very rarely anaphylaxis or immediate hypersensitivity reaction.

[a]Very low risk
[b]Moderate risk
[c]High risk

toms suggest serious illness, immunizations should be delayed after disease recovery.

Vaccinations during pregnancy are not recommended unless specifically indicated. Live vaccines, particularly rubella and varicella vaccine, are contraindicated 3 months before and during pregnancy. However, in non-immune women at imminent risk for yellow fever exposure, vaccination is indicated if risk of exposure is real. Breast-feeding poses no contraindication for either vaccine.

LEGAL ISSUES

Documentation and risk counseling

Vaccinees or parents of under-aged children need to be counseled by the person responsible for vaccine administration about benefits of disease prevention as well as risk of preventive and therapeutic options, including vaccinations. In the USA, the National Childhood Vaccine Injury Act of 1986 requires that the person administering a vaccine covered by this act must provide a copy of the relevant, current edition of the vaccine information material provided by the Centers for Disease Control and Prevention (CDC). It is recommended to document consent, but vaccinees do not need to sign a consent form.

In addition, the liable physician is obligated to keep a record about the exact date of vaccination; occurrence of adverse reactions; vaccine manufacturer; lot number; the site and route of administration; the date of risk-benefit counseling, and vaccine type and date, in case of rejection of a recommended vaccination by the patient. Moreover, mentioned vaccination details need to documented in an official vaccination document.

Vaccinations currently regulated by the World Health Organization (WHO), such as yellow fever vaccination, need to be documented in an internationally standardized immunization certificate.

VACCINE STOCKING AND STORING

Vaccines need to be suitably stored and handled to avoid vaccine failure. Once opened, the remaining doses from a multi-dose vial may be used until the expiration date printed on the vial, providing that the vial has been stored correctly.

Regular temperature monitoring and control (by 'minimum-maximum' thermometer) is essential to guarantee stable temperature. It may be advisable to designate a single person as the vaccine coordinator responsible for safe and careful vaccine storage and handling. Recommendations for handling regulations are usually given in the manufacturers' product information and in publications by the Advisory Committee on Immunization Practices (ACIP) of the Centers for Disease Control and Prevention.[10]

IMMUNIZATIONS IN TRAVELERS

Besides eradication of disease, immunizations can reduce the risk of vaccine-preventable diseases in individuals including travelers. The risk for travelers of contracting infections abroad is variable depending mostly on well-known risk factors such as destination, travel season, duration of stay, and individual travel conditions.

Since most travelers, seeking pre-travel health advice, often just request vaccinations officially required for entry, it appears most reasonable to point out the differentiation between official vaccination regulations and individual vaccination recommendations for the travelers safety:

- The only vaccination currently regulated by the World Health Organization (WHO), yellow fever vaccination, is required for all travelers going to certain endemic countries that have established this requirement under the International Health Regulations. In addition, many countries outside the endemic zone require proof of immunization from travelers arriving from or via an infected country.
- Saudi Arabia requires proof of vaccination against meningococcal meningitis, using quadravalent vaccine in order to procure a Hajj or Umra visa. This is a frequently encountered situation in travel medicine practice, although not recognized under the International Health Regulations.

To compile an individually tailored immunization schedule, selection of travel vaccinations are based on various critical factors including:

- The epidemiological trends in the country of destination: Which vaccine-preventable diseases stand for risk to the traveler? What is the disease incidence? Detailed updated information about disease epidemiology and immunization requirements can be obtained from the Centers for Disease Control and Prevention (CDC) and the World Health Organization (WHO).[11,12] In addition, many countries regularly publish national guidelines regarding travel vaccinations and health requirements.
- Style of travel: detailed itinerary, duration of travel, timing of departure, type of accommodation, adventure travel or luxury tour.
- Purpose of travel: tourism, work, visiting relatives, etc.
- Vaccinations officially required for entry (e.g. yellow fever vaccination).
- Cost/benefit of vaccinations: prioritization of certain immunizations by ability to pay and frequency of traveling.
- Individual contraindications to vaccinations: hypersensitivity, concomitant disease, medication, pregnancy, medical history.
- Personal history of immunizations including primary and booster doses of routine and travel vaccinations.

CONCLUSION

By assisting health professionals in obtaining a deeper understanding of major immunologic as well as practical issues of vaccination, this chapter contributes to the elimination of potential malevolent prejudices concerning vaccine associated harmfulness. It is beyond doubt, that the benefit of immunization, if utilized correctly, outweighs, by far, vaccine-associated risk. Immunization prevents disease. But the best vaccine, however, will have little impact unless promoted and delivered by motivated health professionals and taken up by individuals.

REFERENCES

1. Plotkin S. Immunologic correlates of protection induced by vaccination. *Pediatr Infect Dis J* 2001; **20**:63–75.
2. Chedid L. Adjuvants of immunity. *Ann Immunol Inst Pasteur* 1985; **136D**:283–291.
3. American Academy of Pediatrics, Pickering LK, ed. *Red Book: Report of the Committee on Infectious Diseases.* Elk Grove Village, IL: American Academy of Pediatrics; 2000.
4. Flavo C, Horowitz H. Adverse reactions associated with simultaneous administration of multiple vaccines to travelers. *J Gen Intern Med* 1994; **9**:255–260.
5. King GE, Hadler SC. Simultaneous administration of childhood vaccines: an important public health policy that is safe and efficacious. *Pediatr Infect Dis J* 1994; **13**:394–407.
6. Kaplan JE, Nelson DB, Schonberger LB, *et al.* The effect of immunoglobulin on the response to trivalent oral poliovirus and yellow fever vaccinations. *Bull World Health Organ* 1984; **62**:585–590.
7. Rendi-Wagner P, Kundi M, Stemberger H, *et al.* Antibody-response to three recombinant hepatitis B vaccines: Comparative evaluation of multicenter-travel clinic-based experience. *Vaccine* 2001; **19**:2055–2060.
8. Docci D, Cipolloni PA, Mengozzi S, *et al.* Immunogenicity of a recombinant hepatitis B vaccine in hemodialysis patients: A two-year follow-up. *Nephron* 1992; **61**:352–353.

9. Centers for Disease Control and Prevention. Recommendations of the Advisory Committee on Immunization Practices (ACIP): use of vaccines and immunoglobulins in persons with altered immune competence. *MMWR Morb Mort Wkly Rep* 1993; **42**(RR4):1–18.

10. Centers for Disease Control and Prevention. *Vaccine Management: Recommendations for Handling and Storage of Selected Biologicals.* Atlanta, US: Department of Health and Human Services, Public Health Service; 2001.

11. Centers for Disease Control and Prevention. *Health Information for International Travel 2001–2002.* Atlanta, USA: US Department of Health and Human Services; 2001.

12. World Health Organization. *International Travel and Health: Vaccination requirements and Health Advice.* Geneva, Switzerland: WHO; 2000.

CHAPTER 10 Adult Immunizations

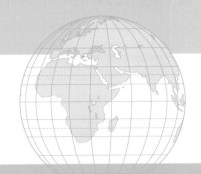

Abinash Virk and Elaine C. Jong

KEYPOINTS

- Vaccine recommendations for travelers are based on the anticipated risks of exposure to vaccine preventable diseases on a given travel itinerary, the severity of the disease if acquired, and any risks of the vaccine itself.

- Risk for each vaccine-preventable disease depends on prevalence of the disease at the destination(s) as well as traveler dependent risk factors which include: recreational and occupational activities, mode of travel and accommodations, duration of travel, degree of close contact (including sexual relations) with local residents, and time of year the travel is undertaken.

- The trip risk assessment is coupled with individual traveler-specific factors, such as age, known allergies, general health, ongoing medications, reproductive status, previous immunization history, and cultural biases to arrive at the set of pre-travel vaccine recommendations.

- Vaccines to be considered are divided into required, routine, and recommended categories: Required vaccines may on certain itineraries include Yellow Fever and meningococcal (Hajj travel only); Recommended vaccines may include hepatitis A, hepatitis B, typhoid, rabies, Japanese encephalitis, tick-borne encephalitis, and cholera; Routine vaccines that may need updating prior to a trip include tetanus/diphtheria, measles, polio, pneumococcal, influenza, and varicella.

INTRODUCTION

Factors that contribute to the pre-travel assessment of the risk of vaccine-preventable diseases in the traveler and influence the priority of vaccines that should be recommended include: environmental and sanitary conditions, presence of insect vectors, and endemic rates of communicable diseases among the local population at the travel destination. A consideration of immunizations against vaccine-preventable diseases for international travelers must take into account both the prevailing standards for routine vaccines in the traveler's home country as well as those in the destination countries. Based on regional patterns of disease transmission, a vaccine considered routine or standard in one country may represent a travel immunization for visitors originating in another country. Examples of this are Japanese encephalitis virus vaccine, Bacillus Calmette-Guerin (BCG) vaccine, and hepatitis A vaccine, each of which may be administered routinely to residents of countries where there is a high risk of transmission of the given disease, but which are considered travel vaccines for visitors to those same countries.

Further complicating the consideration of international immunization practices are the variations that exist in vaccine product formulations, when more than one vaccine against a particular disease is produced by several manufacturers. Some confusion also arises when a given vaccine produced by a single pharmaceutical manufacturer has been licensed under different brand names, dosing schedules and booster intervals in different countries. While most travelers may be able to complete a recommended primary series for a given vaccine before departure from the home country, other travelers – especially long-term travelers, expatriates, and immigrants – may start an immunization series in one country and receive additional doses to complete or boost the primary series in another country. When this is necessary, the fact that vaccine products and practices vary from country to country could impact immunization planning. When available, information on accelerated immunization schedules and vaccine product interchangeability will be provided in this chapter. In general, if a missed or delayed dose in a vaccine series is identified, it is not necessary to repeat the vaccine series from the beginning. The vaccine dose that is due or overdue should be administered and documented, and the immunization schedule should proceed according to age-appropriate standards from that point on in time. The few exceptions to this general approach are noted in the discussion of individual vaccines concerned. Trade names of the commonly used travel vaccines are given in Table 10.1 with those with widespread multinational distribution shown first.

Immunizations against common childhood diseases are usually given during the first 24 months of life, and are often designated the 'routine' immunizations of childhood. The World Health Organization (WHO), through its Expanded Program on Immunizations (EPI) or Global Alliance on Vaccine Initiatives (GAVI) at http://www.vaccinealliance.org has defined global childhood immunization goals for a number of common vaccine-preventable diseases. Detailed information on recommended schedules for the routine immunizations of childhood by country are discussed in Chapter 11 and can also be found on the World Health Organization website: www.who.int/vaccines/GlobalSummary/Immunization/CountryProfileSelect.cfm. The implication for adult travelers from industrialized countries is that when travel is anticipated to areas where the WHO immunization goals (greater than or equal to 80% of the target population vaccinated) for childhood vaccines have not yet been achieved, there can be increased exposure to naturally occurring infections that are not normally transmitted at home. It is important to assure that the adult traveler has completed the primary series of the routine immunizations and received appropriate booster doses. Cases of measles and varicella have been reported as travel-acquired infections among international travelers, and these common childhood infectious diseases are known to cause more serious pathology in infections acquired by adults.

Table 10.1	Trade names of important adult travel-related vaccines worldwide
Cholera (oral)	Orochol, Mutacol, Dukoral
Cholera	Cholera vaccine PH Eur, Freeze-Dried Cholera Vaccine PH Eur
Hepatitis A	Havrix, Vaqta, Avaxim, Epaxal, Nothav, HAVp
Hepatitis B	Engerix-B, Recombivax HB, Gen H-B-Vax, Aunativ, HB VaxII, Euvax-B, Genhevac B, H-B-Vax, Hepaccine-B, HBVax-Dann, Euvax-B, Heprecomb, Bayhep, BayhepB, Heberbiovac, Haptavax HB, HBVaxPro, Hepatect, Hepuman, HepumanB, HevacB, Hepavax-Gene
Hepatitis A/B combination	Twinrix
Hepatitis A/Typhoid combination	Hepatyrix, Viatim
Japanese Encephalitis	JE-Vax, JE-Vaccine
Meningoccocal (polysaccharide):	Antimeningococic A + C, Menomune, Mencevax ACWY, Meningokokken-Impfstoff A + C, AC Vax, ACWY Vax, Imovax Meningo A & C, Mencevax ACW, Mencevax AC, Menpovax A + C, Meningovax A + C, Mengivac A + C, Menpovax 4, Meningitec, Meningococcal Polysaccharide vaccine
Meningoccocal (conjugate)	Menjugate, Neisvac-C, Meningitec
Rabies	Imovax Rabies, Rabies Imovax, Rabavert, VeroRab, Rabipur, Rabies Vaccine Adsorbed, Lyssavac, Lyssavac N, Bayrab, Berirab, Rabuman, Merieux Inactivated Rabies Vaccine, Tollwut-Impfstoff (HDC), Rasilvax,
Typhoid Vi Polysaccharide	Typhim Vi, Typherix, Typhoid Polysaccharide vaccine
Typhoid (oral)	Vivotif Berna, Vac Tab Berna, Typh-Vax, Typhoral L, Taboral, Enterovaccino ISI (Antitifico), Freeze-dried typhoid vaccine
Yellow fever	YF-Vax, Stamaril, Arilvax, Yellow Fever Vaccine (live)
Tick-borne encephalitis	Encepur, FSME-Immun, Tick-borne Encephalitis Vaccine, Ticovac

Most widely distributed trade names listed first. Vaccines are parenteral unless specified.

The WHO develops and adopts the International Health Regulations (IHRs) and recommendations regarding vaccine requirements for international travelers, with annual publication of vaccination requirements and health advice in International Travel and Health (with electronic access through its website www.who.int/ith). Updates on official changes in vaccine requirements for travel to individual WHO member countries are reported by WHO, and also are summarized in the 'Summary of Health Information for International Travel' published biweekly by the Division of Quarantine at the CDC (www.cdc.gov/travel/blusheet.htm).

In the United States, the Advisory Committee on Immunization Practices (ACIP) of the Centers for Disease Control and Prevention (CDC) develops guidelines for childhood and adult immunization standards: www.cdc.gov/nip/acip, in collaboration with professional groups representing various medical specialties. Recently, an immunization schedule for adult immunizations and booster doses has been released (Fig. 10.1). The CDC also develops guidelines and information for international travelers, which are contained in its publication Health Information for International Travel (published on a biannual basis, with electronic access through the CDC website www.cdc.gov/travel). Similar information and guidelines are also published for use in Canada and UK. These can be accessed at http://www.hc-sc.gc.ca/pphb-dgspsp/publicat/cig-gci/ and http://www.archive.official-documents.co.uk/document/doh/hinfo/index.htm respectively.

Health-care providers should consult national public health agencies in the country where they work for current information on the standards of care and vaccine practices appropriate for that country.

Practical vaccine considerations

One of the common practical challenges when advising travelers about pre-travel immunizations is that of scheduling the recommended vaccines in the time available before trip departure. For convenience, a simplified algorithm describing the general approach to considering which vaccines are indicated for an individual traveler is shown in Figure 10.2 as a guide to the more detailed vaccine specific sections, which follow. An overview of commonly administered vaccines for adult travelers, including dosing schedules, accelerated regimens, efficacy estimates, and interchangeability is presented in Table 10.2. The vaccine recipient's immune response to a given vaccine is influenced by multiple factors including age and certain medications, and is likely to be blunted in patients with compromised immunity (Refer to Chapter 25 for a consideration of the traveler with compromised immunity.)

Adverse events

Detailed discussion of vaccine related adverse events will be found below under each individual vaccine. In counseling patients and recommending vaccines, familiarity with numerical data on the risks and benefits of each vaccine are helpful for the provider. Table 10.3 provides a comparison of the estimated risk of acquiring a vaccine preventable disease or being harmed by a complication of that disease with an estimate of the risk of the vaccine for that disease.

Attenuated live vaccines

Live virus vaccines in general are contraindicated in pregnant patients and those with congenital, acquired or pharmacologically-induced immune deficient states because of the concern that an attenuated vaccine virus strain may exhibit increased virulence in immune deficient persons, causing severe disease. When travel to the area of risk cannot be postponed or deferred, decisions regarding vaccination against a particular disease must consider the potential risk of life-threatening illness or death from a disease weighed against the potential risks from the vaccine itself as well as the possibility of the induction of a sub-optimal response to the vaccine itself.

Age group \ Vaccine	19-49 years	50-64 years	65 years and older
Tetanus, Diphtheria (Td)	Booster every 10 years		
Influenza	1 dose annually for persons with medical or occupational indications, or household contacts of persons with indications	1 annual dose	
Pneumococcal (polysaccharide)	1 dose for persons with medical or other indications. (1 dose revaccination for immunosuppressive conditions)		1 dose for unvaccinated persons
			1 dose revaccination
Hepatitis B	3 doses (0, 1-2, 4-6 months) for persons with medical, behavioral, occupational, or other indications		
Hepatitis A	2 doses (0, 6-12 months) for persons with medical, behavioral, occupational, or other indications		
Measles, Mumps, Rubella (MMR)	1 dose if measles, mumps or rubella vaccination history is unreliable; 2 doses for persons with occupational or other indications		
Varicella	2 doses (0, 4-8 weeks) for persons who are susceptible		
Meningococcal (polysaccharide	1 dose for persons with medical or other indications		

Legend: ☐ For all persons in this group   ☐ Catch-up on childhood vaccinations   ☐ For persons with medical/exposure indications

Figure 10.1 Recommended US routine immunization schedule for adults

Intercurrent illness and allergies

Minor febrile illnesses are not a contraindication to any of the routine vaccines. However, it is best to postpone immunizations in the presence of a moderate to severe illness with or without fever. The presence of an illness may potentially decrease the immune response to a given vaccine, and may mask signs and symptoms of an adverse reaction to a given vaccine administered at that time. A history of a serious large localized or systemic hypersensitivity reaction to a previous dose of a vaccine or its components may preclude the use of the same vaccine formulation again. In some cases, other brands or formulations of the vaccine may be available.

Figure 10.2 Immunization algorithm

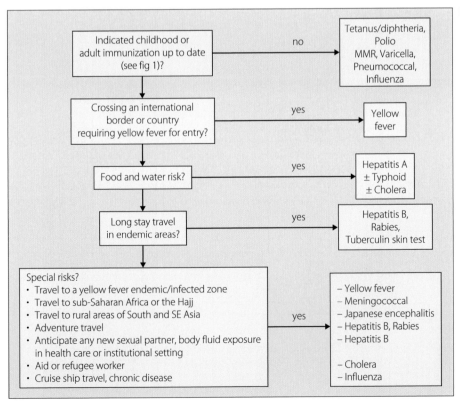

Table 10.2 Summary of commonly used travel vaccines

Disease	Vaccine type; commercial name (Manufacturer)	Efficacy	Primary course – Adult	Boosters	Accelerated schedule	Pregnancy or lactation	Comments
Cholera, oral	Live attenuated bacterial CVD 103-HgR V. cholerae 01; Orochol (Swiss Serum Institute), Mutachol (Berna)	60–100%	Single dose orally for persons 2 years of age or older	Every 6 months	None	Category C. Insufficient data about pregnancy or excretion in breast milk	
Cholera, oral	Killed whole-cell-B subunit vaccine; Dukoral (Powderject; Aventis Pasteur)	85–90%	> 6 years of age: 2 doses orally 7–42 days apart.	Every 2 years for persons over 6 years of age.	None	Category C. Insufficient data about pregnancy or excretion in breast milk	Reported cross-protection against heat-labile toxin of enterotoxigenic E. coli (ETEC) (see text)
Hepatitis A	Inactivated viral antigen; Havrix (GlaxoSmithKline)	~70–80% in 2 weeks; 95% in 4 weeks	Adult ≥ 19 years: 1.0 mL (1440 ELISA units) IM (Intramuscular) Deltoid. One each 0 and 6–12 months. 2nd dose effective as late as 60 months	None	None	Category C. Not contraindicated during lactation	Can be used interchangeably as a second dose in persons previously vaccinated with Avaxim, Epaxal or Vaqta
Hepatitis A	Inactivated viral antigen; VAQTA (Merck)	~70–80% in 2 weeks; 95% in 4 weeks	Adult ≥ 19 years: 1.0 mL (50 units) IM Deltoid (avoid buttock). One each at 0 and 6–18 months	None	None	Category C. Not contraindicated during lactation	Can be used interchangeably as a second dose (booster) in persons previously vaccinated with Avaxim, Epaxal or Havrix
Hepatitis A	Inactivated virosome-formulated antigen; Epaxal (SSI, Berna)	~97% in 2 weeks; 99% in 4 weeks	0.5 mL IM in the deltoid region at 0 and 12 months	None	None	Category C. Not contraindicated during lactation	Can be used interchangeably as a second dose (booster) in persons previously vaccinated with Avaxim, Havrix or Vaqta
Hepatitis A	Inactivated viral antigen; Avaxim (Aventis-Pasteur)	>90% in 2 weeks; 100% in 4 weeks	Adult: 0.5 mL IM in the deltoid region at 0 and 6–12 months	None	None	Category C. Not contraindicated during lactation	Can be used interchangeably as a second dose in persons previously vaccinated with Epaxal, Havrix or Vaqta
Hepatitis A	Immune Globulin for hepatitis A prophylaxis.	85–90% protection	Deep i.m. gluteal muscle For a stay of: < 3 months: 0.02 mL/kg. For a stay of 3–5 months: 0.06 mL/kg. Maximum volume in one site: 5 mL for adults, if more than 5mL then give divided dose in 2 sites	Repeat doses are required with continued exposure. Re-dose every 3–5 months depending on initial dose given	None	Considered safe in pregnancy	See text: wait the required interval after receipt of IG before administration of MMR or Varicella vaccines
Hepatitis A plus Hepatitis B	Inactivated viral antigen;Twinrix (GlaxoSmithKline)	100% protective Hep A Ab levels, 94% protective Hep B Ab levels after 3 doses	Adult >18 years: 1.0 mL IM in Deltoid (720 ELISA units Havrix for Hepatitis A & 20 mcg Engerix B for Hepatitis B). One each at 0, 1 and 6 months	None	Accelerated schedule 0, 7, 21 days plus booster at 1 year, see text	Category C. Not contraindicated during lactation	
Hepatitis A plus Typhoid	Inactivated viral antigen plus Typhoid Vi polysaccharide. Hepatyrix (GlaxoSmithKline) or ViATIM (Aventis-Pasteur)	See monovalent vaccines	See monovalent vaccines	See monovalent vaccines	See monovalent vaccines	See monovalent vaccines	See monovalent vaccines

Continued

Table 10.2 Summary of commonly used travel vaccines—cont'd

Disease	Vaccine type; commercial name (Manufacturer)	Efficacy	Primary course – Adult	Boosters	Accelerated schedule	Pregnancy or lactation	Comments
Hepatitis B	Inactivated viral antigen; Engerix-B Recombinant vaccine. (GlaxoSmithKline)	95% protective Hep B Ab levels after 3 doses	Adult > 19 years: 1.0 ml (20 mcg Hepatitis B surface antigen) IM Deltoid (avoid buttock) at 0, 1 and 6 months. Dialysis patients: use Engerix-B 40 mcg i.m. at 0, 1, 2, and 6 months	Boosters may be necessary in immunocompromised patients with a anti-HBs titer of less than 10 mU/mL.	Accelerated schedule 0, 1, 2 months plus booster, see text	Category C. Not contraindicated during lactation	Can be used interchangeably with Recombivax or Gen H-B Vax doses
Hepatitis B	Inactivated viral antigen; Recombivax Recombinant vaccine. (Merck) or Gen H-B Vax (Aventis-Pasteur)	95% protective Hep B Ab levels after 3 doses	Adult >19 years: 1.0 ml (10 mcg Hepatitis B surface antigen) IM Deltoid (avoid buttock) at 0, 1 and 6 months. Dialysis patients: use Recombivax 40 mcg i.m. at 0, 1, 2, and 6 months.	Boosters may be necessary in immunocompromised patients with a anti-HBs titer of less than 10 mU/mL.	See text	Category C. Not contraindicated during lactation	Can be used interchangeably with Engerix-B doses
Influenza	Inactivated viral vaccine; Influenza (many brands)	Approximately 70–90% effective in healthy persons <65 years of age. Among elderly persons the vaccine is 30–70% effective in preventing hospitalizations and influenza	0.5 ml IM Deltoid	Annually	None	Category C. CDC recommends healthy pregnant women to receive the vaccine in the second and third trimester. Pregnant women with underlying medical problems should receive the vaccine regardless of the stage of pregnancy. Breast feeding not a contraindication for vaccination.	
Japanese B Encephalitis	Inactivated viral vaccine; JE-VAX (Aventis Pasteur)	Single dose: no efficacy. Two doses: 80% efficacy; 3 doses: 99%	Adults and Peds >2 years of age: 1.0 mL SQ (subcutaneous), 0, 7, 30-day schedule	Same dose possibly every at least 3 years	Doses based on age given at a 0, 7, 14-day schedule. If time does not permit, then at least 2 doses 7 days apart provide 80% protection	Category C. Insufficient data about use in pregnancy and during lactation	Administer last vaccine dose at least 10 days before departure in case of rare delayed hypersensitivity reaction (see text)
Measles, mumps, and rubella.	MMR, live attenuated virus vaccine (many brands)	95% response rate per dose	Adults over 18 yrs: 0.5 ml SQ. 1 or 2 doses at least 1 month apart to complete a documented 2-dose series with attenuated live virus vaccine.	None	None	Category C. Not recommended during pregnancy and for 1 month prior to onset of pregnancy because of theoretical risk to the fetus. Inadvertent vaccination not an indication for pregnancy termination. Some risk of transmission via breast milk. Patient should be advised not to breast feed for 1 month after vaccination.	Give on same day as PPD skin test or separate by 28 days

Continued

Table 10.2 Summary of commonly used travel vaccines—cont'd

Disease	Vaccine type; commercial name (Manufacturer)	Efficacy	Primary course – Adult	Boosters	Accelerated schedule	Pregnancy or lactation	Comments
Meningococcal disease	Polysaccharide vaccine. Neisseria meningitidis Groups A, C, Y, W-135. MENOMUNE. (Aventis Pasteur)	85–90% efficacy after 1–2 weeks	Adults: 0.5 mL SQ. Single dose	Same dose. Re-dose every 3–5 years for adults at continued risk of exposure.	None	Category C. No data available during lactation.	
Poliomyelitis	Inactivated viral injectable. IPV (Aventis Pasteur)		0.5 mL SQ 3 doses at 0, 2, 8–14 months	Same dose. If >10 years since completion of the primary vaccine series, boost once in adult life for travel to a polio endemic area.	Primary Series Accelerated: 3 doses at 0, 1, 2 months (minimum 4 weeks apart). Give as many doses as time permits and complete remaining doses as soon as possible thereafter.	Category C. If protection required during pregnancy either OPV or IPV can be given. Not contraindicated during lactation.	
Poliomyelitis, oral	Live attenuated viral vaccine. Oral polio (OPV)		Adult >18 years. Oral dose of 0.5mL at 0, 2, and 10–14 months	See remarks above	Primary series accelerated: Give 3 doses OPV at 0, 1, 2 months (minimum 4 weeks apart). Give as many doses as time permits and complete remaining doses as soon as possible thereafter.	Category C. If protection required during pregnancy either OPV or eIPV can be given. Not contraindicated during lactation.	
Rabies	Inactivated viral vaccine, Human Diploid Cell Vaccine (HDCV). Imovax for IM injection (Aventis Pasteur)		1.0 mL IM Deltoid. Never use gluteal muscle. Pre-exposure schedule of 0, 7, and 21 or 28 days.	Not needed for typical travelers. Possibly 3 years if persistent high risk. Recommend checking serology before boosting.	Days 0, 7, and 21	Category C. No data available during lactation.	
Rabies	Inactivated viral vaccine, Human Diploid Cell Vaccine HDCV). Imovax for ID injection (Aventis Pasteur)		0.1 mL intradermal (ID) on forearm. Pre-exposure schedule of 0, 7, and 21 or 28 days.	See remarks above	Days 0, 7, and 21	Category C. No data available during lactation.	Do not use intramuscular (IM) HDCV for intradermal (ID) immunization, because of efficacy concerns (see text). Imovax ID not currently available in most countries.

Continued

Table 10.2   Summary of commonly used travel vaccines—cont'd

Disease	Vaccine type; commercial name (Manufacturer)	Efficacy	Primary course – Adult	Boosters	Accelerated schedule	Pregnancy or lactation	Comments
Rabies	Inactivated viral vaccine, Purified Chick Embryo Cell vaccine (PCECV). Rabavert (Chiron)	1.0 ml IM Deltoid. Never use gluteal muscle. Pre-exposure schedule of 0, 7, and 21 or 28 days.	See remarks above	Days 0, 7, and 21	Category C. No data available during lactation.		
Rabies	Inactivated viral vaccine, Rabies Vaccine adsorbed (RVA) (GlaxoSmithKline)	1.0 ml IM Deltoid or antero-lateral thigh. Pre-exposure schedule of 0, 7, and 21 or 28 days.	See remarks above	Days 0, 7, and 21	Category C. No data available during lactation.	
Tuberculosis (*Mycobacterium tuberculosis*)	Live attenuated mycobacterial vaccine. BCG [*Bacillus Calmette-Guerin]* vaccine	0–80% efficacy in various trials. More effective in prevent-ing serious disease in children than adults. See text.	0.1mL intradermal (ID)	None	None	Category C. No definite data available about excretion in breast milk.	
Tick-borne encephalitis	Inactivated viral vaccine. FSME-immun (Immuno AG, Baxter AG)	Seroconversion rates of 87–99% after 3 doses.	FSME-immun: 0.5 mL IM Deltoid. Given on day 0, 4–12 weeks, and 9–12 months after the second dose.	Every 3–5 years	0.5 mL on days 0,14, 3rd dose 9–12 months after second. Boosters at 3 years	Category C. Contraindicated in pregnancy and during breast feeding unless the benefits far outweigh any potential risk.	
Tick-borne encephalitis	Inactivated viral vaccine. Encepur (Chiron Behring)	Seroconversion rates of 99% after 3 doses.	0.5 ml IM Deltoid. Given on day 0, 4–12 weeks, and 9–12 months after the second dose.	Every 3–5 years	0.5 mL on days 0, 7, 21 with a booster at 1 year.	Category C. Contraindi-cated in pregnancy and during breast feeding unless the benefits far outweigh any potential risk.	Allergic reaction to gelatin reported at a rate of <1:100 000 vaccine recipients (see text)
Typhoid, oral	Live attenuated bacterial vaccine, capsule. Typhoid TY21a, Vivotif (Berna)	50%–80% effective	3 capsules, 1 capsule taken orally every other day on days 0, 2, 4. In North America, the schedule is 4 capsules, 1 capsule taken orally every other day on days 0, 2, 4, 6.	3–7 years. Wide variation in Package inserts between countries	None	Category C. No clinical studies available in pregnant or lactating women.	The capsules must be refrigerated, and taken on an empty stomach (1 hour before meals) with a cool liquid.
Typhoid, oral	Live attenuated bacterial vaccine, suspension. Typhoid TY21a, Vivotif (Berna)	53%–96% effective	3 doses of suspension taken orally every other day on days 0, 1, 4	5 years	None	Category C. No clinical studies available in pregnant or lactating women.	The vaccine components (sachets of vaccine and buffer) must be refrigerated: each dose is mixed according to directions immediately before use, and taken on an empty stomach (1 h before meals).
Typhoid	Polysaccharide vaccine. Typhoid Injectable. Typhim Vi. (Aventis Pasteur)	63%–96% effective	0.5 mL (25 mcg purified Vi polysaccharide) IM Deltoid	Every 2 years	None	Category C. No clinical studies available in pregnant or lactating women.	

Table 10.2   **Summary of commonly used travel vaccines—cont'd**

Disease	Vaccine type; commercial name (Manufacturer)	Efficacy	Primary course – Adult	Boosters	Accelerated schedule	Pregnancy or lactation	Comments
Varicella	Live attenuated viral vaccine; Varivax (Merck)		Persons aged 13 years or older: 2 doses 1.0 mL vaccine SQ at least 1 month apart.	None	None	Category C. Not recommended during pregnancy and for 1 month prior to onset of pregnancy because of theoretical risk to the fetus. Inadvertent vaccination not an indication for pregnancy termination. Some risk of transmission via breast milk. Patient should be advised not to breast feed for 1 month after vaccination.	Availability limited to a few countries.
Yellow Fever	Live attenuated viral vaccine. YF-VAX, Stamaril (Aventis Pasteur), Arilvax		One dose 0.5 mL SQ	Every 10 years.	None	Category C. Contraindicated in pregnancy except if exposure is unavoidable. Risk of disease exposure to patient versus risk of vaccine strain disease to fetus must be weighed before vaccination. No definite data available about excretion in breast milk.	Observe patient 30 min after vaccine administration in case of immediate hypersensitivity reaction (anaphylaxis) to residual egg components (see text).

Table 10.3   Estimated risk from disease and sequelae versus risk from vaccines

Disease	Risk of acquiring disease or complications from disease	Risk from vaccine
Cholera	Risk of acquiring disease while traveling: 1 in 500 000 traveler	Minimal side-effects from oral cholera vaccines.
Diphtheria	Case fatality rate: 1in 20	Tetanus/Diptheria (Td) vaccine:
Tetanus	Case fatality rate: 3 in 100	Local pain, swelling, and induration at the site of injection are common
Pertussis	Pneumonia: 1 in 8 Encephalitis: 1 in 20 Case fatality rate: 1 in 200	
Hepatitis A	Risk of acquiring disease while traveling: 3–20/1000 persons/ month of travel Case fatality rate: Overall: 0.3% Over 40 years of age: 2%	No serious attributable adverse event reported with hepatitis A vaccines in over 7 million doses including 2.5 million pediatric doses given
Hepatitis B	≥ 8% prevalence of HbsAg carriage in parts of Asia, Africa, and Latin America	
Japanese encephalitis	Risk of JE in highly endemic areas: 1 in 5000 per month of exposure. Risk of JE in highly endemic areas in short-term travelers: <1 per million. Overt encephalitis 1 in 20–1000 cases. Case fatality rate: 25% of encephalitis cases Severe neuropsychiatric sequelae: 30% of encephalitis cases	Vaccine-related neurologic side effects in Japan 1965–1973 (encephalitis, encephalopathy, and peripheral neuropathy): 1 in 2.3 million doses. Severe hypersensitivity reaction: 1–104 per 10 000 vaccinees.
Measles	Pneumonia: 1 in 20 Encephalitis: 1 in 2000 Thrombocytopenia 1 per 30 000–100 000 Death: 1 in 3000	MMR vaccine: Encephalitis or severe allergic reaction: 1 in 1 000 000
Mumps	Encephalitis: 1 in 300	
Rubella	Congenital rubella syndrome (in newborn born to a woman with infection in the early pregnancy): 1 in 4	

Meningococcal disease	Outbreak defined by >6 cases/100 000
	Rates in endemic areas of Africa during epidemics:
	Case fatality rates in industrialized countries:
	  Meningitis – 7%
	  Septicemia – 19%
	Mortality in developing countries during epidemics:
	  Meningitis – 2–10%
	  Septicemia – 50–70%
		Local pain and swelling at the site of injection <3 %

Poliomyelitis	Paralytic cases: 2% of all infections
	Case fatality rate:
	  Children: 2–5% in clinical cases
	  Adults: 15–30% in clinical cases
		Vaccine associated paralytic polio (VAPP): 1 case for every 2-3 million doses of OPV.
		No risk of VAPP with IPV

Rabies	Case fatality rate: 100%	Cell Culture Vaccines (CCV): No risk of vaccine-associated neurologic adverse side-effects; 20% incidence of minor side effects. HDCV: 6% incidence of delayed hypersensitivity reactions
Varicella	Encephalitis: 1.8 in 10 000 Death: 1 in 60 000 cases Age related case fatality rate: 1–14 years: 1 in 100 000 15–19 years: 2.7 in 100 000 30–49 years: 25.2 in 100 000	Generalized varicella-like rash: 4–6% of vaccine recipients. Risk of zoster is 4–5 times LESS in vaccinated than non-vaccinated individuals.
Yellow fever	Case fatality rate: 100%	Type I Hypersensitivity reactions: 1/1 000 000 doses Yellow fever vaccine Associated Neurologic Disease (Yell-AND): 1/8 000 000 Yellow fever vaccine Associated Viscerotrophic Disease (Yell-VTD): Rare

REQUIRED (WHO) TRAVEL VACCINES

Yellow fever vaccine

Yellow fever is an acute viral hemorrhagic disease transmitted to humans by mosquitoes in tropical Africa and South America (see Fig. 10.3). The risk of acquiring yellow fever among travelers is not clearly known. Most experts acknowledge that current surveillance data on yellow fever infections for both traveler and resident populations probably underestimates the true incidence of disease acquired in endemic areas.[1] In the last few years, several cases of yellow fever have been reported among unvaccinated travelers from industrialized countries who had visited endemic areas. The ten cases of imported yellow fever in travelers reported for the period 1979–2002 probably reflects both improved global case reporting and increased travel to destinations where there is risk of exposure.[2–4]

Yellow fever (YF) transmission occurs in jungle and urban cycles in South America, with peak transmission during the months of January through March, particularly in areas recently cleared of trees for habitation and agriculture. The jungle cycle of yellow fever is primarily viral disease of non-human primates in South America, occasionally extending up to Central America and Trinidad. Humans are accidentally infected when they encroach on the jungle environment and are bitten by infected sylvatic mosquito species. In Africa, YF transmission cycles are characterized for the tropical rainforest, moist savannah, and contiguous dry savannah/urban areas, particularly during the rainy and early dry seasons during the months of July through October. Urban outbreaks are thought to result from migratory patterns of human workers who become infected in rural habitats of endemic areas, and serve as reservoirs of infection when they return to the city and become viremic. Currently the urban cycle of YF persists mostly in certain countries and regions in West Africa.

Countries located in YF endemic areas may officially require proof of vaccination against YF as a condition for entry under WHO International Health Regulations (summarized graphically on the Yellow fever Map Fig. 10.3). Only a small number of African countries (Burkina Faso, Cameroon, Congo, Cote D'Ivoire, Democratic Republic of Congo, Gabon, Ghana, Liberia, Mali, Mauritania, Niger, Rwanda, Sao Tome, Togo) and one in South America (French Guiana) require proof of yellow fever vaccination from all arriving travelers. Other countries, both within and outside the endemic zone have more complex requirements, which are summarized graphically on the Yellow Fever Map (Fig. 10.3). While most countries located within endemic areas request proof of YF vaccination for at least some arriving travelers as a requirement for entry, certain countries outside of endemic areas may also designate YF vaccine as a required or mandatory vaccine. Such YF-free countries have the appropriate climatic and entomologic conditions to initiate and maintain a YF transmission cycle, and the purpose of the vaccine requirement in this case is to prevent importation of YF through entry of latent viremic infections in travelers arriving from YF endemic countries.

The vaccine is a live attenuated strain of the yellow fever virus (17D) that was originally developed by Theiler and Smith in 1927. Sub-strains of the WHO-standardized 17D virus seed lot strains in current use are designated 17DD, 17D-204, and 17D-213. WHO currently approves only 5 manufacturers of Yellow Fever vaccine: Aventis Pasteur, France produces 17D-204 vaccine in France (Stamaril) and the US (YF-Vax); Institut Pasteur, Senegal produce 17D-204 yellow fever vaccine; Celltech Group (formerly Medeva, formerly Evans) produces 17D-204 (Arilvax) BioMaguinos, Brazil produces 17DD vaccine and Institute of Poliomyelits and Viral Encephalitides, Russia. Smaller manufacturers of yellow fever vaccine in Germany, and

Colombia either no longer produce it or no longer are WHO approved. 17D-204 and 17DD share 99.9% sequence homology.

Yellow fever vaccination is considered valid if the person received a WHO-approved vaccine and it was administered at an approved Yellow Fever Vaccination Center. The immunization must be given no less than 10 days prior to planned date of entry to meet official requirements and is valid for 10 years. Vaccine administration is documented and stamped on the appropriate page of the *International Certificate of Vaccination*. This proof of vaccination is sometimes required during crossing of international borders, particularly in Africa, or if flying from an infected country to a non-infected country, even if the stay in the endemic country was a brief transit stop. A stamp indicating proof of YF vaccination can be obtained only from an approved Yellow Fever Vaccination Center. A personal signature cannot substitute the official stamp. Individual countries control the number and locations of YF Vaccination Center sites, which may be at either public health clinics or private health centers, depending on the population of the area served, estimated at-risk population, and national vaccine program priorities. In many countries, especially in Latin America, the YF stamp is obtainable only from government clinics that provide the YF vaccine and not from private clinics even if they can purchase and administer the vaccine.

Under WHO regulations, a letter of waiver can be provided to travelers that have medical or other contraindications for receiving the yellow fever vaccination. The waiver letter must be on official letterhead, signed by the person authorized to provide the YF vaccination and bear the stamp of the authorized center. Travelers unable to receive the vaccine and using a letter of waiver to meet the YF vaccine entry requirement for a destination in a YF endemic area need pre-travel counseling about how to decrease the risks of natural disease transmission at destination, through effective use of insect precautions and avoidance of environments where the risk of transmission is likely to be higher.

Indications

The main purpose of vaccination is prevention of disease in individuals at risk. Yellow fever vaccine is approved for use in all persons over 9 months of age who have no YF vaccine contraindication. See Chapter 11 for considerations on immunizing children under the age of 9 months. However, because of rare but possible vaccine-associated adverse side-effects (see below), persons who are not at risk of exposure should not receive the vaccine. In the countries where the disease is endemic and there is a YF vaccine requirement for entry, the risk of disease is usually restricted to limited areas of the country. If a traveler has no possibility to visit that particular area, then YF vaccination may not be warranted on a health risk basis, although YF vaccine certification or an official letter of waiver would be needed to meet the legal requirements for entry. However, if such a traveler then plans to continue travel into another country with YF entry requirements, then vaccination would be required to meet the entry requirements of the second country. It is prudent to vaccinate persons that have anything less than a definite fixed itinerary and/or anticipate travel outside of urban areas in YF endemic countries, regardless of whether the YF vaccine is required.

Contraindications

Since the vaccine virus is grown in chick embryos, it is contraindicated in persons with a history of anaphylaxis or proven hypersensitivity to eggs or egg protein. A history of anaphylaxis to a previous yellow fever vaccine dose or allergy to gelatin precludes use of the vaccine. A person with a questionable history of egg allergy traveling to a highly endemic area may be a candidate for an intradermal test dose according to package insert instructions. Persons who are able to

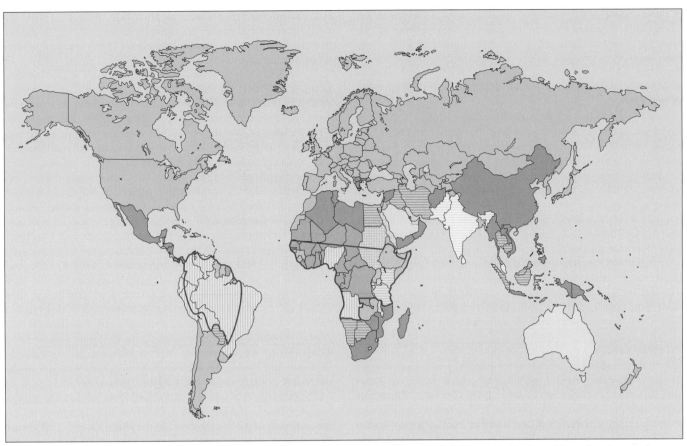

Figure 10.3 Yellow fever map. Areas of South America and Africa where WHO considers travelers to have actual risk of acquiring yellow fever and demarcated by the thick red line* and**. Shading is to be used only in interpreting yellow fever vaccination certificate entry requirements for each country. (1) Infectivity or endemicity of the countries: (a) Currently YF Infected countries (WHO): All those in red and all those in orange with vertical stripes. Infected countries are those that have officially reported current human cases to WHO (2003) See www.cdc.gov/travel/ blusheet.htm for weekly updated lists. (b): Endemic countries (WHO): all those colored red and all those colored orange. A country is considered 'endemic' if the WHO reports there is potential risk of infection on account of the presence of vectors (mosquitoes) and animal reservoirs (non-human primates harboring the yellow fever virus) * and **. (2) Yellow Fever Vaccination Certificate for Entry from All Travelers: All arriving travelers (in accordance with age-related national regulations) to areas of the map that are shown in red. (3) Yellow Fever Vaccination Medically Recommended Because of Risk: Travelers going at anytime outside urban areas of countries depicted in orange and red***. (4) Yellow Fever Vaccination Certificate Only from Certain Travelers: Because of Risk That They are Carrying Yellow Fever: (a): All travelers arriving from infected areas of countries considered infected**** (shown in purple) (b) All travelers arriving from a country any part of which is infected**** with yellow fever (i.e., both red and yellow countries) depicted in green. (c) All travelers arriving from infected countries (whole country or only from an infected area of an infected country) or any endemic country**** (these are the red and orange countries). Countries with these requirements are shown in horizontal stripes either purple or orange or green. These countries may be themselves uninfected countries or infected or endemic countries). *Small forested regions of Argentina and Paraguay that border Brazil are considered by the US CDC to have risk even though they are outside the current WHO endemic zone. **In 2001, Zambia was removed by WHO from the Endemic Zone list, but it may take several years for many maps and lists still in circulation to remove it. *** Many named places marked as cities or towns on maps are more rural than urban. Urban transmission has been documented in cities of Senegal, Ivory Coast, Northern Nigeria, and Amazonian areas of Bolivia. Aedes vectors do not survive above 2300m altitude. ****Minor variations of each country's interpretation of infected and endemic zones for the purposes of enforcing yellow fever vaccine requirements frequently occur. See www.who.int/ith for current updated information.

eat eggs or egg products without side-effects can usually receive the vaccine safely.[5]

The vaccine should not be used in pregnancy unless travel during active yellow fever transmission is unavoidable, based on theoretical concerns about the use of a live attenuated virus vaccine in the relative immune suppressed state of pregnancy, and the possible risk of infection of the fetus during the viremic period that develops in the mother the week following immunization.[6,7] Breast-feeding mothers may receive this immunization. Yellow fever vaccination for immuno-compromised patients is generally contraindicated (see Chapter 25). If administration of the yellow fever vaccine is not prudent given the patient's health status, yet the risk of the disease is high according to the planned travel itinerary and anticipated patient activities, one may advise the patient not to travel to that area because of the risk. If the risk of the disease in the particular travel destination is low, then a letter may be provided to the traveler that requests waiver of the

yellow fever vaccine requirement. HIV patients may be immunized under certain circumstances (see Chapter 25).[8] The need for post-immunization serologic testing in travelers with altered immune states can be discussed with the appropriate public health laboratory testing center.

Precautions

Yellow fever vaccine should be delayed for 8 weeks after having received blood or plasma transfusion but can be received concurrently with immunoglobulin for hepatitis A. Immunoglobulin administration does not interfere with YF response.[9]

Dosing schedules for adults

The primary schedule for yellow fever vaccine in adults is a single 0.5 mL injection given subcutaneously. The duration of immunity from one dose of the vaccine is estimated to last for 10 years or longer.

A booster dose is recommended for persons with continued risk of exposure 10 years from the last dose. The yellow fever vaccine contains no preservative and must be administered within 1 h of reconstitution.

Measures of immune response and duration of immunity/protection

Yellow fever vaccine is extremely immunogenic and induces an immune response in more than 90% of the vaccinees. The vaccine mimics natural infection, and a low level of viremia with the vaccine strain virus is noted in 50–60% of the vaccinees in first week after vaccination. Seroprotective neutralizing antibodies to YF develop within 7–10 days of vaccination. Serum antibodies are measured using a constant serum/varying virus neutralizing test: a log neutralization index of 0.7 or more is considered a positive response. The induced immunity following immunization confers more than 94% protection against YF.

Although the YF certificate is officially valid for 10 years, the true duration of immunity from YF vaccination is probably much longer.[10] The antibodies have been detected in 92–97% of the vaccinees 16–19 years after initial vaccination. In another study, approximately 80% of the vaccinees were seropositive 30 years after a single dose.

Adverse events

Yellow fever vaccine is considered an extremely safe vaccine when given as indicated. Fever, headache, and muscle aches can occur 5–14 days after immunization in about 2–5% of persons. Immediate hypersensitivity reactions are uncommon and tend to occur in persons with egg allergy. The incidence of this type of reaction is estimated to be <1/1 million doses.[5] Most reactions occur within 1 hour of vaccination but some occur as late as 21–24 h. Screening patients for a history of allergy to a previous dose, eggs, chicken or gelatin is important. Those with a positive history of anaphylactic allergies to these may need allergy testing and evaluation, although testing may not be able to detect all patients with a type 1 IgE-mediated hypersensitivity.[11] Package inserts in the USA and some other countries include suggested desensitization regimens.

In the years following 1945, when the seed-lot standardization of yellow fever vaccine strain 17D was accomplished, there have been 27 cases of yellow fever vaccine associated neurotropic disease (YEL-AND), formerly known as postvaccinal encephalitis, reported worldwide mostly in young infants although a few cases of adult disease have been noted. 15 of these cases were in the 1950s, and 13 were in infants less than 4 months old. The YEL-AND typically occurs 7–21 days post immunization and is characterized by neurologic signs, a CSF pleocytosis (100–500 WBC) and increased CSF protein. A brief clinical course with complete recovery was typical. The risk for YEL-AND has been estimated as 1/8 000 000 persons.[8]

Recent case reports of vaccine-associated adverse events among 17D-derived YF vaccine recipients has led to recognition of a new serious adverse reaction, yellow fever vaccine-associated viscerotropic disease (YF-AVD), formerly known as febrile multiple organ system failure. In the period 1996–2002, 13 cases of yellow fever vaccine associated viscerotrophic disease (YEL-AVD) have been reported worldwide on a background of over 100 million doses administered worldwide. The true risk is unclear at present due to incomplete surveillance in most countries but this appears to be a rare event. CDC and WHO have formally stated that no change in vaccine practices or indications is warranted due to these reports. The onset of illness occurs 2-5 days after receiving YF vaccine, and is characterized by fever, myalgia, arthralgia, increased liver enzymes and bilirubin, thrombocytopenia, disseminated intravascular coagulation, lymphopenia, rhabdomyolysis, hypotension, and oliguria. All cases reported so far have

occurred among persons receiving their first YF vaccine dose, and males outnumbered females in a ratio of approximately 2:1. The elderly, over the age of 70 appear more likely to have YF-AVD as well as other severe adverse events.[12–18]

Drug and vaccine interactions

Yellow fever vaccine can be administered concurrently or at any time before or after immune globulin products given for hepatitis A prophylaxis. Studies have shown that the immune response to the vaccine is not altered by the concurrent administration of immunoglobulin. Some data shows that the antibody responses to the oral cholera vaccine and the yellow fever vaccine were lower when the vaccines were administered concurrently. It is preferable, but not mandatory, to give yellow fever vaccine 3 weeks apart from the cholera vaccine. Studies have shown that the yellow fever vaccine can be given concurrently with other live-antigen (MMR, oral typhoid, or OPV) vaccines without a decrease in the vaccine immunogenicity or increased side-effects.[19–21] However, if simultaneous administration of live-virus vaccines is not possible, then it is advisable to separate two live virus vaccines by at least 4 weeks. Clinical trials show that yellow fever vaccine can be administered concurrently with inactivated vaccines such as hepatitis A, hepatitis B, and typhoid polysaccharide vaccines.[22–24] Because of the possibility of live virus vaccinations interfering with the immune response to the tuberculin (PPD) testing, the PPD skin test should be administered either the same day as the yellow fever vaccine or administered 4–6 weeks later.

Experimental data suggests that chloroquine inhibits the replication of yellow fever virus *in vitro*. However, a study in humans has shown that the antibody responses to the yellow fever vaccine are not affected by routine antimalarial doses of chloroquine.[25,26]

RECOMMENDED TRAVEL VACCINES

Hepatitis A vaccine

Hepatitis A (HA), a viral hepatitis transmitted worldwide by the fecal-oral route, has been identified as the most common vaccine-preventable illness acquired by international travelers. The risk of HA among persons from industrialized countries traveling to developing countries had a hepatitis A attack rate estimated at approximately 3/1000 persons per month for the average non-immune traveler or business traveler. A similar rate was noted by the US State Department survey of employees stationed abroad.[27] The attack rate increases significantly to 20/1000 per month of travel for backpackers and budget travelers in highly endemic countries.

The risk of HA infection is highest in developing countries with poor sanitation and food hygiene. Persons traveling in countries in Eastern Europe, Commonwealth of Independent States (including Russia and the Newly Independent States), Greece and Turkey are considered at intermediate risk of acquiring HA. The USA, Canada, Japan, Australia, New Zealand, Scandinavian countries, and developed countries in Europe are all considered areas of low risk[28] (Fig. 10.4).

In addition to geographic risk, the risk of acquiring HA virus (HAV) infection also depends on factors related to the individual travelers – specifically, the country of origin (developed or developing country), age, food habits, duration and type of previous travel or residence in endemic countries, and occupational and recreational exposures. Persons from industrialized countries born after World War II have very low rates of anti-HAV antibodies in serum surveys, therefore such individuals are at significant risk of acquiring HA upon exposure. In one study, less than 20% of persons on the US mainland and Hawaii who were less than 60 years of age were seropositive for anti-HAV antibodies.[29,30] Multivariate analysis showed a higher rate of

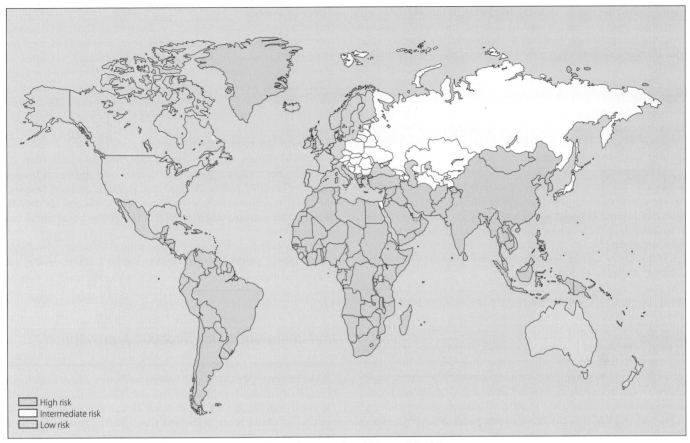

Figure 10.4 Hepatitis A map. Vaccination is indicated for all travelers to high and intermediate risk areas

anti-HAV seropositivity associated with older age, non-white race and birth outside of the USA.[27] The case fatality rate of HAV infection is estimated to be 0.15% but increases to 2% or higher with age over 40 years old.

There are several equally effective inactivated HAV vaccines currently available worldwide (see Table 10.2 for details). China produces a live attenuated hepatitis A virus vaccine, which reportedly is effective but does not seem to induce long-term immunity.

Indications

Hepatitis A vaccine is recommended for persons from a developed country traveling to or working in countries with intermediate or high endemicity of HA, especially for those persons who plan to live in or visit rural areas, trek in back country areas or frequently eat or drink in settings of poor sanitation. This would include essentially every individual traveling outside the USA, Canada, Japan, Australia, New Zealand, Scandinavian countries, and developed countries in Europe. Persons with a history of hepatitis or who previously lived in an endemic country for a prolonged period may benefit from pre-vaccination serum antibody testing.

Hepatitis A vaccine should also be considered when immigrants living in developed countries plan to visit countries with HA risk, since some individuals in this category may be susceptible. Among immigrants from developing countries who immigrated in their second decade of life or later, it is cost-effective to check the patient's hepatitis A serum antibody status since they may already be immune. The traveler should be vaccinated if the hepatitis A IgG serum test is negative, indicating lack of immunity to HA. In one study, 80% of the foreign born nationals were seropositive for HA.[31] History of having had the disease is an unreliable predictor of serum status.

Administration of HA vaccine 2 or more weeks before trip departure and risk of exposure is recommended. The US CDC recommends concurrent administration of immune globulin when the vaccine is administered less than 2 weeks in advance of the anticipated risk of exposure, but this is not a well-accepted practice. The WHO allows that a single dose HA vaccine on the way to the airport may provide protection against disease, and does not recommend IG if the vaccine is administered less than 2 weeks in advance of trip departure. However, patients at higher risk of HA complications, such as those with chronic liver disease, elderly, HIV-infected persons (especially those with low CD4+ T cells), and immunosuppressed patients should be immunized well in advance.

The onset of immunity from vaccination 2–4 weeks after receipt of the first dose of vaccine in relationship to the incubation period of HA, which averages 3 weeks, leads to the consideration of whether or not concurrent administration of immune globulin is necessary at all in travelers departing imminently to areas of risk. Published studies on use of HA vaccine during HA outbreaks suggest that vaccine-induced protection was elicited against manifestations of clinical hepatitis A disease by vaccine doses administered in the midst of ongoing infectious exposures, even among individuals who later showed seroconversion to positive anti-HAV titers.[32,33]

Contraindications

Any HA vaccine should not be given if there has been a serious allergic reaction to a previous dose. Havrix® and Avaxim® should not be given to persons with allergy to aluminum or aluminum hydroxide. Havrix® and Avaxim® also contain the preservative 2-phenoxyethanol. VAQTA® is formulated without preservatives. Avaxim® also contains formaldehyde and trace amounts of neomycin. Epaxal® does not contain aluminum as an adjuvant but has both formaldehyde and thimerosal as ingredients. Vaccination of persons already immune to HA is not indicated. However an inadvertent vaccination of an already immune individual does not increase the risk for adverse effects.

Precautions

Persons with malignancies, congenital or acquired immune disorders or those on immunosuppressive therapy may not mount an adequate immune response to HA vaccine. Such patients may need to have their immune response to the vaccine evaluated by serology before travel or expected exposure. If the serology is negative four or more weeks after the dose, then passive immunity with immunoglobulin may be needed to assure protection against HA (see section on Immune Globulin below). Although the HA vaccines are extremely effective, travelers should still be advised to follow food and water precautions while traveling.

Dosing schedules for adults

The primary schedule for adults consists of one 1 mL dose of inactivated HA vaccine given by intramuscular injection in the deltoid muscle at least 2–4 weeks prior to expected exposure and a second dose is given 6–18 months after first dose. The primary schedule does not need to be re-started if a prolonged delay from the initial dose has occurred. Studies have shown that an inactivated HA vaccine induces an anamnestic booster response and likely induces long-term proliferative T-cell responses in travelers receiving their second booster anywhere from 18 months to 6 years after the single primary dose.[34,35]

Havrix® and VAQTA® can be used interchangeably.[36,37] Avaxim® is interchangeable with VAQTA® or Havrix®, but interchangeability of the other hepatitis A vaccines is unknown.[38,39]

Accepted and possible accelerated schedules

Since seroconversion rates and GMTs at 4 or 6 weeks after a single dose of a HA vaccine are uniformly very high for all available vaccines the need for an accelerated 2-dose schedule prior to the usual 6 month booster is not apparent.

Measures of immune response and duration of immunity/protection

The available HA vaccines are highly immunogenic and safe. The lowest protective antibody level against HAV infection has not been clearly defined. Although the neutralizing antibodies that develop after vaccination are lower than those produced by natural infection, they are protective as evidenced in the low infection rates in the vaccinated individuals in the clinical trials. *In vitro*, animal and clinical studies suggest that HAV antibody levels of 10–20 mIU/mL may be protective.

Protective antibodies develop in 94–100% of immunocompetent adults at 4 weeks and 97–100% in immunocompetent persons aged 2–18 years.[28,33,40–44] After 14 days, 96% of vaccinees have positive anti-HAV titers and after 30 days all vaccinees had seroconverted. Booster doses at 6 months increased the antibody titers by 25-fold.[45] Concurrent administration of immunoglobulin decreased the antibody titers, however the percentage of persons with protective antibody level remained unaltered compared with those that did not receive the immunoglobulin concurrently with hepatitis A.[46,47]

Immune response to the hepatitis A vaccines is diminished in immunocompromised person including those with advanced AIDS,[48] decompensated liver disease and with the presence of advanced disease (Child-Pugh class B/C)[49] and in transplant patients. Booster doses increased seroconversion rates.[50] Other factors that may decrease immune response include older age and increased weight.[51]

Adverse events

Hepatitis A vaccines are extremely well tolerated. The most common side affects reported are injection site pain, warmth, and swelling. Headache is reported in about 14–16% percent of adult recipients. In post-marketing (1995–1998) surveys there have been very few (247) serious adverse events reported with the administration of more than 6.5 million doses (2.3 million pediatric doses) of the two HA vaccines licensed in the USA (Havrix® and VAQTA®).[28]

Drug and vaccine interactions

Accumulated data suggests that concurrent administration of other vaccines such as hepatitis B, tetanus toxoid, diphtheria toxoid, polio, typhoid Vi polysaccharide, oral typhoid, cholera, Japanese encephalitis, rabies or yellow fever vaccines is safe and unlikely to decrease the immune response to the HA or the co-administered vaccines.[24,28,52]

Patients receiving IG concurrently with HA vaccine developed similar seroconversion rates and had protective GMT at week 4, but both the seroconversion and GMT were significantly lower at week 24 when compared with the patients that received the vaccine alone. Responses after second boosters were similar.[53,54]

Immune globulin for hepatitis A prevention

Immune globulin (IG) provides protection against hepatitis A virus (HAV) by passive transfer of pre-formed antibodies. Immune globulin is usually prepared from human serum pools derived from several thousand individuals. Each individual serum sample is tested for evidence of blood borne pathogens (hepatitis B, hepatitis C, HIV), and the pooled sera are then purified by standard biochemical procedures to isolate and purify the IgG fraction. The duration of protection ranges from 3 months to 5 months, depending on the dose administered.[55,56]

Indications

Immunoglobulin is used to provide pre-exposure, short-term prophylaxis for protection against HAV in the following groups: travelers leaving less than 2 weeks after receipt of HA vaccine; children less than 2 years of age in countries where hepatitis A vaccine is not licensed under the age of 2, and others who are unable to receive HA vaccine; persons who are likely to respond poorly to immunization such as compromised hosts, and others who are determined to be seronegative after HA vaccination. Immune globulin is also used for post-exposure prophylaxis against HAV. When administered within 2 weeks following exposure to HAV, IG is >85% effective in preventing Hepatitis A infection.

Contraindications

Anaphylactic reaction to a previous dose contraindicates further IG. Because of the possibility of anaphylaxis, IG should not be given to individuals with isolated immunoglobulin A (IgA) deficiency. The same dose and schedule are used for administration of IG for HAV protection to both immunocompetent and immunocompromised persons. Pregnancy or lactation is not a contraindication to IG; however, IG should be given only when clearly indicated and thimerosal free during pregnancy. If available thimerosal-free IG should be administered for infants or pregnant women.

Dosing schedules for adults

The dose of IG for pre-exposure prophylaxis against HAV for travel of less than 3 months duration is 0.02 mL/kg given by deep intramuscular injection into the gluteus muscle (preferable) or deltoid muscle. For protection against HAV for a trip of 3 months or longer, the dose is 0.06 mL/kg IG given by deep intramuscular injection into the gluteus muscle. Long-stay travelers and persons who are unable to receive the hepatitis A vaccine and remain in an area of exposure beyond the 5 months should receive a repeat IG dose every 5 months.

Adverse events

Because of the volume of the IG, soreness and swelling at the injection site is the most common adverse event. Occasionally, urticaria may occur.

Drug and vaccine interactions

Antibodies contained in IG can interfere with the immune response to live-attenuated vaccines such as measles, mumps, rubella, and chicken pox (see MMR and Varicella sections below). Immune globulin should not be administered concurrently or within a given time preceding or following immunization with such vaccines.

Hepatitis B vaccine

Although hepatitis B (HB) vaccine was incorporated into the schedule of routine childhood immunizations in many countries starting in the late 1980s (see Chapter 11), HB vaccine is a recommended travel vaccine for certain susceptible adult travelers who are going to areas where the disease is endemic. Figure 10.5 divides the world into high, inter-mediate, and low prevalence countries based on seroprevalence of hepatitis B serum markers in the population.

Several HB vaccine formulations are available worldwide. The currently widely used vaccines are the recombinant vaccines which use HBsAg expressed in yeast. The various HB vaccines contain 10–40 ug of HBsAg protein/mL that is adsorption to aluminum hydroxide (0.5 mg/mL) as an adjuvant.[57] Some HB vaccines also contain thimerosal (1:20 000 concentration) as a preservative, although all pediatric HB vaccines in the USA as well as many other countries are now thimerosal free.

Indications

The risk of HB infection for short-term travelers is less than that for long-stay (greater than 1 month) travelers and expatriates. Travelers that anticipate: exposure to blood or body secretions (health care personnel, laboratory workers, relief workers), unprotected sexual exposures with members of the local population or other travelers; accidents (adventure travelers are at higher risk), medical conditions potentially requiring hospitalization or blood transfusion, dental work, intravenous drug use and activities that include needles, such as acupuncture, piercing, or tattooing constitute the highest hepatitis B exposure risk to travelers.[58,59] All individuals anticipating exposure to these risk factors should receive HB vaccine no matter how short the trip or the level of risk at the destination. Vaccination should be highly recommended to all persons traveling for a longer duration –

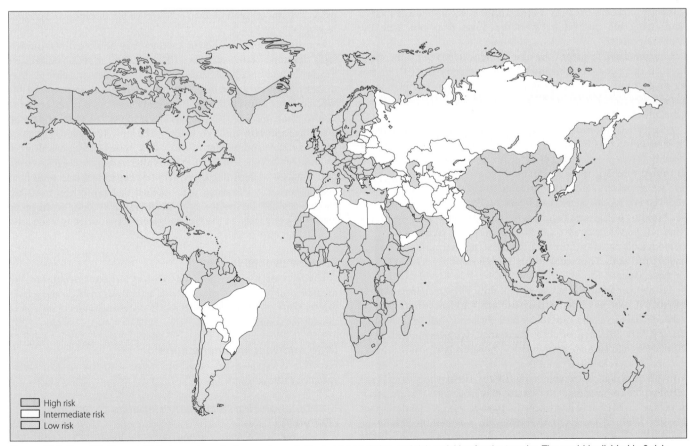

Figure 10.5 Hepatitis B map. Risk depends on both prevalence in the local population and risk activities for the traveler. The world is divided in 3 risk strata according to hepatitis B prevalence in the local population. In high and intermediate risk destinations, vaccine is indicated for all long-stay travelers as well as for all those with frequent short stays. All travelers to these countries with the following risk factors should be vaccinated regardless of duration of stay: adventure travelers, possibility of new sexual partner during stay; extensive travel by road or extensive use of public transportation; possibility of acupuncture, dental work, or tattooing; all health care workers; expected occupational exposure to blood and body fluids. The WHO has recently instituted a recommendation for HB vaccine for all travelers to high and intermediate risk areas

certainly for longer than 4 weeks especially to high and intermediate risk countries. Since HB vaccines are safe and efficacious and accepted into routine childhood vaccination programs in several countries, HB vaccine may be reasonable even for those traveling less than 4 weeks without specific risk factors. The WHO has recently instituted a recommendation for HB vaccine for all travelers to high and intermediate risk areas. Business and other travelers that fly internationally on multiple but short trips should be advised to receive the HB vaccine.

Immigrants from high prevalence countries who are returning home to visit their families may warrant screening for HB disease before vaccination. Similarly children of immigrants planning to visit their home country, should complete HB vaccine before travel. Persons adopting children from these higher prevalence countries should also be vaccinated.

Contraindications

Hypersensitivity to a previous dose, thimerosal, or baker's yeast precludes the use of recombinant HB vaccine. Although most pediatric HB vaccines are thimerosal free, some hepatitis B formulations may still contain small amounts of thimerosal.

Dosing schedules for adults

For adults, the dose of the HB vaccine is 1.0mL (10 mcg of Recombivax HB® or 20 mcg of Engerix B®) given intramuscularly in the deltoid muscle. The primary immunization schedule consists of 3 vaccine doses given on a schedule of 0, 1, and 6 months. The vaccine should be given intramuscularly for best response, but hepatitis B vaccine should not be given in the buttock because this route of administration has been associated with a lower immune response. Prolonging the interval between the doses does not alter the immunogenicity.

In hemodialysis patients, the dose of the vaccine used is increased to 40 mcg (special formulation with the Recombivax HB®, or two 20 mcg in 1mL vials of Engerix B®). Immunization for this special patient population consists of a 4-dose primary series given on a schedule of 0, 1, 2 and 6 months.

Booster recommendations depend on the patient population. In general, boosters of HB vaccine are not recommended at any time for healthy travelers who are not at high risk of exposure. It may be advisable to check titers and boost with a single dose if HB virus surface antibodies (anti-HBs) are undetectable among persons who received HB vaccine more than 10 years ago, who will be at high risk for hepatitis B exposure (e.g., a surgeon planning to do surgery in a high HB prevalent country).[60] Booster doses are recommended for hemodialysis patients if the anti-HBsAg serum test result shows less than 10 mIU/mL. The serum anti-HBsAg should be checked annually in these patients.

A small percentage of apparently healthy HBV recipients do not mount a detectable response to the vaccine. This failure to respond is related to factors such as age (older then 40 years), male sex, smoking, obesity, HIV infection or chronic disease.[61] For persons with these risk factors and who are at high risk of hepatitis B exposure, a post-vaccination serology 1–6 months after the last dose should be done. Patients without detectable anti-HBsAg titers soon after (1–6 months) the completion of the vaccine may need to re-start the series with the dialysis dose (40 mcg) of the vaccine. A standard-dose booster followed by a repeat serology in 1–6 months should be considered for persons who completed vaccination a few years previously and are seronegative now. If the repeat serology is negative, and the person is at high risk, then 2 additional standard doses can be given followed again by serologies. If the patient still remains sero-negative, then repeat HB vaccine series with the dialysis-dose can be performed.[57]

Accelerated schedules

The 3-dose primary series may be accelerated to be administered at 0, 1, and 4 months or 0, 2, and 4 months where the second dose should be given at least 1 month after the first dose and the third dose should be given at least 4 months after the first dose and at least 2 months after the second dose (0, 1, 4 months or 0, 2, 4 months). For persons leaving in less than 3 months for a long trip, an accelerated schedule can be administered, consisting of a standard dose given at 0, 1, and 2, months is followed by a booster in 12 months.

HB vaccine has been studied in a hyper-accelerated schedule of 0, 7, and 21 days followed by a booster in 12 months.[62,63] Although not approved by many regulatory bodies, hyper-accelerated schedules are used widely in practice and may be considered in the all too frequent circumstance where the traveler is leaving in a very short time and is at risk of HB exposure (see above).[64] When accelerated schedules are used for HB immunization, a booster dose at 12 months should be given for a prolonged duration of immunity. A similar 0, 7, 21 days accelerated dosing schedule has been studied and approved for use in Europe with the combination hepatitis A/B vaccine, Twinrix® (GlaxoSmithKline; see below).

Measures of immune response and duration of immunity/protection

The protective efficacy of the HB vaccines is related to the development of the anti-HBs antibody of more than 10 mIU/mL after the primary series. Those patients that developed titers above 10 mIU/mL are essentially 100% protected.[65] The first two doses provide efficacy of 50–90% whereas completing the third dose gives an individual protective efficacy of more then 95% against HB infection and chronic illness.[66,67]

Immune response to the HB vaccines may be altered with underlying immune states such as HIV infection, immunosuppressive medications or conditions such as dialysis or underlying chronic liver diseases.[68] Age is a significant factor for immune response to the vaccine. Persons over the age of 40 years have an immune response <90%, while only 65–75% persons above the age of 65 years develop protective anti-HBs antibody levels.[69] The anti-HBsAg levels decrease gradually after completion of the 3-dose series. The levels drop in 30–60% of the recipients by 9–11 years after vaccination. However, in individuals with declining titers, very few hepatitis B infections have been reported.[69] Therefore, it is believed that protection from HB vaccine should persist for at least 10–12 years despite dropping antibody levels. 76% of the vaccinees were seropositive 10 years after vaccination.[70]

Adverse events

Side-effects of the recombinant HB vaccine are uncommon but include local pain at the injection site, arthralgias/myalgia and a fever greater than 37.7°C.[71] Hepatitis B vaccine does not increase the risk of developing multiple sclerosis.[72]

Drug and vaccine interactions

Hepatitis B vaccines can be administered with live or inactivated vaccines without interference.[73]

Combination Hepatitis A and Hepatitis B vaccine (Twinrix®)

A combination hepatitis A (Havrix®) plus hepatitis B (Engerix B®) vaccine called Twinrix® became available in Europe in the late 1990's and is currently available in most countries including the USA. A pediatric formulation, Twinrix Junior is approved in countries other than the USA. The indications for use of a combined HA and HB vaccine consist of an overlap of indications for the use of the individual vaccines. The combination HA plus HB vaccine is especially suited for patients meeting indications for both vaccines, with special considerations: Long-term (more than 1 month) travelers visiting countries with high HA and HB prevalence; short-term travelers to high HA prevalence countries and likely to participate in activities that place them at high risk for HB exposure (see above); frequent international travelers especially to countries with high prevalence of both diseases; short-term travelers to HA endemic countries who also have non-travel related indications for HBV protection such as fire-fighters, healthcare workers, hemophiliacs, hemodialysis patients or persons living with a HB active carrier, etc.

Contraindications

Hypersensitivity reaction to a previous dose of either Havrix® or Engerix B® or Twinrix® or a known component of either of these vaccines is a contraindication to receiving this vaccine.

Dosing schedules for adults

The adult Twinrix® combination vaccine contains 720 ELISA Units of hepatitis A antigen and 20 mcg of recombinant hepatitis B surface antigen in each 1 mL dose. The primary immunization schedule consists of 3 doses of vaccine given on a schedule of 0, 1 and 6 months. Alternative 2-dose schedules such as 0, 6 months or 0, 12 months have been studied and found to be comparable in immunogenicity.[74,75]

Accelerated schedules

In a randomized controlled study, Twinrix® administered in an accelerated schedule of 0, 7, and 21 days followed by a 12-month booster was compared with monovalent Havrix® and Engerix B® vaccines administered in the same schedule of 0, 7 and 21 days and a 12-month booster. One month after the first dose of Twinrix®, the seroconversion rates of HA were 100% and seroprotective levels against HBV were 83%.[76]

This schedule is currently approved in the EU and increasingly used off-label in other countries including the USA. The accelerated schedule for the combination hepatitis A and B vaccine may prove to be an effective and practical vaccine regimen for travelers at risk of both diseases, who will depart imminently.

Adverse events, and drug and vaccine interactions

Similar to those for the individual component vaccines. The vaccine is extremely well tolerated with minimal side-effects. The most common reactions being allergic-type reactions followed by fever and injection site reactions.[77]

Measures of immune response and duration of immunity/protection

The seroconversion rate after administration of Twinrix® administered on the standard 0, 1, and 6 months schedule was comparable to the responses obtained when each vaccine was administered alone. Monovalent hepatitis A and hepatitis B vaccines are generally interchangeable with Twinrix® at almost any time during the course of the primary regimen.[78]

Typhoid vaccine

Typhoid fever, caused by *Salmonella typhi*, is prevalent worldwide, and is a disease associated with poor sanitation and contaminated food and water supplies. Humans with acute or chronic infections serve as the reservoir of infection. The risk of acquiring typhoid is highest during travel to the Indian subcontinent[79,80] followed by countries in Southeast Asia, western South American countries such as Peru, and parts of north and west Africa and the Middle East (except Kuwait

and Bahrain). The incidence of typhoid among travelers to the Indian subcontinent is 0.3/1000 travelers.[81] Other regions where typhoid fever remains more prevalent are among the less-industrialized countries including those of the former Soviet Union. Annual incidence rates in typhoid endemic countries are estimated to be 227–810 per 10^5 population. The emergence of multi-drug resistant *Salmonella typhi* in the Indian subcontinent and Southeast Asia pose a threat to effective treatment.[82]

Two types of typhoid vaccines are distributed worldwide at the present time: purified Vi capsular polysaccharide vaccines administered by injection, and an oral live attenuated vaccine Ty21a vaccine and (see Tables 10.1 and 10.2 for details of the preparation). Local companies in China, India and Vietnam produce other Vi polysaccharide vaccines. A combination vaccine containing Vi polysaccharide typhoid vaccine and inactivated hepatitis A called Hepatyrix® is available in Europe. Use of the older whole cell heat-inactivated phenol-preserved typhoid vaccine, commonly associated with severe local reactions at the site of injection, has been supplanted by the modern vaccines, although it may still be available in some countries. An acetone-inactivated and dried typhoid vaccine with variable availability was also used in the USA previously, but is no longer in use.

Indications

Typhoid vaccine is recommended for travelers to developing countries in Asia, Africa, and Latin America. Since risk of disease acquisition per person varies with type of travel, duration, and contact with local populations i.e., traveling off usual tourist itineraries, lodging with local people, eating in smaller, more remote areas, vaccine recommendations vary on the travelers' itineraries. Typhoid vaccination should be recommended to all travelers going to very high-risk countries. Short-term travelers to intermediate risk countries may require the vaccination if the traveler is at high risk of acquisition because of activities planned or is risk-averse and prefers complete protection. Food and water precautions should be followed even if a traveler receives typhoid vaccination, as the vaccines are not fully protective and a large oral inoculum may overwhelm even an optimal antibody response.

Contraindications

The live attenuated oral typhoid vaccine is made from the Ty21a strain of *S. typhi*, and contains 2×10^9 CFU (colony forming units) of viable organisms of attenuated *Salmonella typhi* Ty21a. The Ty21a vaccine is contraindicated during pregnancy on theoretical grounds since there is no data for safety in use in pregnant women. Since it is an attenuated live bacterial vaccine, it should not be administered to immunocompromised persons. However, there does not appear to be a risk for an immunocompromised person in the household of a vaccinee as vaccine strain bacteria cannot be isolated from the stools of vacinees.

Persons allergic to a previous dose of the Vi polysaccharide typhoid vaccine or to vaccine components should not receive this vaccine.

The phenol-preserved whole-cell vaccines should be avoided in persons with a history of allergies, due to the vaccine's high incidence of severe local reactions and systemic side-effects. In addition, it is best avoided in debilitated, or chronically ill persons such as those with chronic renal, cardiac disease or malignancy.

Precautions

Ty21a should not be administered in the presence of nausea, vomiting, or diarrhea. The vaccine should be used with caution in persons with inflammatory bowel disease or other ulcerative conditions of the gastrointestinal tract. Although the vaccine should be kept refrigerated at 5 °C ± 3 °C, it maintains its stability even if kept at 25 °C for up to 7 days. Shorter (<24 h) exposure to higher ambient temperature of 37 °C also does not affect its potency. If the Ty21a is accidentally frozen it should be thawed in the refrigerator.[83] During the course of the vaccine and for 48 h before and after, alcohol and antibiotics should be avoided. Ideally, live antigen vaccines should be given at the same time or separated by 4 weeks. However, if necessary, oral typhoid may be administered simultaneously with or at any interval before or after other live-virus vaccines or immune globulin.

Dosing schedules for adults
Vi polysaccharide typhoid vaccine
The Vi polysaccharide typhoid vaccine is approved for use in adults and children 2 years of age or older. The vaccine is given as a single dose of 0.5 mL by intramuscular injection and administration in the travel clinic ensures higher compliance rates in comparison to the multi-dose oral vaccine, which must be self-administered at home by the traveler. The vaccine should be completed at least 2 weeks prior to exposure for optimal immune response. In situations of repeated or continued risk of exposure, the single vaccine dose can be given as a booster every 2 (US labeling) to 3 years (labeling in most other countries).

Ty21a oral typhoid vaccine
The Ty21a oral typhoid vaccine is distributed in two forms: an enteric-coated capsule form which is available in the USA and Canada as well as in Europe, and a suspension form which is available only in Europe at the present time. There are two different immunization schedules used for the oral typhoid vaccine in capsule form. In the USA and Canada, a 4-dose immunization schedule is followed for adults and children 6 years old and above. In Europe and other countries a 3-dose schedule is mostly used. Irrespective of whether 4- or 3-dose series is recommended, the schedule consists of one capsule taken on alternate days. The capsules should be taken on an empty stomach with a cool or lukewarm (not more than 37 °C) water or milk. The capsule form of the vaccine should never be broken open to mix with food and drink. A repeat full 4- or 3-dose series is advised every 3–7 years (varies by national labeling) for persons with continued or repeat exposure. In two studies, the liquid formulation Ty21a was shown to be significantly more efficacious than the capsules.[84,85] A repeat full 3-dose series is advised every 3–4 years for persons with continued or repeat exposure. The doses should be completed at least 1 week prior to exposure.

There is very limited data to guide situations of interrupted Ty21a oral vaccine courses (see below). A general guideline is to complete the course if the course was interrupted less than 3 weeks ago. Persons may need to re-initiate the entire course if not completed and more than 3 weeks have elapsed.

Measures of immune response and duration of immunity/protection
Vi polysaccharide typhoid vaccine
Field trials in Nepal assessing Vi polysaccharide vaccine show an efficacy of 72%, 17 months after the vaccination.[86,87] Another study in South Africa showed 64% efficacy at 21 months and 55% at the 36-month follow-up.[88,89] The repeat doses do not have a booster effect on the primary dose. Typhim Vi and Typherix show equivalent immunogenicity.[90]

Ty21a oral typhoid vaccine
A protective immune response is elicited in approximately 25% of the recipients following one enteric-coated dose. This immune response wanes in 2–3 years. The immune response following 2 enteric-coated doses is 52%. Three doses of the enteric-coated capsules provide 67% protection over a 3-year period.[91] A 4-dose series provided signifi-

cantly higher typhoid protection (62%) compared with the 3-dose series.[92] Protective immunity following the 4-dose series lasts up to 5–7 years in some vacinees. Prolonging the interval between vaccine doses in an immunization series decreases the efficacy of the vaccine. Studies have shown that the liquid formulation is significantly more immunogenic (77% and 53% compared with 33% and 42% in two separate studies) than the capsular formulation (3-dose series).[84,85] A previous study showed the liquid formulation to have efficacy of 96% lasting for 3 years.[93] It conferred 79% protection in the fourth and fifth year of follow-up.[94]

Adverse events
The injectable Vi polysaccharide vaccine is very well tolerated, with fever, flu-like symptoms, or headache reported in less than 1% of vaccine recipients. The most common side-effect associated with the Ty21a is abdominal discomfort and other rare side-effects include nausea, vomiting, rash, urticaria, or headache (0–5%).

Drug and vaccine interactions
Co-administration of other vaccines such as yellow fever, MMR, tetanus, hepatitis A or hepatitis B is safe with the typhoid Vi polysaccharide.[24,95]

The oral Ty21a vaccine should be administered at the same time as other live viral vaccines such as yellow fever or MMR. When given in conjunction with live oral cholera vaccine, both vaccines maintained their immunogenicity, however it may be best to separate the two by at least 8 h.[96,97]

Antibiotics, antimalarials (proguanil, mefloquine and chloroquine) and alcohol may inhibit the Ty21A vaccine if taken concurrently.[98,99] The patient should be off antibiotics at least 24 h and not receive any antibiotics within 72 h after completion of vaccination. Recommendations from WHO suggest waiting 1 week before and after oral Ty21a vaccine course and the ingestion antimalarials and antibiotics. The FDA-approved package insert states that proguanil may interfere with the immune response, but the data was derived from limited studies using a higher dose of proguanil alone than is contained in the present antimalarial combination drug, atovaquone plus proguanil (Malarone®). A study looking at efficacy of the oral Ty21a vaccine taken at the same time as the combination drug Malarone® showed no effect of concurrent Malarone on serum IgA or IgG response to Ty21a so there should be no limitation to the concurrent use of Malarone and Ty21a vaccine.[100]

Mefloquine hydrochloride inhibits the oral vaccine *in vitro*, therefore, the start of prophylactic mefloquine should be separated from oral typhoid vaccine by 24–72 h.

Meningococcal vaccine

Neisseria meningitidis spreads through the air via droplets of contaminated respiratory secretions, or through person-to-person contact (kissing, sharing cigarettes and drinking glasses, etc.). Humans are the only natural reservoir for *N. meningitidis*, and the bacteria may be carried in the nasopharynx of asymptomatic hosts in up to 10% of the population during periods of endemic infection. The carrier prevalence is highest among diverse populations mixing or living in crowded conditions (pilgrims on the Hajj and Umra in Saudi Arabia, military recruits, students living in dormitories, campers at youth camps, participants in rave concerts, etc.).

Of the five meningococcal serogroups: A, B, C, Y, and W-135 serogroups A and C are most often associated with epidemics of meningococcal meningitis especially in sub-Saharan Africa during the dry, winter months from November to June annually.[101] In these select sub-Saharan African countries, referred to as the 'meningitis belt' countries, the annual incidence rates of meningococcal disease are up to 30 cases per 100 000 people.[102,103] In recent years, serogroup W-135 has emerged as a significant epidemic strain in Africa and the Middle East. Group W-135 was identified as causing up to 53% of the meningococcal cases during the 2000–2003 Hajj and Umra, and more recently, an epidemic in Burkina Faso[104,105] may herald its spread throughout Africa (Fig. 10.6 Meningococcal Map) Serogroup A caused epidemics of meningococcal disease in China, Mongolia, India, and Nepal in the 1970s, and also was associated with an epidemic in Mongolia in the early 1990s.

Group B causes 50–90% of the cases of meningococcal disease in Norway, the Netherlands, Germany, and Denmark (with the rest of the cases mostly Group C). Serogroup B epidemics have also been reported from Iceland, Belgium, Spain, Cuba, Colombia, Brazil, and Chile, although infections due to Group B are rare in Africa. In New Zealand, there has been a prolonged epidemic of meningococcal disease due to serogroup B since 1991. Recently, increasing proportions of Group C cases have been reported in the Czech Republic, Slovakia, Greenland, Republic of Ireland, Spain, and the United Kingdom.[103] In the United States, Group B, C, and Y each account for approxi-mately one third of cases of meningococcal disease in adults. Group B is a primary cause of sporadic cases among children and adults. In the 1990s, a rising incidence of Group C infections among young college-aged adults has been noted.

Several meningococcal vaccines are in current use. The two-valent (A+C) meningococcal polysaccharide vaccine is commonly used in Europe, the Middle East, and Africa. The four-valent meningococcal polysaccharide vaccine (A, C, Y, and W-135) has been used in North America since 1982.

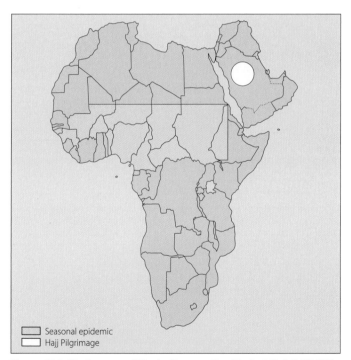

Figure 10.6 Meningococcal Meningitis map. Quadrivalent (A,C,Y, W-135) vaccine is recommended for travelers to Africa's sub-Saharan 'meningitis belt' (in red) during the dry season from December through June. However, out of season epidemics have recently begun to occur in Ethiopia, Somalia and Tanzania. Occasionally, meningococcal epidemics may extend to other 'meningitis-prone' sub-Saharan countries such as Angola, Democratic Republic of Congo, Zambia, Mozambique, Uganda, Rwanda, Burundi and Tanzania. Vaccination is also required for persons traveling to Mecca, Saudi Arabia for the annual Hajj Pilgrimage

Protein conjugate vaccines for Serogroups A, C, and A+C combination are now available in several countries. A meningococcal serogroup C conjugate (MCC) vaccine was approved for use in the UK in 1999.

Indications

Meningococcal vaccine (A+C serogroup vaccine or preferably, the quadrivalent A,C,Y, W-135 vaccine) is recommended for travelers to Africa's sub-Saharan 'meningitis belt' during the dry season from December through June, especially if prolonged contact with the local populace is likely. The countries include Benin, Burkina Faso, Cameroon, Central African Republic, Chad, Cote D'Ivoire, Djibouti, Ethiopia, Gambia, Ghana, Guinea, Guinea Bissau, Mali, Niger, Nigeria, Senegal, Sudan, Somalia, and Togo. Out of season epidemics have recently begun to occur in Ethiopia, Somalia and Tanzania indicating possible changes in epidemiologic trends perhaps due to climatic changes. Occasionally, meningococcal epidemics may extend to other 'meningitis-prone' sub-Saharan countries such as Angola, Democratic Republic of Congo, Zambia, Mozambique, Uganda, Rwanda, Burundi and Tanzania.[102,106] International agencies and NGOs are increasingly recommending vaccination of staff to these 'meningitis-prone' countries and especially for travelers to areas with current outbreaks. Pilgrims participating in the Hajj and Umra pilgrimages in Saudi Arabia are at a higher risk of meningococcal disease. As of 2002, the Saudi Arabia Embassy requires proof of vaccination with the quadrivalent vaccine before issuing the entry visas for the Hajj pilgrimage.

In the USA, entering college freshman (including foreign student/ travelers coming to the USA) that will live in residence halls or dormitories on campus should consider the quadrivalent meningococcal polysaccharide vaccine. A widespread immunization campaign among young adults and college-aged students in the UK using the meningococcal serogroup C conjugate vaccine was implemented in the late 1990s, due to high incidence of predominantly serogroup C disease in this age group, twice the national average.[107,108] Students traveling internationally to the US and UK for study and staying in dormitories should be advised to receive the meningococcal vaccine. Some other countries are beginning to adopt similar guidelines.

Meningococcal vaccine is also recommended for all travelers with anatomical or functional asplenia, and those with component deficiencies in the terminal common complement pathway (C3, C5–C9), since individuals with these conditions are at increased risk of death from overwhelming sepsis from meningococcal infections.

Contraindications

Anaphylactic reaction to thimerosal or a previous dose of the vaccine. Meningococcal vaccine should not be given in pregnancy unless substantial risk exists.

Precautions

Delay vaccination if moderate or severe illness present.

Dosing schedules for adults

The quadrivalent meningococcal polysaccharide vaccine consists of a single dose of 0.5 mL by subcutaneous injection to adults. This vaccine should be administered 1–2 weeks before departure to allow maximum antibody response (estimated efficacy 85–90%). If the vaccine is required for entry into a country, it must be administered at least 10 days prior to entry.

Measures of immune response/duration of immunity/ protection

Immune response to the vaccine is serogroup specific, and consists mainly of polysaccharide antibodies. Adults who received immunization with quadrivalent (A, C, Y, W-135) or bivalent (A+C) meningococcal polysaccharide vaccine and who continue high risk of exposure to meningococcal disease may be considered for revaccination within 3–5 years. Similarly, young college-aged adults may be given a booster dose at 3 years for continued risk of exposure.

The polysaccharide vaccines do not appear to decrease meningococcal carriage among vaccine recipients. Thus, during an outbreak, close contacts and others with significant exposure to diagnosed cases of meningococcal disease should be given antibiotic prophylaxis (ciprofloxacin or rifampin) even if they have been previously immunized with a meningococcal polysaccharide vaccine in order to control transmission. However, in a one year follow-up study among a population of young adults <18 years of age who were immunized with the meningococcal serogroup C protein conjugate vaccine, carriage of meningococci serogroup C was reduced by 66% one year later.[107]

Adverse events

Minor side-effects consisting of local pain, swelling and erythema at the site of injection, and rarely, a low-grade fever, have been reported.

Drug and vaccine interactions

There are no specific drug or vaccine interactions.

Rabies vaccine

Rabies is transmitted in most countries of the world. The difference among countries is in the degree of the endemicity. Countries with higher prevalence of rabies include countries in South Asia (the Indian subcontinent), Southeast Asian countries especially Thailand, and countries in Central and South America such as Brazil, Bolivia, Colombia, Ecuador, El Salvador, and Guatemala (Fig. 10.7). Absence of rabies is reported from selected countries in Europe, Oceania, Australia, New Zealand, and some countries in Asia and Africa (Table 10.4)

WHO defines a rabies-free country as one with no animal or human cases for two consecutive years. Some rabies-free countries have had no cases in 100 or more years while others have been considered rabies free for much shorter periods of time so that the list may change slightly on an ongoing basis. Surveillance is better in more developed countries than in less developed countries. Small numbers of fatal human case of bat Lyssavirus infection have occurred in Scotland and in Australia, both considered rabies-free, in recent years. Bat Lyssaviruses (5 or more species) and rabies virus are closely related members of the Lyssavirus family and several of them may cause clinical rabies in terrestrial mammals including humans. European bat Lyssavirus is carried by insectivorous bats in several European countries, some of which are considered rabies-free, and does not transmit readily to terrestrial species so that human infection is rare. Risk to travelers from these Lyssaviruses is virtually non-existent and rabies pre-exposure immunization is not recommended. Post-exposure rabies prophylaxis may be considered for documented bat bites in rabies-free countries with known endemicity of bat Lyssaviruses. Regular occupational exposure to bats might be considered an indication for rabies pre-exposure vaccination even in rabies-free countries.

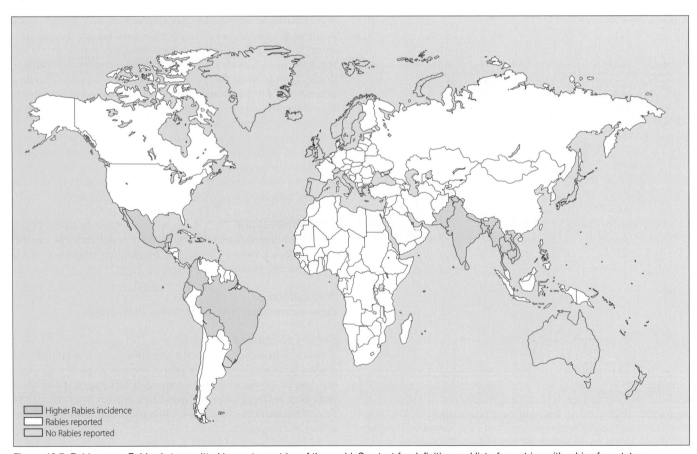

Higher Rabies incidence
Rabies reported
No Rabies reported

Figure 10.7 Rabies map. Rabies is transmitted in most countries of the world. See text for definition and list of countries with rabies free status. Countries with the highest prevalence of rabies include countries in South Asia and the Indian Subcontinent. Countries in Central and South America especially Bolivia, Colombia, Ecuador, El Salvador, and Guatemala and most countries in Africa are thought to have somewhat higher risk than most developed countries but surveillance is poor. In most developing countries with rabies vaccine is recommended for all prolonged stays as well as for shorter stays at locations more than 24 hours travel from a reliable source of post-exposure rabies vaccine; occupational exposure; all children; all adventure travelers, cave explorers and backpackers

Table 10.4	Rabies-free countries of the world. Adapted from the World Survey for Rabies No. 35. 2002. World Health Organization. Geneva and Office International des Epizooties (OIE) www.oie.int accessed November 2002				
North America	**Central and South America**	**Europe, Eastern Europe and the Independent Soviet States**	**Africa**	**Asia**	**Western Pacific**
Bermuda	Anguilla, Antigua and Barbuda, Bahamas, Barbados, Cayman Is., Dominica, Falkland Is., Guadeloupe, Jamaica, Martinique, Montserrat, Netherlands Antilles (Bonaire, Curaçao, Saba, Sint Maarten, and Saint Eustatius), Saint Kitts (Saint Christopher) and Nevis, St-Helena, Saint Lucia, Saint Vincent and Grenadines, and Virgin Is., (U.K. and U.S.). Turks-Caicos, Uruguay, and Wake Is.	Andorra, Azores, Belgium, Canary Is., Channel Is., Cyprus Faroe Is., Finland, Gibraltar, Greece, Iceland, Ireland, Italy, Liechtenstein, Luxembourg, Madeira Is., Malta, Monaco, Norway, Portugal, San-Marino, Sweden, Switzerland#, United Kingdom# and Vatican-City	Cape Verde, Mauritius, Réunion, and Seychelles	Armenia, Bahrain, Brunei-Darussalam, Comoros, Cyprus, Hong Kong, Japan, Kuwait, Macao, Maldives, Qatar, Singapore, and Taiwan.	American-Samoa, Australia#*, Christmas Is, Cook Is, Fiji, French Polynesia, Guam, Kiribati, Marshall Is., Micronesia, New Caledonia, New Zealand, Nauru, Northern-Mariana Is., Niue, Palau, Papua New Guinea, Pitcairn, Samoa, Sao-tome-Principe, Solomon Is., Tonga, Tuvalu and Vanuatu

*Bat rabies may exist. # Rabies free in terrestrial animals.

Transmission is primarily by dogs in Asia, Africa, and Latin America. However other animals implicated in transmission of rabies include cats, monkeys, tigers, rabbits, rats, mongoose and squirrels. Small rodents, although highly susceptible to rabies, transmit rabies poorly to humans and therefore are not major vectors. Bats play an important role in rabies transmission in the USA and increasing in other parts of the world. Important vectors in Europe, Canada, Alaska, and the former Soviet Union include foxes and the raccoon dog.

There are many different rabies vaccine formulations available throughout the world. Among all the rabies vaccine products, the modern cell culture vaccines (CCV) are the safest and the most immunogenic.[109] The vaccine strain may be grown in either cultured human diploid or other animal cell lines and then inactivated by beta-propiolactone, or by formalin. HDCV (human diploid cell vaccine) and PCECV (chick embryo cell vaccine) vaccines are the CCV distributed the most widely. Distribution of RVA (fetal rheus cell) is more limited. The commonly used human diploid cell vaccine (HDC) contains <150 mcg of neomycin and may contain phenolsulfonphthalein. Rabavert (Chiron) a PCECV uses a different rabies strain and contains chlortet-racycline, amphotericin B and gelatin in addition to the components in HDCV.

The production cost of these cultured cell vaccines is high, making the CCV vaccines relatively unaffordable and thus not always easily available in many developing countries. Partial doses of the CCV manufactured for intramuscular use have been used in some developing countries as multi-site intradermal doses at one sitting to decrease costs.[110] While this is an area of intense investigation by WHO and others, the vaccine antigen has not been standardized for this application, such practices are not approved or condoned, and carry the risk of suboptimal or negligible protection in the vaccine recipient. Only rabies vaccine specifically formulated and standardized for intradermal immunization should be administered by this route to travelers. In case of an animal exposure during travel, the immune status of a traveler pre-immunized with an unapproved intradermal regimen cannot be assessed and they must be considered unimmunized and given a full post-exposure rabies regimen anyway.

Indications

Rabies is not a common travel acquired infection but has potentially long latency and uniformly fatal outcome. Advice on avoiding animal contact is essential for pre-travel counseling. Expatriates and young children who are less likely to report animal bites are at higher risk.[111] Pre-exposure vaccination should be recommended for the following groups below.

■ Long-term travelers or expatriates going to countries where rabies is a threat, including most countries in Asia (except Taiwan and Japan), Africa, and Latin America.

■ Shorter-duration travelers at high-risk for exposure during travel, such as those who are very likely to come in contact with animals in dog rabies enzootic areas (see risk groups above) and where immediate access to appropriate medical care, including CCV vaccine and rabies immunoglobulin (RIG), might be limited. Risk groups include, adventure travelers, bikers, hikers, cave explorers, or busi-ness travelers who travel for short but frequent trips and plan to go running outdoors on these trips.

■ Persons with potential occupational exposure.

All travelers going to rabies endemic areas should be advised to immediately cleanse the animal bite wounds, scratches or saliva contact by vigorous scrubbing with soap and water, followed by an immediate evaluation at a local hospital. The protocol shown in Figure 10.8 should be followed. If pre-exposure rabies immunization was with a non-cell culture derived vaccine or the bitten individual has any underlying health condition which might compromise the immune response to vaccination, and the bite injury/risk of exposure is considered severe, then such persons should receive a full 5-dose series of CCV rabies vaccine for post-exposure treatment in addition to rabies immune globulin (RIG).[112] Increasingly human RIG (HRIG) which is necessary if there is no history of pre-exposure immunization, is either scarce or only rabies immune globulin of equine origin is available (ERIG). Although the adverse event rate (serum sickness) is low with purified ERIG, unpurified ERIG may carry a higher risk of reactions. The availability and purity of these products is difficult to verify in advance.

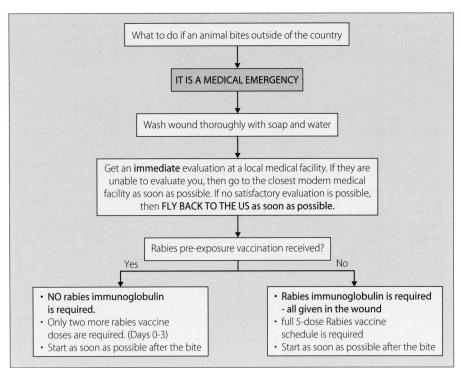

Figure 10.8 Algorithm regarding advise to traveler in the event of an animal bite in a rabies-endemic country

Contraindications

Hypersensitivity to a previous dose of the vaccine or any of the components of the vaccine used is a contraindication for rabies vaccination. Persons with a history of 'immune-complex-like' hypersensitivity from a HDCV rabies vaccine dose should not get more doses of HDCV unless a high risk bite has occurred, and RVA or PCEC vaccines are not available.

Precautions

The earlier rabies vaccines were derived from infected brain/neural tissue of animals (Semple vaccines) or cultured in embryonated duck eggs (duck embryo vaccine or DEV). These older vaccines were less efficacious than the modern CCVs and were associated with potentially severe adverse effects. The neural tissue derived vaccines contained myelin basic protein, which has been associated with the development of myeloencephalitis. Because of cost, the older types of vaccines are available and still commonly used in Asia, Africa and Latin America. Travelers should be specifically advised to avoid these vaccines should post-exposure immunization be required during travel to developing countries.

Immunosuppression can interfere with the development of immunity after rabies immunization. Immune compromised individuals should consider postponing activities for which rabies pre-exposure prophylaxis is indicated, if possible. At-risk immune compromised persons should be vaccinated only by the IM route and response confirmed by antibody titers.

Dosing schedules for adults

The widely available CCV against rabies are considered interchangeable. The standard primary pre-exposure cell culture vaccine (CCV) series consists of 3 doses of 1.0 mL each given intramuscularly in the deltoid on days 0, 7, and 21 or 28. An approved regimen of primary rabies immunization using a formulation of HDCV (Imovax) for intradermal use and consisting of 3 doses of 0.1 mL over 28 days is no longer manufactured.

In case of continuous occupational risk a single intramuscular booster dose of 1.0 mL of CCV may be given every 2 years. Serology can be done to assess need for boosters or the individual simply boosted. A booster is recommended if the titer falls below 1:5 serum dilution by the rapid fluorescent focus inhibition test.[113] However, for the majority of travelers that do receive the rabies pre-exposure prophylaxis such as expatriates to endemic countries, the risk is infrequent enough not to need a booster or need serologic testing. This is based on data showing good anamnestic responses to the 2 post exposure rabies booster doses in those who had been vaccinated remotely. The imme-diate post-exposure care of the wound and evaluation by a local facility is critical to the appropriate management of bites in pre-vaccinated individuals while in endemic areas.

Accepted and possible accelerated schedules

For persons traveling imminently, the rabies pre-exposure vaccination can be accelerated to a schedule of three injections given on days 0, 7 and 21 days.

Measures of immune response and duration of immunity/protection

There have been no placebo controlled randomized studies on efficacy. However, three doses given during 21–28 day schedule induce antibodies in 100% of individuals. An estimated 50 000 persons per year receive pre-exposure vaccination in the USA, with no reported rabies cases in persons receiving adequate post-exposure immunization. The approved intradermal HDCV rabies vaccine series formerly used is less immunogenic than the intramuscular series but is still generally considered adequate. For post-exposure immunization, there is 100% protective efficacy if the patient received RIG appropriately (see Fig. 10.8) and the first HDCV dose soon after the bite.

Adverse events

Injection site pain is observed in 25% of the recipients. Other adverse effects noted with the CCV rabies vaccine include headache, nausea, abdominal pain, muscle aches, and dizziness (occurring in approximately 20%). Urticaria, pruritus, and malaise or other 'immune-complex-like' illness may be experienced by 6% of persons receiving HDCV booster vaccinations. Urticaria was noted in a small number of recipients of PCECV.

Inactivated nerve tissue vaccines made from the brains of adult animals or suckling mice (Semple vaccines) that are available in many developing countries may induce neuroparalytic reactions among approximately 1/200 to 1/2000 persons and 1/8000 persons vaccinated respective. Travelers need avoid these vaccines.

Drug and vaccine interactions

The intramuscular formulations of the rabies CCV do not have any specific drug interaction. Concurrent use of chloroquine phosphate and possibly other structurally related antimalarials such as mefloquine may interfere with antibody response to intradermal HDCV. In situations where the antimalarials need to be started before travel, intramuscular HDCV should be administered.

Japanese encephalitis vaccine

Japanese encephalitis (JE) is a mosquito (*Culex* species) transmitted flavivirus infection that is endemic in Asia (Fig. 10.9 Japanese Encephalitis Map). In temperate regions the transmission season generally extends from April through November with a peak in July–September. In tropical or subtropical regions of Oceania and Southeast Asia transmission may occur year round. JE is mostly a disease in rural areas where enzootic cycle exits between the mosquitoes and domestic livestock. Humans become infected incidentally in these rural surroundings, as a result of deforestation and development. Increased risk is associated with monsoons and increased irrigation of rice-paddy fields. Occasionally, epidemics have been reported in suburban areas of large cities in these countries such as from Hanoi (Vietnam), Lucknow (India), Bangkok (Thailand), Beijing and Shanghai (China).[113]

The most widely available JE vaccine (JEV) is the formalin inactivated mouse brain derived vaccine that is produced by the Research Institute of Osaka University (Biken) and distributed in most other countries by Aventis Pasteur. The killed vaccine is produced from JE virus infected mouse brain and undergoes a process of purification, inactivation and precipitation. Gelatin is used as a stabilizer and thimerosal is the preservative used in the vaccine. The vaccine contains no detectable myelin basic protein. A Beijing-1 strain vaccine is mostly used in Japan whereas the Nakayama virus strain vaccine is used worldwide. Although the Beijing-1 strain JEV produces higher neutralizing titers and confers broader antibody response to the JE strains, the Nakayama strain JEV is equally effective and meets standard of efficacy. JEV is also produced in People's Republic of China (Taiwan), India, Japan, the Republic of Korea, Thailand and Vietnam. China produces both an inactivated and a live attenuated Japanese encephalitis vaccine.

Indications

Factors for considering the JEV are the duration of stay in endemic area, extent of outdoor activities especially in rural areas, and season of travel. Extremes of age are associated with a higher likelihood of developing symptomatic disease. Japanese encephalitis infection in a pregnant woman may potentially cause an intra-uterine fetal infection or death.

An average short-term traveler's risk of acquiring JE during travel to endemic countries is extremely low. The following traveler itineraries may justify JE vaccination of travelers:
- Persons expatriating to JE endemic countries
- Consider JEV for travelers who plan to spend two (WHO guideline) to 4 (CDC guideline) weeks or more in endemic areas particularly in rural areas during the transmission season. Travelers planning extensive unprotected outdoor, evening and night time exposure in rural areas may be at risk even if the trip is very short. Risk of transmission is higher in rural areas, especially where pigs are raised and where rice fields, marshes and standing pools of water provide breeding grounds for mosquitoes and feed for birds
- Since there is no clear data on the duration of immune response from natural infection, immigrants returning to their home countries should be vaccinated with the same guidelines as natives of industrialized countries

Regardless of vaccination status, travelers should be counseled to take precautions against mosquito bites.

Contraindications

Because of the risk of allergic reactions with the JEV (see Adverse events below) this vaccine should not be used or used cautiously in persons with a history of urticaria, asthma, allergic rhinitis, multiple allergies and allergies to bee stings. The vaccine is contraindicated in persons who have had a reaction to a previous dose of the vaccine or a history of anaphylaxis to any of the components of the vaccine such as thimerosal. JEV should not be given in pregnancy.

Precautions

Since JEV has been associated with delayed hypersensitivity reactions, the manufacturer recommends it should be completed at least 10 days prior to departure although most but not all of the reported delayed reactions occur within the first 48 h. Vaccine recipients should be advised about allergic signs and symptoms that should prompt early care at an appropriate health care facility.

Dosing schedules for adults

The primary schedule in adults is a series of 3 doses of 1.0 mL of JEV administered by subcutaneous injection on a schedule of 0, 7, and 30 days. At the present time it is estimated that the immunity should last for at least 3 years after primary immunization series. In some Asian countries, the primary JEV series includes only two vaccine doses (separated by 4 weeks) followed by a booster dose in 1 year and every 2 years until 15 years of age.

Accepted and possible accelerated schedules

Patients leaving the country imminently can receive an accelerated schedule of vaccine doses on days 0, 7, and 14, so that immunization can be completed in 14 days. However the patient should still remain in the country for 10 days after the last vaccine dose because of the potential of delayed reactions.

Two JEV doses given 1 week apart will induce immunity in about 80% of recipients. This schedule should be used where adherence to the recommended schedules is not possible, such as a person expected to have a high-risk exposure but leaving imminently. Due to the risk of delayed reactions, observation time after the second dose should still be kept in mind when deciding to give 2 doses in someone leaving soon. Single JEV dose yields minimal efficacy and therefore is not helpful.

Measures of immune response and duration of immunity/protection

The immunogenicity to the JEV varies slightly with the vaccine viral strain used, the schedule (2-dose versus 3-dose) and interval between the doses. The 2-dose schedule as used in some Asian countries induces neutralizing antibodies in approximately 94–100% of the vaccinees. Antibody levels decline in the first 12 months after vaccination. However, antibody response increases to 100% after boosters at 1 year.[114,115]

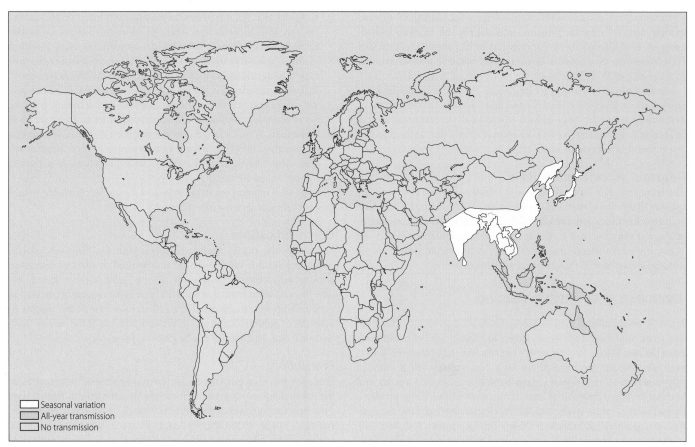

Seasonal variation
All-year transmission
No transmission

Figure 10.9 Japanese Encephalitis map. Yellow shading indicates areas where transmission is seasonal generally May to November with a July to September peak. Red shading indicates year-round transmission. Transmission to humans on mainland Australia probably does not occur. Vaccination is indicated for all persons expatriating to JE endemic countries even if they will be primarily urban dwellers. Consider vaccination for travelers who plan to spend two (WHO guideline) to 4 (CDC guideline) weeks or more in endemic areas particularly in rural areas during the transmission season. Travelers such as bicyclists, hikers and adventure travelers planning extensive unprotected outdoor, evening and night time exposure in rural areas may be at risk even if the trip is very short

The 3-dose series provides higher neutralizing antibody levels. The 3-dose schedule induces antibody responses in more than 90% of the recipients.[116,117] The antibody levels are higher in patients receiving the non-accelerated schedules (i.e., 0, 7, 28 day versus 0, 7 and 14 day).[113] Vaccination with 1 dose does not provide adequate protection. Two doses of the JEV results in 80% protection from JE infection in the first year after vaccination.[118] Three doses provide close to 100% protection.[119,120] With the 3-dose primary series as advised in most countries outside Asia, the protective levels at 12 months were similar to those at 3 years after vaccination.[120] Vaccination with JEV may also provide some cross-immunity against other flaviviruses infections such as dengue, and possibly West Nile virus.[121] Persons with immunodeficiency such as HIV/AIDS may not mount an adequate response to the JEV.[122]

Adverse events

Injection site pain and redness has been reported in approximately 20% of the vaccinees. The occurrence of some side effects was reported in up to 50% of the vaccinees, which included fever, headache, malaise, rash, myalgias, nausea, emesis and dizziness.[123] Overall, the estimated risk of reaction to the JEV is 2.8 and 15/100 000 doses in Japan and the USA respectively.

Neurological side-effects including encephalitis, encephalopathy, seizures and peripheral neuropathy in the order of 1–2.3 per million vaccinees occur.[124,125]

In rare cases, anaphylaxis or respiratory distress has occurred. The rates of these reactions with the JEV vary from 1–64/10 000 doses. In Japan rates of hypersensitivity (9.4 million doses given between 1996–1998) and the USA (more than 813 000 doses distributed from 1993–1998) are 0.8 and 6.3/100 000 doses respectively.[125] In the US data of the 42 reports of allergic reactions, 22 (52%) required an emergency room visit and six required hospitalization for 1–2 days. The etiology of the reactions is not clear however gelatin has been implicated due to presence of serum anti-gelatin IgE in children with immediate-type allergic reactions with JEV. Reactions did not vary by amount or type of gelatin present in the vaccines.

Drug and vaccine interactions

Co-administration of other travel vaccines is not considered a risk factor for increasing adverse reactions to JEV.

Tick-borne encephalitis vaccine

Tick-borne encephalitis (TBE) is one of the most prominent tick transmitted *Flavivirus* central nervous system infections in Europe and parts of Asia. In Europe, TBE prevalence extends from Belgium to Austria. European countries with higher prevalence include The Czech Republic, Slovakia, Hungary, Austria, Switzerland, Germany, Poland, Lithuania, Estonia, Latvia and Sweden. TBE is prevalent focally in the Scandinavian countries and extends east to Siberia in former Russia.

There are 2 subtypes – the central European subtype in central Europe (Central European Encephalitis, CEE), and the Far Eastern subtype found mainly in the Asian part of the Russian Federation (Russian Spring and Summer Encephalitis, RSSE). TBE occurs mainly in the rural, forested regions and up to altitudes of 1000 m. It occurs seasonally May/June to September/October in areas of endemicity. The European disease is milder (case fatality 1–2%) than the RSSE (case fatality of 20%). Symptoms of the disease range from meningitis to severe meningoencephalitis with significant residual neurologic sequelae (see Fig. 10.10).

Currently there are two chick-cell culture derived formalin inactivated TBE vaccines in use in Europe, Encepur® (Chiron) and FSME-IMMUN® (Baxter AG), manufactured in Germany and Austria respectively. These vaccines are not available in the US, but the FSME-IMMUN® is available by special release in Canada and both vaccines are available in the UK on a named patient basis. A Russian mouse brain derived inactivated TBE vaccine is not used any more because of myelin associated adverse effects. An immune globulin (IG) preparation (FSME-BULIN®) against TBE for passive immunization was discontinued in 2002.

Indications

Risk to travelers is low unless extensive outdoor activities are planned in forested regions of countries where TBE is prevalent. In endemic areas, including parts of Germany and Austria, the vaccine is incorporated into the routine pediatric schedule.

Criteria

- Active immunization with the TBE is recommended for persons planning to expatriate or live for an extended period of time in endemic countries with ongoing transmission in non-urban forested areas. Transmission does occur in some wooded sections of urban areas especially in the Baltic countries.
- Travelers going to work (e.g., farmers, woodcutters, field work) or planning on adventure travel, extensive outdoors exposure, or camping in the forests of the endemic countries during the endemic season.

Contraindications

TBE is contraindicated in persons with hypersensitivity to thimerosal (FSME-IMMUN®), gelatin (Encepur®), and eggs (both). Persons with a history of allergies or a reaction to a previous dose are at higher risk of developing a hypersensitivity reaction to the vaccine therefore should not receive it. Pregnant or lactating women, or persons with history of autoimmune diseases should undergo vaccination only if the risk of TBE disease is high and the vaccine is considered necessary.

Dosing schedules for adults

The active immunization schedule for TBE (Encepur® and FSME-IMMUN®) consists of 3 doses. The first dose of 0.5 ml is initially followed by a second dose in 4–12 weeks. The second dose should be completed at least 2 weeks before departure. A booster dose in 9–12 months from the second dose will give protection for up to 3 years. Reinforcing booster doses every 3–5 years are recommended for those at continued risk of exposure. The adult formulations of Encepur® and FSME-IMMUN can be used in adults and children older than 12 years. Due to risk of allergic reaction with these vaccines, patients should be observed for 30–60 minutes after vaccination.

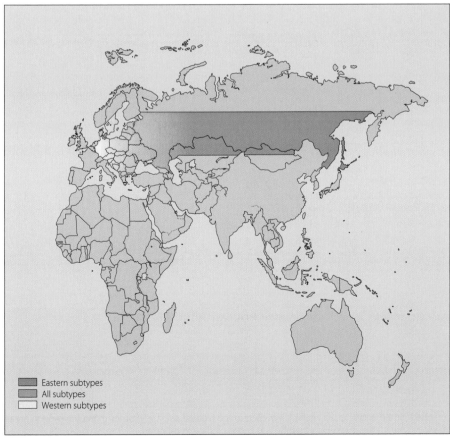

Figure 10.10 Tick-borne encephalitis map. The map shows the overall distribution of the tick-borne encephalitis. Risk to travelers is low unless extensive outdoor activities are planned in forested regions of endemic areas. Vaccine is recommended for persons planning to expatriate or live for an extended period of time in endemic countries with ongoing transmission in non-urban forested areas. Short stay travelers travelers anticipating extensive outdoors exposure such as hiking, biking or camping in the forested areas should also consider vaccine. Transmission occurs in some wooded sections of urban areas especially in the Baltic countries. Disease is more severe with the Eastern sub-type

Eastern subtypes
All subtypes
Western subtypes

Accepted and possible accelerated schedules

In limited time availability before travel, Encepur® has a registered accelerated schedule of 3 TBE vaccine doses given at days 0, 7, and 21 days with a booster at 1 year. The second dose of the FSME-IMMUN® can be given 2 weeks after the first with the third dose still 9–12 months after the second. However, these patients should receive a booster in 12–18 months after the third dose. Additional boosters every 3–5 years may be required in continued exposure.

Measures of immune response and duration of immunity/protection

Both the TBE vaccines induce seroconversion rate of 87%.[126] Seroconversion with Encepur® is 50% after the first dose, 98% and 99% after the second and third dose respectively. The antibodies induced are protective towards all strains of the TBE.[127] Thus far there have been no reported cases of TBE in vaccinated individuals. Persons previously vaccinated against yellow fever may have an enhanced antibody response to the TBE.

Adverse events

Local reactions can occur with both. Occasionally fatigue, nausea, lymphadenitis or headaches occur.[128] Fever and rash may be seen. Rarely neurological side-effects such as neuritis have been reported however causal relationship is not clear. Aggravation of underlying autoimmune diseases such as multiple sclerosis and iridocyclitis has also been reported with TBE vaccination. The Encepur® was associated with a higher risk of allergic reactions, especially in children. The allergic reactions are potentially IgE mediated reactions against the gelatin. Post-marketing surveillance of the Encepur® has shown that allergic reactions following vaccination were less than 1 for every 100 000 doses sold.

Drug and vaccine interactions

Limited data is available about concomitant administration of other medications or vaccinations. Manufacturer information states that persons who have received their primary vaccination with FSME-immun® mount an adequate (4-fold) response to booster with Encepur®. No time interval separation is required for other live or inactivated vaccinations.

Cholera vaccine

The risk of cholera to an average traveler is extremely low (0.01 to 0.001% per month of stay in a developing country).[129] The highest incidence (72%) of the cholera cases in the world, occur in Africa (Fig. 10.11). The large numbers of cases currently being reported are from Africa predominantly from South African and Democratic Republic of Congo, Mozambique, and Malawi. The current pandemic is showing signs of waning in Latin America and the Middle East since 1998 but still ongoing in other affected regions of the world. In Bangladesh and India a substantial number of cases are also caused by *V. cholerae* O139 which is not affected by current vaccines.

Cholera occurs mainly in countries with poor sanitation, and inadequate food and water hygiene. Contaminated water transmission of cholera may be through municipal water in a city with an ongoing epidemic, water from ponds and rivers or other standing water bodies, ice made of contaminated water, or water stored in large open containers. Host factors such as history of achlorhydria, *H. pylori* infection, and persons with blood group O may increase the risk of acquiring cholera.

Newer cholera vaccines include live attenuated oral vaccines and killed whole cell (KWC) oral vaccines (see Tables 10.1 and 10.2). The

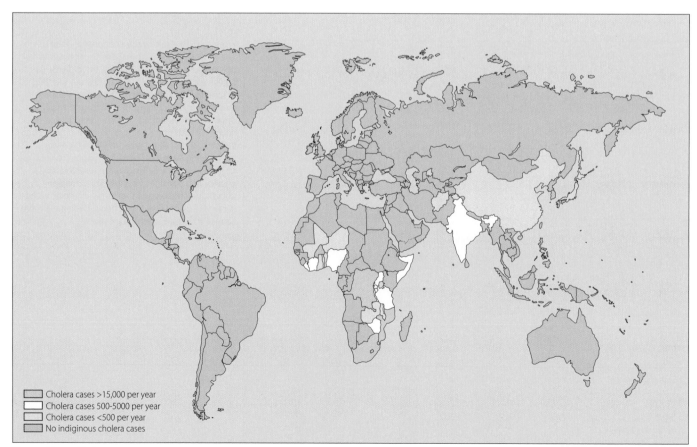

Cholera cases >15,000 per year
Cholera cases 500-5000 per year
Cholera cases <500 per year
No indiginous cholera cases

Figure 10.11 Cholera map. Vaccination is only recommended for aid and refugee workers traveling to the highest risk areas or for those traveling to areas with a current epidemic. Although epidemic in Latin America in the 1990s, there are currently few cases of cholera reported.

CVD 103 HgR oral cholera vaccine contains a genetically engineered mutant *V. cholerae* Inaba strain, but although it has the genes for the cholera toxin B subunit, it does not produce the cholera toxin.[130]

The KWC oral vaccines contain the formalin and heat-inactivated whole bacterial cells from the *V. cholerae* O1 Inaba, Ogawa and El Tor strains and either a nontoxic B subunit of the cholera toxin or a recombinant B subunit of the toxin (Dukoral®). Aside from Dukoral®, another KWC vaccine without the B subunit is produced in Vietnam for local use that is found to be safe in children and adults and also being produced in Indonesia.[131]

The parenteral cholera inactivated vaccine used in many years past is currently not widely available or used. Immunization with that vaccine resulted in short-lived and incomplete protection, as it was only about 50% effective in reducing clinical illness with the O1-type cholera strain for 3–6 months after vaccine administration. It did not provide protection against the new Bengal strain (O139 type).

Indications

Cholera vaccine is not required for entry into any country under current WHO International Health Regulations. Cholera vaccine is not recommended for the short-term tourists traveling to an endemic country. Immunization may be recommended for travelers who plan extensive travel or work in highly endemic/epidemic areas under unsanitary conditions and without access to Western style medical care. Persons particularly at risk are healthcare providers and aid workers in epidemic areas.

Contraindications

The live attenuated oral cholera CVD-103 HgR vaccine is extremely safe. As with other live attenuated vaccines, the vaccine should not be given to immunosuppressed patients or those with chronic liver disease. There is no data on safety in pregnant women. The killed whole cell recombinant B subunit (KWCbS) oral cholera vaccine also appears to be extremely safe, and the only contraindication is intolerance to a previously administered dose. The inactivated parenteral cholera vaccine has no specific contraindications except pregnancy, where data is lacking. It is contraindicated for simultaneous use with yellow fever since it may interfere with the immune response against the latter.

Dosing schedules for adults

The CVD 103-HgR vaccine is given in a single dose of 5×10^9 CFU of lyophilized CVD 103-HgR, provided in a sachet. In addition, a buffer made of sodium bicarbonate and ascorbic acid with aspartame (sweetener) is also provided. The contents of the buffer are mixed in 100 ml of clean cold or lukewarm water before the vaccine is added. It is taken at least 1 h before a meal. Boosters are recommended every 6 months.

The KWC B-subunit oral cholera vaccine (Dukoral®) is taken in 2 doses, separated by 7–42 days. The series should be restarted if more than 42 days elapse. Each dose consists of 1 mg nontoxic subunit B and 10^{11} killed *V. cholerae* taken with an alkaline buffer mixed in a glass of water. The vaccine is taken on an empty stomach (1 h before or 2 h after a meal). A booster of the same dose is recommended every 2 years for repeated exposure.

Measures of immune response and duration of immunity/protection

CVD 103-HgR oral cholera vaccine

The immune response with the old parenteral killed vaccine is approximately 50% for 6 months. Vibriocidal titers decrease significantly after the first year of the initial vaccination. However, the protective efficacy can be maintained for 3–4 years with 6 monthly boosters.

Although the duration of immunity with the live attenuated cholera vaccines is not much better than the inactivated parenteral vaccine, the efficacy of the CVD 103-HgR is considerably improved.[132] A single dose of CVD 103-HgR vaccine confers approximately 95% protection against moderate to severe cholera and approximately 80% protection from any cholera diarrhea. A study of CVD 103-HgR among US volunteers, showed a protective efficacy of 91% in preventing moderate to severe diarrhea and an overall efficacy of 80%, suggesting that it should be effective among travelers from industrialized countries to areas of cholera endemicity.[133] The onset of protection is as early as 8 days and remaining at the same level for at least 6 months. It provides protection against cholera caused by either Classical, El Tor biotypes irrespective of the serotypes of *V. cholerae*.

The oral KWC-recombinant B subunit toxin vaccine has a protective efficacy of about 85–90% in the first 6 months, 58% at the end of 1 year however, it drops to less than 50% after that.[134–137] The protective efficacy against Classical and El Tor cholera is similar in the first 6 months however, it is lower against El Tor than classical biotype 3 years following the initial series. The oral KWC-B subunit toxin vaccine has some protective efficacy (approx. 50%) against enterotoxigenic *E. coli* (ETEC) infection, a common cause of traveler's diarrhea.[138,139]

The basis of this is immunologic cross reactivity between the b subunit of cholera toxin and the LT toxin (heat labile) of ETEC.

Dukoral® is registered for protection against travelers' diarrhea in Canada, Sweden, and Norway. Licenses for this indication is pending in the EU and many other countries as of 2003. ETEC is responsible for less than 50% of the cases of travelers' diarrhea. After a primary series boosters need to be given every 3 months.

Adverse events

Both the CVD 103-HgR and oral KWC vaccines are safe and appear to be well-tolerated in adults without a significant difference of reported side-effects compared with placebo.

Drug and vaccine interactions

The live attenuated CVD 103-HgR vaccine efficacy may be decreased by the concurrent use of antibiotics, proguanil and chloroquine, and therefore should be separated by at least 1 week before and after vaccination. However, mefloquine has not shown to have a similar effect. Additionally, because of the different buffers in the CVD 103-HgR vaccine and the oral live attenuated typhoid vaccine, it is recommended that the 2 vaccines be separated by at least 8 h. It can be administered with yellow fever concurrently.[140]

Vaccine response may be decreased with concurrent administration of the KWC parenteral cholera and the yellow fever vaccines. When possible, these should be separated by an interval of 3 weeks. However, due to time constraints, they may be administered simultaneously with the realization that protection may be limited against both diseases.

ROUTINE VACCINES

Tetanus and diphtheria

Tetanus is ubiquitous worldwide. Diphtheria transmission is likely to be increased in areas of the world where immunization programs have not yet reached coverage goals and socio-economic conditions favor disease transmission. The tetanus and diphtheria (Td) combined vaccine is recommended for primary immunization and booster doses in children >7 years and in adults (Fig. 10.1). The diphtheria toxoid content in Td vaccine is lower than in the pediatric DTaP, DTP or DT vaccines for children less than 7 years old, to decrease the likelihood of local side-effects at the site of injection. In some countries, the Td combination vaccine is not available, and monovalent tetanus toxoid vaccine is used to booster adult immunity against tetanus. Travelers receiving tetanus only boosters would be unprotected against diphtheria.

Indications

All adult and pediatric travelers should be up-to-date on tetanus and diphtheria immunizations, appropriate for age, because of the possibility of accidental injury and ubiquitous risk of tetanus inoculation into wounds and potential exposure to diphtheria. In particular, travelers to the former Soviet Union, Albania, Haiti, Dominican Republic, Ecuador, Brazil, Philippines, Indonesia, and countries in Africa and Asia should be updated.

Short-term and long-term travelers should at least have completed their primary series before travel. Particular attention should be paid to persons likely to engage in high risk activities such as construction, adventure travel, back-packing and low-budget travel, and living with local people.

Contraindications

Contraindications to immunization with Td include the presence of a moderate or severe illness with or without fever, the history of a neurologic or severe hypersensitivity reaction following a prior dose of Td, or known allergy to a vaccine component such as thimerosal or gelatin.

Precautions

Vaccination should be deferred for 3 months if immunosuppressive medications will be discontinued shortly. Immune deficiency disorders and immunosuppressive therapies may reduce the immune response to the vaccine. A prolonged interval between doses does not require reinitiating the primary series.

Dosing schedules for adults and children >7 years old

Adults should receive at least three or preferably four primary Td doses before travel to area of risk. The 0.5 ml Td dose is given by intramuscular injection in the deltoid area. The first two doses are given 4–8 weeks apart, followed by a third dose, 6–12 months later. The same brand should be used to complete the primary series as much as possible, especially for the first three doses. In case of imminent departure at least two doses should be completed, if possible. Travelers should be advised to complete the series in their destination country in situations of prolonged expatriation and inability to complete the primary Td series before departure.

If the primary series has been completed but 10 years or more have elapsed since the last dose, a booster Td should be given before departure to cover diphtheria risk, even in countries where routine tetanus immunization is not recommended as frequently as on a 10 year basis.

Children and adolescents who completed a primary series before age 7 years should receive the first booster dose with Td vaccine starting in adolescence 10 years after the last primary dose. In the USA only, the first Td booster dose is recommend at 11–12 years of age provided at least 5 years have passed since last primary dose of DTP, DTaP, or DT.

Measures of immune response and duration of immunity/protection

Tests to measure serum antibody levels against tetanus, diphtheria, and pertussis are not routinely available.

Adverse effects

Local adverse effects including injection site redness, swelling, tenderness, and/or induration are common. Painful swelling from elbow to shoulder may occur 2–8 h after injection, most often in adults who have received frequent booster doses of Td. Rarely, anaphylaxis, generalized rash/itching, fever, systemic symptoms, occurrences of brachial neuritis and Guillain-Barré syndrome have been reported.

Polio vaccine: oral (OPV) and inactivated (IPV)

Poliovirus is an enteric virus transmitted by oral-fecal contamination of food and water in areas of poor sanitation. Thus, immunization against polio is recommended for travel to all developing countries where poliovirus is still transmitted. Due to the current global eradication program, polio has been eradicated from most countries in the world while being near eradication in most others (Fig. 10.12). Polio is considered eradicated from all parts of the world except on the Indian sub-continent and in Africa and adult boosters therefore would be advised for those going to these. Although most African countries do not report current polio cases, possible under-reporting or inadequate surveillance would make it prudent to boost travelers to all African countries until the WHO African region is certified polio-free. The current target for worldwide polio eradication is 2005.

Indications for polio vaccines

Persons traveling to currently polio-endemic countries and have previously completed a 3-dose primary vaccine series should receive a one-time single dose of polio vaccine as a booster if the last dose or booster dose was at least 10 years or more. Either inactivated polio vaccine (IPV) or oral live attenuated polio vaccine (OPV) (if available) may be used for the booster regardless of the type of polio vaccine used for primary immunization. Persons who previously received less than the full 3-dose primary series of polio vaccine should be given the remaining doses in the series with either IPV or OPV, regardless of the interval since the last dose and the type of vaccine previously administered. If possible, non-immune adults should receive the full 3-dose primary series of IPV before traveling to countries with endemic or epidemic wild poliovirus circulation.

Dosing schedules for both IPV and OPV

The primary immunization schedule for adults consists of 3 doses of 0.5 mL IPV administered by i.m. injection at 0, 2, and 8–14 months.

The OPV prepackaged liquid dose is administered orally according to package insert directions. The schedules for OPV in adults are the same as the IPV above. The use of the OPV, when available, is reserved for outbreak situations, or recommended when an unimmunized traveler is unable to get two doses of the inactivated vaccine.

Accelerated schedules for both IPV and OPV

Previously unimmunized travelers and/or those whose immunization status is unknown should complete the primary 3-dose IPV series before travel to a polio endemic or epidemic area. The minimum recommended interval between OPV or IPV doses is 4 weeks. When the traveler is leaving imminently and time is short, the following schedules can be used:

- If at least 8 weeks available: three doses of IPV given 4 weeks apart.
- If 4–8 weeks available: two doses of IPV given 4 weeks apart.
- If less than 4 weeks available: a single dose of OPV or IPV is recommended and the remaining doses should be completed at the travel destination if the traveler remains at risk.

Inactivated polio vaccine

Contraindications

IPV should not be given to persons with a history of anaphylactic reaction to neomycin, polymyxin B or streptomycin.

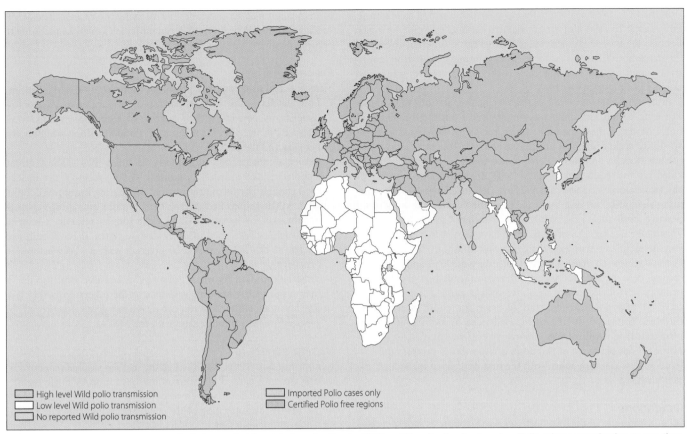

Legend:
- High level Wild polio transmission
- Low level Wild polio transmission
- No reported Wild polio transmission
- Imported Polio cases only
- Certified Polio free regions

Figure 10.12 Poliomyelitis 2002 map. Polio is targeted for global eradication by 2005 and the situation is changing. Polio primary vaccination or one-time adult boosters are recommended for persons traveling to areas not certified to be polio-free yet. In addition, vaccine related polio cases in the Philippines Haiti and Dominican Republic warrant polio vaccination for travel to these areas.

Precautions

Vaccination should be delayed if moderate or severe illness present, and caution used in vaccinating persons with bleeding disorders or on anticoagulants. Breast-feeding mothers may receive IPV.

Side-effects

Injection site pain, fever; rarely: anaphylaxis or other systemic effects.

Oral polio vaccine

Oral polio vaccine (OPV) is used for primary polio immunization or booster doses when IPV is unavailable or contraindicated. Many countries still use the OPV in their vaccination programs. Among travelers, OPV can be used (when available) for immunization of travelers to a polio endemic or epidemic area. In particular it can be administered if travel has to be started before the completion of the primary immunization with IPV. OPV is no longer in use in the USA.

Contraindications

OPV should not be given to patients with immune deficiency diseases. IPV should be used to vaccinate immunodeficient persons and their household contacts. OPV should not be used in family members or close contacts of persons with compromised immunity.

Precautions

OPV may be given on the same day or 30 days after other live-virus vaccines. OPV is a live virus and guidelines for administering live viral vaccines to immunocompromised individuals need to be follow-ed (See Chapter 25). Tuberculin testing should be done either on the same day that oral polio vaccine is given or 4–6 weeks later. OPV and oral typhoid vaccine can be administered concurrently. OPV can be given to breast-feeding mothers.

Adverse events

All vaccine recipients should be informed of the exceedingly rare risk of vaccine-associated paralytic poliomyelitis (VAPP) from OPV. The estimated risk of VAPP is 1 in 2.4 million OPV doses.

Drug and vaccine interactions

Oral polio vaccine can be taken concurrently or without a waiting interval after having received gamma globulin for hepatitis A prevention. OPV may be given concurrently with other live viral or bacterial vaccines, and with inactivated or toxoid vaccines.

Measles, mumps, and rubella vaccine (MMR)

Documented immunity to measles is highly recommended for all international travelers, as this infection, like other common childhood viral diseases, is characterized by higher rates of complications when contracted by susceptible adults. Measles transmission has been higher in certain tropical developing countries because of the lack of sufficient childhood immunization programs, and the necessity of maintaining cold storage of vaccine doses for retention of vaccine potency. The incidence of measles in developing countries in temperate climates has also been affected by the status of childhood immunization programs. The World Health Organization is actively working on global eradication of measles.

In the USA, persons born before 1957 are presumed to have immunity against measles and do not require vaccination prior to travel. Because the measles epidemiology is different in different countries, the presumptive cutoff year for measles immunity varies from country to country. For example 1970 is the cutoff year for presumed measles immunity in Canada.

Prior to 1967, inactivated measles vaccine preparations were in use, and long-lasting immunity was not assured from these immunizations. Many of these measles vaccine recipients developed a severe syndrome called atypical measles when subsequently exposed to natural measles infection. Persons previously vaccinated with the killed vaccine require revaccination with the live vaccine to gain reliable protection. Vaccines employing live attenuated measles virus came into use in 1963, but were not used in routine childhood vaccination practice until the 1970s. While these vaccines appear to be more immunogenic, decades of experience have shown that up to 5% of vaccine recipients may experience waning immunity in adult years. For this reason, in many countries including the USA and Canada, a second dose of measles vaccine is recommended at the time of primary school, secondary school or college entry if not previously received and documented, and likewise for adult international travelers. Immunity to measles is evidenced by documentation of physician-diagnosed measles, laboratory evidence of measles immunity, or proof of receipt of two doses of live measles vaccine administered at least 1 month apart, with the first dose given on or after the first birthday.

Indications

All non-immune adults traveling to endemic countries should receive the MMR or monovalent measles vaccine before leaving, particularly those that are staying for longer duration in developing countries. MMR has a higher rate of adverse events, secondary to the rubella component, so that if induction of measles immunity is the goal, then many clinicians prefer to administer monovalent measles vaccine. Immigrants who return to their home countries and have no documentation of the disease or clear clinical history should have their serologies tested and managed according to the immune status.

Contraindications

The MMR or monovalent measles vaccine should not be given if there has been a serious allergic reaction to a previous dose or if there is a history of anaphylaxis to neomycin. Persons with a history of anaphylactic reactions to gelatin containing products should be immunized with caution under close supervision. There have been several case reports of severe allergic reactions following receipt of MMR vaccine among persons with a history of gelatin allergy. Allergy to eggs or egg protein is not a contraindication to receiving the vaccine. The MMR vaccine should not be given to pregnant females or those planning to become pregnant within 1 month

Precautions

Three unusual situations exist regarding administration of this vaccine:

1 Low platelets – The measles portion of the vaccine may cause low platelets in persons with a history of thrombocytopenia (low platelets) in the past. Immunization should be done weighing the benefits and the possible risks.

2 Recent administration of Immune Globulin (IG) – The immune response to the measles component of the vaccine is diminished for a variable period of time after administering Immune Globulin (IG). MMR should be deferred for 3 months after post-exposure prophylaxis for hepatitis A and for a longer, undefined interval after higher doses used in other disease states. If IG is indicated for travel, the MMR should be given at least 2 weeks before IG. (Table 10.5)

3 Tuberculosis skin testing – Because this is a live viral vaccine, it may suppress the immune response to the tuberculosis skin test. The Mantoux (PPD) skin test can be reliably given concurrently or 4–6 weeks after immunization with the MMR.

Dosing schedule

In non-immune adults, two doses of the measles vaccine separated by at least 1 month is used for primary immunization. A single measles or MMR vaccine dose is given to complete the 2-dose series, if the initial MMR immunization with a live attenuated measles vaccine after 1963 is documented.

Adverse effects

The MMR vaccine is generally well tolerated. Ten to fourteen days after vaccination, 1 in 15 recipients can develop a red maculopapular, often confluent rash, a fever and a flu-like syndrome, with fever lasting 1–2 days, due to the vaccination. These persons are not contagious for measles. Minor side-effects include local discomfort at the site of injection, headache and malaise. Side-effects from the second dose are less frequent than with the first dose.

There is a rare risk of rubella vaccine-associated arthritis reported among women of reproductive age groups.

Measures of immune response and duration of immunity/protection

Serum antibody tests for measles, mumps, and rubella are used to measure immunity to each individual disease, and are widely available through public and private laboratories.

Table 10.5	Interaction between immune globulin with MMR and varicella vaccines		
	Recommended time intervals between receipt of immune globulin (IG) and MMR vaccine		
Sequence of IG administration	If IG for hepatitis A has been received *before* the Measles MMR vaccine:	If high-dose IG or measles IG has been received *before* the Measles or MMR vaccine:	If IG for hepatitis A must be administered *after* the measles or MMR vaccine:
Measles or MMR (Measles–Mumps–Rubella) vaccine	Wait 3 months	Wait 5–11 months	Wait at least 2 weeks
	Recommended time intervals between receipt of immune globulin (IG) and varicella vaccine		
Sequence of IG administration	If IG for Hepatitis A or IG or VZIG has been received *before* Varicella vaccine:	If IG for Hepatitis A must be administered *after* varicella vaccine	If high-dose IG or VZIG must be administered *after* varicella vaccine
Varicella vaccine (chickenpox)	Wait 5 months	Wait at least 3 weeks	Wait at least 2 months

Varicella vaccine (chickenpox vaccine)

There is no data to date on the incidence of varicella infection in travelers. It is known, however, that varicella is a disease of adolescents and young adults in tropical, non-industrialized countries, as opposed to being a disease of childhood in temperate climates. The susceptible traveling adult or adolescent may therefore be at increased risk when traveling to these areas.[141,142] Traveling adults who have not had a definitive case of varicella should strongly consider vaccination. People who are unsure about whether or not they have had the disease should consider having their blood tested to determine immunity. Varicella vaccine is only available in a limited number of countries.

Indications

All healthy, non-pregnant international travelers without evidence of varicella immunity, particularly those who plan to have close personal contact with local populations, should consider immunization. Susceptible individuals age 13 or older should be immunized because the disease can be more severe and have more complications in this age group. Varicella vaccine is also recommended for non-immune non-pregnant adults who live in households with children, who work in daycare facilities, or are exposed to settings of high transmission risk (colleges, military or correctional institutions).

Contraindications

Varicella vaccine is a live attenuated virus vaccine, and the usual precautions in pregnant women and compromised hosts apply (see Chapters 20 and 25). It is, however, permissible to vaccinate any household members living with a pregnant or lactating woman. Contraindications to immunization are a history of an anaphylactic reaction to neomycin or gelatin, or to a previous varicella vaccine dose. Active, untreated tuberculosis is a contraindication. Vaccination should be delayed for 6 months following the prior receipt of IG or varicella zoster immune globulin (VZIG) (See Table 10.5). For optimal efficacy, the vaccine must be stored frozen and be reconstituted within 30 min prior to administration or the vaccine must be discarded.

Precautions

Vaccine recipients should not become pregnant for 1–3 months after vaccination. PPD tests should be done either the same day or 4–6 weeks after receiving varicella vaccination. Vaccine candidates should be asked if there is a family history of immunodeficiency or if they are living in a household with high-risk persons. Vaccinees should avoid household contact with pregnant women lacking documented immunity to varicella and any immunocompromised individual for 6 weeks after receiving varicella vaccine especially if rash develops after the vaccine. Patients who are transplantation candidates should receive the varicella vaccine (at least 6 weeks before transplantation). Aspirin therapy, particularly in children and adolescents, should be withheld for 6 weeks after immunization.

Dosing schedules for adults

The varicella vaccine schedule for individuals aged 13 years or older consists of 2 doses of 0.5 mL administered by subcutaneous injection in the deltoid area, given 4–8 weeks apart (if more than 8 weeks elapse following first dose, the second dose can be administered without restarting the schedule).

Measures of immune response and duration of immunity/protection

The varicella vaccine is highly effective, giving 97–99% protection against varicella when dosing recommendations are followed. Booster doses are not recommended at this time. However, there are ongoing clinical trials investigating the efficacy of giving varicella vaccine to older individuals to boost immunity to varicella-zoster virus, to prevent onset and recurrence of shingles.[142]

Varicella vaccination is effective in preventing or modifying the varicella disease severity if given to a non-immune individual within 72 h (or even within 5 days) of exposure to someone with varicella. The vaccine should be administered on the standard schedule given above.

Adverse events

Side-effects are reported to be mild and may include redness, induration, swelling and transient pain at injection site, and fever. A varicella-like rash (local or generalized) may develop in 3–6% of vaccinees, with the occasional reaction typically noted within 2 days of vaccination and the generalized reaction typically noted within 2–3 weeks of vaccination. Herpes zoster following vaccination in healthy children is a rare occurrence (18/100 000 person-years of follow-up) and has been mild and without complications.

Drug and vaccine interactions

Varicella vaccine should be delayed by 5 months after having received immunoglobulin for hepatitis A (both 0.02 ml/kg or 0.06 ml/kg doses). Intervals for live attenuated vaccines and PPD testing should be followed.

Influenza vaccine

For international travelers, the decision about influenza vaccination is dependent on several risk factors: general health status, travel destination, and availability of the vaccine. Travelers with medical conditions placing them at high risk of complications from influenza should receive the vaccine regardless of destination or duration of travel. After diarrhea, respiratory illness is the most common cause of morbidity in travelers, likely due to close contact travelers have with large numbers of other people in close quarters. The recent SARS epidemic has illustrated this point. Evidence from the occupational medicine literature suggests that annual influenza illness ameliorates absenteeism due to all respiratory illness and not just influenza. Thus, influenza vaccination may be considered for all other travelers if they are going to a temperate zone during the influenza season, or to the tropics irrespective of the time of the year (since influenza is non-seasonal in the tropics). An increased risk of influenza has been reported among cruise ship passengers particularly during the summer Alaska cruise season, possibly because of other passengers and travel personnel originating in the Southern Hemisphere.

If the planned travel is during the influenza season and if the current year's vaccine is available, then that particular vaccine should be used. For travelers from the temperate Northern Hemisphere going to the subtropical Southern Hemisphere from May through October, the most recent influenza vaccine should be used if they were not vaccinated the previous fall or winter.

Indications

Annual influenza vaccination is recommended for adults at risk because immunity declines in the year following vaccination, and the vaccine antigens are changed annually in order to increase antigenic similarity between the vaccine and strains of influenza that are in circulation.[143] In the USA, the influenza vaccine is recommended as part of the routine adult immunization schedule for persons over 50 years of age without specific risk factors. Persons below 50 years of age may receive the influenza vaccine as desired. In most other countries with routine influenza vaccine programs vaccination is recommended for those over age 65 and those with chronic disease at any age.

The antiviral drugs rimantadine or amantadine may be used for prevention of type A influenza when influenza vaccine is unavailable, and to augment protection for immunodeficient persons, who may have a poor antibody response to the vaccine. The antiviral drug oseltamivir provides protection against types A and B influenza, and may be similarly used for chemoprophylaxis. However, antiviral chemoprophylaxis should not be substituted for vaccination unless vaccination is contraindicated or unavailable.

Contraindications

Influenza vaccination is contraindicated in patients with a history of anaphylaxis or hypersensitivity to a previous dose, to egg or egg protein. Allergy to vaccine components such as gelatin or thimerosal is a contraindication. Do not use influenza vaccine in persons with a past history of Guillain-Barré syndrome. Breast-feeding is not a contraindication for vaccination.

Immunization schedules for adults and children

For adults and children over 12 years of age, the influenza vaccine schedule consists of a single dose of the current year's vaccine given as an intramuscular injection, annually. The vaccine dose may possibly vary with manufacturer.

Measures of immune response and duration of immunity/protection

Immune response to influenza vaccination is both humoral and cell-mediated. Hemagglutination-inhibition antibodies correlate with protection against disease. Immune response among healthy adults less than 65 years of age varies approximately 70–90%. This response varies with age being lower among persons older than 65 years. Nonetheless, the influenza vaccine is effective in preventing secondary complications and decreasing the risk for influenza-related hospitalization and death.[144]

Adverse events

Most commonly reported side-effects of the influenza vaccine are injection site pain and swelling.[145] Fever, malaise, muscle pain infrequently occur 6–12 h after vaccination. Hypersensitivity reactions (hives, angioedema, allergic asthma, and systemic anaphylaxis) are rare and when they occur, may be related to remnant egg protein.

Pneumococcal polysaccharide vaccine (23-valent)

Streptococcus pneumoniae is a major cause of mortality and morbidity worldwide, affecting both children and adults. The estimated incidence of pneumococcal infections in travelers is not clearly defined. However, in numerous studies 25–30% of travelers suffer from respiratory illnesses related to travel. While it is probable that most are viral in nature however; pneumococcal infections are probably included in such estimates. The global emergence of penicillin or multi-drug resistant *S. pneumoniae* (PRSP or DRSP) coupled with potentially limited antimicrobial availability in numerous countries also needs to be considered when reviewing the need for pneumococcal vaccination for the traveler.[146,147]

Indications

The pneumococcal polysaccharide vaccine is recommended for persons aged 65 and older, including previously unvaccinated persons and persons who have not received vaccine within 5 years (and were <65 years of age at the time of vaccination).[148] Others at higher risk for severe pneumococcal disease such as the elderly, immunocompromised persons including those with AIDS, asplenia, sickle cell disease and those with chronic liver disease or other chronic diseases such as chronic renal failure, chronic liver disease (cirrhosis), diabetes mellitus, and chronic pulmonary disease should receive the vaccine before travel.

The vaccine may be considered for healthy persons 2–64 years of age if they are planning to expatriate for a prolonged duration of time to a country with high PRSP rates. Otherwise healthy persons with cochlear implants should also receive the pneumococcal vaccine for prevention of pneumococcal meningitis.[149]

Contraindications

The vaccine is contraindicated in persons with a history of anaphylactic reaction to thimerosal or a previous dose of pneumococcal polysaccharide 23-valent vaccine. Pneumococcal vaccine may be used in pregnancy if clearly indicated.

Precautions

Vaccination should be delayed if moderate or severe illness present (oral penicillin chemoprophylaxis is another method of preventing pneumococcal infection). Use caution in vaccinating persons with bleeding disorders or on anticoagulation.

Dosing schedules

Primary immunization consists of a single dose of 0.5 mL given by either intramuscular or subcutaneous injection. Booster doses are not routinely recommended, except in the following circumstances:

- For persons aged ≥65, give booster dose of vaccine if patient received vaccine ≥5 years previously and was <65 years of age at the time of vaccination.
- For persons aged 2–64 years with functional or anatomic asplenia; for persons >10 years of age, give a single booster ≥5 years after previous dose
- For immunocompromised persons, give single booster dose if ≥5 years have elapsed since receipt of first dose.

Measures of immune response and duration of immunity/protection

The 23-valent pneumococcal polysaccharide vaccine induces type-specific antibody responses to the capsular polysaccharide antigens of 23 serotypes of *S. pneumoniae*. The type-specific antibodies are induced in 3–4 weeks in >80% of healthy recipients. The vaccine efficacy is estimated to be 50–70% in case control studies. Vaccination is associated with decrease in hospitalization and mortality.[150]

Adverse events

Injection site pain, redness, swelling; rarely fever, myalgias, or severe systemic effects.

Bacillus of Calmette Guerin (BCG) vaccine

Bacillus of Calmette Guerin (BCG) vaccine is a live attenuated mycobacterial vaccine utilized by many countries as a part of the childhood immunization programs. BCG immunization appears to offer some protection against extra-pulmonary tuberculosis disease in infants less than 1 year old. It is not significantly protective against pulmonary tuberculosis. In countries with a high incidence of tuberculosis, infants are routinely immunized at birth with a single dose. In countries with low incidence of tuberculosis, a single dose is often given during adolescence. Other countries, like the USA, rely on screening, case identification and treatment.

Occasionally, schools or colleges in countries where BCG is still a routine childhood vaccine require proof of vaccination for entry of students coming from countries that no longer have BCG as part of the childhood vaccination. In such circumstances, a letter explaining the home country's national immunization policy with regard to BCG vaccine may suffice. In rare circumstances, BCG vaccination may still be required. If administration of BCG vaccine is planned, information on the lack of protective efficacy in adults, risk of misinterpretation of PPD testing after BCG vaccine, and risk (although small) of vaccine-related disease in the event of immune dysfunction should be discussed with the traveler. The vaccine is contraindicated in immunocompromised individuals.[151] Some national guidelines, particularly in the UK and some British Commonwealth countries still include the use of BCG for particularly high risk travelers such as healthcare workers, aid workers, and those who expect to be living in close quarters with local people in extremely tuberculosis high risk countries.

VACCINES USED IN SPECIAL CIRCUMSTANCES

Anthrax vaccine

Although anthrax is uncommon in industrialized countries and the true global estimate is unknown, it still occurs in rural agricultural parts of many countries. Anthrax is reported from Southern and Eastern Europe, Asia, Africa, Middle East, Caribbean, Central and South America as an occupational disease among persons who work in close contact with livestock, hides, and wool, and the majority of the cases are cutaneous. Anthrax spores were used as an agent of bioterrorism in 2001. The risk of anthrax to the international traveler is negligible, not enough to warrant vaccination.

The availability of anthrax vaccine products and their formulation are variable worldwide. In the USA, the vaccine is currently available only through restricted governmental agencies. The anthrax vaccine adsorbed (AVA) was licensed for use in the USA in 1965. It is administered in 6 doses – one dose subcutaneously at 0, 2 and 4 weeks followed by a dose at 6, 12 and 18 months with annual boosters thereafter. Approximately 95% of the vaccinees demonstrate a response as measured by an indirect hemagglutination serology after three doses. The protective efficacy of the AVA is approximately 92% in preventing disease. There is no data for use of AVA in persons less than 18 years or more than 65 years of age. The duration of the efficacy is unknown. The most common side-effects of the AVA are local reactions. Severe local reactions (erythema and induration >20mm) occurred in less than 1% of the vaccinees, while moderate and mild local reactions occurred in 3% and 20% of recipients, respectively. Systemic reactions are reported in less than 0.06%. Studies are in progress evaluating side-effects, alternative routes and schedules. In case of known and documented exposure to aerosolized spores, prophylaxis with ciprofloxacin or doxycycline for 60 days should be initiated.[152]

Smallpox vaccine

Naturally occurring smallpox, caused by variola virus, was declared eradicated by the WHO in 1980. Global eradication of smallpox followed a successful WHO immunization campaign utilizing vaccinia vaccine in the preceding decades. The last case of naturally occurring smallpox was reported from Somalia in 1977. Currently, smallpox is not considered a risk for international travelers.

Supplies of the vaccinia vaccine and vaccinia immune globulin are officially controlled by national governments and existing stocks as of 2002 were all manufactured in the 1970s and 1980s. In the USA, the CDC retains a restricted supply of both products for use in individuals at high risk of exposure (such as the military, research laboratory workers, and health-care workers likely to serve as first responders in the event of a bio-terrorism attack).

Existing vaccines, such as Dryvax (Wyeth), are all crude homogenates made using bovine lymph extracted from scraped pustules on calves inoculated with vaccinia virus. The vaccine is a live attenuated virus vaccine that is administered by a unique percutaneous multiple-puncture technique with a bifurcated needle. Other routes of administration have been proven ineffective. More than 95% of vaccinees develop neutralizing antibodies within days after vaccination, with persistence of protective immunity for 5–10 years. Titers persist longer with revaccination. Adverse effects following immunization include development of a pustule, erythema, induration and tenderness at the vaccine site, and regional lymphadenitis. Inadvertent autoinoculation of the vaccine virus can result in a severe vaccinia virus infection involving the face, eyes, and other body sites. More severe side-effects include eczema vaccinatum, progressive vaccinia (vaccinia necrosum) infection, post-vaccination encephalitis, myocarditis and keratitis. The vaccine is contraindicated in persons with eczema, pregnancy, or immunodeficient states such as HIV/AIDS or other. During an outbreak of documented smallpox, the risk of exposure to smallpox versus the risks of vaccine-related complications must be weighed between the vaccine candidate and the health care provider. Vaccinia immune globulin (VIG) and cidofovir are being studied for investigational use in the management of severe adverse reactions to vaccinia vaccine. At least several hundred million doses of a new vaccinia virus vaccines, produced by Acambis and Baxter in partnership and using the same viral strain as was used in Dryvax and produced using current cell culture techniques will be ready during 2003. Proper clinical trials will need to be done prior to registration or widespread routine preventive use.[153]

Plague vaccine

Yersinia pestis, the bacterium causing plague is prevalent in many countries of Asia, Africa, Central and South America, and in parts of North America and Southeastern Europe. Disease transmission can occur through bites of infectious rat fleas, direct exposure to body fluids of infected rodents, or rarely by aerosolization. Usual short-term and long-term travelers are at negligible risk of exposure to plague. However, the risk increases with travel to rural, semi-arid and mountainous regions among travelers that hike or camp in rural locations or that handle dead or infected animals as part of their work in countries where plague is enzootic.

Access to plague vaccine is subject to regional availability and product formulations worldwide. Most plague vaccines are formalin-inactivated whole-cell bacterial vaccine. Vaccine efficacy as measured by antibodies to fraction 1 capsular antigen and the mouse protection index is only approximately 55–72% for the product commercially available in the USA up until 1999. There are limited controlled human studies evaluating vaccine efficacy, and it is not clear whether the vaccine is protective against aerosolized pulmonary infections. Plague vaccine is administered intramuscularly (in the deltoid area) in a 3-dose series. The first dose is 1.0 mL, followed by a 0.2 mL dose given 1–3 months after the first dose and 5–6 months after the second dose. Thereafter, boosters can be given every 6 months for 18 months, and every 1–2 years if the person continues to be in high exposure risk. The vaccine is approved for use only in persons 18–61 years of age. Adverse effects include local erythema, lymphadenopathy and pain (~29% of recipients). The vaccine is contraindicated in persons with a previous reaction to a dose or any of the components.

Due to lack of clear efficacy, and low risk of exposure for most travelers, plague vaccine is not routinely recommended. It may be considered for persons who are likely to work with animals such as field workers, ecologist etc. Persons at risk should be advised to use personal protective measures against flea bites, avoid contact with rodents, dead or ill animals. They should also avoid areas with ongoing epidemic. In case of a potential exposure, a seven-day course of antibiotics (tetracycline, doxycycline or trimethoprim/sulfamethoxazole) at therapeutic doses against *Yersina pestis* may be prescribed as post-exposure prophylaxis.[154]

REFERENCES

1. Monath TP, Cetron MS. Prevention of yellow fever in persons traveling to the tropics. *Clin Infect Dis* 2002; **34**(10):1369–1378.
2. McFarland JM, Baddour LM, Nelson JE *et al.* Imported yellow fever in a United States citizen. *Clin Infect Dis* 1997; **25**(5):1143–1147.
3. CDC-Anonymous. Fatal yellow fever in a traveler returning from Venezuela, 1999. *MMWR* 2000; **49**(14):303–305.
4. CDC. Fatal yellow fever in a traveler returning from Amazonas, Brazil, 2002. *MMWR* 2002; **51**(15):324–325.
5. CDC. Yellow fever vaccine. Recommendations of the Immunization Practices Advisory Committee (ACIP). *MMWR* 1990; **39**(RR-6):1–6.
6. Nasidi A, Monath TP, Vandenberg J *et al.* Yellow fever vaccination and pregnancy: a four-year prospective study. *Trans R Soc Trop Med Hyg* 1993; **87**(3):337–339.
7. Nishioka S, Nunes-Araujo FR, Pires WP, *et al.* Yellow fever vaccination during pregnancy and spontaneous abortion: a case-control study. *Trop Med Int Health* 1998; **3**(1):29–33.
8. Cetron MS, Marfin AA, Julian KG, *et al.* Yellow fever vaccine. Recommendations of the Advisory Committee on Immunization Practices (ACIP). *MMWR* 2002; **51**(RR-17):1–11.
9. Kaplan JE, Nelson DB, Schonberger LB, *et al.* The effect of immune globulin on the response to trivalent oral poliovirus and yellow fever vaccinations. *Bull World Health Organ* 1984; **62**(4):585–590.
10. Niedrig M, Lademann M, Emmerich P, Lafrenz M. Assessment of IgG antibodies against yellow fever virus after vaccination with 17D by different assays: neutralization test, haemagglutination inhibition test, immuno-fluorescence assay and ELISA. *Trop Med Int Health* 1999; **4**(12):867–871.
11. Mosimann B, Stoll B, Francillon C, *et al.* Yellow fever vaccine and egg allergy. *All Clin Immunol* 1995; **95**(5 Pt 1):1064.
12. CDC, Anonymous. Adverse events associated with 17D-derived yellow fever vaccination – United States, 2001–2002. *MMWR* 2002; **51**(44):989–993.
13. Martin M, Tsai TF, Cropp B, *et al.* Fever and multisystem organ failure associated with 17D-204 yellow fever vaccination: a report of four cases. *Lancet* 2001; **358**(9276):98–104.
14. WHO Adverse events following yellow fever vaccination. *Weekly Epidemiological Record* 2001; **76**(29):217–218.
15. Martin M, Weld LH, Tsai TF, Mootrey GT, Chen RT, Niu M, Cetron MS and the GeoSentinel Yellow Fever Working Group. Advanced age a risk factor for illness temporally associated with yellow fever vaccination. *Emerg Infect Dis* 2001; **7**(6):945–951.
16. Receveur MC, Thiebaut R, Vedy S *et al.* Yellow fever vaccination of human immunodeficiency virus-infected patients: report of 2 cases. *Clin Infect Dis* 2000; **31**(3):E7–E8.
17. Vasconcelos PF, Luna EJ, Galler R *et al.* Serious adverse events associated with yellow fever 17DD vaccine in Brazil: a report of two cases. *Lancet* 2001; **358**(9276):91–97.
18. Chan RC, Penney DJ, Little D, *et al.* Hepatitis and death following vaccination with 17D-204 yellow fever vaccine. *Lancet* 2001; **358**(9276): 121–122.
19. Adu FD, Omotade OO, Oyedele OI, *et al.* Field trial of combined yellow fever and measles vaccines among children in Nigeria. *East Af Med J* 1996; **73**(9):579–582.
20. Ambrosch F, Fritzell B, Gregor J *et al.* Combined vaccination against yellow fever and typhoid fever: a comparative trial. *Vaccine* 1994; **12**(7): 625–628.
21. Tsai, T. F., Kollaritsch H, Que JU *et al.* Compatible concurrent administration of yellow fever 17D vaccine with oral, live, attenuated cholera CVD103-HgR and typhoid ty21a vaccines. *J Infect Dis* 1999;179(2): 522–524.
22. Dumas R, Forrat R, Lang J, Farinelli T *et al.* Safety and immunogenicity of a new inactivated hepatitis A vaccine in concurrent administration with a typhoid fever vaccine or a typhoid fever + yellow fever vaccine. *Adv Therapy* 1997; 14:160–167
23. Yvonnet B, Coursaget P, Deubel V, *et al.* Simultaneous administration of hepatitis B and yellow fever vaccines. *J Med Virol* 1986; 19(4):307–311.
24. Jong EC, Kaplan KM, Eves KA *et al.* An open randomized study of inactivated hepatitis A vaccine administered concomitantly with typhoid fever and yellow fever vaccines. *J Travel Med* 2002; **9**(2):66–70.
25. Tsai TF, Bolin RA, Lazuick JS, Miller KD. Chloroquine does not adversely affect the antibody response to yellow fever vaccine. *J Infect Dis* 1986; 154(4):726-7
26. Barry M, Patterson JE, Tirrell S, *et al.* The effect of chloroquine prophylaxis on yellow fever vaccine antibody response: comparison of plaque reduction neutralization test and enzyme-linked immunosorbent assay. *Am J Trop Med Hyg* 1991; 44:79-82
27. Steffen R, Kane MA, Shapiro CN, *et al.* Epidemiology and prevention of hepatitis A in travelers. [see comments]. *JAMA* 1994; 272:885-9.
28. CDC, Anonymous. Prevention of hepatitis A through active or passive immunization: Recommendations of the Advisory Committee on Immunization Practices (ACIP). *MMWR: Recommendations & Reports.* 1999; 48(RR-12):1–37.
29. Ansdell V. Prevalence of hepatitis A antibody in travelers from Hawaii. *J Trav Med* 1994; **3**(1):27–31.
30. Hyams KC, Struewing JP, Gray GC. Seroprevalence of hepatitis A, B, and C in a United States military recruit population. *Military Med.* 1992; 157:579-82.
31. Lee KK, Beyer-Blodget J. Screening travelers for hepatitis A antibodies: an observational cost-comparison study of vaccine use. *Western J of Med* 2000; 173:325-9.
32. Werzberger A, Kuter B, Shouval D, *et al.* Anatomy of a trial: a historical view of the Monroe inactivated hepatitis A protective efficacy trial. [Review]. *J Hepatol* 1993; 18:S46-50.
33. Innis BL, Snitbhan R, Kunasol P, *et al.* Protection against hepatitis A by an inactivated vaccine. *JAMA* 1994; 271:1328-34.
34. Iwarson S, Lindh M, Widerstrom L. Excellent booster response 4-6 y after a single primary dose of an inactivated hepatitis A vaccine. *Scandinavian J Infect Dis* 2002; 34:110-1
35. Hornick R, Tucker R, Kaplan KM, *et al.* A randomized study of a flexible booster dosing regimen of VAQTA in adults: safety, tolerability, and immunogenicity. *Vaccine* 2001; 19:4727-31.
36. Bryan JP, Henry CH, Hoffman AG, *et al.* Randomized, cross-over, controlled comparison of two inactivated hepatitis A vaccines. *Vaccine* 2000; 19:743-50.
37. Connor BA, Phair J, Sack D, *et al.* Randomized, double-blind study in healthy adults to assess the boosting effect of Vaqta or Havrix after a single dose of Havrix. *Clin Infect Dis* 2001; 32:396-401.
38. Clarke P, Kitchin N, Souverbie F. A randomised comparison of two inactivated hepatitis A vaccines, Avaxim and Vaqta, given as a booster to subjects primed with Avaxim. *Vaccine* 2001; 19:4429-33.
39. Zuckerman JN, Kirkpatrick CT, Huang M. Immunogenicity and reactogenicity of Avaxim (160 AU) as compared with Havrix (1440 EL.U) as a booster following primary immunization with Havrix (1440 EL.U) against hepatitis A. [erratum appears in *J Travel Med* 1998 Sep;5(3):inside front cov.]. *J Travel Med* 1998; 5:18-22.
40. Vidor E, Xueref C, Blondeau C, *et al.* Analysis of the antibody response in humans with a new inactivated hepatitis A vaccine. *Biologicals* 1996; 24:235-42.
41. Fisch A, Cadilhac P, Vidor E, Prazuck T, Dublanchet A, Lafaix C. Immunogenicity and safety of a new inactivated hepatitis A vaccine: a clinical trial with comparison of administration route. *Vaccine* 1996; 14:1132-6.
42. Goilav C, Zuckerman J, Lafrenz M, *et al.* Immunogenicity and safety of a new inactivated hepatitis A vaccine in a comparative study. *J Med Virol* 1995; 46:287-92.
43. Van Damme P, Thoelen S, Cramm M, De Groote K, Safary A, Meheus A. Inactivated hepatitis A vaccine: reactogenicity, immunogenicity, and long-term antibody persistence. *J Med Virol* 1994; 44:446-51.
44. Briem Hp, Safary Ap. Immunogenicity and safety in adults of hepatitis A virus vaccine administered as a single dose with a booster 6 months later. *J Med Virol* 1994; 44:443-5.
45. Victor J, Knudsen JD, Nielsen LP, *et al.* Hepatitis A vaccine. A new convenient single-dose schedule with booster when long-term immunization is warranted. [see comments.]. *Vaccine* 1994; 12:1327-9.
46. Leentvaar-Kuijpers, A., Coutinho, R. Brulein V, Safary A. Simultaneous passive and active immunization against hepatitis A. *Vaccine* 1992; 10: S138-41
47. Shouval D, Ashur Y, Adler R, *et al.* Safety, tolerability, and immunogenicity of an inactivated hepatitis A vaccine: effects of single and booster injections, and comparison to administration of immune globulin. *J Hepatol* 1993; 18:S32-7.
48. Tilzey AJ, Palmer SJ, Harrington C, O'Doherty MJ. Hepatitis A vaccine responses in HIV-positive persons with haemophilia. *Vaccine* 1996; 14:1039-41.
49. Arguedas MR, Johnson A, Eloubeidi MA, Fallon MB. Immunogenicity of hepatitis A vaccination in decompensated cirrhotic patients. *Hepatology* 2001; 34:28-31.

50. Stark K, Gunther M, Neuhaus R, *et al.* Immunogenicity and safety of hepatitis A vaccine in liver and renal transplant recipients. *J Infect Dis* 1999; 180:2014-7.

51. Nalin DR, Kuter BJ, Brown L, *et al.* Worldwide experience with the CR326F-derived inactivated hepatitis A virus vaccine in pediatric and adult populations: an overview. [Review]. *J Hepatol* 1993; 18:S51-5.

52. Bock HL, Kruppenbacher JP, Bienzle U, De Clercq NA, Hofmann F, Clemens RL. Does the concurrent administration of an inactivated hepatitis A vaccine influence the immune response to other travelers vaccine. *J Travel Med* 2000; 7:74-8.

53. Walter EB, Hornick RB, Poland GA, *et al.* Concurrent administration of inactivated hepatitis A vaccine with immune globulin in healthy adults. *Vaccine* 1999; 17:1468-73.

54. Zanetti A, Pregliasco F, Andreassi A, *et al.* Does immunoglobulin interfere with the immunogenicity to Pasteur Merieux inactivated hepatitis A vaccine? *J Hepatol* 1997; 26:25-30.

55. Shouval D, Ashur Y, Adler R, *et al.* Single and booster dose responses to an inactivated hepatitis A virus vaccine: comparison with immune serum globulin prophylaxis. *Vaccine* 1993; 11:S9-14.

56. Zaaijer H, Leentvaar-Kuijpers A, Rotman H, Lelie P. Hepatitis A antibody titres after infection and immunization: implications for passive and active immunization. *J Med Virol* 1993; 40:22-7.

57. CDC Anonymous. Hepatitis B virus: a comprehensive strategy for eliminating transmission in the United States through universal childhood vaccination. Recommendations of the Immunization Practices Advisory Committee (ACIP). *MMWR. Recommendations & Reports* 1991; 40:1-25.

58. Zuckerman, J. N. and R. Steffen. Risks of hepatitis B in travelers as compared with immunization status. *J Travel Med.* 2000; 7(4):170-174.

59. Steffen, R. Risks of hepatitis B for travellers. *Vaccine* 1990; 8(suppl):S31-S32; discussion S41-S43.

60. Zuckerman JN, Sabin C, Craig FM, Williams A, Zuckerman AJ. Immune response to a new hepatitis B vaccine in healthcare workers who had not responded to standard vaccine: randomised double blind dose-response study. *BMJ* 1997; 314:329-33.

61. Poland GA. Hepatitis B immunization in health care workers. Dealing with vaccine nonresponse. *Am J Prev Med* 1998; 15:73-7.

62. Engler SH, Sauer PW, Golling M, *et al.* Immunogenicity of two accelerated hepatitis B vaccination protocols in liver transplant candidates. *Eur J of Gastroenterology & Hepatology* 2001; 13:363-7.

63. Marchou B, Excler JL, Bourderioux C, *et al.* A 3-week hepatitis B vaccination schedule provides rapid and persistent protective immunity: a multicenter, randomized trial comparing accelerated and classic vaccination schedules. *J Infect Dis* 1995; 172:258-60.

64. Anonymous (CDC) Health Information for International Travel. US Department of Health and Human Services, 2002.

65. Jack AD, Hall AJ, Maine N, Mendy M, Whittle HC. What level of hepatitis B antibody is protective? *J Infect Dis* 1999; 179:489-92.

66. Francis DP, Hadler SC, Thompson SE, *et al.* The prevention of hepatitis B with vaccine. Report of the centers for disease control multi-center efficacy trial among homosexual men. *Ann of Int Med* 1982; 97:362-6.

67. Krugman S, Holley HPJ, Davidson M, Simberkoff MS, Matsaniotis N. Immunogenic effect of inactivated hepatitis B vaccine: comparison of 20 microgram and 40 microgram doses. *J Med Virol* 1981; 8:119-21.

68. Horlander JC, Boyle N, Manam R, *et al.* Vaccination against hepatitis B in patients with chronic liver disease awaiting liver transplantation. *Am J Med Sci* 1999; 318:304-7.

69. Mahoney F, Kane M. Hepatitis B Vaccine. In: Plotkin S, WA O, eds. *Vaccines.* Philadelphia, PA: WA Saunders, 1999.

70. Wainwright RB, Bulkow LR, Parkinson AJ, Zanis C, McMahon BJ. Protection provided by hepatitis B vaccine in a Yupik Eskimo population—results of a 10-year study. *J Infect Dis* 1997; 175:674-7.

71. McMahon BJ, Helminiak C, Wainwright RB, Bulkow L, Trimble BA, Wainwright K. Frequency of adverse reactions to hepatitis B vaccine in 43,618 persons. *Am J Med* 1992; **92**(3):254-256.

72. Confavreux C, Suissa S, Saddier P, Bourdes V, Vukusic S, Vaccines in Multiple Sclerosis Study Gp. Vaccinations and the risk of relapse in multiple sclerosis. Vaccines in Multiple Sclerosis Study Group. *N Eng J Med* 2001; 344:319-26.

73. Coursaget P, Fritzell B, Blondeau C, Saliou P, Diop-Mar I. Simultaneous injection of plasma-derived or recombinant hepatitis B vaccines with yellow fever and killed polio vaccines. *Vaccine* 1995; 13:109-11.

74. Burgess MA, Rodger AJ, Waite SA, Collard F. Comparative immunogenicity and safety of two dosing schedules of a combined hepatitis A and B vaccine in healthy adolescent volunteers: an open, randomised study. *Vaccine* 2001; 19:4835-41.

75. Greub G, Genton B, Safary A, Thoelen S, Frei PC. Comparison of the reactogenicity and immunogenicity of a two injection combined high-dose hepatitis A and hepatitis B vaccine to those of Twinrix. *Vaccine* 2000; 19:1113-7.

76. Nothdurft HD, Dietrich M, Zuckerman JN, *et al.* A new accelerated vaccination schedule for rapid protection against hepatitis A and B. *Vaccine* 2002; 20:1157-62.

77. Van Damme P, Leroux-Roels G, Law B, *et al.* Long-term persistence of antibodies induced by vaccination and safety follow-up, with the first combined vaccine against hepatitis A and B in children and adults. *J Med Virol* 2001; 65:6-13.

78. Kallinowski B, Knoll A, Lindner E, *et al.* Can monovalent hepatitis A and B vaccines be replaced by a combined hepatitis A/B vaccine during the primary immunization course?. *Vaccine* 2000; 19:16-22.

79. Caumes E, Ehya N, Nguyen J, Bricaire F. Typhoid and paratyphoid fever: a 10-year retrospective study of 41 cases in a Parisian hospital. *J Travel Med* 2001; 8:293-7.

80. Ackers ML, Puhr ND, Tauxe RV, Mintz ED. Laboratory-based surveillance of Salmonella serotype Typhi infections in the United States: antimicrobial resistance on the rise. *JAMA* 2000; 283:2668-73.

81. Steffen, R. Hepatitis A and hepatitis B: risks compared with other vaccine preventable diseases and immunization recommendations. *Vaccine* 1993; **11**(5):518-520.

82. Rowe B, Ward LR, Threlfall EJ. Multidrug-resistant Salmonella typhi: a worldwide epidemic. [Review]. *Clin Infect Dis* 1997; 24:S106-9.

83. Cryz SJJ, Pasteris O, Varallyay SJ, Furer E. Factors influencing the stability of live oral attenuated bacterial vaccines. Developments in *Biological Standardization* 1996; 87:277-81.

84. Simanjuntak CH, Paleologo FP, Punjabi NH, *et al.* Oral immunisation against typhoid fever in Indonesia with Ty21a vaccine. *Lancet* 1991; 338:1055-9.

85. Levine MM, Ferreccio C, Cryz S, Ortiz E. Comparison of enteric-coated capsules and liquid formulation of Ty21a typhoid vaccine in randomised controlled field trial. *Lancet* 1990; 336:891-4.

86. Acharya IL, Lowe CU, Thapa R, *et al.* Prevention of typhoid fever in Nepal with the Vi capsular polysaccharide of Salmonella typhi. A preliminary report. *N Eng J Med* 1987; 317:1101-4.

87. Engels EA, Falagas ME, Lau J, Bennish ML. Typhoid fever vaccines: a meta-analysis of studies on efficacy and toxicity. *BMJ* 1998; 316:110-6.

88. Klugman KP, Gilbertson IT, Koornhof HJ, *et al.* Protective activity of Vi capsular polysaccharide vaccine against typhoid fever. *Lancet* 1987; 2:1165-9.

89. Plotkin SA, Bouveret-Le Cam N. A new typhoid vaccine composed of the Vi capsular polysaccharide. *Arch Intern Med* 1995; 155:2293-9.

90. Lebacq E. Comparative tolerability and immunogenicity of Typherix or Typhim Vi in healthy adults: 0, 12-month and 0, 24-month administration. *Biodrugs* 2001; 15:5-12.

91. Levine MM, Ferreccio C, Black RE, Germanier R. Large-scale field trial of Ty21a live oral typhoid vaccine in enteric-coated capsule formulation. *Lancet* 1987; 1:1049-52.

92. Ferreccio C, Levine MM, Rodriguez H, Contreras R. Comparative efficacy of two, three, or four doses of TY21A live oral typhoid vaccine in enteric-coated capsules: a field trial in an endemic area. *J Infect Dis* 1989; 159:766-9.

93. Wahdan MH, Serie C, Cerisier Y, Sallam S, Germanier R. A controlled field trial of live Salmonella typhi strain Ty 21a oral vaccine against typhoid: three-year results. *J Infect Dis* 1982; 145:292-5.

94. Levine, M. M. Typhoid Fever Vaccines. *Vaccine.* S. Plotkin and O. WA. Philadelphia, PA., W.B. Saunders: 1999; 781-814.

95. Cryz, S. J. Post-marketing experience with live oral Ty21a vaccine. *Lancet* 1993; 341(8836):49-50.

96. Cryz SJJ, Que JU, Levine MM, Wiedermann G, Kollaritsch H. Safety and immunogenicity of a live oral bivalent typhoid fever (Salmonella typhi Ty21a)-cholera (Vibrio cholerae CVD 103-HgR) vaccine in healthy adults. *Infect Immun* 1995; 63:1336-9.

97. Kollaritsch H, Furer E, Herzog C, Wiedermann G, Que JU, Cryz SJJ. Randomized, double-blind placebo-controlled trial to evaluate the safety and immunogenicity of combined Salmonella typhi Ty21a and Vibrio cholerae CVD 103-HgR live oral vaccines. *Infect Immun* 1996; 64:1454-7.

98. Kollaritsch H, Que JU, Kunz C, Wiedermann G, Herzog C, Cryz SJ. Safety and immunogenicity of live oral cholera and typhoid vaccines administered alone or in combination with antimalarial drugs, oral polio vaccine, or yellow fever vaccine. *J Infect Dis* 1997; 175:871-5.

99. Horowitz H, Carbonaro CA. Inhibition of the Salmonella typhi oral vaccine strain, Ty21a, by mefloquine and chloroquine. *J Infect Dis* 1992; 166:1462-4.

100. Faucher JF, Binder R, Missinou MA, Matsiegui PB, Gruss H, Neubauer R, Lell B, Que JU, Miller GB, Kremsner PG. Efficacy of atovaquone/proguanil for malaria prophylaxis in children and itseffect on the immunogenicity of live oral typhoid and cholera vaccines. *Clin Infect Dis* 2002; 35(10):1147-1154.

101. Pollard, A. J. and D. R. Shlim. Epidemic meningococcal disease and travel. *J Travel Med* 2002; 9(1):29-33.

102. Molesworth AM, Thomson MC, Connor SJ, *et al.* Where is the meningitis belt? Defining an area at risk of epidemic meningitis in Africa. *Trans R Soc Trop Med Hyg* 2002; 96:242-9.

103. Memish, Z. A. Meningococcal disease and travel. *Clin Infect Dis* 2002; 34(1):84–90.

104. Aguilera JF, Perrocheau A, Meffre C, Hahne S, Group WW. Outbreak of serogroup W135 meningococcal disease after the Hajj pilgrimage, Europe, 2000. *Emerging Infect Dis* 2002; 8:761-7.

105. WHO, Anonymous. Meningococcal disease, serogroup W135, Burkina Faso. Preliminary report, 2002. *Weekly Epidemiological Record.* 2002; 77(18):152–155.

106. WHO Anonymous. Meningococcal disease, Great Lakes area (Burundi, Rwanda, United Republic of Tanzania) – update. *Weekly Epidemiological Record* 2002; 77(38):317.

107. Maiden M, Stuart J, Group. TUMC. Carriage of serogroup C meningococci 1 year after meningococcal C conjugate polysaccharide vaccination. *Lancet* 359(9320):1829-31 2002; 359:1829-31.

108. Salisbury, D. Introduction of a conjugate meningococcal type C vaccine programme in the UK. *J Ped & Child Health* 2001; 37(5):S34–S36; discussion 37.

109. Plotkin, S. A. Rabies. *Clin Infect Dis.* 2000; 30(1):4–12.

110. Plotkin S, Rupprecht C, Koprowski H. Rabies Vaccine. In: Plotkin S, Orenstein W, eds. *Vaccines.* Philadelphia, PA: W. B Saunders, 1999:743-767.

111. Pandey P, Shlim DR, Cave W, Springer MF. Risk of possible exposure to rabies among tourists and foreign residents in Nepal. *J Travel Med* 2002; 9:127-31.

112. CDC, Anonymous. Human rabies prevention – United States, 1999. Recommendations of the Advisory Committee on Immunization Practices (ACIP). *MMWR* 1999; 48(RR-1):1–21.

113. CDC, Anonymous. Inactivated Japanese encephalitis virus vaccine. Recommendations of the Advisory Committee on Immunization Practices (ACIP). *MMWR* 1993 ;42(RR-1):1–15.

114. Rojanasuphot S, Charoensuk O, Kitprayura D, *et al.* A field trial of Japanese encephalitis vaccine produced in Thailand. *Southeast Asian J Trop Med & Pub Health* 1989; 20:653-4.

115. Tsai T, Chang G, Yu Y. Japanese Encephalitis Vaccines. In: Plotkin S, WA O, eds. *Vaccines.* Philadelphia, PA: WA Saunders, 1999.

116. Hsu TC, Chow LP, Wei HY, Chen CL, Hsu ST. A controlled field trial for an evaluation of effectiveness of mouse-brain Japanese encephalitis vaccine. Taiwan I Hsueh Hui Tsa Chih - *J of the Formosan Med Association* 1971; 70:55-62.

117. Poland JD, Cropp CB, Craven RB, Monath TP. Evaluation of the potency and safety of inactivated Japanese encephalitis vaccine in US inhabitants. *J Infect Dis* 1990;161(5):878–882.

118. Defraites RF, Gambel JM, Hoke CHJ, *et al.* Japanese encephalitis vaccine (inactivated, BIKEN) in U.S. soldiers: immunogenicity and safety of vaccine administered in two dosing regimens. *Am J Trop Med & Hyg* 1999; 61:288-93.

119. Sanchez JL, Hoke CH, McCown J, *et al.* Further experience with Japanese encephalitis vaccine. *Lancet* 1990; 335:972-3.

120. Gambel JM, DeFraites R, Hoke CJ, *et al.* Japanese encephalitis vaccine: persistence of antibody up to 3 years after a three-dose primary series. *J Infect Dis* 1995; 171:1074.

121. Hoke CH, Nisalak A, Sangawhipa N, *et al.* Protection against Japanese encephalitis by inactivated vaccines. *N Engl J Med* 1988; 319:608-14.

122. Rojanasuphot S, Shaffer N, Chotpitayasunondh T, *et al.* Response to JE vaccine among HIV-infected children, Bangkok, Thailand. *Southeast Asian J Trop Med & Pub Health* 1998; 29:443-50.

123. Nothdurft HD, Jelinek T, Marschang A, Maiwald H, Kapaun A, Loscher T. Adverse reactions to Japanese encephalitis vaccine in travellers. *J Infect* 1996; 32:119-22.

124. Jelinek, T and H. D. Nothdurft. Japanese encephalitis vaccine in travellers. Is wider use prudent? *Drug Safety* 1997; 16(3):153–156.

125. Takahashi H, Pool V, Tsai TF, Chen RT. Adverse events after Japanese encephalitis vaccination: review of post-marketing surveillance data from Japan and the United States. The VAERS Working Group. *Vaccine* 2000; 18:2963-9.

126. Demicheli V, Graves P, Pratt M, Jefferson T. Vaccines for preventing tick-borne encephalitis. *Cochrane Database of Systematic Reviews* 2000:CD000977.

127. Hayasaka D, Goto A, Yoshii K, Mizutani T, Kariwa H, Takashima I. Evaluation of European tick-borne encephalitis virus vaccine against recent Siberian and far-eastern subtype strains. *Vaccine* 2001; 19:4774-9.

128. Grzeszczuk A, Sokolewicz-Bobrowska E, Prokopowicz D. Adverse reactions to tick-borne encephalitis vaccine: FSME-Immun. *Infection* 1998; 26:385-8.

129. Ryan, E. T. and S. B. Calderwood. Cholera vaccines. *Clin Infect Dis* 2000; 31(2):561–565.

130. Levine, M. M. and J. B. Kaper. Live oral vaccines against cholera: an update. *Vaccine* 1993; 11(2):207–212.

131. Trach D, Cam P, Ke. N, *et al.* Investigations into the safety and immunogenicity of a killed oral cholera vaccine developed in Viet Nam. *Bull of the WHO.* 2002; 80:2-8.

132. Cryz SJJ, Levine MM, Kaper JB, Furer E, Althaus B. Randomized double-blind placebo controlled trial to evaluate the safety and immunogenicity of the live oral cholera vaccine strain CVD 103-HgR in Swiss adults. *Vaccine* 1990; 8:577-80.

133. Tacket CO, Kotloff KL, Losonsky G, *et al.* Volunteer studies investigating the safety and efficacy of live oral El Tor Vibrio cholerae O1 vaccine strain CVD 111. *Am J Trop Med Hyg* 1997; 56:533-7.

134. van Loon FP, Clemens JD, Chakraborty J, *et al.* Field trial of inactivated oral cholera vaccines in Bangladesh: results from 5 years of follow-up. *Vaccine* 1996; 14:162-6.

135. Graves P, Deeks J, Demicheli V, Pratt M, Jefferson T. Vaccines for preventing cholera. *Cochrane Database of Systematic Reviews.* 2000:CD000974.

136. Sanchez JL, Trofa AF, Taylor DN, *et al.* Safety and immunogenicity of the oral, whole cell/recombinant B subunit cholera vaccine in North American volunteers. *J Infect Dis* 1993; 167:1446-9.

137. Sanchez JL, Vasquez B, Begue RE *et al.* Protective efficacy of oral whole-cell/recombinant-B-subunit cholera vaccine in Peruvian military recruits. *Lancet* 1994; 344:1273-6.

138. Holmgren J, Svennerholm A. Development of oral vaccines against cholera and enterotoxinogenic Escherichia coli diarrhea. *Scandinavian J Infect Dis* 1990; 76(suppl):47–53.

139. Clemens. J, Sack D, Harris J, *et al.* Cross-protection by B subunit-whole cell cholera vaccine against diarrhea associated with heat-labile toxin-producing enterotoxigenic Escherichia coli: results of a large-scale field trial. *J Infect Dis* 1988; 158:372-7.

140. Tsai TF, Kollaritsch H, Que JU, *et al.* Compatible concurrent administration of yellow fever 17D vaccine with oral, live, attenuated p6olera CVD103-HgR and typhoid ty21a vaccines. *J Infect Dis* 1999; 179:522-4.

141. Lee BW. Review of varicella zoster seroepidemiology in India and *Southeast Asia. Trop Med Int Health* 1998; 3(11):886–890.

142. CDC, Anonymous. Prevention of varicella: Recommendations of the Advisory Committee on Immunization Practices (ACIP). Centers for Disease Control and Prevention. *MMWR. Recommendations & Reports* 1996; 45(RR-11):1–36.

143. Poland GA, Rottinghaus ST, Jacobson RM. Influenza vaccines: a review and rationale for use in developed and underdeveloped countries. *Vaccine* 2001; 19:2216-20.

144. Gross PA, Hermogenes AW, Sacks HS, Lau J, Levandowski RA. The efficacy of influenza vaccine in elderly persons. A meta-analysis and review of the literature. *Ann Intern Med* 1995; 123:518-27.

145. Margolis KL, Nichol KL, Poland GA, Pluhar RE. Frequency of adverse reactions to influenza vaccine in the elderly. A randomized, placebo-controlled trial. *JAMA* 1990; 264:1139-41.

146. Song JH, Lee NY, Ichiyama S, *et al.* Spread of drug-resistant Streptococcus pneumoniae in Asian countries: Asian Network for Surveillance of Resistant Pathogens (ANSORP) Study. *Clin Infect Dis* 1999; 28:1206-11.

147. Di Fabio JL, Castaneda E, Agudelo CI, *et al.* Evolution of Streptococcus pneumoniae serotypes and penicillin susceptibility in Latin America, Sireva-Vigia Group, 1993 to 1999. PAHO Sireva-Vigia Study Group. Pan American Health Organization. *Ped Infect Dis J* 2001; 20:959-67.

148. Poland, G. A. The prevention of pneumococcal disease by vaccines: promises and challenges. *Infect Dis Clin of N Am* 2001; 15(1):97–122.

149. CDC, Anonymous. Pneumococcal Vaccination for Cochlear Implant Recipients. *MMWR- Recommendations & Reports* 2002; 51(41):931.

150. Nichol KL, Baken L, Wuorenma J, Nelson A. The health and economic benefits associated with pneumococcal vaccination of elderly persons with chronic lung disease. *Arch Intern Med* 1999; 159:2437-42.

151. CDC, Anonymous. The role of BCG vaccine in the prevention and control of tuberculosis in the United States. A joint statement by the Advisory Council for the Elimination of Tuberculosis and the Advisory Committee on Immunization Practices. *MMWR - Recommendations & Reports* 1996; 45(RR-4):1–18.

152. CDC, Anonymous (). Use of Anthrax Vaccine in the US. Recommendations of the Adivsory Committe of Immunization Practices. *MMWR - Recommendations & Reports* 2000; 49(RR-15):1–22.

153. Breman, J. G. and D. A. Henderson. Diagnosis and management of small-pox. *N Engl J Med* 2002; 346(17):1300–1308.

154. CDC, Anonymous. Prevention of Plague. Recommendations of the Advisory Committee of Immunization Practices. *MMWR - Recommendations & Reports* 1996; 45(RR-14):1–15.

CHAPTER 11   Pediatric Vaccinations

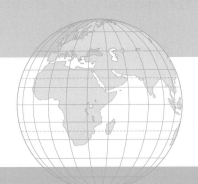

Sheila M. Mackell

KEYPOINTS

- Current recommendations for routine childhood vaccination in the USA are shown in detail as an example, but most industrialized countries follow similar schedules. Detailed information on routine recommended childhood schedules by country may be found at: www-nt.who.int/vaccines/GlobalSummary/Immunization/Country-ProfileSelect.cfm

- Polysaccharides are T-cell independent antigens, therefore, poorly immunogenic and mostly ineffective in children less than 2 years old. The most important examples are the vaccines against meningococcal meningitis (standard A+C or A/C/Y/W-135 vaccines) and typhoid (Vi polysaccharide vaccines)

- Routine pediatric vaccinations may need to be accelerated if the traveling child is departing before the primary series can be completed and he/she will be at high risk. A table showing the earliest possible age of administration and recommended minimum amount of time between doses is provided (Table 11.1)

- Safety issues generally preclude the use of yellow fever vaccine below the age of 9 months and Tick-borne encephalitis vaccines below the age of 1 year. Safety data is lacking for Japanese Encephalitis vaccine use below the age of 1 year

- Travel related vaccines for which special pediatric formulations or doses need to be used for certain age groups are: Hepatitis A, Hepatitis B, Hepatitis A/B, Tick-borne encephalitis, Japanese encephalitis, and varicella

INTRODUCTION

Vaccinating children for travel requires consideration of differences in the pediatric immune response from that of adults, the rationale for vaccine usage or omission at certain ages, and a working knowledge of the current recommendations for routine vaccinations for children. This Chapter will address vaccination considerations particular to traveling children when compared with the adult recommendations described in Chapter 10 (Table 11.1). Recommendations for updating and/or accelerating routine pediatric vaccinations as dictated by specific travel plans will be emphasized.

VACCINE CONSIDERATIONS IN INFANTS AND CHILDREN

The immune response begins *in utero*. Immunoglobulins are transferred via the placenta during the third trimester and form the beginnings of antigen response-recognition. Premature infants lack the late gestational maternal antibodies, thus are incapable of fighting many post-natally acquired infections, yet they are able to respond to vaccine antigens at an acceptable rate. Schedules for vaccinating former premature infants are identical to those of full term infants.

Vaccine response in infants and children is characterized by several factors impacting efficacy. The age of the infant or child determines the type of response. The infant immune system is characterized by impaired T-cell function. There is decreased collaboration between B and T cells and the immunoglobulin repertoire is restricted. Antibody response is also of low affinity.[1]

Role of maternal antibody

Passively transferred maternal antibody to specific diseases can influence the outcome of vaccine response. The nature and dose of antigen, the number of vaccine doses, the age at immunization, and the level of residual maternal antibody at the time of immunization all affect the vaccine response.[2] Maternal antibody has been measured in infants to pertussis, mumps and polio. The antibodies are present transiently, for a variable duration of time and generally gone within the first 4–6 months of life. Little or no protection is conferred to hepatitis A, typhoid fever, polio, Japanese encephalitis, yellow fever, pertussis, mumps, rubella and measles despite the presence of antibodies to these organisms. Nevertheless, antibody presence interferes with the ability to respond to vaccine associated antigens to differing degrees.

Polysaccharide vaccines

Polysaccharides are T-cell independent antigens and poorly immunogenic in young children and infants. In addition, children less than 2 years old are unable to make IgG_2 subclass and this is the main response elicited by the polysaccharide vaccines.[3] Examples of polysaccharide vaccines are those against meningococcal meningitis (standard A+C or A/C/Y/W-135 vaccines) and typhoid (Vi polysaccharide vaccines). Age limitations for these vaccines are based on an ineffective response under the licensed age, which is generally 2 years.

Table 11.1	Vaccine considerations that may be unique to infants and children
Adverse event profile	
Interfering maternal antibody	
Ineffective response	
No data on safety and/or efficacy	
Off label usage	

Conjugate vaccines

Developments in vaccinology have led to improvements in ways to stimulate the immune response in both infants and adults. Oligosaccharide-protein conjugate vaccines are being introduced for a variety of diseases.[4] These vaccines produce a T-cell dependent response to a polysaccharide that normally induces a T-cell independent response. This allows children under the age of 2 years to respond to important antigens and also induces immunologic memory that is important for robust booster responses to future doses. Meningococcal conjugate vaccines, now made by several manufacturers and available in several countries (not including the USA), are the most developed example of this advance in vaccinology.

Intercurrent illness and vaccination

Minor febrile illnesses are not a contraindication to any of the routine or travel vaccines and should not lead to postponement of indicated doses. Simultaneous administration of vaccines is acceptable and does not diminish antibody response. As with adults, live viral vaccines should be given together or, if separate, at least 30 days apart.

ROUTINE PEDIATRIC VACCINES

Immunization against common vaccine-preventable diseases occurs routinely throughout the first 24 months of life. The current recommendations for routine childhood vaccination in the USA are shown in detail in Figure 11.1. Most industrialized countries follow similar schedules with some variations that are mostly in the timing of each initial and serial dose. A few vaccines, most notably Varicella may not be routinely recommended or available in some countries. Detailed information on routine recommended childhood schedules by

country may be found at: www-nt.who.int/vaccines/GlobalSummary/ Immunization/CountryProfileSelect.cfm. More relevant to developing countries, the World Health Organization sponsored Global Alliance for Vaccines and Immunizations (GAVI) focuses on six core vaccine-preventable diseases in formulating recommendations for worldwide childhood vaccination schedules: polio, diphtheria, tuberculosis, pertussis, measles and tetanus. As additional options, hepatitis B vaccine is recommended globally, hemophilus influenza B vaccine is recommended in Latin America, the Middle East and where other evidence of disease exists, and yellow fever vaccine is recommended in Africa and South America in endemic areas. GAVI recommendations for childhood vaccination are summarized in Table 11.2.

Diphtheria-tetanus-acellular pertussis

The combination of diphtheria, tetanus and pertussis is recommended for all children in the sequence shown in Table 11.2. Refinements in the pertussis component of the vaccine in the past decade have improved the side-effect profile. The acellular pertussis component is minimally reactogenic compared with the whole cell pertussis vaccine and is the preferred product. There is ongoing research on the use of an additional dose of pertussis vaccine in adolescence and adults is indicated, but, at this time, the use of pertussis containing vaccine should be limited to children under the age of 7 years.

Contraindications to subsequent DTaP vaccination include an immediate anaphylactic reaction or encephalopathy within 7 days of an earlier dose. Adverse events, including a seizure with or without fever within 3 days of the vaccine, persistent, inconsolable crying for 3 or more hours, collapse or shock-like state within 48 h, and otherwise unexplained fever greater than or equal to 40.5 °C (104.9 °F) are considered precautions, not absolute contraindications to further vaccination. Decisions on further doses of vaccine must be weighed

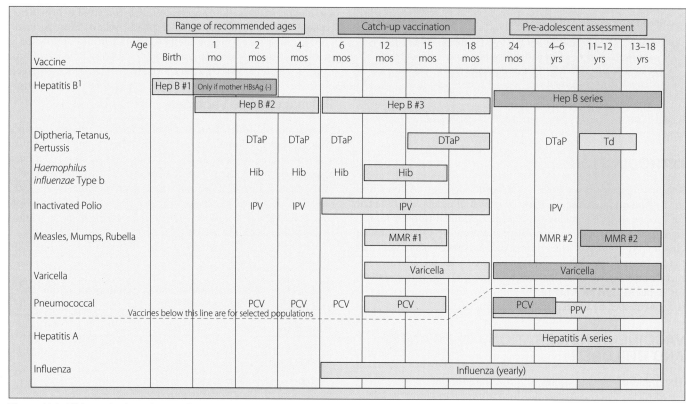

Figure 11.1 USA vaccination schedule. Source: http://www.aap.org/policy/2003lmm.pdf

Table 11.2   WHO GAVI immunization schedule

Age	Vaccine
Birth	BCG, OPV-0, HBV-1
6 weeks	DPT-1, OPV-1, HBV-2 (HBV-1)*
10 weeks	DPT-2, OPV-2 (HBV-2)
14 weeks	DPT-3, OPV-3, HBV-3
9 months	Measles, Yellow fever

*HBV, Schedule option

individually. The whole cell pertussis vaccine (DTP) should be avoided in infants and children at increased risk of convulsions and those who have underlying conditions that predispose to seizures.[5]

The diphtheria toxoid content in Td vaccine is lower than in DTaP, DTP or DT vaccines, to decrease the likelihood of local side effects at the site of injection. Children greater than 7 years old should receive Td for primary doses, if unimmunized previously, or booster doses to reduce the incidence of these side-effects.

Measles-mumps-rubella

Measles remains the leading cause of vaccine preventable death in children worldwide and an active WHO initiative for the global eradication of measles is ongoing. Vaccination programs are aimed at protecting young children from the severe consequences of infection.

Outbreaks of measles occur in developed, as well as developing countries (Fig. 11.2). Child travelers need particular attention to the status of their measles immunity if traveling to developing countries.

The first dose of measles/mumps/rubella (MMR) vaccine is recommended at 12–15 months of age in most industrialized countries. By this age, the effect of maternal antibody to measles is waning and an adequate immune response to the vaccine is likely. The first dose of the MMR vaccine gives protective immunity in approximately 95% of recipients. The second dose is not a booster dose, but induces immunity in the remainder of those who may not have responded. The second dose can be given as soon as 1 month after the first dose. In the routine pediatric vaccine schedule in many countries, it is given at 4–5 years old at kindergarten entry.

In view of the risk of measles during travel, infants between the ages of 6 and 12 months traveling to the developing world should be vaccinated with an extra dose of the monovalent measles vaccine, or, if unavailable, MMR.[6] This will provide immediate protection for several months or more but not a durable or lasting immune response. Thus, any dose given before the age of 12 months is not considered countable towards the routine immunization schedule and the child still requires the two routine MMR vaccines after the age of 12 months. Any child between the age of 12 months and 4–5 years traveling to measles endemic areas should receive their second MMR vaccine before departure as long as it is at least 4 weeks since the first dose. This second dose is a countable dose towards their routine immunization schedule.

The MMR vaccine is well tolerated. Ten to fourteen days after vaccination, 1 in 15 recipients will develop a red maculopapular, often confluent rash, a fever and a flu-like syndrome, with fever lasting

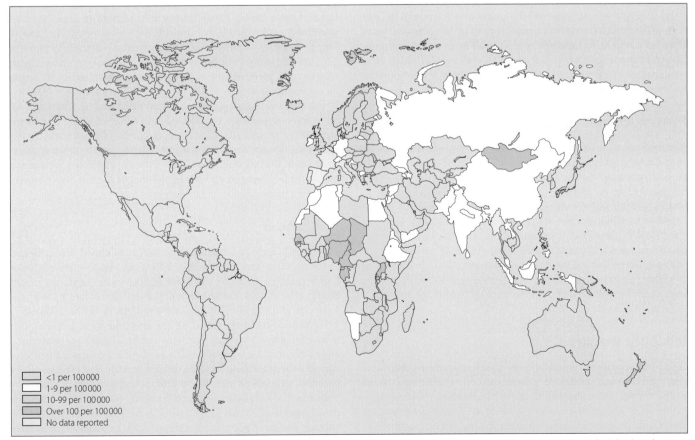

Figure 11.2 Reported measles incidence rates, 1999. WHO, available from: http://www.who.int/vaccines-surveillance/graphics/htmls/meainc.htm (now updated to 2001).

1–2 days, due to the vaccination. These persons are not contagious for measles. Minor side effects include local discomfort at the site of injection, headache and malaise. Side-effects from the second dose are less frequent than with the first dose.

The MMR vaccine should not be given if there has been a serious allergic reaction to a previous dose or if there is a history of anaphylaxis to neomycin. Persons with a history of anaphylactic reactions to gelatin containing products should be immunized with caution under close supervision. There have been several case reports of persons with gelatin allergy having a severe allergic reaction to the MMR vaccine, which contains small amount of gelatin in the formulation. Allergy to eggs or egg protein is not a contraindication to receiving the vaccine.

Polio vaccine

The recommendations for the primary polio vaccine series have been modified in many industrialized countries in recent years. The injectable inactivated polio vaccine is now recommended for the primary series instead of the oral polio vaccine, which is still the standard in the WHO Polio eradication program. The relative risk of vaccine-associated poliomyelitis, while very low with the oral vaccine, is non-existent with the all-inactivated schedule. The use of the oral polio vaccine is reserved for control programs, for outbreak situations, or recommended when an unimmunized traveler is unable to get two doses of the inactivated vaccine. Oral Polio Vaccine (OPV) production has ceased in several countries including the USA. Traveling infants can begin the IPV series as soon as 6 weeks of age.[7] Maternal antibody presence limits its effectiveness at earlier ages.[1] The second dose of IPV should be given at least 4 weeks later. For infants traveling sooner than 6 weeks, the OPV is preferred, if available. The OPV can be started as early as birth and subsequent doses can be given 4 and 8 weeks later. A single booster dose of the inactivated vaccine is recommended for travelers to polio endemic regions in the adolescent years. Data do not exist to indicate the exact waning of polio immunity, however, approximately 10 years after the primary series has been suggested as an appropriate interval to administer the IPV booster if indicated for travel.

Pneumococcal vaccine

The most common cause of otitis media and invasive bacterial disease in children is pneumococcal infection. The seven-valent pneumo-cocccal conjugate vaccine (PCV7) was introduced into the United States schedule in February 2000. The vaccine is immunogenic in infants and recommended routinely at 2, 4 and 6 months of age. Infants and children older than 6 months and under 5 years are vaccinated at the schedule outlined in Figure 11.2. The serogroups present in the seven-valent vaccine are those which cause disease in young children and are most commonly resistant to penicillin. The 23-valent pneumococcal vaccine is recommended for children older than 2 years with under-lying chronic medical conditions, and adults, as noted in Chapter 10.

Influenza vaccine

Influenza vaccination should be considered in all children older than 6 months traveling during the influenza season, which is year-round in the tropics, December–April in the Northern Hemisphere temperate zones and April–October in Southern Hemisphere temperate zones. Infants younger than 6 months do not respond well to the current vaccine.[8] Infants and children less than 12 years old should receive the split virus preparation, which is less reactogenic than the

whole virus product. Children older than 12 years can receive the whole cell vaccine. Any child less than 8 years old receiving the influenza vaccine for the first time should receive two doses of the vaccine, 1 month apart. Influenza vaccine is a live virus vaccine and thus should be avoided in immunocompromised individuals. All children 6–23 months of age, regardless of travel plans, should be considered for influenza vaccine because of a higher incidence of complications and hospitalization associated with influenza infections. An intranasal influenza vaccine against both Influenza A and B was approved for use in children older than 5 years in the United States in June of 2003.

Varicella

According to the Centers for Disease Control and Prevention, 90% of varicella in the USA occurs in children. Child and adult travelers from tropical countries to temperate climates may be at risk of acquiring varicella. Testing for immunity, if there is no definitive history of the disease, and vaccinating those susceptible is recommended.

Varicella vaccination was licensed in the USA in March 1995 and is recommended for all susceptible children and adolescents over 12 months of age, who should receive a single dose of vaccine.[9] Children over the age of 12 years should receive two doses spaced by 4–8 weeks. It is also recommended for international travelers, and non-pregnant adults who live in households with children, who work in daycare settings, or are exposed to settings of high transmission risk (colleges, military or correctional institutions). Susceptible adolescents are strongly encouraged to obtain vaccination, as they are more likely to experience complications of the disease. Varicella vaccine should not be used by most immunocompromised people.

The varicella vaccine is highly effective, giving 97–99% protection against varicella when dosing recommendations are followed. This vaccine is very well tolerated and so far no major side-effects have been demonstrated. 7-8% of those vaccinated develop a mild vaccine-associated rash, often consisting of 2–5 chicken-pox-like lesions. Some 20–35% of vaccinees report pain or redness at the injection site. This vaccine should not be given if there has been a serious allergic reaction to a previous dose or if there is a history of allergy to gelatin or neomycin.

The manufacturer recommends that salicylates not be administered for 6 weeks after varicella vaccine administration, due to the association of varicella virus (*not* vaccine), salicylates and Reye's syndrome. Reye's Syndrome was first described in the 1970s as severe brain and liver failure associated with an unknown interaction between salicylates and varicella in children. It has not been reported with the vaccine.

Hepatitis B

Hepatitis B vaccine is increasingly a routine childhood vaccination in many countries and is part of the WHO GAVI recommendations for highly endemic countries. The three dose series can be started immediately at birth, with a schedule of 0, 1 month and 6 months. Alternatively, they can be given at 2, 4, and 6 months of age, with dose two being at least 1 month after dose one and dose three being at least 4 months after dose one. Pre-term infants should be immunized before hospital discharge if weighing at least 2 kg, or at 2 months of age. The vaccine should be given intramuscularly for best response. A two dose schedule (0 and 4–6 months) is in use for adolescents 11–15 years old.[10] As for adults, vaccine efficacy is between 90–95%. Routine post-immunization serologic testing is not recommended for the routine pediatric population. Infants born to Hepatitis B surface antigen positive mothers are recommended to have serology performed 1-2 months after the third dose of vaccine. Side effects of the

Hepatitis B vaccine include local pain at the injection site and a low-grade fever. It is estimated that 1–6% of vaccine recipients experience fever. Allergic reactions are rare.

Accelerating routine vaccines

Routine pediatric vaccinations may need to be accelerated if the traveling child is departing before the primary series can be completed and he/she will be at high risk. The recommended minimum amount of time between doses is listed in Table 11.3. Earliest age of vaccination recommendations are derived due to either interfering maternal antibodies, lack of effective immune response, or lack of data. The minimum interval noted is required to produce an immunologic response. Longer intervals are preferable.[11]

PEDIATRIC TRAVEL VACCINATIONS

Required vaccinations

Yellow fever vaccine

Itineraries involving travel to Sub-Saharan Africa or the Amazonia region of South America may require the yellow fever vaccine for entry to the country. For most countries in the endemic or infected zone, vaccination is medically recommended on the basis of risk of yellow fever rather than because of legal requirements (see Chapter 10 for general advice on risk areas). Some 300 million people have been vaccinated with yellow fever (YF) vaccine in the past 50 years. Initial experience with the vaccine revealed an increased incidence of yellow fever encephalitis in young infants. Twenty-one cases of 17D encephalitis have been reported since 1952. Fifteen of these cases were in the 1950s, and 13 were in infants less than 4 months old.

The vaccine associated encephalitis syndrome typically occurs 7–21 days post immunization and is characterized by a reversion to wild-type virus. Neurologic signs and cerebrospinal fluid pleocytosis (100–500 WBC) with increased protein were noted clinically. Brief clinical course with complete recovery was typical. The basis for this increased risk in infants is unknown. Theories include the immature blood–brain barrier, a possible prolonged or higher viremia, and these factors combined with a delayed clearance of vaccine related infection.[12]

In 1960, an age restriction (9 months) was placed on the use of the vaccine and is generally adhered to internationally. Current advice is for infants less than 9 months to avoid travel to very high areas or those with ongoing epidemics or current cases. The vaccine is absolutely contraindicated in infants less than 6 months old. If travel is unavoidable for infants between 6 and 9 months, an expert in the current epidemiology of transmission should be consulted to assess the real risk at the particular destination (Table 11.4).[13] The incidence of vaccine associated encephalitis in young infants has been estimated at 0.5–4 per 1000.[12] Booster doses are recommended every 10 years, as for adults.

Recommended vaccinations

Hepatitis A vaccine

Hepatitis A in young children is usually a mild disease. Young children can serve as reservoirs and transmit the infection to adults and caregivers while they are shedding the virus asymptomatically. Vaccination in this age group is indicated to control the disease in both the child traveler and contacts both during travel and after return.

Hepatitis A vaccination is recommended for travel to developing countries as it is for adults. In addition, routine vaccination with Hepatitis A vaccine is recommended in certain high-risk regions of developed countries such as the USA and Canada.

Data exists to show that infants as young as 6 months will respond to Hepatitis A vaccination if they do not have interfering maternal antibody present.[14,15] Maternal antibody, if present, interferes with seroconversion response for a variable amount of time. Seropositive infants respond well at 1 year of age or older, once the maternal antibody levels decline. Specific reduced dose pediatric formulations of hepatitis A vaccines exist and are currently licensed in the USA for children older than 2 years. In most other countries, the vaccine is licensed for use in infants at 1 year of age and WHO recommends use in children older than 1 year.

For children unable, or unwilling (in the case of off-label use), to receive the vaccine, immune globulin, if available, can be given as passive Hepatitis A prophylaxis. The dose of IG for pre-exposure prophylaxis against Hepatitis A infection for travel of less than 3 months duration is 0.02 mL/kg given by deep intramuscular injection into the gluteus muscle (preferable) or deltoid muscle. For protection against Hepatitis A infection for a trip of 3 months or longer, the dose is 0.06 mL/kg IG given by deep intramuscular injection into the gluteus muscle.[13]

Hepatitis A–Hepatitis B combination vaccine

A Hepatitis A–Hepatitis B combination vaccine, Twinrix (GlaxoSmithKline) is now widely used for adults. The adult formulation is licensed for use in adolescents older than 18 years in the USA and older than 16 years in Europe and Canada. For children of 1–15 years, Twinrix-Junior (GlaxoSmithKline) is widely available and licensed for use in Europe and Canada.[16] It is also administered in a three dose series at 0, 1 and 6 months. An accelerated regimen of the adult formulation of Twinrix (0, 7, 21 days and 1 year) is licensed in the European Union and widely used off-label in other countries. No data on accelerated pediatric regimens are available.

Table 11.3	Accelerating routine pediatric vaccinations	
	Earliest age	Minimum interval (weeks)
DTaP	6 weeks	4
IPV	6 weeks	4
OPV	birth	4
Hib	6 weeks	4
Hepatitis B	birth	4
PCV7	6 weeks	4
Measles (single antigen) preferred, MMR if unavailable	6–11 months, followed by MMR at 12 months	4
Measles (single antigen) 6–11 months, followed by MMR at 12 months old		

Table 11.4	Age limitations to the use of yellow fever vaccine[16a]
Age	Recommendation
<6 months	Never
6–9 months	Consult with experts
>9 months	Travel to yellow fever endemic or infected areas

Meningococcal meningitis vaccine

Children traveling to the meningitis prone areas in equatorial Africa during the December–June dry season or to the Hajj in Saudi Arabia, should receive the quadravalent A/C/Y/W-135 meningococcal meningitis vaccine. It is a polysaccharide vaccine and therefore confers little immunity to children less than 2 years old. Infants as young as 3 months old will respond to serogroup A (the most common serogroup in epidemics) to a limited extent, when two doses are given.[17] Children younger than 2 years of age making a single trip to a high-risk area should be vaccinated, as there will be some short-term benefit of vaccination. Children vaccinated before the age of 4 years should be re-vaccinated at least once per year if they remain at risk. The vaccine is less immunogenic in children under 4 years compared with older children. Infants are unable to make significant antibody response to serogroup C.

In the USA, the quadrivalent vaccine has been recommended for US-born college freshman living in dormitories. This recommendation should be extended to non-US born students studying in the USA. Serogroups C and Y have emerged as significant causes of meningococcal meningitis. While group B remains a serious cause of disease, a vaccine to this serogroup has been difficult to develop due to its resemblance to human neural tissue. The incidence of meningococcal disease in college freshman residing in dormitories is modestly increased at 4.6 per 100 000, compared with 1.4 per 100 000 in all 18–23 year olds in the USA. Vaccination will decrease but not eliminate the disease in this group.[18]

Meningococcal meningitis conjugate vaccines

Protein conjugate vaccines for Serogroups A, C, and A/C combination are now available in several countries. The conjugate vaccine produces a T-cell dependent response, thus is immunogenic in infants.[19] The meningococcal C conjugate vaccines (e.g., Menjugate, Chiron or NeisVac-C, Baxter) have been licensed for use in infants less than 2 years in Canada, the UK and several other EU countries. It is routinely recommended in these countries on a schedule of 2, 4, and 6 months in infancy (three doses, at least 4 weeks apart). A single dose is recommended for children between 1 and 4 years old. College students in the UK (as well as foreign students attending college in the UK), receive the Meningococcal A+C conjugate vaccine due to an incidence (2/100 000) disease, predominantly serogroup C, twice the national average.

Typhoid vaccine

Both live attenuated oral Ty21a *S. typhi* and injectable killed Vi polysaccharide vaccines are available for pediatric use. The capsule form of Ty21a is licensed widely for use in children older than 6 years, who can swallow the capsules whole. The capsules need to be swallowed intact in order that the contained liquid suspension of live bacteria pass undisturbed through the acid milieu of the stomach. In many countries, but not the USA, a lyophilized preparation that is reconstituted in water is available in a 3-dose regimen for children older than 3 years.

The Vi polysaccharide vaccine is poorly immunogenic in children less than 2 years old.[20] It can be given as a single injection to children older than 2 years and confers protection for 2–3 years. Boosters are recommended if exposure or travel warrants.

Whole cell killed parenteral phenol inactivated typhoid vaccine was licensed for use in infants as young as 6 months, but is no longer available in most countries. This vaccination had significant systemic side-effects, which limited its usefulness.

Children under 2 years old currently have no available vaccine for protection, therefore, recommending meticulous food and water precautions is prudent. Efforts are underway to convert the Vi antigen into a T-cell dependent antigen and produce an immunogenic vaccine for infants.

Rabies vaccine

Rabies is highly endemic in many countries worldwide. Given its potentially long latency and uniformly fatal outcome, advice on avoiding animal contact is essential for pre-travel counseling whether for children or adults. Pre- and post-exposure algorithms are found in Chapter 10 and do not differ in dose or timing between children and adults. Nevertheless children may be more likely to contact animals and may not report encounters,[21] therefore, the pre-exposure rabies vaccine series should be considered for ambulatory children who will travel extensively or live in rural villages in countries where rabies is endemic even when parents refuse it for themselves. High cost is an issue for rabies pre-exposure immunization so that prioritization for young children is an important consideration. Infants and children respond well to the vaccine and no age limitations exist to its administration. The Vero cell vaccine has been studied in combination with the DTP and IPV vaccines and no interference exists.[22] Limited data exist to support its safety and efficacy with routine pediatric immunizations.

Japanese B encephalitis

Japanese encephalitis (JE) is rarely a disease of travelers; however, indications for vaccination exist, as with adults. JE vaccine is primarily indicated for long-stay travel in rural areas of risk. Worldwide JE primary vaccination occurs in many Asian countries (see Chapter 10). Table 11.5 shows countries with routine usage of JE vaccine for children. Published and true incidence rates for human cases of JE may be low in such countries due to high vaccination coverage and will mask a significant risk of infection in rural farming areas.

Limited data exists on vaccine safety and efficacy in infants less than 1 year old and it should not be used in this age group. The role of maternal antibody in endemic areas is unknown, but may account for the rarity of Japanese B encephalitis in infants less than 1 year old. Children going to live in endemic areas or spend a significant amount of time in Japanese B encephalitis endemic environments should be considered for vaccination.[13,23] The vaccine schedule is identical to that of adults and dosage is listed in Table 11.6. The dose for children between 1–3 years of age is half the normal adult dose. Delayed anaphylactic reactions have been documented in adults and in the absence of specific pediatric data the same considerations should apply in children (see Chapter 10).

Table 11.5	Routine Japanese B encephalitis vaccination
Country	**Age**
China	1 year
Korea	3 years
Japan	3 years (6–90 months)
Thailand	18 months
Taiwan	15–27 months

Table 11.6 **Summary of travel vaccinations for children. See text for specific vaccine details**[a]

Vaccine	Age	Primary series	Booster interval/comments
Cholera, oral (CVD103-HgR)[b]	>2 years	1 dose oral, in buffered solution	Optimal interval not established; manufacturer recommends 6 months.
Hepatitis A	>2 years[a] >12 years	Havrix (GSK): 2 doses (0.5 mL i.m.) at 0, 6–18 months later Vaqta (Merck): 2 doses (0.5 mL i.m.) at 0 and 6 months Avaxim (AventisPasteurMerieux) Europe and Canada Epaxal (Berna Biotech): >1 year old Switzerland	See text
Immune globulin	Birth	0.02mL/kg i.m.	See text
Japanese B encephalitis	>1 year	1–3 year: 3 doses (0.5 mL s.c.) at 0, 7, 14 or 30 days >3 year: 3 doses (1.0mL s.c.) at 0, 7, 14 or 30 days	3 years
Meningococcal meningitis (ACYW-135)	> 2 years	1 dose (0.5 mL s.c.)	Boost annually if first dose was given before 4 years old. See text for age <2.
Plague vaccine	>18 years	Not for use in children	
Rabies vaccine	Any age	3 doses (1 mL i.m., deltoid/anterolateral thigh for infants, or 0.1 mL ID) at 0, 7, 21 or 28 days	Only HDCV approved for intradermal use (not presently marketed)
Tick-borne encephalitis	1–11 years	EncepurKinder (Chiron Behring): 3 doses (0.25 mL i.m.) at 0, 1–3 months and 9–12 months FSME-IMMUN Junior (Baxter): 3 doses (0.25 mL i.m.) at 0, 1–3 months and 9–12 months	Booster dose recommended 3 years after the primary series for the standard dosing regimen of either vaccine. See text for accelerated schedules.
Typhoid, oral Ty21a	>3 years[b] >6 years	3 doses: 1 sachet PO in 100 mL water every other day 4 doses: 1 capsule PO every other day	Liquid vaccine[b] booster: 7 year Capsule vaccine: 5 year
Typhoid, Vi, parenteral	>2 years	1 dose (0.5 mL i.m.)	Boost after 2 year for continued risk of exposure
Yellow fever	>9 months	1 dose (0.5 mL s.c.)	10 year; see text for <9 months

[a]Manufacturer's package insert for recommendations on dosage.
[b]Not approved in the USA. Available in Canada and Europe.
Adapted from: Mackell S. Travel advice for pediatric travelers: infants, children and adolescents, in Jong EC and McMullin R, eds. *The Travel and Tropical Medicine Manual*, 3rd edn., London: Saunders; 2003.

Tick-borne encephalitis vaccine

Tick-borne encephalitis (TBE) is transmitted by the bite of the Ixodes ricinus tick, present in forested areas of central and Eastern Europe. It can also rarely be acquired by consuming unpasteurized milk from infected cows, goats and sheep. Symptoms of TBE range from meningitis to severe meningoencephalitis with significant residual neurologic sequelae. It is seasonally (summer) acquired in endemic areas (see Chapter 10). In endemic areas, the vaccine is incorporated into the routine pediatric schedule. There are two available vaccines licensed for use in children. EncepurKinder (Chiron) is manufactured in Germany. It is an inactivated viral vaccine and can be used in children 1–11 years, while children 12 years and older should receive the adult vaccine. An accelerated schedule of 0.25 ml given on days 0, 7 and 21 is recommended if rapid immunization is required. Seroconversion can be expected no sooner than 14 days after the second vaccination. A booster is recommended 12–18 months later.[24]

Although generalized flu-like symptoms may occur after the first vaccine, an increased incidence of febrile reactions greater than 38 °C is reported in children between 1 and 2 years old, therefore, vaccination in this age group must be considered on an individual basis.[24] See Chapter 10 for a discussion of adult TBE vaccine preparations.

In some countries, FSME-IMMUN Junior (Baxter, Austria), formulated for children 1–12 years old, is available with the same dosing regimens as for EncepurKinder. The adult formulation is recommended for those older than 12 years.[25] Dosages are listed in Table 11.4. FSME-IMMUN is available in Canada and in the UK by a special release mechanism. No TBE vaccine is available in the USA.

BCG

Vaccination against the tuberculosis bacteria is not routinely recommended or used in children in the USA or Canada. The available vaccine, Bacille Calmette-Guerin (BCG), is a live bacterial vaccine and confers protection to extra-pulmonary tuberculous disease in infants less than 1 year old. It is not significantly protective against pulmonary tuberculosis. In countries with a high incidence of tuberculosis and some others such as the UK, infants are routinely immunized at birth with a single dose. In countries with low incidence of tuberculosis, a single dose is often given during adolescence. Other countries, like the USA, rely on screening, case identification and treatment. The vaccine is contraindicated in immunocompromised individuals. Although there is wide disagreement across national boundaries, BCG can be considered in infants and children under the age of 5, traveling for extended periods of time to areas of very high tuberculosis incidence with expected contact with the local population. Post-travel testing for tuberculosis should be done on an individual basis.[26]

CONCLUSION

Pediatric travelers require special attention to appropriately immunize them from disease. Advances in vaccine development have led to many recent changes and additions to the routine childhood immunization schedule. Immunizing child necessitates knowledge of the indications and immunologic actions of all available travel vaccines. Published age limitations to pediatric vaccination are based on the development of the child's immune system, potential adverse events, the presence of interfering maternal antibodies, and, in some cases, the lack of adequate data on safety and/or efficacy. Informed parental consent is recommended for the use of vaccinations outside of recommended limits and licensure.

REFERENCES

1. Siegrist CA. Vaccination in the neonatal period and early infancy. *Int Rev Immunol* 2000; **19**(2–3):195–219.
2. Siegrist CA, Cordova M, Brandt C, *et al.* Determinants of infant responses to vaccines in presence of maternal antibodies. *Vaccine* 1998; Aug–Sep; **16**(14–15):1409–1414.
3. Plotkin SA. Immunologic correlates of protection induced by vaccination: *Pediatr Infect Dis J* 2001; **20**(1): 63–74.
4. Plotkin SA. Vaccine recommendations: challenges and controversies. *Infect Dis Clin N Am* 2001; **15**(1): March.
5. American Academy of Pediatrics, Pickering LK, ed. *2000 Red Book: Report of the Committee on Infectious Diseases.* 25th edn. Elk Grove Village, IL: American Academy of Pediatrics; 2000.
6. American Academy of Pediatrics. Measles. In: Pickering LK, ed. *2000 Red Book: Report of the Committee on Infectious Diseases.* 25th edn. Elk Grove Village, IL: American Academy of Pediatrics; 2000:392.
7. American Academy of Pediatrics. Poliovirus infections. In: Pickering LK, ed. *2000 Red Book: Report of the Committee on Infectious Diseases.* 25th edn. Elk Grove Village, IL: American Academy of Pediatrics; 2000: 468.
8. Centers for Disease Control and Prevention: Prevention and control of influenza. Recommendations of the Advisory Committee on Immunization Practices (ACIP). *MMWR Recomm Rep.* 2002: Apr 12; **51**(RR–3):1–31.
9. Centers for Disease Control and Prevention: Prevention of varicella: Recommendations of the Advisory Committee on Immunization Practices (ACIP). *MMWR Recomm Rep.* 1996: Jul 12; **45**(RR–11):1–36.
10. Cassidy WM, Watson B, Ioli VA, Williams K, Bird S, West DJ. A randomized trial of alternative two- and three-dose hepatitis B vaccination regimens in adolescents: antibody responses, safety, and immunologic memory. *Pediatrics* 2001; **107**(4):626–631.
11. American Academy of Pediatrics. Immunizations in special clinical circumstances. In: Pickering LK, ed. *2000 Red Book: Report of the Committee on Infectious Diseases.* 25th edn. Elk Grove Village, IL. American Academy of Pediatrics; 2000:77–78.
12. Monath TP, Yellow Fever. In: Plotkin SA, Orenstein W, eds. *Vaccines,* 3rd edn. Philadelphia: W.B. Saunders, 1999:858–863.
13. Centers for Disease Control and Prevention. *Health Information for International Travel, 2003–2004*, US Department of Health and Human Services, 2001.
14. Dagan R, Amir J, Mijalovsky A, *et al.* Immunization against hepatitis A in the first year of life: priming despite the presence of maternal antibody. *Pediatr Infect Dis J.* 2000; **19**(11):1045–1052.
15. Troisi CL, Hollinger FB, Krause DS, Pickering LK. Immunization of seronegative infants with hepatitis A vaccine (HAVRIX; SKB): a comparative study of two dosing schedules. *Vaccine* 1997; Oct. **15**(15):1613–1617.
16. Diaz-Mitoma F, Law B, Parsons J. A combined vaccine against hepatitis A and B in children and adolescents. *Pediatr Infect Dis J* 1999 Feb; **18**(2): 109–114
16a. Cetron MS, Marfin AA, Julian KG, *et al.* Yellow fever vaccine. Recommendations of the Advisory Committee on Immunization Practices (ACIP), 2002. *MMR Recomm Rep* 2002; **8**:51(RR–17): 1–11.
17. Lepow ML, Perkins BA, Hughes PA, Poolman JT. Meningococcal Vaccines. In: Plotkin SA and Orenstein W, eds. *Vaccines,* 3rd edn., Philadelphia: W.B. Saunders; 1999: 718–721.
18. Centers for Disease Control and Prevention. Prevention and Control of Meningococcal Disease: Recommendations of the Advisory Committee on Immunization Practice. *MMWR* June 30, 2000; **49**(RR07):1–10.
19. Pollard, AJ, Levin M. Vaccines for prevention of meningococcal disease. *Pediatr Infect Dis J.* 2000; **19**(4):333–345.
20. Plotkin SA. A new typhoid vaccine composed of the Vi capsular polysaccharide. *Arch Internal Medicine* 1995; **155**:2293–2299.
21. Fisher DJ. Resurgence of rabies. A historical perspective on rabies in children. *Arch Pediatr Adolesc Med* 1995; **149**(3):306–312.
22. Lang J, Duong GH, Nguyen VG, Le TT, Nguyen CV, Kesmedjian V, Plotkin SA. Randomised feasibility trial of pre-exposure rabies vaccination with DTP-IPV in infants. *Lancet* 1997 349(9066):1663–1665.
23. World Health Organization: *International Travel and Health Recommendations,* 2003. Available at http://www.who.int/ith/
24. Chiron Behring Co. Encepur-Kinder (TBE) vaccine; Package insert 10/01.
25. Baxter Vaccines. FSME-Immun package insert. Available at http://www.baxter-ag.at/presseforum/pressematerial_fsme/presskit/PIFSME-IMMUN14.02.02.htm
26. Centers for Disease Control and Prevention. The role of BCG vaccine in the prevention and control of tuberculosis in the United States: a joint statement by the Advisory Committee on Immunization Practices and Advisory Council for the Elimination of Tuberculosis, *MMWR* 1996; 45(RR–4):1

CHAPTER 12

Malaria: Epidemiology and Risk to the Traveler

Alan J. Magill

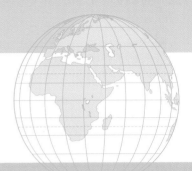

KEYPOINTS

■ Travelers to sub-Saharan Africa and Oceania are at highest risk of acquiring malaria

■ Particular groups, such as visiting friends and relatives (VFRs), have a higher risk

■ Failure to use personal protection measures to prevent mosquito bites and use of sub-optimal chemoprophylaxis agents or non-compliance with recommended regimens for efficacious chemoprophylaxis agents is the cause of most cases of malaria in travelers

■ Drug resistance patterns determine the use of suitable antimalarial drugs. Never prescribe chloroquine or chloroquine containing regimens for travel to sub-Saharan Africa

INTRODUCTION

Malaria is no longer an endemic infectious disease in the industrialized countries of North America, Europe, Australia, New Zealand, and Japan. However, the marked increase in pleasure and business travelers to malaria endemic areas and immigration and refugee migrations into non-endemic areas has led to a large number of imported cases of malaria in the industrialized countries. Between 1990 and 2000, international tourist arrivals to sub-Saharan Africa, the geographic destination at highest risk, saw an increase from 6.7 million to 17.1 million arrivals. (World Tourism Organization, http://www.worldtourism.org/market_research/facts&figures/menu.htm). Table 12.1 shows reported malaria cases in the industrialized countries between 1985 and 1995.[1] Although reporting methods and the accuracy and completeness of surveillance vary between countries,[2] over 100 000 cases were reported in the 11-year period. Trends have been relatively stable in some countries to modestly increasing in others.

The UK alone represented about a fifth of the total cases, possibly reflecting a large immigrant population who frequently visit their country of birth and a large traveling population. For non-European countries, there were almost 25 000 cases, with the USA having just over 10 000 cases. Since 1980, the number of imported cases in the USA has ranged from a low of 803 in 1983 to 1544 in 1997.[3] Canada and Australia had fewer total cases but much larger per capita rates of disease.

WHO IS AT RISK?

Although any non-immune person not taking efficacious chemoprophylaxis is likely to develop clinical malaria if bitten by an infected mosquito, some groups are at higher risk, based on their exposures and habits. It is clear that infection rates, based on the appearance of antibodies to malaria proteins, are different from disease rates. Travelers who fail to take chemoprophylaxis, use inadequate regimens, or are noncompliant with prevention measures routinely develop clinical symptoms at higher rates than those who do. Particular groups, such as those returning to homes and families in endemic countries ('visiting friends and relatives' or VFRs), seem to be at much higher risk. Hospital-based studies in Europe, the USA, and Canada reveal an increasing percentage of cases in immigrants and the foreign born. VFRs in Britain have a 3-fold higher risk than short-term travelers to Africa and an 8-fold increased risk over travelers to Asia.[4,5] When migrants return to their home countries, they often spend more time, may return to rather simple country villages of their youth, and often bring their children with them, who may be completely non-immune. Adults may have left their home country, such as India, at a time when malaria transmission was relatively low, only to return years later when transmission is much higher. Many never used chemoprophylaxis as a youth, and are unaware that clinical immunity to malaria wanes over a few years. Table 12.2 shows the primary reason for travel for cases of imported malaria as reported by the US CDC in their annual surveillance summaries between 1996–2000. The trend shows cases of imported malaria in VFRs to be increasing while other categories remain little changed. Immigrants and VFRs are less likely to be aware of and use effective chemoprophylaxis when returning to their home countries for a visit. In a study of imported cases in Italian travelers from 1989–1997, only 4% of foreign-born immigrants or VFRs, mostly Africans, used regular chemoprophylaxis compared to 36% of Italian citizens.[6] Similarly, in a comparison of the epidemiology of imported malaria into Belgium in 1988/89–1997, African patients took chemoprophylaxis significantly less frequently than Caucasian patients (1988/89: 18% versus 64%; 1997: 7% versus 51%).[7] Clearly, the VFR group is at much higher relative risk of acquiring malaria.

Although age itself should not be a risk factor for acquiring malaria, activities that different age groups may participate in could pre-dispose certain age groups to more infections. For example, the young backpacker may be at increased risk of infection based on more exotic destinations and activities, less controlled sleeping arrangements, and longer duration of travel. Once infection occurs, older travelers are at higher risk of poor clinical outcomes and death. The case fatality rate of *P. falciparum* malaria in US travelers from 1966–1987 was 3.8% (66 deaths/1760 cases). The case fatality rate increased dramatically with age. For persons from 0 to age 19 years of age, it was 0.4%; from 20–39 years of age it was 2.2%; from 40–69 years of age, it was 5.8%; and for those aged 70–79, it was 30.3% (10 deaths/33 cases).[8]

Activities and sleeping arrangements can dramatically affect infection risk. For example, individual travelers were at almost a 9-fold greater risk of infection than those on package tours to sub-Saharan Africa.[9] This increased risk seen in German travelers was possibly related to longer stay and more rough and casual travel and sleeping conditions.

Table 12.1 Reported malaria cases in industrialized countries, 1985–1995

Country	1985	1986	1987	1988	1989	1990	1991	1992	1993	1994	1995	Annual Mean	Total Cases
							Europe						
Australia	421	696	574	601	770	874	939	743	670	710	610	692	7608
Austria	82	92	52	83	98	112	111	58	89	75	80	85	932
Belgium	208	298	258	271	272	264	314	249	320	423	304	289	3181
Canada	314	436	515	307	284	417	674	407	483	n/a	637	447	4474
Czechoslovakia	9	11	20	26	28	7	8	7	8	n/a	n/a	14	124
Denmark	128	178	138	142	125	114	110	110	113	136	175	134	1469
Finland	30	28	19	n/a	52	46	33	39	31	49	31	36	358
France	631	1125	1143	1664	1863	1491	1165	905	769	824	1167	1159*	12747
Germany	591	1137	794	1030	1143	976	900	773	732	830	941	895	9847
Greece	34	39	47	52	48	28	45	29	35	27	24	37	408
Ireland	22	21	28	30	23	12	11	15	9	12	9	17	192
Italy	178	191	287	350	468	521	471	499	688	782	743	471	5178
Japan	53	50	40	48	49	49	52	49	51	64	n/a	51	505
Luxembourg	7	3	5	n/a	8	7	5	1	4	6	6	5	52
Malta	4	5	2	2	10	3	5	0	4	2	6	4	43
Netherlands	137	167	153	259	244	248	272	179	223	236	312	221	2430
New Zealand	n/a	n/a	n/a	n/a	27	32	39	29	58	34	41	37	260
Norway	53	68	47	53	52	60	71	36	76	73	80	61	669
Poland	15	14	16	21	22	21	16	17	27	18	20	19	207
Portugal	62	95	119	113	161	129	108	61	49	67	n/a	96	964
Romania	10	8	13	n/a	5	9	11	19	21	20	30	15	146
Spain	112	179	166	176	118	161	159	154	171	268	263	175	1927
Sweden	140	147	155	172	180	205	149	124	143	160	161	158	1736
Switzerland	200	196	192	322	340	295	322	261	285	310	289	274	3012
UK	2212	2309	1816	1674	1987	2096	2332	1629	1922	1887	2055	1993	21919
USA	1045	1091	932	1023	1102	1098	1046	910	1275	1014	n/a	1054	10536
USSR (former)	1918	1686	1323	1580	1145	356	254	188	293	485	548	889	9776
Yugoslavia	57	75	64	53	46	23	18	10	20	n/a	n/a	41	366
Total	8673	10345	8918	10052	10670	9654	9640	7501	8569	8512	8532	—	101666

*True mean figure is estimated at 3900 cases per annum.

WHERE ARE TRAVELERS AT RISK OF ACQUIRING MALARIA?

Figure 12.1 shows current malaria endemic areas and the global distribution of drug resistant malaria. The impact of the disease on persons who live in endemic areas has increased significantly over the past 3 decades. From a nadir in the early 1960s following the eradication efforts of the 1950s, malaria, and especially drug resistant malaria, has reclaimed historic geographic distributions in the Amazon and the Indian sub-continent. However, the geographic locations where persons acquire imported malaria may vary depending on the reason for travel and the prevention measures used by the traveler.

Sub-Saharan Africa is the destination where the vast majority of malaria infections are acquired. Five to 49% of travelers to sub-Saharan Africa develop antibodies to malaria proteins following return indicating exposure to infective mosquitoes.[9–11] Shorter stays in coastal Kenyan hotels were associated with the lower infection rates,[10] while longer travel in independent travelers was associated with a remark-able infection rate of 49% in one study.[9] Figure 12.2 shows the risk of infection, based on detection of antibodies to a parasite protein, from 2131 German travelers. More recent seroepidemiology studies of returning travelers confirm the high relative risk of infection to Africa.[11,12] Infection rates increased with length of stay and with more rural exposure.[9] Without chemoprophylaxis, the risk of symptomatic malaria is estimated at 2.4% per month in West Africa and 1.5% per month in East Africa.[13] In Italian travelers between 1989–1997, a relatively stable incidence of acquiring malaria was calculated as 1.5/1000 in Africa, 0.11/1000 in Asia, and 0.04 in Central-South America, despite a significant increase in travel to Asia and Central-South America.[6] The incidence in Africa was 10–20-fold higher than Asia and 30–40-fold higher than in the Americas. This is similar to other studies showing morbidity, mortality and relative risk of infection for travel to the Americas, Southeast Asia, and the Indian sub-continent is much lower than Africa.[10,12,14] Risk varies for specific localities and traveler activities, even for travel to Africa, New Guinea, and the Pacific Islands at highest risk. For most popular tourist destinations,

Table 12.2 Number of imported malaria cases among US civilians by purpose of travel at the time of acquisition – US, 1996–2000. Data from US Centers for Disease Control and Prevention (CDC). Surveillance Summaries. *MMWR.* Available at http://www.cdc.gov/mmwr/mmwr_ss.html

Category	Imported Cases No. (%)				
	1996	1997	1998	1999	2000
Teacher/student	85 (14)	63 (9)	46 (7)	48 (6)	48 (6)
Visiting friends or relatives	72 (12)	157 (23)	245 (39)	325 (39)	296 (36)
Tourist	50 (8)	80 (12)	74 (12)	89 (11)	85 (10)
Missionary	59 (10)	76 (11)	46 (7)	76 (9)	84 (10)
Business representative	39 (6)	65 (9)	64 (10)	58 (7)	60 (7)
Peace Corps volunteer	12 (2)	14 (2)	8 (1.3)	17 (2)	21 (3)
Sailor/Air crew	4 (1)	4 (0.6)	5 (0.8)	3 (0.4)	3 (0.4)
Refugee/immigrant	4 (1)	10 (1.4)	NR	5 (0.6)	1 (0.1)
Unknown/other	289 (48)	226 (33)	141 (22)	165 (20)	190 (23)
Total	614 (100)	695 (100)	629 (100)	831 (100)	825 (100)

the risk of infection is non-existent or extremely low and chemoprophylaxis is not indicated.

Travel medicine practitioners can access destination risk information from many sources. *Health Information for International Health 2003–2004* (the CDC yellow book) is a very common source for many USA-based practitioners. The hardcopy is available from the Public Health Foundation (Tel: 1 877 252 1200 or 301 645 7773 or order Online at http://bookstore.phf.org). An online version and a free download in pdf format are available at http://www.cdc.gov/travel/yb/index.htm.

There are two types of malaria risk information in the yellow book. Geographic risk is described at the country level with clarification in some cases of specific risk areas based on elevation above sea level, focal areas within countries, and some popular tourist destinations. This information is limited by the infrequent consideration of seasonal

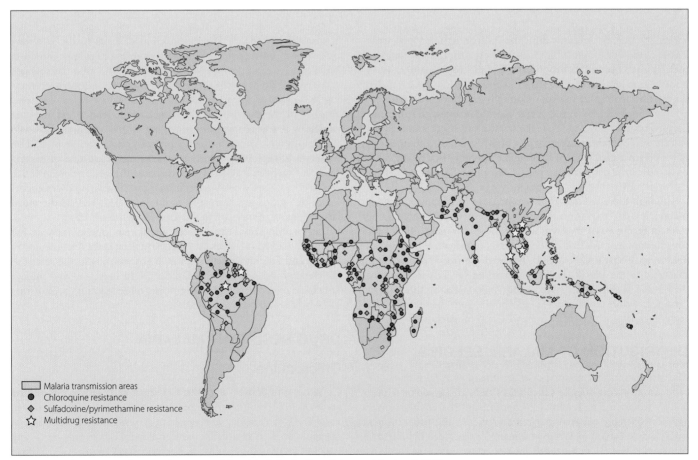

Figure 12.1 Current malaria endemic areas and the global distribution of drug resistant malaria.[24]

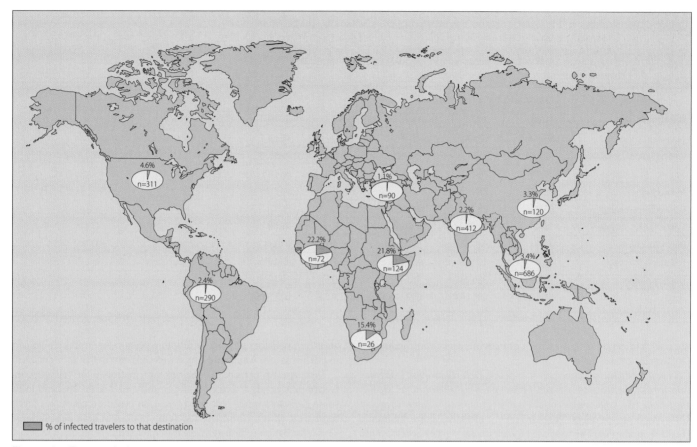

Figure 12.2 The risk of infection, based on detection of antibodies to a parasite protein. (Data from US Centers for Disease Control and Prevention (CDC). Surveillance Summaries MMWR at http:www.cdc.gov/mmwr/mmwr_ss.html).

variability and the inherent difficulty in quantitating actual transmission risk. For example, in much of West Africa, transmission of malaria is intense and year round, while in the tropical Americas, the transmission risk is focal, seasonal, and often very low. Since much of the specific geographic risk information is listed by political boundaries within countries, it is imperative to have access to sufficiently detailed maps in order to locate the travel destinations and the listed risk areas. Along with geographic area of risk, specific mention is made of the presence or absence of chloroquine resistant malaria. The yellow book also provides malaria specific recommendations concerning chemoprophylactic drugs licensed for use in the USA.

Although there are many other sources of geographic risk information, it is challenging for the infrequent or non-expert practitioner to identify and assess the credibility of these sources in a busy practice environment. Malaria destination risk information is also available online from the CDC at http://www.cdc.gov/travel/diseases.htm#malaria and the World Health Organization (WHO) International Travel and Health home page at http://www.who.int/ith/chapter07_01.html. North American readers should note that some WHO recommendations may differ from CDC recommendations.

DISTRIBUTION OF MALARIA SPECIES

The vast majority of imported cases are caused by *P. falciparum* or *P. vivax*. In most countries, less than 5% of cases are caused by *P. ovale* and *P. malariae*. The reported proportions of Plasmodium species vary considerably between geographic regions. The proportion of malaria cases caused by *P. falciparum* and *P. vivax* seen in individual countries reflect the destinations travelers choose for travel and to a larger extent the nature of the immigrant communities. For example,

historically a relatively large proportion of cases in the UK were caused by *P. vivax*, reflecting the large number of immigrants from India and Pakistan, former British colonies.[4] The ratio has changed more recently to over 50% of the cases caused by *P. falciparum* reflecting the increased falciparum transmission in East Asia.[15] Likewise, 70–80% of the cases of imported malaria in France and Italy are caused by *P. falciparum*, most occurring in African immigrants who visit family and friends in their country of origin and become ill on return to Europe.[2,16–18] Figure 12.3 shows the proportion of malaria cases in American travelers by species over the last 6 years, in which complete data are available. *P. falciparum* malaria is now predominant, but still is less than 50% of the total. This reflects the much larger number of travelers to the Americas from the USA.

Species proportions can also vary at different times of the year. For example, marked increases in *P. falciparum* cases are documented in France and Italy in September, which corresponds to the return of travelers following the August holidays.[2,6] In Italy, a second peak in January is seen reflecting Italian tourists returning from a Christmas holiday in a warm tropical locale.[6]

DRUG RESISTANT MALARIA

Chloroquine

Countries and destinations with CQ sensitive *P. falciparum* malaria are Mexico, all countries of Central America west of the Panama Canal, rural areas of Paraguay and northern Argentina, and the island of Hispaniola (Haiti and the Dominican Republic), the only remaining endemic focus in the Caribbean. There are focal areas of CQ sensitive malaria in North Africa (Egypt, Algeria, Morocco), the Caucasus

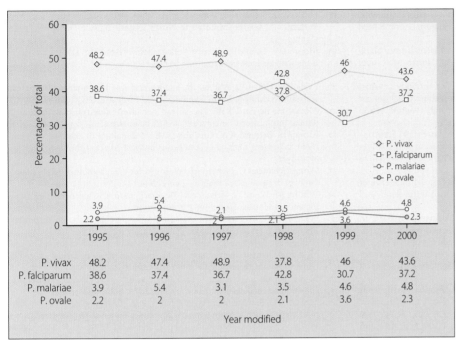

Figure 12.3 Percentage of malaria cases, by Plasmodium species (USA, 1995–2000).

	1995	1996	1997	1998	1999	2000
P. vivax	48.2	47.4	48.9	37.8	46	43.6
P. falciparum	38.6	37.4	36.7	42.8	30.7	37.2
P. malariae	3.9	5.4	3.1	3.5	4.6	4.8
P. ovale	2.2	2	2	2.1	3.6	2.3

Year modified

(Armenia, Azerbaijan, Georgia), Turkey, Turkmenistan, some island nations (Mauritius, Cape Verde), the Middle East (Iraq, Syria) and Korea (North and South near the Demilitarized Zone). The risk in these countries is often seasonal, focal, unpredictable, and quite low. Occasionally, small epidemic outbreaks can occur. Many of these risk areas are destinations seldom visited by short-term tourists on holiday, but may be visited by other types of travelers such as soldiers, diplomats, construction workers, and aid or relief workers. The risk of acquiring *P. vivax* malaria is much higher than *P. falciparum* malaria in many of these countries with CQ sensitive malaria, especially the Americas. Unfortunately, this list of countries and locations with CQ-sensitive *P. falciparum* malaria excludes most of the malarious world.

CQ-resistant *P. falciparum* (CRPf) malaria is now found throughout the rest of the endemic areas to include all of Sub-Saharan Africa, South America, the Indian sub-continent and Southeast Asia, and Oceania. CRPf was first recognized in the early 1960s in Columbia,[19] spreading throughout the Amazon Basin within a decade and Cambodia[20] spreading through south Asia and into East Africa in 1978. CRPF was widely distributed throughout Sub-Saharan Africa by the late 1980s.[21-23]

CQ-resistant *P. vivax* (CRPv) malaria was first described in an Australian soldier returning from Papua New Guinea in 1987.[24] Since that initial recognized case, studies have shown that CRPv is relatively widespread in Indonesia, and Papua New Guinea with more sporadic reports from Borneo, Thailand, Mynamar (Burma), and India in the Old World[25] and Guyana.[26] Therapeutic failures without documentation of therapeutic blood levels for chloroquine have also been seen in Colombia[27] and Brazil. Since all of these areas are also co-endemic with CRPf, this has minimal impact on the traveler, as the chemoprophylaxis choice for these areas is not CQ.

Two cases of CQ-resistant P. malariae were recently reported from Indonesia, but the clinical significance and distribution of this entity remains undefined.[28]

Mefloquine

The only destinations with known risk of MQ resistance are border areas of western Thailand and eastern Burma (Myanmar) and eastern Thailand and western Cambodia.[23,29] More extensive MQ resistance may occur in Burma and Cambodia, but these areas are not common tourist destinations. Sporadic cases of MQ prophylaxis failures have been reported from other locations in Africa and South America, but these few cases do not alter routine travel chemoprophylaxis recommendations.

Doxycycline

There are no known geographic areas where doxycycline should not be recommended because of drug resistance. In fact, resistance to doxycycline had not been reported.

Atovaquone/proguanil

Resistance to either atovaquone or proguanil is based on single point mutations in the cytochrome B gene or the dihydro-folate reductase (DHFR) gene, respectively. Drug resistant parasites emerge rather quickly with treatment when either drug is used separately. In combination, drug resistance is much less common. However, a single case of late treatment failure has been reported in a returning traveler treated with Atovaquone/Proguanil recently[30] but no cases of breakthroughs in prophylaxis have been reported to date.

REFERENCES

1. Schlagenhauf P, Muentner P. Imported Malaria. In: Schlagenhauf P, ed. *Travelers' Malaria*. Hamilton: BC Decker; 2001:495–508.
2. Legros F, Gay F, Belkaid M, Danis M. Imported malaria in continental France on 1996. *Eurosurveillance* 1998; **3**(4):37–38.
3. Causer L, Newman R, Barber A, *et al*. Malaria Surveillance – United States, 2000. Surveillance Summaries. *Morb Mortal Wkly Rep* 2002; **51**(SS-5):9–23.
4. Phillips-Howard PA, Bradley DJ, Blaze M, Hurn M. Malaria in Britain: 1977–86. *BMJ (Clin Res Ed)* 1988; **296**(6617):245–248.
5. Phillips-Howard PA, Radalowicz A, Mitchell J, Bradley DJ. Risk of malaria in British residents returning from malarious areas. *BMJ* 1990; **300**(6723): 499–503.
6. Romi R, Sabatinelli G, Majori G. Malaria epidemiological situation in Italy and evaluation of malaria incidence in Italian travelers. *J Travel Med* 2001; **8**(1):6–11.

7. Ende J Van den, Morales I, Abbeele K Van den, *et al.* Changing epidemiological and clinical aspects of imported malaria in Belgium. *J Travel Med* 2001; **8**(1):19–25.

8. Greenberg AE, Lobel HO. Mortality from Plasmodium falciparum malaria in travelers from the United States, 1959 to 1987. *Ann Intern Med* 1990; **113**(4):326–327.

9. Jelinek T, Loscher T, Nothdurft HD. High prevalence of antibodies against circumsporozoite antigen of Plasmodium falciparum without development of symptomatic malaria in travelers returning from sub-Saharan Africa. *J Infect Dis* 1996; **174**(6):1376–1379.

10. Nothdurft HD, Jelinek T, Bluml A, Sonnenburg F von, Loscher T. Seroconversion to circumsporozoite antigen of Plasmodium falciparum demonstrates a high risk of malaria transmission in travelers to East Africa. *Clin Infect Dis* 1999; **28**(3):641–642.

11. Jelinek T, Bluml A, Loscher T, Nothdurft HD. Assessing the incidence of infection with Plasmodium falciparum among international travelers. *Am J Trop Med Hyg* 1998; **59**(1):35–37.

12. Jelinek T, Schulte C, Behrens R, *et al.* Imported Falciparum malaria in Europe: sentinel surveillance data from the European network on surveillance of imported infectious diseases. *Clin Infect Dis* 2002; **34**(5):572–576.

13. Steffen R, Fuchs E, Schildknecht J, *et al.* Mefloquine compared with other malaria chemoprophylactic regimens in tourists visiting east Africa. *Lancet* 1993; **341**(8856):1299–1303.

14. Jelinek T, Grobusch MP, Loscher T. Patterns of Plasmodium falciparum drug resistance in nonimmune travellers to Africa. *Eur J Clin Microbiol Infect Dis* 2001; **20**(4):284–286.

15. Bradley DJ. Current trends in malaria in Britain. *J R Soc Med* 1989; **82**(suppl **17**):8–13.

16. Talarmin F, Sicard JM, Mounem M, Verrot D, Husser JA. Imported malaria in Moselle: 75 cases in three years. *Rev Med Interne* 2000; **21**(3):242–246.

17. Raglio A, Parea M, Lorenzi N, *et al.* Ten-year experience with imported malaria in Bergamo, Italy. *J Travel Med* 1994; **1**(3):152–155.

18. Di Perri G, Solbiati M, Vento S, *et al.* West African Immigrants and New Patterns of Malaria Imported to North Eastern Italy. *J Travel Med* 1994; **1**(3):147–151.

19. Moore DV, Lanier JE. Observations on two Plasmodum falciparum infections with an abnormal response to chloroquine. *Am J Trop Med Hyg* 1961; **10**:5.

20. Eyles DE, Hoo CC, Warren M, Sandosham AA. Plasmodium falciparum resistant to chloroquine in Cambodia. *AM J trop Med Hyg* 1963; **12**:840.

21. Moran JS, Bernard KW. The spread of chloroquine-resistant malaria in Africa. Implications for travelers. *JAMA* 1989; **262**(2):245–248.

22. Moran JS, Bernard KW, Greenberg AE, *et al.* Failure of chloroquine treatment to prevent malaria in Americans in West Africa. *JAMA* 1987; **258**(17):2376–2377.

23. Wongsrichanalai C, Pickard AL, Wernsdorfer WH, Meshnick SR. Epidemiology of drug-resistant malaria. *Lancet Infect Dis* 2002; **2**(4):209–218.

24. Whitby M, Wood G, Veenendaal JR, Rieckmann K. Chloroquine-resistant Plasmodium vivax. *Lancet* 1989; **2**(8676):1395.

25. Whitby M. Drug resistant Plasmodium vivax malaria. *J Antimicrob Chemother* 1997; **40**(6):749–752.

26. Phillips EJ, Keystone JS, Kain KC. Failure of combined chloroquine and high-dose primaquine therapy for Plasmodium vivax malaria acquired in Guyana, South America. *Clin Infect Dis* 1996; **23**(5):1171–1173.

27. Soto J, Toledo J, Gutierrez P, et al. Plasmodium vivax clinically resistant to chloroquine in Colombia. *Am J Trop Med Hyg* 2001; **65**(2):90–93.

28. Maguire JD, Sumawinata IW, Masbar S, *et al.* Chloroquine-resistant Plasmodium malariae in south Sumatra, Indonesia. *Lancet* 2002; **360**(9326):58–60.

29. Wongsrichanalai C, Sirichaisinthop J, Karwacki JJ, *et al.* Drug resistant malaria on the Thai-Myanmar and Thai-Cambodian borders. *Southeast Asian J Trop Med Public Health* 2001; **32**(1):41–49.

30. Fivelman QL, Butcher GA, Adagu IS, Warhurst DC, Pasvol G. Malarone treatment failure and in vitro confirmation of resistance of Plasmodium falciparum isolate from Lagos, Nigeria. *Malar J* 2002; **1**(1):1.

CHAPTER 13 Malaria Chemoprophylaxis

Patricia Schlagenhauf, Carrie Beallor and Kevin C. Kain

KEYPOINTS

All travelers to malaria-endemic areas need to:

■ be aware of the risk of malaria and understand that it is a serious, potentially fatal infection

■ know how to best prevent it with insect protection measures and chemoprophylaxis (where appropriate)

■ seek medical attention urgently should they develop a fever during or after travel

■ The use of antimalarial drug regimens should be carefully directed at high-risk travelers where their benefit most clearly outweighs the risk of adverse events

■ None of the available regimens are ideal for all travelers and the travel medicine practitioner should attempt to match the individual's risk of exposure to malaria to the appropriate regimen based on drug efficacy, tolerability, safety, and cost

INTRODUCTION

The development and spread of drug-resistant malaria parasites and insecticide-resistant mosquitoes have led to the resurgence of malaria as a global health problem. In 1998, The World Health Organization estimated that there were 273 million cases and more than 1 million deaths due to malaria.[1] Although the burden of malaria is primarily borne by individuals in developing nations, the dramatic increase in international travel now exposes an estimated 50–70 million Western travelers to infection annually.[2] Approximately 30 000 travelers from industrialized countries are reported to contract malaria each year and between 1–4% of travelers who acquire *Plasmodium falciparum* malaria will die. Record numbers of imported malaria cases have recently been documented in North America and Europe, with an increasing number caused by drug-resistant *P. falciparum*.[4–9] However, the incidence of malaria in travelers is likely to be an underestimate since it does not include those diagnosed and treated abroad and because it is estimated that 40–70% of imported malaria cases are not reported to health authorities.

The overall case fatality rate of imported *P. falciparum* malaria varies from 0.6 to 3.8%, but may be 20% or greater in the elderly or in cases of severe malaria even when optimally managed in modern intensive care units.[4–9] Case fatality rates for malaria complicated by adult respiratory distress syndrome (ARDS) often exceed 80%.[8] However, malaria infection and associated fatalities are largely preventable. In nearly all reported fatal cases of imported malaria, travelers failed to use or comply with appropriate chemoprophylactic regimens. Recent reports of fatal cases of malaria in North America and Europe highlight problems in these areas.[5–8] In nearly all fatal outcomes, patients were using either no chemoprophylaxis or an inappropriate regimen, had a delay or errors in the diagnosis of malaria by physicians and laboratories, or received incorrect initial chemotherapy.

APPROACH TO MALARIA PREVENTION

All travelers to malaria-endemic areas need to be:
■ aware of the risk of malaria and understand that it is a serious, potentially fatal infection;
■ know how to best prevent it with insect protection measures and chemoprophylaxis (where appropriate);
■ seek medical attention urgently should they develop a fever during or after travel.

This section will highlight the important principles of malaria prevention. The reader is also referred to other sources[11–14] and websites listed in Table 13.1 for additional information on country specific malaria risk.

Protection against malaria can be summarized into four principles.

Assessing individual risk

Estimating a traveler's risk is based on a detailed travel itinerary and specific risk behaviors of the traveler. The risk of acquiring malaria will vary according to the geographic area visited (e.g. Africa versus Southeast Asia), the travel destination within different geographic areas (e.g. urban versus rural travel), type of accommodations (camping versus well-screened or air conditioned), duration of stay (1 week business travel versus 3 month overland trek), time of travel (high or low malaria transmission season; risk usually is highest during and immediately after the rainy season), efficacy of and compliance with preventive measures used (e.g. treated bednets, chemoprophylactic drugs), and elevation of destination (malaria transmission is rare above 2000 m).

There have been recent reports of a resurgence of malaria at higher elevations, particularly in the highlands of East Africa. Although there was initial speculation that this was attributable to climate change, more recent data has not supported this contention.[10] Escalating drug resistance and population movements are a more plausible explanation for these highland epidemics. Country specific altitude limitations to malaria can generally be found in destination references[11–14] and websites in Table 13.1. It should be noted that the starting points and base camps for many higher altitude hikes, for example Mount Kilimanjaro, are at altitudes where there may be a high risk for malaria.

Additional information can be obtained from studies that estimate risk of malaria in travelers using malaria surveillance data and the numbers of travelers to specific destinations. These studies demon-

Table 13.1 Selected websites for information about country-specific malaria risk

Site sponsor (URL)	Comments
US Centers for Disease Control and Prevention (http://www.cdc.gov)	See Travelers' Health Section. Online references include full-text *Health Information for International Travel*, 2001–2002, with full adult and pediatric recommendations, including malaria risks and recommendations. Information is also available via telephone (877-FYI-TRIP) or fax (888-232-3299)
World Health Organization (http://www.who.int/ith)	See *International Travel and Health* information resource page for travelers. Includes updates on country-specific malaria risk.
Switzerland (http://www.safetravel.ch)	Provides recommendations and updates for preventing and treating malaria in travelers in French and German.
Health Canada (http://www.hc-sc.gc.ca/pphb-dgspsp/tmp-pmv/)	See recommendations and updates for preventing and treating malaria in travelers.

strate a higher risk of infection, particularly with *P. falciparum*, in Africa and New Guinea compared with Asia or Latin America. Risk of infection if no chemoprophylaxis is used varies from >20% per month in regions of Papua (formerly Irian Jaya), to 1.7–2.4% per month in West Africa, to 0.01% per month in Central America.[7,15,16] Of note, the estimated risk of malaria for travelers to Thailand in one study was 1:12 254 that may be less than the risk of a serious adverse event secondary to malaria chemoprophylaxis.[17] Such data can help provide an estimate of the risk-benefit ratio for the use of various chemoprophylactic drugs in different geographic areas. Updated malaria information and country specific risk are available on line from several sources including the Centers for Disease Control and Prevention (CDC), the World Health Organization (WHO), and Health Canada (see Table 13.1).

Preventing mosquito bites (personal protection measures)

All travelers to malaria-endemic areas need to be instructed how best to avoid bites from *Anopheles* mosquitoes which transmit malaria. Any measure that reduces exposure to the evening and night-time feeding female *Anopheles* mosquito will reduce the risk of acquiring malaria. Recent studies have demonstrated that only DEET-based repellents provide adequate protection against mosquito bites.[18] Controlled trials have also shown that DEET-based insect repellents are effective at preventing vector-borne diseases such as malaria.[19] A recent randomized placebo controlled trial examined the use of DEET-based repellents (20% DEET) during 2nd and 3rd trimester of pregnancy. No adverse effects were identified in mother or fetus, providing some reassurance regarding the use of low concentration DEET-based repellents by pregnant women.[20] Insecticide-impregnated bed nets (permethrin or similarly treated) are safe for children and pregnant women and are an effective prevention strategy that is under utilized by travelers (Chapter 7).

Use of chemoprophylactic drugs where appropriate

The use of antimalarial drugs and their potential adverse effects must be weighed against the risk of acquiring malaria (as described above). The following questions should be addressed before prescribing any antimalarial.
- Will the traveler be exposed to malaria? The risk of malaria exists in urban and rural areas of sub-Saharan Africa and the Indian sub-continent, whereas most urban areas, beach and tourist resort areas of Southeast Asia, Central and South America do not have sufficient risk of malaria to warrant routine use of chemoprophylaxis.
- What type of malaria predominates at the destination; *P. falciparum* or *P. vivax* or other
- Will the traveler be in a drug-resistant *P. falciparum* zone? See Figure 13.1 and Table 13.2.
- Will the traveler have prompt access to medical care (including blood smears prepared with sterile equipment and then properly interpreted) if symptoms of malaria were to occur?
- Are there any contraindications to the use of a particular antimalarial drug? Several issues including underlying health conditions, drug interactions, pregnancy, and breastfeeding must be considered. It is also important to determine whether a woman is planning on becoming pregnant while traveling.

An overview of antimalarial drug regimens based on drug-resistance zones is provided in Figure 13.1 and Table 13.2. It is important to note that a number of travelers to low risk areas such as urban areas and tourist resorts of Southeast Asia, continue to be inappropriately prescribed antimalarial drugs that result in unnecessary adverse events but little protection. Improved traveler adherence with antimalarials will likely result when travel medicine practitioners make a concerted effort to identify and carefully council the high-risk traveler and avoid unnecessary drugs in the low risk individual.

Seeking early diagnosis and treatment if fever develops during or after travel

Travelers should be informed that although personal protection measures and antimalarials can markedly decrease the risk of contracting malaria, these interventions do not guarantee complete protection. Symptoms due to malaria may occur as early as 1 week after first exposure, and as late as several years after leaving a malaria zone whether or not chemosuppression has been used. Approximately 90% of malaria-infected travelers do not become symptomatic until they return home.[21–23] Most travelers who acquire falciparum malaria will develop symptoms within 3 months of exposure.[21–23] Falciparum malaria can be effectively treated early in its course, but delays in therapy may result in a serious and even fatal outcome. The most important factors that determine outcome are early diagnosis and appropriate therapy. Travelers and health-care providers alike must consider and urgently rule out malaria in any febrile illness that occurs during or after travel to a malaria-endemic area.

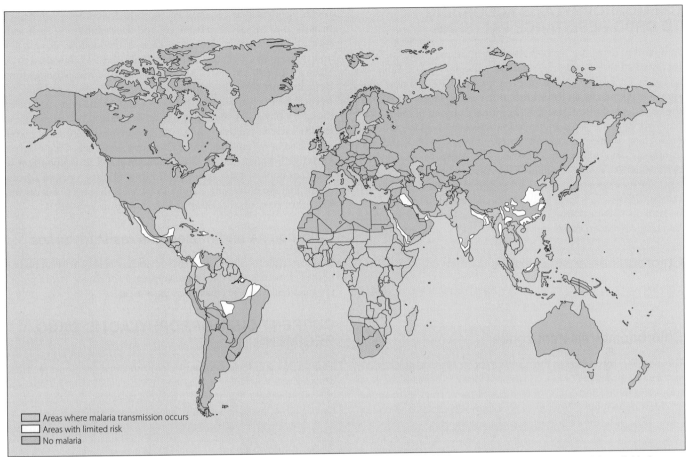

Figure 13.1 Map of malaria-endemic areas and zones of resistance. Intended as a guide *only* (see detailed country specific malaria risk available from sources listed in Table 13.1).

Table 13.2	Malaria chemoprophylactic regimens for persons at risk by zone[a]	
Zone	**Drug(s) of choice[b]**	**Alternatives**
No Chloroquine resistance	Chloroquine	Mefloquine, Doxycycline or Atovaquone/proguanil
Chloroquine resistance	Mefloquine or Atovaquone/proguanil or Doxycycline	1st Choice: Primaquine[c]; 2nd Choice: Chloroquine plus Proguanil[d]
Chloroquine and Mefloquine resistance	Doxycycline	Atovaquone/proguanil
Adult doses Chloroquine phosphate: Mefloquine: Atovaquone/proguanil: Doxycycline: Primaquine: Proguanil:	300 mg (base) weekly 250 mg (salt in USA; base elsewhere) weekly One tablet daily (250 mg/100 mg) 100 mg daily 30 mg (base) daily[c] 200 mg daily	

[a]*IMPORTANT NOTE*: Protection from mosquito bites (insecticide-treated bednets, DEET-based insect repellents, etc.) is the first line of defense against malaria for *all* travelers. In the Americas and Southeast Asia, chemoprophylaxis is recommended *only* for travelers who will be exposed outdoors during evening or night time in rural areas.
[b]Chloroquine and Mefloquine are to be taken once weekly, beginning 1 week before entering the malarial area, during the stay and for 4 weeks after leaving. Doxycycline and proguanil are taken daily, starting 1 day before entering malarial areas, during the stay and for 4 weeks after departure. Atovaquone/proguanil and primaquine are taken once daily, starting one day before entering the malarial area, during the stay and may be discontinued 7 days after leaving the endemic area.
[c]Contraindicated in G6PD (glucose-6-phosphate dehydrogenase) deficiency and during pregnancy. *Not* presently licensed for this use. A G6PD level must be performed before prescribing.
[d]Chloroquine plus proguanil is less efficacious than Mefloquine, doxycycline or AP in these areas.

CHEMOPROPHYLAXIS ACCORDING TO DRUG RESISTANCE PATTERNS

Antimalarial drugs are selected based on individual risk assessment (as discussed above) and drug-resistance patterns (Fig. 13.1, Tables 13.1 and 13.2). Chloroquine-resistant *P. falciparum* (CRPF) is now widespread in all malaria-endemic areas of the world, except for Mexico, the Caribbean, Central America, Argentina, and parts of the Middle-East and China. *P. falciparum* malaria resistant to chloroquine and mefloquine is still rare except on the borders of Thailand with Cambodia and Myanmar (Burma). Resistance to sulfadoxine-pyrimethamine is now common in the Amazon basin and Southeast Asia and is emerging in various regions of Africa. Chloroquine-resistant *Plasmodium vivax* is also becoming an important problem, particularly in Papua New Guinea, West Papua (formerly Irian Jaya), Vanuatu, Myanmar, and Guyana.

Chloroquine-sensitive zones

Chloroquine is the drug of choice for travel to areas where chloroquine resistance has *not* been described.

Chloroquine-resistant zones

For most at risk travelers to these areas a choice between mefloquine, atovaquone-proguanil , or doxycycline will have to be made. In those with contraindications to or intolerance of these drugs, primaquine or chloroquine plus proguanil may occasionally be used. Deciding

which agent is best requires an individual assessment of risk of malaria and the specific advantages and disadvantages of each regimen (Tables 13.1–13.7). For drugs such as mefloquine, doxycycline and chloroquine/proguanil to be optimally effective, they need to be taken for 4 weeks after leaving a malaria-endemic area, although traveler adherence with this component has traditionally been poor.[21–23] Agents such as atovaquone-proguanil and primaquine are called causal prophylactics since they kill act on malaria parasites early in the life-cycle in the liver, and therefore may be discontinued 1 week after leaving an endemic area. This advantage makes these agents attractive for high-risk but short duration travel. It is important to note that none of these agents is ideal and all carry a risk of adverse events that are distressing enough to travelers that 1–7% will discontinue their prescribed chemoprophylactic regimen.[3,11–13,21–23]

Chloroquine and mefloquine resistant zones

In these regions along the Thai-Myanmar and Thai-Cambodian border, doxycycline is the chemosuppressive of choice. Atovaquone-proguanil may also be effective in these areas.[11–13]

CURRENT CHEMOPROPHYLACTIC DRUG REGIMENS

This section will review currently recommended chemoprophylactic drug regimens including indications, adverse effects, precautions, and contraindications. The reader is referred elsewhere for other important details of management of malaria-infected patients.[11–13,24]

Table 13.3 Incidence of *any* adverse event during malaria chemoprophylaxis in non-immune travelers

Study	Population	MQ	C+P	DX	A+P
Steffen 1993	Travelers	24	35	–	–
Boudreau 1993	US Marines	43	46	–	–
Barrett 1996	Travelers	41	41		
Nasveld 2000	Austral. Defense	–	–	58	38
Hogh[a] 2000	Travelers	–	28	–	22
Overbosch 2001	Travelers	68	–	–	71
Schlagenhauf 2002	Travelers	88	86	84	82

MQ, Mefloquine; C+P, Chloroquine/proguanil; DX, Doxycycline; A+P, Atovaquone/proguanil
[a]Drug associated.

Table 13.4 Incidence of *severe[a]* events during malaria chemoprophylaxis in travelers

Study	Population	MQ	C+P	DX	A+P
Phillips 1996	Australian	11.2	–	6.5	–
Schlagenhauf 1996	Swiss	11.2	–	–	–
Barrett 1996	UK	17	16	–	–
Steffen 1993	European	13	16		
Hogh[b] 2000	International		2		0.2
Overbosch[b] 2001	International	5	–		1
Schlagenhauf[c] 2002	International	10.5	12.4	5.9	6.7

MQ, Mefloquine; C+P, Chloroquine/proguanil; DX, Doxycycline; A+P, Atovaquone/proguanil
[a]Interferes with daily activity
[b]Stopped taking antimalarials
[c]Sought medical attention in context of the study

Table 13.5 Incidence of *serious*[a] adverse events during malaria chemoprophylaxis

Report	Population	MQ	C+P	DX	A+P
MacPhearson 1992	Canadian	1/20 000		?	?
Steffen 1993	European	1/10 000	1/13 600		
Croft 1996	UK soldiers	1/ 6000			
Barrett 1996	UK	1/600	1/1200		
Roche Drug Safety 1997	Worldwide	1/20 000			

MQ, Mefloquine; C+P, Chloroquine/proguanil; DX, Doxycycline; A+P, Atovaquone/proguanil
[a]Hospitalization

Chloroquine, chloroquine/proguanil

Description, pharmacology and mode of action

Chloroquine was initially developed in Germany in the 1930s and further evaluated by the Allied powers in the 1940s. It was found to be an outstanding anti-malaria drug and has been in continuous use for over 50 years. Although still widely consumed in endemic areas, widespread resistance (Fig. 13.1) limits the use of chloroquine and its combinations by travelers. This 4-aminoquinoline drug is chemically a racemate and both enantiomers have equivalent anti-malaria activity. Preparations are available as phosphate, sulfate and hydrochloride salts under a wide variety of trade names. The combination of proguanil-200 mg (usually as Paludrine®) daily and chloroquine base-300 mg weekly has been used extensively. In some countries, a combined tablet is now available that contains chloroquine 100 mg base and proguanil hydrochloride 200 mg (Savarine®).

Chloroquine is a potent blood schizonticide active against the erythrocytic forms of sensitive strains of all four species of malaria and it is also gametocidal against *P. vivax*, *P. malariae* and *P. ovale*.[24] The site of action of chloroquine is within the lysosome of the blood stage parasite[25] where it complexes with hemin and prevents its conversion to the non-toxic hemozoin.[26] Proguanil is converted to the active cycloguanil which is a dihydrofolate reductase inhibitor that acts by interfering with folic-folinic acid systems. Proguanil is effective against the primary exo-erythrocyctic hepatic forms and is therefore a causal prophylactic. It is also a slow-acting blood schizonticide and has sporonticidal effects against *P. falciparum*.

Efficacy and drug resistance

Chloroquine resistant malaria began to appear in Southeast Asia and South America in 1960 and reached East Africa in 1978 and West Africa in 1985.[27] Proguanil-resistant *P. falciparum* is widespread and this agent is not recommended as a mono-prophylaxis. Chloroquine-resistant *P. falciparum* (CRPF) is now widespread in many malaria-endemic areas of the world. It is believed that resistance prevents access of chloroquine to the digestive process in the parasite's lysosome and this process is primarily modulated by mutations in the gene PfCRT that encodes a transmembrane digestive vacuole protein. Mutations in PfCRT permit the parasite to persist in chloroquine concentrations that kill sensitive parasites.[29-31] Chloroquine-resistant *P. vivax* has been reported in 1989 in New Guinea and later elsewhere in Oceania, India, Asia and parts of South America but resistance in this species does not appear to be mediated through mutations in PvCRT.[28]

Only one published randomized controlled trial (RCT) examining the efficacy of chloroquine as a malaria chemoprophylaxis for travelers is available. This compares chloroquine with the combination sulfadoxine/pyrimethamine in Austrian workers based in Nigeria.[32] The study found no significant difference in malaria incidence between medication groups. In the years 1990–1992 Peace Corps Volunteers stationed in West Africa had a monthly malaria incidence of 3.8 cases/100 volunteers when they used chloroquine alone. Chloroquine/proguanil users had a monthly incidence of 1.7 cases and mefloquine 0.2 cases/100 volunteers.[33] Croft and Geary[34] recently reviewed studies of chloroquine plus proguanil and found two published RCTs on the use of chloroquine plus proguanil in non-immune, general travelers where the chloroquine/proguanil combination was not significantly more effective than proguanil alone[35] or a combination of chloroquine with sulfadoxine/pyrimethamine.[36] A recent study[37] found superior efficacy for atovaquone/proguanil (1 *P. ovale* case in 511 travelers) compared with 3 *P. falciparum* cases in 511 travelers using chloroquine/proguanil. Using the combination tablet Savarine®, French soldiers in Central Africa had a 4.8% incidence of *P. falciparum* malaria compared with 0.6% of doxycycline users.[38]

Tolerability

Croft and Geary have summarized the tolerability evidence of the chloroquine/proguanil combination based on five studies[39-43] conducted in the late 1990s. They found a 1–5% incidence of mild adverse effects (AE) such as depression, dizziness, headache, mouth ulcers, sleeping difficulties, vivid dreams, visual difficulties, vomiting, 6–10% incidence of mainly gastrointestinal AE and a high incidence >10% of anorexia. A recent RCT has shown that atovaquone/proguanil is significantly better tolerated than chloroquine/proguanil[37] and the most recent RCT[44] has shown poor tolerability of chloroquine/proguanil (as Savarine®) compared with doxycycline, mefloquine or atovaquone/proguanil. Serious AE such as psychotic episodes,[16] have been reported in ~1/13 600 users of the chloroquine/proguanil regimen. Keratopathy and retinopathy have been reported in chloroquine users particularly during long-term use of the drug. Six-monthly, ophthalmologic checks are recommended particularly when the cumulative dose exceeds 100 g.

Contraindications, precautions and drug interactions[45]

According to the manufacturer, chloroquine is contraindicated in persons hypersensitive to the 4-aminoquinoline compounds and in G-6-PD deficient individuals (although significant hemolysis is rare when given at prophylactic and therapeutic doses). Other contraindications are: pre-existing retinopathy, diseases of the central nervous system, myasthenia gravis, disorders of the blood producing organs, persons with a history of epilepsy or psychosis. Dosage reduction may be required in patients with hepatic function impairments. Chloroquine and chloroquine/proguanil may be used in pregnancy. During lactation, the drug is present in breast milk, but not in suffi-

Table 13.6 Antimalarial drugs, doses[a], and adverse effects (listed alphabetically) (see text for contraindications)

Generic name	Trade name	Packaging	Adult dose	Pediatric dose	Adverse effects
Atovaquone/ proguanil	Malarone®	250 mg atovaquone *and* 100 mg proguanil (adult tablet)	See text 1 tablet daily	See text[b] 11–20 kg ¼ adult tablet or 1 pediatric tablet 21–30 kg ½ adult tablet or 2 pediatric tablets 31–40 kg ¾ adult tablet or 3 pediatric tablets > 40 kg 1 adult tablet	Nausea, vomiting, abdominal pain, diarrhea, increased transaminases, seizures, rash
Chloroquine[c] phosphate or sulfate	Aralen® Avochlot® Nivaquine® Resochia®	150 mg base	300 mg base once weekly	5 mg base once weekly 5–6 kg; 25 mg base 7–10 kg; 50 mg base 11–14 kg; 75 mg base 15–18 kg; 100 mg base 19–24 kg; 125 mg base 25–35 kg; 200 mg base 36–50 kg; 250 mg base >50 kg or if ≥14 years: 300 mg base	Pruritus in black-skinned individuals, nausea, headache, skin eruptions, reversible corneal opacity, nail and mucous membrane discoloration, nerve deafness, photophobia, myopathy, retinopathy with daily use, blood dyscrasias, psychosis, seizures, alopecia
Doxycycline	Vibramycin® Vibra-Tabs® Doryx®	100 mg	100 mg once daily	1.5 mg/kg once daily (max 100 mg daily) <25 kg or if <8 years: contraindicated 25–35 kg; 50 mg 36–50 kg; 75 mg >50 kg or if ≥14 years: 100 mg	GI upset, vaginal candidiasis, photosensitivity, allergic reactions, blood dyscrasias, azotemia in renal diseases, hepatitis
Mefloquine	Lariam® Mephaquin®	250 mg base (salt in USA)	250 mg base once weekly	<5 kg: no data 5–15 kg; 5 mg/kg once weekly 15–19 kg; ¼ tablet 20–30 kg; ½ tablet 31–45 kg; ¾ tablet >45 kg; 1 tablet once weekly	Dizziness, diarrhea, nausea, vivid dreams, nightmares, irritability, mood alterations, headache, insomnia, anxiety, seizures, psychosis
Primaquine		15 mg base	30 mg base/day Terminal prophylaxis or radical cure: 15 mg base/day for 14 days[d]	0.5 mg base/day to max of 30 mg base/day Terminal prophylaxis or radical cure: 0.3 mg base/kg/day for 14 days[e]	GI upset, hemolysis in G6PD deficiency, methemoglobinemia
Proguanil	Paludrine®	100 mg	200 mg daily *Note*: Not recommended as a single agent for prophylaxis	5–8 kg; 25 mg (¼ tablet) 9–16 kg; 50 mg (½ tablet) 7–24 kg; 75 mg (¾ tablet) 25–35 kg: 100 mg (1 tablet) 36–50 kg: 150 mg (1½ tablets) >50 kg or if ≥14 years: 200 mg (2 tablets)	Anorexia, nausea, mouth ulcers

[a]Dose for chemoprophylaxis.
[b]In the USA and EU, a pediatric formulation is available (Quarter strength = 62.5 mg atovaquone and 25 mg proguanil)
[c]Chloroquine sulfate (Nivaquine®) is not available in USA and Canada, but is available in most malaria-endemic countries in both tablet and syrup form.
[d]Doses are increased to 30 mg base/day for primaquine-resistant *P. vivax*.
[e]Doses are increased to 0.5 mg base/kg per day for primaquine-resistant or tolerant *P vivax*.

Table 13.7	Clinical utility score for current malaria chemoprophylactic regimens					
Drug	Efficacy[a]	Tolerance[b]	Convenience[c]	Causal[d]	Cost[e]	Total
Mefloquine	3	1	3	0	2	9
Doxycycline	3	2	2	0	3	10
Chloroquine/ proguanil	1	2	1	0	2	6
Primaquine	2	2	1[f]	2	3	10
Atovaquone/ proguanil	3	3	2	2	1	11

NOTE: Scores and weighting are arbitrary and can be modified/individualized to specific travelers and itineraries.
[a]Efficacy: 1 = <75%; 2 = 75–89%; 3 = ≥90%.
[b]Tolerance: 1 = occasional disabling side-effects; 2 = rare disabling side-effects; 3 = rare minor side-effects.
[c]Convenience: 1 = daily and weekly dosing required; 2 = daily dosing required; 3 = weekly dosing required.
[d]Causal: 0 = no causal activity; 2 = causal prophylactic (may be discontinued within 1 week of leaving risk area).
[e]Cost: 1 = >US$100 for 1 month of travel; 2 = US$50–100; 3 = <US$50.
[f]Requires a pre-travel G6PD level resulting in a lower convenience score.

cient quantities to harm or protect the infant. There is no known absolute contraindication for proguanil. Concomitant use of chloroquine and proguanil has been shown to increase the incidence of mouth ulcers. Administration of the oral live typhoid vaccine and live cholera vaccine should be completed 3 days before chloroquine use and chloroquine may suppress the antibody response to intradermal primary pre-exposure rabies vaccine. Other possible interactions can occur with gold salts, MAO inhibitors, digoxin and corticosteroids. The activity of methotrexate and other folic acid antagonists is increased by chloroquine use.

Indications and administration

Chloroquine is the drug of choice in the few malaria endemic areas free of CRPF. Combining chloroquine and proguanil is an option for CRPF when other 1st line antimalarials are contraindicated. The adult chloroquine dose is 300 mg base weekly (or in some countries 100 mg base daily). Pediatric preparations are available. The recommended childrens' dosage of chloroquine is 1.5 mg/kg body weight daily. The adult dose of proguanil is 200 mg daily when combined with chloroquine (or 100 mg daily when combined with atovaquone). For children the WHO recommended dosage is 3 mg/kg daily. The combination Savarine® is now registered in several European countries and contains 100 mg chloroquine base and 200 mg proguanil.

Mefloquine

Description, pharmacology and mode of action

Mefloquine was selected in the 1960s by the Walter Reed Army Institute of Research from nearly 300 quinoline methanol compounds for further investigation because of its high antimalarial activity in animal models.[46] Today, mefloquine is used clinically as a 50:50 racemic mixture of the erythro isomers and all clinical studies with the drug have used this mixture. The commercial form is available as tablets containing 250 mg mefloquine base. The mefloquine formulation available in the USA contains 250 mg mefloquine hydrochloride (equivalent to 228 mg mefloquine base). Mefloquine is available for malaria chemoprophylaxis in non-immunes since 1985 in Europe; since 1990 in the USA and has been used by more than 25 million travelers for this indication.

Mefloquine is a potent, long acting blood schizontocide (Fig. 13.1) and is effective against all malarial species including *P. falciparum* resistant to chloroquine and pyrimethamine-sulfonamide combinations. The exact mechanism of activity is unclear but mefloquine is thought to compete with the complexing protein for haem binding and the resulting drug-haem complex is toxic to the parasite.[47]

Efficacy and drug resistance

Mefloquine is currently recognized as a highly effective malaria chemoprophylaxis for non-immune travelers to high risk CRPF areas (Table 13.3). The first report of mefloquine resistance came from Thailand in 1982 and this region remains a focus of resistance particularly on the Thai-Cambodian and Thai-Burmese borders where prophylaxis breakdown has been observed. As reviewed by Mockenhaupt[48] reports of mefloquine treatment or prophylactic failures have been reported from distinct foci in Asia and to a lesser extent, from Africa and the Amazon Basin in South America. Studies in 1993 showed high efficacy of mefloquine in travelers. The protective effectiveness of mefloquine in a large cohort of travelers to East Africa was 91% that was significantly higher than other regimens used at that time: chloroquine/proguanil (72%), and chloroquine monoprophylaxis at various doses (10–42%).[16] Long-term prophylaxis with mefloquine proved highly effective in Peace Corps volunteers stationed in sub-Saharan Africa with an incidence of 0.2 infections per month in 100 volunteers. Weekly mefloquine was considered 94% more effective than prophylaxis with chloroquine and 86% more effective than prophylaxis with the chloroquine/proguanil combination regimen.[49] Mefloquine was shown to be highly efficacious (100%) in the prevention of malaria in Indonesian soldiers in Papua[15] and Rieckmann[50] found mefloquine to be 100% effective against *P. falciparum* in Australian soldiers deployed in Papua New Guinea (PNG). Pergallo[51] reported on the effective use of mefloquine by Italian troops in Mozambique, 1992–1994. When chloroquine/proguanil was the recommended regimen, an attack rate of 17 cases per 1000 soldiers per month was noted. The rate dropped significantly to 1.8 cases/1000 per month when chloroquine/proguanil was replaced by mefloquine. The effectiveness of long-term mefloquine in United Nations Peace Keeping Forces in Cambodia in 1993 was 91.4%.[52] Conversely, mefloquine was found to be incompletely effective in the prevention of malaria in Dutch Marines in Western Cambodia during the period 1992–1993. The attack rate in Marines varied significantly according to the geographical location of the battalions. Of 260 persons assigned to the area Sok San, 43 developed malaria (16%, 6.4/1000 person weeks) compared with 21 of 2029 stationed elsewhere (1%, 0.5/1000 person weeks). Mefloquine resistant parasites were isolated from Dutch and

Khmer patients.[53] The use of antimalarials by American troops during Operation Restore Hope in Somalia in 1992–1993 showed high prophylactic efficacy in mefloquine users. Sanchez *et al.*[54] reported the prophylactic efficacy in an uncontrolled cross-sectional survey of troops at one location (Bale Dogle). Mefloquine users had a malaria rate of 1.15 cases/10 000 person weeks compared with 5.49 cases/10 000 person weeks in doxycycline users. From this and other reports,[55] mefloquine was shown to be more effective than doxycycline in US troops deployed in Somalia. The lower efficacy of doxycycline was attributed to poorer compliance. Mefloquine was shown to provide a high degree of protection in Dutch service men (*n* = 125) deployed as part of a disaster relief operation to Goma, Zaire (1994). Despite evidence of exposure to *P. falciparum* as shown by the presence of circumsporozoite antibodies in 11.2% of the group, none developed overt malaria that was attributed to their use of mefloquine prophylaxis.[56] In a German population-based case-control study, mefloquine was considered to be 94.5% effective in preventing malaria in tourists to Kenya.[57]

Prophylactic failures and resistance

In many geographic regions, mapping of prophylactic failures, mainly in non-immune individuals has been used to detect early resistance development although it should be emphasized that prophylactic failures do not prove resistance. Mefloquine blood concentrations of 620 ng/ml are generally considered necessary to achieve 95% prophylactic efficacy. As defined by Lobel, a prophylactic failure is defined as a confirmed *P. falciparum* infection in persons with mefloquine blood levels in excess of this protective level.[49,58] Using this definition, an analysis of 44 confirmed *P. falciparum* cases, acquired in sub-Saharan Africa[58] showed five volunteers with mefloquine-resistant *P. falciparum* malaria. Other confirmed cases were attributed to poor compliance and the authors concluded that prevalence of mefloquine-resistant malaria in sub-Saharan Africa is still low. With regard to cross-resistance, there is recent evidence that exposure of parasite populations to antimalarial drug pressure may select for resistance not only to the drug providing the pressure but also to other novel drugs. This was clearly illustrated in the northern part of Cameroon, West Africa, where the detection of a high level of resistance to mefloquine was attributed to cross resistance with quinine[59] a drug that had been widely deployed for therapy in the area. Resistance to mefloquine appears to be distinct from chloroquine resistance, as shown by the activity of mefloquine against CRPF and by the inefficacy of verapamil to reverse mefloquine resistance although it does modulate chloroquine resistance. Moreover, *in vitro* studies have documented an inverse relationship between chloroquine and mefloquine resistance. Mefloquine resistance is however associated with halofantrine resistance[60] and quinine resistance.[59-60] Innate resistance, i.e. the existence of small sub-populations of intrinsically resistant malarial parasites within any infecting parasite biomass, is still controversial and may to some extent be explained by cross resistance to other drugs.[48] The molecular basis of mefloquine resistance is currently unknown but may be the result of mutation or amplification of certain gene products such as Pgh1, an energy-dependent transporter encoded by the mdr (multi-drug resistant) homolog *Pfmdr1*. Recent transfection studies demonstrate that mutations in *pfmdr1* may confer mefloquine resistance to sensitive parasites.[61] Penfluridol, a psychotropic drug has been reported to reverse mefloquine resistance in *P. falciparum in vitro.*[62]

Tolerability

There is considerable controversy among international experts regarding the tolerability of mefloquine prophylaxis versus alternative regimens such as doxycycline, chloroquine/proguanil, and more recently, the combination of atovaquone/proguanil. An overview of the studies and databases comparing use of malaria chemoprophylactic agents in travelers (Tables 13.3–13.5) shows largely disparate results due to differing designs, definitions and methodologies and differing study populations. Regarding the reporting of any AE, the incidence during use of mefloquine lies in the range 24–88% and when there is a comparator, is usually equivalent to the incidence reported for almost all chemoprophylactic regimens. A recent study however, showed that the tolerability of atovaquone/proguanil and doxycycline is superior to that of mefloquine.[44]

Meta-analysis

A meta-analysis evaluating the efficacy and tolerability of mefloquine prophylaxis included 10 trials in which 2750 nonimmune adult participants were randomized to mefloquine or placebo or an alternative chemoprophylaxis.[64] Rates of withdrawal and overall incidence of AE with mefloquine were not significantly higher than that observed with comparator regimens and the authors concluded that no difference in tolerability between mefloquine and comparator regimens was detected. This meta-analysis will need updating with the results of newer studies.

Moderate/severe adverse events

Although often a subjective report by the traveler, when some measure of severity is applied to AE reporting, it appears that between 11–17%[16,66-68] of travelers using mefloquine are, to some extent, incapacitated by adverse events. The extent of this incapacitation is often difficult to quantify and a good measure of the impact of adverse events is the extent of chemoprophylaxis curtailment. In a study of 5120 Italian soldiers, using either chloroquine/proguanil (C+P) or mefloquine, deployed in Somalia and Mozambique in 1992–1994, the rate of prophylaxis discontinuation in the C+P users was 1.5% compared with a significantly lower rate of discontinuation in mefloquine users (0.9%).[51] This contrasts with a recent study comparing mefloquine and atovaquone/proguanil (A+P) where subjects receiving the A+P combination regimen had a significantly lower rate of drug related adverse events that caused discontinuation of prophylaxis (5% versus 1%).[65] A recent controlled tolerability study showed intermediate withdrawal rates for mefloquine (3.9%) and doxycycline (3.9%) versus chloroquine/proguanil (5.2%) compared with atovaquone/proguanil which had the lowest withdrawal rate (1.8%).[44]

Serious adverse events

These are adverse events that constitute an apparent threat to life, which require or prolong hospitalization or which result in severe disability.[69] With mefloquine the incidence range is estimated between 1/6000–1/10 600[16,70-71] compared with a rate in chloroquine users of 1/13 600. In a retrospective cohort analysis, serious neuropsychiatric AE were noted for 1/607 mefloquine users versus 1/1181 chloroquine/proguanil users.[66]

Neuropsychiatric adverse events

This is the main area of controversy in the tolerability of mefloquine. Neuropsychiatric disorders include two broad categories of symptoms namely central and peripheral nervous system disorders (including headache, dizziness, vertigo, seizures) and psychiatric disorders (including major psychiatric disorders, affective disorders, anxiety and sleep disturbances). Lobel *et al.*[49] found an incidence of strange dreams (25%), insomnia (9%) and dizziness (8.4%) in Peace Corps volunteers using long-term mefloquine prophylaxis similar to those reported by users of chloroquine (corresponding incidence 26%, 6.5%, 10%). No severe neuropsychiatric reactions were causally associated with mefloquine use in this study. Steffen *et al.*[16] reported similar findings in an analysis of tourists ($n = 139\ 164$) returning from East Africa. Headache was observed in 6.2% of mefloquine users versus 7.6% of chloroquine/proguanil users, and dizziness, depression and insomnia by 7.6%, 1.8% and 4.2% of mefloquine users versus 5.5%, 1.7% and 6.3% of the chloroquine/proguanil group. In this same large cohort study, serious neuropsychiatric AE were observed at a rate of 1/10 600. A total of five probably associated hospitalizations were reported: two cases of seizures, two psychotic episodes and one case of vertigo. The rate of such events in chloroquine users was 1/13 600 with three associated hospitalizations for neuropsychiatric events (one seizure and two psychotic episodes). Croft[72] reported on the experience of the British army with mefloquine which indicated that the incidence of severe neuropsychiatric reactions arising during a period of prophylaxis lasting 3 months, is not higher than 1/6000. In a randomized, double-blind, placebo-controlled ongoing monitoring of AE in Canadian travelers using mefloquine ($n = 251$) or placebo ($n = 238$) there was no significant difference in the number or severity of AE reported by the mefloquine or placebo users. One clinically significant neuropsychiatric AE, a moderate to severe anxiety attack occurred in one of the 251 mefloquine users.[70] In the UK retrospective survey with telephone interviews[66] significantly more neuropsychiatric AE were reported by mefloquine users compared with travelers taking the chloroquine/proguanil combination. Neuropsychiatric events classified as disabling were reported by 0.7% of mefloquine and 0.09% chloroquine/proguanil users, respectively ($P = 0.021$). Two travelers taking mefloquine (1/607) versus one traveler using chloroquine/proguanil (1/1181) were hospitalized for such events. A retrospective survey of returned travelers suggested a causal relationship between neuropsychiatric events during travel and the use of mefloquine prophylaxis.[73] Two recent studies have shown a significant excess of neuropsychiatric events in mefloquine users versus comparators.[44,65] The precise role of antimalarial drugs in neuropsychiatric adverse events is difficult to define and the role of travel as a catalyst for such events should be considered together with other confounding factors such as gender predisposition and the use of recreational drugs and alcohol.[74] The WHO recommends that mefloquine be contraindicated for persons with a personal or family history of such psychiatric disorders. In terms of all AE, studies have shown that women are significantly more likely to experience AE.[66–68,75] This might be due to dose-related toxicity although studies have shown no association between body weight and AE in malaria prophylaxis.[67–68] It might be due to reporting bias, greater compliance with prescription[76] or to gender related differences in drug absorption, metabolism[67] or CNS distribution. Computer simulations suggest that reduced dosage in women would be effective and may result in improved tolerability.[67,77] An earlier tolerability study aimed to correlate nonserious AE occurring during routine chemoprophylaxis with concentrations of racemic mefloquine, its enantiomers or the carboxylic acid metabolite.[68] The disposition of mefloquine was found to be highly selective but neither the concentrations of enantiomers, nor total mefloquine nor metabolite were found to be significantly related to the occurrence of non-serious AE.[74] A role has been suggested for the concomitant use of mefloquine and recreational drugs[67,73] or an interaction between mefloquine and large quantities of alcohol[77] although concomitant use of small quantities of alcohol does not appear to adversely affect tolerability.[78] Children tolerate mefloquine well as do elderly travelers who report significantly fewer AE than younger counterparts.[79] One report suggests that subjects with AE have slower elimination of mefloquine than the population in general.[80] Careful screening of travelers with particular attention to contraindications such as personal or family history of epilepsy/seizures or psychiatric disorders, should minimize the occurrence of serious AE.

Contraindications, precautions and drug interactions

Mefloquine is contraindicated in persons with a history of hypersensitivity to mefloquine or related substances such as quinine. Persons with a history of epilepsy or psychiatric disorders including active depression shouldn't use the drug and concomitant treatment with halofantrine is contraindicated.[11–13,81]

Use of mefloquine for pregnant women in the second and third trimester who cannot defer travel to high-risk areas, has been sanctioned by the WHO and CDC[11–13]. It has been suggested that pregnancy should be avoided for 3 months after completing prophylaxis due to mefloquine`s long half-life although inadvertent pregnancy while using mefloquine is not considered grounds for pregnancy termination. Mefloquine is secreted into breast milk in small quantities. The effect, if any, on breast-fed infants is unknown.

A retrospective analysis of a database of antimalarial tolerability data showed that co-medications commonly used by travelers have had no significant clinical impact on the safety of prophylaxis with mefloquine.[82] The co-administration of mefloquine with cardioactive drugs might contribute to the prolongation of QTc intervals, although, in the light of the information currently available, co-administration of mefloquine with such drugs is not contraindicated but should be monitored. Vaccination with oral live typhoid or cholera vaccines should be completed at least three days before the first dose of mefloquine. Caution is indicated in persons performing tasks requiring fine coordination[11–13,81] but a review of performance impact of mefloquine[82–84] suggests that if mefloquine is tolerated by an individual then his or her performance is not undermined by use of the drug.

Indications and administration

Mefloquine is effective in the prevention of CRPF malaria, except in clearly defined Thai border regions of multidrug resistance. It is a priority antimalarial for travelers to high risk malaria endemic areas. The recommended adult dose for chemoprophylaxis is 250 mg base weekly as a single dose (US 228 mg base). Adults weighing less than 45 kg and children >5 kg require a weekly dose of 5 mg base/kg.

In order to reach steady-state levels of mefloquine in a reduced time-frame (4 days rather than 7–9 weeks with the regular 250 mg per week regimen) some studies[70,78,83,84] have used a loading dose strategy of 250 mg mefloquine daily for 3 days followed thereafter by weekly mefloquine dosage. This strategy has also been suggested for last minute travelers to high-risk areas with chloroquine-resistant CRPF. The advantage being rapid attainment of mefloquine protective levels (620 ng/ml) within 4 days but this is offset to some extent by a higher proportion of individuals with AE using the loading dose strategy.[83]

Mefloquine and its metabolite are not appreciably removed by hemodialysis.[85] No special dosage adjustments are indicated for dialysis patients to achieve concentrations in plasma similar to those in healthy volunteers.

Doxycycline

Description

The tetracyclines form a class of broad spectrum antimicrobial agents with activity against gram-positive and gram-negative aerobic and anaerobic bacteria, mycoplasma, rickettsia, chlamydiae, and protozoa, including those that cause malaria. Doxycycline and minocycline were derived semi-synthetically in 1967 and 1972, respectively.[86,87]

Pharmacology and mode of action

Tetracyclines, including doxycycline, are relatively slow-acting schizonticidal agents and are therefore not used alone for treatment. However, numerous studies have established the efficacy of doxycycline as a solo chemoprophylactic agent against *P. vivax* and *P. falci-*

parum malaria. In addition to its activity against the erythrocytic stage of the parasite, doxycycline is thought to possess some pre-erythrocytic (causal) activity. However, studies examining its efficacy as a causal agent had unacceptable high failure rates, and doxycycline needs to be taken as a chemosuppressive for 4 weeks after leaving a malaria-endemic area to be optimally effective.[11,12,88,89]

The mechanism of action of tetracyclines in bacteria has been examined in detail and is presumed to be similar in protozoa. Tetracyclines reversibly bind primarily to the 30S ribosomal subunit thereby inhibiting protein synthesis by preventing the incorporation of new amino acids into the growing peptide chain.[86] Doxycycline has several advantages over first-generation tetracyclines, including improved absorption, a broader spectrum, a longer half-life, and an improved safety profile. Doxycycline is well absorbed from the proximal small bowel (>90% oral absorption), and in contrast to other tetracyclines, its uptake does not change significantly with food intake. Doxycycline may be taken with food or milk, and this approach decreases the gastrointestinal irritation occasionally associated with this drug. Doxycycline is highly protein-bound (93%), has a small volume of distribution (0.7 L/kg), and is lipid soluble. These features may explain its high blood levels and prolonged half-life, permitting a once-daily dosing regimen. Doxycycline has a half-life of approximately 15 to 22 h that is unaffected by renal impairment. Doxycycline is eliminated unchanged in the urine by glomerular filtration and largely unchanged in the faeces by biliary and gastro-intestinal (GI) secretion. About 40% of the dose is eliminated in the urine in individuals with normal kidney function whereas those with renal dysfunction are able to eliminate it via the liver-biliary-GI route. Therefore, unlike other tetracyclines, doxycycline may be used in renal failure, and the dose does not need to be adjusted in cases of renal impairment. The drug is not effectively removed by peritoneal dialysis or hemodialysis.[86,87]

Efficacy and drug resistance

A number of randomized trials have examined the efficacy of doxycycline as a chemoprophylactic against *Plasmodium* sp.[15,89-97] Four of these studies were randomized, double blind, and placebo controlled. Two of these trials evaluated semi-immune children or adults in Kenya, and three trials examined non-immune populations in Oceania. The reported protective efficacy in these trials was excellent, ranging from 92% to 100% against *P. falciparum* and *P. vivax* malaria. In comparative trials in areas with chloroquine-resistant *P. falciparum* malaria, doxycycline has been shown to be equivalent to mefloquine and atovaquone-proguanil and superior to azithromycin and chloroquine-proguanil.[15,93-97] Parasite resistance to doxycycline has not been reported to be an operational problem in any malaria-endemic area thus far.

Tolerability

The most commonly reported adverse events related to doxycycline use are GI effects, including nausea, vomiting, abdominal pain, and diarrhea. These adverse effects are less frequent with doxycycline than with other tetracyclines. Esophageal ulceration is a rare but well-described adverse event associated with doxycycline use that generally presents with retrosternal burning and odynophagia 1 to 7 days after therapy is initiated.[55,98] In a study of ~10 000 US troops deployed in Somalia, esophageal ulceration due to doxycycline was the most frequent cause of hospitalization attributed to the use of malaria chemoprophylaxis.[55] Taking doxycycline with food and plentiful fluids, in an upright position can reduce GI adverse effects.

Dermatologic reactions are also a frequent adverse event associated with doxycycline use. These reactions range from mild paresthesias or exaggerated sunburn in exposed skin to photo-onycholysis (sun-

induced separation of nails), severe erythema, bulla formation, and (rarely) Stevens-Johnson syndrome.[86] The reported rate of photosensitivity varies from ~4% to 16% or more of users, and the reaction is mild in the majority of cases.[97,100] The risk of photosensitivity may be reduced by the use of appropriate sunscreens (>SPF 15 and protective against both ultraviolet A [UVA] and ultraviolet B [UVB] radiation).[97,99]

Although doxycycline has a lesser effect on normal bacterial flora than other tetracyclines, it still increases the risk of oral and vaginal candidiasis in predisposed individuals. Travelers with a past history of these problems who are prescribed doxycycline should be advised to carry an appropriate treatment course of antifungal therapy.

Other uncommon adverse events occasionally attributed to doxycycline include dizziness, lightheadedness, darkening or discoloration of the tongue, and (rarely) hepatotoxicity, pancreatitis, or benign intracranial hypertension.[100]

Overall, a number of comparative studies have shown that doxycycline used as a chemoprophylactic agent is generally well tolerated and has relatively few reported side-effects.[15,55,90,91,94-97] In clinical trials, doxycycline was tolerated as well as or better than placebo or the comparator drug with few serious adverse events reported. Randomized controlled trials comparing the tolerability of mefloquine and doxycycline in soldiers deployed in Thailand, and primaquine, doxycycline, proguanil/chloroquine, and mefloquine compared with placebo in semi-immune children in Kenya found no significant differences in tolerability between these agents.[94,101] Ohrt and colleagues compared mefloquine and doxycycline in a randomized placebo-controlled field trial in non-immune soldiers in Papua (Irian Jaya). In this trial, both drugs were well tolerated, but doxycycline was better tolerated than mefloquine or placebo, with respect to the frequency of reported symptoms.[15] The authors attributed this to the potential of doxycycline to prevent other infectious processes. Anderson and colleagues compared doxycycline and azithromycin in a field trial in semi-immune adults in western Kenya.[95] Both drugs were well tolerated compared with placebo, but there was one case of doxycycline withdrawal due to recurrent vaginitis. There were no significant differences observed in adverse event profiles between the treatment arms, except that azithromycin was protective against dysentery. More recently, a randomized comparative trial of doxycycline versus atovaquone/proguanil was performed in Australian military personnel deployed in Oceania. There were no malaria breakthrough infections in either arm of this trial. Both drugs were well tolerated; however, atovaquone/proguanil was significantly better tolerated, with less reported GI (29% versus 53%) adverse events.[97] A recent randomized comparative trial of antimalarials tolerability has reported that doxycycline was well tolerated compared with other commonly used agents and significantly better tolerated than chloroquine/proguanil.[44]

Adherence with doxycycline, despite its daily dosing schedule, has been reported to be relatively good in studies examining short-term use.[15,91,92,95] Estimating adherence rates in travelers is difficult because such studies require close daily monitoring. Ohrt and colleagues extended their initial comparative study of doxycycline and mefloquine but did not enforce adherence as they did in the first phase of the study.[15] This resulted in a drop in the protective efficacy of doxycycline from 99% (95% CI: 94% to 100%) to 89% (95% CI: 78% to 96%) against all malaria, suggesting a decrease in drug adherence if close monitoring is not done. Similar experience of declining effectiveness over time due to adherence issues has been reported by the US military deployed in Somalia and in Dutch troops deployed in Cambodia.[53-55] US troops in Somalia using doxycycline had five-fold higher attack rates by *P. falciparum* than did mefloquine users. These differences were attributed to poor adherence with daily use rather than to doxycycline resistance.[55] Collectively, these studies suggest that adherence with daily doxycycline may be challenging, especially for long-term travelers.

Contraindications, precautions, and drug interactions

Doxycycline administration is not recommended in the following situations[11–13,86,87]:

- Allergy or hypersensitivity to doxycycline or any member of the tetracycline class.
- Infants and children under 8 years of age. Tetracyclines bind calcium and may cause permanent yellow-brown discoloration of teeth, damage to tooth enamel, and impairment of skeletal bone growth in this population. Doxycycline binds calcium less than other tetracyclines, and short courses of doxycycline (such as in the treatment of Rocky Mountain spotted fever) have not been reported to cause clinically significant staining of teeth.[102]
- Pregnancy. Doxycycline crosses the placenta and therefore may cause permanent discoloration of teeth, damage to tooth enamel, and impairment of skeletal growth in the fetus.
- Breast-feeding. Doxycycline is excreted in breast milk and therefore may cause permanent discoloration of teeth, damage to tooth enamel, impairment of skeletal growth, and photosensitivity in breast-fed infants.

Precautions should be taken when using doxycycline in individuals who are susceptible to photosensitivity reactions or who have vaginal yeast infections or thrush. In addition, certain susceptible individuals with asthma may experience an allergic-type reaction to sulfite, which is formed with the oxidation of doxycycline calcium oral suspension. Doxycycline is partially metabolized by the liver; in individuals with significant hepatic dysfunction, there may be a prolonged half-life, and a dose adjustment may be required.[86,87]

The safety of long-term use of doxycycline (> 3months) has not been adequately studied.[99] Because lower doses of doxycycline and minocycline (a related tetracycline) are frequently used for extended periods to treat acne, it has been presumed that long-term use of doxycycline at an adult dose of 100 mg/day is safe. However, serious adverse events, including autoimmune hepatitis, fulminant hepatic failure, a serum-sickness-like illness, and drug-induced lupus erythematosus, have recently been reported with the use of minocycline for acne.[103] It is not known whether doxycycline causes similar adverse events. A number of potentially important drug interactions have been associated with doxycycline use,[86,87] including those involving the following drugs and substances:

- Antacids containing divalent or trivalent cations (calcium, aluminium, and magnesium). Doxycycline binds cations, and concomitant administration of antacids will decrease serum levels of doxycycline.
- Oral iron, bismuth salts, calcium, cholestyramine or colestipol, and laxatives that contain magnesium. Concomitant ingestion of these compounds may decrease doxycycline absorption. The above agents should not be taken within 1–3 h of doxycycline ingestion.
- Barbiturates, phenytoin, and carbamazepine. These drugs induce hepatic microsomal enzyme activity and, if used concurrently with doxycycline, may decrease doxycycline serum levels and half-life and may necessitate a dosage adjustment.
- Oral contraceptives. Concurrent use of doxycycline with estrogen-containing birth control pills may result in decreased contraceptive efficacy; generally, an additional method of birth control is advised. However, there are few examples of oral contraceptive failure attributable to doxycycline use, and serum hormone levels in patients taking oral contraceptives have been reported to be unaffected by co-administration of doxycycline.[104]
- Warfarin. By an unknown mechanism, the anticoagulant activity of warfarin compounds may be enhanced with concurrent use of doxycycline. Close monitoring of prothrombin time is advised if these drugs are used together.
- Vitamin A. The use of tetracyclines with vitamin A has been reported to be associated with benign intracranial hypertension.[87]

Indications and administration

Doxycycline is currently indicated as an agent of choice for prevention of mefloquine-resistant *P. falciparum* malaria (evening or overnight exposure in rural border areas of Thailand with Myanmar [Burma] or Cambodia) or an alternative to mefloquine or atovaquone/proguanil for the prevention of CRPF malaria.[11–13] Doxycycline has a long half-life that permits once-daily dosing. The dosage of doxycycline recommended for chemoprophylaxis against drug-sensitive and drug-resistant malaria is 2 mg base/kg of body weight, up to 100 mg base daily. Studies have examined lower-dose regimens, but such regimens have provided inadequate protective efficacy.[91,92] Doxycycline should be taken once daily, beginning 1 to 2 days before entering a malarious area, and should be continued while there. Because of its poor causal effect, it must be continued for 4 weeks after leaving the risk area. To decrease the occurrence of GI adverse events, it should be taken in an upright position with food and at least 100 mL of fluid. Doxycycline should not be taken within 1 to 3 h of administering an oral antacid or iron.

Atovaquone/proguanil

Introduction

Atovaquone/proguanil (AP), a fixed drug combination, is the newest antimalarial to become available although its individual components have been used for years. AP was first approved in Switzerland in August 1997 and is now available in several countries for the treatment and prophylaxis of *P. falciparum* malaria.

Description

AP is effective for both the prevention and treatment of malaria. Atovaquone is a hydroxynaphthoquinone compound and combined with proguanil, an antifolate drug, works synergistically against the erythrocytic stages of all the *Plasmodia* parasites and the liver-stage (causal prophylaxis) of *P. falciparum*.[105–107] AP is not active against hypnozoites in *P. vivax and P. ovale* and does not prevent relapse infections.

Pharmacology and mode of action

Atovaquone acts by inhibition of parasite mitochondrial electron transport at the level of the cytochrome bc1 complex and collapses mitochondrial membrane potential.[108] The plasmodial electron transport system is a thousand-fold more sensitive to atovaquone than the mammalian electron transport system, which likely explains the selective action and limited side effects of this drug. Proguanil, as described above, is metabolized to cycloguanil, which acts by inhibiting dihydrofolate reductase (DHFR). The inhibition of DHFR impedes the synthesis of folate cofactors required for parasite DNA synthesis. However, it appears that the mechanism of synergy of proguanil with atovaquone is not mediated through its cycloguanil metabolite. In studies, proguanil alone had no effect on mitochondrial membrane potential or electron transport, but significantly enhanced the ability of atovaquone to collapse mitochondrial membrane potential when used in combination. This might explain why proguanil displays synergistic activity with atovaquone even in the presence of documented proguanil resistance or in patient populations who are deficient in cytochrome P450 enzymes required for the conversion of proguanil to cycloguanil.[108]

Atovaquone is a highly lipophilic compound with poor bioavailability. Taking atovaquone with dietary fat increases its absorption and therefore tablets should be taken with a meal or a milky beverage. Atovaquone is greater than 99% protein bound. It is eliminated almost exclusively by biliary excretion. Greater than 94% can be recovered unchanged in the faeces over 21 days and less than 0.6% in the urine. The elimination half-life is about 2–3 days in adults and 1–2 days in children.[109,110] Pharmacokinetic studies in elderly patients and those with renal and hepatic impairment indicate that no dosage adjustment is require for the elderly, those with moderate hepatic or mild to moderate renal impairment. However, those with severe renal insufficiency (creatinine clearance <30 mL/min) should not use atovaquone/proguanil due to potential elevated cycloguanil levels and decreased atovaquone levels.

Efficacy and drug resistance

Atovaquone/proguanil is effective against malaria isolates resistant to a variety of other antimalarial drugs. Resistance to atovaquone develops rapidly if this drug is used alone.[111] Resistance to the combination of atovaquone plus proguanil, although uncommon, has been documented in a small number of cases following therapeutic courses of AP. Resistance in these cases was associated with mutations in the cytochrome b gene of *P. falciparum,* particularly around position 268.[112–114]

Several volunteers challenge studies have confirmed that atovaquone, proguanil and the combination have causal activity (they kill parasites as they develop in the liver).[105,107] In the most recent studies, none of 18 participants randomized to receive atovaquone or atovaquone/proguanil developed falciparum malaria following infected mosquito challenge, compared with eight of eight placebo recipients.

Three double-blind, randomized, placebo-controlled chemoprophylaxis trials have been conducted in semi-immune residents in Kenya, Zambia and Gabon.[115–117] The overall efficacy of AP in the prevention of *P. falciparum* malaria in these trials was 98% (95% CI 91.9–99.9%). The most common reported adverse events attributed to the study drug were headache, abdominal pain, dyspepsia, and diarrhea. However, of note, all adverse events occurred with similar frequency in subjects treated with placebo or AP and there were no serious adverse events.

Studies among non-immune travelers have recently been completed. In randomized, double-blind studies, ~2000 non-immune subjects traveling to a malaria-endemic area received either AP, daily for 1–2 days before travel until 7 days after travel, mefloquine or chloroquine/proguanil, from 1–3 weeks before travel until 4 weeks after travel.[37,65] No confirmed diagnosis of falciparum malaria occurred with either AP or mefloquine, but three documented cases of falciparum malaria occurred in travelers using chloroquine/proguanil. All drugs were well tolerated, but AP was significantly better tolerated than either mefloquine or chloroquine/proguanil in these studies. Drug-related discontinuation rates for AP versus mefloquine were 1.2% versus 5% (*P* = 0.001) and for AP versus chloroquine/proguanil were 0.2% versus 2% (*P* = 0.015).[37,65] In a comparative trial of AP versus doxycycline in 175 Australian military participants, there were no prophylactic failures in either arm but AP was better tolerated with a significantly lower rate of gastrointestinal (29% versus 53%) adverse events.[97]

Taken together, these studies indicate that AP is an efficacious chemoprophylactic regimen for *P. falciparum*. Additional data are required to establish the efficacy against non-falciparum malaria but these trials are underway. Preliminary data from a randomized-controlled trial in non-immune transmigrants in Papua, indicate a protective efficacy of 84% (95% CI, 45–95%) against *P. vivax* and 96% (95% CI, 71–99) against *P. falciparum*.[118]

Tolerability

Collectively, the controlled trials indicate that AP at prophylactic doses is well-tolerated by adults and children with drug discontinuation rates of 0–2%. The most commonly reported adverse events are gastrointestinal which can often be reduced by taking AP with food. According to the product monograph, when used as prevention of malaria the most commonly reported adverse events possibly attributed to AP were headache and abdominal pain; however in placebo controlled trials these occurred at similar rates as placebo recipients. In the non-immune traveler studies described above, compared with mefloquine, participants receiving AP reported significantly lower rates of neuropsychiatric adverse events (14% versus 29%) and lower drug discontinuation rates (1.2% versus 5%).[65] Compared with CP, AP users reported significantly lower GI adverse events (12% versus 20%) and lower discontinuation rates (0.2% versus 2%).[37] In a recent randomized trial in travelers, AP was the best-tolerated chemoprophylactic with discontinuation rates of 1.8% versus 3.9% for mefloquine and doxycycline and 5.2% for chloroquine/proguanil.[44]

Efficacy and tolerability have also been examined in a randomized comparative trial of AP versus CP in pediatric travelers.[119] There were no prophylactic failures but AP was better tolerated with no premature discontinuation of AP due to an adverse event compared with 2% of pediatric travelers using CP.

Contraindications, precautions and drug interactions

AP is contraindicated in those with severe renal impairment (creatinine clearance of less than 30 mL/min) and in those with a history of hypersensitivity to any of the drug components. AP should not be used to treat an individual who has failed AP chemoprophylaxis.

Safety in children less than 11 kg, in pregnant women and in lactating women has not been established.[120]

AP should not be given with other proguanil containing medications. Concomitant use with tetracycline has been associated with a 40% decrease in plasma concentrations of atovaquone. Similarly, rifampin, rifabutin, and metoclopramide significantly reduce the level of atovaquone and should not be used concurrently.[120]

Indications and administration

AP is currently indicated for short-term prophylaxis and treatment of *P. falciparum* malaria including areas where chloroquine resistance has been reported. Ongoing studies are evaluating its efficacy against other forms of malaria. Travelers who have experienced intense exposure to *P. vivax* and *P. ovale* should be considered for radical treatment with primaquine upon leaving the malaria-endemic area. Because of its causal activity, AP is taken one day prior to travel in a malarious zone, daily while exposed, and for 7 days upon leaving.

Primaquine

Introduction and description

Primaquine is an 8-aminoquinoline that has been used for over 50 years for the terminal prophylaxis or radical cure of relapsing forms of malaria (*P. vivax* and *P. ovale*) due to its ability to eradicate liver hypnozoite stages. Primaquine was re-discovered as a malaria chemoprophylactic agent in the 1990s based on its ability to eliminate developing liver stages of *P. falciparum* and *P. vivax* (causal prophylaxis).[121,122] Primaquine also has gametocidal activity against, and has been used to decrease the transmission of *P. falciparum* in malaria endemic areas (see Fig. 13.2).

Pharmacology and mode of action

The precise mechanisms of action of 8-aminoquinoline drugs are unknown. Primaquine localizes within the plasmodial mitochondria

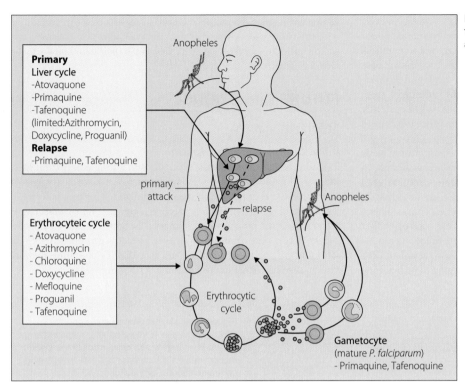

Figure 13.2 The life-cycle of malaria parasites in the human host showing sites of action of antimalarial drugs.

Within the figure:

Primary
Liver cycle
-Atovaquone
-Primaquine
-Tafenoquine
(limited:Azithromycin,
Doxycycline, Proguanil)
Relapse
-Primaquine, Tafenoquine

Erythrocyteic cycle
- Atovaquone
- Azithromycin
- Chloroquine
- Doxycycline
- Mefloquine
- Proguanil
- Tafenoquine

Anopheles

primary attack

relapse

Anopheles

Erythrocytic cycle

Gametocyte
(mature *P. falciparum*)
- Primaquine, Tafenoquine

suggesting drug-induced mitochondrial dysfunction as one potential mechanism of action. It is rapidly absorbed from the gastrointestinal tract and rapidly excreted. Peak plasma levels occur within 2–3 h and the mean half-life is approximately 4–5 h. Primaquine is metabolized to a carboxylic acid derivative of unknown antimalarial activity that has a half-life of 24–30 h.[123,124]

Efficacy and drug resistance

There have been five recent randomized controlled field trials, two in Indonesia, two in Colombia, and one in Africa, have convincingly demonstrated the prophylactic potential of primaquine. In four studies, adults with little previous experience of malaria were given 30 mg base of daily primaquine for between 12–52 weeks. Non-immune immigrants to Papua are intensively exposed to both *P. falciparum* and *P. vivax* malaria. In 1995 a randomized placebo controlled trial indicated that daily primaquine for up to one year had a protective efficacy of 95% (95% CI, 57%–99%) against *P. falciparum* malaria and 90% (95% CI, 58%–98%) against *P. vivax* malaria.[125] A subsequent trial in the same region in 1999/2000 over 20 weeks showed a protective efficacy of 88% (48%–97%) for *P. falciparum* and >92% (95% CI, >37%–99%) for *P. vivax*.[126] In placebo-controlled field studies in Colombian soldiers, primaquine was 94% efficacious (95% CI, 78%–99%) against *P. falciparum* and 85% (95% CI, 57%–95%) against *P. vivax*.[127] In an attempt to improve the efficacy rate against *P. vivax* malaria, weekly chloroquine was added to the daily primaquine in a subsequent field trial; however the results were similar to that of primaquine alone.[128]

Relapses of *P. vivax* malaria following standard courses of primaquine (15 mg base/day for 14 days) are commonly reported from Papua New Guinea, Papua, Thailand and other parts of Southeast Asia and Oceania (failure rates ~35%), and less commonly from India and Colombia. Smoak *et al.*[129] reported high relapse rates in American soldiers deployed to Somalia. Of 60 *P. vivax*-infected

soldiers treated with standard doses of chloroquine and primaquine (15 mg base/day for 14 days), 26 relapsed for a failure rate of 43%. Eight soldiers had a second relapse following another course of chloroquine plus primaquine therapy including several who completed a higher dose primaquine regimen (30 mg base/day × 14 days).

Tolerability

Randomized controlled trials have shown that daily primaquine is well tolerated with reported discontinuation rates generally ≤2%. The most commonly identified adverse event has been minor gastrointestinal disturbances, which are minimized by taking the drug with food. In the recent study by Baird the primaquine was as well tolerated as placebo.[126]

Contraindications and precautions

The adverse events of greatest concern with primaquine are methemoglobinemia and hemolysis in glucose 6 phosphate dehydrogenase (G6PD) deficient persons. Primaquine-induced hemolysis can be life threatening in a severely deficient person. Methemoglobinemia is generally not a serious concern when <20% hemoglobin is in the methemoglobin form; only rarely will testing for methemoglobinemia be indicated on clinical grounds such as with cyanosis, dizziness or dyspnea. Controlled trials have demonstrated that methemoglobinemia levels after 20 or 52 weeks of 30 mg base of primaquine daily were no higher than those following standard 15 mg base daily for 14 days.[125,126] Methemoglobin levels have remained below 8.5% in recent trials, well below the 20–30% associated with symptoms.

Primaquine is contraindicated in G6PD deficiency and during pregnancy because of the risk of hemolysis in the fetus. There is no experience with the prophylactic use of primaquine in children. Prior to receiving primaquine individuals should be confirmed to have a normal G6PD status by laboratory testing.

Indications and administration

Randomized controlled trials of 339 participants in Indonesia, South America and Africa have demonstrated that primaquine is an efficacious and well-tolerated chemoprophylactic agent (0.5 mg/kg base per day; adult dose 30 mg base/day) against *P. vivax* and *P. falciparum*. Because of its causal activity it may be discontinued 1 week after leaving an endemic area. However, primaquine is not currently licensed for this indication. Current pivotal trials may be sufficient to meet regulatory requirements for this indication.

For individuals, not taking primaquine as a chemoprophylactic agent, for whom exposure to *P. vivax* or *P. ovale* malaria is thought to have been particularly high (e.g. long-term expatriates, soldiers etc.) consideration may be given to the use of primaquine to eliminate latent hepatic parasites by administering a two week course of primaquine (0.3 mg/kg base per day; adult dose 15 mg base/day) after return to a non-endemic area. Patients who relapse following a standard course of primaquine should receive two times the standard dose (30 mg base/day for 14 days) or a total dose of 6 mg/kg of primaquine

to prevent further relapse.[130,131] Based on reports of frequent failures with the 15 mg base dosing regimen, many experts now routinely use 30 mg primaquine base/day × 14 days in individuals known to be G6PD normal.

FUTURE DIRECTIONS

Tafenoquine

Introduction and description

Tafenoquine is a primaquine analogue with a long elimination half-life (14–28 days versus 4–6 h for primaquine). It has activity against liver, blood and transmission stages of malaria. The long half-life of Tafenoquine allows infrequent dosing regimens. When the drug is taken with food, absorption is increased by approximately 50%, and the severity of gastrointestinal adverse effects is diminished.[132,133] *In vitro* and *in vivo* animal studies indicate that Tafenoquine is more potent and less toxic than primaquine.[130] (See Fig. 13.3).

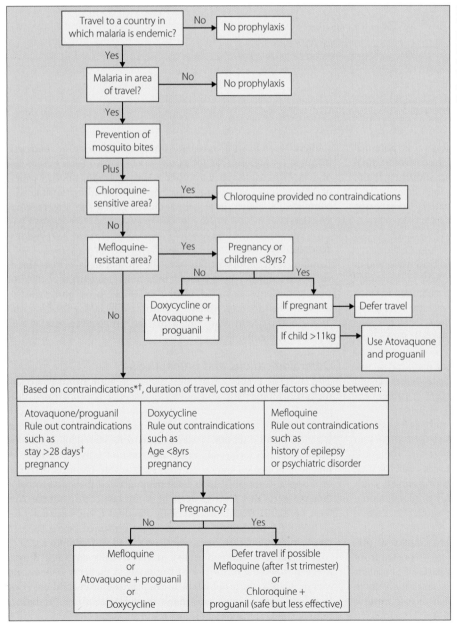

Figure 13.3 Malaria prophylaxis algorithm.
*Note: This figure is intended as a *visual aid* only. Please refer to text and product/package insert monograph for other important details regarding contraindications, precautions, and drug tolerability. †At present in Europe (except the UK), atovaquone/proguanil is only registered for a maximum period of 28 days.

Efficacy and drug resistance

To date, four field trials have assessed prophylactic efficacy of Tafenoquine in malaria endemic areas.[134–137] A randomized dose-ranging study of Tafenoquine was performed in Gabon in older children and young adults. A loading dose strategy using 25 mg base to 200 mg base of Tafenoquine once daily for 3 days was evaluated. Doses of 50 mg, 100 mg, and 200 mg daily for 3 days all showed substantial protective efficacy through 10 weeks of follow up. Compared with placebo, Tafenoquine 200 mg base daily for 3 days provided 100% protection out to week 11.[136] This suggested that a 'fire-and-forget' strategy of three daily doses of Tafenoquine might be sufficient to protect exposed short-term travelers.

In a randomized placebo-controlled trial in semi-immune adults in western Kenya, 200 mg base daily for 3 days followed by 200 mg weekly for 13 weeks resulted in a protective efficacy of 87% (95% CI, 73%–93%); 400 mg daily for 3 days followed by 400 mg weekly had a protective efficacy of 89% (98% (95% CI, 77%–95%). One group receiving only 400 mg for 3 days at the beginning of the study followed by placebo. The protective efficacy at week 15 in this group was 68% (95% CI, 53%–79%), however, there were equivalent malaria rates to the weekly treated groups out to study week 7, again supporting a fire-and forget dosing strategy.[134]

A randomized trial examined Tafenoquine's prophylactic efficacy against *P. falciparum* in semi-immune adults in Ghana.[135] Volunteers received a loading dose of study drug on each of 3 consecutive days, then a single weekly dose for 12 weeks. Doses of Tafenoquine 200 mg base afforded a protective efficacy of approximately 86%, similar to protection afforded by 250 mg mefloquine weekly.

The prophylactic efficacy against *P. vivax* was evaluated in a placebo-controlled trial in 205 non-immune soldiers in the northeastern border regions of Thailand. Using 400 mg base of Tafenoquine daily for three consecutive days followed by a single monthly dose of 400 mg resulted in a 95% protective efficacy against *P. vivax*.[137] Additional field trials using a 200 mg base weekly dosing regimen are currently underway in East Timor by the Australian Armed Forces.

Tolerability

The most commonly reported adverse event noted during Tafenoquine prevention trials has been mild gastrointestinal upset that was not statistically different from the placebo groups. Other adverse effects have included dermatologic problems, headaches, and mild transient elevations in serum liver transaminases.

Contraindications, precautions and drug interactions

The potential toxicities of concern with Tafenoquine are the same as primaquine: methemoglobinemia or hemolysis in G6PD deficient persons. During the Kenyan field trial two G6PD deficient individuals were inadvertently given Tafenoquine which resulted in significant intravascular hemolysis requiring blood transfusion in one case. Hemolysis resolved and no renal compromise was observed in spite of hemoglobinuria ('blackwater').[134]

Although methemoglobinemia has been documented in persons receiving Tafenoquine, it has not resulted in levels sufficient to induce symptoms or require treatment.[134]

Indications and administration

The indications for the use of Tafenoquine in the treatment or prevention of malaria have yet to be established. Most recent field trials are exploring a weekly dosing schedule, but of particular interest for short term travelers (<1 month) is a fire-and-forget approach with a 3-day loading dose (3 doses over 3 days). Tafenoquine may also be an alternative for terminal prophylaxis and a substitute for primaquine in the therapy of vivax malaria.[133] Tafenoquine's ability to kill sexual stages suggests it might also have an important public health application in transmission blocking.[138]

DRUGS NOT RECOMMENDED FOR CHEMOPROPHYLAXIS

A number of agents, not mentioned above, are occasionally used or recommended to travelers to prevent malaria. While some of these agents are effective drugs for malaria treatment, their pharmacokinetics, adverse events or toxicities make them inappropriate drugs to prevent malaria.[11–13] Below is a list of drugs that are not recommended for chemoprophylaxis.

Amodiaquine is a 4-aminoquinalone drug that has been available since the 1940s and is structurally similar to chloroquine. It is currently still used for therapy in some sub-Saharan African countries; however its potential adverse effects include agranulocytosis and hepatitis and it is not recommended as a chemoprophylactic agent.[124,130]

Pyrimethamine/sulfadoxine (Fansidar) is widely used for the treatment of falciparum malaria in sub-Saharan Africa and occasionally as standby treatment of malaria in travelers. It is not used in a prophylactic setting due to the risk of severe cutaneous adverse reactions including Steven's-Johnson syndrome and toxic epidermal necrolysis [124,130]. Other forms of pyrimethamine alone (for example Daraprim™) are also not recommended due to widespread resistance.

Quinine remains a first line therapeutic agent for chloroquine resistant malaria. It is not used as a prophylactic drug due to its short half-life and its frequent treatment-associated adverse effects including nausea, vomiting, headache, tinnitus, cardiovascular toxicity and risk of blackwater fever with prolonged use.

Azithromycin is an azalide antimicrobial agent that has been evaluated as a chemosuppressive agent. Although protective against *P. vivax* (>90%), protective efficacy against *P. falciparum* (70–83%) is generally considered to be too low to rely on azithromycin as a single agent to prevent falciparum malaria.[11–13,95,96]

Artemisinin or Qinghaosu derivatives, including Artesunate, are a class of extremely effective therapeutic agents; however there is currently no role for these drugs as chemoprophylactics.[130,139]

Halofantrine is a 9-phenanthrene-methanol drug that continues to be used in some countries as a therapeutic agent for malaria. It is not recommended for the prevention or treatment of malaria due to its potential to cause potentially fatal cardiac arrhythmias and prolongation of the QTc intervals. These cardiac changes can be especially accentuated when used in combination with other cardiac altering antimalarials such as mefloquine.[81,140]

CHEMOPROPHYLAXIS IN SPECIAL POPULATIONS

Pregnancy, lactation and conception

Falciparum malaria in a pregnant woman represents a serious medical condition. Falciparum malaria is associated with an increased risk of spontaneous abortion and stillbirth, intrauterine growth retardation, premature delivery, and maternal mortality. Travel by pregnant women or women who might become pregnant to destinations where CRPF malaria is transmitted should be avoided or deferred when possible. This advice is based on the fact that the most effective antimalarial regimens against CRPF are neither recommended nor adequately studied during pregnancy, especially in the first trimester.

If a pregnant woman must travel to a CRPF malarial endemic area, the use of insect repellents and insecticide treated-bednets should be strongly encouraged[11–13] and chemoprophylaxis should be used.

Chloroquine alone or in combination with proguanil is safe in pregnancy and lactation; however these agents only offer partial protection in areas with transmission of CRPF. If the travel is to an area where there is intense transmission of CRPF with high-grade chloroquine resistance and travel cannot be deferred, mefloquine may be considered for chemoprophylaxis, especially after the first trimester of pregnancy. For areas with less intense transmission, chloroquine and proguanil chemoprophylaxis can be considered. Some sources recommend supplementation with folic acid for pregnant women taking proguanil.

When possible conception should be delayed for 3 months from the time of completion of mefloquine; however inadvertent conception while on mefloquine is not an indication for termination of pregnancy.[12]

At present there is insufficient data available on the use of AP in pregnancy or breast-feeding and therefore it is not recommended unless the potential benefit outweighs the potential risk to the fetus.[11,120] AP is currently licensed for use in children greater than 11 kg, however current studies are evaluating it in children down to 5 kg.

Doxycycline is contraindicated in pregnancy and breast-feeding. Conception should be delayed until one week after completion of doxycycline. Primaquine is contraindicated in pregnancy though is considered safe in breastfeeding provided that the infant and mother are both screened for G6PD deficiency.[11] There is currently no safe and effective chemoprophylaxis regimen for pregnant women at risk of mefloquine-resistant *P. falciparum* malaria (see Chapter 20).

Infants and children

Young children are at special risk for malaria because of their inability to protect themselves from mosquitoes, the difficulty in administering antimalarial drugs and the rapidity at which they become severely ill. Parents and guardians must pay particular attention to insect protection measures including repellents and treated bednets.

Malaria chemoprophylaxis in the very young infant is difficult to achieve. Although most antimalarials taken by the mother will be present in breast milk, the drug concentrations are not considered high enough to provide an adequate protective dose to the nursing infant. Thus, malaria prevention in the nursing infant must be addressed separately from what is recommended to the mother.

For pediatric travelers to malarious areas where chloroquine is still effective, the chloroquine dose can be adjusted based on weight (Table 13.6). Chloroquine phosphate pediatric suspension is available in some destination countries, but not in the USA or Canada. If the suspension is not available, chloroquine phosphate tablets (250 mg salt = 150 mg chloroquine base) can be ground up by the pharmacist, and the weight-adjusted dose plus a filler can be put into capsules. Once a week, the capsule can be opened and the chloroquine powder mixed into a syrup to be given to a child. Chocolate syrup is recommended over fruit syrups and jams, as chocolate can effectively mask the bitter taste of the chloroquine and make the mixture palatable to a child. Tablets should also be kept out of sunlight and humidity once removed from the protective packaging. All medication should be kept out of reach from children to avoid over-doses which may be fatal.

The dosage of proguanil can also be adjusted based on weight. AP (available in a one-quarter strength pediatric tablet) and mefloquine dosage for children can be adjusted based on weight for those weighing more than 11 kg for AP and 5 kg for mefloquine. There is currently no safe and effective chemoprophylaxis regimen for (<11 kg) at risk of mefloquine-resistant *P. falciparum* malaria. Doxycycline is contraindicated in children less than 8 years of age.

In general children should not rely on standby treatment for malaria, rather they should be prescribed appropriate chemoprophylaxis

and seek medical attention if any febrile illness occurs when traveling (see Chapter 21).

Immunocompromised travelers

Plasmodium falciparum malaria has been shown to increase HIV-1 replication and proviral loads and may cause faster progression of HIV-1 disease. HIV-1 infection also appears to make malaria worse and is associated with higher parasitemia infections and an increase in clinical malaria.[141] Therefore malaria prevention is particularly important in this population.

The special concern is the possible interaction between antimalarial drugs and anti-retroviral agents. Both mefloquine and protease inhibitors are metabolized by cytochrome P450. Inducers or inhibitors of cytochrome P450 might be expected to alter drug levels of these agents. Mefloquine has been shown to decrease the drug levels of ritonavir, but ritonavir had little effect on mefloquine.[142] There is reported to be less interaction between mefloquine and other protease inhibitors such as nelfinavir or indinavir.[143] Evafirenze is an anti-retroviral with potential neuropsychiatric adverse events including dizziness, altered concentration, insomnia, abnormal dreaming, sleepiness, confusion, abnormal thinking, memory loss and hallucinations. Although unknown, it is possible that agents like mefloquine might potentiate these effects. There are little available data on the inter-action of other antiretrovirals with mefloquine.[142–144]

Atovaquone increases the level of some nucleoside reverse transcriptase inhibitors (NRTIs) such as stavudine as well as the level of zidovudine plus AZT. Whether this increases the risk of adverse drug events is unknown. There are also little data available regarding the potential interaction of proguanil and antiretroviral agents.[145]

Doxycycline may cause photosensitivity, similar to anti-retrovirals like abacavir, and predispose to candidiasis, potential problems for HIV-infected individuals.

Because of potential or unknown interactions between antiretroviral and antimalarial drugs, it may be advantageous to start an antimalarial drug in advance of the recommended start date in order to monitor for any adverse effects.

ILLUSTRATIVE CASES

Case 1

A 23-year-old female is about to travel to sub-Saharan Africa for a two-month safari. She is concerned that she might develop adverse events related to mefloquine while away. She is wondering if there is a way to reassure her that she will be able to tolerate mefloquine before leaving.

Approach

This is a common and appropriate concern voiced by many potential travelers. No-one wants to experience adverse drug events particularly when they are far from home. This concern most commonly arises with mefloquine use and there are at least two approaches one might want to consider. (1) Begin mefloquine prophylaxis 2.5 to 3 weeks before departure. Since the majority of side-effects occur within the first three doses this will allow an opportunity to assess adverse events before departure. However, if the individual tolerates three doses of mefloquine, they may be reassured that they will likely tolerate this drug. (2) Another strategy is to consider the use of a loading dose of mefloquine. In this case, one tablet of mefloquine is used each day for 3 consecutive days, followed by the typical once weekly dosing regimen. For many travelers who will be intolerant to mefloquine it will come evident during the week of the loading dose. Both the above strategies allow an assessment of drug tolerability prior to departure and permit a change to a suitable alternative agent if necessary.

Case 2

A business executive in Bangkok is required to take several short (3–5 day) trips to rural Cambodia and rural Laos over the course of the next 3 months. Since standard chemoprophylactic drugs like doxycycline and mefloquine require use for 4 weeks after malaria exposure, he notes that he will constantly be on antimalarials for many months. He is wondering if there is another option.

Approach

Short and repeated trips to malaria endemic areas are ideal situations to consider the use of causal antimalarials such as AP and primaquine. Since these drugs only need to be taken for a short time (1 week) after leaving the malaria endemic area they are more user-friendly for this type of travel. A similar situation exists in Nairobi, Kenya (one of few malaria-free areas in East Africa) where travel outside of the city places individuals at risk of chloroquine resistant *P. falciparum* malaria.

Case 3

A microbiologist brings her 6-year-old daughter to your travel clinic for advice regarding antimalarial prophylaxis and immunizations for travel to sub-Saharan Africa. The mother elects to use AP for malaria and also requests oral typhoid vaccine. She asks you whether the AP will inhibit the immune response to the live oral vaccine.

Approach

Antimicrobial agents can theoretically effect host immune response to live vaccines. Recent data in Gabonese children showed that AP did not affect the seroconversion rates to live oral typhoid and cholera vaccines (Faucher *et al.* Prophylaxis with Malarone in combination with typhoid and cholera vaccines in Gabonese children. *Amer Soc Trop Med Hyg* 2001. abstract 580).

Case 4

A 36-year-old client e-mails you from Cambodia. He indicates he is having difficulty tolerating doxycycline. He has been able to acquire AP and wants to switch. He wishes to know whether he can discontinue AP 1 week after leaving Cambodia.

Approach

As a causal prophylactic agent AP is normally discontinued 1 week after leaving a malaria endemic area. However all studies have examined the use of AP prior to malaria exposure. It is unknown whether it will work as a causal agent when started after exposure. For this reason, people switching to AP should use the drug as a suppressive rather than a causal agent and therefore continue it for 4 weeks after leaving the endemic area.

Case 5

A 39-year-old female visits Papua and uses AP as a chemoprophylactic agent. Three months after returning home she develops *P. vivax* malaria. She asks you why she has developed malaria despite using a antimalarial prophylactic agent.

Approach

AP is an efficacious drug to prevent *P. falciparum* and *P. vivax* malaria. However, AP has no activity against liver stage hypnozoites and therefore cannot prevent relapses of *P. vivax* and *P. ovale* malaria. For individuals who have had extensive exposure to relapsing forms of malaria, consideration should be given to the use of terminal prophylaxis with primaquine upon leaving the malaria endemic area.

CONCLUSION

In summary, the use of antimalarial drug regimens should be carefully directed at high-risk travelers where their benefit most clearly outweighs the risk of adverse events. None of the available regimens are ideal for all travelers and the travel medicine practitioner should attempt to match the individual's risk of exposure to malaria to the appropriate regimen based on drug efficacy, tolerance, safety, and cost. One strategy to facilitate clinical decision making is the use of a Clinical Utility Score,[131] in which different attributes of each drug regimen, such as efficacy, tolerance, convenience, cost etc. are weighted based on clinical trials and experience with these drugs (Table 13.7). The pros and cons are discussed with the client in reaching a suitable choice. This may help provide an objective approach in identifying the 'best choice' drug for an individual traveler. The scores assigned are arbitrary and users may weigh each variable somewhat differently depending on the specific needs and risk of drug-resistant malaria.

REFERENCES

1. World Health Organization. *The World Report 1999: Making a Difference*. Geneva, Switzerland: World Health Organization; 1999.
2. World Tourism Organization. *WTO news*. 2nd quarter. World Tourism Organization; 2000. Available: http://www.worldtourism.org/newlett/aprjunoo/results.html, accessed 10 May 2001.
3. Ryan ET, Kain KC. Health advice and immunizations for travelers. *N Engl J Med* 2000; **342**:1716–1725.
4. Kain KC. Prophylactic drugs for malaria: why do we need another one? *J Travel Med* 1999; **6(suppl 1)**:S2–S7.
5. Greenberg AE, Lobel HO. Mortality from Plasmodium Falciparum malaria in travelers from the United States, 1959 to 1987. *Ann Intern Med* 1990; **113**:326–327.
6. Newman RD, Barber AM, Roberts J, *et al*. Malaria surveillance – United States, 1999. CDC Surveillance Summaries, 29 March, 2002. *MMWR* 2002; **55**:15–28.
7. Bradley DJ, Warhurst DC, Blaze M, *et al*. Malaria imported into the United Kingdom in 1996. *Eurosurveillance* 1998; **3**:40–42.
8. Kain KC, Macpherson DW, Kelton T, *et al*. Malaria deaths in visitors to Canada and in Canadian travelers: a case series. *CMAJ* 2001; **164**:654–659.
9. Reid AJ, Whitty CJ, Ayles HM, *et al*. Malaria at Christmas: Risks of Prophylaxis Versus Risks of Malaria. *BMJ* 1998; **317**:1506–1508.
10. Hay SI, Cox J, Rogers DJ, *et al*. Climate change and the resurgence of malaria in the East African highlands. *Nature* 2002; **415**:905–909.
11. Centers for Disease Control and Prevention. Health Information for international travel: 2001–2002. Atlanta: US Department of Health and Human Services; 2001.
12. Canadian recommendations for the prevention and treatment of malaria among international travelers. Committee to Advise on Tropical Medicine and Travel (CATMAT), Laboratory for Disease Control. *Can Commun Dis Rep* 2000; **26(suppl 2)**:1–42.
13. World Health Organization (WHO). *International Travel and Health*. Geneva, Switzerland: WHO; 2002:2002.
14. Funk-Baumann M. Geographic Distribution of Malaria at Traveler Destinations. In: Schlagenhauf P., ed. *Travelers' Malaria*. Hamilton, OH: BC Decker Inc; 2001:56–94.
15. Ohrt C. Ritchie Tl, Widjaja H, *et al*. Mefloquine compared with doxycycline for the prophylaxis of malaria in Indonesian soldiers. *Ann Intern Med* 1997; **126**:963–972.
16. Steffen R, Fuchs E, Schildknecht J, *et al*. Mefloquine compared with other malaria chemoprophylactic regimens in tourists visiting East Africa. *Lancet* 1993; **341**:1299–1303.
17. Hill DR, Behrens RH, Bradley DJ. The risk of malaria in travelers to Thailand. *Trans Roy Soc Trop Med Hyg* 1996; **90**:680–681.
18. Fradin MS, Day JF. Comparative efficacy of insect repellents against mosquito bites. *N Engl J Med* 2002; **347**:13–18.

19. Soto J, Medina F, Dember N, Berman J. Efficacy of permethrin-impregnated uniforms in the prevention of malaria and leishmaniasis in Colombian soldiers. *Clin Infect Dis* 1995; **21**:599–602.

20. McGready R. Safety of the insect repellent N, N-diethyl-m-toluamide (DEET) in pregnancy. *Am J Trop Med Hyg* 2001; **65**:285–289.

21. Kain KC, Keystone JS. Malaria in travelers. Epidemiology, disease and prevention. *Infect Dis Clin North Am* 1998; **12**:267–284.

22. Baird JK, Hoffman SL. Prevention of malaria in travelers. *Med Clin North Am* 1999; **83**:923–944.

23. Behrens RH, Curtis CF. Malaria in travelers: epidemiology and prevention. *Br Med Bull* 1993; **49**:363–366.

24. World Health Organization. Severe falciparum malaria. *Trans R Soc Trop Med Hyg* 2000; **94(suppl 1)**:S1–S90.

25. Warhurst DC, Hockley DJ. Mode of action of chloroquine on Plasmodium berghei and P. cynomolgi. *Nature* 1967; **214**:935–936.

26. Slater AF, Cerami A. Inhibition by chloroquine of a novel haem polymerase enzyme activity in malaria trophozoites. *Nature* 1992; **355**:167–169.

27. Peters W. *Chemotherapy and Drug Resistance in Malaria.* London: Academic Press; 1987.

28. Rieckmann KH, Davis DR, Hutton DC. Plasmodium vivax resistance to chloroquine? *Lancet* 1989; **2**:1183–1184.

29. Fidock DA, Nomura T, Talley A, et al. Mutations in the P. falciparum lysosome trans-membrane protein PfCRT and evidence for their role in chloroquine resistance. *Mol Cell* 2000; **6**:861–871.

30. Djimde A, Doumbo OK, Cortese JF, et al. A molecular marker for chloroquine-resistant falciparum malaria. *N Engl J Med* 2001; **344**: 257–263.

31. Warhurst DC. A molecular marker for chloroquine-resistant malaria. *N Eng J Med* 2000; **344**:299–302.

32. Stemberger H, Leimer R, Widermann G. Tolerability of long-term prophylaxis with Fansidar: a randomized double-blind study in Nigeria. *Acta Trop* 1984; **41**:391–399.

33. Lobel HO, Gerber RA. Malaria prevention for long-term travelers. In: Schlagenhauf P, ed. *Travelers' Malaria.* Hamilton, OH: BC Decker; 2001:261–269.

34. Croft AM, Geary KG. Chloroquine and combinations. In: Schlagenhauf P, ed. *Traveller's Malaria.* Hamilton, OH: BC Decker; 2001:163–182.

35. Wetsteyn JCFM, Geus A de. Comparison of three regimens for malaria prophylaxis in travelers to east, central and southern Africa. *BMJ* 1993; **307**:1041–1043.

36. Fogh S, Schapira A, Bygbjerg IC, et al. Malaria chemoprophylaxis in travelers to east Africa: a comparative, prospective study of chloroquine plus proguanil with chloroquine plus sulfadoxine-pyrimethamine. *BMJ* 1988; **296**:820–822.

37. Hogh B, Clarke P, Camus D, et al. Atovaquone/proguanil versus chloroquine/proguanil for malaria prophylaxis in non-immune travelers: Results from a randomized, double-blind study. *Lancet* 2000; **356**:1888–1894.

38. Baudon D, Martet G, Pascal B, et al. Efficacy of daily antimalarial chemoprophylaxis in tropical Africa using either doxycycline or chloroquine-proguanil; a study conducted in 1996 in the French Army. *Trans R Soc Trop Med Hyg* 1999; **93**:302–303.

39. Huzly D, Schönfeld C, Beurle W, et al. Malaria chemoprophylaxis in German tourists: a prospective study on compliance and adverse reactions. *J Travel Med* 1996; **3**:148–155.

40. Corominas N, Gascon J, Mejias T, et al. Reacciones adversas asociadas a la quimioprofilaxis antipaludica. *Med Clin (Barc)* 1997; **108**:772–775.

41. Durrheim DN, Gammon S, Waner S, et al. Antimalarial prophylaxis-use and adverse events in visitors to the Kruger National Park. *S Afr Med J* 1999; **89**:170–175.

42. Peterson E, Ronne T, Ronn A, et al. Reported side-effects to chloroquine, chloroquine plus proguanil, and mefloquine as chemoprophylaxis against malaria in Danish travelers. *J Travel Med* 2000; **7**:79–84.

43. Carme B, Péguet C, Nevez G. Chimioprophlaxie du paludisme: tolerance et observance de la mefloquine et de l'association proguanil/chloroquine chez des touristes francais. *Bull Soc Pathol Exot* 1997; **90**:273–276.

44. Schlagenhauf P, Tschopp A, Johnson R, et al. Randomized, double-blind, four-arm study of the adverse event profiles of malaria chemoprophylaxis in non-immune travelers to sub-Saharan Africa [Abstract]. Denver: ASTMH; 2002.

45. Steffen R, DuPont HL, eds. *Manual of Travel Medicine and Health.* Hamilton, OH: BC Decker; 1999.

46. Schmidt LH, Crosby R, Rasco J, et al. Antimalarial activities of various 4–quinolinemethanols with special attention to WR-142,490 (Mefloquine). *Antimicrobial Agents and Chemotherapy* 1978; **13**:1011–1030.

47. Warhurst DC. Antimalarial interaction with ferriprotoporphyrin IX monomer and it's relationship to the activity of the blood schizonticides. *Ann Trop Med Parasitol* 1987; **81**:65–67.

48. Mockenhaupt FP. Mefloquine resistance in Plasmodium falciparum. *Parasitol Today* 1995; **11**:248–253.

49. Lobel HO, Miani M, Eng T, et al. Long term malaria prophylaxis with weekly mefloquine. *Lancet* 1993; **341**:848–851.

50. Rieckmann KH, Yeo AE, Davis DR, et al. Recent military experience with malaria chemoprophylaxis. *Med J Aust* 1993; **158**:446–449.

51. Pergallo MS, Sabatinelli G, Majori G, et al. Prevention and morbidity in non-immune subjects; a case-control study among Italian troops in Somalia and Mozambique, 1992–1994. *Trans R Soc Trop Med Hyg* 1997; **91**:343–346.

52. Axmann A, Félegyhazi CS, Huszar A, Juhasz P. Long term malaria prophylaxis with Lariam in Cambodia, 1993. *Travel Med Int* 1994; **12**(1):13–18.

53. Hopperus Buma AP, Thiel PP van, Lobel HO, et al. Long-term prophylaxis with mefloquine in Dutch marines in Cambodia. *J Infect Dis* 1996; **173**:1506–1509.

54. Sanchez JL, DeFraites RF, Sharp TW, et al. Mefloquine or doxycycline prophylaxis in US troops in Somalia. *Lancet* 1993; **341**:1021–1022.

55. Wallace MR, Sharp TW, Smoak B, et al. Malaria among United States troops in Somalia. *Am J Med* 1996; **100**:49–55.

56. Bwire R, Slootman EJH, Verhave JP, et al. Malaria anticircumsporozoite antibodies in Dutch soldiers returning from sub-Saharan Africa. *Trop Med Int Health* 1998; **3**(1):66–69.

57. Muehlberger N, Jelinek T, Schlipkoeter U, et al. Effectiveness of chemoprophylaxis and other determinants of malaria in travelers to Kenya. *Trop Med Int Health* 1998; **3**(5):357–363.

58. Lobel HO, Varma JK, Miani N, et al. Monitoring for mefloquine-resistant Plasmodium falciparum in Africa: implications for travelers health. *Am J Trop Med Hyg* 1998; **59**:129–132.

59. Brasseur P, Kouamouo J, Moyou-Somo R, Druilhe P. Multi-drug resistant falciparum malaria in Cameroon in 1987–1988. II Mefloquine resistance confirmed in vivo and in vitro and its correlation with quinine resistance. *Am J Trop Med Hyg* 1992; **46**:8–14.

60. Cowman AF, Galatis D, Thompson JK. Selection for mefloquine resistance in Plasmodium falciparum is linked to amplification of the pfmdr1 gene and cross resistance to halofantrine and quinine. *Proc Nat Acad Sci USA* 1994; **91**:1143–1147.

61. Reed MB, Saliba KJ, Caruana SR, Kirk K, Cowman AF. Pgh1 modulates sensitivity and resistance to multiple antimalarials in Plasmodium falciparum. *Nature* 2000; **403**:906–909.

62. Oduola AMJ, Omitowoju GO, Gerena L, Kyle DE, et al. Reversal of mefloquine resistance with penfluridol in isolates of Plasmodium falciparum from south-west Nigeria. *Trans R Soc Trop Med Hyg* 1993; **87**:81–83.

63. Wallace MR, Sharp TW, Romajzl PJ, et al. Malaria among US troops in Somalia. *Clin Infect Dis* 1994; **3**:101, 580.

64. Croft A, Garner P. Mefloquine for preventing malaria in non-immune adult travelers. Cochrane Collaboration. Cochrane Database of Systematic Reviews. Issue 2001; **1**

65. Overbosch D, Schilthuis HS, Bienzle U, et al. Atovaquone/proguanil versus mefloquine for malaria prophylaxis in non-immune travelers: results from a randomized, double-blind study. *Clin Infect Dis* 2001; **33**:1015–1021.

66. Barrett PJ, Emmins PD, Clarke PD, et al. Comparison of adverse events associated with the use of mefloquine and combination of chloroquine and proguanil as antimalarial prophylaxis: postal and telephone survey of travelers. *BMJ* 1996; **313**:525–528.

67. Phillips MA, Kass RB. User acceptability patterns for mefloquine and doxycycline malaria chemoprophylaxis. *J Travel Med* 1996; **3**:40–45.

68. Schlagenhauf P, Steffen R, Lobel H, et al. Mefloquine tolerability during chemoprophylaxis: focus on adverse event assessments, stereochemistry and compliance. *Trop Med Int Health* 1996; **1**(4):485–494.

69. CIOMS Working Group. *International reporting of adverse drug reactions.* CIOMS Working Group Report. Geneva: World Health Organization; 1987.

70. MacPherson D, Gamble K, Tessier P, et al. Mefloquine tolerance-randomized, double-blinded, placebo-controlled study using a loading dose of mefloquine in pre-exposed travelers. *Program and Abstracts of the Fifth International Conference on Travel Medicine*, Geneva, Switzerland, 24–27 March 1997.

71. Jaspers CA, Hopperus Buma AP, Thiel PP van, et al. Tolerance of mefloquine prophylaxis in Dutch military personnel. *Am J Trop Med Hyg* 1996; **55**:230–234.

72. Croft AJM. World MJ. Neuropsychiatric reactions with mefloquine chemoprophylaxis. *Lancet* 1996; **347**(326)

73. Potasman I, Beny A, Seligmann H. Neuropsychiatric problems in 2,500 long-term travelers to the tropics. *J Travel Med* 1999; **6**:122–133.

74. Schlagenhauf P, Steffen R. Neuropsychiatric events and travel: do antimalarials play a role? *J Travel Med* 2000; **7**(5):225–226.

75. Schwartz E, Potasman I, Rotenberg M, et al. Serious adverse events of mefloquine in relation to blood level and gender. *Am J Trop Med Hyg* 2001; **65**:189–192.

76. Howard PA, Kuile FO ter. CNS adverse events associated with antimalarial agents. Fact or fiction? *Drug Safety* 1995; **12**:370–383.

77. Wittes RC, Sagmur R. Adverse reactions to mefloquine associated with ethanol ingestion. *Can Med Assoc J* 1995; **152**:515–517.

78. Vuurman EFPM, Muntjewerff ND, Uiterwijk MMC, *et al.* Effects of mefloquine alone and with alcohol on psychomotor and driving performance. *Eur J Clin Pharm* 1996; **50**:475–482.

79. Mittelholzer ML, Wall M, Steffen R, *et al.* Malaria prophylaxis in different age groups. *J Travel Med* 1996; **4**:219–223.

80. Jerling M, Rombo L, Hellgren U, *et al. Evaluation of mefloquine adverse effects in relation to the plasma concentration.* Fourth International Conference on Travel Medicine, Acapulco, Mexico, 23–27 April 1995.

81. Sudden death in a traveler following halofantrine administration – Togo, 2000. *Morb Mortal Wkly Rep* 2001; **50**(9):169–170, 179.

82. Handschin JC, Wall M, Steffen R, *et al.* Tolerability and effectiveness of malaria chemoprophylaxis with mefloquine or chloroquine with or without co-medication. *J Travel Med* 1997; **4**(3):121–127.

83. Boudreau E, Schuster B, Sanchez J, *et al.* Tolerability of prophylactic Lariam regimens. *Trop Med Parasit* 1993; **44**:257–265.

84. Schlagenhauf P, Lobel HO, Steffen R, *et al.* Tolerability of mefloquine in Swissair trainee pilots. *Am J Trop Med Hyg* 1997; **56**:235–240.

85. Crevoisier C, Joseph I, Fischer M, *et al.* Influence of hemodialysis on plasma concentration-time profiles of mefloquine in two patients with end-stage renal disease: a prophylactic drug monitoring study. *Antimicrob Agents Chemother* 1995; **39**:1892–1895.

86. Joshi N, Miller DQ. Doxycycline revisited. *Arch Intern Med* 1997; **157**:1421–1426.

87. USP DI. *Drug Information for the Health Professional.* 1st edn. Vol. 1. Englewood, CO: Micromedex, Inc; 2001:2801–2812.

88. Shmuklarsky MJ, Boudreau EF, Pang LW, *et al.* Failure of doxycycline as a causal prophylactic against Plasmodium falciparum malaria in healthy nonimmune volunteers. *Ann Intern Med* 1994; **120**:294–299.

89. Shanks DG, Barnett A, Edstein MD, *et al.* Effectiveness of doxycycline combined with primaquine for malaria prophylaxis. *Med J Aust* 1995; **162**:306–310.

90. Pang LW, Limsomwong N, Boudreau EF, *et al.* Doxycycline prophylaxis for falciparum malaria. *Lancet* 1987; **1**:1161–1164.

91. Pang LW, Limsomwong N, Singharaj P. Prophylactic treatment of vivax and falciparum malaria with low-dose doxycycline. *J Infect Dis* 1988; **158**:1124–1127.

92. Watanasook C, Singharaj P, Suriyamongkol V, *et al.* Malaria prophylaxis with doxycycline in soldiers deployed to the Thai-Kampuchean border. *Southeast Asian J Trop Med Public Health* 1989; **20**:61–64.

93. Baudon D, Martet G, Pascal B, *et al.* Efficacy of daily antimalarial chemoprophylaxis in tropical Africa using either doxycycline or chloroquine-proguanil; a study conducted in 1996 in the French Army. *Trans R Soc Trop Med Hyg* 1999; **93**:302–303.

94. Weiss WR, Oloo AJ, Johnson A, *et al.* Daily primaquine is effective for prophylaxis against falciparum malaria in Kenya: comparison with mefloquine, doxycycline, and chloroquine/proguanil. *J Infect Dis* 1995; **171**:1569–1575.

95. Anderson SL, Oloo AJ, Gordon DM, *et al.* Successful double-blinded, randomized, placebo-controlled field trial of azithromycin and doxycycline as prophylaxis for malaria in western Kenya. *Clin Infect Dis* 1998; **26**:146–150.

96. Taylor WRJ, Richie TL, Fryauff DJ, *et al.* Malaria prophylaxis using azithromycin: a double-blind, placebo controlled trial in Irian Jaya, Indonesia. *Clin Infect Dis* 1999; **28**:74–81.

97. Nasveld PE, Edstein MD, Kitchener SJ, *et al.* Comparison of the effectiveness of atovaquone/proguanil combination and doxycycline in the chemoprophylaxis of malaria in Australian Defense Force personnel. *Program and Abstracts of the 49th Annual Meeting of the American Society of Tropical Medicine and Hygiene*; Houston, TX 2000; **62**(3):139.

98. Adverse Drug Reactions Advisory Committee. Doxycycline-induced esophageal ulceration. *Med J Aust* 1994; **161**:490.

99. Schuhwerk M, Behrens RH. Doxycycline as first line malarial prophylaxis: how safe is it? *J Travel Med* 1998; **5**:102.

100. Westermann GW, Bohm M, Bonsmann G, *et al.* Chronic intoxication by doxycycline use for more than 12 years. *J Intern Med* 1999; **246**:591–592.

101. Arthur JD, Echeverria P, Shanks GD, *et al.* A comparative study of gastrointestinal infections in United States soldiers receiving doxycycline or mefloquine for malaria prophylaxis. *Am J Trop Med Hyg* 1990; **43**:606–618.

102. Lochary ME, Lockhart PB, Williams WT. Doxycycline and staining of permanent teeth. *Pediatr Infect Dis J* 1998; **17**:429–431.

103. Gottlieb A. Safety of minocycline for acne. *Lancet* 1997; **349**:374.

104. Neeley JL, Abate M, Swinker M, *et al.* The effect of doxycycline on serum levels of ethinyl estradiol, norethindrone, and endogenous progesterone. *Obstet Gynecol* 1991; **77**:416–420.

105. Shapiro TA, Ranasinha CD, Kumar N, *et al.* Prophylactic activity of atovaquone against Plasmodium falciparum in humans. *Am J Trop Med Hyg* 1999; **60**:831–836.

106. Radloff PD, Philipps J, Hutchinson D, *et al.* Atovaquone proguanil is an effective treatment for P. ovale and P. malariae malaria. *Trans R Soc Trop Med Hyg* 1996; **90**:682.

107. Berman JD, Chulay JD, Dowler M, *et al.* Causal prophylactic efficacy of Malarone in a human challenge model. *Trans R Soc Trop Med Hyg* 2001; **95**:429–432.

108. Srivastava IK, Vaidya AB. A mechanism for the synergistic antimalarial action of atovaquone and proguanil. *Antimicrob Agents Chemother* 1999; **43**:1334–1339.

109. Beerahee M. Clinical pharmacology of atovaquone and proguanil hydrochloride. *J Travel Med* 1999; **6**(suppl 1):S13–S17.

110. Pudney M, Gutterage W, Zeman A, *et al.* Atovaquone and proguanil hydrochloride: a review of nonclinical studies. *J Travel Med* 1999; **6**(suppl 1):S8–S12.

111. Looareesuwan S, Viravan C, Webster HK, *et al.* Clinical studies of atovaquone, alone or in combination with other antimalarial drugs, for treatment of acute uncomplicated malaria in Thailand. *Am J Trop Med Hyg* 1996; **54**:62–66.

112. Srivastava IK, Morrisey JM, Darrouzet E, *et al.* Resistance mutations reveal the atovaquone-binding domain of cytochrome b in malaria parasites. *Mol Microbiol* 1999; **33**:704–711.

113. Korsinczky MCN, Kotecka B, Saul A, *et al.* Mutations in plasmodium falciparum cytochrome b that are associated with atovaquone resistance are located at a putative drug-binding site. *Antimicrob Agents Chemother* 2000; **6**(suppl):2100–2108.

114. Fivelman QL, Butcher GA, Adagu IS, *et al.* Malarone treatment failure and in vitro confirmation of resistance of Plasmodium falciparum isolate from Lagos, Nigeria. *Malar J* 2002; **1**:1.

115. Shanks GD, Gordon DM, Klotz FW, *et al.* Efficacy and safety of atovaquone/proguanil as suppressive prophylaxis for Plasmodium falciparum malaria. *Clin Infect Dis* 1998; **27**:494–499.

116. Lell B, Luckner D, Ndjave M, *et al.* Randomized placebo-controlled study of atovaquone plus proguanil for malaria prophylaxis in children. *Lancet* 1998; **351**:709–713.

117. Sukwa TY, Mulenga M, Chisdaka N, *et al.* A randomized, double-blind, placebo-controlled field trial to determine the efficacy and safety of Malarone (atovaquone/proguanil) for the prophylaxis of malaria in Zambia. *Am J Trop Med Hyg* 1999; **60**:521–525.

118. Baird K, Lacy M, Sismadi P, *et al.* Randomized, double-blind, placebo-controlled evaluation of Malarone for prophylaxis of P. vivax and P. falciparum malaria in non-immune transmigrants to Papua. *Clin Infect Dis* 2002; in press.

119. Camus D, Djossou F, Hogh B, *et al.* Malarone versus chloroquine/proguanil for malaria prophylaxis in pediatric travelers. *Abstr Am Soc Trop Med Hyg* 2001; poster 579.

120. Malarone product monograph; 2000.

121. Arnold JAA, Hockwald RS. The effect of continuous and intermittent primaquine therapy on the relapse rate of Chesson strain vivax malaria. *J Lab Clin Med* 1954; **44**:429–438.

122. Arnold JAA, Hockwald RS. The antimalarial action of primaquine against the blood and tissue stages of falciparum malaria (Panama, P-F-6 strain). *J Lab Clin Med* 1955; **46**:391–397.

123. Ward SA, Mihaly GW, Edwards G, *et al.* Pharmacokinetics of Primaquine in man. Comparison of acute versus chronic dosage in Thai subjects. *Br J Clin Pharm* 1985; **19**:751–755.

124. Taylor T, Strickland, T. Malaria. In: Strickland, T, ed. *Hunter's Tropical Medicine and Emerging Infectious Diseases,* 8th ed. Philadelphia: WB Saunders; 2000.

125. Fryauff DJBJ, Basri H, Sumawinata I, *et al.* Randomized placebo-controlled trial of primaquine for prophylaxis of falciparum an vivax malaria. *Lancet* 1995; **346**:1190–1193.

126. Baird KLM, Sismadi P, Gramzinski R, *et al.* Randomized pivotal trial of primaquine for prophylaxis against malaria in Javanese adults in Papua, Indonesia. *Clin Infect Dis* 2001; **33**:1990–1997.

127. Soto JTJ, Rodriquez M, Sanchez J, *et al.* Primaquine prophylaxis against malaria in nonimmune Colombian soldiers: efficacy and toxicity. A randomized, double-blind, placebo-controlled trial. *Ann Intern Med* 1998; **129**:241–244.

128. Soto JTJ, Rodriquez M, Sanchez J, *et al.* Double-blind, randomized, placebo-controlled assessment of chloroquine/primaquine prophylaxis for malaria in nonimmune Colombian soldiers. *Clin Infect Dis* 1999; **29**:199–201.

129. Smoak BL, DeFraites RF, Magill AJ, *et al.* Plasmodium vivax infections in U.S. Army troops: failure of primaquine to prevent relapse in studies from Somalia. *Am J Trop Med Hyg* 1997; **56**:231–234.

130. Shanks GD, Kain KC, Keystone JS. Malaria chemoprophylaxis in an age of drug resistance II. Drugs that may be available in the future. *Clin Infect Dis* 2001; **33**:381–385.

131. Kain KC, Shanks GD, Keystone JS. Malaria chemoprophylaxis in an age of drug resistance I. Currently recommended drug regimens. *Clin Infect Dis* 2001; **33**:226–234.

132. Brueckner RPLK, Lin ET, Schuster BG. First-time-in-humans safety and pharmacokinetics of WR 238605, a new antimalarial. *Am J Trop Med Hyg* 1998; **58**:645–649.

133. Walsh DS Loodreesuwan S, Wilairatana P, Heppner DG Jr, *et al.* Randomized dose-ranging study of the safety and efficacy of WR 238605 (Tafenoquine) in the prevention of relapse of Plasmodium vivax malaria in Thailand. *J Infect Dis* 1999; **180**:1282–1287.

134. Shanks GD, Klotz FW, Aleman GM. GM *et al.* A new primaquine analogue, Tafenoquine (WR238605), for prophylaxis against Plasmodium falciparum malaria. *Clin Infect Dis* 2001; **33**:1968–1974.

135. Hale BR, Koram KA, Adjuik M, *et al.* A randomized, double-blinded, placebo-controlled trial of Tafenoquine for prophylaxis against Plasmodium falciparum in Ghana [abstract]. *Am J Trop Med Hyg* 2000; **62**:139–140.

136. Lell BFJ, Missinou MA, Borrmann S, *et al.* Malaria chemoprophylaxis with Tafenoquine: a randomized study. *Lancet* 2000; **355**:2041–2045.

137. Walsh DSEC, Sangkharomya S. Randomized, double-blind, placebo controlled evaluation of monthly WR 238605 (Tafenoquine) for prophylaxis of Plasmodium falciparum and P. vivax in Royal Thai Army soldiers. *Am J Trop Med Hyg* 1999; **61**(502)

138. Coleman RECA, Milhous WK. Gametocytocidal and sporontocidal activity of antimalarials against Plasmodium berghei ANKA in ICR Mice and Anopheles stephensi mosquitoes. *Am J Trop Med Hyg* 1992; **46**:169–182.

139. Brewer TG, Grate SJ, Peggins JO, *et al.* Fatal neurotoxicity of arteether and artemether. *Am J Trop Med Hyg* 1994; **51**:251–259.

140. World Health Organization. Drug Alert: halofantrine. *Wkly Epidemiol Rec* 1993; **68**:268–270.

141. Whitworth J, Morgan D, Quigley M, *et al.* Effect of HIV-1 and increasing immunosuppression on malaria parasitemia and clinical episodes in adults in rural Uganda: a cohort study. *Lancet* 2000; **356**:1051–1056.

142. Khaliq Y, Gallicano K, Tisdale C, *et al.* Pharmacokinetic interaction between mefloquine and ritonavir in healthy volunteers. *Br J Clin Pharm* 2001; **51**:591–600.

143. Schippers EF, Hugen PW, Hartigh J den, *et al.* No drug-drug interaction between nelfinavir or indinavir and mefloquine in HIV-1-infected patients. *AIDS* 2000; **14**:2794–2795.

144. Colebunders R, Nachega J, Gompel A Van. Antiretroviral treatment and travel to developing countries. *J Trav Med* 1999; **6**:27–31.

145. Tessier D. Immunocompromised travelers. In: Schlagenhauf, P, ed. *Travelers' Malaria.* Hamilton, OH: BC Decker Inc; 2001:324–335.

CHAPTER 14 # Self-diagnosis and Self-treatment of Malaria by the Traveler

Martin P. Grobusch

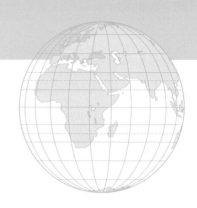

KEYPOINTS

- Inspite of the availability of chemoprophylaxis, malaria can occur in travelers

- 10 years ago the concept of stand-by emergency treatment (SBET) was introduced

- The principle of SBET: early treatment of malaria is life-saving

- Rapid diagnostic tests are not fully reliable as decision-making tools for SBET in the hands of travelers

- The choice of drugs for SBET is dependent on drug resistance and tolerability

INTRODUCTION

Despite the availability of prophylactic measures,[1,2] a considerable number of travelers contract malaria every year.[3–6] The majority of cases are due to *Plasmodium falciparum*, which causes the potentially life-threatening 'malignant tertian', or falciparum malaria, in non-immune patients. In Europe, with an estimated number of 11 000 malaria cases per year, 8000 of which were caused by *Plasmodium falciparum*,[7,8] mortality rates within recent years were estimated to be as high as 3.6%.[7–9] In the USA, 3555 cases of falciparum malaria with 47 deaths (1.3%) were recorded among civilians from 1985 to 1998. However, exact data on the morbidity and mortality of travel-related malaria are currently unavailable,[4,8] since not all cases are reported to national registries.

Currently, a comprehensive, single, safe and highly effective method (ideally a vaccine) to prevent malaria in travelers to endemic areas is neither available nor in sight.[10] Recommendations for the prevention of malaria in travelers are therefore predominantly based on the combination of avoidance of mosquito bites ('exposure prophylaxis') and an appropriate chemoprophylactic regimen.[2] Even a combination, however, does not provide 100% protection. More importantly, only a minority of travelers make use of available protective measures. For example, in a cohort of 1659 malaria patients observed in Europe, 60.4% of the European travelers and 72.4% of VFR's traveled without using chemoprophylaxis,[8] and only a small number of individuals tried to adhere fully to the prevention of insect bites.

Among those individuals who chose to use appropriate chemoprophylaxis, the protection rate varied between 70–95% in various prospective and case control studies.[11,12] This applied not only to established drugs, but also to recently introduced compounds such as atovaquone/proguanil or tafenoquine.[13,14] There are many reasons for chemoprophylaxis failures. Apart from a reduced sensitivity of *Plasmodium* spp. against the antimalarials used, the main reasons for failure are a lack of adherence to the recommended regimen (particularly early cessation of prophylaxis), drug resorption problems (e.g., due to vomiting or diarrhea) and prolonged exoerythrocytic phase times of malaria (i.e., exceeding the period of drug intake).

Each chemoprophylactic agent is linked to a risk of adverse events, with frequencies ranging from 10–30%.[12] Apart from taking individual contraindications and intolerances into account, the general risk of adverse events should be weighted against the risk of infection at the destination. This applies particularly to certain groups of travelers and occupational groups, such as airline crews who make frequent short visits to endemic areas over prolonged periods of time, as well as to a larger group of travelers with prolonged duration of travel. It also applies to those with a low to moderate risk of contracting malaria (Fig. 14.1).

Regardless of the prophylactic used, one has to keep in mind that infection with *P. falciparum* may lead to very severe disease within a short period of time. This is particularly true for non-immune individuals, such as children in endemic areas and travelers who live in malaria-free regions.[1,4,5]

Complications and deaths are predominantly the result of a delay in the initiation of treatment or in the provision of inappropriate therapy. The early diagnosis and treatment of malaria are the critical factors in reducing malaria-related morbidity and mortality.[5,15]

In developing countries where malaria is endemic, health-care facilities may be readily available for the management of severe illness. In fact, most febrile illnesses are treated as malaria regardless of the blood film results (which are not infrequently falsely positive). However, in many remote areas optimal medical care is not readily accessible within a reasonable period of time.

For this reason, more than 10 years ago, the concept of standby-emergency treatment (SBET) was introduced[16] and recently updated.[2] Travelers are provided with a treatment dose of an appropriate antimalarial drug to be carried and taken in case of a febrile illness, when medical care cannot be reached promptly.

The current recommendations of WHO in accordance with various national expert committees[2,17,18] contain the option to abandon chemoprophylaxis in favor of SBET for particular situations, assuming that the traveler will maintain rigorous protection measures against mosquito bites.[19] In Europe, SBET is often recommended in low malaria risk

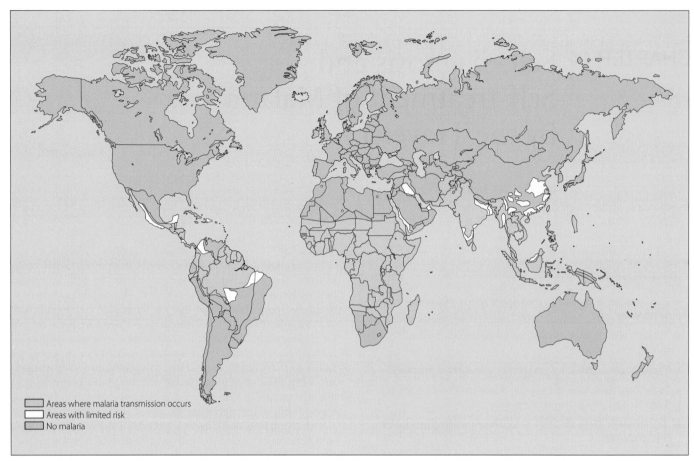

Figure 14.1 Overview on malarious areas of the world and approximate risk of malaria transmission. (Adapted with kind permission from WHO, Geneva, 2002.)

situations such as travel to Thailand and to Central and South America. The malaria branch of the Centers for Diseases Control and Prevention in the USA takes a more conservative approach and recommends SBET only to those travelers who do not wish to take chemoprophylaxis or who choose a suboptimal prophylaxis regimen. In such cases, SBET is recommended when illness is suspected to be malaria and the traveler cannot reach medical care within 24 hours.[2]

A major problem with SBET is the difficulty that travelers have in making a self-diagnosis of malaria on the basis of clinical symptoms. Since the introduction of new, rapid immunochromatographic tests to detect plasmodial antigens, the question now arises as to whether these tests are suitable for self-diagnosis.

RAPID DIAGNOSTIC TESTS FOR MALARIA

Rationale

Despite a rapid development of alternative methods for the diagnosis of malaria in recent years, expert examination of thick and thin Giemsa-stained blood smears still remains the diagnostic standard for malaria in both malaria-endemic and non-endemic countries. Various authors[20–23] have reviewed new diagnostic approaches for malaria in detail. Microscopy with fluorescent stains,[24] polymerase chain reaction assays[25] and some automated blood cell analyzers[26] offer, to a varying extent, alternatives for laboratory-based diagnostic, epidemiological and research applications for *Plasmodium* spp. detection. However, in theory, novel rapid antigen detection techniques might be recommended for use by laypersons for self-

diagnosis of malaria, since they do not require a laboratory or medical expertise to use them.

Principle

The so-called rapid diagnostic tests (RDTs) for malaria are based on the immunochromatographical detection of plasmodial proteins, namely histidine-rich protein II (HRP-2), and in some tests in combination with parasite-specific aldolase, or parasite-specific lactate dehydrogenase (pLDH).

Test principles and procedures vary depending on the manufacturer. The ready-to-use test kits contain nitrocellulose test strips onto which monoclonal antibodies against HRP-2 or pLDH are immobilized. A small amount of whole blood is applied to the test strip, together with a diluent which hemolyzes the red cells. A detecting antibody attached to colloidal gold or an enzyme against HRP-2, parasite-specific aldolase or pLDH is applied later, or is already integrated in the test strip. After the addition of a buffer solution, the reagents migrate along the test strip.

In a positive case, the complex of parasite protein and detecting antibody is bound to an immobilizing antibody. The colloidal gold, or substrate-enzyme produces a visible line which can be read with the naked eye. A control line with the antibody against the detecting antibody indicates whether the test was performed correctly. All tests can be performed within 5–15 minutes. Figure 14.2 illustrates the test principle, Figures 14.3 and 14.4 demonstrate test results, and Table 14.1[22,27–33] details the variety of test formats, which have been, or are currently, available.

Commercially available test kits

Rapid tests for HRP-2 detection are commercially available from various manufacturers. The best known and most extensively tested are the ParaSight-F® test (Becton Dickinson),[27] which is no longer available, and the ICT Malaria P.f.® test (ICT Diagnostics, now Binax),[28] which has also been marketed under the name of MalaQuick®. As HRP-2 antigen is only produced and released by *P. falciparum*, these rapid tests are not suitable for diagnosis of the other plasmodial species. Recently, several test kits of other manufacturers based on HRP-2 detection have been produced with the aim of lowering costs. Although published studies are few so far, these products appear to have the same quality as the original test formats.[29–32]

In the meantime, the test kit now named ICT Malaria P.f./P.v.® (or RIDA MalaQuick Kombi) includes the detection of a malaria-specific aldolase[34] dubbed 'panmalarial antigen', which is in theory occurring in all four human *Plasmodia* species.

Rapid immunochromatographic tests for pLDH detection are marketed under the name OptiMal® (Flow Inc.). Since pLDH occurs in antigenically slightly different isoforms in the various *Plasmodia* species, monoclonal antibodies with different specificity have been developed.[35] The currently available OptiMal® test is able to detect a *P. falciparum*- and a panspecific pLDH (predominantly occurring with *P. falciparum* and *P. vivax*). A more sophisticated OptiMal®-2 test that is able to differentiate all four *Plasmodia* species is not yet available.[22,36]

The cost for the original test formats was estimated to be 3–5 USD per test, an acceptable price in the context of self-diagnosis by travelers as discussed here.

Performance of RDTs for laboratory diagnosis of malaria

More than 50 studies that evaluate the different RDTs in various populations have been published and reviewed.[21–23,36] In comparison to microscopical diagnosis the sensitivity for detecting symptomatic *P. falciparum* infections was high with all rapid tests having a sensitivity of 85%–100% in the majority of studies. In a few cases with proven falciparum malaria rapid tests were already positive at a time when it was impossible to detect parasites microscopically. With low para-sitemias, predominantly occurring in semi-immunes, the sensitivity of all tests was significantly lower and reached only 50–70% with parasitemias less than 100/μL.[36,37]

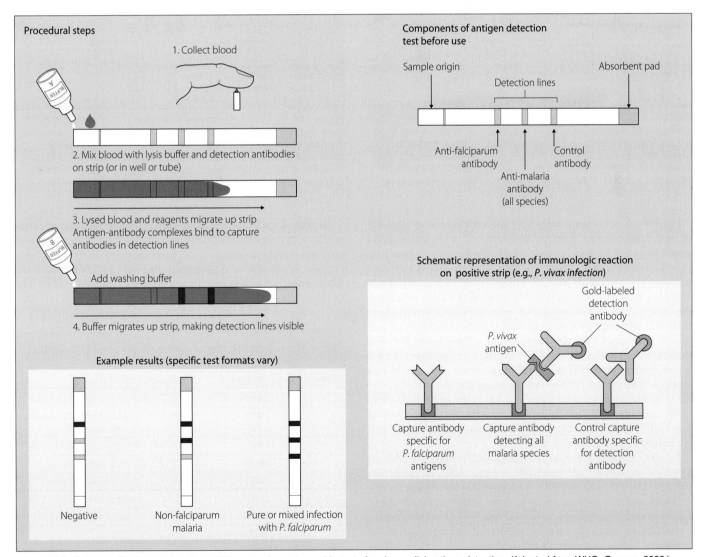

Figure 14.2 Scheme of test procedure in rapid immunochromatographic tests for plasmodial antigen detection. (Adapted from WHO, Geneva, 2000.)

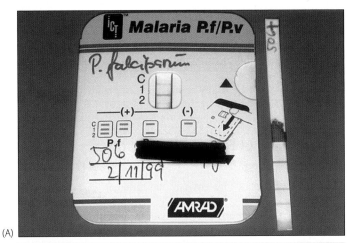

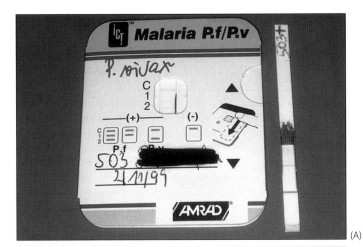

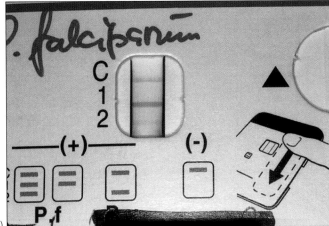

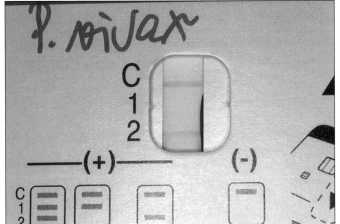

Figure 14.3 (A) RDTs for combined detection of *P. falciparum* and *P. vivax* displaying test results positive for *P. falciparum*. Left side, test format for the detection of histidine-rich protein-2 (HRP-2) in combination with plasmodial aldolase (ICT Malaria P.f./P.v.®); right side, test format for the detection of parasite-specific lactate dehydrogenase (pLDH) (OptiMal®). (B) Close-up view of 'A' to illustrate test result as seen by the examiner.

Figure 14.4 (A) – RDTs for combined detection of *P. falciparum* and *P. vivax* displaying test results positive for *P. vivax*. Left side, test format for the detection of histidine-rich protein-2 (HRP-2) in combination with plasmodial aldolase (ICT Malaria P.f./P.v.®); right side, test format for the detection of parasite-specific lactate dehydrogenase (pLDH) (OptiMal®). (B) Close-up view of 'A' to illustrate test result as seen by the examiner.

However, false negative results have also been occasionally recorded with higher parasitemias (>500–1000/µL).[38–41] A false-negative MalaQuick® test, in which the *P. falciparum* parasitemia was 30%, became positive after a 1:10 dilution of the patient's blood; a prozone phenomenon with high antigen concentrations was postulated.[40] More importantly it is estimated that 2–3% of all isolates might lack the HRP-2 gene, thus making these infections undetectable when using this antigen.[42–44] Also since mature gametocytes do not produce HRP-2; cases with gametocytes alone will be missed.[45,46] This finding, as well as the fact that HRP-2 antigenemia persists for up to 4 weeks' following clinical and parasitological cure[23,47] is of relevance when considering test methods for follow-up after therapy.

The specificity in most investigations was in the range of 90–100% in the majority of studies. False-positive results are possible with all tests. They were observed in patients with rheumatoid factor,[48–50] particularly with the ParaSight-F test®.

For the detection of *P. vivax* infections, pLDH detection with the OptiMal® yielded a high sensitivity and specificity of more than 90%.[51–53] The ICT Malaria P.f/P.v.® test (or RIDA® MalaQuick Kombi) showed a similarly high specificity of >90% with *P. vivax* infections, but the overall sensitivity (72–75%) was lower.[33,54] At low parasitemias, (<500/µL), as frequently seen in patients with tertian malaria, the sensitivity decreases significantly with both tests, making them inferior to microscopy.[53,55,56]

For the diagnosis of *P. ovale* and *P. malariae*, comprehensive studies with both antigens (aldolase and pLDH) are lacking. For both tests false-negative results have been reported in patients with established *P. ovale* or *P. malariae* infections,[52,57–59] the diagnostic value appears to be low with these infections, using the test systems

Table 14.1 Dipstick tests for malaria diagnosis

Generation	Antigen(s)	Species	Brand name
1	HRP2	P.f.	ParaSight-F[27]
1	HRP2	P.f.	Binax Malaria P.f. alias MalaQuick[28]
1	HRP2	P.f.	PATH falciparum malaria[29]
1	HRP2	P.f.	Paracheck-P.f.[30]
1	HRP2	P.f.	Determine Malaria P.f.[31]
1	HRP2	P.f.	Quorum RTM[32]
2	HRP2 + PMA	P.f. + P.v.	Binax Malaria P.f./P.v.[33]
2	pLDH isoforms	P.f. + P.v.	OptiMal[22]

P.f., P. falciparum; P.v., P. vivax.

currently available. Table 14.2 summarizes characteristic findings for the various test systems.

Performance of RDTs for self-use by travelers

After the introduction of rapid tests, which can be performed without additional technical devices and under field conditions, the question arises whether the self-use of these tests would be a feasible option for travelers to help them decide whether or not to embark on SBET.

In an open, comparative trial to determine whether travelers can successfully use and interpret the ParaSight-F test, 160 visitors to a large travel clinic in Zurich, Switzerland, were asked to test their own blood and to interpret five pre-prepared test strips of the ParaSight-F® test. Seventy-five percent succeeded with self-testing after receiving written instructions only, whereas 90% managed to handle the test correctly after having received combined written and oral instructions.[60] However, the interpretation of pre-prepared tests was not satisfactory (only 70.6% correct interpretations) and yielded a high rate of false-negative results (14.1%). A comparative study between ParaSight-F® and MalaQuick® with 164 participants yielded no significant difference regarding self-testing with both systems, but the MalaQuick® test with its cardboard format was considered easier to perform by the laypersons than the test strip format of the ParaSight-F®.[61] Reliable results were obtained with both test strips from specimens with parasitemias between 0.1–2.0%. Interestingly, in *low* parasitemias-ParaSight-F® test strips were correctly read by 52.1% versus 10.8% with MalaQuick®, but in *high* parasitemias-ParaSight-F® test strips were correctly read by only 33.8% versus 96.8% with MalaQuick®. Overall, both test systems were associated with unacceptably high levels of false-negative interpretations. The authors concluded that major improvements to assist lay individuals in test performance would be necessary to justify its use by travelers. When asking volunteers for a judgment on the technique, about 67.5% considered self-testing a helpful concept, 31.9% found it indispensable, and only 0.6% judged it as superfluous.

In an investigation of 98 European tourists with febrile disease in Kenya under 'field conditions,' only 68% of patients were able to complete the MalaQuick® correctly. Most importantly, 10 out of 11 patients with microscopically confirmed falciparum malaria were unable to self-diagnose their condition by rapid testing (see Table 14.3 for details). On the other hand, when these tests were performed by medical personnel, sensitivity and specificity reached 100%. The authors concluded that a considerable proportion of patients might be too sick to correctly diagnose malaria by RDT's and subsequently, to start treatment by themselves.[62]

In a prospective study carried out in the UK with 153 returning travelers with an acute febrile illness, only 14 (9%) failed to carry out a MalaQuick® test correctly on presentation, using an improved test instruction leaflet. All 22 patients with microscopically confirmed falciparum malaria completed self-testing successfully, and the overall sensitivity reached 95%, with 97% specificity.[63] The authors argued that differences in the various studies were possibly due to the poor quality of the manufacturer's instruction sheet, and the customized test procedure. If appropriately validated, a more user-friendly kit could be implemented for travelers, without additional instruction and training. Table 14.4[62] summarizes the studies dealing with this subject so far. Table 14.5 gives the pros and cons of self-diagnosis.

Stand-by emergency self-treatment for malaria

Principle and rationale for use

SBET as defined by the WHO[6] is the self-administration of antimalarial drugs when malaria is suspected, and when prompt medical attention is unavailable within 24 h following the onset of symptoms. In her comprehensive review of SBET by travelers, Schlagenhauf[65] points out that presumptive self-treatment is indicated only in emergency situations, and that it must be followed by medical consultation as soon as possible. This implies that a careful risk-benefit analysis, based on an individual's travel, should be carried out before departure. SBET is not indicated for sojourns in areas where travelers

---

Table 14.2   Quality of malaria dipstick tests

Species to be detected	P. falciparum	P. vivax (combined with P.f.)	P. ovale + malariae (combined with P.f. and P.v.)
Antigen(s)	HRP2, pLDH	PMA, pLDH	PMA, pLDH
Product(s)	Binax Malaria P.f. *alias* Malaquick[a], ParaSight-F[a] and others; OptiMal[b]	Binax Malaria P.f./P.v. *alias* Malaquick[c]; OptiMal[b]	Binax Malaria P.f./P.v. *alias* Malaquick[c]; OptiMal[b]
Size of database	Large	Intermediate	Small
Study area(s)	Endemic/nonendemic areas	Endemic/nonendemic areas	Endemic/nonendemic areas
Sensitivity versus GS	85–100% in majority of studies	80–95% in majority of studies	Database too small
Specificity versus GS	90–100% in majority of studies	90–100% in majority of studies	Database too small
Tests in direct comparison	No significant differences	OptiMal superior?	Database too small
State-of-the-art	Established knowledge, 'me-too' products work probably equally well	Issue unsettled so far	Issue unsettled so far; detection/differentiation appears unreliable

[a]Using HRP2 plasmodial antigen
[b]Using pLDH plasmodial antigen
[c]Using plasmodium-specific aldolase and HRP2 plasmodial antigen
GS, gold standard

Table 14.3	Self-use of rapid diagnostic tests by travelers	
Setting	**Test used**	**Main findings**
Healthy Swiss travelers: dry run before travel[60]	ParaSight F (n = 160)	75% success after oral instruction; 90% success after additional oral/written instruction 14% false-negative interpretation of pre-prepared test Major technical modifications recommended
Healthy Swiss travelers: dry run prior to travel[61]	ParaSight F, ICT P.f. (n = 164)	Interpretation problems at low parasitemias (< 0.1%) High level of false-negative interpretations Technical improvement and instruction required
Febrile travelers (Kenya)[62]	ICT P.f (n = 98)	68% success with manufacturer's instructions only Only 1 out of 11 patients with confirmed falciparum malaria tested successfully Intensive training/instruction required
Febrile returning travelers (London)[63]	ICT P.f (n = 153)	91% success after intensive instruction and assistance obtaining sample In 22 patients with confirmed falciparum malaria: 100% success, sensitivity 95%, specificity 97%

Data reproduced from Nothdurft and Jelinek[64]

Table 14.4	Reasons for failure of tourists to obtain valid results with rapid test for falciparum malaria	
Reasons for failure		**Number of patients[a]**
Unable to draw blood (finger prick)		22 (71%)
Unable to place the blood drop appropriately on the test kit		8 (26%)
Did not wait for the recommended period (8 min)		12 (39%)
Unable to identify the bands indicating the test result		18 (58%)
Unable to interpret the result		27 (87%)

[a]Of a total of 31 patients; some patients failed on more than one point.
Data reproduced from Jelinek, Amsler and Grobusch et al.[62]

Table 14.5	Pros and cons of self-diagnosis	
Pros	**Cons**
Diagnosis following immediately after onset of symptoms is possible	Test performance and interpretation of results possibly impaired in those already compromised by illness, and in the poorly trained
Relatively inexpensive procedure	Depending on travel conditions, quality of test can be impaired by high humidity and temperature
No loss of transfer time to doctor/waiting time	Risk of 'false security' feeling following false-positive or false-negative test
SBET can be initiated on the grounds of a (preliminary) diagnosis rather than 'blind' treatment based solely on clinical suspicion	

have access to good medical care. An indication for SBET may be independent of whether or not a chemoprophylactic agent is being used. Since chemoprophylaxis failures are possible with any of the currently available drugs, particularly in areas with high transmission rates and known resistance.

Whereas current recommendations of WHO[2] and CDC[3] emphasize the benefits of chemoprophylaxis, other national expert committees take a different approach with regard to the estimated real risk of contracting malaria in defined areas. A current Swiss recommendation, for example, is to carry SBET rather than to use chemoprophylaxis in areas with a low risk of malaria, since the adverse effects of the drug may outweight, by far, the risk of malaria. Since malaria symptoms are not specific at the onset of illness, every acute febrile episode occurring after seventh day in an endemic area must be considered as possible malaria.

The traveler should be informed that malaria can occur in spite of strict adherence to a recommended prophylactic regimen. The traveler must know that SBET is not an alternative to early medical treatment. Still, if a decision for the administration of SBET is made, regardless of the reason, medical help should be sought as soon as possible under all circumstances, to confirm – or rule out – suspected malaria, control the success of therapy and, if necessary, to search for other illnesses.

When counseling the traveler, health-care providers should keep in mind that SBET should be considered for about 4–8 weeks after the end of the exposure period, to ensure swift intervention in case of a delayed *Plasmodium falciparum* infection.

Possible indications for considering SBET are given in Table 14.6[65]; guidelines for use of SBET are given in Table 14.7. Table 14.8 summarizes the essentials to be discussed when counseling travelers with regard to SBET.

RECOMMENDATIONS FOR CHOICE OF DRUGS

Table 14.9[65] provides a list of drugs suitable for SBET depending on whether or not, drugs are used for chemoprophylaxis. Some drugs listed are not, or are no longer, available or registered in all countries, such as sulfadoxine/pyrimethamine combinations (e.g., Fansidar®)

Table 14.6	Possible indications for SBET[a]

Stay in areas with low risk of malaria (e.g., beach holiday in Mexico)

No, or suboptimal use of chemoprophylaxis and visit of a remote malaria-endemic area without health care facilities within reach (e.g., adventure trekking in Sumatra)

Changing itineraries, perhaps with visits to foci with multidrug resistance not, or inadequately covered by the chosen prophylactic regimen (e.g., traveling in Cambodia using mefloquine prophylaxis or no prophylaxis

Sojourn in malaria-free areas, therefore no continuous chemoprophylaxis, with brief occasional visit(s) to malaria-endemic area(s) (e.g., touring South-Africa for 3 weeks including 2 nights in Kruger Park)

Frequent stays in malarious areas for short periods (e.g., air crew weekly 1 overnight stay in New Delhi)

Contraindications, or known intolerance towards recommended chemoprophylactics, therefore no/only 'suboptimal' chemoprophylaxis

Travel for a prolonged period (exceeding 3 months) or residency in malarious areas

Poor motivation towards any chemoprophylaxis

Use of adequate chemoprophylaxis, but feared risk of breakthrough malaria e.g. on the grounds of low drug levels due to reduced absorption (e.g., because of diarrhea, vomiting) and absence of health service facilities in reach within 24 h

[a]Modified from Schlagenhauf (2001)[65]

Table 14.7	Guidelines for starting SBET

Onset of acute febrile disease suggestive for malaria

Sojourn in malaria-endemic area for more than 6 days

Qualified medical care probably not available within next 24h

Table 14.8	Points to be discussed or trained when counseling travelers considering SBET (with or without chemoprophylaxis)

SBET is a measure for emergency situations only

Recognition of malaria-suggesting symptoms, stress unspecific character

Indications to self-initiate treatment (see Table 14.7)

Necessity to take a full therapeutic dose

Possibility of adverse events following SBET

Possibility of SBET failure

Necessity to seek medical advice despite initiation of SBET

Necessity to carry SBET for approximately 4 weeks after the end of exposure

or those which are less suitable for SBET due to dosage scheme and side effects profile (e.g., quinine or quinine/tetracycline). Novel drugs – atovaquone/proguanil (Malarone®), artemether-lumefantrine (Riamet®) – which are only registered and marketed in a limited number of countries, are listed. Halofantrine (Halfan®) is not listed, as it is no longer recommended for use because of reports that predisposed patients with Q-Tc interval prolongation and ventricular dysrhythmias can have a life-threatening outcome.[66,67]

The recommendations of the various national expert groups are guided by the report by WHO[2] (Fig. 14.1), in which SBET with chloroquine (Nivaquine®, Resochin® and other trademarks) is only recommended in zones of limited risk. In those zones of considerable malaria risk, particularly mefloquine (Lariam®, Mephaquine®), atovaquone/proguanil (Malarone®) and artemether/lumefantrine (Riamet®) ought to be considered as suitable compounds. Due to increasing mefloquine resistance in the West of Cambodia and along

Table 14.9	Available options for stand-by emergency treatment (SBET)			
Generic name	Trade name(s)	Amount per dosage	SBET[a] dosage (adult)	
Chloroquine	Aralen, Avlochlor, Nivaquine, Resochin	Tablet: 100 or 150 mg (base); syrups available	600 mg on days 1 and 2, followed by 300 mg on day 3	
Sulfadoxine/pyrimethamine	Fansidar	Tablet: 500 mg/25 mg	3 tablets in a single dose	
Sulfadoxine/pyrimethamine/ mefloquine	Fansimef	Tablet: 500 mg/25 mg/250 mg	3 tablets in a single dose	
Sulfalene/pyrimethamine	Metakelfin	Tablet: 500 mg/25 mg	3 tablets in a single dose	
Mefloquine	Lariam, Mephaquin	Tablet: 250 mg (US, 228 mg)	5–6 tablets in divided doses,[b] depending on body weight	
Quinine (sulfate, bisulfate, dihydrochloride, hydrochl.)	Tablet: 300 mg (salt)	600 mg (2 tablets) t.i.d.[c] for 7 days (total of 42 tablets)		
Atovaquone/Proguanil	Malarone	Tablet: 250 mg/100 mg	4 tablets daily as a single dose on 3 consecutive days (total of 12 tablets)	
Artemether/Lumefantrin[d]	Riamet	Tablet: 20 mg/120 mg	4 tablets initially on day 1, followed by a further 4 tablets 8 h later; 4 tablets twice daily on days 2 and 3 (total of 24 tablets)	

[a]SBET, stand-by emergency treatment; [b]Manufacturer's recommendation: 25 mg/kg for non-immunes, WHO recommendation: 15 mg/kg (25 mg/kg for certain areas on Thailand border); [c]t.i.d., three times daily; [d]There is a paucity of data regarding the efficacy and tolerability of these newer combinations in non-immune travelers.
Note: halofantrine is no longer on the WHO-recommended list; for use under medical supervision only.
Data reproduced from Schlagenhauf.[65]

the Thai-Cambodian, -Laotian and -Burmese borders, for those and adjacent areas atovaquone/proguanil and artemether/lumefantrine are preferred.

For specific contraindications and adverse events profile of particular drugs, see Chapters 13 and 15 and Table 14.10 for factors influencing SBET.

SBET recommendations for pregnant women, children, and chronically ill patients

Pregnant women and non-immune children are at particular risk of severe malaria. Therefore, if possible, sojourns in areas with high malaria risk should be avoided. In case of a febrile episode, all efforts should be made to seek medical attention as soon as possible. In pregnant women, quinine is the drug of choice for SBET. Mefloquine should only be used after careful risk-benefit analysis but not in the first trimester. Sufficient experience with atovaquone/proguanil and artemether/lumefantrine are not yet available. For children heavier than 5 kg, atovaquone/proguanil (above 10 kg) and artemether/lumefantrine are suitable for SBET. For newborns lighter than 5 kg, quinine is the drug of choice. Table 14.11[65] details drug regimens for SBET suitable for use in children.

For travelers with chronic illnesses who are on medication, a suitable regimen for both chemoprophylaxis and/or SBET has to be tailored carefully to their individual needs. The profile of contraindications, expected drug interactions, and adverse events must be taken into consideration on the background of their underlying illness. For example, mefloquine should be strictly avoided for both prophylaxis and SBET in individuals with a past medical history of neuropsychiatric disorders of any kind.[65]

Balancing of recommendations

The diagnosis of malaria solely on clinical grounds is unreliable and difficult even for trained medical staff. Fever is the most common and reliable symptom. Even on short trips to developing countries, it is observed with a frequency of 3.8–10%.[68]

Travelers appear to have difficulty implementing SBET appropriately. It is particularly feared that the frequency of febrile diseases of varying origin leads to an uncontrolled over-treatment of malaria with combined risk of delayed diagnosis of another illness and antimalarial adverse events.[69] Finally, it has been speculated that SBET recommendations might encourage travelers to abandon chemoprophylaxis altogether.[69–71]

So far, two prospective studies have investigated the practical aspects of implementing SBET recommendations. A Swiss study[72] investigated 1187 travelers who received only SBET recommendations without simultaneous chemoprophylaxis (predominantly for journeys to Asia and Latin America). In another study of 2867 German travelers to highly malaria-endemic areas in sub-Saharan Africa chemoprophylaxis and SBET were recommended.[70] Both studies confirmed the high incidence of febrile illness among travelers

(8.1% versus 10.4%, respectively) even for short trips to malarious regions (average duration of stay 4 weeks). However, only a small proportion of travelers took SBET in both studies (0.5%, or 1.4% respectively, of all travelers; 4.9%, or 17% respectively, of febrile travelers). In only 10.8%, or 16.7%, respectively, of the latter group, was malaria confirmed retrospectively. A total of 100 (57%) patients sought medical advice after SBET. Out of 30, or 15%, of all patients, respectively but predominantly those who took mefloquine or mefloquine–sulphadoxin/pyrimethamine as SBET, one required hospitalization for adverse events, in conjunction with SBET. For travelers who adhered both to advice for chemoprophylaxis and SBET, adherence to chemoprophylaxis was not worse than in comparable studies of chemoprophylaxis alone.[11,12] Both studies pointed out the importance of counseling during which detailed advice in both written and oral form is necessary to ensure a responsible and adequate handling of SBET recommendations by travelers. Table 14.12[65] summarizes studies on travelers' use of malaria SBET.

As concluded by Schlagenhauf,[65] the knowledge and behavior of travelers are difficult to predict. In the Swiss study, despite awareness of the need for rapid diagnosis and treatment of malaria, approximately 66% of travelers with a febrile illness failed to seek prompt medical advice.[72] In a UK survey almost 25% of participants would have acted inappropriately while having malaria-like symptoms, predominantly by resting at home and waiting for resolution of symptoms.[73] On the other hand, the difficulty in deciding correctly – in absence of diagnostic tools and medical formation – that an acute febrile illness is malaria, is highlighted by a German study in which only four (10.4%) of 37 SBET treatment users were found to have significant antibody levels against *Plasmodium falciparum*.[71]

Airline crews may be an ideal group to assess efficacy and safety of SBET alone. After abandoning mefloquine chemoprophylaxis for SBET among Swissair crews traveling to destinations in highly malaria-endemic areas, there was no significant increase in malaria cases observed, although only approximately 1% of crew members took SBET per year.[65,74] Table 14.13 gives the pros and cons of self-treatment.

SUMMARY AND LOOK INTO THE FUTURE

For rational use of SBET, a reliable tool is crucial for rapid self-diagnosis – or exclusion – of malaria in travelers. If performed in the laboratory, sensitivity and specificity of rapid immunochromatographic 'dipstick' tests almost equal the quality of microscopy results obtained by trained staff. In the only cohort of travelers for which field study data are available, however, serious problems with test performance and interpretation arose particularly in those individuals who were seriously ill. Although it has been demonstrated that test performance can be improved considerably by adequate information and training, inherent problems of immunochromatographic antigen detection such as false-negative results even with high parasitemias, cannot be ignored or overcome easily.

CONCLUSION

Rapid tests do not appear to be of great help for making appropriate decisions on the use of SBET and it remains mandatory that travelers with acute febrile illness should seek medical help as soon as possible in any case. If this is not feasible within a day, the indication for SBET should be independent of a malaria dipstick test result.

The concept of SBET has proven itself to be a valuable additional tool for reducing malaria illness among travelers. The indication for SBET should be clearly and unambiguously stated by the travel medicine advisor, and the traveler should be informed meticulously. When

Table 14.10	Factors influencing choice of SBET
The intake of chemoprophylaxis and the drugs used therefore	
The expected local plasmodial resistance pattern	
Simplicity/complexity of application (tolerability, handling)	
Individual contraindications and expected/previously experienced intolerances	

Table 14.11 Drug regimens for stand-by emergency treatment (SBET): Children's dosages[a]

Mefloquine[b]			Sulfadoxine/ Pyrimethamine (500 mg/25 mg)		Chloroquine[c] (100 mg base)				Artemether/ Lumefantrine[d,e] (20 mg/120 mg)				Atovaquone/ Proguanil[d] (250 mg/100 mg)			
Weight (kg)	h 1	h[e]6–24	Weight (kg)	Single dose	Weight (kg)	Day 1	Day 2	Day 3	Weight (kg)	Day 1	Day 2	Day 3	Weight (kg)	Day 1	Day 2	Day 3
5–6	¼	¼	5–6	¼	5–6	½	½	½	–	–	–	–	–	–	–	–
7–8	½	¼	7–10	½	7–10	1	1	½	–	–	–	–	–	–	–	–
9–12	¾	½	11–14	¾	11–14	1½	1½	½	10–15	2 × 1	2 × 1	2 × 1	11–20	1	1	1
13–16	1	½	15–18	1	15–18	2	2	½	–	–	–	–	–	–	–	–
17–24	1½	1	19–29	1½	19–24	2½	2½	1	15–25	2 × 2	2 × 2	2 × 2	21–30	2	2	2
25–35	2	1½	30–39	2½	25–35	3½	3½	2	25–34	2 × 3	2 × 3	2 × 3	–	–	–	–
36–50	3	2	40–49	2½	36–50	5	5	2½	–	–	–	–	31–40	3	3	3

[a] Given as tablet fractions. [b] The total dosage (25 mg [base]/ kg) is divided into two doses: 15 mg (base)/kg, followed by 10 mg (base)/kg 6–24 h later. [c] The total dosage is 25 mg (base)/kg divided over 3 days (Tablets usually contain either 100 mg or 150 mg chloroquine base). [d] There is a paucity of data on efficacy and tolerability of this drug combination in non-immune travelers. [e] On day 1, the tablets should be taken at 8-h intervals; on days 2 and 3, at 12-h intervals. [f] h = hour(s).
Data reproduced from Schlagenhauf.[65]

Table 14.12 Traveler's use of malaria stand-by emergency treatment

Year	Agent	Traveler's origin	Destination	Use (%)
1987/1988	SDX/PYR	Swiss	Africa	5.4
1989	MQ	Swiss	Africa	3.6
1991	MQ/SDX/PYR	French	Africa	2.1
1992	MQ/SDX/PYR	Swiss	Asia, Americas	0.5
1992/1993	H, MQ, CL SDX/PYR	German	Asia Africa	0.3 1.0
1994	H, MQ, SDX/PYR	German	Asia Africa	1.0 5.0

CL, chloroquine; H, halofantrine; MQ, mefloquine; MQ/SDX/PYR, mefloquine/sulfadoxine/ pyrimethamine (Fansimef); SDX/PYR, sulfadoxine/pyrimethamine (Fansidar).
Data reproduced with kind permission from Schlagenhauf[65]

Table 14.13 Pros and cons of self-treatment

Pros	Cons
Swift initiation of therapy, possibly avoiding progression to more severe disease	False treatment based on misdiagnosis, with possible risk of missing underlying, severe, non-malarious condition
Of use if prophylaxis fails	Risk of inappropriate dosages (both too low or too high) or inappropriate drug used
Of use for travelers for whom prophylaxis is inappropriate	Medical advice following initiation of SBET still ought to be sought

adequate oral and written instructions, along with comprehensive practical advice have been provided to the traveler, it appears that most travelers can make responsible use of the recommendations. The fear of abandoning a chemoprophylaxis in favour of SBET or the risk of antimalarial drug adverse events, however, cannot be confirmed.

New drugs with better tolerability and efficacy, in multidrug resistance areas, will ensure that SBET is a useful additional tool for the safety of travelers to malarious areas.

REFERENCES

1. Fischer PR, Bialek R. Prevention of malaria in children. *Clin Inf Dis* 2002; **34**:493–498.
2. World Health Organization. Malaria. In: International travel and health: situation as on 1 January 2002. Geneva: World Health Organization 2002; pp.130–148.
3. Centers for Disease Control and Prevention (CDC). *Health Information for the International Traveler 2001–2002*. Atlanta: US Department of Health and Human Services, Public Health Service; 2001.
4. Legros F, Danis M and Eurosurveillance Editorial Board. Surveillance of malaria in European Union countries. *Eurosurveillance* 1998; **3**:45–47.
5. Steffen R, Behrens RH. Traveller's malaria. *Parasitol Today* 1992; **8**:61–66.
6. World Health Organization. Malaria 1982–1997. *Weekly Epidem Rec* 1999; **74**:265–272.
7. Surveillance of malaria in European Union countries. *Eurosurveillance* 1998; **3**:45–47.
8. Jelinek T, Schulte C, Behrens R, *et al.* Imported falciparum malaria in Europe: Sentinel surveillance data from the European network on surveillance of imported infectious disease. *Clin Inf Dis* 2002; **34**:572–576.
9. Muentener P, Schlagenhauf P, Steffen R. Imported malaria (1985–95): trends and perspectives. Bull World Health Organ 1999; **77**:560–566.
10. Richie TL, Saul A. Progress and challenges for malaria vaccines. *Nature* 1998; **415**:694–701.
11. Mühlberger N, Jelinek T, Schlipkoeter U, *et al.* Effectiveness of chemoprophylaxis and other determinants of malaria in travellers to Kenya. *Trop Med Int Health* 1998; **3**:357–363.
12. Steffen R, Fuchs E, Schildknecht J, *et al.* Mefloquine compared with other chemoprophylactic regimens in tourists visiting East Africa. *Lancet* 1993; **341**:1299–1303.
13. Lell B, Luckner D, Ndjave M, *et al.* Randomized placebo-controlled study of atovaquone plus proguanil for malaria prophylaxis in children. *Lancet* 1998; **351**:709–713.
14. Lell B, Faucher JF, Missinou MA, *et al.* Malaria chemoprophylaxis with tafenoquine: a randomized study. *Lancet* 2000; **355**:2041–2045.
15. World Health Organization. New Perspectives – Malaria Diagnosis. Report of a joint workshop WHO/USAID informal consultation 25–27 October 1999. World Health Organization, Geneva 2000.
16. World Health Organization. Development of recommendations for the protection of short-stay travellers to malaria-endemic areas: Memorandum from two WHO Meetings. *Bull WHO* 1988; **66**:177–196.
17. DTG (Deutsche Gesellschaft für Tropenmedizin und Internationale Gesundheit). *Empfehlungen zur Malariavorbeugung für beratende Ärzte, June 2001*. Online. Available at: http://www.tropmed.dtg.org. DTG-Infoservice, P.B. 400466, D-80704 Munich, Germany.
18. Hatz CFR, Beck B, Blum J, *et al.* Malaria-Chemoprophylaxe 2001. *Therap Umschau* **58**:347–351.
19. Connor BA. Expert recommendations for antimalarial prophylaxis. *J Travel Med* 2001; **8(suppl 3)**: S57–S64.
20. Bain BJ, Chiodini PL, England JM, *et al.* The laboratory diagnosis of malaria. *Clin Lab Haematol* 1997; **19**:165–170.
21. Hänscheid T. Diagnosis of malaria: a review of alternatives to conventional microscopy. *Clin Lab Haematol* 1999; **21**:235–245.
22. Makler MT, Palmer CJ, Ager AL. A review of practical techniques for the diagnosis of malaria. *Ann Trop Med Parasitol* 1998; **92**:419–433.
23. Moody A. Rapid diagnostic tests for malaria parasites. *Clin Microbiol Rev* 2002; **15**:66–78.

24. Lowe BS, Jfa NK, Pederson C, *et al.* Acridine orange fluorescence techniques as alternatives to traditional Giemsa staining for the diagnosis of malaria in developing countries. *Trans R Soc Trop Med Hyg* 1996; **90**:34–36.

25. Snounou G, Viriyakosol S, Jarra W, *et al.* Identification of the four human malaria parasite species in field samples by the polymerase-chain-reaction and detection of a high prevalence of mixed infections. *Molecular Biochem Parasitol* 1993; **58**:283–292.

26. Hänscheid T, Valadas E, Grobusch MP. Automated malaria diagnosis using pigment detection. *Parasitol Today* 2000; **16**:549–551.

27. Shiff CJ, Minjas JN, Premji Z. The ParaSight-F® test: a simple rapid manual dipstick test to detect Plasmodium falciparum infection. *Parasitol Today* 1994; **10**:494–495.

28. Garcia M, Kirimoama S, Marlborough D, *et al.* Immunochromatographic test for malaria diagnosis. *Lancet* 1996; **347**:1549.

29. Gaye O, Diouf M, Diallo S. A comparison of thick smears, QBC malaria, PCR and PATH falciparum malaria test strip in Plasmodium falciparum diagnosis. *Parasite* 1999; **6**:273–275.

30. Proux S, Hkirijareon L, Ngamngonkiri C, *et al.* Paracheck-Pf: a new, inexpensive and reliable rapid test for diagnosis of falciparum malaria. *Trop Med Int Health* 2001; **6**:99–101.

31. Singh N, Valecha N. Evaluation of a rapid diagnostic test, 'Determine malaria pf', in epidemic-prone, forest villages of central India (Madhya Pradesh). *Ann Trop Med Parasitol* 2000; **94**:421–427.

32. Wolday D, Balcha F, Fessehaye G, *et al.* Field trial of the RTM dipstick method for the rapid diagnosis of malaria based on the detection of Plasmodium HRP2 antigen in whole blood. *Trop Doct* 2001; **31**:19–21.

33. Tjitra E, Suprianto S, Dyer M, *et al.* Field evaluation of the ICT malaria P.f./P.v. immunochromatographic test for detection of Plasmodium falciparum and Plasmodium vivax in patients with a presumptive clinical diagnosis of malaria in Eastern Indonesia. *J Clin Microbiol* 1999; **37**:2412–2417.

34. Meier B, Dobeli H, Certa U. Stage-specific expression of aldolase iso-enzymes in the rodent malaria parasite Plasmodium berghei. *Mol Biochem Parasitol* 1992; **52**:15–27.

35. Makler MT, Piper RC, Milhous WK. Lactate dehydrogenase and the diagnosis of malaria. *Parasitol Today* 1998; 14, 376–377.

36. Burchard GD. Malariaschnelltests. *Bundesgesundheitsbl Gesundheitsforsch Gesundheitsschutz* 1999; **42**:643–649.

37. Ricci L, Viani I, Piccolo G, *et al.* Evaluation of OptiMal assay to detect imported malaria in Italy. *New Microbiol* 2000; **23**:391–398.

38. Beadle C, Long GW, Weiss WR, *et al.* Diagnosis of malaria by detection of Plasmodium falciparum HRP-2 antigen with a rapid dipstick antigen-capture assay. *Lancet* 1994; **343**:564–568.

39. Kodisinghe HM, Perera KLRL, Premawansa S, *et al.* The ParaSight-F® dipstick test as a routine diagnostic tool for malaria in Sri Lanka. *Trans R Soc Trop Med Hyg* 1997; **91**:398–402.

40. Risch L, Bader M, Huber AR. Self-use of rapid tests for malaria diagnosis. *Lancet* 2000; **335**:237.

41. Stow NW, Torrens JK, Walker J. An assessment of the accuracy of clinical diagnosis, local microscopy and a rapid immunochromatographic card test in comparison with expert microscopy in the diagnosis of malaria in rural Kenya. *Trans R Soc Trop Med Hyg* 1999; **93**:519–520.

42. Pieroni P, Mills CD, Ohrt C, *et al.* Comparison of the Parasight-F® test and the ICT Malaria P.f.® test with the polymerase chain reaction for the diagnosis of Plasmodium falciparum in travelers. *Trans R Soc Trop Med Hyg* 1998; **92**:166–169.

43. Trarore I, Koita O, Doumbo O. Field studies of the ParaSight-F® test in a malaria-endemic area: cost, feasibility, sensitivity, specificity, predictive value and the deletion of the HRP-2 gene among wild type Plasmodium falciparum in Mali [Poster SO2]. *Am J Trop Med Hyg* 1997; **57**:272.

44. Uguen C, Rabodonirina M, De Pina JJ, *et al.* ParaSight-F rapid manual diagnostic test of Plasmodium falciparum infections. *Bull World Health Organization* 1995; **73**:643–649.

45. Banchongaksorn T, Yomokgul P, Panyim S, *et al.* A field trial of the ParaSight-F® test for the diagnosis of Plasmodium falciparum infection. *Trans R Soc Trop Med Hyg* 1996; **90**:244–245.

46. Craig MH and Sharp BL. Comparative evaluation of four techniques for the diagnosis of Plasmodium falciparum infections. *Trans R Soc Trop Med Hyg* 1997; **91**:279–282.

47. Humar A, Ohrt C, Harrington MA, *et al.* ParaSight-F® test compared with the polymerase chain reaction and microscopy for the diagnosis of Plasmodium falciparum malaria in travelers. *Am J Trop Med Hyg* 1997; **56**:44–48.

48. Grobusch MP, Alpermann U, Schwenke S, *et al.* False-positive rapid tests for malaria in patients with rheumatoid factor. *Lancet* 1999; **353**:297.

49. Iqbal J, Sher A, Rub A. Plasmodium falciparum histidine-rich protein 2–based immunocapture diagnostic assay for malaria: cross-reactivity with rheumatoid factors. *J Clin Microbiol* 2000; **38**:1184–1186.

50. Laferl H, Kandel K, Pichler H. False-positive dipstick test for malaria. *N Engl J Med* 1997; **337**:1635–1636.

51. Lee MA, Aw LT, Singh M. A comparison of antigen dipstick assays with polymerase chain reaction (PCR) technique and blood film examination in the rapid diagnosis of malaria. *Ann Acad Med Singapore* 1999; **28**:498–501.

52. Moody A, Hunt-Cooke A, Gabbett E, *et al.* Performance of the OptiMal® malaria antigen capture dipstick for malaria diagnosis and treatment monitoring at the Hospital for Tropical Diseases, London. *Br J Haematol* 2000; **109**:891–894.

53. Palmer CJ, Lindo JF, Klaskala WI, *et al.* Evaluation of the OptiMal test for rapid diagnosis of Plasmodium vivax and Plasmodium falciparum malaria. *J Clin Microbiol* 1998; **36**:203–206.

54. Singh N, Saxena A, Valecha N. Field evaluation of the ICT malaria P.f./P.v. immunochromatographic test for diagnosis of Plasmodium falciparum and P.vivax infection in forest villages of Chhindwara, central India. *Trop Med Int Health* 2000; **5**:765–770.

55. Iqbal J, Sher A, Hira PR, *et al.* Comparison of the OptiMal test with PCR for diagnosis of malaria in immigrants. *J Clin Microbiol* 1999; **37**:3644–3646.

56. Jelinek T, Grobusch MP, Schwenke S, *et al.* Sensitivity and specificity of dipstick tests for rapid diagnosis of malaria in nonimmune travelers. *J Clin Microbiol* 1999; **37**:721–723.

57. Dyer ME, Tjitra E, Currie BJ, *et al.* Failure of the 'panmalarial' antibody of the ICT Malaria P.f./P.v. immunochromatographic test to detect symptomatic Plasmodium malariae infection. *Trans R Soc Trop Med Hyg* 2000; **94**:518.

58. Hunt-Cooke A, Chiodini PL, Doherty T, Moody AH, Ries J, Pinder M. Comparison of a parasite lactate dehydrogenase-based immunochromatographic antigen detection assay (OptiMal) with microscopy for the detection of malaria parasites in human blood samples. *Am J Trop Med Hyg* 1999; **60**:173–176.

59. John SM, Sudarsanam A, Sitaram U, *et al.* Evaluation of OptiMal, a dipstick test for the diagnosis of malaria. *Ann Trop Med Parasitol* 1998; **92**:621–622.

60. Trachsler M, Schlagenhauf P, Steffen R. Feasibility of a rapid dipstick antigen-capture assay for self-testing of traveller's malaria. *Trop Med Int Health* 1999; **4**:442–447.

61. Funk M, Schlagenhauf P, Tschopp A, *et al.* MalaQuick versus ParaSight F as a diagnostic aid in traveller's malaria. *Trans R Soc Trop Med Hyg* 1999; **93**:268–272.

62. Jelinek T, Amsler L, Grobusch MP, Nothdurft HD. Self-use of rapid tests for malaria diagnosis by tourists. *Lancet* 1999; **354**:1609.

63. Behrens RH, Whitty CJ. Self-use of rapid tests for malaria diagnosis. *Lancet* 2000; **355**:237.

64. Nothdurft HD, Jelinek T. Use of rapid tests for and by travelers. In: Schlagenhauf P, ed. *Travelers' Malaria*. London: BC Decker; 2001: 423–430.

65. Schlagenhauf P. Stand-by emergency treatment by travelers. In: Schlagenhauf P, ed. *Travelers' Malaria*. Hamilton, London: BC Decker; 2001:446–462.

66. Matson PA, Luby SP, Redd SC, *et al.* Cardiac effects of standard-dose halofantrine therapy. *Am J Trop Med Hyg* 1996; **54**:229–231.

67. World Health Organization 1993. Drug alert: halofantrine. *Wkly Epidemiol Rec* 1993; **68**:268–270.

68. Steffen R, Lobel HO. Epidemiologic basis for the practice of travel medicine. *J Wilderness Med* 1994; **5**:56–66.

69. Schlagenhauf P, Steffen R. Stand-by treatment of malaria in travellers: a review. *J Trop Med Hyg* 1994; **97**:151–160.

70. Löscher T, Nothdurft HD. Malaria – rapid diagnostic tests and emergency self-treatment. *Ther Umsch* 2001; **58**:352–361.

71. Nothdurft HD, Jelinek T, Pechel SM, *et al.* Stand-by treatment of suspected malaria in travellers. *Trop Med Parasitol* 1995; **46**:161–163.

72. Schlagenhauf P, Steffen R, Tschopp A, *et al.* Behavioural aspects of travellers in their use of malaria presumptive treatment. *Bull World Health Organization* 1995; **73**:215–221.

73. Behrens RH, Phillips-Howard PA. What do travellers know about malaria? *Lancet* 1989; **ii**:1395–1396.

74. Steffen R, Holdener F, Wyss R, *et al.* Malaria prophylaxis and self-therapy in airline crews. *Aviat Space Environ Med* 1990; **61**:942–945.

CHAPTER 15   # Approach to the Patient with Malaria

Urban Hellgren

KEYPOINTS

- Patients with any fever pattern should be considered to have malaria until proven otherwise when they have been to endemic areas

- Symptoms of malaria are dependent on the plasmodium species, the immune status and the age of the patient

- As a rule non-immune adults or children suffer from more severe clinical symptoms than semi-immune adults

- Immediate diagnosis and treatment are the key factors in reducing fatalities from malaria

- Malaria treatment options are determined by the species involved, the severity of disease and the expected resistance pattern

INTRODUCTION

Malaria remains a significant health problem in travelers to endemic areas. Each year, at least 10 000 travelers fall ill.[1] Falciparum malaria is by far the most dangerous species and carries a high mortality rate if left untreated in a previously non-immune individual. The pattern of imported malaria has changed during recent decades and *Plasmodium falciparum* has become the dominant species. One probable reason for this is the increasing resistance to chloroquine in sub-Saharan Africa. Falciparum malaria is a medical emergency. The risk of dying is very low during the first 1–2 days, but then increases rapidly with time. This underlines the importance of early diagnosis to avoid 'Doctors Delay'. Fortunately, the other three human malaria species pathogenic to man, *Plasmodium vivax*, *Plasmodium ovale* and *Plasmodium malariae* are usually not lethal in otherwise healthy individuals.

DEVELOPMENT OF MALARIA IMMUNITY

The immunity to malaria is a combination of cellular and humoural mechanisms. It is not an absolute, protective, sterilizing immunity, but rather a more suppressive type. Individuals born and raised in highly malaria-endemic areas, who during several years are repeatedly exposed to malaria, develop a relative immunity. As the immunity gets stronger, the parasite multiplication is inhibited more and more. A balance between the suppressive effect of the immune system and the capacity of the parasites to multiply is gradually established. The individual becomes an asymptomatic carrier of malaria parasites while they are still present in the blood but at very low densities. However, the parasites do not cause any harm to the semi-immune individual. The time to develop this disease-protecting immunity depends on the level of transmission and the exposure to malaria infection. In highly endemic (holoendemic) areas, children older than 5 years of age rarely suffer from acute malaria. In areas with less endemicity, acute malaria is common also in older children. In areas with low endemicity or epidemic outbreaks only, such a disease-protecting immunity may never develop.

Expatriates who live in malarious areas are not exposed to malaria to the same extent as indigenous populations, and therefore do not develop any significant malaria immunity; they should be considered to be non-immune. A more difficult question is the immune status of individuals who have grown up in highly endemic areas (i.e., most of Africa south of the Sahara or on Papua New Guinea), but who have lived for long periods in non endemic countries. When they return to their countries of origin they may still develop symptomatic malaria but the remaining immunity might protect them from severe disease. However, the time it takes for the immunity to disappear in previously semi-immune individuals is not well documented.

SYMPTOMATOLOGY OF *P. FALCIPARUM* INFECTIONS IN NON-IMMUNE INDIVIDUALS

The symptomatology of malaria depends on the species involved, the immune status and the age of the patient. In several western European countries, the fatality rate among imported falciparum malaria cases (mostly non-immune adult patients) has been as high as 1.5–7%.[2] These unacceptable high figures suggest both a delayed diagnosis and inadequate management of the disease. Overall, about 1% of the patients with *P. falciparum* malaria die from the disease.[1]

Uncomplicated falciparum malaria

The symptomatology in uncomplicated malaria is not specific for the disease. The vast majority of patients complain of fever. The onset is usually abrupt and often accompanied by shivering. The pattern is irregular and the stated typical malaria fever with peaks every 48 h is not seen in *P. falciparum* infections. The false expectation that patients with falciparum malaria should have a so-called regular tertian fever pattern may lead to a missed diagnosis. High fever (39–40°C) is especially common in children. At our department, 86% of the patients treated for falciparum malaria had an elevated body temperature during the first 24 h after admission. Travelers to malaria endemic countries are mainly healthy adults with male dominance. In those who take NSAIDs or paracetamol, the antipyretic effect of these compounds should be considered.

Children more often have anorexia, vomiting, and diarrhea. Gastrointestinal symptoms are less frequent in adults. Except for a dry cough which is noted in a few patient's, acute respiratory symptoms are not seen and suggest another diagnosis i.e. influenza or pneumonia. In a summary of reported symptoms from several different studies, the most common were fever (97%) followed by chills (79%), headache (70%) sweating (64%) myalgia (36%) nausea (27%) and vomiting (27%).[3]

On physical examination an increased body temperature is usually present but of little differential diagnostic value. The spleen might become enlarged in patients who present with a longer duration of disease but is usually not palpable during the first few days of illness. Slight jaundice and a tender hepatomegaly or pallor is sometimes also found in patients without severe manifestations. Neck rigidity or other signs of meningism are rarely seen.

Severe and complicated malaria in adults

In adults, the time for the development to severe disease after onset of symptoms is usually 3–7 days. There are, however, reports of non-immune patients dying within 24 h.[4]

Severe manifestations of *P. falciparum* malaria are listed in Table 15.1. The prognosis is determined by the number and extent of vital organ systems involved.[4] Some important underlying conditions that can predispose to development of severe malaria are splenectomy, pregnancy, treatment with corticosteroids or cytotoxic drugs or other immunosuppression including HIV infection.

Cerebral malaria is the most common cause of death in adults with severe malaria. It often starts dramatically with generalized convulsions. The strict definition is unrousable coma with a score of nine or less on the Glasgow Coma Scale.[4] To distinguish cerebral malaria from transient postictal coma, unconsciousness should persist for at least 30 min after a convulsion. Other infectious etiologies should be excluded (meningitis or encephalitis) and *P. falciparum* parasites must be found in the blood. The Glasgow Coma Scale emphasizes, however, that 'In clinical practice, patients with any degree of impaired consciousness and any other sign of cerebral dysfunction should be treated with utmost urgency'.[4] The mechanism of cerebral malaria is still not fully known. One hypothesis is microcirculatory obstruction in the brain. This could be due to decreased deformability of parasitized red blood cells. Another, perhaps more probable explanation, is that parasitized erythrocytes bind to non-infected erythrocytes. This so-called 'rosetting' results in microvascular blood flow obstruction and local hypoxia. Parasitized erythrocytes might also cause capillary blood flow impairment by direct binding to endothelial cell receptors. Undoubtedly, cytokine production and possibly nitric oxide play a role in the severe manifestations of malaria. The mortality in cerebral malaria is around 20%, but permanent neurological sequelae are rare in survivors.

The occurrence of severe anemia is correlated with the level of parasitemia. A parasitemia with more than 4% parasitized erythrocytes should be treated as severe malaria in non-immune subjects.[4] In cerebral malaria, a parasitemia more than 5% indicates a poor prognosis. Hemoglobinuria due to hyperparasitemia related hemolysis is sometimes present. Another mechanism is immune mediated lysis of quinine sensitized erythrocytes as a result of previous repeated self-treatment with inadequate doses. Jaundice is common in adults with severe malaria; however, clinical signs of liver failure are not seen. Milder forms may be caused by hemolysis alone but very high bilirubin values (predominantly unconjugated type) indicate hepatic dysfunction.

Acute renal failure is often one component of multi-organ failure seen in patients with severe malaria. In patients successfully treated with antimalarials, renal failure can still develop. In these patients the prognosis is good provided that facilities for dialysis are available.

Pulmonary edema is often a fatal manifestation of severe malaria. It is usually not caused by fluid overload or cardiac failure, but rather is a result of increased pulmonary capillary permeability. The condition resembles adult respiratory distress syndrome (ARDS). The onset is sudden and may occur after several days of therapy parasites have disappeared and everyone thought the danger was over.

Hypoglycemia can be related to the malaria infection itself or be a consequence of increased insulin release due to quinine treatment. All patients, in particularly those with cerebral malaria, should have repeated determinations of blood glucose. Inspite of the very common finding of low platelet counts and laboratory signs of activated intravascular coagulation, a clinically evident bleeding tendency is rare in severe malaria.[4]

FALCIPARUM MALARIA IN THE INDIGENOUS POPULATION IN ENDEMIC AREAS

Approximately 90% of the clinical cases of malaria occur in Africa south of the Sahara. Each year, about 1 million children under the age of 5 years die from malaria in that part of the world. Malaria-related mortality constitutes nearly one-quarter of the total childhood mortality in Africa, with cerebral malaria and severe anemia as the major causes of death.[2]

Fever is the most common symptom in African children. The pattern is non-specific. Gastrointestinal complaints with diarrhea and vomiting are also quite common, but, unlike primary infectious gastroenteritis the symptoms do not dominate the clinical picture and diarrhea is usually mild. Older children might complain of headache or myalgia. A dry cough is sometimes also present. Due to the lack of

Table 15.1	Severe manifestations of *P. falciparum* malaria in adults[4]		
		Frequency	Prognostic value
Clinical manifestation	Jaundice	+++	+
	Prostration	+++	?
	Impaired consciousness	++	+
	Respiratory distress	+	+++
	Circulatory collapse	+	+++
	Pulmonary edema (X-ray)	+	+++
	Multiple convulsions	+	++
	Abnormal bleeding	+	++
	Hemoglobinuria	+	+
Laboratory findings	Renal impairment	+++	++
	Hypoglycemia	++	+++
	Acidosis	++	+++
	Hyperlactatemia	++	+++
	Hyperparasitemia	+	++
	Severe anemia	+	+
Modified from[4]			

specific diagnostic facilities and the fact that malaria is a common and severe disease, it is often recommended to regard any febrile episode as a possible malaria infection and give treatment accordingly for the worst case scenario, chloroquine resistant *P. Falciparum*.[2] This is also called presumptive treatment. Even when a good quality microscopic examination can be performed, it is difficult to establish if a low parasitemia is the cause of the illness or if the child merely is an asymptomatic carrier with fever due to another reason. In high parasitemias a symptomatic infection is more probable.

The symptoms of severe falciparum malaria varies according to the level of malaria transmission. In highly endemic areas, the dominating symptom is severe anemia in 1–3-year-old children. In areas with lower transmission, cerebral malaria in children between 3 and 7 years of age is a major manifestation of severe disease. Older children and adults still have low numbers of malaria parasites in the blood but they rarely cause any clinical symptoms. Pregnant women experience a partial loss of malaria immunity. This can result in maternal anemia and an increased frequency of low birth weight.[5]

CLINICAL PRESENTATION OF NON-FALCIPARUM MALARIA

Acute onset of fever is the initial symptom also in non-falciparum malaria. In patients with their first malaria attack caused by *P. vivax* or *P. ovale*, typically a regular fever pattern may develop with time. Relapse occurs in approximately half of the patients after the first initial infection if primaquine is not taken to eradicate dormant liver hypnozoites. When the patient has a relapse, regular fever might be present from onset of symptoms. The regular pattern with fever every second day is called tertian fever. The onset is usually abrupt. The body temperature rises to high levels within a few hours. During this increase in body temperature, the patient often experiences intense shivering and chills, together with headache and muscular discomfort. The temperature stays high for a few hours before it decreases. Profuse sweating starts and gradually the patient recovers. The total duration from the onset of paroxysm to recovery is 6–12 h. The next day, the patient feels quite well before a new paroxysm starts around 48 h after the last one. In typical cases the diagnosis may be confirmed just by looking at the pattern on the temperature chart. With time, as the infection continues, splenomegaly and anemia develop. Eventually after a few weeks without treatment the infection gradually resolves.

P. vivax and *P. ovale* can only invade young erythrocytes and therefore do not cause high parasitemias.[7] This is one major reason why they are less dangerous than *P. falciparum* which can invade erythrocytes of all ages with hyperparasitemia as a feared consequence. Pulmonary edema, rarely, may occur in vivax malaria. Other severe complications such as cerebral malaria are not seen in non-falciparum infections.

LABORATORY PARAMETERS IN NON-IMMUNES WITH ACUTE MALARIA

All patients with fever after a visit to malaria endemic areas must be examined for malaria parasites. They should also have a routine biochemical and hematological laboratory examination including hemoglobin value, white blood cell and platelet counts, liver function tests, and determination of serum creatinine and electrolytes if signs of dehydration are noticed. In patients with impaired general condition or other signs of severe malaria a much more thorough laboratory examination must be performed.

Anemia, contrary to what one would expect, is not a hallmark in uncomplicated malaria. In one study, 32% of adult men and 44% of adult women with malaria had a hemoglobin level below reference values. Most of the patients were non-immune. There was no difference between falciparum and non falciparum (mostly vivax) malaria in the frequency of acute anemia.[8]

The most common laboratory abnormality is thrombocytopenia (platelets <150 x 10^9/L) which can be found in up to 80% of the malaria patients irrespective of the etiology.[8] Commonly, a further decrease in platelet counts are noted during the first few days after initiation of therapy before they are normalized or even overcompensated with transient thrombocytosis as a result. A profound thrombocytopenia is more common in severely ill malaria patients in accordance with septicemia where a low platelet count also is a negative prognostic factor.

C-reactive protein (CRP) has successfully been used in differentiating between bacterial and viral infections. In malaria patients, CRP is almost always elevated and one study has reported higher values in patients with high parasitemia.[9] The diagnostic value of CRP is limited as other acute febrile illnesses also frequently have elevated levels. Very high levels (>200 mg/L) are rarely seen and should turn one's attention towards a severe bacterial infection (lobar pneumonia, pyelonephritis, or septicemia) as a more probable explanation.

Moderate leukopenia is a common finding in malaria patients whereas leukocytosis is rare. A slight increase of liver enzyme levels is often present. Due to hemolysis, both bilirubin and lactate dehydrogenase levels are frequently elevated.

Compared with a control group of patients with other febrile illnesses after visiting endemic areas, thrombocytopenia was much more common in those with malaria (80% versus 13%). The malaria patients also had lower white blood cell counts and marginally lower hemoglobin values.[8] In a patient with normal platelets and leukocytosis the malaria diagnosis is less probable but a specific parasitological examination must still be undertaken. The later is found in only 5% of patients.

IMPORTANT DIFFERENTIAL DIAGNOSIS

The complaints in patients with acute malaria are not specific for the disease and many other differential diagnoses can be considered. During colder months, the most common differential diagnosis is acute influenza. Patients with flu also have high-grade fever, but almost invariably have respiratory complaints in particular a dry cough often combined with retrosternal pain. Dengue fever is a frequent illness in many malaria endemic areas. Patients with dengue usually complain of severe myalgia (break bone fever) and headache. Unlike malaria, there is often an nonspecific skin eruption, sometimes in combination with conjunctivitis. The laboratory findings are similar, with thrombocytopenia and leucopenia occuring frequently.

Patients with pneumococcal pneumonia often have an acute onset with high-grade fever and do not always suffer from respiratory symptoms during the first days. Febrile upper urinary tract infections, particularly in elderly patients, are often not accompanied with urinary complaints or low back pain. Travelers to developing countries have an increased risk of septicemia due to salmonella typhi or other salmonella strains. Gastrointestinal symptoms are often lacking but the onset is usually more gradual than in malaria. In patients with severe malaria the most important differential diagnoses are bacterial meningitis and septicemia with multi organ involvement.

HOW TO AVOID 'DOCTORS DELAY'

It is very important to ask all patients where they have been and if they have taken any malaria prophylaxis. It is also important to determine the drug, regularity of intake and, whether the individual, is still on the medication. In all those who have visited a malaria endemic area who present with fever starting between 1 week after the first possible exposure and 3 months (or even later in rare cases) after the last possible exposure, a diagnosis of malaria has to be excluded.[1] This is valid even if the symptomatology or the actual epidemiological situation suggests another more probable explanation. Unfortunately, there are many reports of febrile patients who have initially got a probable flu diagnosis over the phone, or even after a medical examination, and later developed severe malaria. If treated early, even falciparum malaria is a readily manageable disease that does not always need hospitalization. To reduce the risk of unnecessary delay, health-care providers must be informed about when to suspect malaria and to where the patient can be referred. It is also recommended that travelers be urged to demand that malaria be excluded if they experience a febrile illness after their return and directly seek medical care at an institution where a good quality microscopic examination can be performed. As part of the pre-travel counseling, every traveler should get written information about the symptoms of malaria and what to do if the diagnosis is suspected.

INCUBATION PERIODS AND RECURRENCE

Falciparum malaria

Information about incubation times have been obtained from studies of malaria treatment in neurosyphilis and from inoculation of volunteers. In a summary of these old data, the average incubation period for P. falciparum from sporozoite inoculation by the female mosquito to appearance of erythrocytic parasite stages in the blood was 11 days. Fever was usually present 2 days later on day 13.[6] The incubation period for P. falciparum is between 1 week and 2 months, or even later in rare cases.[1] A total of 65–95% of non-immune travelers develop their symptoms of falciparum malaria within 1 month after leaving an endemic area.[4]

When P. falciparum parasites have developed low-grade resistance, partially effective chemoprophylaxis can prolong the incubation period. During ongoing prophylaxis the parasite multiplication is inhibited but parasites survive in low numbers. When drug levels decrease after discontinuation cf prophylaxis the parasites are able to multiply and cause clinical malaria.

In falciparum malaria, the cause of recurrent infection is also usually a low-grade resistance with failure to eradicate parasites (RI resistance). The time to recurrence depends on the initial parasite density, the degree of resistance, and the half life of the antimalarial drug used, it occurs most frequently within 2–4 weeks after initial treatment.

Non-falciparum malaria

In the case of P. vivax and P. ovale malaria, the mean incubation period after inoculation is 13–14 days. However, some strains of P. vivax can remain in the liver for 9–12 months or even longer (P. vivax hibernans) before release and subsequent multiplication in the blood will cause symptoms. With the exception of vivax malaria from North India these strains, previously present in temperate climates, are now nearly extinct.

After the first symptomatic infection, relapse of P. vivax and P. ovale caused by release of liver forms can occur on several occasions but eventually after 3–4 years the infection usually dies out. A relapse is noted in approximately half of those infected with P. vivax. The onset is usually within the first 2–3 months.[6] In P. malariae infection, relapse has been reported 30–40 years after the original infection.[10] The mechanism for this phenomenon is still not established.

MICROSCOPIC DIAGNOSIS

Microscopic examination remains the gold standard for detecting and identifying malaria parasites.[11] One advantage with microscopic examination is the high sensitivity. By carefully examining the thick film a parasite density as low as 5–10 parasites/microliter blood can be detected. Contrary to rapid diagnostic tests based on antigen detection, a microscopic examination enables the quantification of the parasitemia. This is necessary for classification of both disease severity and parasite response to treatment.

Microscopic examination begins with the collection of a finger prick or venepuncture blood sample. Both thick and thin blood films are prepared on standard microscopic slides. The thin film, but not the thick film, is fixed with methanol. The slides are then stained, usually with 3–4% Giemsa, rinsed and dried before examination. Preferably a ×100 oil-immersion lens is used together with a ×10 eye piece giving a total magnification of ×1000. The thick film is examined for detection of malaria parasites. Before a thick film is considered negative at least 100 fields should be examined. This takes an experienced microscopist 7–10 min. The sensitivity is 10–20 times higher examining the thick film: if it is negative, the thin can be discarded.

In the thin film the erythrocytes are preserved and the size, shape and appearance of the parasitized red blood cells can be studied. This is usually necessary for correct species determination. If the parasitemia is intermediate to high, the percentage of parasitized red blood cells should be counted. The total time required from finger prick to the result of the microscopic examination is in the order of not more than 30 minutes.

Non-immune patients with malaria can sometimes have symptoms before the number of parasites are above the level of detection by microscopic examination. If there is a clinical suspicion of malaria and the examination of a thick film is negative, a microscopic examination should be repeated twice more at 6- to 12-hour intervals to rule out malaria. Some laborations now screen for malaria with rapid antigen detection assays since microscopic examination requires a high degree of expertise, often lacking in many clinical laboratories.[1]

SOME ASPECTS ON CHEMOTHERAPY IN NON-IMMUNE PATIENTS

The treatment of malaria depends mainly on the malaria species involved the degree of parasitemia, the patient's ability to tolerate oral medication, and the drug susceptibility pattern. Chloroquine is still the drug of choice for P. ovale and P. malariae infections. In parts of the world (Irian Jaya, Myanmar, Papua New Guinea, and Vanuatu), P. vivax has developed resistance to chloroquine and primaquine. In these areas, mefloquine has become the treatment of choice.[1] In non-falciparum malaria, severe disease is rare and oral treatment is usually possible.

Treatment of P. falciparum malaria has become increasingly difficult because of the development of resistance to chloroquine and anti-folates such as sulfadoxine/pyrimethamine. In parts of South East Asia (Trat and Tak provinces in Thailand together with adjacent areas in Burma and Cambodia) reduced susceptibility to mefloquine and quinine is also present. If the patient has contracted falciparum malaria despite regular prophylaxis, this is more or less a proof of resistance and implies that another compound should be used for treatment. Major disadvantages and advantages of the antimalarials used in treatment of P. falciparum infections are seen in Table 15.2.

In the last decade, artemisinin derivatives have been made available outside China for treatment of multi-drug resistant falciparum malaria. These compounds all originate from the herb quinghao (Artemisia annua) that has been used in traditional Chinese medicine for over 2000 years to control fever. They are all rapidly hydrolyzed in the body to the active metabolite dihydroartemisinin. Development of resistance has not been a problem, but they have not yet been used on a large scale in highly endemic areas in Africa. The only major disad-

Table 15.2 Advantages and disadvantages for antimalarials commonly used for treatment of *P. falciparum* infections

Compound	Advantages	Disadvantages
Chloroquine	Parenteral preparations. Inexpensive	Resistance in all malarious areas except north of the Panama channel
Sulphadoxine/ Pyrimethamine	Single dose, usually well tolerated	Increasing resistance in most malarious areas Slow acting No parenteral preparation
Mefloquine	Effective in Africa and most other malarious areas*	No parenteral preparation Side-effects (not lethal)
Quinine	Effective in Africa and most other malarious areas* Parenteral preparations	Concentration dependent side-effects (cinchonism) Long treatment duration (7 days)
Atovaquone/ proguanil	Probably effective in most malarious areas Probably well tolerated	Limited experience No parenteral preparation Expensive
Artemisinine** derivatives	Effective in all areas Rapid action Parenteral preparations	Long treatment duration (7 days) if not combined
Artemether/ Lumefantrine	Probably effective in most malarious areas Probably well tolerated	Limited experience No parenteral preparation Expensive

*Not in areas of Thailand near the borders with Cambodia and Myanmar as well as in western Cambodia
**Artemether, arteether, artesunate and artemisinin

vantage is that due to their short half lives, they have to be administered for 5–7 days when used as a monotherapy. To reduce the duration of treatment and possibly the risk for development of resistance these compounds are often combined with mefloquine or more recently with lumefantrine (Riamet).

Because of lack of parenteral preparations many antimalarials can only be given orally and thus cannot be used in severely ill patients or in those with repeated vomiting. Of the several artemisinin derivatives that can be given parenterally, only artemether and artesunate are in extensive clinical use. For treatment of severely ill patients with falciparum malaria, either parenteral quinine/quindine or a parenteral artemisinin preparation is preferred, unless the disease was contracted in an area with reduced quinine susceptibility (Table 15.2). In a recent meta-analysis in patients with severe falciparum malaria, no difference was found between artemether and quinine in mortality, (14% versus 17%), coma recovery or development of neurological sequelae. It was concluded that artemether is at least as effective as quinine in terms of mortality and superior to quinine in terms of overall serious adverse events.[12]

MONITORING PARASITOLOGICAL RESPONSE AND CLASSIFICATION OF RESISTANCE

Drug resistance in malaria has been defined as 'the ability of parasite strains to survive and to multiply despite the administration of a drug given in equal doses or higher than those usually recommended'.[13] The response to chloroquine and other 4-aminoquinolines can be classified according to Table 15.3, using 28 days of follow-up.[14] This classification has also been widely used for other antimalarials with the modification of a longer follow up period in drugs with longer half lives (mefloquine and sulfadoxine/pyrimethamine).[15] The clinical consequence is that a patient with falciparum malaria and sensitive parasites is permanently cured. In the case of low grade resistance (RI) the patient improves and becomes afebrile but will experience a clinical relapse during follow-up. Intermediate resistance (RII) is characterized by temporary clinical improvement and in high-grade resistance (RIII) no clinical effect is seen.

In the present situation with varying resistance to most commonly used antimalarials and insufficient data about the performance of

Table 15.3 Classification of parasitological response[14]

Response	Definition
S, sensitive	Asexual parasites cleared by day 7 and no recrudescence during 28 days of follow-up
RI, resistance grade I	Asexual parasites cleared for at least two consecutive days, latest on day 7, followed by recrudescence during follow-up
RII, resistance grade II	Marked reduction of asexual parasites to less than 25% of the pre-treatment value within 48 h but parasites do not disappear
RIII, resistance grade III	No marked reduction in parasites during the initial 48 h and no subsequent disappearance of parasites

Modified from[14]

new drugs (Malarone, Riamet) in non-immune populations it is advised to always monitor the parasite response after treatment. The most crucial time for a repeat parasite count is 48 h after initiation of treatment. If the number of parasites at this time is more than 25% of the initial number high grade resistance should be suspected and treatment immediately switched to another drug. If the initial parasite count approaches 5%, repeat films should be carried out twice daily until the trend has been determined.

CONCLUSION

Acute malaria must be suspected in all travellers who complain of fever after a stay in an endemic area. Severe and complicated *P. falciparum* malaria can develop within a few days after onset of symptoms. Early diagnosis and prompt treatment are of utmost importance to reduce morbidity and mortality from this preventable infection.

REFERENCES

1. *International Travel and Health*. Geneva, Switzerland: WHO; 2003.
2. Expert committee on malaria. *Technical Report Series* No. 892. Geneva: WHO; 2000.
3. Genton B, D'Acremont V. Clinical features of malaria in returning travelers and migrants. In: Schlagenhauf-Lawlor P, ed. *Travellers' Malaria*. Hamilton: BC Decker; 2001:371–392.
4. WHO. Severe falciparum malaria. *Trans Roy Soc Trop Med Hyg* 2000; **94(suppl 1)**: 1–90.
5. Marsh K. Clinical features of Malaria. In: Wahlgren M, Perlman P, eds. *Malaria - Molecular and Clinical Aspects*. Amsterdam: Harwood; 1999:87–117.
6. White NJ. Malaria. In: Cook, GC and Zumla, A. *Manson's Tropical Diseases*. 21st edn. London: WB Saunders; 2003:1205–1295.
7. The biology of malaria parasites. *Technical Report Series* No. 743. Geneva: WHO; 1987.
8. Eriksson B, Hellgren U, Rombo L. Changes in erythrocyte sedimentation rate, C-reactive protein and hematological parameters in patients with acute malaria. *Scand J Infect Dis* 1989; **21**:435–441.
9. Naik P, Voller A. Serum C-reactive protein levels and falciparum malaria. *Trans Roy Soc Trop Med Hyg* 1984; **78**:812–813.
10. WHO. Chemotherapy of malaria. Revised 2nd edn. *Monograph Series* No. 27. Geneva, Switzerland: WHO; 1986.
11. Malaria Diagnosis. Report of a joint WHO/USAID informal consultation 25–27 October 1999. Geneva, Switzerland: WHO; 2000.
12. The Arthemether – Quinine Meta-analysis Study Group. A meta-analysis using individual patient data of trials comparing artemether with quinine in the treatment of severe falciparum malaria. *Trans Roy Soc Trop Med Hyg* 2001; **95**:637–650.
13. Resistance of malaria parasites to drugs. *Technical Report Series* No. 296. Geneva: WHO; 1965.
14. Chemotherapy of malaria and resistance to antimalarials. *Technical Report Series* No. 529. Geneva: WHO; 1973.
15. Wernsdorfer WH, Payne D. Drug sensitivity tests in malaria parasites. In: Wernsdorfer WH, Mcgregor I, eds. *Malaria. Principles and Practice of Malariology*. Edinburgh, UK: Churchill Livingstone; 1988:1765–1800.

CHAPTER 16 Epidemiology of Travelers' Diarrhea

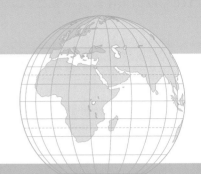

Steven J. Brewster and David N. Taylor

KEYPOINTS

- Travelers' diarrhea (TD) is the most common travel-related health problem

- A major leap in our understanding of travelers' diarrhea occurred when Enterotoxigenic *E. Coli* (ETEC) was discovered to be a cause of the illness

- Bacteria are the most common cause of TD and ETEC is the most common bacterial pathogen

- Host factors such as age, pre-existing immunity, and underlying medical conditions play a role in susceptibility to TD

- Avoidance of high risk foods, although advisable, is not enough to completely eliminate the risk of acquiring TD

INTRODUCTION

Over 50 million travelers from the industrialized nations visit tropical and developing areas of the world each year.[1] A quarter to more than half of these international travelers are afflicted with diarrhea during their trips abroad,[2–7] making this illness the most common travel-related health problem[8,9] (Table 16.1). Diarrheal illness has long been a problem for military forces as well, affecting more than 50% of troops in some initially deployed units to the Persian Gulf.[10] Travelers' diarrhea (TD) usually presents as an acute illness that lasts less than a week, until full recovery. About 10% of cases may last up to 2 weeks.[3] Travelers' diarrhea is, for the most part, a mild, self-limited illness; however, even a day of relative incapacitation can disrupt a carefully planned vacation. A 1999 study estimated the average cost for medication, treatment, and missed activities to be $116.50 per patient with diarrhea on a vacation in Jamaica.[11] Tourists are not the only ones who feel the economic burden of this illness. In addition to the morbidity and mortality of diarrhea, developing nations suffer losses in tourism revenue. Diarrhea-wary travelers often remove high-risk countries from their itinerary.[12] TD is caused by a myriad of food and water-borne organisms that include bacteria, viruses and parasites. Clarifying the epidemiology and etiology of traveler's diarrhea has potential for reducing risk in the traveler and lowering the endemicity of disease in developing nations.

HISTORY

For as long as there have been travelers, there has been travelers' diarrhea. Diarrhea, dysentery and enteric fever, the triad of gastroin-

testinal infectious diseases, have determined the outcome of wars, have shortened the lives of poets and artists seeking inspiration on foreign shores, and have been the subject of literature. In the twenty-first century, travel no longer occurs on a grand scale, but on a global scale. Whether traveling for business or pleasure, travel brings change in environment, time zone, diet, and inevitably change in exposure to microbial pathogens. Studies of Peace Corps volunteers have shown altered bowel flora within days after flying into, e.g., Thailand.[13] On arrival these westerners were colonized with *E. coli* that were susceptible to antibiotics. After a few days these *E. coli* were gradually replaced with resistant ones indigenous to Thailand. We are constantly ingesting *E. coli* and, for the most part, these organisms harmlessly colonize the gut.

Dr. Ben Kean was one of the first researchers to conclude that 'tourista' or travelers' diarrhea was 'possibly related to shifts in the bacterial population or introduction of 'foreign' bacterial strains into the intestinal tract'.[14] He defined travelers' diarrhea as a clinical syndrome. His vivid description of the sudden onset of profuse watery diarrhea remains one of the classic descriptions of an illness. For most of his career the exact cause of travelers' diarrhea eluded him, but he ruled out all of the known causes and correctly surmised that the primary cause was bacterial because pre-exposure antibiotic use prevented many of the illnesses. In 1970 Rowe *et al.* isolated a new serotype of *E. coli*, O148: H28, from a majority of soldiers with diarrhea in Aden, Yemen. A technician working with their organism in a London lab later developed a severe attack of diarrhea, from which, subsequently, *E. coli* O148: H28 was recovered in pure culture.[15] SL Gorbach, RB Sack and others first associated *E. coli* with an enterotoxin in patients with acute undifferentiated diarrhea in the Indian subcontinent where it was found to be the most common cause of non-vibrio cholera (profuse watery diarrhea).[16,17] Dupont *et al.* were able to isolate this enterotoxigenic *E. coli* (ETEC) from US soldiers who became ill in Vietnam.[18] Kean, in collaboration with Gorbach, repeated the studies in Mexico and found ETEC was the major cause of travelers' diarrhea in this country.[19] Studies performed since this time have confirmed that ETEC remains the single most important diarrheal pathogen world-wide. Clinicians should be aware in today's global economy that exposure to microorganisms responsible for travelers' diarrhea can occur when food from a developing country is imported into Western nations.[20,21] Moreover, passengers aboard airlines and cruise ships who have never been to a developing nation may unknowingly be exposed to food prepared in a high-risk country.[22,23]

CLINICAL CHARACTERISTICS

A case of travelers' diarrhea is described as the sudden onset of loose, watery stools associated with abdominal pain, fever, or tenesmus. Rigid criteria for frequency, duration and severity are academic. The

Table 16.1 Incidence of various health problems among European travelers during a short stay in various climatic zones[8]

New or worsened disease	Incidence of health problem during travel (%)		
	Tropics (n = 10 555)	USA/Canada (n = 1300)	Significance, USA and Canada used as control group
Diarrhea	33.9	5.8	P<0.001
Respiratory infections	13.3	8.5	P<0.001
Insomnia	10.6	7.0	P<0.001
Headache	7.8	7.6	Not significant
Dermatosis	5.7	3.4	P<0.001
Fever of any origin	3.8	1.2	P<0.001
Cardiovascular disease	1.6	1.2	Not significant
Accidents	0.3	0.1	Not significant

sense of urgency can be profound and there may be a few prodromal symptoms such as stomach gurgling or queasiness. Nausea and vomiting are also common in the first few hours adding to the discomfort and water loss. Often, the stool will begin as a mixture of stool and water and later become entirely watery. Dehydration in adults is rarely life threatening but mild dehydration leads to dry lips and mucous membranes. Malaise or a tired washed out feeling is also common and may be the result of dehydration.

Dependent upon the type and location of travel, the onset of diarrhea usually occurs within the first 2 weeks of travel and symptoms usually resolve within 3–4 days.[4,24] Approximately one-quarter of travelers with diarrhea will have to alter their activities, however the majority of these will be incapacitated for less than 24 h. A survey among soldiers over a 4-month period during Operation Desert Shield found that 20% reported they were temporarily unable to perform their duties because of diarrheal symptoms.[10]

Like most clinical syndromes, there is a spectrum of illness both in severity and type of clinical symptoms. Clinical features and laboratory parameters have proven to be either too insensitive or too nonspecific to be of use in differentiating between pathologic organisms.[25,26] In general, ETEC has tended to cause a milder form of diarrhea than other bacterial agents such as *Campylobacter*.[24] Those who have a mild clinical presentation usually recover more quickly, regardless of the etiology. Health-care providers are often challenged to offer appropriate counseling to their patients before they travel. Diarrhea occurs in travelers when two conditions are met. The traveler must be exposed to the infectious agent and the traveler must be susceptible to it. Travelers coming from developed countries have not been exposed to many of the common infectious agents in the tropics or areas where inadequate sanitation ensures that the infectious agent reaches a susceptible host. Individuals or groups stepping outside of their normal sanitary environment develop diarrhea to varying degrees while traveling, dependent upon their unique combination of etiologic agent, host and environmental factors. These three factors serve as categories under which we may examine the determinants and distribution of diarrheal illness. With such knowledge, practitioners can more readily prepare their patients for travel.

ETIOLOGY

Isolation rates for pathologic agents among travelers' diarrhea studies have roughly varied from 30–60%.[11,27–31] In 1974, Merson *et al.* iden-

tified a pathogen in 63% of travelers who developed TD while traveling in Mexico.[3] Twenty years later, Jiang *et al.* conducted a longitudinal study in travelers to Guadalajara, Mexico that isolated an organism in only 44% of diarrheal cases.[31] Despite advances in laboratory methods and improvements in the handling of stool specimens we have not significantly improved upon these isolation rates. There are a number of variables that might explain why an organism is not isolated from the stool or why rates vary for specific agents. Antibiotics and bismuth compounds may have been used prior to stool collection; the illness may have waned to the point where few numbers of organisms were shed; the stool specimen may have been inadequate to detect the organism; moreover, the appropriate diagnostic tool may not have even been used to identify the pathogen. Further complicating the search for infectious etiology, asymptomatic travelers often shed pathogenic organisms in their stool and about 15% of ill travelers have multiple enteric pathogens.[29] Nonetheless, one consistency remains throughout these studies: Enterotoxigenic *Escherichia coli* (ETEC) is the most commonly isolated pathogen (see Table 16.2). Future studies are likely to uncover new etiologic agents. The fact that travelers usually respond to antibiotics, even if a bac-terial pathogen is not isolated, suggests that most undiagnosed cases of travelers' diarrhea are bacterial in origin.

Table 16.2 Distribution of enteropathogens among patients with TD in Guadalajara, Mexico, 1992–1997 (modified)[31a]

Pathogen	Isolates (%)					
	1992	1993	1994	1996	1997	Total
n	382	163	140	157	86	928
ETEC[a]	22.2	18.4	17.9	19.1	27.9	19.9
Shigella	15.4	19.0	9.0	3.2	10.0	12.6
Salmonella	7.3	4.9	1.4	3.8	4.6	5.2
Campylobacter	1.0	1.8	5.0	1.9	0	1.8
Giardia	0.8	0	0.7	1.3	0	0.6
Undetected	50	56	65	69	50	56

[a]ETEC, enterotoxigenic *Escherichia coli*.

BACTERIA

Enterotoxigenic *Escherichia coli* (ETEC)

Bacteria are the most common causes of travelers' diarrhea and ETEC is the most common bacterial cause. Salmonella, Shigella and Campylobacter make up the majority of remaining bacterial pathogens (Table 16.3). All of these are important causes of diarrheal disease in the United States and all are commonly acquired domestically, except ETEC. There is no routine method available to microbiology laboratories for the diagnosis of ETEC. In order to identify an *E. coli* as enterotoxigenic, one must identify the toxin as it is released from bacterial culture or one must identify the genes for the heat-labile (LT) or heat-stable (ST) toxin produced by strains of ETEC. Neither test is commercially available.

A high number of ETEC organisms are necessary to induce diarrhea.[18] In contrast to an infectious dose of less than 200 cells for *Shigella*, Dupont et al. demonstrated that 10^6 organisms are required for ETEC to cause diarrhea. These high inoculums suggest that a marked breakdown in sanitation, as often happens in developing nations, must occur in order for such high bacterial loads to be ingested. An occasional outbreak of ETEC has occurred in the USA. In 1975, a large water-borne outbreak presented at Crater Lake National Park, when raw sewage entered park water, affecting more than 2000 people.[32] Dupont's study also showed that ETEC pathogenic for animals did not cause disease in humans.[18] This, coupled with ETEC's inability to easily colonize livestock further support the suspicion that humans are the main reservoir for ETEC.

In addition to ETEC, there are at least four other groups of *E. coli* that distinctly cause diarrheal illness.[33,34] The role of these groups in travelers' diarrhea is less clear, though future research may provide clarification. Enteroinvasive *E. coli* (EIEC) is closely related to *Shigella sp.* and causes a similar clinical picture of dysentery but is not a significant cause of TD. Enterohemorrhagic *E. coli* (EHEC) causes hemorrhagic colitis and hemolytic uremic syndrome via shiga-like toxin (SLT). Although EHEC is a significant cause of illness in the USA, Europe, and Japan, it has rarely been acquired in tropical destinations. This is significant because antibiotics are contraindicated for EHEC

infections but are commonly used to treat travelers' diarrhea.[35] Enteropathogenic *E. coli* (EPEC) is an important cause of infant diarrhea through an 'attaching and effacing' adherence[36] though does not appear affect travelers to a significant degree. Finally, there is entero-aggregative *E. coli* (EAEC), a recently recognized pathogen that is likely to be a major etiologic agent in travelers' diarrhea. At present, there is no clear understanding of the pathogenesis of diarrhea caused by EAEC. However, in a recent study, EAEC was isolated in 26% of cases of travelers' diarrhea and was second only to ETEC as the most common enteropathogen.[37] It is interesting that this organism explained 28% of cases with unknown etiology, illustrating the importance of bacteria as prominent etiologies of travelers' diarrhea and the need for further study in this area.

Campylobacter spp.

While *Campylobacter* infections are common in the USA and other developed nations, the incidence of disease is many fold higher in developing nations.[38] In such countries, constant, heavy exposure eventually induces an immunity that becomes apparent after the first year of life. Travelers have a high risk of acquiring *Campylobacter* that may reach 10% of total cases on a 2-week trip. Resistance to fluoroquinolones is >70% in Spain and Thailand.[28,39,40] Erythromycin and the newer macrolides have once again become the drugs of choice for treating TD in these regions.[40]

Salmonella spp.

An average of 240 cases of Salmonella serotype Typhi occur in the USA each year. Over 70% of these cases of typhoid fever had traveled internationally before their illness.[41] Fortunately, *S. typhi* is still rare, with an overall rate of 2.2 per 1 million American travelers, due in part to the availability of an effective vaccine. The risk for acquiring *S. typhi* is highest on the Indian subcontinent, where the incidence is 812 per million travelers. Non-typhi *salmonella* infections have been increasingly common in the USA and other developed countries but are a relatively infrequent cause of TD in developing countries.[38]

Table 16.3 Enteropathogens identified among westerners presenting with diarrhea to Western clinics in Nepal 1986–1987[29]

Enteropathogen	CIWEC[a] Clinic, (*n* = 191)	Peace Corps Medical Clinic (*n* = 137)	Total (*n* = 328)
ETEC	27	20	24
Shigella	16	10	14
Campylobacter	14	4	9
Salmonella	3	3	3
Enteroinvasive *E. coli*	3	1	2
Enteroadherent *E. coli*	1	0	1
Any bacterial pathogen	55	34	47
Rotavirus	8	6	8
Entamoeba histolytica	6	5	5
Giardia lamblia	14	9	12
Cryptosporidium	5	4	5

[a]CIWEC, Canadian International Water and Energy Consultants.

Shigella spp.

Shigella becomes more prevalent as sanitary conditions decline. It has been a problem for the US military during deployments in Saudi Arabia and Somalia.[10,42] As the length of deployment increases *Shigella* holds increasing importance as a cause of diarrhea and dysentery. The low infectious dose increases the incidence of person-to-person transmission and fly-borne disease. Because *Shigella* is a fastidious organism, the true incidence of this organism may be underestimated in conditions where prompt processing of fresh fecal material is not always possible.[43]

Vibrio spp.

Vibrio parahaemolyticus and non-O1 *Vibrio cholerae* have been associated with seafood and have been a problem in hotels that offer seafood buffets.[44] *Vibrio cholerae* O1 has in general been a rare cause of TD, but reports from Americans working in Lima, Peru and Japanese returning from Bali, Indonesia suggest that westerners can get cholera in endemic areas.[45] The symptoms are the same as other causes of TD and the pathogens cannot be differentiated without culture.

VIRUSES

Viruses such as adenovirus, astrovirus, rotavirus, and calicivirus have been documented as etiologic agents for TD.[10,11,26,29] Most studies have not specifically looked for viral causes of TD. In those that have, many have used electron microscopy or enzyme immunoassay (EIA), which are insensitive, labor intensive and operator dependent.[46] Newer studies are incorporating polymerase chain reaction (PCR) and reverse-transcriptase PCR to look for viruses and the specific strains responsible for TD.[47–49] The calicivirus family, which includes Noroviruses Norwalk virus and Norwalk-like viruses, are increasingly recognized as etiologic agents for foodborne, water-borne and person-to-person diarrheal outbreaks that present with nausea, vomiting and diarrhea. Outbreaks have occurred aboard cruise ships and in hotels.[23,50–53] These viruses are transmitted by the fecal-oral and aerosol route and are believed to be the most common cause of non-bacterial TD. During the Gulf War, Norwalk virus was a significant cause of diarrhea during the winter months. Once this virus was introduced, person-to-person transmission was believed to have been an important mode of spread, causing substantial morbidity among deployed service members.[54]

PARASITES

The most common agents for protracted diarrhea in returning travelers are parasitic infections. The likelihood of parasitic etiology rises commensurately with the duration of diarrheal symptoms. Among travelers in Nepal with diarrhea for more than 14 days, 27% were diagnosed with Giardia in contrast to only 10% who had diarrhea for less than 14 days.[29] The differential for parasitic diarrhea is most likely to include *Giardia lamblia*, *Entamoeba histolytica*, *Cryptosporidium parvum*, and *Cyclospora cayetanensis*. *Microsporidia* and *Dientamoeba fragilis* are rare causes of persistent low-grade gastrointestinal symptoms.[55–58] While the risk factors for intestinal parasites are not well defined, it appears that duration of stay is a major factor in acquiring a parasitic pathogen[59] and that this risk is associated with a traveler's continual exposure to human fecal material in drinking water and food.[60]

Giardia lamblia

The most common protozoal infection in returning travelers is *Giardia lamblia*.[61,62] This organism causes a clinical picture that ranges from the asymptomatic to an acute self-limited illness. If untreated, chronic, intermittent diarrhea characterized by flatulence, fatigue and weight loss can persist for months.[63,64] Chlorination is ineffective in preventing water-borne infection. Reliance upon this method of water treatment at a Greek resort hotel resulted in a large Giardia outbreak[65] among UK tourists in 1997. Filtration or boiling of drinking water will help to prevent infections in such cases, though other possible water-borne sources include recreational water sources. Diagnosis is usually made by stool examination, but multiple careful exams may be necessary to demonstrate the organism. Stool antigen test kits for *G. lamblia* are available, but have not replaced stool examination.[66] A duodenal string test has fallen out of favor in recent years.[67]

Entamoeba spp.

In recent years, some of the issues in diagnosing and treating *Entamoeba histolytica* infections have been clarified. It is now clear that there are two distinct, but morphologically identical strains of amoebae.[68] *E. histololytica* is a pathogen, whose symptoms can range from a mild chronic infection to severe and even fatal colitis. *E. dispar* is a non-pathogen that often presents in patients who are 'asymptomatic cyst passers'.[69] The organisms cannot be distinguished microscopically, but non-microscopic tests are being developed.

Cyclospora

Cyclospora cayetanensis, along with *Isospora belli*, is a coccidian in the Eimeria family of protozoa. Seasonal *Cyclospora* outbreaks have caused up to a third of diarrheal illness in Nepal during the rainy summer months.[60,70] Imported Guatemalan raspberries have carried *Cyclospora* into the USA, causing outbreaks in summer months.[20] Fatigue and anorexia are extremely prominent, and help distinguish *Cyclospora* infection from other pathogens. Untreated, the illness lasts for an average of 6 weeks.

Isospora belli

Isospora belli is endemic in tropical and subtropical countries. Healthy travelers to the Caribbean, India and Africa have returned to the USA with *Isospora* infection. After traveling extensively in West Africa, an American developed chronic diarrhea and cramping abdominal pain.[71] Multiple stool examinations over a 5-week period finally revealed *Isospora belli* in this patient.

Cryptosporidium parvum

Scattered reports of cases in immunocompetent persons led to this organism's classification as a pathogen about 10 years ago. Its resistance to chlorine has led to numerous water-borne outbreaks in US cities, most notably a huge outbreak in Milwaukee, Wisconsin in 1993.[72] In 34 Finnish students who made a weekend trip to Leningrad, seven returned with symptomatic *Cryptosporidium*, four with *Giardia*, and two with both.[73] In contrast to a mean incubation period of 16 days for *Giardia*, *Cryptosporidium* had a mean incubation of 6 days, and symptoms that lasted 9–23 days. Immunocompromised HIV-infected travelers are particularly susceptible to Cryptosporidiosis and should be cautious while traveling abroad.[63]

Blastocystis hominis

There has long been debate whether this organism causes diarrhea, though the consensus appears to be that it is not a pathogen. A careful case-control study in Katmandu in 1995 showed that *B. hominis* was found equally often in the stools of diarrhea patients as in control patients with no diarrheal symptoms.[74] It is sensible to continue to look for a recognized pathogen in symptomatic returned travelers who have *B. hominis* in the stool.

HOST FACTORS

People from Europe, the USA, Australia and Japan comprise the majority of individuals who travel from a developed to a less developed country. They consist of vacationers, business employees, the military and aid workers. From the developing world, refugees and other displaced persons make up another important at risk group. Groups and individuals have different demographic and behavioral characteristics that play a role in determining their risk of developing diarrhea.

Age/gender

Numerous studies have shown that increasing age is significantly protective.[4,7,8,14,27,75] This association persisted even after controlling for preference of adventurous travel, duration of stay and travel experience. One study found each additional year of age decreased the incidence of diarrhea by 1%.[4] Younger travelers may be at increased risk for a number of reasons. They eat a larger amount of food and therefore pathogen, and they tend to be less selective in the source and type of their food. Additionally, their immune responses to pathogens may differ from that of older travelers. Gender has consistently been shown not to be a factor in developing diarrhea.[11,14,24]

Travelers' diarrhea in children

Travelers' diarrhea in children is a relatively neglected area, but it is clear that more adults are now traveling with children and infants. Pitzinger conducted a retrospective study in Zurich to assess the incidence of diarrhea in children. She found that adolescents had a 38% rate of TD, which was as high as in young adults 20–29 years old. Rates declined to 20% in children 7–14 years old and were lowest (8%) in children 3–6 years old. Most notable, children 0–2 years old had the highest diarrhea rates of 40%[76] (Fig. 16.1). In small children,

the clinical course tended to be severe and prolonged. In these children, 40% of parents reported that they had consistently practiced dietary preventive measures.

Infants still breast-feeding may be an exception. Breast-feeding is the safest nourishment in the absence of other diseases and has saved the lives of millions of children in less developed countries. Infant formula and baby food is available in most urban areas and can be prepared safely. Families moving to a developing country should quickly find a place to live that has a kitchen. The best way to decrease the risk of diarrhea is to have control of how the food is prepared. It is difficult to provide safe foods when trekking with infants. Parents may be able to carry toddlers while trekking but they must remember that the risk of diarrhea is high. Children's hands will become contaminated and the dose of organisms necessary to cause disease may be significantly lower in children. Parents who must travel with children merit detailed education regarding dietary prevention, self-treatment, and oral rehydration.

There are few direct data comparing etiology of TD among children and adults. There is some data describing causes of diarrhea among children returning to developing countries. Available data suggest that the etiology in traveling children is very similar to that in traveling adults. This is understandable since causes of diarrhea in children living in lesser-developed countries are the same as those that afflict traveling adults from developed countries.

Country of origin

A traveler's country of origin appears to be a risk factor for diarrheal illness. While traveling in less developed regions, residents from more developed countries have the highest attack rates,[8] whereas travelers from lesser developing nations have lower or similar rates than that found in the host population.[77] When traveling to developing nations, persons residing in northern countries show significantly higher TD attack rates than those from more southern countries.[11,78] These observations support the observation that attack rates correlate directly with socioeconomic status, as was noted when a diverse group of Panamanians visited Mexico.[79]

Immunity

Protective immunity develops after natural infection with ETEC. The role of specific antigens, such as colonization factors or toxins, or of specific components of the immune system, such as gut IgA or serum IgG in protective immunity is not well defined. Humans who have

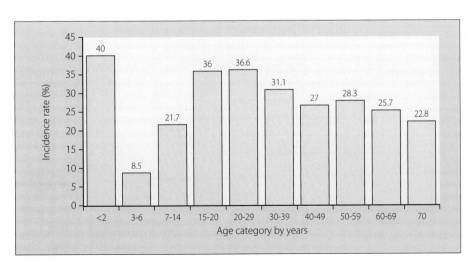

Figure 16.1 Age specific incidence rates of diarrhea among travelers to the tropics.[76]

recovered from natural infection are protected from challenge with the homologous strain,[18,80,81] so immunity clearly occurs. The decreasing rate of infection associated with increasing age and length of stay in a host nation support these findings.[82,83] However, the duration of protection stemming from induced immunity is not known. Little protective benefit is derived from having previously visited a specific high-risk country or having traveled in another developing nation.[8,84] Several case series studies have demonstrated that the risk for diarrheal illness in developing nations remains for years after arrival, though there is a demonstrable decrease over time[27,29,82,83] (Fig. 16.2). In particularly high endemic environments, this risk may be more persistent. A prospective study in Nepal demonstrated no diminution in diarrhea risk within the first year of residence and a high monthly incidence that persisted up to 2 years after arrival.[60]

Underlying medical conditions

Low gastric acidity is thought to be a risk factor for TD.[18] Individuals who are post-gastrectomy and those using antacids such as proton pump inhibitors are thought to be at increased risk. Other chronic gastrointestinal problems may worsen during travel and contribute to increased diarrheal symptoms.[84] Underlying medical conditions do not otherwise appear to affect the risk of acquiring diarrhea.[4] The exception to this may be in immunocompromised travelers. Patients with AIDS are prone to infection from a myriad of travel-related organisms, ranging from parasites such as *Cryptosproridium*, *Microsporidium* and *Isosopora belli* to bacteria such as *Salmonella* and *Campylobacter*.[85]

ENVIRONMENTAL FACTORS

While traveling in developing nations, environmental risks for TD are omnipresent and often unavoidable. For example, various foods and drinks in lesser-developed countries have been associated with diarrheal illness (Table 16.4). Data also indicates that eating at smaller restaurants or street vendors might put a person at increased risk for TD.[83,86] This suggests that travelers would benefit from avoiding certain foods and eating venues. In Somalia, the US military limited its service members to prepackaged meals from the USA and to water from strictly monitored sources. Vectors for pathogens such as flies

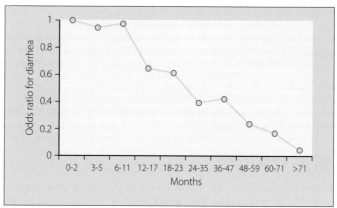

Figure 16.2 Decrease in OR of diarrhea (relative to baseline) for increasing duration of time living in Nepal.[27]

were aggressively controlled, and field sanitation facilities were constructed. These tremendous efforts led to a low diarrheal incidence of 4.5% over an 8-week period in a highly endemic region.[42] Most travelers do not find themselves in a position to benefit from such prevention measures, nor would they necessarily want to. However, well-advised travelers may be able to modify their behavior to the extent that risk is significantly reduced

Pre-travel advice

Typically, travelers are urged to follow precautionary recommendations such as 'boil it, cook it, peel it, or forget it'. The benefits of following this sensible advice have been difficult to demonstrate.[3,7,11,78] In a study from 1991, Hill personally provided 784 travelers with detailed counseling and written instructions on the prevention of travelers' diarrhea and the use of empiric therapy according to accepted guidelines. Despite this aggressive education, 34% of the travelers reported significant clinical diarrhea during their trip and nearly a quarter of these cases experienced fever and vomiting. Of these, 35% had to alter their travel plans.[4] One prospective study has illustrated some benefit to pre-travel dietary advice.[87] The degree to which patients adhere to this advice and whether it is

Table 16.4	Case-control study of risk factors for diarrheal disease in Nepal[27]			
	Resident cases	Resident controls	Odds ratio	P
n	69	87		
Age <30	41	15	3.9	<0.001
Median time in country (months)	9 (4.5–19.5)	23 (8–67)		<0.001
Drank untreated water	9	9	1.5	ns
Unpeeled fresh fruit	39	37	1.1	ns
Ate at least once in restaurant in 1 week	96	83	4.5	<0.01
Median number of meals at restaurants in week	4 (2–7)	2 (1–5)		=0.03
Type of food eaten in Restaurant				
Ate reheated food	22	7	3.8	<0.007
Blended fruit drinks	32	9	4.7	<0.001
Fruit salad	34	32	1.1	ns
Raw vegetables	38	33	1.2	ns
Ice	9	11	0.8	ns

All numbers expressed as percent except for *n*, age and time in country. ns, not significant.

effective are still matters of debate. It does appear that pre-travel counseling reduces the need for medical assistance while abroad and reduces physician workload in terms of post-travel health visits with returning travelers by 50%.[88]

Travel packages and meals

Travelers who chose to travel under an 'all-inclusive package' or with partial board are at higher risk for developing TD than those who chose their own meals.[11,89] A protective effect is seen when one is able to cook their own meals, or eat at the homes of friends or family.[27,86,90] Food appears to be the primary mode of transmission for *E. coli*, *Shigella* and *Salmonella* and caliciviruses, while water seems to be the primary vehicle through which rotavirus is transmitted.[91,92] Tjoa *et al.* conducted a study in Mexico in 1975 that recovered *E. coli* from food prepared by 39% of restaurants, 55% of street vendors and 40% of small grocery stores. The highest counts of *E. coli* were found in dairy products. The potential perils in dining are further illustrated in the fact that four *Shigella* carriers were found among kitchen personnel in this study.[86]

In a case-control among expatriate residents of Katmandu in 1992–1993, foods that required reheating and blended drinks held the highest risk of diarrhea.[27] There is conflicting data as to the benefits of bottled water or the risks associated with eating raw vegetables, salads, fresh fruit or ice served in restaurants.[3,27,78] The present data support cooking one's own meals whenever possible, and choosing reputable, safe restaurants able to serve hot, steaming meals if one eats out. Bottled, carbonated beverages should be chosen over juices and fountain drinks. One should also avoid eating salads or other cold dishes that have a higher risk of containing enteric pathogens.

Cruise ships have the task of preparing food for large numbers of travelers, but have limited space for food storage and preparation. Buffet lines are a common means of serving meals aboard ships and often food is left at room temperature for hours before serving, allowing time for pathogen propagation. ETEC, *Salmonella*, and caliciviruses are among those agents found to be causes of food-borne outbreaks aboard ships. As previously noted, the caliciviruses have increasingly been implicated in the literature. Suspect transmission vehicles include shellfish, ice, salads, cake icing and even bottled water. Time reveals the insidious means by which travelers acquire diarrhea. Ill food-handlers and inappropriate handling, hygiene and storage have been at the root of viral outbreaks. Many of these cases can be averted aboard ships if travelers choose a line that cooks food thoroughly, uses pasteurized eggs, and avoids onshore caterers for off-ship excursions.[23]

Person-to-person transmission has come to light as a probable means of acquiring illness as well. In a study of diarrhea aboard a cruise ship in which a calicivirus was implicated, passengers who had shared toilet facilities were twice as likely to acquire gastroenteritis than those who had a private bathroom.[93] Kean found an association between developing diarrhea and having a roommate with similar symptoms.[14] Once an outbreak has begun, it is difficult to interrupt the cycle of transmission. Classic preventive measures such as hand washing, chlorinated water, and flush toilets are less than effective in preventing calicivirus illness in such cases.[46] Among soldiers deployed to Operation Desert Storm, Norwalk virus was a significant cause of diarrheal illness. In this study, canteen use was strongly associated with developing diarrhea. The military typically uses chlorine to treat water, and the CDC has recommended high-level chlorination (10 ppm or 10 mg/L for 30 min or more) as a protective measure, although acknowledges that even this method may be inadequate.[94]

Lodging

Guests in luxury four or five star hotels often assume that they are protected from developing TD, if eating their meals in the hotel restaurant or from the room service menu. Steffen found that four-star hotels did not offer protection from TD over lesser-rated establishments.[7,84] Travelers should not assume guaranteed protection based on the rating of any establishment. Nonetheless, those undertaking adventurous travel (backpacking, camping, or trekking through rural areas) should be especially cautious, as their risk is higher than that of travelers staying in hotels.[76,84]

Risk by geographic region

There are regional differences in the risk and etiology of diarrhea. Black reviewed 34 studies among travelers to Latin America, Asia and Africa. He found attack rates (median values) for travelers in these three regions to be remarkably similar: Latin America, 53% (range 21–100%); Asia 54% (range 21–57%); and Africa, 54% (range, 36–62%).[12] Dupont has distinguished three grades of risk (high, moderate and low) for travelers' diarrhea.[91] He classifies the above three regions as 'high risk'. Low risk countries include the USA Canada, north and central Europe, Australia, and New Zealand. In these countries the risk does not usually rise above 8%.[8,84] Intermediate risk make up the remaining regions to include the Caribbean (except Haiti), and the major resorts in Pacific and northern Mediterranean. Presumably, countries of the former Soviet Union would be included in this category, though data is lacking in this region. See Figure 16.3.

If we consider specific etiologies within some of these regions, ETEC is the predominant cause of diarrheal illness in Latin America, Africa, and South Asia,[6,97] but appears to be less common in SE Asia.[98] From a series of studies in Latin America and Africa, Black concluded that these two regions hold remarkable similarity in the prevalence of differing etiologic agents.[97] In order of lessening prevalence after ETEC, he noted that rotavirus, Norwalk virus, *Shigella*, *Salmonella*, *G. lambia* and *E. histolytica* were identified most frequently. *Campylobacter* has been noted to be the predominant pathogen among US troops on military exercises in Thailand.[99] It was also the most common pathogen in Morocco during the winter.[100] See Table 16.5.

Within more temperate regions there may be seasonal variation of diarrheal etiology. In Nepal, for example, the greatest number of diarrheal cases occurs during the hot months just before and during monsoon season when TD rates typically double. This is the time of year when the fly population is greatest and when indigenous food-borne cases of diarrhea peak among Nepalese.[27] Seasonality is further demonstrated by *Cyclospora* infection rates in Nepal, which consistently peak during the monsoon season and drop to negligible levels throughout the rest of the year, suggesting a water-borne transmission.[60,70] Rotavirus and Norwalk virus infections have typically displayed higher infection rates during the cooler months.[29,108] Other large retrospective studies have failed to demonstrate a seasonal influence on the overall incidence of diarrhea.[7]

CONSEQUENCES OF TRAVELERS' DIARRHEA

Chronic diarrhea has been estimated to affect 1% of all travelers.[100] Steffan's study among Swiss travelers in the 1980s showed that 11% of travelers who developed acute diarrhea, went on to experience chronic diarrhea.[7] Twenty of the 73 cases of chronic diarrhea were associated with protozoa such as amoeba or *Giardia*; the rest were undiagnosed. The highest rate of chronic diarrhea was noted after travel in West Africa and East Asia. One-third of the patients became symptomatic only after returning home some after more than a month long delay.

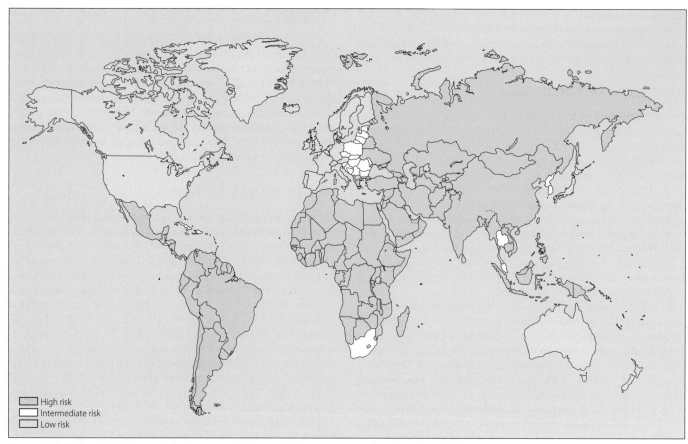

Figure 16.3 Estimated incidence of diarrhea over a 14 day period for western travelers by region visited.

Table 16.5	(%) Isolation rates of suspected etiologic pathogens by travel destination in Westerners with travelers' diarrhea							
Organism	**Jamaica**[95,96]	**Morocco**	**India**[95]	**Egypt**[97,98,99]	**Thailand**[100,101]	**Mexico**[102]	**Nepal**	**Kenya**
Bacterial Etiology								
ETEC	12–30	13	24–39	27–57	0–37	20–40	20–28	33–35
Other Ecoli spp. (EIEC, EHEC, EPEC EAEC)	5–19			42	13	4–33	4–24	
Campylobacter spp.	6	10–29	2–11	0–3	2–17	2	4–28	5
Salmonella spp.	4–8	10	6–13	2–3	8–33	3–10	3	3
Shigella spp.	0.3–4	<1	10–17	0–9	7–13	6–15	10–23	9
Aeromonas spp.	0	6	3	<1	10–31	<1	3	2
Vibrio spp.	0–0.3		1–5	0–2	1–3	0–2	0	3
Viral Etiology								
Astrovirus							2	6
Rotavirus	9	3	5		3–4	10	6–11	
Calicivirus (Norwalk)					7			
Adenovirus	4		2					3
Parasitic Etiology								
Giardia lamblia	0.6		2			1–3	0–16	0
Entamoeba spp.	0.6		5	0–11		<1	3–6	0
Cyclospora							11	
Cryptosporidum parvum	0.8		2	0–5		1–3	4	0
No Pathogen Identified	42–68	40	36–45	36–51	10–53	22–37	17	47

Chronic diarrhea ranked second of all travel related illness in days of inability to work.

Antibiotic-associated diarrhea may affect 2–5% of those treated with fluoroquinolones or macrolides.[101] This clinical diagnosis should be considered in the differential among TD patients who are treated with antibiotics yet who have persistent or worsening symptoms. Other notable complications of TD include reactive arthritis and *Campylobacter jejuni* associated Guillain-Barré syndrome.

CONCLUSION

TD is a common illness that affects up to a half of travelers during their first two weeks abroad. Symptoms are, for the most part short-lived, but may incapacitate and lay ruin to a carefully planned vacation or business trip. Effective pre-travel counseling may motivate some travelers to modify their travel plans. This, in turn is likely to reduce diarrheal incidence, but does not obviate the need for continued vigilance while traveling.

REFERENCES

1. Ryan ET, Kain KC. Health advice and immunizations for travelers. *N Engl J Med* 2000; **342**(23):1716–1725.
2. Guerrant RL, Rouse JD, Hughes JM, *et al.* Turista among members of the Yale Glee Club in Latin America. *Am J Trop Med Hyg* 1980; **29**(5):895–900.
3. Merson MH, Morris GK, Sack DA, *et al.* Travelers' diarrhea in Mexico. A prospective study of physicians and family members attending a congress. *N Engl J Med* 1976; **294**(24):1299–1305.
4. Hill DR. Occurrence and self-treatment of diarrhea in a large cohort of Americans traveling to developing countries. *Am J Trop Med Hyg* 2000; **62**(5):585–589.
5. Echeverria P, Blacklow NR, Sanford LB, *et al.* Travelers' diarrhea among American Peace Corps volunteers in rural Thailand. *J Infect Dis* 1981; **143**(6):767–771.
6. Sonnenburg F von, Tornieporth N, Waiyaki P, *et al.* Risk and aetiology of diarrhoea at various tourist destinations. *Lancet* 2000; **356**(9224):133–134.
7. Steffen R, Linde F van der, Gyr K, *et al.* Epidemiology of diarrhea in travelers. *JAMA* 1983; **249**(9):1176–1180.
8. Steffen R. Epidemiology of travellers' diarrhoea. *Scand J Gastroenterol Suppl* 1983; **84**:5–17.
9. Steffen R, Rickenbach M, Wilhelm U, *et al.* Health problems after travel to developing countries. *J Infect Dis* 1987; **156**(1):84–91.
10. Hyams KC, Bourgeois AL, Merrell BR, *et al.* Diarrheal disease during Operation Desert Shield. *N Engl J Med* 1991; **325**(20):1423–1428.
11. Steffen R, Collard F, Tornieporth N, *et al.* Epidemiology, etiology, and impact of traveler's diarrhea in Jamaica. *JAMA* 1999; **281**(9):811–817.
12. Black R. Epidemiology of travelers' diarrhea and relative importance of various pathogens. *Rev Infect Dis* 1990; **12**(**suppl** 1):S73–S79.
13. Echeverria P, Sack RB, Blacklow NR, *et al.* Prophylactic doxycycline for travelers' diarrhea in Thailand. Further supportive evidence of Aeromonas hydrophila as an enteric pathogen. *Am J Epidemiol* 1984; **120**(6):912–921.
14. Kean BH. The Diarrhea of Travelers to Mexico: Summary of Five-Year Study. *Ann Intern Med* 1963; **59**(5):605–614.
15. Rowe B, Taylor J, Bettelheim KA. An investigation of traveller's diarrhoea. *Lancet* 1970; **1**(7636):1–5.
16. Gorbach SL, Banwell JG, Chatterjee BD, *et al.* Acute undifferentiated human diarrhea in the tropics. I. Alterations in intestinal microflora. *J Clin Invest* 1971; **50**(4):881–889.
17. Sack RB, Gorbach SL, Banwell JG, *et al.* Enterotoxigenic Escherichia coli isolated from patients with severe cholera-like disease. *J Infect Dis* 1971; **123**(4):378–385.
18. DuPont HL, Formal SB, Hornick RB, *et al.* Pathogenesis of Escherichia coli diarrhea. *N Engl J Med* 1971; **285**(1):1–9.
19. Gorbach SL, Kean BH, Evans DG, *et al.* Travelers' diarrhea and toxigenic Escherichia coli. *N Engl J Med* 1975; **292**:933–936.
20. Herwaldt BL, Ackers ML. An outbreak in 1996 of cyclosporiasis associated with imported raspberries. *Cyclospora Work Group N Engl J Med* 1997; **336**(22):1548–1556.
21. CDC. Cholera associated with imported frozen coconut milk – Maryland, 1991. *MMWR* 1991; **40**(49):844–845.
22. Eberhart-Phillips J, Besser RE, Tormey MP, *et al.* An outbreak of cholera from food served on an international aircraft. *Epidemiol Infect* 1996; **116**(1):9–13.
23. Koo D, Maloney K, Tauxe R. Epidemiology of diarrheal disease outbreaks on cruise ships, 1986 through 1993. *JAMA* 1996; **275**(7):545–547.
24. Mattila L. Clinical features and duration of traveler's diarrhea in relation to its etiology. *Clin Infect Dis* 1994; **19**(4):728–734.
25. Ericsson C, Patterson T, Dupont H. Clinical presentation as a guide to therapy for travelers' diarrhea. *Am J Med Sci* 1987; **294**(2):91–96.
26. Svenungsson B, Lagergren A, Ekwall E, *et al.* Enteropathogens in adult patients with diarrhea and healthy control subjects: a 1-year prospective study in a Swedish clinic for infectious diseases. *Clin Infect Dis* 2000; **30**(5):770–778.
27. Hoge C, Shlim D, Echeverria P, *et al.* Epidemiology of diarrhea among expatriate residents living in a highly endemic environment. *JAMA* 1996; **275**(7):533–538.
28. Hoge CW, Gambel JM, Srijan A, *et al.* Trends in antibiotic resistance among diarrheal pathogens isolated in Thailand over 15 years. *Clin Infect Dis* 1998; **26**:341–345.
29. Taylor D, Houston R, Shlim D, *et al.* Etiology of diarrhea among travelers and foreign residents in Nepal. *JAMA* 1988; **260**(9):1245–1248.
30. Keskimaki M, Mattila L, Peltola H, *et al.* Prevalence of diarrheagenic Escherichia coli in finns with or without diarrhea during a round-the-world trip. *J Clin Microbiol* 2000; **38**(12):4425–4429.
31. Jiang ZD, Mathewson JJ, Ericsson CD, *et al.* Characterization of enterotoxigenic Escherichia coli strains in patients with travelers' diarrhea acquired in Guadalajara, Mexico, 1992–1997. *J Infect Dis* 2000; **181**(2):779–782.
32. Rosenberg ML, Koplan JP, Wachsmuth IK, *et al.* Epidemic diarrhea at Crater Lake from enterotoxigenic Escherichia. coli. A large water-borne outbreak. *Ann Intern Med* 1977; **86**:714–718.
33. Levine MM. Escherichia coli that cause diarrhea: enterotoxigenic, enteropathogenic, enteroinvasive, enterohemorrhagic, and enteroadherent. *J Infect Dis* 1987; **155**(3):377–389.
34. Wanke CA. To know Escherichia coli is to know bacterial diarrheal disease. *Clin Infect Dis* 2001; **32**(12):1710–1712.
35. Wong CS, Jelacic S, Habeeb RL, *et al.* The risk of the hemolytic-uremic syndrome after antibiotic treatment of Escherichia coli O157: H7 infections. *N Engl J Med* 2000; **342**(26):1930–1936.
36. Knutton S, Baldwin T, Williams PH, *et al.* Actin accumulation at sites of bacterial adhesion to tissue culture cells: basis of a new diagnostic test for enteropathogenic and enterohemorrhagic Escherichia coli. *Infect Immun* 1989; **57**(4):1290–1298.
37. Adachi JA, Jiang ZD, Mathewson JJ, *et al.* Enteroaggregative Escherichia coli as a major etiologic agent in traveler's diarrhea in 3 regions of the world. *Clin Infect Dis* 2001; **32**(12):1706–1709.
38. Taylor DN. Campylobacter Infections in Developing Countries. In: Nachamkin I, Blaser MJ, Tompkins LS, eds. *Campylobacter jejuni: current status and future trends.* Washington DC: American Society for Microbiology; 1992:20–30.
39. Allos BM. Campylobacter jejuni infections: update on emerging issues and trends. *Clin Infect Dis* 2001; **32**(8):1201–1206.
40. Kuschner RA, Trofa AF, Thomas RJ, *et al.* Use of azithromycin for the treatment of Campylobacter enteritis in travelers to Thailand, an area where ciprofloxacin resistance is prevalent. *Clin Infect Dis* 1995; **21**(3):536–541.
41. Mermin JH, Townes JM, Gerber M, *et al.* Typhoid fever in the United States, 1985–1994: changing risks of international travel and increasing antimicrobial resistance. *Arch Intern Med* 1998; **158**(6):633–638.
42. Sharp TW, Thornton SA, Wallace MR, *et al.* Diarrheal disease among military personnel during Operation Restore Hope, Somalia, 1992–1993. *Am J Trop Med Hyg* 1995; **52**(2):188–193.
43. Kotloff KL, Winickoff JP, Ivanoff B, *et al.* Global burden of Shigella infections: implications for vaccine development and implementation of control strategies. *Bull World Health Organ* 1999; **77**(8):651–666.
44. Sriratanaban A, Reinprayoon S. Vibrio parahaemolyticus: a major cause of travelers' diarrhea in Bangkok. *Am J Trop Med Hyg* 1982; **31**:128–130.
45. Taylor DN, Rizzo J, Meza R, *et al.* Cholera among Americans living in Peru. *Clin Infect Dis* 1996; **22**(6):1108–1109.
46. Greenberg HB, Matsui SM. Astroviruses and caliciviruses: emerging enteric pathogens. *Infect Agents Dis* 1992; **1**(2):71–91.
47. Moe CL, Gentsch J, Ando T, *et al.* Application of PCR to detect Norwalk virus in fecal specimens from outbreaks of gastroenteritis. *J Clin Microbiol* 1994; **32**(3):642–648.
48. Schwab KJ, Neill FH, Fankhauser RL, *et al.* Development of methods to detect 'Norwalk-like viruses' (NLVs) and hepatitis A virus in delicatessen foods: application to a food-borne NLV outbreak. *Appl Environ Microbiol* 2000; **66**(1):213–218.
49. Deneen VC, Hunt JM, Paule CR, *et al.* The impact of foodborne calicivirus disease: the Minnesota experience. *J Infect Dis* 2000; **181**(**suppl 2**):S281–S283.
50. Khan AS, Moe CL, Glass RI, *et al.* Norwalk virus-associated gastroenteritis traced to ice consumption aboard a cruise ship in Hawaii: comparison and

application of molecular method-based assays. *J Clin Microbiol* 1994; **32**(2):318–322.

51. Herwaldt BL, Lew JF, Moe CL, *et al*. Characterization of a variant strain of Norwalk virus from a food-borne outbreak of gastroenteritis on a cruise ship in Hawaii. *J Clin Microbiol* 1994; **32**(4):861–866.

52. McEvoy M, Blake W, Brown D, *et al*. An outbreak of viral gastroenteritis on a cruise ship. *Commun Dis Rep CDR Rev* 1996; **6**(13):R188–R192.

53. Sekla L, Stackiw W, Dzogan S, *et al*. Foodborne gastroenteritis due to Norwalk virus in a Winnipeg hotel. *CMAJ* 1989; **140**(12):1461–1464.

54. Hyams KC, Malone JD, Kapikian AZ, *et al*. Norwalk virus infection among Desert Storm Troops. *J Infect Dis* 1993; **167**:986–987.

55. Cuffari C, Oligny L, Seidman EG. Dientamoeba fragilis masquerading as allergic colitis. *J Pediatr Gastroenterol Nutr* 1998; **26**(1):16–20.

56. Raynaud L, Delbac F, Broussolle V, *et al*. Identification of Encephalitozoon intestinalis in travelers with chronic diarrhea by specific PCR amplification. *J Clin Microbiol* 1998; **36**(1):37–40.

57. Thielman NM, Guerrant RL. Persistent diarrhea in the returned traveler. *Infect Dis Clin North Am* 1998; **12**(2):489–501.

58. Wanke CA, DeGirolami P, Federman M. Enterocytozoon bieneusi infection and diarrheal disease in patients who were not infected with human immunodeficiency virus: case report and review. *Clin Infect Dis* 1996; **23**(4):816–818.

59. Herwaldt BL, Arroyave KR de, Wahlquist SP, *et al*. Multiyear prospective study of intestinal parasitism in a cohort of Peace Corps volunteers in Guatemala. *J Clin Microbiol* 2001; **39**(1):34–42.

60. Shlim D, Hoge C, Rajah R, *et al*. Persistent high risk of diarrhea among foreigners in Nepal during the first 2 years of residence. *Clin Infect Dis* 1999; **29**(3):613–616.

61. Tomkins AM, James WP, Walters JH, *et al*. Malabsorption in overland travellers to India. *Br Med J* 1974; **3**(927):380–384.

62. Wright SG, Tomkins AM, Ridley DS. Giardiasis: clinical and therapeutic aspects. *Gut* 1977; **18**(5):343–350.

63. Okhuysen PC. Traveler's diarrhea due to intestinal protozoa. *Clin Infect Dis* 2001; **33**(1):110–114.

64. Nash TE, Herrington DA, Losonsky GA, *et al*. Experimental human infections with Giardia lamblia. *J Infect Dis* 1987; **156**(6):974–984.

65. Hardie RM, Wall PG, Gott P, *et al*. Infectious diarrhea in tourists staying in a resort hotel. *Emerg Infect Dis* 1999; **5**(1):168–171.

66. Marshall MM, Naumovitz D, Ortega Y, *et al*. Water-borne protozoan pathogens. *Clin Microbiol Rev* 1997; **10**(1):67–85.

67. Goka AK, Rolston DD, Mathan VI, *et al*. The relative merits of faecal and duodenal juice microscopy in the diagnosis of giardiasis. *Trans R Soc Trop Med Hyg* 1990; **84**(1):66–67.

68. Jackson TF. Entamoeba histolytica and Entamoeba dispar are distinct species; clinical, epidemiological and serological evidence. *Int J Parasitol* 1998; **28**(1):181–186.

69. Nanda R, Baveja U, Anand BS. Entamoeba histolytica cyst passers: clinical features and outcome in untreated subjects. *Lancet* 1984; **2**(8398):301–303.

70. Hoge C, Shlim D, Rajah R, *et al*. Epidemiology of diarrhoeal illness associated with coccidian-like organism among travellers and foreign residents in Nepal. *Lancet* 1993; **341**(8854):1175–1179.

71. Shaffer N, Moore L. Chronic travelers' diarrhea in a normal host due to Isospora belli. *J Infect Dis* 1989; **159**(3):596–597.

72. MacKenzie WR, Schell WL, Blair KA, *et al*. Massive outbreak of water-borne cryptosporidium infection in Milwaukee, Wisconsin: recurrence of illness and risk of secondary transmission. *Clin Infect Dis* 1995; **21**(1):57–62.

73. Jokipii AM, Hemila M, Jokipii L. Prospective study of acquisition of Cryptosporidium, Giardia lamblia, and gastrointestinal illness. *Lancet* 1985; **2**(8453):487–489.

74. Shlim D, Hoge C, Rajah R, *et al*. Is Blastocystis hominis a cause of diarrhea in travelers? A prospective controlled study in Nepal. *Clin Infect Dis* 1995; **21**(1):97–101.

75. Black RE, Merson MH, Rowe B, *et al*. Enterotoxigenic Escherichia coli diarrhoea: acquired immunity and transmission in an endemic area. *Bull World Health Organ* 1981; **59**(2):263–268.

76. Pitzinger B, Steffen R, Tschopp A. Incidence and clinical features of traveler's diarrhea in infants and children. *Pediatr Infect Dis J* 1991; **10**(10):719–723.

77. Ryder RW, Wells JG, Gangarosa EJ. A study of travelers' diarrhea in foreign visitors to the United States. *J Infect Dis* 1977; **136**:605–607.

78. Loewenstein MS, Balows A, Gangarosa EJ. Turista at an international congress in Mexico. *Lancet* 1973; **1**(7802):529–531.

79. Ryder RW, Oquist CA, Greenberg H, *et al*. Travelers' diarrhea in Panamanian tourists in Mexico. *J Infect Dis* 1981; **144**(5):442–448.

80. Levine MM, Nalin DR, Hoover DL, *et al*. Immunity to enterotoxigenic Escherichia coli. *Infect Immun* 1979; **23**(3):729–736.

81. Levine MM, Rennels MB, Cisneros L, *et al*. Lack of person-to-person transmission of enterotoxigenic Escherichia coli despite close contact. *Am J Epidemiol* 1980; **111**(3):347–355.

82. Dupont HL, Haynes GA, Pickering LK, *et al*. Diarrhea of travelers to Mexico. Relative susceptibility of United States and Latin American students attending a Mexican University. *Am J Epidemiol* 1977; **105**(1):37–41.

83. Herwaldt BL, Arroyave KR de, Roberts JM, *et al*. A multiyear prospective study of the risk factors for and incidence of diarrheal illness in a cohort of Peace Corps volunteers in Guatemala. *Ann Intern Med* 2000; **132**(12):982–988.

84. Steffen R. Epidemiologic studies of travelers' diarrhea, severe gastrointestinal infections, and cholera. *Rev Infect Dis* 1986; **8**(suppl 2):S122–S130.

85. Guerrant RL, Hughes JM, Lima NL, *et al*. Diarrhea in developed and developing countries: magnitude, special settings, and etiologies. *Rev Infect Dis* 1990; **12**(suppl 1):S41–S50.

86. Tjoa WS, DuPont HL, Sullivan P, *et al*. Location of food consumption and travelers' diarrhea. *Am J Epidemiol* 1977; **106**(1):61–66.

87. Kozicki M, Steffen R, Schar M. Boil it, cook it, peel it, or forget it. *Int J Epidemiol* 1985; **14**:169–172.

88. McIntosh I, Reed J, Power K. Travellers' diarrhoea and the effect of pre-travel health advice in general practice. *Br J Gen Pr* 1997; **47**(415):71–75.

89. Yazdanpanah Y, Beaugerie L, Boelle P, *et al*. Risk factors of acute diarrhoea in summer – a nation-wide French case-control study. *Epidemiol Infect* 2000; **124**(3):409–416.

90. Ericsson CD, Pickering LK, Sullivan P, *et al*. The role of location of food consumption in the prevention of travelers' diarrhea in Mexico. *Gastroenterology* 1980; **79**(5 Pt 1):812–816.

91. Dupont H. Travellers' Diarrhoea. *Clin Res Rev* 1981; **1**(suppl 1):225–234.

92. Glass RI, Noel J, Ando T, *et al*. The epidemiology of enteric caliciviruses from humans: a reassessment using new diagnostics. *J Infect Dis* 2000; **181**(suppl 2):S254–S261.

93. Ho MS, Glass RI, Monroe SS, *et al*. Viral gastroenteritis aboard a cruise ship. *Lancet* 1989; **2**(8669):961–965.

94. CDC. 'Norwalk-Like Viruses' Public Health Consequences and Outbreak Management. *MMWR* 2001; **50**(RR-9):1–18.

95. Echeverria P, Hodge FA, Blacklow NR, *et al*. Travelers' diarrhea among United States Marines in South Korea. *Am J Epidemiol* 1978; **108**(1):68–73

96. Cobelens FG, Leentvaar-Kuijpers A, Kleijnen J, Coutinho RA. Incidence and risk factors of diarrhoea in Dutch travellers: consequences for priorities in pre-travel health advice. *Trop Med Int Health* 1998; **3**(11):896–903.

97. Black R. Pathogens that cause travelers' diarrhea in Latin America and Africa. *Rev Infect Dis* 1986; **8**(suppl 2):S131–S135.

98. Taylor D, Echeverria P. Etiology and epidemiology of travelers' diarrhea in Asia. *Rev Infect Dis* 1986; **8**(suppl 2):S136–S141.

99. Echeverria P, Jackson LR, Hoge CW, *et al*. Diarrhea in U.S. troops deployed to Thailand. *J Clin Microbiol* 1993; **31**(12):3351–3352.

100. Mattila L, Siitonen A, *et al*. Seasonal variation in etiology of travelers' diarrhea. *J Infect Dis* 1992; **165**:385–388.

101. Jiang ZD, Lowe B, Verenkar MP, *et al*. Prevalence of enteric pathogens among international travelers with diarrhea acquired in Kenya (Mombasa), India (Goa), or Jamaica (Montego Bay). *J Infect Dis* 2002; **185**(4): 497–502.

102. Paredes P, Campbell-Forrester S, Mathewson JJ, *et al*. Etiology of travelers' diarrhea on a Caribbean island. *J Travel Med* 2000; **7**(1): 15-8.

103. Haberberger RL, Mikhail IA, Burans JP, *et al*. Travelers' diarrhea among United States military personnel during joint American-Egyptian armed forces exercises in Cairo, Egypt. *Mil Med* 1995; **160**(7): 331-4.

104. Oyofo BA, Peruski LF, Ismail TF, *et al*. Enteropathogens associated with diarrhea among military personnel during Operation Bright Star 96, in Alexandria, Egypt. *Mil Med* 1997; **162**(6): 396-400.

105. Oyofo BA, el-Gendy A, Wasfy MO, et al. A survey of enteropathogens among United States military personnel during Operation Bright Star '94, in Cairo, Egypt. *Mil Med* 1995; **160**(7): p331-4.

104. Sanders JW, Isenbarger DW, Walz SE, *et al*. An observational clinic-based study of diarrheal illness in deployed United States military personnel in Thailand: presentation and outcome of Campylobacter infection. *Am J Trop Med Hyg* 2002; **67**(5): 533-8.

106. Taylor DN, Echeverria P, Blaser MJ, *et al*. Polymicrobial aetiology of travellers' diarrhoea. *Lancet* 1985; **1**(8425): 381-3.

107. Bouckenooghe AR, Jiang ZD, De La Cabada FJ, *et al*. Enterotoxigenic Escherichia coli as cause of diarrhea among Mexican adults and US travelers in Mexico. *J Travel Med* 2002; **9**(3): 137-40

108. Mounts AW, Ando T, Koopmans M, *et al*. Cold weather seasonality of gastroenteritis associated with Norwalk-like viruses. *J Infect Dis* 2000; **181**(suppl 2):S284–S287.

109. DuPont HL, Capsuto EG. Persistent diarrhea in travelers. *Clin Infect Dis* 1996; **22**(1):124–128.

110. Bartlett JG. Clinical practice. Antibiotic-associated diarrhea. *N Engl J Med* 2002; **346**(5):334–339.

CHAPTER 17 # Prevention of Travelers' Diarrhea

Luis Ostrosky-Zeichner and Charles D. Ericsson

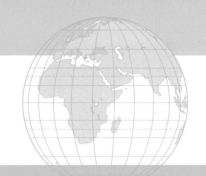

KEYPOINTS

- Effective prophylactic measures to prevent travelers' diarrhea include behavior modification and the use of prophylactic agents like bismuth subsalicylate and antimicrobials

- While prophylaxis is an attractive and effective strategy to prevent disease, it is not free of risks and side-effects

- Prophylaxis may induce complacency and an increase in risky behavior

- Prophylaxis should be considered for short-term travelers who are high-risk hosts or are taking critical trips

- The comparative advantages of prophylaxis versus early treatment of travelers' diarrhea are largely unknown, but early treatment seems a useful strategy that prevents morbidity while not exposing large numbers of subjects to the potential side-effects of prophylactic measures

INTRODUCTION

The impact and frequency of travelers' diarrhea have been discussed in previous chapters. Given the prevalence and morbidity of the syndrome, the logical question is: is there any way to prevent it? As a rule, preventive measures are more cost-effective and practical than treating a disease and its complications. This fully applies to travelers' diarrhea, but the benefits of early self-treatment need to be considered in the equation. Prevention of this syndrome has been accomplished by several measures including educational interventions for risk avoidance and chemoprophylaxis with antimicrobials and other agents. Currently available prevention strategies are summarized in Table 17.1. If one prescribes an efficacious prophylactic regimen to a host at risk, a degree of success is likely. One must carefully balance the risks and potential benefits of such an intervention. However, the decision to use prophylaxis is not simple, because another strategy, namely early empiric treatment, has also proven to be highly efficacious. This chapter will discuss the available preventive measures for travelers' diarrhea, contrasting them with empiric treatment. Vaccination as a prevention strategy is discussed in more detail in Section 3 of this volume.

THE IMPACT OF PREVENTION

While some experts argue that travelers' diarrhea is a trivial, self-limiting disease, we prefer to approach it as a disease of high prevalence, with a high potential for vexatious morbidity. Travelers' diarrhea affects up to 30–70% of the 50 million travelers moving from developed to developing countries.[1] While rarely lethal, or hospitalization-requiring, it may put one to bed for a day, and it may just plainly ruin a trip. A measure that could prevent a reasonable fraction of the disease would be justified in the minds of the millions of travelers whose trips were 'saved'.

When the predominant cause of the syndrome was determined to be bacterial enteropathogens, prophylaxis studies focused on antimicrobials. Some 80–90% protection against diarrhea could be realized when local strains were susceptible to the antimicrobial agent studied.[2] Bismuth subsalicylate (BSS) afforded 40–65% protection.[3] Other interventions have shown variable but generally disappointing results (e.g., probiotics), or simply have not been adequately studied (e.g., behavior modification).

A measure that can prevent even 40% of 10 million cases of diarrhea should be seriously considered. However, prophylaxis is not risk free and will not be desired by everyone, yet, the travel medicine expert must be conversant with the issues and prepared to discuss the pros and cons with certain high risk or interested travelers.

PREVENTION STRATEGIES

Identifying hosts at risk

Perhaps the most important factors when considering prophylaxis are knowledge of the epidemiology of travelers' diarrhea and host risk factors. A high-risk profile makes prophylaxis worth considering. Known epidemiologic risk factors are: resident of a developed country traveling to a developing country, no travel to a tropical area in the past six months, adventure or 'extreme' travel, higher socio-economic status, and disregard of food and water recommendations. Host factors include those for whom the incidence of diarrhea can be predicted to be higher, or those with higher risks of complications, such as young age (<6 years of age) and conditions that reduce gastric acidity or host defenses (chronic gastrointestinal disease). Host factors can also associate with a worse course of diarrhea (e.g., immune deficiency associated with malignancy, transplantation and HIV infection), a concern for the fetus (pregnancy), and worry that the ill traveler might not treat themselves adequately, such as the elderly.[1,2,4–8] Risk factors and hosts are summarized in Table 17.2.

Not all epidemiologic factors can be influenced by education. One factor to be considered is the nature of the trip. Since by definition adventure or 'extreme' travelers are more likely to engage in risky behaviors and are unlikely to respond to attempts at behavior modification, so prophylaxis should be more readily considered than in the average traveler. Another group that might benefit from prophylaxis is the business traveler on a short critical trip, who is too frequently exposed to high-risk meals offered by well meaning hosts and for whom a severe episode of diarrhea could have serious economic consequences.

Table 17.1	Current strategies for the prevention of travelers' diarrhea	
Strategy	Reported success rates	Comments
Risk behavior modification	Generally low	Always thought of as the cornerstone of prevention. While it may prevent disease, advice is often hard to follow or ignored. Must be simple and practical.
Chemoprophylaxis with bismuth subsalicylate	40–65%	Dose is two tablets four times a day. May cause dark stools and 'black tongue'. Salicylate intoxication rare but possible. Should not be used with coumadin and NSAIDs.
Antimicrobial use	80–90%	Highly effective when regional microbiology and susceptibilities are considered. May cause side-effects and induce resistance.
Probiotics	Variable	Clinical trial evidence is conflictive. Relatively safe.

The concept of 'criticality' is sometimes invoked in the decision to prescribe chemoprophylaxis. In our minds 'critical' is a negotiation between the travel medicine provider and the traveler. Who is really to say that an Olympic athlete or a president or a honeymooning couple have more or less critical trips?

Education and behavior modification

Education and risk behavior modification have always been regarded as one of the pillars in the prevention of travelers' diarrhea. While 'Boil it, cook it, peel it or forget it!' is popular, simple and generally does make sense, several studies have shown that few travelers actually comply with these kinds of directives. Furthermore, studies have shown conflicting results in the value of following such strict advice.[9] We consider food and drinks to fall into three general categories: safe, probably safe, and unsafe. Examples of these are shown in Table 17.3. Travelers can be instructed in these categories, and probably should be made aware of how food choices affect their likelihood of experiencing diarrhea, but such education is still no guarantee that the traveler will comply with prudent culinary advice

'Water paranoia' is common among travelers; however, beverage choices, while important, contribute to travelers' diarrhea much less than contaminated foods. Carbonated beverages can be considered safe. Bottled natural water is generally safe especially if a seal must be broken before consumption. Water supplied in large containers cannot be considered automatically safe; sometimes it is no more than bottled local water from the regular municipal source. Cans and bottles should be cleaned and dried before consuming their contents. While boiling water is a very effective way to assure water safety, this is highly impractical for the short-term traveler. Chemical disinfection with iodine is a practical way to purify water, but the ensuing chemical

taste may discourage its use, and iodine should not be used in the pregnant traveler and the traveler with thyroid disease. Also, care must be taken to clarify water before iodine disinfection and close attention must be paid to the amount of iodine to use, the ambient temperature and duration of disinfection. Chlorine disinfection is less reliable than iodine since cysts of parasites like *Giardia* might survive the process.

Commercially available filters exist to supply both a large and small supply of water. Filters are adequate to remove bacteria and parasitic cysts, but viruses will pass through the filter. The combination of a filter with an iodine resin not only removes bacteria and cysts but probably removes many viruses as well.

Water must be kept pure after it has been disinfected. Container handling is of paramount importance, since a contaminated container may defeat the purpose of disinfection, and put the traveler at increased risk (see Chapter 6).

Contaminated food is much more of a problem than water. Food may be contaminated at its source (such as with the use of fecal fertilizers on crops), or during preparation due to poor personal hygiene of the cook or food preparer or inadequate food handling and storage practices. The best advice is to eat food that has been thoroughly and recently cooked, and served piping hot. Temperatures in the range of 160°F are necessary, and such food is too hot to eat. Cold foods like salads, and raw vegetables and fruits, should be avoided. Fresh sauces and condiments (such as 'salsa') that sit on restaurant counters for long periods of time are ideal culture media, and likewise should be avoided. A recent study of salsas from popular restaurants in Guadalajara, Mexico showed a high rate of *E. coli* contamination.[10] Unpasteurized milk products, as well as uncooked seafood, are high-risk foods that should not be consumed.

Choice of where food is obtained and consumed also makes a difference. While not a guarantee, eating meals at a private residence

Table 17.2	Travelers at risk of travelers' diarrhea
Hosts with increased risk of disease	Host with increased risk of complications
Travel from developed to underdeveloped countries	<6 years old and the elderly
No travel to tropical areas in the past semester	Immunocompromised hosts
Higher socio-economic status	Chronic gastrointestinal disease
Adventure or 'extreme' travel	Pregnancy
Low gastric acidity	

Table 17.3	**Food and beverage recommendations for travelers**		
Category	Safe	Probably safe	Unsafe
Beverages	Carbonated soft drinks	Fresh citric juices	Tap water
	Carbonated water	Bottled water	Chipped ice
	Boiled water	Packaged (machine-made) ice	Unpasteurized milk
	Purified water (iodine or chlorine)		
Food	Hot, thoroughly grilled, boiled	Dry items	Salads
	Processed and packaged	Hyperosmolar items (such as jam and syrup)	Sauces and 'salsas'
	Cooked vegetables and peeled fruits	Washed vegetables and fruits	Uncooked seafood Raw or poorly cooked meats Unpeeled fruits Unpasteurized dairy products Cold desserts
Setting	Recommended restaurants	Local homes	Street vendors

is generally safer than eating out. Also, eating at a luxury hotel may not be safer than eating at an economy or standard hotel, because many fancy foods are hand-prepared, uncooked, and intentionally served cold. The highest risk comes from food purchased from street vendors. Such food may not be well prepared to start with. The personal hygiene of the vendor is critical, as are food storage practices and the cleanliness of the plates and utensils.

Behavior modification through food and water advice should be as dynamic and candid as possible. Dogmatic advice and long lists of 'bad' foods are likely to be unsuccessful. In our own clinic we try to simplify the message. Safe beverages are anything carbonated and water from a container with a sealed cap. Safe food is hot, dry or peeled. Avoid cold, raw or unpasteurized foods. However, the impact of even such simple education appears to be minimal. Especially if one identifies a high-risk traveler with a poor attitude toward behavioral modification, the focus should probably be less on education and more on prophylaxis or empiric treatment strategy.[11]

Chemoprophylaxis

A few earlier studies of the prevention of travelers' diarrhea focused on bulk forming (polycarbophil) or adsorption agents (activated charcoal). While these substances may have other GI indications, their use for the prevention of travelers' diarrhea cannot be recommended since they lack effectiveness and might interfere with the absorption of other drugs.

Considerable research has been done on bismuth subsalicylate, the active ingredient of Pepto Bismol®. Bismuth subsalicylate disassociates in gastric acid to form bismuth salts like bismuth oxychloride. Bismuth subsalicylate has antimicrobial and anti-secretory properties and a potential for toxin adsorption. Salicylic acid is released as a by-product of the reaction and is nearly completely absorbed. Chewing a total of eight Pepto Bismol® tablets/day is equivalent to taking 3–4 adult aspirin tablets. Although salicylic acid does not have the same anticoagulant properties as acetylsalicylic acid, travelers taking coumadin or NSAIDs should avoid bismuth subsalicylate.

Bismuth subsalicylate is an effective and safe agent for the prevention and treatment of travelers' diarrhea. Protection ranges from 40–65%, according to the amount and frequency of the dose. Ideally it should be taken as two tablets chewed four times a day.[3,12,13]

Blackening of the stools due to the black bismuth salts can mimic melena. Travelers should be advised to rinse their mouths thoroughly after each dose and after the bedtime dose. Tongue brushing is recommended to help avoid the otherwise purely aesthetic problem of black tongue. Theoretically, the absorbed salicylate may cause tinnitus, but in studies this occurred no more frequently in bismuth subsalicylate-treated patients than in placebo-treated patients. Care should be exercised when using bismuth subsalicylate in patients with impaired renal function. Bismuth subsalicylate can contribute to salicylate intoxication, so it should not be taken with aspirin. Encephalopathy has been anecdotally reported, but the bismuth in bismuth subsalicylate is essentially not absorbed compared to other bismuth compounds, so such reports are exceedingly rare.

Antimicrobials

Much of the early work on travelers' diarrhea prevention focused on the use of prophylactic antimicrobials, so a large body of data exists on the subject. While use of antimicrobials has demonstrated clear efficacy for the prevention of the disease, the side-effect profile, along with ecological and practical considerations make this a highly controversial area. Table 17.4 shows currently recommended antimicrobials with the suggested dosing regimens.

Classic studies by Ben Kean[14] noted the utility of the antibiotic, neomycin, in the prevention of travelers' diarrhea. Then studies with doxycycline dosed at 100 mg/day showed it to be a highly protective agent. Increasing resistance to tetracyclines in developing regions have made it an obsolete approach. Doxycycline remains an alternative choice for malaria prevention, but travelers should be cautioned not to use it with bismuth subsalicylate, because the bivalent cations in bismuth subsalicylate preparations can lower the bioavailability of doxycycline.

Trimethoprim and the combination of trimethoprim and sulfamethoxazole (TMP/SMX) were historically the next generation of antimicrobials used for prevention of diarrhea. These agents provided 71–95% protection in areas where resistance was low; however, rising resistance around the world has compromised the usefulness of these antimicrobials as well.[2] TMP/SMX is ineffective against *Campylobacter jejuni*, an important cause of travelers' diarrhea, particularly in Southeast Asia. While TMP/SMX is relatively inexpensive, easy to

Table 17.4	Currently recommended antimicrobials for the prevention of travelers' diarrhea	
Antimicrobial	Dose	Comments
Trimethoprim-sulfamethoxazole	160/800 mg p.o. q.d.	Global resistance is increasing. Must consider regional patterns to use. Ineffective against *C. jejuni*. May rarely cause severe hypersensitivity reactions.
Quinolones Ofloxacin Norfloxacin Ciprofloxacin Levofloxacin	300 mg p.o. q.d. 400 mg p.o. q.d. 500 mg p.o. q.d. 500 mg p.o. q.d.	Over 90% effective. Currently the best choice for prophylaxis, although we prefer to reserve them for self-therapy. Side-effects include dizziness, insomnia, and anxiety. Promotion of resistance is a concern.

administer, and can be used in children, its major disadvantages include rashes, hypersensitivity reactions (including Stevens-Johnson syndrome), bone marrow depression, and gastrointestinal disturbances. Serious side-effects are rare, but need to be considered when prescribing this drug for purposes of prophylaxis.

Quinolones are, as a group, currently the most popular, effective and safe agents for the prevention and treatment of travelers' diarrhea. Efficacy has been reported over 90%.[2,15] Unfortunately, quinolone resistance, particularly among *C. jejuni*, is increasingly being reported. Adverse reactions are uncommon, but can include rash, GI intolerance and central nervous system stimulation manifested as insomnia, nervousness or dizziness. Quinolones should not be used in pregnant women. Data on their safety in children is accumulating. It is for this class of drugs that induction of resistance in the community is critical, since their broad spectrum of activity, including respiratory tract pathogens, has given them a wide range of clinical applications.

Newer antibiotics with efficacy in the treatment of travelers' diarrhea, but for which prophylaxis data are not available, include azithromycin and rifaximin. These agents are attractive for their broad spectrum of activity against enteropathogens including *C. jejuni* and availability (or at least presumed safety) for use in children and pregnant women. Rifaximin has exclusively intraluminal action with no gastrointestinal absorption, documented low potential for generating cross resistance, and a profile of clinical use that is limited to GI syndromes or hepatic encephalopathy.

Probiotics and other forms of prophylaxis

Use of probiotics for the protection of travelers from diarrhea has long been an attractive idea. The premise behind probiotics is the colonization of the gastrointestinal tract by non-pathogenic microorganisms so as to displace or prevent infection by pathogenic organisms. Some claims of local immunomodulation effects have also been made. Other authors postulate a change in the intestinal pH, which in turn inhibits growth of enteropathogens. Early studies of probiotics were significantly limited by the lack of standardized organisms, delivery vehicles, and solid clinical trial design. Later clinical trials with standardized organisms (genetically engineered strains like *Lactobacillus* GG) have added to the confusion by showing conflicting results. Only three out of seven trials have shown modest positive effects.[16–19] Other probiotics, such as *Saccharomyces boulardii*, that have shown good activity against other forms of diarrhea (like antibi-otic-associated diarrhea) are promising in preliminary clinical expe-rience.[20] At this time, we do not feel that probiotic therapy can be routinely recommended for the prevention of travelers' diarrhea. However, because probiotics are safe, we have

no objection if travelers wish to use the products, while they also exercise careful choices of foods and beverages.

The use of antimotility agents such as loperamide or diphenoxylate/atropine, anticholinergic agents and calmodulin inhibitors for the prevention of travelers' diarrhea should be strongly discouraged. They may cause constipation or even ileus, and in the case of diphenoxylate, dependence.

Vaccine development for the agents of travelers' diarrhea has been slow since there are multiple organisms that can cause it. Vaccines are available at this time to cover *Shigella* spp, *Salmonella typhi*, *Vibrio cholerae* and enterotoxigenic *E. coli*.[21] All are live-attenuated vaccines, except for *E. coli*, which is an inactivated vaccine. All are given orally, except for *Salmonella*, which has both an oral and an inactivated preparation. The efficacy rates are: 73–74% for *Shigella*, 64–72% for *Salmonella* (parenteral), 85% for *Vibrio*, and >70% for *E. coli*. Despite initial problems (like intussusception and diarrhea), Rotavirus vaccines are being further developed. These vaccines should be carefully considered for special situations, in which the prevalence of a particular disease makes them useful.[6,22,23]

PROPHYLAXIS VERSUS EARLY TREATMENT

So what is the most effective, safe and worthwhile approach to travelers' diarrhea: prophylaxis or early treatment? Prophylaxis requires the administration of antibiotics or other potentially toxic substances to a large number of patients to prevent about 80% of cases. While this may be cost effective in terms of saving trips in a population where the disease prevalence is extremely high, it carries significant potential for toxicities, drug interactions, promotion of bacterial resistance, and engagement in risk behaviors. Furthermore, a consensus conference at the National Institutes of Health in 1985 mentioned that while antimicrobial drugs and bismuth subsalicylate are clearly effective for the prevention of travelers' diarrhea, routine use of these agents for any group of travelers was not recommended because of the potential for known and unknown side-effects.[1,24] This negative approach fails to deal effectively with certain high risk hosts who might be at risk only for a short time and who can easily understand the pros and cons of chemoprophylaxis followed by empiric therapy as necessary. In this approach, we have generally favored the use of bismuth subsalicylate for prophylaxis and have reserved the quinolones for treatment. With the availability of both rifaximin and azithromycin as treatment options, perhaps the quinolones now can be used as the prophylactic antimicrobial agent of choice.

Early treatment however, has proven to be a highly effective strategy for the management of the disease, since if used correctly, it controls symptoms and significantly shortens duration of the disease to a matter of hours, in most cases with the use of a single dose of an antibiotic.[25] Nevertheless, it involves actually experiencing the disease, with some degree of discomfort, and potential for progression and complications.

Our current approach includes simplified recommendations for behavior modification with specific instructions for early treatment for most travelers. We generally consider and recommend antimicrobial prophylaxis only for high risk hosts and travelers on critical, high risk trips, when experiencing even a few hours of intense disease would be undesirable. Figure 17.1 presents an algorithm of our proposed approach to TD prevention.

CONCLUSION

- Effective prophylactic measures to prevent travelers' diarrhea include behavior modification and the use of prophylactic agents like bismuth subsalicylate and antimicrobials.
- While they are not especially active, agents like *Lactobacillus* GG are safe, but they may induce food complacency.
- While prophylaxis is an attractive and effective strategy to prevent disease, it is not free of risks and side-effects.
- Prophylaxis may induce complacency and an increase in risky behavior.
- Prophylaxis should be considered for short-term travelers who are high-risk hosts or are taking critical trips.
- The comparative advantages of prophylaxis versus early treatment of travelers' diarrhea are largely unknown, but early treatment seems a useful strategy that prevents morbidity while not exposing large numbers of subjects to the potential side-effects of prophylactic measures.

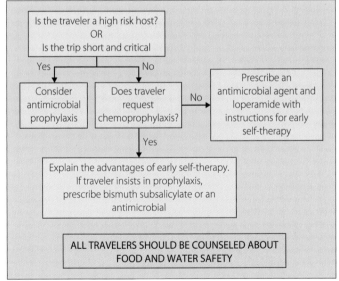

Figure 17.1 Algorithm for the prevention of travelers' diarrhea.

REFERENCES

1. DuPont HL, Ericsson CD. Prevention and treatment of traveler's diarrhea. *N Engl J Med* 1993; **328**(25):1821–1827.
2. Ansdell VE, Ericsson CD. Prevention and empiric treatment of traveler's diarrhea. *Med Clin North Am* 1999; **83**(4):945–973.
3. DuPont HL. Bismuth subsalicylate in the treatment and prevention of diarrheal disease. *Drug Intell Clin Pharm* 1987; **21**(9):687–693.
4. Ericsson CD, DuPont HL, Mathewson IJ. Epidemiologic Observations on Diarrhea Developing in U.S. and Mexican Students Living in Guadalajara, Mexico. *J Travel Med* 1995; **2**(1):6–10.
5. Ericsson CD. Travelers' diarrhea. Epidemiology, prevention, and self-treatment. *Infect Dis Clin North Am* 1998; **12**(2):285–303.
6. Juckett G. Prevention and treatment of traveler's diarrhea. *Am Fam Physician* 1999; **60**(1):119–124, 135–136.
7. Mathews DS, Pust RE, Cordes DH. Prevention and treatment of travel-related illness. *Am Fam Physician* 1991; **44**(4):1343–1358.
8. Virk A. Medical advice for international travelers. *Mayo Clin Proc* 2001; **76**(8):831–840.
9. Steffen R, Van der Linde F, Gyr K, Schar M. Epidemiology of diarrhea in travelers. *JAMA* 1983; **249**(9):1176–1180.
10. Adachi JA, Mathewson JJ, Jiang ZD, Ericsson CD, DuPont HL. Enteric pathogens in Mexican sauces of popular restaurants in Guadalajara, Mexico, and Houston, Texas. *Ann Intern Med* 2002; **136**(12):884–887.
11. Ericsson CD, DuPont HL. Travelers' diarrhea: approaches to prevention and treatment. *Clin Infect Dis* 1993; **16**(5):616–624.
12. Graham DY, Estes MK, Gentry LO. Double-blind comparison of bismuth subsalicylate and placebo in the prevention and treatment of enterotoxigenic Escherichia coli-induced diarrhea in volunteers. *Gastroenterology* 1983; **85**(5):1017–1022.
13. Steffen R, DuPont HL, Heusser R, Helminger A, Witassek F, Manhart MD, Schar M. Prevention of traveler's diarrhea by the tablet form of bismuth subsalicylate. *Antimicrob Agents Chemother* 1986; **29**(4):625–627.
14. Kean BH. Travelers' diarrhea: an overview. *Rev Infect Dis* 1986; **8**(suppl 2):S111–S116.
15. Parry H, Howard AJ, Galpin OP, Hassan SP. The prophylaxis of travellers' diarrhoea; a double blind placebo controlled trial of ciprofloxacin during a Himalayan expedition. *J Infect* 1994; **28**(3):337–338.
16. de dios Pozo-Olano, J, Warram JH Jr., Gomez RG, Cavazos MG. Effect of a lactobacilli preparation on traveler's diarrhea. A randomized, double blind clinical trial. *Gastroenterology* 1978; **74**(5 Pt. 1):829–830.
17. Gorbach SL. Probiotics and gastrointestinal health. *Am J Gastroenterol* 2000; **95**(suppl 1):S2–S4.
18. Katelaris PH, Salam I, Farthing MJ. Lactobacilli to prevent traveler's diarrhea? *N Engl J Med* 1995; **333**(20):1360–1361.
19. Marteau PR, de Vrese M, Cellier CJ, Schrezenmeir J. Protection from gastrointestinal diseases with the use of probiotics. *Am J Clin Nutr* 2001; **73**(suppl 2):430S–436S.
20. D'Souza AL, Rajkumar C, Cooke J, Bulpitt CJ. Probiotics in prevention of antibiotic associated diarrhoea: meta-analysis. *BMJ* 2002; **324**(7350):1361.
21. Lindberg AA. Vaccination against enteric pathogens: from science to vaccine trials. *Curr Opin Microbiol* 1998; **1**(1):116–124.
22. Clarke SC. Diarrhoeagenic Escherichia coli – an emerging problem? *Diagn Microbiol Infect Dis* 2001; **41**(3):93–98.
23. Ryan ET, Calderwood SB. Cholera vaccines. *Clin Infect Dis* 2000; **31**(2):561–565.
24. Gorbach SL, Edelman R, eds. Travelers' diarrhea: National Institutes of Health Consensus Development Conference. Bethesda, MD, 28–30 January, 1985. *Rev Infect Dis* 1986; **8**(suppl 2):S109–S233.
25. Adachi JA, Ostrosky-Zeichner L, DuPont HL, Ericsson CD. Empirical antimicrobial therapy for traveler's diarrhea. *Clin Infect Dis* 2000; **31**(4):1079–1083.

CHAPTER 18   # Clinical Presentation and Treatment of Travelers' Diarrhea

Thomas Löscher and Bradley A. Connor

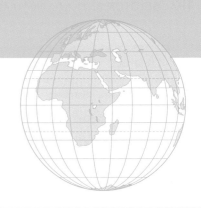

KEYPOINTS

- Clinical course and severity of travelers' diarrhea may be varied and precise definitions based on number or frequency of bowel movements in a 24 hour period are arbitrary

- The mean duration of untreated TD is 3 to 5 days, however in 8-15% a prolonged course (>1 week) occurs and in 1-3% chronic diarrhea (>4 weeks) will develop

- 50% of patients with TD will be incapacitated for at least 1 day, 20% are confined to bed for 1-2 days and 5-15% seek professional medical help

- Risk groups prone to more severe and complicated illness are the very young, the old, the immunocompromised and those suffering from certain underlying chronic medical conditions

- Diarrhea in travelers might be the initial presentation of other potentially dangerous diseases such as falciparum malaria

DEFINITION AND SPECTRUM

Most studies define travelers' diarrhea (TD) as the passing of three or more loose stools in a 24 h period, in association with at least one symptom of enteric disease[1,2] such as nausea, vomiting, cramps, fever, fecal urgency, tenesmus or the passage of bloody, mucoid stools (Table 18.1).

However, TD is not a distinct disease, but a poly-etiological syndrome covering a broad spectrum of mainly infectious enteric diseases caused by a considerable number of various pathogens. In addition, a small part of diarrhea in travelers may be due to non-infectious causes like travel-related stress, jet lag, change in diet (e.g., food of high fat/oil content, hot spices, increased alcohol consumption). Therefore, in every day practice, the limits of TD definition are not absolutely precise. Even bowel disturbances that do not fulfill the definition of classic TD (Table 18.1) may be of relevance to the health of the traveler (mild and moderate TD), and can disrupt a business commitment or other travel plans significantly.[3,4] On the other hand, diarrhea in travelers may be a symptom of severe or systemic disease (Table 18.2), which can be difficult to distinguish clinically from TD, at least in the beginning. In particular, it is important to remember that diarrhea may be a symptom of falciparum malaria and that TD may be a fatal misdiagnosis in those patients.[5]

Signs and symptoms

Clinical course and severity of TD vary considerably between studies depending on geographical differences and variation of the microbial spectrum. TD usually does not start immediately upon arrival, it typically begins after 3-4 days.[3,4] Most cases, in some studies up to 90%, manifest during the first 2 weeks.[3,4,6] Depending on duration, purpose, and destination of travel, two or more separate episodes of TD were reported in 5-30% of travelers,[4,7,8] representing new infections or relapses.

The typical attack begins abruptly. However, in some patients gastrointestinal symptoms start insidiously (seen more often in TD of protozoal origin). The majority of patients has 3-5 diarrheal stools per day. At least 20% of cases have more frequent bowel movements with up to 20 and more stools per 24 h.[3,4] In most patients the stool is watery. Visible blood in stool or the presence of bloody, mucoid stools (Fig. 18.1) has been reported in 3-15% of classic TD.[1,2,4] Concomitant symptoms are frequent and often more disturbing than diarrhea itself. Fecal urgency, nausea, abdominal pain or tenesmus are experienced by almost all patients (Table 18.1). Urgency can be so strong that fecal incontinence occurs. Vomiting does occur most often within the first hours of disease. Frequent vomiting may be very debilitating and can contribute to significant electrolyte imbalance and fluid loss, especially in infants.

Initial fever lasting for 1-2 days is common (Table 18.1) and has been found at some destinations in up to 40% of patients with classic TD.[3] High-grade fever (sometimes with chills) or fever lasting longer than 2 days is more common in classic TD and in cases with an identified pathogen.[3,9] In addition to gastrointestinal symptoms and fever, a variety of general symptoms may occur (i.e. myalgia, arthralgia, cephalgia).

The majority of cases has a self-limited and uncomplicated course. More severe and complicated disease requiring fluid or electrolyte substitution and/or dysentery has been observed in 3-15% in different studies.[1,4,6,7] Fatalities from TD are exceedingly rare, and are seen almost only in high risk groups (see complications) or in severe or enteroinvasive diseases that are beyond the definition of TD (e.g., cholera, shigella or amebic dysentery).

Mild and moderate TD often last for 1-2 days only.[3,4] Untreated the mean duration of classical TD in various studies has been 3-5 days. However, in 8-15% a prolonged course (>1 week) is observed, and in 1-3% chronic diarrhea (≥ 4 weeks) will develop.[3,9]

Almost half the patients with classical TD are incapacitated (defined as inability to pursue planned activities) for a mean duration of one day.[4] Approximately 20% of patients are confined to bed for 1-2 days, and 5-15% seek professional medical help.[3,4] The hospitalization rate

Table 18.1	Definition of travelers' diarrhea[1-4]
Mild travelers' diarrhea:	One or two unformed stools per 24 h, no additional symptoms
Moderate travelers' diarrhea:	One or two unformed stools per 24 h plus at least one of the following symptoms[a]
Classic travelers' diarrhea:	≥ 3 unformed stools per 24 h plus at least one of the following symptoms[a]

[a]Symptom	Frequency (in %) in various studies
Nausea	10–70
Vomiting	4–36
Cramps	60
Fever	10–30
Urgency	>90
Abdominal pain or tenesmus	80
Blood in stool	5–15

is low and usually below 2%, but it may increase up to 10% and more depending on the medical circumstances and the microbial spectrum at the destination.[3]

Complications

Risk groups, prone to more severe and complicated illness, are the very young, the old, the immunocompromised, and patients suffering from underlying conditions with special sensitivity to fluid loss or electrolyte imbalance (i.e., diabetes, cardiac or renal insufficiency).

In patients with profuse watery diarrhea and/or severe and frequent vomiting, the pronounced loss of fluids and electrolytes may cause dehydration, and if not treated adequately, hypotonia, muscle cramps, oliguria, cardiac arrhythmias, coma, and shock may develop. Especially infants who can develop severe dehydration rapidly (Fig. 18.2), and the same pathogens found in TD are leading causes of mortality in under-fives in developing countries.[10]

Enteroinvasive and/or cytotoxin-producing pathogens (Table 18.2)[11] may cause significant mucosal injury presenting as dysentery (Fig. 18.1), mucosal inflammation and ulceration (Fig. 18.3) that can be associated with the risks of severe bleeding or perforation. In addition, invasive pathogens and some absorbable cytotoxins may cause sepsis syndromes and various extraintestinal manifestations like hemolytic-uremic syndrome (enterohemorrhagic *E. coli*, *Shigella dysenteriae* 1), arthritis, and organ abscesses (e.g., amebic liver abscess, extraintestinal salmonella infection).

Some bacterial pathogens (i.e., *Shigella* spp., *Salmonella* spp., *Yersinia* spp., *Campylobacter* spp.) are associated with the development of reactive arthritis (Reiter's syndrome) up to several weeks after acute diarrheal disease. Reiter's syndrome is seen predominantly in patients with the HLA-B27 haplotype and can also manifest as urethritis, conjunctivitis, uveitis, and various skin and mucocutaneous lesions.

In patients with AIDS and others immunocompromised, more severe and chronic courses of TD have been observed.[12,13] In addition, there is an extended spectrum of potential pathogens and various opportunistic pathogens have to be considered (e.g., CMV, mycobacteria, *Cryptosporidium* spp., microsporidia, *Isospora*, *Cyclospora cayetanensis*).

Differential diagnosis

Significant information concerning probable etiological spectrum, severity, and appropriate management can be concluded from clinical

Table 18.2	Pathogenic mechanisms of diarrhea (modified)[11]		
Pathogenesis	Mode of action	Clinical presentation	Pathogens (examples)
Mucosal adherence	Attachment, colonization and effacement of mucosa	Secretory diarrhea	EPEC[a], EaggEC[a], diffuse adhering *E. coli*, ETEC[a], *Giardia lamblia*
Toxin production			
Neurotoxin	Action on the autonomous system	Enteric symptoms	Staphylococcal enterotoxin B, *Clostridium botulinum*, *Bacillus cereus*
Enterotoxin	Fluid secretion without damage to the mucosa	Watery diarrhea (secretory diarrhea)	*Vibrio cholerae*, ETEC[a] *Salmonella* spp., *Campylobacter* spp., *Clostridium difficile* toxin A, *Clostridium perfringens* type A
Cytotoxin	Damage to the mucosa	Inflammatory colitis, dysentery	*Shigella dysenteriae* serotype 1, EHEC[a], *C. difficile* toxin B, *Salmonella* spp., *Campylobacter* spp.
Mucosal invasiveness	Penetration into the mucosa and destruction of epithelial cells	Dysenteric syndrome	*Shigella* spp., EIEC[a], *Campylobacter* spp., *Yersinia* spp., *Entamoeba histolytica*

[a]EPEC, enteropathogenic *Escherichia coli*; EaggEC, enteroaggregative *E. coli*; ETEC, enterotoxic *E. coli*; EHEC, enterohemorrhagic *E. coli*; EIEC, enteroinvasive *E. coli*.

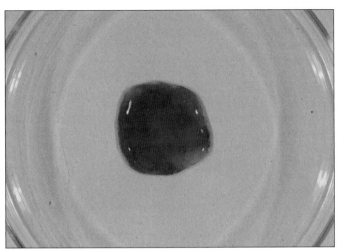

Figure 18.1 Bloody, mucoid diarrhea in a patient with shigellosis.

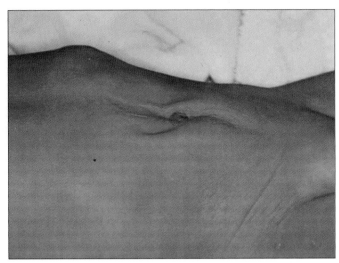

Figure 18.2 'Standing skin folds' as a clinical sign of dehydration in a 7-year-old child with acute water diarrhea.

presentation and anamnestic data (Table 18.3). However, it is not possible to predict the etiological agent from the clinical presentation because the clinical spectrum of the various pathogens causing TD is overlapping considerably:

- Bloody, mucoid stools (Fig. 18.1), abdominal cramps, tenesmus and fever are typical for shigellosis. However, full blown dysentery may also occur in infections with *Campylobacter jejuni*, enteroinvasive and enterohemorrhagic *E. coli*, salmonella, yersinia or *Clostridium difficile*. In amebic dysentery, diarrhea often is mucoid and blood-stained, high fever and abdominal cramps are less common.
- Profuse watery diarrhea might suggest cholera, which is rarely a cause of TD. However, enterotoxigenic *E. coli* and many other pathogens can cause a cholera-like syndrome.
- Malabsorptive diarrhea with hyperperistaltic, meteorism, flatulence and urgent, often postprandial bowel movements of voluminous liquid stools without blood or mucus is typical for giardiasis, but can be observed in infections due to enteropathogenic and entero-aggregative *E. coli*, cryptosporidium, Isospora, or Cyclospora.

Protozoa at most destinations are less frequent causes of TD. However, in persisting gastrointestinal disorders of returning travelers they play a more important role. Diarrhea caused by helminth infec-

tions (strongyloidiasis, trichuriasis, fasciolopsiasis, schistosomiasis and other) is common in children in developing countries but rare in travelers. Blood eosinophilia is frequently present.

Diarrhea after previous treatment with antibiotics (incl. chemotherapy of TD) may be caused by toxinogenic *Clostridium difficile*.

Clinical clues for the management

The management of TD is guided by the severity of disease, age and underlying conditions of the patient, and eventually by any pathogens isolated (Fig. 18.4).

Most cases of TD in otherwise healthy adults are uncomplicated and self-limited, and respond well to symptomatic treatment. A further diagnostic work-up is neither necessary for appropriate management nor cost-effective.[14] The key point for advising travelers as well as for the medical management is the timely recognition of:

- severe and complicated TD, and
- other potentially dangerous diseases, that might present as TD initially.

Table 18.3   Clinical presentation and specific enteropathogens

Symptoms	Fever	Incubation period	Fecal leukocytes and erythrocytes	Enteropathogens
Nausea, vomiting, watery diarrhea	Ø	1–18 h	Negative	ETEC[a], *Staph. aureus* (toxin), *Bacillus cereus* (toxin), *Clostridium perfringens*
Profuse watery diarrhea, atonic vomiting	Ø	5 h–3 days	Negative	*Vibrio cholerae*, ETEC[a]
Nausea, vomiting, diarrhea, myalgias, cephalgia	+	12 h–3 days	Negative	Rotavirus, Norwalk virus, Norwalk-like viruses
Dysentery (bloody, mucoid stools), abdominal cramps	+	1–3 days	Positive	*Shigella* spp., *Campylobacter jejuni*, *Salmonella* spp. *Yersinia* spp., *Clostridium difficile*
Dysentery	Ø/+	Variable	Positive	*Entamoeba histolytica*
Gastrointestinal bleeding	Ø/+	1–3 days	Blood	EHEC[a], cytomegalovirus[b]
Malabsorptive diarrhea, meteorism, flatulence	Ø	1–2 weeks	Negative	*Giardia lamblia*, *Cryptosporidium parvum*, *Cyclospora cayetanensis*, microsporidia[b]

[a]ETEC, enterotoxic *Escherichia coli*; EHEC, enterohemorrhagic *Escherichia coli*.
[b]Almost only in immunocompromised.

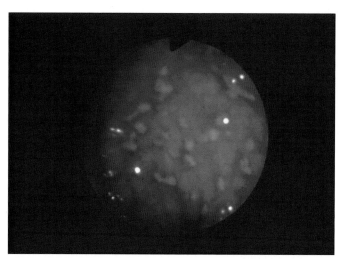

Figure 18.3 Amebic colitis with multiple small (3–5 mm) ulcers of the colon with yellowish exudate and hyperemic borders, and almost normal mucosa between ulcers.

This can be done on the basis of clinical clues by evaluating signs and symptoms as well as anamnestic data appropriately.

Danger signs, indicating severe or complicated disease are:

- profuse watery diarrhea and/or severe and frequent vomiting
- blood in stool and/or bloody, mucoid diarrhea (dysentery)
- high and/or continuing fever
- severe disease (i.e., clinical signs of dehydration, hypotonia).

If one or more of these signs are present, further medical evaluation is warranted, and in case of signs of invasive disease (i.e., dysentery, fever), empirical antibacterial therapy may be indicated initially. Additional indications for microbiological diagnostic work-up are:

- diarrheal disease of epidemiological relevance (outbreaks, epidemics)
- chronic diarrhea, and
- diarrhea in the immunocompromised.

In addition, it has to be considered in each case that diarrhea and other gastrointestinal symptoms may be manifestations of other diseases (Table 18.4), including potentially dangerous ones. For example, diarrhea has been reported in 14% of non-immune travelers with falciparum malaria in a recent study.[5] Therefore, during or after a stay in malaria endemic areas, a timely microscopic investigation for malaria has to be done in all patients with fever and diarrhea.

Persistent and chronic TD (≥ 4 weeks) is seen in 1–3% of patients and may last in some cases for more than one year.[2,3,9] Chronic TD can be a considerable diagnostic challenge (see Chapter 54).

TRAVELERS' DIARRHEA TREATMENT

Antibiotics are the mainstay of therapy of travelers' diarrhea (TD). As bacterial etiologies of TD far outnumber other microbial etiologies, treatment with an antibiotic directed at enteric bacterial pathogens remains the best empiric therapy for TD. Both as empiric therapy or for treatment of a specific bacterial pathogen, first line antibiotics include those of the fluoroquinolone class such as ciprofloxacin (Table 18.5).[1] Antimicrobials have been shown to shorten the illness associated with specific bacterial enteropathogens but also ameliorate cases of TD for which no specific pathogen has been identified, providing evidence that bacterial agents are responsible for the large majority of cases of TD. The optimal duration of antimicrobial therapy in TD has not been established. Historically treatment was recommended for 7 days but over the past two decades treatment courses have been shortened to 5 days, 3 days, 2 days and in some instances single dose therapy has been used successfully.[15] Single dose therapy

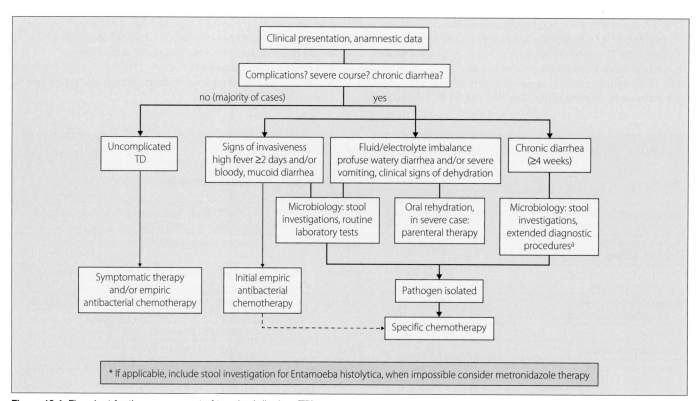

Figure 18.4 Flowchart for the management of travelers' diarrhea (TD).
[a]See Chapter 54 in this volume.

Table 18.4	Diarrhea as a symptom of systemic infections
Acute infections	**Chronic infections**
Katayama syndrome[a]	African Trypanosomiasis
Legionellosis	Chagas disease (chronic stage)
Listeriosis	Cytomegaly[b]
Malaria	Intestinal tuberculosis
Measles	Histoplasmosis
Ornithosis	HIV infection
Rickettsioses	Lymphogranuloma venereum
Sepsis	*Mycobacterium avium-intracelluare* infection[b]
Toxin shock syndrome	Schistosomiasis (intestinal)
Trichinellosis	Visceral leishmaniasis
Typhoid / paratyphoid fever	Whipple's disease
Viral hepatitis (esp. A and E)	

[a]Acute schistosomiasis
[b]Usually only in immunocompromised patients

has not yet become standard of care but there is almost no reason to treat beyond three days.[16]

In the 1970s and early 1980s, doxycycline and trimethoprim-sulfamethoxazole were the drugs of choice for treatment of TD. However, by the early 1980s, an unacceptably high rate of resistant Shigella and ETEC became increasingly identified worldwide.[17] Along with this was the recognition of *Campylobacter jejuni* as an important etiologic agent of TD, a bacteria known to be resistant to these agents.[18] As a result, fluoroquinolones became the standard therapy for TD. Fluoroquinolones are safe and efficacious against a broad spectrum of bacterial enteric pathogens. Fluoroquinolones are well-absorbed after oral administration and reach peak tissue levels quickly. The most well studied of the fluoroquinolones in the treatment of TD have been ciprofloxacin and norfloxacin, however, other fluoroquinolones such as ofloxacin and levofloxacin appear to be efficacious as well.[19]

An effective alternative to the fluoroquinolones in the treatment of enteric bacterial pathogens is azithromycin, a macrolide antibiotic. Azithromycin achieves very high tissue levels in the intestinal mucosa,

Table 18.5	Drug treatment for bacterial pathogens in adults
Antibiotic	**Dose**
Fluoroquinolones	
Ciprofloxacin	500 mg p.o. b.i.d. × 1–3 days
Norfloxacin	400 mg p.o. b.i.d. × 1–3 days
Ofloxacin	400 mg p.o. b.i.d. × 1–3 days
Levofloxacin	500 mg p.o. q.d. × 1–3 days
Gatifloxacin	400 mg p.o. q.d. × 1–3 days
Lomefloxacin	400 mg p.o. q.d. × 1–3 days
Moxifloxacin	400 mg p.o. q.d. × 1–3 days
Macrolides	
Azithromycin	500 mg p.o. b.i.d. × 3 days. Consider first line for countries with quinolone resistant Campylobacter (e.g., Thailand)
Rifamycin derivatives	
Rifaximin	400 mg p.o b.i.d. × 3 days

and appears to have fewer gastrointestinal motility side-effects than erythromycin. In addition, azithromycin has been shown to be effective in treatment of Campylobacter infections resistant to fluoroquinolones.[20] In some areas of the world, such as Thailand, quinolone resistant *Campylobacter jejuni* are prevalent and treatment failures may occur with the use of fluoroquinolones. Azithromycin might be considered first line treatment for travelers returning from such areas.[21,22]

A new approach to the treatment of TD has been the development of antimicrobial agents, which are poorly absorbed from the gut, reducing the possibility of medication related systemic effects or adverse events. Rifaximin, a rifamycin derivative with broad spectrum antibacterial properties, is an example of such an agent. Rifaximin is a nonabsorbable, locally active antibacterial with a broad-spectrum antimicrobial activity selectively used against pathogens inside the gastrointestinal tract. A unique characteristic of this agent is that it remains virtually unabsorbed after oral administration, not only in healthy volunteers but also in those with damaged intestinal mucosa such as those affected by inflammatory bowel disease. Rifaximin treatment minimizes the risk of systemic adverse events as well as pharmacological interactions while ensuring a high concentration of antibacterial reaches the intestinal site of infection. Rifaximin has been shown to be more effective than trimethoprim-sulfa, and equivalent to ciprofloxacin, in treating TD.[23] Rifaximin is given at a dose of 400 mg twice a day for 3 days.

Other non-absorbable antimicrobials such as bicozamycin and aztreonam have demonstrated in vitro activity against bacterial pathogens and have been shown to be effective as well in the treatment of TD. These agents are currently in clinical trials and unavailable commercially.

Oral rehydration therapy

Fluid and electrolytes are lost in cases of TD and replenishment is important to consider, especially in young children or adults with chronic medical illnesses or in situations where shifts in fluid-electrolyte balance may exacerbate underlying medical problems. In travelers who are otherwise healthy, severe dehydration resulting from TD is unusual. Nonetheless replacement of fluid losses remains an important adjunctive measure to other forms of therapy. Most healthy adults with travelers' diarrhea can consume hypotonic glucose-containing solution along with other clear liquids such as soups, broths, and saltine crackers to meet fluid and salt losses. For those with chronic medical problems or in young infants, more aggressive measures may be needed, including standardized oral rehydration therapy (Table 18.6). Oral rehydration solutions (ORS) can also be used in cases of diarrhea associated with vomiting. Standard WHO ORS salts or modified, more palatable versions are available from travel medicine and travel gear supply houses or web sites. Rice based

Table 18.6	Composition of World Health Organization oral rehydration solution (ORS) for diarrheal illness		
Ingredient	**Amount**	**Measurement**
Sodium chloride	3.5 g/L	½ tsp
Potassium chloride	1.5 g/L	¼ tsp
Glucose	20.0 g/L	2 tbsp
Trisodium citrate or Sodium bicarbonate	2.9 g/L 2.5 g/L	½ tsp
H_2O	1000 g	1 L

solutions such as Ceralyte may also be used. If commercial ORS are not available, home-made versions can often be concocted without difficulty by travelers by mixing six level teaspoons of sugar plus one level teaspoon of salt in 1 L of safe drinking water.[24]

Nonantibiotic treatments

Although the primary goal of treatment of TD is eradication of the underlying infection, antisecretory agents, anti-motility agents, and water-absorbing agents may play some role as well in the treatment of some of the symptoms associated with TD. Some patients may benefit from symptomatic therapy alone where as others will be best served by a combination of antimicrobial therapy and antisecretory or antimotility agents. (Table 18.7)

Antisecretory agents

Bismuth subsalicylate (BSS or Pepto-Bismol): With its antisecretory as well as anti-inflammatory and antibacterial properties, bismuth subsalicylate has been shown to bind toxins associated with Vibrio cholerae and ETEC.[25] A salicylate-dependent antisecretory mechanism reduces intestinal secretions. There is some evidence that bismuth subsalicylate exhibits some antimicrobial properties but it is unclear whether this has any effect on the treatment of TD. A dose of bismuth subsalicylate of 524 mg (two tablets or 30 mL) taken every 30 min for eight doses has been shown to reduce the number of stools and duration of illness by 50% compared with placebo.[26] Side-effects of bismuth subsalicylate include black tongue, black stool, tinnitus, and decreased absorption of antibiotics taken within 6 h.

Investigations are ongoing to find novel effective antisecretory compounds with which to treat TD. Taking advantage of the fact that some toxigenic organisms such as ETEC cause diarrhea by calmodulin mediated pathways, an intestinal calmodulin inhibitor, zaldaride maleate, was developed and was found to be effective as antisecretory therapy of TD.[27] Zaldaride maleate at a dose of 20 mg four times daily for 2 days reduces the duration of diarrhea from 42–28 h.

Another antisecretory agent, Racecadotril has been studied in adults with acute diarrhea.[28] Racecadotril (acetorphan) is a specific enkephalinase inhibitor with a selective antisecretory mode of action. Studies in adults and children have shown this agent to be effective. It is not yet commercially available.

Antimotility agents

Antimotility agents act by modulating intestinal contractions and reducing frequency of bowel movements. The most effective antimotility agents are synthetic opiates, diphenoxylate with atropine, (Lomotil), and loperamide (Imodium). Historically, opiates such as paregoric, tincture of opium, and codeine were noted to be effective

in the short-term treatment of diarrhea, but their effects on the central nervous system and potential for drug dependency limited their use. The first of the synthetic opiates, diphenoxylate with atropine (Lomotil), has been shown effective in treating TD, however, because of the anticholinergic properties associated with atropine, can cause dry mouth and blurred vision. Loperamide has little if any central opiate effects and is more gut specific than diphenoxylate.[29] In addition, it may possess additional antisecretory properties.[30] Loperamide reduces by 60% the number of stools passed and the duration of diarrhea at a dose of 4 mg (two capsules) initially, followed by 2 mg (one capsule) after each unformed stool. A dose of eight capsules or 16 mg is considered maximal therapy in a 24 h period.[31] By slowing the intestinal transit, increased reabsorption of water and electrolytes is thought to occur. Antimotility agents can cause bloating and gas, increase abdominal cramping, and cause constipation for variable lengths of time following treatment.

Antimotility agents should not be used in infants, since abdominal distention, paralytic ileus, and systemic side-effects (e.g., lethargy) have been observed more frequently in some studies.[32,33]

In a retrospective cohort study, the use of antimotility agents was associated with a higher risk of hemolytic uremic syndrome in children with Escherichia coli 0157: H7 infection.[34]

Antimotility agents are sometimes recommended in combination with antibiotic therapy.[35] Antimotility agents serve to reduce symptoms during the initial period before bacterial eradication has been completed. The combination of loperamide and an antibiotic often resolves symptoms in a shorter time than with an antibiotic alone. This might be especially useful for a traveler who has to catch a bus or continue a trek before the antibiotic has had a chance to kick in.

An area which is still subject to some controversy is whether antimotility agents should be used in cases of invasive diarrhea. The concern resulted from one study where diphenoxylate and atropine (Lomotil) was shown to cause prolonged carriage of Shigella and decreased effectiveness of concomitant antibiotic therapy.[36] Subsequent studies using loperamide alone, even without an antibiotic, appeared to be safe and unassociated with prolongation of disease. In a double-blind placebo controlled study of ciprofloxacin plus loperamide compared with ciprofloxacin alone for the treatment of dysentery caused by Shigella, no adverse effects were seen with combination therapy and this group recovered more quickly than the group receiving antibiotics alone.[37] Thus, for most cases of TD in adults, antimotility agents or antimotility agents in combination with an antibiotic appears to be a rational and effective therapeutic approach. A note of caution however is warranted in patients with severe dysenteric disease as it is still unclear whether antimotility agents are to be recommended in this setting.

Water-absorbing and hydrophilic agents

Although heavily marketed, these are probably the least effective agents in the treatment of TD. Because they are not absorbed by intestinal mucosa, they are, however, probably very safe agents. Absorbants are thought to act by binding toxins or microbial agents or by coating the mucosa. Attapulgite and kaolin with pectin are agents in this category. They may add more bulk to stool, reducing the watery nature of bowel movements, however, they have very little true value and are not to be recommended.

Probiotic agents

Although probiotic agents such as Lactobacillus GG and Saccharomyces boulardii have been used in several trials to study their effectiveness in the prevention of TD, controlled treatment trials have been limited.[38] Both Lactobacillus GG and Saccharomyces boulardii

Table 18.7	Non antibiotic therapies
Agent	**Dose**
Antimotility agents	
Loperamide (Imodium)	2 capsules (4 mg) initially followed by 2 mg after each unformed stool up to 16 mg/day
Diphenoxylate with atropine (Lomotil)	2 tablet (4 mg) q.i.d. for 2 days
Antisecretory agents	
Bismuth subsalicylate (Pepto-Bismol)	30 ml or 2 tablets every 30 min for up to eight doses
Zaldaride maleate	20 mg q.i.d. × 2 days

have been used to treat Clostridium difficile diarrhea. In addition, Saccharomyces boulardii was investigated in the treatment of acute diarrhea in adults and children, showing some promise in a small number of subjects.[39]

TREATMENT OF PARASITIC CAUSES OF TRAVELERS' DIARRHEA

Pathogenic intestinal protozoa such as *Giardia lamblia* and *Entamoeba histolytica* generally cause a more insidious onset of diarrhea with fewer constitutional symptoms. Differences in clinical presentation between bacterial and protozoan pathogens are well described in the subsequent chapter.

The most common parasitic cause of TD is the protozoan Giardia lamblia.[40] Treatment options (Table 18.8) include metronidazole 250 mg t.i.d. for 7 days or tinidazole at a single dose of 2 g. Recent treatment failures with these agents have been reported. Albendazole at a dose of 400 mg daily for 7 days has been used as an alternative but despite some promise in the treatment of Giardia in children, it has shown more limited success in adult travelers. Quinacrine, a medication used for many years for the treatment of Giardia infections but unavailable for the past few years, has recently become available once again. Doses of quinacrine 100 mg t.i.d. for seven days appear to be effective therapy. Refractory cases of giardiasis have been treated using regimens involving combinations of quinacrine and metronidazole or with prolonged courses of nitazoxanide.[41]

Entamoeba histolytica has probably historically been overestimated as a cause of TD. Frequently overdiagnosed in destination laboratories and with the recent discovery of the two morphologically identical but pathogenically disparate strains it has become clear that the risk of E. histolytica infections in travelers is not great. Entamoeba dispar, the nonpathogenic strain, is ten times more prevalent than the pathogenic Entamoeba histolytica. Although molecular methods are available for distinguishing these two morphologically indistinguishable species, diagnosis can also be made by finding hematophagous trophozoites on stool microscopy. Clinical presentation with amebiasis usually takes one of three forms. The first is asymptomatic cyst passage detected in screening stool specimens. Nondysenteric amebiasis, the second form, often presents with cyclical alterations of diarrhea and constipation with fatigue and the third, amebic colitis is manifested by dysentery, crampy abdominal pain, and tenesmus. Patients with asymptomatic cyst passage may be treated with a luminal cystocidal agent alone, such as paromomycin 500 mg t.i.d. for 10 days, iodoquinol 650 mg t.i.d. for 20 days or diloxanide furoate.

For patients with nondysenteric amebiasis or amebic colitis, treatment consists of metronidazole 750 mg t.i.d. for 10 days or tinidazole 2 g daily for 3 days followed by a luminal cystocidal agent. (Table 18.9)[42]

Cyclospora cayetanensis, a coccidian protozoan responsible for syndromes of acute and chronic diarrhea, was first described in outbreaks in Nepal and Peru in the early 1990s. The organism, unrecognized at the time, was probably seen earlier in reports of diarrhea in travelers to Papua New Guinea, Haiti, and Mexico. Reports of Cyclospora in returned travelers from many countries worldwide have now been documented. The organism produces a recognizable syndrome of profound fatigue and anorexia in addition to the gastrointestinal symptoms. Currently, trimethoprim sulfamethoxazole one double strength tablet b.i.d. for 10 days is the only antimicrobial therapy proven to be effective against Cyclospora infections.[43]

Cryptosporidium parvum was first described as an opportunistic pathogen causing diarrhea in AIDS patients, however, reports of cases in returned travelers and a large water-borne outbreak in Milwaukee, Wisconsin, demonstrated that the immunocompetent were also at risk. Although usually a self-limited illness in the immunocompetent, symptoms can still last several weeks. Nitazoxanide holds some promise as therapy based on a study of a small number of patients.[44]

Other parasitic causes of TD and treatment regimens are listed in Table 18.10.

Table 18.8	Drugs for treatment of giardiasis
Drugs	**Dosage**
Adults	
Metronidazole	250 mg p.o. t.i.d. for 5–7 days
Tinidazole	2 g once by p.o.
Quinacrine	100 mg p.o. t.i.d. for 5–7 days
Albendazole	400 mg p.o. once a day for 5 days
Furazolidone	100 mg p.o. q.i.d. for 7–10 days
Paromomycin	500 mg p.o. t.i.d. for 7 days
Refractory cases	
Metronidazole *and*	750 mg p.o. t.i.d. for 14 days
Quinacrine	100 mg p.o. t.i.d. for 14 days
Nitazoxanide	500 mg p.o. b.i.d. for 3 days

Table 18.9	Drug treatment of Entameba histolytica infections
Syndrome	**Dose**
Asymptomatic cyst passer	
E. dispar	No treatment
E. histolytica	Luminal agent: iodoquinol 650 mg p.o. t.i.d. for 20 days paromomycin 500 mg p.o. t.i.d. for 7 days diloxanide furoate 500 mg p.o. t.i.d. for 10 days
Non-dysenteric or amebic colitis:	Metronidazole 750 mg p.o. t.i.d. for 10 days *or* Tinidazole 2 g p.o. once a day for 3 days *or* Ornidazole 1 g p.o. once a day for 5 days *plus* Luminal agent (above)

Table 18.10   **Treatment of other intestinal protozoan causes of travelers' diarrhea**

Pathogen	Drug/dosage
Balantidium coli	Tetracycline 500 mg p.o. q.i.d. for 10 days *or* Metronidazole 750 mg p.o. t.i.d. for 5 days *or* Iodoquinol 650 mg p.o. t.i.d. for 20 days
Cryptosporidium parvum	Nitazoxanide 500 mg p.o. b.i.d. for 3 days
Cyclospora cayetanensis	Trimethoprim/sulfamethoxazole DS (160/320 mg) p.o. b.i.d. for 10 days
Dientamoeba fragilis	Iodoquinol 650 mg p.o. t.i.d. for 20 days *or* Tetracycline 500 mg p.o. q.i.d. for 10days *or* Doxycycline 100 mg p.o. b.i.d. for 10 days *or* Paromomycin 500 mg p.o. t.i.d. for 7 days
Enterocytozoon bieneusi	Fumagillin 20 mg p.o. t.i.d. for 14 days
Encephalitozoon intestinalis	Albendazole 400 mg p.o. b.i.d. for 3 weeks
Isospora belli	TMP/SMX DS (160/320 mg) p.o. q.i.d. for 10 days followed by b.i.d. for 21 days

REFERENCES

1. DuPont HL, Ericsson CD. Prevention and treatment of travelers' diarrhea. *New Engl J Med* 1993; **328**:1821–1837.
2. Peltola H, Gorbach SL. Travelers' diarrhea – Epidemiology and clinical aspects. In: DuPont HL, Steffen R, eds. *Textbook of Travel Medicine and Health*. Hamilton/London: BC Decker; 2001:151–159.
3. Steffen R, Collard F, Tornieporth N, *et al*. Epidemiology, etiology, and impact of travelers' diarrhea in Jamaica. *JAMA* 1999; **281**:811–817.
4. Sonnenburg F von, Tornieporth N, Waiyaki P, *et al*. Risk and aetiology of diarrhoea at various tourist destinations. *Lancet* 2000; **356**:133–134.
5. Jelinek T, Schulte C, Behrens R, *et al*. Imported Falciparum malaria in Europe: sentinel surveillance data from the European network on surveillance of imported infectious diseases. *Clin Infect Dis* 2002; **34**:572–576.
6. Steffen R. Epidemiologic studies of travelers' diarrhea, severe gastrointestinal infections, and cholera. *Rev Inf Dis* 1986; **8**:S122–S130.
7. Cobelens FG, Leentvaar-Kuijpers A, Kleijnen J, *et al*. Incidence and risk factors of diarrhoea in Dutch travellers: consequences for priorities in pretravel health advice. *Trop Med Int Health* 1998; **3**:896–903.
8. Hyams KC, Bourgeois AL, Merrell BR, *et al*. Diarrheal disease during Operation Desert Shield. *N Engl J Med* 1991; **325**:1423–1428.
9. Mattila L. Clinical features and duration of travelers' diarrhea in relation to its etiology. *Clin Inf Dis* 1994; **19**:728–734.
10. World Health Organization. The World Health Report 2001. Geneva, Switzerland: WHO; 2001.
11. Arduino RC. DuPont HL. Enteritis, Enterocolitis and Infectious Diarrhea Syndromes. In: Armstrong D, Cohen J, eds. *Infectious Diseases*. London/Philadelphia: Mosby; 1999:2.35.1–2.35.10.
12. Baer JT, Vugia DJ, Reingold AL, *et al*. HIV infection as a risk factor for shigellosis. *Emerg Infect Dis* 1999; **5**:820–823.
13. Furrer H, Chan P, Weber R, Egger M, Cohort Study SHIV. Increased risk of wasting syndrome in HIV-infected travellers: prospective multicentre study. *Trans R Soc Trop Med Hyg* 2001; **95**:484–486.
14. Guerrant RL, Shields DS, Thorson SM, *et al*. Evaluation and diagnosis of acute infectious diarrhea. *Am J Med* 1985; **78**:91–99.
15. Dupont HL, Ericsson CD, Mathewson JJ, *et al*. Five versus three days of ofloxacin therapy for travelers' diarrhea: a placebo-controlled study. *Antimicrob Agents Chemother* 1992; **36**(87–91):2821–2824.
16. Salam I, Katelaris P, Leigh-Smith S, *et al*. Randomized trial of single-dose ciprofloxacin for travelers' diarrhoea. *Lancet* 1994; **344**:1537–1539.
17. Echeverria P, Verhaert L, Ulyangco CV, *et al*. Antimicrobial resistance and enterotoxin production among isolates of Escherichia coli in the Far East. *Lancet* 1978; **2**:589–592.
18. Sack RB, Rahman M, Yunus M, Khan EH. Antimicrobial resistance in organisms causing diarrheal disease. *Clin Infect Dis* 1997; **24**(**suppl 1**): S102–S105.
19. Wiström J, Jertborn M, Ekwall E, *et al*. Empiric treatment of acute diarrheal disease with norfloxacin: a randomized, placebo-controlled study. *Ann Intern Med* 1992; **117**:202–208.
20. Piddock LJ. Quinolone resistance and Campylobacter spp. *J Antimicrob Chemother* 1995; **36**:891–898.
21. Hoge CW, Gambel JM, Srijan A, *et al*. Trends in antimicrobial resistance among diarrheal pathogens isolated in Thailand over 15 years. *Clin Infect Dis* 1998; **26**:341–345.
22. Kuschner RA, Trofa AF, Thomas RJ, *et al*. The use of azithromycin for the treatment of Campylobacter enteritis in travelers to Thailand, an area where ciprofloxacin resistance is prevalent. *Clin Infec Dis* 1995; **21**:536–541.
23. DuPont HL, Jiang ZD, Ericsson CD, *et al*. Rifaximin versus ciprofloxacin for the treatment of travelers' diarrhea: A randomized, double-blind clinical trial. *Clin Infect Dis* 2001; **33**:1807–1815.
24. Greenough WB. Oral rehydration therapy: something new, something old. *Infect Dis Clin Pr* 1998; **7**:97–100.
25. Ericsson CD, Tannenbaum C, Charles TT. Antisecretory and anti-inflammatory properties of bismuth subsalicylate. *Rev Infect Dis* 1990; **12**(**suppl 1**):S16–S20.
26. Steffen R. World wide efficacy of bismuth subsalicylate in the treatment of travelers' diarrhea. *Rev infect Dis* 1990; **12**(**suppl 1**):S80–S86.
27. Okhuysen PC, DuPont HL, Ericsson CD, *et al*. Zaldaride maleate (a new calmodulin antagonist) versus loperamide in the treatment of travelers' diarrhea: randomized, placebo-controlled trial. *Clin Infect Dis* 1995; **21**(2):341–344.
28. Cezard JP, Duhamel JF, Meyer M, *et al*. Efficacy and tolerability of racecadotril in acute diarrhea in children. *Gastroenterology* 2001; **120**:799–805.
29. Ericsson CD, Johnson PC. Safety and Efficacy of Loperamide. *Am J Med* 1990; **88**(**suppl 6A**):10S–14S.
30. Schiller LR, Santa Ana CA, Morawski SG, *et al*. Mechanism of the anti-diarrheal effect of loperamide. *Gastroenterology* 1984; **86**:1475–1480.
31. Johnson PC, Ericsson CD, DuPont HL, *et al*. Comparison of loperamide with bismuth subsalicylate for the treatment of acute travelers' diarrhea. *JAMA* 1986; **255**:757–760.
32. Murtaza A, Khan SR, Butt KS, *et al*. Paralytic ileus, a serious complication in acute diarrhoea disease among infants in developing countries. *Acta Paediatr Scand* 1989; **78**(5):701–705.
33. Heap J, Macnair A. Loperamide in childhood diarrhoea. *Lancet* 1980; **i**:1085–1086.
34. Bell BP, Griffin PM, Lozano P, *et al*. Predictors of hemolytic uremic syndrome in children during a large outbreak of Escherichia coli O157: H7 infections. *Pediatrics* 1997; **100**:E12.
35. Ericsson CD, DuPont HL, Mathewson JJ. Single dose ofloxacin plus loperamide compared with single dose or three days of ofloxacin in the treatment of travelers' diarrhea. *J Travel Med* 1997; **4**:3–7.

36. DuPont HL, Hornick RB. Adverse effect of Lomotil therapy in shigellosis. *JAMA* 1973; **226**:1525–1528.

37. Petruccelli BP, Murphy GS, Sanchez JL, *et al.* Treatment of travelers' diarrhea with ciprofloxacin and loperamide. *J Infect Dis* 1992; **165**:557–560.

38. Reid G. Probiotics in the Treatment of Diarrheal Diseases. *Curr Infect Dis Rep* 2000; **2**:78–83.

39. Hochter W, Chase D, Hagenhoff G. Saccharomyces boulardii in acute adult diarrhoea. *Munch Med Wochenschr* 1990; **132**:188–192.

40. Ortega YR. Adam RD. Giardia: overview and update. *Clin Infect Dis* 1997; **25**:545–550.

41. Nash TE, Ohl CA, Thomas E, *et al.* Treatment of patients with refractory giardiasis. *Clin Infect Dis* 2001; **33**:22–28.

42. Petri WA Jr, Singh U. Diagnosis and management of amebiasis. *Clin Infect Dis* 1999; **29**:1117–1125.

43. Connor BA, Reidy J. Soave, Cyclosporiasis: clinical and histopathologic correlates. *Clin Infect Dis* 1999; **28**:1216–1222.

44. Doumbo O, Rossignol JF, Pichard E, *et al.* Nitazoxanide in the treatment of cryptosporidial diarrhea and other intestinal parasitic infections associated with acquired immunodeficiency syndrome in tropical Africa. *Am J Trop Med Hyg* 1997; **56**:637–639.

CHAPTER 19 # Self-diagnosis and Treatment of Travelers' Diarrhea

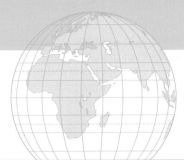

David R. Shlim

KEYPOINTS

- As preventive measures can reduce but never completely eliminate the risk of travelers' diarrhea (TD), the focus has shifted to how the traveler might accurately and safely self diagnose and treat their diarrheal illness when it occurs

- The abrupt onset of relatively uncomfortable diarrhea is bacterial in origin, and can be treated with an antibiotic as soon as the illness is clearly demonstrated to be present

- The treatment of bacterial diarrhea is with a fluoroquinolone or azithromycin for 1–2 days only

- The gradual onset of not so troublesome diarrhea is usually protozoal in origin. Empiric treatment with tinidazole or metronidazole can be offered to travelers on trips of a month or longer, or who may be traveling in a very remote area

- If the patient experiences a subsequent episode of diarrhea after the first episode has cleared, it can be treated with a repeat dose of the same antibiotic, as the etiology is almost certainly a new bacteria

INTRODUCTION

Diarrhea is the most frequent illness associated with travel to developing countries, affecting 30–70% of travelers in the first 2 weeks of their trip.[1,2] Historically, the focus of travel medicine advice as been on how the traveler might take precautions that could prevent travelers' diarrhea (TD) in the first place. Despite the emphasis on these personal hygiene measures (often abbreviated as 'boil it, peel it, or forget it'), the rate of TD in travelers has not diminished in the past 50 years. In addition, there are no scientific studies that support that travelers are able to actively prevent TD through being cautious with what they eat. Thus, the focus has shifted to how the traveler might accurately and safely self-diagnose and treat their diarrheal illness when it occurs. Treatment is now so effective that this method can often limit the duration of illness to less than a day. Therefore, travel medicine practitioners should make it a part of their practice to teach travelers how to treat diarrheal illness when it occurs. The following chapter will review the history of travelers' diarrhea, the etiology, and the reasons that self-diagnosis and treatment can be safely and effectively used in travelers.

ETIOLOGY AND HISTORY OF TRAVELERS' DIARRHEA

The rate of infection with pathogens causing travelers' diarrhea in Mexico was initially determined to be around 30% when the syndrome was first recognized in the 1950s.[3] Subsequent studies have confirmed a rate of TD that varies between 30–70%, depending on the destination. When studies gradually included longer-term travelers, the risk of TD was found to be constant for the first one to two years of travel or residence in a high risk country.[4] The cumulative chance of getting diarrhea during 1–3 months of travel in a high risk destination approaches 100%. Despite dozens of published books aimed at helping travelers prevent diarrhea, and the growth of travel medicine as a specialty from the late 1980's, the rate of diarrhea in travelers has not diminished.

When diarrhea was first determined to be a risk of travel from developed countries to developing countries, the etiology was still unknown. Laboratories were only able to culture for *Salmonella* or *Shigella* spp, and these were almost always negative. Attempts to explain TD by invoking protozoal parasites or viruses also failed to find enough of these organisms to account for the prevalence of TD.[5] The use of prophylactic antibiotics, however, did decrease the risk of TD, suggesting that the syndrome was probably caused by as yet unrecognized bacteria.[6]

In the early 1970s, several papers were published describing a new form of *Escherischii coli* that could produce enterotoxins that caused diarrhea.[7] These organisms became known as enterotoxigenic *E. coli*, or ETEC. ETEC has proved to be the major cause of diarrhea in all surveys of travelers' diarrhea, but the rate varies in different parts of the world, from a maximum of 37% in Asian studies, to 70% in Latin American studies.[8] The discovery of another bacteria capable of causing diarrhea came in the late 1970s with the recognition of *Campylobacter* species.[9,10] *Campylobacter* species accounts for an additional 10–18% of TD.[11,12]

Rotavirus, discovered in 1973, became known as a prominent cause of severe diarrhea in hospitalized children in developing countries.[13] However, the median incidence of rotavirus in 14 studies of TD was 2.5%, and other pathogens were often present.[14] The cumulative incidence of gastrointestinal viruses rarely exceeds 8%.[13] Protozoan infections are rare in the short-term traveler, and account for less than 15% of infections even in longer term travelers and expatriates. Thus, TD has proven to be a disease of predominantly bacterial origin.

PREVENTION OF TRAVELERS' DIARRHEA

When effective antibiotics became available, studies were done to see if they could prevent TD. Early studies were done in Peace Corps volunteers in Kenya and Morocco using doxycycline 100 mg/day. The rates of protection were 86% and 83% respectively.[15,16] Subsequent studies utilizing co-trimoxazole and later ciprofloxacin were performed, and found a protective efficacy of over 90%.[17]

In spite of these studies, travel medicine experts have been reluctant to prescribe antibiotics widely for prevention of TD. There are several reasons for this reluctance. The disease was felt to be benign and self-limited, and the risk of adverse reactions from widespread use of antibiotics in healthy travelers was felt to not be justified. Thus, although antibiotics are effective at preventing TD, they have not been widely utilized in this way.

SELF-DIAGNOSIS AND TREATMENT OF TRAVELERS' DIARRHEA

If preventive measures have not been effective, and if prophylactic antibiotics are considered effective, but not suitable for most travel, then the only remaining strategy is to treat those individuals who have already acquired diarrhea. Initially, this strategy was not encouraged because TD was felt to be a mild, self-limited infection.[18] With growing recognition that TD disrupts travel plans, frequently lasts for 7 days or more, and often causes severe discomfort, this advice was no longer acceptable for most people. Even when therapy was considered to be indicated, physicians felt that treatment could not be initiated without having a culture-proven etiology. Since bacterial cultures are not readily available, and it often takes 3–4 days to get results, the reluctance to recommend empiric treatment based on symptoms led to few people actually being treated with antibiotics. Now that bacterial pathogens have been confirmed as the predominant etiology of TD, and certain antibiotics proved to have a wide spectrum of activity against enteric pathogens, the concept of travelers treating themselves based on symptoms has become more acceptable.

A strategy of self-diagnosis and treatment with antibiotics was promoted directly to travelers in Nepal in the 1980s, as part of medical advice given to trekkers heading into remote areas with no possibility of medical care for weeks at a time.[19] People who became ill were forced to diagnose and treat their own ailments, and instructions needed to be tailored to this specific group. The growing acceptance of self-diagnosis and treatment of TD coincided with shortening the length of empiric treatment. What initially had been a 7–10 day course of antibiotics was shortened first to 5 days,[20] then 3 days,[21] and now to a 1 day course, or even a single dose.[22] The availability of such a simplified treatment lowered the threshold for travelers to decide to treat themselves. This strategy has become so effective that it can now be used safely and effectively wherever TD is a risk, even if medical care were theoretically available. Indeed, a study of domestically acquired diarrhea in Chicago demonstrated a significant shortening of illness with the use of empiric ciprofloxacin.[23]

THE RATIONALE FOR SELF-DIAGNOSIS AND TREATMENT

In order to be confident that travelers can self-diagnose and treat an illness effectively, three criteria should be met. These are:
1. The etiology of the disease should be well known.
2. The diagnosis should have a simple, clinical definition.
3. The treatment should be simple, effective, and low risk.

In the case of TD, the etiology became clear in 30 years of studies that proved that bacterial pathogens are the predominant cause of TD, particularly in the first 1–2 weeks of travel. Bacterial pathogens account for up to 90% of all episodes of TD in the first week of travel.

Experience in treating over 20 000 people for TD at the CIWEC Clinic Travel Medicine Center in Katmandu, Nepal, confirmed a simple, clinical definition of bacterial TD: 'The sudden onset of relatively uncomfortable diarrhea.' This definition highlights the two consistent features of bacterial diarrhea pathogens: they cause a relatively abrupt onset of symptoms, and the symptoms are bothersome from the very beginning. This definition stands in contrast to the clinical definition of protozoal-caused diarrhea: 'The gradual onset of not so severe diarrhea.'

Once the traveler can ascertain whether they most likely have a bacterial pathogen, the choice of treatment has been simple, and getting simpler. Fluoroquinolones became the drug of choice in the 1990s, with ciprofloxacin being the most popular choice. Treatment is now generally recognized as effective with either a single dose of ciprofloxacin, or twice-daily doses, for 1–2 days. Side-effects from fluoroquinolones used in a short course tend to be rare and mild, with virtually no risk of a life-threatening reaction. Azithromycin is an alternative choice in areas known to have fluoroquinolone-resistance Campylobacter.

SYMPTOMS OF BACTERIAL DIARRHEA

Bacterial diarrhea can present with a wide spectrum of severity, from a few urgent loose stools, to profound prostration associated with fever, abdominal pain, blood in the stool, and vomiting. If vomiting is present, it almost always occurs at the beginning of the illness, and usually ends after 6–12 h, at which point the diarrhea continues alone. Bacterial diarrhea can be either predominantly secretory, or invasive. The presence of fever, white blood cells or frank blood in the stool suggests an invasive form of bacterial pathogen. The predominance of watery stool without pus or blood suggests a secretory diarrhea, mediated by a toxin. Either form of diarrhea can be equally distressing to the patient and require treatment.

The mean duration of diarrhea without antibiotic treatment is 4–5 days, but 8–15% of cases can last 7 days or more, and 2% of cases can last for a month or more.[24]

DIAGNOSIS OF TRAVELERS' DIARRHEA

Stool examination provides useful information when done in a reliable lab. White blood cells in the stool are highly correlated with the presence of a bacterial pathogen. Rarely, an unsuspected protozoal pathogen might be present, such as *Giardia lamblia*, *Cyclospora cayetanensis*, or Cryptosporidium spp. Depending on the history, these protozoal pathogens may be co-infections. Studies at the CIWEC Clinic Travel Medicine Center found an incidence of 17% of diarrhea patients who had more than one pathogen in their stool exam.[12]

Stool examination in an unreliable lab can be worse than no exam at all, with false positive findings the most common error. Thus, someone with bacterial diarrhea may be told that they have *E histolytica* (a very common error in local labs in Nepal), and multiple courses of drugs may be prescribed that will not treat the actual bacterial diarrheal infection.

Cultures are the only way to determine the presence of specific bacterial pathogens. However, one only finds what one seeks, so unless the lab is particularly interested in the etiology of bacterial diarrhea, they may not be able to diagnose ETEC, and they may not use enriched agar plates to detect other pathogens. On top of that, stool culture can take three days or more to make a definitive diagnosis. Therefore, empiric treatment for suspected bacterial diarrhea is still more practical.

TREATMENT OF BACTERIAL DIARRHEA

The current drug of choice is a fluoroquinolone, of which ciprofloxacin is the most popular. Length of treatment ranges from a single dose,[22] to b.i.d. for 3 days. The usual dose is 500 mg every 12 h, for 1–2 days. Single dose treatment with either norfloxacin 800 mg, ciprofloxacin 1000 mg, or ciprofloxacin 500 mg, have all been shown to be effective treatment for bacterial TD.[25] Studies in Thailand have found a high percentage of quinolone-resistant Campylobacter, and azithromycin has been used empirically in that country.[26] Subsequent spread of quinolone resistance may lead to wider use of azithromycin as empiric treatment. The dosing regimen has not been well-confirmed in studies. Most authors use 500 mg as a single dose per day, for 2 days, for adults and 10mg/kg per dose once a day for 2 days for children.

The use of diphenoxylate (Lomotil) and later loperamide (Imodium) as a treatment of TD has been controversial. One study suggested that volunteers infected with *Shigella* had a prolongation of fever and diarrhea compared to a placebo group.[27] This led to caution about using a bowel paralyzing agent in the presence of signs and symptoms of dysentery. However, in the presence of an antibiotic, loperamide appears to be safe to use, even with dysenteric symptoms.[28] Travelers can be advised that it is safe to use loperamide in the presence of severe diarrhea if they have already started an antibiotic. The combination of trimethoprim-sulfamethoxazole and loperamide in a study among American students in Mexico shortened the illness to 1 h.[29] Loperamide is particularly useful if travel is necessary on the days that one is ill with diarrhea.

Anti-emetics can have a role to play in the treatment of TD. They are usually ineffective when given orally to a person who is actively vomiting. However, they can help speed rehydration and return to nutrition when taken while nausea persists but active vomiting has stopped.

Children are equally, if not more, susceptible to TD. Since ciprofloxacin is contraindicated, at present, for children under age 18 (although some travel medicine experts feel that it can be safely used in children in light of the favorable experience of using ciprofloxacin in children with cystic fibrosis), the drug of choice for treatment of TD in children is now azithromycin, in a dose of 10 mg/kg per day as a single dose for 2 days. The drug is available in a powder form, which can be reconstituted with water when the drug is needed.

Nalidixic acid, in either liquid or pill form, is an alternative treatment for children, in a dose of 50mg/kg per day in three divided doses for one to two days. (Note: this regimen is different from the published regimen of 55 mg/kg per day in four divided doses. However, the simpler regimen has been proven effective over many years at the CIWEC Clinic Travel Medicine Center). This drug is difficult to obtain in the USA, but is available in many developing countries.

Trimethoprim-sulfamethoxazole should not be used as empiric treatment of TD anymore because the rates of resistance are consistently over 50% in all developing countries.

Some travel medicine practitioners have expressed concern that the frequent use of antibiotics in travelers might accelerate the development of resistant bacteria. However, experience has shown that travelers make an insignificant contribution to exposing all the bacteria of a subcontinent to antibiotics. Only when the same antibiotic is used widely by local people have resistant bacteria been shown to emerge.

Another concern that has arisen more recently is the observation that the outcome of *E coli* 0157:H7 infection in children may be worsened by the use of antibiotics.[30] Although this situation needs to be monitored, *E coli* 0157:H7 is almost never encountered in travel situations to developing countries, even though numerous etiologic studies have specifically looked for it.

OTHER PATHOGENS ASSOCIATED WITH TRAVELERS' DIARRHEA

The most frequently identified protozoa in travelers' diarrhea is *Giardia lamblia*, found in 5–12% of travelers who acquire diarrhea in a developing country. With an incubation period of 1–2 weeks, Giardia is rarely the cause of diarrhea in short-term travelers. Other protozoal pathogens that are found less than 5% of the time are *E histolytica* and *Cryptosporidium*. *Cyclospora cayetanensis* is a coccidian pathogen that can present with the sudden onset of relatively uncomfortable diarrhea.[31] The initial symptoms diminish after a few days, and the patient experiences persistent anorexia, fatigue, and low-grade diarrhea with a mean of 6 weeks duration. Cyclospora is common in Nepal, Peru, and Guatemala, but tends to be highly seasonal.

Protozoal infections other than Cyclospora tend to have a gradual onset, with the patient noting some loose stools, increased gas, or abdominal cramping, but not being incapacitated by the symptoms. The symptoms persist, however, and the patient begins to feel fatigue, occasional urgent loose bowel movements, and decreased interest in food. In a study at the CIWEC Clinic, patients who proved to have a bacterial pathogen in their stool presented for evaluation within 3 days of the onset of their illness. In contrast, those who proved to have a protozoal pathogen causing their symptoms did not present for evaluation until two weeks after the onset of their illness.[12] Travelers without access to reliable medical care who suspect that they have a protozoal infection are most often infected with *G lamblia*. Empiric treatment consists of tinidazole 2000 mg/day as a single dose, for 2 days. An alternative is metronidazole, 250 mg three times per day for 7 days. Treatment for the main pathogens associated with travelers' diarrhea is summarized in Table 19.1.

Toxic gastroenteritis, or food poisoning, can also present with sudden onset of diarrhea and/or vomiting. This syndrome is recognizable when the symptoms abruptly end after 6–12 h. The patient who presents with toxic gastroenteritis will often appear ill, but talk

---

Table 19.1   A list of selected pathogens along with their characteristic presentations and empiric treatment

Pathogen	Characteristic symptoms	Empiric treatment
Bacterial pathogens	Abrupt onset of relatively uncomfortable diarrhea	Ciprofloxacin 500 mg q.12 h for 1 day. Other fluoroquinolones are also acceptable.
Giardia lamblia	Gradual onset of not so troublesome diarrhea associated with increased gas and 'churning' intestines	Tinidazole 2000 mg/day as a single dose for 2 days; Metronidazole 250 mg t.i.d. for 7 days
Entamoeba histolytica	Crampy, frequent small stools for 1–2 days, alternating with 1–2 days of no diarrhea	Tinidazole 2000 mg/day as a single dose for 3 days. Ideally should be followed by diloxanide furoate or paromomycin for 10 days.
Cyclospora cayetanensis	Sudden onset of uncomfortable diarrhea for 2–3 days. Followed by decreased diarrhea, but increasing fatigue and anorexia	Co-trimoxazole DS b.i.d. for 7–10 days

about their symptoms in the past tense: 'I was so ill last night.' There are no tests to confirm the presence of a toxin in the patient, so this syndrome can only be diagnosed clinically.

Viral gastroenteritis is not reliably distinguishable from bacterial diarrhea by symptoms. However, since viral pathogens are found in less than 5–8% of travelers with diarrhea, the impact on treatment decisions is minimal.

CONCLUSION

All travelers headed to developing countries with a risk of TD should be taught the following:

- The abrupt onset of relatively uncomfortable diarrhea is bacterial, and can be treated with an antibiotic as soon as the illness is clearly determined to be present.
- The treatment of bacterial diarrhea is with a fluoroquinolone or azithromycin for 1–2 days only.
- The gradual onset of not so troublesome diarrhea is usually protozoal in origin. Empiric treatment with tinidazole or metronidazole can be offered to travelers on longer journeys (>1 month), or who may be in a very remote area.
- If the patient experiences a subsequent episode of diarrhea after the first episode has cleared, it can be treated with a repeat dose of the same antibiotic, as the etiology is almost certainly new bacteria.

REFERENCES

1. Merson MH, Morris GK, Sack DA, *et al.* Travelers' diarrhea in Mexico: A prospective study of physicians and family members attending a congress. *N Engl J Med* 1976; **294**:1279–1305.
2. Steffen R, Linde F van der, Gyr K, Schar M. Epidemiology of diarrhea in travelers. *J Am Med Assoc* 1983; **249**:1176–1180.
3. Kean BH. The diarrhea of travelers to Mexico: summary of a five-year study. *Ann Intern Med* 1963; **59**:605–614.
4. Shlim DR, Hoge CW, Rajah R. Scott R McN, Pandey P, Echeverria P. Persistent high risk of diarrhea among foreigners in Nepal during the first two years of residence. *Clin Infect Dis* 1999; **29**:613–616.
5. Kean BH. The diarrhea of travelers to Mexico. *Ann Intern Med* 1963; **59**:605–614.
6. Kean B, Schaffner W, Brennan RW, Waters SR. The diarrhea of travelers: V. Prophylaxis with phthalylsulfathiazole and neomycin sulphate. *JAMA* 1962; **180**:107–111.
7. Gorbach SL, Kean BH, Evans DG, Evans DJ, Bessudo D. Travelers' diarrhea and toxigenic Escherichia coli. *N Engl J Med* 1975; **292**:933–936.
8. Peltola H, Gorbach SL. Travelers' diarrhea: Epidemiology and clinical aspects. In: DuPont HL, Steffen R, eds. *Textbook of Travel Medicine and Health.* 2nd edn. Hamilton: BC Decker; 2001:151–159.
9. Butzler JP, Dekeyser P, Detrain M, Dehaen F. Related vibrio in stools. *J Pediatr* 1973; **83**:493–495.
10. Skirrow MB. Campylobacter enteritis: a 'new' disease. *BMJ* 1977; **2**:9–11.
11. Taylor DN, Echeverria P, Blaser MJ, *et al.* Polymicrobial aetiology of travellers' diarrhoea. *Lancet* 1985; **1**(8425):381–383.
12. Taylor DN, Houston R, Shlim DR, *et al.* Etiology of diarrhea among travelers and foreign residents in Nepal. *J Am Med Assoc* 1988; **260**:1245–1248.
13. Blacklow NR, Greenberg HB. Viral gastroenteritis. *N Engl J Med* 1991; **325**:252–264.
14. Midthun K, Black RE. Viral diarrheas. In: Strickland GT, ed. *Hunter's Tropical Medicine and Emerging Infectious Diseases.* 8th edn. Philadelphia: WB Saunders; 2000:220–223.
15. Sack DA, Kaminsky DC, Sack RB, *et al.* Prophylactic doxycycline for travelers' diarrhea: results of a prospective double-blind study of Peace Corps volunteers in Kenya. *N Engl J Med* 1978; **298**:758–763.
16. Sack RB, Froehlich JL, Zulich AW, *et al.* Prophylactic doxycycline for travelers' diarrhea: results of a prospective double-blind study of Peace Corps volunteers in Morocco. *Gastroenterology* 1979; **76**:1368–1373.
17. Taylor DN. Quinolones as chemoprophylactic agents for travelers' diarrhea (editorial). *J Travel Med* 1994; **1**:119–121.
18. Gorbach SL. Bacterial diarrhoea and its treatment. *Lancet* 1987; **2**(8572):1378–1382.
19. Shlim DR. Safety and health. In: Armington S, ed. *Trekking in the Nepal Himalaya.* 4th edn. South Yarra, Australia: Lonely Planet Publications; 1985:52–69.
20. Pichler HET, Diridl G, Stickler K, Wolf D. Clinical efficacy of ciprofloxacin compared with placebo in bacterial diarrhea. *Am J Med* 1987; **83**(suppl 4A):329–332.
21. Bassily S, Hyams KC, El-Masry NA, *et al.* Short-course norfloxacin and trimethoprim sulfamethoxazole treatment of shigellosis and salmonellosis in Egypt. *Am J Trop Med Hyg* 1994; **51**:219–223.
22. Salam I, Katelaris P, Leigh-Smith S, Farthing MJG. Randomized trial of single-dose ciprofloxacin for travellers' diarrhoea. *Lancet* 1994; **344**:1537–1539.
23. Goodman LJ, Trenholme GM, Kaplan RL, *et al.* Empiric antimicrobial therapy of domestically acquired acute diarrhea in urban adults. *Arch Intern Med* 1990; **150**:541–546.
24. Ericsson CD, Dupont HL. Travelers' diarrhea: approaches to prevention and treatment. *Clin Infect Dis* 1993; **16**:616–624.
25. Gotuzzo E, Oberhelman RA, Maguina C, *et al.* Comparison of single-dose treatment with norfloxacin and standard 5-day treatment with trimethoprim-sulfamethoxazole for acute shigellosis in adults. *Antimicrob Agents Chemother* 1989; **33**:1101–1104.
26. Kuschner RA, Trofa AF, Thomas RJ, *et al.* Use of azithromycin for the treatment of campylobacter enteritis in travelers to Thailand, an area where ciprofloxacin resistance is prevalent. *Clin Infect Dis* 1995; **21**:536–541.
27. DuPont HL, Hornick RB. Adverse effect of Lomotil therapy in shifellosis. *JAMA* 1973; **226**:1525–1528.
28. Murphy GS, Bedhidatta L, Echeverria P, *et al.* Ciprofloxacin and loperamide in the treatment of bacillary dysentery. *Ann Intern Med* 1993; **118**:582–586.
29. Ericsson CD, DuPont HL, Mathewson JJ, *et al.* Treatment of traveler's diarrhea with sulfamethoxazole and trimethoprim and loperamide. *J Am Med Assoc* 1990; **263**:257–261.
30. O'Ryan M, Prado V. Risk of the hemolytic-uremic syndrome after antibiotic treatment of Escherichia coli O157: H7 infections. *N Engl J Med* 2000; **26**(343):1271.
31. Shlim DR, Cohen MT, Eaton M, *et al.* An alga-like organism associated with an outbreak of prolonged diarrhea among foreigners in Nepal. *Am J Trop Med Hyg* 1991; **45**:383–389.

CHAPTER 20 The Pregnant and Breast-feeding Traveler

Sheila M. Mackell and Susan A. Anderson

KEYPOINTS

- Assessment of the pregnant traveler includes a detailed obstetrical history, contraindications to travel, access to medical care abroad and possible risk activities such as travel modalities, physical recreation and travel at altitude

- With few exceptions, live vaccines are contraindicated during pregnancy

- Since malaria poses a considerable hazard to mother and child, prevention measures, including chemoprophylaxis, are paramount

- Food and water precautions are essential in the prevention of pathogens that are of particular high risk during pregnancy (e.g., hepatitis E, listeriosis and toxoplasmosis)

- As a general rule, the advantages of breast-feeding outweigh the low risks to the infant that maternal drug therapy might entail

INTRODUCTION

The availability of convenient international and domestic travel has opened up the possibilities for pregnant women who have any reason to travel. As many working women have chosen to delay childbearing, business travel during pregnancy becomes a reality for many.

Much of the information on the pregnant traveler is based on small studies, anecdotal information, and extrapolation from non-pregnant travelers. While evidence based recommendations are ideal, they are lacking for pregnant women. This chapter will summarize available data and experience in this growing field of travel medicine.

PREGNANCY

Routine obstetric care starts at approximately 10–12 weeks gestation, and continues monthly until the seventh month. Then pregnancy is followed every 2 weeks until 36 weeks, when weekly monitoring is standard.

Mild to moderate exercise is not associated with increased pregnancy loss.[1] Since running and high impact aerobics may divert blood from the uterus, they must be done with care as the pregnancy progresses. American College of Obstetrics and Gynecology (ACOG) recommen-dations for exercise during pregnancy are as follows[2]:

- Maternal heart rate <140 bpm during exercise
- Strenuous activity <15 mins
- Avoid core temperature >38 °C (101.4 °F)
- No exercise in the supine position after the fourth month.

These recommendations are somewhat controversial.[3] Current studies are looking at modification of these recommendations for the woman who was a moderate to competitive athlete prior to pregnancy. Many pregnant women in this group have exceeded the recommendations in the ACOG guidelines without known harm to the fetus.

PRE-TRAVEL PREPARATION

Pre-travel preparation for the traveler who is pregnant starts with a review of her obstetric and medical history. Any history of pregnancy problems, bleeding, pre-term labor, or chronic illness warrants consultation with an obstetrician regarding the advisability of the proposed itinerary. Contraindications to travel are listed in Table 20.1.[4]

Counseling on the timing of travel should be done. According to the American Academy of Obstetrics and Gynecology, the safest time for a pregnant woman to travel is the second trimester. The pregnancy is established and the extra weight is not usually a functional limitation for the mother. The risk of miscarriage is highest in all women in the first trimester. First trimester vaccination is not recommended due to unknown effects on the developing fetal organs. In addition, antimalarial chemoprophylaxis carries more uncertainties during the first trimester. Obstetric risks during the third trimester include pregnancy complications such as bleeding, pre-eclampsia, and pre-term labor and delivery.

Table 20.1	Potential contraindications for travel during pregnancy

Medical risk factors
Valvular heart disease
Chronic organ system dysfunction requiring ongoing assessment and medication
Severe anemia

Obstetric risk factors
History of miscarriage
Threatened abortion or vaginal bleeding during present pregnancy
Incompetent cervix
Premature labor, premature rupture of membranes, or existing placental abnormalities
History of ectopic pregnancy (should be ruled out prior to travel with ultrasound)
Multiple gestations in present pregnancy
History of toxemia, hypertension, diabetes with any pregnancy
Primigravida ≤35 or ≥15 years old

Travel to destination that may be hazardous
High altitude
Areas endemic for or where epidemics are occurring of life threatening food or insect borne infections
Areas where chloroquine resistant *Plasmodium falciparum* is endemic
Areas where live vaccines are required and recommended

Adapted from the CDC Health Information for International Travel 2003–2004.[4]

The physiologic changes of pregnancy may impact travel. Reduced exercise and heat tolerance, the elevated heart rate from increased plasma volume, and physiologic anemia may exaggerate travel-related discomforts.

Access to medical care abroad

Awareness of local medical resources and qualified obstetric care at the destination is essential knowledge for the pregnant traveler. She should be encouraged to consider in advance how she may feel if pregnancy complications or adverse outcomes occur during or because of her travel. Any sign of an obstetric problem, such as bleeding, abdominal pain, premature rupture of membranes, severe or recurrent headaches, or high blood pressure should prompt an evaluation by a qualified physician. Investigating the blood supply and screening procedures at the destination (HIV, hepatitis), and knowing her blood type is wise. While many travel itineraries require focus on the risk of infectious diseases, maternal trauma remains the leading cause of fetal death. Motor vehicle accidents and falls can cause placental abruption or preterm labor. Extra care needs to be taken later in pregnancy, when balance and position are more difficult to maintain.[5]

Personal health insurance should be checked for limitations to coverage. Unanticipated delivery away from home or approved health-care providers may not be covered under some insurance policies. Evacuation insurance that will specifically cover any pregnancy or delivery problem is advisable. Exclusions to insurance benefits should be carefully scrutinized.

Travel by air

Airline regulations vary. Most United States air carriers require a physician letter beyond the 36th week of gestation for domestic travel and at the 35th week for international travel. The letter should document the status of the pregnancy and the expected delivery date.

Aircraft cabins are routinely pressurized to an altitude of 6500–8000 feet (2000–2400 meters). The corresponding partial pressure of oxygen lowers the maternal oxygenation to a far greater extent than the fetus. Fetal oxygenation is affected to a much lesser degree due to presence of fetal hemoglobin, which binds more tightly to oxygen molecules. The hemoglobin-oxygen dissociation curve permits the fetus to remain oxygenated at a wide fluctuation of maternal oxygen values.[6] Hence, the risk of travel to the fetus is not hypoxia.

Because of the expanded plasma volume and demands of the developing fetus, mild anemia is common during pregnancy. Iron supplementation is recommended for all pregnant women. If the anemia is more pronounced, and travel is essential, supplemental oxygen can be considered at hemoglobin levels of <8.5 g/dL. Air travel by pregnant women with sickle cell anemia should be considered only after careful review of overall pregnancy status and close consultation with the obstetrician involved.

Cabin humidity aboard the airplane is approximately 8%. In this relatively dry environment, increased fluid intake over normal is recommended to maintain placental blood flow. Six to eight glasses of non-caffeine containing fluid are the recommended amount for normal daily intake during pregnancy.

During long flights, thrombophlebitis may occur in any traveler due to venous stasis from immobility. A pregnant woman is at increased risk of thrombophlebitis due to the hormones of pregnancy and the pressure of the uterus on the veins, impeding flow.[1] Although no randomized, controlled studies have been done, it is recommended that pregnant women sit in an aisle seat, stand up and move, or walk hourly while on long flights. Isometric lower leg exercises can also be done while seated to promote venous return. Aspirin is not recommended for routine use in pregnancy, particularly during the last three months, when increased bleeding and adverse fetal effects may occur.

Radiation exposure during pregnancy should be limited. The eighth to fourteenth week of gestation are considered the most radiation sensitive for the fetus, as brain and nervous system development occur. The fetus is exposed to the same amount of radiation as the mother since a mother's body does not provide an effective shield from radiation exposure. Current Federal Aviation Administration recommendations[7] are for a total pregnancy exposure of 1 mSv, regardless of the number of months flying, or a monthly limit of 0.5 mSv. The amount of radiation exposure per flight depends on the airplane cruising altitude and the duration of the flight. Further details on these recommendations can be obtained from the United States Department of Transportation, Office of Aviation Medicine.[7] Additional suggestions include avoiding travel on the Concorde, which flies at a higher altitude and involves more radiation exposure, and limiting travel along polar routes. Magnetometers at security check points pose no risk of radiation exposure.

Water sports and travel by boat

Pregnant women contemplating a cruise should research the availability of medical care and equipment and trained personnel on board, should pregnancy complications arise. Choices for the treatment of motion sickness are limited by pregnancy.

The risks of water-skiing during pregnancy are external genital lacerations and forceful water entry into the abdominal cavity via the cervix. Miscarriage or peritonitis may result.

Little data exist on scuba diving and pregnancy. Scuba diving is generally considered unsafe at any stage of pregnancy. The potential risks to the fetus of decompression sickness, congenital abnormalities, and hyperbaric oxygen exposure, should decompression sickness occur, are unknown.

Travel by automobile

Recommendations regarding automobile travel include limiting driving to 6 h/day, with stops of 10 min every 2 h.[7] Care should be taken to position the seat belt low on the abdomen to prevent fetal compression in a rapid stop. Lap belts alone are not sufficient restraints and a shoulder-lap belt combination is recommended.

IMMUNIZATIONS

Immunization during pregnancy requires a careful evaluation of the potential risk of a vaccine-preventable disease versus the possible risks of vaccination for both the mother and the fetus. Vaccination during pregnancy is indicated in situations where exposure is highly probable and the disease poses a greater risk to the woman or fetus than the vaccination (risk-benefit ratio). Ideally, all women should be vaccinated before pregnancy as part of preconception care. Whenever possible, the pre-travel visit should be used to update the vaccination status of non-pregnant women of reproductive age.

The risks of immunization during pregnancy are largely theoretical (Table 20.2). There have been no well-controlled studies of vaccine effects on the fetus. Case reports and post-exposure data comprise the knowledge currently available on vaccinating pregnant women.

In general, vaccinations should be avoided in the first trimester of pregnancy due to the uncertain effect of the vaccine on the developing fetus. Live virus vaccines should be avoided in all trimesters, except in special circumstances. Yellow fever vaccine can be given during pregnancy if travel to a high-risk area is unavoidable.[4] Small numbers of pregnant women inadvertently vaccinated with the yellow fever vaccine have been studied.[8] The vaccine did not appear to adversely affect the fetal or maternal outcomes. A letter of waiver can

Table 20.2   **Immunizations during pregnancy**

Immunobiologic agent	Type of vaccine	Issues in pregnancy
Measles; Mumps; Rubella	Live-attenuated	Contraindicated Pregnancy should be delayed for 3 months after MMR is given Check titer if immunity unknown May give immune globulin if exposure
Polio	Trivalent live attenuated (OPV) Killed (IPV)	Avoid in previously non-immune individuals due to risk of vaccine associated paralysis ACIP recommends use in outbreak situation Preferred over OPV in pregnancy
Varicella	Live attenuated	Contraindicated in pregnancy Check titer if exposed to infection during pregnancy; Give VZIG if not immune by history or titer For severe symptoms (pneumonitis/encephalitis) treat with Acyclovir i.v. or p.o. Although no teratogenic effects of the vaccine have been documented, pregnancies occurring within 3 months of the vaccine or vaccinations given inadvertently during pregnancy should be reported to the Varivax registry (800-986-8999).
Tetanus diphtheria	Combined toxoid	Safe in pregnancy Use if lack of primary series or no booster within 10 years
Influenza	Inactivated vaccine	Recommended for all pregnant women in their second or third trimester during influenza season Indicated for pregnant women in any trimester if history of high risk medical condition
Pneumococcus	Polysaccharide	Vaccine used only in high risk pregnancies Post splenectomy
Meningococcal meningitis	Polysaccharide	Administer for high risk exposure
Hemophilus B conjugate	Polysaccharide	For high risk persons
Typhoid (Ty21a)	Live-attenuated bacterial, oral	No data in pregnancy Use should reflect actual risk of disease Avoid in pregnancy on theoretical grounds (live vaccine)
Typhoid Vi	Vi capsular polysaccharide, parental	If indicated
Hepatitis A	Formalin inactivated vaccine	Data on safety in pregnancy are not available; the theoretical risk of vaccination should be weighed against the risk of disease Consider immune globulin rather than vaccine Consider checking titer if prior exposure
Hepatitis B	Recombinant purified hepatitis B surface antigen	Pre-exposure and post-exposure prophylaxis indicated in pregnant women at risk for infection
Yellow fever	Live attenuated	Contraindicated except if exposure unavoidable Give letter of waiver for travel to low risk area
Japanese encephalitis	Killed vaccine	Should reflect actual risk of disease and probable benefit of vaccine JE virus infection acquired during first or second trimester of pregnancy may result in uterine infection and fetal mortality
Tick-borne encephalitis	Inactivated	Not recommended in pregnancy Practice strict tick-bite precautions
Rabies	Killed virus Human diploid cell rabies vaccine (HDCV) or Rabies vaccine adsorbed (RVA)	Post-exposure prophylaxis is indicated during pregnancy. Pre-exposure prophylaxis only when substantial risk for exposure exists
Immune globulins (IG) Pooled or hyperimmune	Immune globulins or specific antitoxin serum including antivenin for snakebite, spider-bite, diphtheria antitoxin, HBIG, rabies IG, tetanus IG, RH *(D) IG, varicella zoster IG	Give appropriate immunoglobulin or antitoxin as indicated for exposure
Cholera	Inactivated whole cell vaccine Killed oral cholera toxin B subunit whole cell (BS-WC) Live attenuated oral cholera vaccine (CVD 103 HgR strain)	Not recommended for any travelers due to low efficacy Not available in the USA. Available in Canada and Europe No live organisms. May be efficacious in high risk situations but not recommended during pregnancy at this time Not recommended in pregnancy Not available in the USA Available in Canada and Europe

Adapted from CDC Information for International Travel, 2003–2004.

be considered for the pregnant traveler going to a low risk destination, where yellow fever vaccine may be required for entry into the country or for travel between certain countries but the actual risk of acquiring the disease is low.

MALARIA AND PREGNANCY

Malaria affects between 300–500 million people a year resulting in over 3 million deaths.[9] Morbidity and mortality are the greatest in children and pregnant women. Malaria during pregnancy may have severe consequences. Data indicate that women are more susceptible to malaria during pregnancy and the immediate postpartum period.[10,11] Pregnancy increases the clinical severity of *Plasmodium falciparum* malaria in women with and without existing immunity.[12] There is preferential sequestration of parasitized red blood cells in the placenta, along with suppression of selected components of the immune system during pregnancy. This can result in intrauterine growth retardation, premature delivery, anemia, fetal loss, maternal death, and/or congenital malaria. Maternal and perinatal mortality markedly increase with infection.

Pregnant travelers need to scrutinize their itinerary and be aware of the increased risk to themselves and their fetus. If a woman is pregnant or plans to become pregnant and cannot defer travel to a high-risk area, appropriate chemoprophylaxis and maximal personal protective measures are essential. Travel to areas where chloroquine resistant strains of plasmodium falciparum exists poses increased risk due to limited data on treatment options. Women who plan to become pregnant while traveling or shortly after also need to be aware of existing information regarding the potential effects of prophylactic or treatment medications on the fetus, and availability of appropriate medical care, should they contract malaria.

Plasmodium vivax malaria occurs more commonly than *P. falciparum* in many parts of the tropics outside Africa.[9] The effects of *P. vivax* infection in pregnancy have not been as well characterized as those of *P. falciparum*. *P. vivax* malaria during pregnancy is associated with maternal anemia and low birthweight but does not appear to be associated with miscarriage, stillbirth or with a shortened duration of pregnancy.[13] Though the effects of *P. vivax* infection are less striking than those of *P. falciparum* infection during pregnancy, antimalarial chemoprophylaxis for travel to predominantly *P. vivax* endemic areas is recommended. Most of the research studies have been conducted on pregnant women living in endemic areas and may not necessarily be extrapolated to non-immune pregnant travelers who are at higher risk of illness.

Guidelines for prevention

Personal protective measures

The pregnant traveler should use a combination of physical and chemical barriers to reduce the risk of contracting malaria. Permethrin-treated bednets should be recommended. They have been studied on pregnant women in Africa and have not caused any harmful effects on the pregnancy. Prudent application of DEET (diethyl-meta-toluamide) in a concentration of upto 35 % can be used during pregnancy. The safety of DEET has been assessed in a single study of women in the second and third trimester of pregnancy in Thailand.[14] There were no neurologic, gastrointestinal, or dermatologic adverse effects reported in the group that applied DEET. DEET was detected in the cord blood of 8% of the infants. There was no effect on survival, development, growth or status at one year of age in this group of infants.

Chemoprophylaxis

In recommending pharmacologic prophylaxis to a pregnant woman, the risk of malaria must be weighed with the benefit of the medica-

tion. For travel to chloroquine sensitive areas, chloroquine may be prescribed safely in the usual adult doses. Chloroquine has been used for decades for both prophylaxis and treatment of malaria during pregnancy without adverse fetal or maternal effects.

If at all possible, travel to areas of chloroquine resistant *P. falciparum* should be deferred during pregnancy. Mefloquine is currently the only available recommended antimalarial for use in chloroquine resistant *P. falciparum* areas. If travel is unavoidable, there are data to support the use of mefloquine in second and third trimesters. A double-blind, placebo controlled study in 339 pregnant women in the second half of pregnancy was done on Thai-Myanmar border. Mefloquine provided 86% protection against *P. falciparum* and 100% protection against *P. vivax*. The study was done in two phases. Excess stillbirths were noted in study Phase I. This finding was not confirmed, however, in the larger Phase II segment of the study.[15]

Phillips-Howard, *et al.* reported on mefloquine use in the first trimester.[16] They looked at first trimester exposures to chloroquine plus proguanil, sulfa plus pyrimethamine and mefloquine. Exposure to mefloquine was not associated with a spontaneous abortion rate above background population rate. In addition, they reviewed a pharmaceutical database of first trimester mefloquine exposures. The overall rate of abnormal outcomes was not significantly different from women taking sulfadoxine-pyrimethamine. Spontaneous abortions were significantly higher with mefloquine than sulfadoxine-pyrimethamine (9.1% versus 2.6%), but the higher rate was comparable to background rates of 7–11%. They concluded that there is no indication that the risk of taking mefloquine in the first trimester of pregnancy is greater than that from any of the other antimalarials studied. The risk of infection with falciparum malaria is considerably greater than that noted to date with the use of mefloquine.

The combination of weekly chloroquine and daily proguanil is safe during pregnancy; however, it is no longer recommended as a first line due to low efficacy in areas of chloroquine resistance. Doxycycline is contraindicated for use in pregnancy due to staining of the fetal teeth. Tetracyclines cross the placenta and can adversely affect fetal skeletal development.[17] The combination of atovaquone plus proguanil (Malarone) is not recommended to date for chemoprophylaxis in pregnancy due to lack of data on the effects of atovaquone use. It is currently classified as Pregnancy Category C (Table 20.3).[18]

Treatment

There is no convincing evidence that the treatment of malaria during pregnancy adversely affects the pregnancy outcome. Quinine has been used for treatment in the third trimester and is probably the safest option if prophylaxis has failed. Stillbirths and congenital malformations have been reported. Hypoglycemia commonly occurs with quinine treatment during pregnancy and blood glucose should be followed closely.

Fansidar (Pyrimethamine/sulfadoxine) has been used for treatment during pregnancy.[19] Infantile jaundice can occur if used close to delivery and the risk of Stevens-Johnson syndrome from the sulfa component must be taken into account. Mefloquine has been used for treatment during pregnancy, but is not approved by the United States Food and Drug Administration for this use.

Atovaquone/Proguanil has not been studied for malaria treatment of pregnant women. It is currently considered an option for treatment in multi-drug resistant *P. falciparum* infections.

The quinghosu derivatives, artesunate and artemether have been used to treat malaria in women in all trimesters of pregnancy in Thailand. They are well tolerated and no adverse pregnancy outcomes have been reported in a case report of 441 women in Thailand. Further study is needed of the use of these compounds in preg-

Table 20.3   Malaria chemoprophylaxis in pregnant travelers

Antimalarials	Dose	Comments
Chloroquine sensitive areas Chloroquine (CQ)	300 mg base (equal to 500 mg of phosphate salt) Start 1 week before travel and continue for 4 weeks after travel to malarious zone	Safe Reactions rare
Chloroquine resistant areas (options for Chemoprophylaxis) Mefloquine (MQ)	250 mg weekly Start 1 week before travel and continue for 4 weeks after travel to malarious zone	Safety in first trimester not fully established although CDC recommended Possible trend in stillbirths noted in some studies Severe neuropsychiatric reactions 1:15 000 to 20 000 in adults
Atovaquone-proguanil (Malarone)	Atovaquone 250 mg + Proguanil 100 mg 1 tablet daily for 1–2 days before travel and for week after leaving malarious area	Safety of atovaquone in pregnancy *not* established It is not known whether atovaquone is excreted into human milk Proguanil is excreted into human milk in small quantities Because data are not yet available on safety and efficacy, Malarone should not be given to a woman who breast-feeds an infant who weighs less than 11 kg, unless the potential benefit to the woman outweighs the potential risk to the child (e.g., for a lactating woman who had acquired *P. falciparum* malaria in an area of multi-drug resistance who could not tolerate other treatment options).
Proguanil + Chloroquine	Proguanil 200 mg per day *and* CQ 300 mg base per week Start 1 week before travel and continue for 4 weeks after travel to malarious zone	Anecdotally safe in pregnancy Only 70% effective Folate supplements recommended Limited use due to increasing drug resistance
Pyrimethamine-dapsone (Maloprim)	Pyrimethamine 12.5 mg and Dapsone 100 mg 1 tablet once a week	Restricted use only Not FDA approved Pyrimethamine should be avoided in the first trimester Folinic acid supplement needed Side-effects of dapsone include dose-related hemolytic anemia, more severe in G6PD deficient individuals, methemoglobinemia, agranulocytosis 1:20 000
Pyrimethamine-sulfadoxine (Fansidar)	Pyrimethamine 25 mg + Sulfadoxine 500 mg; 1 tablet once a week	Generally *not* recommended Severe cutaneous reactions 1:5000 to 1:10 000
Azithromycin	250 mg daily	More data needed Effectiveness only 70–80% Not recommended for prophylaxis Treatment studies during pregnancy are in progress

Adapted from Samuel and Barry.[18]

nancy.[20] Studies are underway to evaluate the use of azithromycin to treat malaria during pregnancy.

FOOD AND WATER PRECAUTIONS

Travelers' diarrhea

The pregnant traveler needs to make every effort to avoid travelers' diarrhea. Travelers' diarrhea is reported in 33–50% of all travelers on a short-term trip to a developing country. All travelers should take meticulous food and water precautions. Food should be thoroughly cooked to avoid the usual bacterial, viral and protozoaen pathogens. Pharmacologic prophylaxis, either with antibiotics or bismuth, is not recommended for the pregnant traveler. The fever and dehydration that accompany many travelers' diarrhea syndromes may compromise placental blood flow and potentially adversely effect the fetus. Decreased stomach acidity during pregnancy may theoretically increase susceptibility. In addition, some pathogens (listeria, toxoplasma, hepatitis E) pose unusually high risk during pregnancy.

Congenital toxoplasmosis can occur if a woman is acutely infected during pregnancy. Approximately 3/1000 infants show evidence of congenital toxoplasmosis. Congenital infection is most likely to occur when maternal infection develops in the third trimester. Less than half of affected infants are symptomatic at birth. The risk for severe abnormalities may be 5–6% and includes seizures, mental retardation, cerebral palsy, deafness and blindness in the infant. Latent infection (before pregnancy) is unlikely to cause fetal injury in an other-wise healthy mother.[21] The risk of contracting toxoplasmosis can be diminished by thoroughly cooking meat and wearing gloves for contact with dirt (putting up a tent or other activities that involve dirt contact). Preg-nant women should not change a cat's litter box.

Infection with listeria during pregnancy may cause miscarriage, stillbirth, premature labor and death of the fetus. Listeria may be in unpasteurized milk and other soft cheeses. Pregnant women should avoid feta, Brie, Camembert, Mexican style and blue veined cheeses, and deli meats.

Enterically transmitted hepatitis E infection in pregnancy may cause serious illness. It is a major cause of hepatitis outbreaks in India, Nepal, China, Pakistan, Africa, and the former Soviet Union and has been reported from Central America and Southeast Asia. Transmis-sion of the virus occurs through fecal-oral exposure. Most outbreaks occur due to fecal contamination of drinking water. This infection is most common in persons of childbearing age, 15–40 years old. Clinical illness can range from mild to severe. Hepatitis E acquired during pregnancy has a particularly high maternal fatality rate (15–30%). In non-pregnant women, severe disease occurs in less than 1% of individuals. In pregnant women, however, 20–30% may experience fulminant disease.[22] Studies have demonstrated that the maternal fatality rate during pregnancy due to hepatitis E may increase from 2% during the first trimester to 20–30% during the third trimester. The causes of increased severity during pregnancy are not known. Hepatitis E infection acquired during the third trimester is also associated with fetal morbidity and mortality. A vaccine is in clinical trials but not available at this time. Pregnant women should avoid travel to areas with a high rate of hepatitis E, if at all possible. Passive immunization with immune globulin is not effective in preventing infection.

Water purification

A clean water source should be assured. Boiling water for 1 min at sea level kills all organisms. The manufacture of bottled water is not regulated. Bottled water should be inspected for a factory-sealed cap. Commercially available ceramic water purifiers remove bacteria and 99–99.9% of viruses. Filters alone do not remove viruses and are not recommended. Heavily contaminated ground water should be pre-treated with chlorine or iodine, then filtered. Chemically treating water with iodine tablets can be used for short-term travel (2–3 weeks). Higher, though undefined, amounts of iodine ingested while pregnant may cause fetal goiter and hypothyroidism. The World Health Organization (WHO) recommends 200 μg iodine/day for pregnant women.[23] The pregnant traveler should investigate residual iodine from iodine tablets.

Treatment

The treatment of travelers' diarrhea during pregnancy must first stress the importance of oral rehydration. World Health Organization (WHO) oral rehydration solution (ORS) should be used in sufficient quantities to avoid dehydration. Pre-packaged electrolyte or rice-based ORS should be part of the pregnant traveler's medical kit.

Pharmacologic treatment is limited by pregnancy and the potential harm to the fetus. There is not a single ideal drug. Ciprofloxacin, the drug of choice for non-pregnant adults, is theoretically contraindicated for use in pregnancy due to the potential adverse effects on the developing fetal skeleton. There have been no reports to date of adverse fetal outcomes in pregnant women who were inadvertently exposed to ciprofloxacin. In a single controlled study of 200 women exposed during pregnancy, the rates of spontaneous abortions, fetal distress, and prematurity and the birth weight did not differ from the control group. In addition, there was no clinically significant musculoskeletal dysfunction in the exposed children.[24] Until more data are available ciprofloxacin is not universally recommended unless the risk of the infection outweighs the risk of the medication. A single dose of ciprofloxacin can be considered with informed consent, given the severity of potential infection in pregnancy. Of note, ciprofloxacin is recommended in pregnancy if exposure to anthrax is suspected. Azithromycin is a Category B (see Table 20.4) drug and has good efficacy against Campylobacter and ETEC. Cefixime is an oral third generation drug that may be used in pregnancy. While it covers *E. coli* and Salmonella, it is not an optimal choice for shigellosis or Campylobacter.[25] Ampicillin and erythromycin are safe to use in pregnancy, but lack efficacy against common travelers' diarrhea pathogens. Clarithromycin should be avoided. Likewise, furizolidone should be avoided, as it may cause problems in the presence of fetal glucose-6-phosphate dehydrogenase (G6PD) deficiency. Metronidazole may be used when indicated after the first trimester. Paromomycin, a non-absorbed intraluminal amebicide, is safe for use in pregnancy.[26]

Pepto-Bismol is relatively contraindicated due to data on bismuth toxicity in sheep and the salicylate component which may cause fetal bleeding. Loperamide may be used in pregnancy, in conjunction with oral rehydration. Medications that may be used in pregnancy are listed in Table 20.5.[27]

ALTITUDE AND PREGNANCY

Significant issues to consider in contemplating this type of adventure travel while pregnant include the availability of adequate medical care for the mother or fetus, transport risks, and the treatment of enteric infections. Emergency transport may pose risks to the fetus if an unpressurized aircraft is used, or if delivery occurs during transport. Enteric infections should be treated appropriately to avoid maternal dehydration and the possible onset of preterm labor. The limitations of choices for treatment have been described above.

Little data are published on the pregnant woman traveling to altitude for a short trip. Advice to pregnant women wishing to exercise at altitude is based on isolated observations and several systematic studies. Few studies have explored the limits of combined exercise and altitude exposure in human pregnancy. Consideration should be given to known physiologic changes of residence at high altitude, the

Table 20.4	Food and drug administration use in pregnancy ratings
FDA Category/rating	**Description**
Category A	Adequate and well-controlled studies in women show no risk to fetus.
Category B	No evidence of risk in humans. Studies in animals show risk, but human findings do not, or, in the absence of human studies, animal findings are negative.
Category C	Risk cannot be ruled out. No adequate and well-controlled studies in humans, or animal studies are either positive for fetal risk or lacking as well. Drugs should be given only if the potential benefit justifies the potential risk to the fetus.
Category D	There is positive evidence of human fetal risk. Nevertheless, potential benefits may outweigh the potential risks.
Category X	Contraindicated in pregnancy. Studies in animals or humans or investigational or post-marketing reports have shown fetal risk that far outweighs any potential benefit to the patient.

Table 20.5   Medications for travel use during pregnancy and lactation[27]

Medication	FDA Class	Issues during pregnancy	Issues during lactation
Analgesics/antipyretics		Try non-pharmaceutical methods first to treat pain such as rest, heat, massage.	
Acetaminophen	B	Safe in low doses short term.	Safe
Aspirin	C/D	Avoid last trimester. Has been associated with premature closure of ductus arteriosus in fetus and excessive bleeding. Low dose aspirin (60–80 mg) may be used for pre-eclampsia.	Unknown
Non-steroidal anti-inflammatory (ibuprofen, naproxen)	B/D (last trimester)	Should not be used in last trimester due to effects on premature closure of ductus arteriosus in fetus and effects on clotting Not teratogenic	Safe
Codeine	B	Use cautiously. May cause respiratory depression and withdrawal symptoms in fetus if used near term.	
Hydrocodone	B	Use cautiously. May cause respiratory depression in infant if used near term.	
Antibiotics		Treat symptomatically Only use antibiotics if evidence of bacterial infection.	
Amoxicillin, amoxicillin/Clavulanic acid (Augmentin)	B	Safe. Use for treatment of otitis media, sinusitis, strep throat.	Safe
Amoxicillin/sulbactam (Unasyn) Azithromycin	B	Safe. Use for bronchitis, pneumonia, Campylobacter, shigella, salmonella, *E. coli*.	Safe
Cephalosporins	B	Safe. Use for otitis, strep, sinusitis, pharyngitis.	Safe
Clindamycin oral or vaginal cream	B	Safe Treat bacterial vaginosis orally or locally in second or third trimester Avoid in first trimester Alternative for malaria treatment when used orally with quinine or quinidine.	Safe
Ciprofloxacin, other quinolones	C	Controversial Some use for short-term use in severe infections and/or long term use in life threatening infections (anthrax). Should be used if potential benefit justifies risk to fetus.	Avoid
Dicloxacillin	B	Safe. Use for skin infections.	Safe Used to treat mastitis
Doxycycline/tetracycline	D	May cause permanent discoloration of the teeth during tooth development, including the last half of pregnancy and children <8 years old. May be used in combination with quinine for life threatening situations such a treatment of malaria.	Avoid
Erythromycin (base)	B	Safe. Treatment of bacterial causes URI.	Safe
Nitrofurantoin	B	Drug of choice for UTI in Pregnancy. Avoid if G6PD deficient and near term.	Safe
Penicillin	B	Safe.	Safe
Sulfisoxazole	C/D	Safe. Not recommended last trimester due to risk of hyperbilirubinemia.	Avoid due to infant risk of kernicterus
Trimethoprim	C	Safe.	safe
Gastrointestinal Antidiarrheal Atropine sulfate diphenoxylatehydrochloride (Lomotil)	C	Replace fluids Avoid during pregnancy.	Avoid
Loperamide (Imodium) Antiemetics for nausea, heartburn, esophageal reflux	B	Use if severe symptoms Encourage supportive measures first such as crackers upon arising, frequent small meals, protein meal at bedtime, rather than medications.	Safe
Antacids	B	May use sparingly for symptoms as needed.	Safe
Bismuth subsalicylate Pepto Bismol)	D	Avoid Contains salicylate.	avoid
Cimetidine, ranitidine, omeprazole	B	A cohort study involving a total of 2236 pregnancies demonstrated that the use of acid-suppressing agents (i.e., cimetidine, ranitidine, and omeprazole) during the first trimester is not associated with an increase in congenital malformations.	Safe
Metoclopramide (Reglan)	B	Safe in small doses.	Safe
Dimenhydrinate(dramamine)	B	Safe for severe nausea.	Safe

Table 20.5   Medications for travel use during pregnancy and lactation[27]—cont'd

Medication	FDA Class	Issues during pregnancy	Issues during lactation
Phenothiazines (Compazine)	C	Rare cases of congenital malformations have occurred with use durng pregnancy.	avoid
Acupressure (SeaBands)		Safe.	Safe
Emetrol (fluid replacement)	B	Emetrol is an oral solution containing balanced amounts of dextrose (glucose) and Levulose (fructose) and phosphoric acid with controlled hydrogen ion concentration.	Safe
Ginger	B	Safe	Safe
Meclizine	B	Safe for treatment of severe nausea and vomiting.	Safe
Pyridoxine (B$_6$)	A	Safe. Used for nausea.	Safe
Constipation		Increase fiber + fluid in diet first.	
Bisacodyl	B	Safe to use occasionally.	Safe
Milk of magnesia	B	Safe in small amounts.	Safe
Psyllium hydrophilic mucilloid	B	Safe.	Safe
Hemorrhoids		Increase fiber + fluid in diet.	
Anusol HC suppositories	B	Safe occasionally.	
Antihistamines			
Chlorpheniramine	B	Use cautiously for severe sx.	Unknown
Cetirizine (Zyrtec)	B	Safe, non-sedating, use cautiously.	Unknown
Diphenhydramine (Benadryl)	B	Safe, use cautiously.	Avoid
Loratadine (Claritin)	B	Safe, non-sedating, use cautiously.	Unknown
Dextromethorphan	C	Probably safe, use in small amounts.	Unknown
Guaifenesin	C	Probably safe, use only if needed.	Unknown
Pseudoephedrine (Sudafed)	C	Avoid first trimester, use cautiously.	Unknown
Saline nasal spray	A	Safe.	Safe
Topical nasal decongestants	C	Safe, do not use more then 3 days.	Safe
Oxymetazoline (Afrin)			
Asthma/allergy			
Inhaled bronchodilators	C	Safe for use of wheezing during pregnancy.	Unknown
Inhaled steroids	C	Use if indicated.	Safe
Nasal steroids	C	Use if indicated.	safe
URI/congestion/cough		Symptomatic RX steam, rest, fluids.	
Antimalarials			
Mefloquine	C	Avoid during first trimester unless unavoidable travel to high-risk area. Safe in second and third trimester for high-risk travel. May also be used for treatment if not used for prophylaxis.	Unknown effect. Is excreted in breast milk in very small amounts. Infant also needs prophylaxis.
Chloroquine	C	Safe on basis of empirical data.	Safe. Is excreted in small amounts. Infant needs prophylaxis.
Atovaquone/proguanil (Malarone)	C	Avoid in first trimester. Studies underway to evaluate safety in pregnancy.	No data
Doxycycline	D	Contraindicated. May be considered for treatment of severe infections.	Avoid
Halofantrine	C	Avoid embryotoxic.	Avoid
Primaquine	C	Do not administer during pregnancy because of the possibility the fetus may be G6PD-deficient. Continue suppressive treatment until delivery.	
Proguanil	C	Not associated with teratogenicity	Unknown
Pyrimethamine/sulfadoxine (Fansidar)	C	May use for treatment in high-risk situations with no access to care. Do not use near term or if G6PD deficient.	Safe short term
Quinine sulfate	C	Do not use unless life-threatening infection. May induce severe hypoglycemia.	
Quinidine	C	*No* case reports of teratogenicity to date resulting from quinidine use. Relatively safe in pregnancy, but excessive doses may lead to premature labor and overdoses have lead to abortions. Quinidine has been used in obstetrics since the 1930s.	
Azithromycin	B	Studies underway to evaluate use during pregnancy for malaria treatment.	
Insect repellent			
DEET		Safe, use sparingly as directed.	Safe
Antiparasitics			
Albendazole	C	Teratogenic in animal studies. Avoid first trimester. Treat after delivery if possible. May be indicated for serious infections.	Unsafe
Furazolidone	C	Use only if indicated for severe infection.	Unsafe
Iodoquinol	C	Use only if indicated for severe infection.	Unknown

Table 20.5 **Medications for travel use during pregnancy and lactation[27]—cont'd**

Medication	FDA Class	Issues during pregnancy	Issues during lactation
Metronidazole	B	Avoid first trimester. Use only if clearly indicated.	Use caution. Best to use one dose therapy and delay breast-feeding for 12–24 h.
Paromomycin	B	Minimal systemic absorption occurs following oral administration. Recommended for the treatment of severe infections with Giardia lamblia. *Entamoeba histolytica* and tapeworm infestations during pregnancy.	
Praziquantel	B	Used in treatment of severe schistosomiasis. Preferable to delay treatment during pregnancy until after delivery, unless absolutely essential.	Do not breast-feed on day of treatment and for 72 h following dose
Antivirals Acyclovir	B	Use only for severe infections.	Safe
Altitude sickness Acetazolamide (Diamox)	C	Do not use during first trimester. Use only if benefit outweighs risk.	Discontinue nursing while on drug
Dexamethasone (Decadron)	C	May use if needed for treatment for altitude illness.	Avoid breast-feeding during therapy
Calcium Channel blockers (Nifedipine)	C	Use only to treat severe symptoms pulmonary edema	Safe
Water purification Iodine	D	Avoid, except for short term (2–3 weeks). May lead to goiter and fetal hypothyroidism.	Avoid

degree of physiologic adaptations to both pregnancy and altitude, and data from the few systematic studies in human preg-nancy. Because individual altitude tolerance and exercise capacity cannot be reliably determined at sea level, advice should err on the side of caution and recognize the limitations of the available data.

Short-term travel to moderate altitude does not seem to have nega-tive effects on pregnancy. For women living at altitude, pregnancy-induced hypertension and pre-eclampsia are more common. Infant birth weights are lower at altitude compared with infants born at sea level.[28] Chronic placental changes occur at altitude, but have not been seen or conclusively studied in the short-term traveler. Low oxygen tension and pressure changes result in intrauterine growth retarda-tion and an increased risk of premature labor in women who spend most of their pregnancy above 8000 ft (2400 meters).[29]

Studies on pregnant women at altitude show that the human fetus develops normally under low-oxygen conditions. Exposure of a preg-nant woman to the hypoxia of high altitude results in acclimatization responses, which act to preserve the fetal oxygen supply. The fetus also utilizes several compensatory mechanisms to survive brief periods of hypoxia. While fetal heart rate monitoring data during air travel sug-gest no compromise of fetal oxygenation, exercise at high alti-tude may place further stress on oxygen delivery to the fetus. Thus, a preg-nant woman who goes to altitude must take time to acclima-tize and avoid high altitude pulmonary edema or additional hypoxic stress.

The risks of high altitude trekking to the mother and fetus are not well-defined physiologically, though fetal bradycardia has been seen with exposure to extreme altitudes.[30] It is reassuring that there have been no reports of injury, pregnancy complications or losses asso-ciated with exercise at altitude (skiing, running, mountain bicycling, trekking, etc). Studies to date, however, have been conducted at mod-erate altitudes for short periods and low intensities. Until more data are available, it is recommended that pregnant women avoid the additional hypoxic stress of extreme altitude.[31]

PREGNANCY PLANNING

Women considering conception should take into account the poten-tial effects of certain vaccinations and medications and plan accord-ingly, if possible.

Attempts to conceive should be deferred until 3 months after receiv-ing the measles-mumps-rubella (MMR) vaccine. The precaution is based on the theoretical risk of fetal infection with a live viral vacci-nation. No congenital defects have been reported, and receiving any component of the vaccine singly or in combination is not an indica-tion for pregnancy termination.

Pregnancy should likewise be avoided for one month after admin-istration of the varicella vaccine. The VARIVAX pregnancy registry (800-986-8999) is monitoring the maternal and fetal outcomes of women inadvertently vaccinated with varicella vaccine while preg-nant or during the 3 months before pregnancy.

Antimalarial chemoprophylaxis with mefloquine is not recom-mended within 3 months of becoming pregnant. Data on inadvertent exposure, however, does not indicate that peri-conceptual mefloquine exposure is an indication for pregnancy termination. Limited data indicate that there is no increase in fetal malformations over the background rate.

Atovaquone/proguanil, doxycycline, and chloroquine do not carry these pre-conceptual precautions.

BREAST-FEEDING

Drugs in breast milk

Because no randomized controlled trials exist on the safety of medica-tions during lactation, any medication given to a lactating woman should be carefully considered. Most routinely prescribed drugs are safe to use during lactation. Short-acting drugs administered after a feeding have the least opportunity to be excreted into milk. Few drugs are absolutely contraindicated while breast-feeding. Quinolones are currently contraindicated for use in children less than 18 year old.

Ciprofloxacin is excreted into breast milk in small quantities, but there have been no adverse reports regarding any effect on breast-fed infants.

Malaria prevention

Mefloquine, chloroquine, tetracyclines and proguanil are excreted into human milk in small amounts. It is not known whether atovaquone or doxycycline is excreted in breast milk. The amount of any of the drugs studied is insufficient to protect the nursing infant. There is no evidence that amounts excreted in human milk are harmful to a nursing infant.[27] Therefore, the infant should also receive appropriate antimalarial chemoprophylaxis.

Immunizations

Lactating mothers may safely receive all vaccinations. Strains of live virus vaccines are not known to be transmitted in breast milk, with the exception of attenuated rubella virus. The infants are usually not infected by the vaccine strain of rubella.[32] There is no contraindication to yellow fever vaccine in the nursing mother.[4]

Practicalities

Good breast hygiene should be practiced by the nursing mother while traveling. Human milk protects the infant from many enteric diseases and breast-feeding should be strongly supported for the traveling newborn infant.

For the nursing mother who is traveling without her infant, meticulous attention should be given to maintaining the breast pump. Both manual and electric pumps should be washed after use with clean water and soap and dried in a fly-free environment. Breast milk can be kept at room temperature for 4 h before use, or refrigerated for use within 72 h. Frozen breast milk can be stored for up to 4 months.

Women should use the breast pump nearly as frequently as they would nurse the infant, to avoid painful engorgement or the development of mastitis. If mastitis develops, more frequent pumping, analgesics and an anti-staphylococcal antibiotic (dicloxacillin or cephalexin) are treatments to consider.

MEDICATIONS

General principles to consider when prescribing a medication to a pregnant woman include:
- How do the pharmacokinetics of the medication differ during pregnancy?
- Are the adverse reactions or side-effects more common during pregnancy than in the non-pregnant woman?
- What is the potential risk of the medication used to treat or prevent the disease versus the risk of acquiring the disease to the developing fetus?

The US Food and Drug Administration (FDA) categorizes each medication and immunization used in the USA. As most medications and immunizations have not been tested during pregnancy or lactation, they are categorized as FDA category C (see Table 20.5). There are other classification systems which have been developed in other countries, such as Sweden, Australia, Netherlands and Denmark, to estimate fetal risk. There are also a number of website resources with information on possible teratogen risk of a particular medication or vaccine.

The American College of Obstetrics and Gynecology has released recommendations regarding use of antimicrobial therapy during pregnancy.[33] They classify the commonly used antibiotics as:

- those considered safe (i.e., penicillin and erythromycin base, stearate or ethylsuccinate);
- those that probably are safe (but to be used with caution: i.e., azithromycin, metronidazole, nitrofurantoin)
- those that are contraindicated in (i.e., tetracycline, fluroquinones, and erythromycin estolate).

Table 20.4 reviews some of the commonly used medications in travel during pregnancy.

OTHER ISSUES

Alternative medications

The use of herbal remedies has increased over the last several years in all areas of medicine, especially in the area of women's health. Some of these remedies have shown promising application, such as the use of ginger or acupressure for nausea during pregnancy. Women travelers may be tempted to try traditional healing practices or local remedies for symptoms. Pregnant women should be advised that some medicinal herbs may have unknown side-effects, such as inducing uterine contractions or fetal teratogenicity. Until more data are available, all herbal remedies should be used with caution especially in the first trimester.

REFERENCES

1. Ryan KJ, Berkowitz RS, Barbieri RL, Dunaif A, eds. *Kistner's Gynecology and Women's Health.* 7th edn. St. Louis, MO: Mosby, Inc; 1999.
2. American College of Obstetricians and Gynecologists Exercise during pregnancy and the postpartum period. *Technical Bulletin* 1994; No. 189.
3. Clapp JF 3rd. Exercise during pregnancy. A clinical update. *Clin Sports Med* 2000; **19**(2):273–286.
4. Center for Disease Control. *Health Information for International Travel, 2003–2004.* US Department of Health and Human Services; 2001.
5. Rose, SR. Pregnancy and travel. *Emerg Med Clin N Am* **15**(1):95–111.
6. Huch R, Baumann H, Fallenstein F, Schneider KT, Holdener F, Huch A. Physiologic changes in pregnant women and their fetuses during jet travel. *Am J Ob Gyn* **154**(5):996–999.
7. United States Department of Transportation, Office of Aviation Medicine. http://www.hf.faa.gov/docs/cami/00_33.pdf.
8. Robert E, Vial T, Schaefer C, Arnon J, Reuvers M. Exposure to yellow fever vaccine in early pregnancy. *Vaccine* 1999; **17**(3):283–285.
9. Kain KC, Keystone JS. Malaria in travelers. Epidemiology, disease, and prevention. *Infect Dis Clin North Am* 1998; **12**(2):267–284.
10. Diagne N. Increased susceptibility to malaria during the early postpartum period. *N Engl J Med* 2000; **343**(9):598–603.
11. Lindsay S, Ansell J, Selman C, Cox V, Hamilton K, Walraven G. Effect of pregnancy on exposure to malaria mosquitoes. *Lancet* 2000; **355**(9219):1972.
12. Nathwani D, Currie PF, Douglas JG, Green ST, Smith NC. *Plasmodium falciparum* malaria in pregnancy: a review. *Br J Ob Gyn* 1992; **99**:118–121.
13. Nosten F, McGready R, Simpson JA, et al. Effects of *Plasmodium vivax* malaria in pregnancy. *Lancet* 1999; **354**(9178):546–549.
14. McGready R, Hamilton KA, Simpson JA, et al. Safety of the insect repellent N,N-diethyl-M-toluamide (DEET) in pregnancy. *Am J Trop Med Hyg* 2001; **65**(4):285–289.
15. Nosten F, ter Kuile F, Maelankiri L, et al. Mefloquine prophylaxis prevents malaria during pregnancy: a double-blind, placebo-controlled study. *J Infect Dis* 1994; **169**:595–603.
16. Phillips-Howard PA, Steffen R, Kerr L, et al. Safety of mefloquine and other antimalarial agents in the first trimester of pregnancy. *J Travel Med* 1998; **5**(3):121–126.
17. Mortola JP. Birth weight and altitude: a study in Peruvian communities. *J Pediatr* 2000; **136**(3):324–329.
18. Samuel BU, Barry M. The pregnant traveler. *Infect Dis Clin North Am* 1998; **12**(2):325–354.
19. Nissen D. *Mosby's Drug Consult 2002.* St. Louis, MO: Mosby.
20. McGready R. Artemisinin antimalarials in pregnancy: a prospective treatment study of 539 episodes of multidrug-resistant *Plasmodium falciparum. Clin Infect Dis* 2001; **33**(12):2009–2016.
21. Gabbe SG, Neibyl JR, Simpson, JL, eds. *Obstetrics – Normal and Problem Pregnancies.* 4th edn. London: Churchill Livingstone; 2002.

22. Aggarwal R, Krawczynski K, Hepatitis E. an overview and recent advances in clinical and laboratory research. *J Gastroenterol Hepatol* 2000; **15**(1):9–20.

23. WHO. *Bulletin of the World Health Organization 1996*, 74(1):1–3. Reprint 5665; also available at: http://whqlibdoc.who.int/hq/1996/WHO_NUT_96.5.pdf

24. Loebstein R, Addis A, Ho E, *et al.* Pregnancy outcome following gestational exposure to fluoroquinolones: a multicenter prospective controlled study. *Antimicrob Agents Chemother* 1998; **42**(6):1336–1339.

25. Salam MA, Seas C, Khan WA, Bennish ML. Treatment of shigellosis: IV. Cefixime is ineffective in shigellosis in adults. *Ann Intern Med* 1995; **123**(7):505–508.

26. Rosenblatt JE. Antiparasitic agents. *Mayo Clin Proc* 1999; **74**(11):1161–1175.

27. Briggs GG, Freeman RK, Yaffe SJ. *Drugs in Pregnancy and Lactation: A Reference Guide to Fetal and Neonatal Risk.* 5th edn. Baltimore MD: Williams & Wilkins; 1998.

28. Niermeyer, S. The pregnant altitude visitor. *Adv Exp Med Biol* 1999; **474**:65–77.

29. Ali, KZ, Ali ME, Khalid ME. High altitude and spontaneous preterm birth. *Int J Gynaecol Obstet* 1996; **54**(1):11–15.

30. Hackett PH. High altitude and common medical conditions. In: Hornbein T and Schoene R, eds. *High Altitude: An Exploration of Human Adaptation.* New York, NY: Dekker; 2001; **161**:839–86.

31. Huch, R. Physical activity at altitude in pregnancy. *Sem Perinatol* 1996: **20**(4):303–314.

32. American Academy of Pediatrics. Rubella. In: Pickering LK, eds. *2000 Red Book: Report of the Committee on Infectious Diseases.* 25th edn. Elk Grove Village, IL: American Academy of Pediatrics; 2000:499.

33. American College of Obstetricians and Gynecologists: Antimicrobial Therapy for Obstetric Patients. *ACOG Educational Bulletin* No 245. Washington, DC: ACOG; 1998.

CHAPTER 21 Pediatric, Neonatal and Adolescent Travelers

Philip R. Fischer

KEYPOINTS

- With appropriate planning and preparation, frequent rest stops, and liberal food and hydration, travel with children can be very rewarding

- Safety considerations include motor vehicle and aircraft restraints, and vigilant supervision during water and land activities

- Sun and insect protection and avoidance of animals, are particularly important for children

- When used appropriately, DEET is safe for use in children

- Self-treatments of travelers' diarrhea with antibiotics should be considered, but antimotility agents should be avoided

- It is reasonable to screen long-term travelers upon return from high-risk areas particularly for exposure to tuberculosis

INTRODUCTION

Travel with children offers family fun, cultural broadening, development of worldviews, and opportunities for service. Despite obvious benefits, though, international travel also opens families to the possibility of inconvenience, injury, and illness. Families, children, and adolescents should all appropriately prepared[1,2] so that they can maximize the benefits of international travel while avoiding undue risks.

Indeed, the Bible tells of Cain, the first human child, in the fourth chapter of Genesis. Accepting his fate of being a 'restless wanderer on the earth,' Cain was aware of the risks of travel (fearing that 'whoever finds me will kill me'). God took preventive action ('put a mark on Cain') prior to Cain's trip in an effort to decrease the risk of travel-associated injury and death. Similarly, pre-travel counsel and intervention can help current-day travelers prepare for safe, healthy, and beneficial experiences in a variety of locations.

Pediatric travel medicine is a dynamic process. Supported by four moving 'wheels' (safety and comfort, immunization, avoidance of insect-borne diseases, and diarrhea management), pediatric travelers are carried along on their journeys. The age, health status, and itinerary of the child determine whether all four 'wheels' are powered and how they are used. Health behaviors in each of these four domains are incorporated into the child's trip even as the wheels of the landing gear are raised into an aircraft. The child is then safely propelled on a life-enhancing voyage. Practitioners of pediatric travel medicine have the privilege of preparing children and their families for valuable international experiences.

SAFETY AND COMFORT

Contraindications to travel

Is it safe for children to travel internationally?

Whether going across a street for minutes or across an ocean for months, all travel carries at least some risk. Those responsible for a child must be convinced that the benefit of the trip outweighs whatever risks the trip might entail. Furthermore, responsible adults should help the traveling child take reasonable precautions to decrease the risks of adverse consequences that might come with the planned travel.

For instance, should a 9-month-old accompany his or her parents on a hike to the summit of Mount Kilimanjaro? One would be hard pressed to identify benefits to the child that would outweigh the risk of mountain sickness that could harm the child and cause the parents to abort their ascent. Should missionary parents take their 2-month-old daughter to their home in rural Kenya? The eternal value that the parents perceive in their ministry might prompt them to accept the risk of insect-borne diseases in their baby; at the same time they should take appropriate precautions with insect repellents, insecticide-impregnated bednets, malarial chemoprophylaxis, and, when the child is a few months older, yellow fever vaccine. A travel medicine practitioner can help parents wisely choose the timing and destination of proposed trips in light of a risk-benefit balance with the child in mind.

Parents and trip organizers should also be advised to schedule activities with a view toward the child's perspective. Running rapidly from museum to museum might not be in a 4-year-old child's best interest, although a visit to a museum between other activities along with appropriate rest might give a pre-school-aged child a good, age-appropriate view of history and art. Popular books can guide parents in preparing for travel with children.[3,4]

The benefits (indications) to travel must always be balanced with the risks (potential contraindications) for individual children. But, are there absolute contraindications to travel? There probably are no *absolute* contraindications to travel, but medical conditions can impose *relative* contraindications that would provide a practitioner with compelling reasons to advise against undertaking certain proposed trips. With adequate planning and with access to medical resources and means of transportation, any trip could probably be arranged. Nonetheless, common sense (which is not actually always common) should help guide decisions. Travel medicine practitioners, particularly those seasoned with their own travel experience, can help inform families of both the risks and benefits of trips and can then help suggest interventions to decrease risks. Traveling families can also get good advice about local resources and risks by contacting peers who reside in or have traveled to their destinations. Adequately informed, most families will adjust plans and make preparations to avoid undue risks.

What precautions should be taken for children with chronic medical conditions?

Pediatric patients with anemia, serious respiratory problems, or congenital heart disease should know how to quickly gain access to oxygen and emergency medications during long trips. Even children with asthma should carry an adequate supply of the medications that they would use for a severe exacerbation. Immunodeficient children should carry appropriate antibiotics with which to begin presumptive therapy while seeking good medical care in inconvenient settings. Health insurance and evacuation insurance are important considerations for all travelers, but they are especially critical for chronically compromised pediatric travelers.

Schedules

Having carefully considered an itinerary with the children in mind, parents can make sure they have ready access to plenty of food and drink. Adjusting to new climatic areas, children often need to increase their fluid intake. In addition, children should be provided with plenty of rest breaks during their trips.

Motor vehicles

Traumatic injury accounts for more deaths in travelers than do infectious diseases.[5] Motor vehicle accidents are a leading cause of traumatic injury among traveling children.

Families should be reminded to supervise their children around streets and roads. Children should be counseled about specific areas to avoid unfamiliar destinations when cars and children can otherwise share the same space.

Rates of motor vehicle crashes and deaths are higher in many travel destination countries than they are in many home countries. Families should be particularly careful as they plan road trips; in many areas, road travel after dark is dangerous and should be avoided. Pre-travel counsel sessions should also include advice about the appropriate restraints for children in cars (Table 21.1.). The use of appropriate restraints limits distraction of the driver and, thus, decreases the risk of collisions. The use of restraints also limits the extent of the injuries incurred by children who are in collisions. During the first year of life, children should be restrained in a harness style safety seat that is strapped securely into the car's backseat. Children are at decreased risk of neck injury when they are facing backwards until reaching at least 1 year of age *and* 20 pounds of body weight.[6] Harness restraints are recommended until reaching 4 years of age and 40 pounds of body weight. 'Booster seats', which provide either a harness strap or a barrier across the level of the chest are recommended until the child is at least 8 years old and weighs at least 80 pounds.[7] Families can be reminded that the inconvenience of ensuring the availability of appropriate car seat restraints is less than the 'inconvenience' of life-threatening traumatic injuries. Since child safety seats are often not readily available in foreign sites, families traveling with children should seriously consider taking their own safety seats along. When appropriate restraints are not available, the middle of a rear seat is usually the least dangerous place in a car. A child should not face forward in a car seat that is not attached with a seat belt to the car, but an unrestrained rear-facing safety seat might prevent some crash-related injuries. As for traveling adults, children should be transported only in safe vehicles, and travel should be limited to times when road conditions and driver ability are adequate.

Water

In both domestic and foreign destinations, water-related activities are associated with serious injury in travelers.[8,9] Avoidable risk factors for boating injuries include alcohol use by drivers and leaving propellers running while people are either swimming near the boat or climbing in or out of the boat. Families planning to use boats during their trips should be counseled about good boating safety practices.

Safety near the water's edge is also important for children. No child should be unsupervised near water, and an adult 'buddy' should always be available in the water near a child playing in the water. Abrasions by coral and injuries by marine animals are managed in children as they are in adults.

Swimming raises other questions for some pediatric travelers.

Should children with tympanostomy tubes (ventilation tubes through the eardrums, sometimes referred to as 'pressure equalization' tubes) swim?

Surface swimming might moisten the external ear canal but should not push fluid into the middle ear. Thus, splashing and playing at the water's surface is not contraindicated by the presence of tympanostomy tubes.[10] Holding the ears underwater, however, provides enough hydrostatic pressure to force water through the tubes into the middle ears. Therefore, individuals whose eardrums are not intact, whether by recent perforation or by tympanostomy tube placement, should not dive or hold their ears under water unless they have customized plugs to completely occlude the external ear canals.

What about 'swimmer's ear'?

Swimmer's ear, or otitis externa, is a superficial infection of the external ear canal that is most common in people who spend significant amounts of time in the water with wet ears. This is not a dangerous condition, and infections can be easily treated (with topical acetic acid or anti-inflammatory drops); concern about swimmer's ear need not limit water activities during travel.

Two medical conditions, long QT[11] syndrome and epilepsy,[12] may increase the risk of drowning in traveling children who choose to play or swim in water. Children with a history of having lost consciousness during water activity should consider evaluation for these possible problems prior to international travel. Parents of pediatric travelers known to have either of these conditions should make sure that the underlying condition is adequately treated and that their child is not more than a couple of arms' lengths from someone who can help should the child lose consciousness in the water.

Air travel

Is it safe for infants to travel in commercial airplanes or go to high altitudes?

Data are limited on this and many other aspects of pediatric travel medicine. Nonetheless, available evidence suggests that even though young age has been linked to respiratory and cardiovascular changes

Table 21.1	Vehicle restraints for children
Age	Recommended restraint
Birth to 1 year and 9 kg	Harnessed in carseat, facing backwards in rear seat
1–4 years (and 9–18 kg)	Harnessed in carseat, facing frontwards in rear seat
5–8 years (and 18–38 kg)	Belted booster seat in rear seat
>8 years	Seat belt

in high altitude – like environments, young age is not a contra-indication to air travel.

Travel in commercial aircraft includes spending time in a pressurized cabin similar to an environment at ~2700 m above sea level. The oxygen content of the room air at this elevation is similar to that of 15% oxygen at sea level. Would this relative hypoxia be a problem for infants or children? There has been concern that newborns might not tolerate this relative hypoxia due to a relative immaturity of their alveoli,[13] but there is no actual evidence that young alveoli pose a problem for otherwise healthy infants. Pending further data, healthy newborns, infants, and children need not be restricted from air travel based on concerns about alveolar development. Children with pulmonary and cardiac problems and resultant concerns about hypoxia, however, might not tolerate prolonged air travel without supplemental oxygen.

Might the relative hypoxia of aircraft cabins change normal breathing patterns in infants?

After noting an anecdotal association between air travel and sudden infant death syndrome, researchers studied breathing patterns in babies exposed overnight to 15% oxygen. Babies had lower oxygen saturations in low oxygen environments (mean 93% versus normal means of 98%) and also had more irregular breathing patterns with more respiratory pauses. None of the respiratory pauses constituted true apnea (considered to be a lack of respiration for at least 20 s), and no adverse clinical outcomes were noted. Neither genetic (relative of a victim of sudden infant death) nor other identified predisposing factors were predictive of which individual infants would have prolonged oxygen desaturations. It seems that long air flights (or visits/residence at high elevation locations) might indeed be associated with changes in infant respiratory control.[14] It is not clear, however, that these changes are linked to significant health consequences.

What about the risk of injury during air travel?

There is active debate over the use of restraints for children during routine air travel, and at least one group advocates mandatory use of restraints.[15] During automobile travel, safety seats are clearly effective in reducing crash-related injury. Per mile traveled, air crashes are much less frequent than car crashes, and the cost (a ticket for an additional seat) and discomfort (crying with prolonged restraint in a harnessed seat) are not clearly overcome by the benefit (less chance of injury in some sorts of crashes). Also, in air crashes and during time of air turbulence, the forces applied to an infant's body are not as easily predicted as with the more two-dimensional forward deceleration/acceleration movements of car crashes. It is thus not clear just what sort of a restraining system might best protect a baby during an air crash. It is clear that sharing an adult's seat belt might cause dangerous abdominal compression in a child who is squeezed between the belt and an adult during sudden deceleration; a child would be safer in an individual belt attached to the adult's seat belt. Since the use of a car safety seat confers at least some theoretical protection, a family might choose to use this seat on a plane even though cost-effectiveness data are not available to support legislation regarding the use of such restraints. Many families reasonably accept the limited benefit data as a reason not to pay the extra expense of a separate seat for an infant. At the present time, there is not widespread agreement to mandate the use of in-flight safety seats for infants.

Assuming that reasonable safety precautions are in order, what can be done to ensure comfort for a child and family traveling by air?

As noted in front-row ('bulkhead') seats on most inter-continental flights provide wall hanging beds that allow horizontal sleep for infants. Aisle access allows an accompanying family member to take 'walks' with a child who tires of prolonged sitting. Parents should help children with seats and trays while food and, especially, hot drinks are being served so that spills and burns do not occur. Clothing should be comfortable, and fresh clothes should be available when accidental spills and soiling do occur. Fluids should be available to maintain hydration in a fairly dry air environment. Age-appropriate books, toys, and games can be used to provide entertainment, especially for children who aren't able to see a movie screen. Views of specific landmarks from windows, changes of outside lighting, or progress on in-flight maps can be triggers to open surprise packages of new toys to help a child maintain anticipation and enthusiasm for a long voyage. Appropriate scheduling with the child's interests in mind can help maximize the value of airport layovers and breaks in travel during long voyages.

Should children be sedated during long flights?

Medicines are used to sedate or anesthetize children for painful medical procedures; is a long air trip a 'painful procedure' that should qualify for medical intervention? If so, would this intervention be aimed at helping the child or would it be using pediatric medicine to help the comfort of adult traveling companions? Different families answer these questions differently, and some do choose to sedate their children. Understanding that there are no studies measuring outcomes using pre-flight or in-flight sedation while realizing, nonetheless, that diphenhydramine (1 mg/kg per dose given every 4–6 h as needed) is a relatively safe medication, most experts do not advise sedation for traveling children. In fact, pharmacologists have noted a peculiar excitatory response to antihistaminics in children less than 2 years old. Parents wanting to avoid this paradoxical excitatory response during travel could use a test dose prior to the trip to ensure that the child is not predisposed to an undesired response.

Painful earaches bother some children (and those sitting near them) during the ascent and descent of commercial aircraft as cabin pressures are adjusted. With ascent, approximately 6% of children experience bothersome pain, and about 10% have pain with descent. Adults who have such pains find preventive efficacy in the use of pseudoephedrine,[16] but a single study of this product in young pediatric travelers showed no decrease in apparent pain.[17] Though untested, physical maneuvers such as sucking, chewing, and swallowing in an effort to open the Eustachian tubes can be suggested. Infants should have something to drink readily available during ascent and descent when flight attendants are often not available to get drinks.

Skin protection

Whether vacationing or moving to a new foreign residence, traveling children often have increased outdoor activities with a resultant increase in sun exposure, sometimes at beaches with limited skin coverage and sometimes closer to the equator where sunlight comes more directly. Sun exposure is clearly linked to acute burns and to subsequent increases in wrinkling, pigmentary changes, and skin cancer. In fact, a blistering sunburn during childhood is a key risk factor predisposing to later malignant melanoma.[18] Sunscreen is both safe and effective at reducing the adverse consequences of sun exposure, but avoidance of both direct and reflective sunlight exposure, especially during the mid-day hours, is important for maximal protection. Potency of sunscreen is measured in terms of sun protection factor ('SPF') which is the ratio of the time required to produce minimal erythema on sunscreen-covered skin to the time required to produce the same erythema on uncovered skin under artificial testing conditions. A sunscreen with SPF 15 blocks approximately 93% of damaging ultraviolet light, and a sunscreen with SPF 30 blocks about

96%.[19] Children should use sunscreen of at least SPF 15. Though knowledge of increasing skin cancer incidences has increased in recent years, many children still fail to use sunscreen appropriately.[20] Sunscreen should be applied 15–30 minutes before exposure and then can be reapplied 15–30 min after exposure begins as well as after washing, swimming, and excessive sweating. Subsequent reapplication after a few hours of ongoing sun exposure is not needed.[21] Sunscreen use is no longer thought to be contraindicated during the first six months of life, but young children are better kept in shaded areas or covered than in either reflective or direct sunlight. Clothing provides only partial protection from the penetration of sunlight, and sunscreen can be helpful even for children wearing light clothes in shaded areas.

Clothes and shoes can also protect the skin from injury and from microbiologic contamination. Comfortable clothes that cover most of the skin are particularly useful in areas of insect-borne illnesses, and protective footwear helps prevent penetration by hookworm larvae in areas of poor sanitation.

High altitude

Acute mountain sickness is a potential problem for children as for adults.[22] The exact incidence of acute mountain sickness in children is unknown. Whether headache and malaise are effects of travel or effects of altitude exposure is not always easily discerned. One study suggested that 28% of school-aged children developed signs of acute mountain sickness when vacationing at 2835 m elevation, but 21% of similar children vacationing at sea level had similar symptoms.[23] In another study of preverbal children aged 3–36 months, 22% developed what seemed truly to be acute mountain sickness, suggesting that the risk of children developing symptoms at high altitude is similar to that in adults.[24] Acetazolamide has not been specifically studied as a mountain sickness prophylactic in children, but the medicine is safe in children when used at similar doses for other indications. As for adults, the mainstay of treatment of severe altitude-related illnesses (high-altitude pulmonary edema, high-altitude cerebral edema) is prompt descent. Dexamethasone (for high-altitude cerebral edema, which has not actually been reported in children[25,26]) and nifedipine (for high-altitude pulmonary edema) could be helpful adjuncts to treatment of severely affected children.

Staying at high altitude, children undergo physiologic adaption.[27,28] Acutely, oxygen saturation drops. Over time, however, oxygen saturation seems to rise as oxygen uptake is enhanced related to increases in ventilation, lung compliance, and pulmonary diffusion. Chest volumes and hemoglobin concentrations also rise. These changes help children grow to tolerate high altitude and to thrive in those environments.

Not all children, however, tolerate continued exposure to high altitude environments, and some develop life-threatening pulmonary hypertension. Initially, elevated pulmonary artery pressures are provoked by decreased oxygen delivery, but subsequently, pulmonary hypertension can be detrimental. While the incidence of life-threatening pulmonary hypertension in children at high altitude is not known, a study of 15 infant autopsies in Tibet (3600 m elevation) suggested that children of a non-indigenous ethnic group were at a higher risk than were indigenous children and that most deaths occurred in children who had recently immigrated to the high altitude setting.[29] Similarly, pulmonary hypertension occurred in some children at high altitude in Colorado, and symptoms resolved with descent and relocation to lower environments.[30] In a catheterization study in Peru, asymptomatic pulmonary hypertension was not uncommon but became less significant with increasing age.[31] The pulmonary hypertension seen in children at high altitude is not completely understood but seems to be a real occurrence in some children with newly arrived children of some genetic backgrounds being at

greater risk than some other children. Clearly, any child with cardio-respiratory symptoms at high altitude should be carefully evaluated; descent to a lower altitude might be a major part of the treatment plan.

Is sudden infant death syndrome (SIDS, 'crib death,' or 'cot death') more common at high altitude than in children residing at lower elevations? There are no clear data suggesting that sudden infant death is more common at higher elevations, and various studies are not comparable due to variations in diagnostic criteria. Nonetheless, one study in a relatively low-lying area of the USA suggested that SIDS might occur more commonly in babies residing at higher elevations.[32] At any altitude, the mainstays of SIDS prevention are to have infants sleep in a supine position and to keep infants away from cigarette smoke.[33]

Animal contact

One of the pleasures of foreign travel is seeing new varieties of animals. Whether casually viewing different sorts of backyard birds in Europe or going on a wildlife safari in Africa, childhood exposures to animals can bring either pleasures or problems. Safety precautions are vitally important around animals.

Obviously, animal bites are to be avoided. Children, especially young children, should not play around unknown animals, and wildlife viewing should always be from a safe distance. Animal bites should prompt a traveling family to visit a physician in view of injury, bacterial contamination, and rabies.

Even without biting, animals can unwittingly transmit illnesses to children. This can vary from family dogs sharing *Toxocara* to raccoons leaving *Baylisascaris*-laden stool in pediatric play areas to cats carrying plague-infected fleas. Children should be kept safe in areas that are shared with animals, and parents should help traveling children stay clean during and after contact with animals.

Since not all animal bites are easily avoided, families should have ready access to cleaning supplies and water to wash and vigorously irrigate any animal bite. Prophylactic antibiotics can be considered for animal bites as well, especially those on the hands or face. Rabies vaccine is sadly neglected by families traveling with children,[34] and pre-exposure rabies vaccination should be considered for all children going to places such as Asia and Africa where rabies is not uncommon, especially when the trip is of more than a month or two.

Risk-taking behaviors

Substance use during travel can represent a significant risk for traveling children. Occasionally, this occurs accidentally as parents unknowingly give a young child a glass of orange juice without realizing that the orange juice in some Caribbean locales always comes with vodka in it. More often, pediatric substance abuse involves adolescents. Traveling teenagers sometimes find themselves with a new sense of freedom. They might be on 'Spring Break' with inexpensive drugs of abuse and partying peers, or they might be imagining that 'When in Rome, do as the Romans' means that they should drink excessively during a European study trip. Pre-travel counsel should remind adolescents and their parents/supervisors to set up careful safety limits to avoid unsafe use of alcohol and other illicit substances during foreign travel (Table 21.2).

Body fluid exposures provide other risks for adolescents and, sometimes, younger children. Children needing injections, such as children with diabetes taking insulin, should carry an adequate supply of sterile equipment and medication. They should also carry adequate documentation about these medical supplies to satisfy curious immigration officials. Travelers should insist that medical testing and treatment involve only sterile supplies. Blood transfusions should

Table 21.2	Caring for adolescent travelers

What to tell them
Have a great time!
Why food and water selection matters
How insect avoidance prevents sickness

What to give them:
Update routinely recommended immunizations
Give appropriate travel vaccines

What they should take along:
Medical kit (see other table)
Water purifier if bottled water not available

What they should do:
Learn lots
Use seat belts and helmets appropriately
Avoid mind-altering substance use
Avoid potential body fluid contact:
    Tattooing, piercing, non-sterile medical care
    Sexual contact
Only swim or boat with a friend along
Use sunscreen
Avoid stray animals
Choose food and drink wisely
Drink lots of pure fluid in case of diarrhea
Take suggested malaria medicine as directed

Table 21.3	Medical kit for traveling children: items for potential inclusion

Information card noting:
Name
Birthdate
Chronic medical conditions, if any
Regular medications, if any
Medical allergies, if any
Blood type, if known
Immunization record
Emergency contact(s)

Supplies:
Bandages
Adhesive tape
Gauze
Antiseptic cleaning solution

Medications
Acetaminophen
Ibuprofen
Diphenhydramine
Topical antibiotic cream or ointment such as mupirocin
Antibiotic such as azithromycin or ciprofloxacin if risk of severe travelers' diarrhea
Loperamide if older child
Regular medications, if any

Products:
Oral hydration salts
Sunscreen, SPF 15 or 30
Insect repellent
Permethrin

only be accepted for life-threatening conditions and hopefully when safe blood is available. Sexual contact is a significant risk for teenage travelers, whether it occurs with traveling companions or new acquaintances. Abstinence is the safest plan; non-abstinent individuals can be provided with barrier methods to decrease the risk of dangerous sharing of body fluids. Body piercing and tattooing, especially when needles are not sterilized between subjects or when a common tattoo dye source is used for multiple recipients,[35] is well known to transmit hepatitis viruses and human immunodeficiency virus. Teen travelers should be advised to avoid any piercing or tattooing.

Medical kit for families with children

Realizing that proactive safety measures are not always completely successful, responsible adults should carry a medical kit that includes supplies of use to traveling children. A sampling of items that might be included is noted in Table 21.3. This includes documentation of health situations, first aid supplies, common medications, and some hygienic supplies. Children with chronic or underlying medical conditions could certainly have additional supplies or products included.

IMMUNIZATION

Pre-travel consultation provides an opportunity to ensure that the child is current on vaccinations for the home environment. With changing schedules, additional immunizations might be appropriate for some traveling children. Various agencies around the world publicize their 'routine' immunization schedules, and the American Academy of Pediatrics updates vaccine recommendations and information regularly.[36,37] Young travelers might be helped by 'accelerating' the schedule of routine immunizations to provide maximal coverage during their trip (see Chapter 11). Immunization plans should be individualized for special needs children. Prematurely delivered babies are generally immunized according to their chronologic age without changing their immunization schedule in view of their young gestational age.[36] Immunocompromised children should usually avoid live vaccines, but pre-symptomatic children with HIV can still benefit

from vacci-nation against measles, mumps, and rubella.[36] Finally, the selection of specific vaccines for children should be based on careful considera-tion of the child's activities, age, and medical condition. Children have increased risk for getting some diseases such as rabies, and young children mount incomplete responses to some vaccines such as that against meningococcus. Details about vaccines can be found in Chapters 10 and 11.

INSECT-BORNE DISEASES

More than a million children die each year due to malaria and other insect-borne diseases. Traveling children should be adequately protected from insect bites, especially in areas where vector-borne diseases are prevalent. Bite avoidance measures include activity scheduling, environmental manipulation, physical barriers, chemical repellents, and insecticides.[38]

Armed with knowledge of insect biting habits, families traveling with children can help schedule activities is such a way that children will decrease their risk of dangerous bites. Tick bites in central Europe, for instance, are more common in the summer than in the winter. Malaria-transmitting mosquitoes bite most in the evening and at night and can bite either inside or outside. In some areas, malaria transmission varies seasonally with the dry season typically being safer than the rainy season. Some dengue vectors are adapted for urban, indoor, daytime biting; since dengue may be life-threatening in children, families should be careful to avoid even the mosquitoes that are active during the morning and late afternoon hours. Sandflies transmitting leishmaniasis usually bite during the daytime. In areas of leishmaniasis endemicity, children should not camp or play near rodent burrows where sandflies are more active in disease transmission. Families who must share environments at seasons or times when disease transmission can occur should be particularly careful about applying personal protection measures to limit bites.

Mosquitoes like aquatic environments. They live and breed around water and do not necessarily require much more than a small puddle to support ongoing generations. When possible, children should be kept away from stagnant water, especially during evening and night hours when malaria-carrying mosquitoes are active. Residences, especially when windows are not perfectly screened, should not be surrounded by open water storage containers, puddles, or even plants that can hold water between leaves and stems. Cleaning the environment around dwelling places can markedly reduce the risk of transmission of malaria. When living or social obligations require children to be around untreated fresh water in the evening (such as during picnics near a river or lake), other insect protection measures should be fortified.

Clothes and bednets are useful barriers to block many insect bites. During times of insect activity in disease-endemic areas, children are advised to wear long sleeves and long pants or skirts. These clothes should be lightweight for comfort in tropical climates and should be lightly colored to make them less attractive to mosquitoes and other insects.

Bednets are highly effective in blocking insects' access to the skin of sleeping children. In areas where mosquitoes and other insects transmit pathogens at night, children should either sleep inside closed, screened, or air-conditioned rooms or else be placed under bednets. Bednets should be free of tears and should adequately cover the sleeping area so that the child will not sleep with body parts pressed up against the net. Bednets are most effective when they are impregnated with an insecticide such as permethrin.

DEET (N,N,diethyl-meta-toluamide or N,N-diethyl-3-methylbenzamide) is the best insect repellent available. This product has been used safely and effectively in millions of children for more than four decades.[39,40] Increased concentrations of DEET provide prolonged durations of effective repellent activity with 5–7% DEET protecting for one to 2 hours and 24% DEET protecting for 5 hours.[41] Polymerized formulations of DEET and near pure concentrations of DEET seem to provide slightly longer durations of protection from bites, but comparative data are limited. Recent popular pressure and concern about rare tragic outcomes in association with DEET use have stimulated controversy about the use of DEET in children. DEET can cause irritation of the eyes on local contact, and ingested DEET can have systemic complications. There have been 13 serious problems reported in children who were using DEET. Full details of these cases are not known, but the DEET was used inappropriately (more than ten times a day, licked off the skin) in at least some of the involved children. There has not actually been any good data to support a link between DEET concentration and the risk of adverse outcomes.[42] In the USA, both the Environmental Protection Agency[43] and, more recently, the American Academy of Pediatrics[44] have withdrawn restrictions about DEET concentration for use in children. In areas where life-threatening diseases may be transmitted, children can safely use DEET (Table 21.4) in a concentration (or with reapplication) to provide adequate protection from bites during the entire duration of their exposure to insects. DEET should not, however, be put near the eyes of young children who might rub it into their eyes, and DEET should not be put on the hands and forearms of children who have the habit of biting or licking those body parts. 'Natural,' botanical repellents containing citronella, eucalyptus, or other products are generally less effective than DEET as they provide only very short term (30 min) protection. Perfumed repellents smell nice but might actually attract insects. Newer repellents such as 1-pipetidinecarboxylic acid (Bayrepel) are being evaluated and hold promise of being at least as effective as DEET. Environmental insecticides including those that slowly release insecticide through gradually burning coils have some (50–75%) protective efficacy.[38] Ultrasonic buzzers and insect electrocuters are not effective in reducing insect bites.

Table 21.4	Use of DEET by children
Concentration	30–35%
Location	Use on exposed skin
	Avoid ocular contact (and hands and faces of children who rub eyes)
	Avoid oral ingestion (and hands of children who lick hands)
Technique	Light layer on exposed skin
	Reapply after 4–6 h if ongoing exposure

Permethrin and related pyrethroid compounds actually kill a variety of insects on contact. These products are effective against mosquitoes and ticks. They can be sprayed widely in communities, impregnated into bednets, or applied to clothes. Bednets and clothes lightly moistened with a 0.5% solution or spray of permethrin should be air-dried for about six hours before coming into contact with children. These nets and clothes are then protective for several weeks, even if laundered. Bednets immersed in and impregnated by more concentrated forms of insecticide can maintain their protective role for six to 12 months. The use of impregnated bednets decreases bites to children sleeping under the nets as well as to other individuals living in the same area.

Treatment of bites

Even with good bite avoidance efforts, however, insects do sometimes bite children. Uncomfortable swelling and itching can be relieved with the use of topical or systemic antihistamines such as diphenhydramine (given at a dose of about 1 mg/kg/dose every 4 to 6 h when used orally, sedation is not an uncommon side-effect). Bite sites should be kept clean, and scratching should be avoided to prevent the introduction of bacterial pathogens into the inflamed skin. The erythema and induration caused from the bite can increase for 24 h and can persist for ≥48 h. Swelling and redness that are still increasing after 24–48 h could be due to a superimposed secondary bacterial infec-tion. These bacterial infections might be helped by an oral antibiotic to cover against *Staphylococcus* and *Streptococcus* (such as cephalexin dosed at 15 mg/kg per dose three times daily or amoxicillin-clavulanate with the amoxicillin component dosed at 20 mg/kg per dose given twice daily). Red streaks extending from a bite could represent lymphangitic spread of a bacterial infection and could necessitate more aggressive antibiotic therapy.

For bothersome bites, systemic steroid therapy is reserved for very severe reactions such as those involving anaphylaxis. When a child has a true allergy to bites with systemic findings such as altered mental status, hypotension, or respiratory obstruction, epinephrine (0.01 ml/kg up to a maximum dose of 0.3 to 0.5 ml of the 1:1000 solution, repeated after 15 min if needed) and, possibly, glucocorticoids can be used.

Additional preventive strategies for specific insect-borne diseases

Malaria

Realizing that malaria[38] may be rapidly life threatening in children, chemoprophylaxis is usually incorporated into the preventive health-care plan of children traveling to malaria-endemic areas. The selection of medications depends on the travel itinerary and local resistance patterns as is discussed in Section 4. One of the high-risk groups for getting malaria during overseas trips includes families who previously came from the destination country and who are returning to visit friends and relatives. Such travelers sometimes bring their children in for pre-travel counsel. The child-based visit can serve as a good opportunity to offer necessary intervention to older traveling companions who might otherwise neglect their own care.

Children, especially those living in endemic areas, get sicker and get sick more quickly with malaria than their adult counterparts do. Prevention is, thus, vitally important. Even though some of a mother's chemoprophylaxis is distributed into breast milk, the effective dose reaching the child is very low and even nursing children need their own chemoprophylaxis.

Mefloquine is safe and effective in children irrespective of age and size. In general, side-effects with mefloquine in prophylactic doses seem to be similar to the effects in adults. But, vomiting, perhaps related to the taste, is frequently reported by people administering mefloquine to children. Mefloquine is given weekly as prophylaxis to children with a dose approximating 5 mg/kg. The weekly dose may be compounded into capsules to open at the time of administration, or the dose may be approximated upward to the nearest one-quarter pill amount. Either way, the tablet may be swallowed quickly by the older child or given crushed to a younger child. The crushed tablet does not taste good and may be mixed with a small volume of an age appropriate, tasty material, such as breast milk, chocolate pudding or syrup, or a cola drink. Emesis within 30 min of administration should prompt the re-administration of a full dose. As in adults, children should be encouraged to drink plenty of fluid as they take mefloquine. Also, as in adults, children with known psychiatric problems, cardiac rhythm disturbances, or an active seizure disorder should take an alternative agent. Children with attention deficit disorders or a remote history of a febrile convulsion should be able to take mefloquine without concern.

The combination of atovaquone and proguanil is, by all available evidence, safe and effective in traveling children. Again, since this product is not available in a liquid formulation, pills can be cut and crushed as needed to provide the appropriate dosing. The smaller 'pediatric' pills provide for ease in dosing in children. Compliance with daily administration and cost with longer-term travelers are issues, but the product seems as valuable in children as in adults. The 11 kg lower weight limit for the use of atovaquone-proguanil is based only on lack of supportive data and is not representative of any particular concern about safety or efficacy. When other chemoprophylactic agents are problematic in small children, the 'off-label' use of atovaquone-proguanil could be considered.

Daily doxycycline is useful in malaria prophylaxis of older children who are unable to take other products or who are going to areas of mefloquine resistant malaria. Doxycycline is generally not given to children less than 8 years of age due to concerns with the staining of growing teeth. There is also theoretical concern about altering long bone growth, but this does not seem to be a practical problem in children after fetal life. Use of doxycycline is accepted for the short-term treatment of life-threatening rickettsioses in young children, but the use of doxycycline for malaria prophylaxis prior to the eighth birthday is not widely accepted – even though the risk is 'only' dental discoloration. Use of sunscreen blocking both UVA and UVB light is advised, especially in those known to have photosensitivity reactions. Adolescent girls using doxycycline might benefit from having antifungal agents available in case vaginal candidosis becomes symptomatic.

For children traveling to an area where chloroquine-resistant falciparum malaria occurs, prophylaxis is usually with mefloquine, atovaquone-proguanil, or doxycycline. The choice between these agents depends on health history, age, and personal choice. For children who can not use any of these options and who have been tested and found to have normal glucose-6-dehydrogenase activity, primaquine could be another option for prophylaxis.

Chloroquine is safe in children of any age and size and can be used when indicated. Liquid formulations of chloroquine sulfate are available in some countries. Otherwise, compounded or crushed chloroquine pills (easiest if not the enteric-coated type) can be used to adjust doses to approximate 5 mg/kg dose of chloroquine base given orally each week. Despite a very low risk of retinopathy, periodic eye exams would be advised for children using prophylactic chloroquine for more than five years. See Section 4 for further details and dosages.

Tick-borne diseases[45]

Tick-borne diseases such as Lyme disease, rickettsioses, and tick paralysis, are problems for children in some areas. Tick bites, like mosquito bites are successfully prevented by the use of DEET on exposed skin with permethrin impregnation of clothes.

Most tick-borne illnesses do not develop until the ticks have been attached for more than 24 h. Thus, daily skin exams while in tick-laden environments are advised. Special attention should be paid to the neck and groin. Ticks may be removed by grasping them at the skin surface and pulling perpendicularly to the skin.

The risk of Lyme disease is possibly decreased by the use of post-bite doxycycline. When particularly large ticks (suggesting a prolonged attachment by the time of discovery) are identified in Lyme-endemic areas, a single 200 mg dose of doxycycline may be given to children 8 years of age and older. Prophylactic antibiotics are not otherwise indicated following tick removal.[45,46]

The Lyme vaccine previously used in the USA did not seem to protect against borreliosis in other parts of the world. Vaccines are not available for other tick-borne diseases.

Yellow fever and Japanese encephalitis

Mosquitoes transmit both yellow fever and Japanese encephalitis. Mosquito precautions are effective in preventing many bites. Vaccines, as discussed above and in Section 3, are effective for children at risk of contracting these illnesses during travel.

DIARRHEA

Food and water hygiene

The principles of preventing fecal-oral transmission of microbes through food and water hygiene are similar for adults and for children. Nonetheless, several pediatric-specific points are important.[47]

Breast-feeding provides good infant nutrition and some anti-infective protection. With exclusive breast-feeding during the first 4–6 months of life, traveling infants will have less exposure to potentially contaminated water/formula. Normal cleaning of the mothers' breasts is adequate.

Travelers' diarrhea seems to be more common in infants than in older children.[48] Food and water hygiene should be emphasized to parents of traveling infants. Many children have a habit of putting their hands in their mouths – either to suck, bite nails, or pick teeth. Parents of such children should be advised to be particularly careful about keeping hands washed. All children should be reminded to wash their hands before eating.

Children, perhaps even more than adults, sometimes forget to wisely select water sources during trips. Children in areas of incomplete water purification should be supervised and, as needed, reminded not to use tap water for drinking or for brushing teeth.

Epidemiology of diarrhea in pediatric travelers

The incidence of travelers' diarrhea, in at least one study,[48] varied with age. Forty percent of infants 0–2 years of age developed diarrhea during international travel, while only 9% of 3–6 year olds, 22% of 7–14 year olds, and 36% of 15–20 year olds did so. Infants also seemed to have travelers' diarrhea of longer duration and of greater severity than did older children.

The etiologic agents responsible for travelers' diarrhea do not seem to vary between children and adults. Thus, enterotoxigenic *Escherichia coli*, *Campylobacter*, *Salmonella*, and *Shigella* would all be potential bacterial pathogens in traveling children with diarrhea.

Treatment

Medications to prevent diarrhea are generally not indicated for children. Bismuth subsalicylate has some efficacy, but the link between salicylate use and Reye syndrome adds a pediatric-specific risk to the use of this product. Prophylactic antibiotics are generally not used in an effort to avoid the development of resistant bacterial strains among the nasopharyngeal and gastrointestinal flora.

For children with diarrhea, the major risk is dehydration. Therapy should center on oral hydration. When children are not dehydrated, water and routine drinks may be used for hydration. The child should take in a normal 'maintenance' amount of fluid along with enough to fully replace the extra gastrointestinal losses incurred during the illness. When dehydration is present, electrolyte solutions containing ~2% sugar and plenty of salt are best absorbed. To this end, the WHO rehydration solution, commercial products such as Pedialyte or Infalyte, or home-made solutions (2 tablespoons of table sugar and a quarter teaspoon of salt with, if possible, a quarter teaspoon of baking soda mixed in a liter of pure water) are effective. Fluids may be given via cup, spoon, or syringe. The child can continue with a regular, age-appropriate diet during the diarrheal illness once dehydration is corrected.[49,50]

Antimotility agents are used for adult travelers with bothersome diarrhea. These medications decrease the frequency of stool evacuation, but there is no clear evidence that they actually decrease intestinal fluid loss. Parents of children on antimotility agents should not be fooled into thinking that oral hydration efforts can be relaxed. Some antimotility agents such as diphenoxylate are absorbed and can have toxic systemic effects so are best avoided in young children. Loperamide has minimal systemic effects, though some adverse outcomes have been seen in young children. Loperamide did not decrease the need for rehydration in one infant study[51] but was effective in decreasing the severity and duration of diarrhea in children aged two to 11 years in others.[52] In general, the use of loperamide in infants and young children is not advised due to the risks of distracting families from needed oral hydration and of slowing the passage of invasive bacterial that might be causing the diarrhea.[49]

Bulking agents such as kaolin change the character of the stool but do not change the net fluid loss. They have not been shown to actually decrease the severity of diarrhea or the incidence of dehydration. Similarly, binding agents designed to attach to intestinal toxins are of unproven efficacy in children with travelers' diarrhea. Probiotics are being studied and hold some potential for developing a future indication in the treatment of children with travelers' diarrhea.[53]

Travelers' diarrhea, with good oral hydration, is a self-limited illness. Nonetheless, using systemic antibiotics can decrease the duration of symptoms. The agents responsible for travelers' diarrhea in adults and children have become increasingly resistant to sulfa antibiotics. Presumptive antibiotic therapy can shorten the duration of diarrhea in travelers. In areas such as industrialized nations where *E. coli*

O157:H7 is common, the risk of facilitating the development of hemolytic uremic syndrome precludes presumptive antibiotic therapy in children with bloody diarrhea.[54] For the typical child with travelers' diarrhea in a non-industrialized area, the benefit of a shortened illness often outweighs the minimal risks of antibiotic therapy.

Which antibiotic should be used in children?

Azithromycin (10 mg/kg once and 5–10 mg/kg on the subsequent 1–2 days as needed is often suggested, but no detailed studies comparing dosing regimens have been done) is effective against the pathogens causing travelers' diarrhea[47], is safe in children, and is available in convenient child-friendly dosing formulations. Ciprofloxacin (10 mg/kg twice daily for 1–3 days), is often effective against the causes of travelers' diarrhea and, despite early concerns about joint cartilage toxicity, seems safe in children.[55] Amoxicillin, co-trimoxazole, and erythromycin are of less effectiveness against the causal microorganisms in most traveling children.

RETURNED/IMMIGRATING TRAVELERS

What should be done for children returning from international journeys?

After short trips, an asymptomatic child would not require any specific medical intervention. After longer exposures overseas, even asymptomatic children can benefit from screening for common medical conditions. All returned pediatric travelers and immigrating children should be integrated into ongoing health care maintenance and supervision.

After international trips of longer than 3 months duration, one could consider several screening tests for the returned child.[56] Skin testing for tuberculosis would be useful if the child has been in an area where tuberculosis is common, but an asymptomatic child ideally should wait for 3 months after travel to be tested to avoid a falsely negative result during the 'window' between exposure and skin test positivity. If the child has been in an area of poor hygiene where intestinal parasitoses are common, stool microscopy for ova and parasites is useful. If the child was exposed to fresh water in a schistosomiasis-endemic area, urine and stool tests could be considered, but negative tests do not fully rule out infection; serology could be performed.

An immigrating child who is newly settling in to an industrialized nation could be a candidate for further health screening. A diet history and anthropomorphic measurements would help guide dietary counsel. Vision and hearing screening could help pick up mild deficits. Dental evaluation is useful to prevent asymptomatic dental caries from progressing to more serious conditions. Depending on the overseas situation from which the child came, there might be value in screening for HIV, hepatitis B antigenemia, hepatitis C antibodies, anemia, and lead toxicity in addition to screening for tuberculosis and intestinal and/or urinary parasites. Vaccination can be initiated or updated. Social workers can also help with adaptation to a new area. Psychologic referral can help children coming from particularly traumatic situations.

A febrile child who has been in a malaria-endemic area within the preceding couple of months should be immediately evaluated for malaria, even if appropriate prophylactic measures had been used. A complete blood count may give evidence of anemia or thrombocytopenia. Thick and thin malaria smears may provide a definitive diagnosis but should be repeated six to eight hours later if initially negative with significant concern for the possibility of malaria. A child with typhoid fever may present with fever in the absence of localizing physical signs and might have a mild leukopenia; cultures of blood and stool might give a definitive diagnosis. The specific and supportive care measures needed for a febrile returned traveler are similar to those in adults as long as weight-adjusted medication doses are used. Details of malaria treatment are discussed in Chapter 13.

Diarrhea is not uncommon in returned travelers. Diarrhea containing blood and mucus should prompt stool culture for invasive bacterial pathogens (*Campylobacter*, *Escherichia coli* O157:H7, *Shigella*, *Salmonella*, and, sometimes, *Yersinia*) as well as stool microscopy for amoeba. Antibiotics should be withheld pending culture results (to avoid treatment that is unnecessary or risky for prolonged carriage with *Salmonella* or risky for the development of hemolytic uremic syndrome such as with *E. coli* O157:H7). Hydration and routine feeding should be continued for a returned pediatric traveler with diarrhea. A child with chronic diarrhea should be tested for infectious causes (such as *Giardia* and *Cyclospora*) in addition to being evaluated for inflammatory bowel disease if that seemed likely. However, children may suffer from the same transient post-infectious bowel disorders as adults, namely, lactose intolerance and irritable bowel syndrome.

Dermatologic problems seem more common in returned pediatric travelers than in their adult companions, possibly because of the child's increased skin contact with the environment. Dermatitis from irritation or specific contacts can be treated with humidifying lotions and, when severe, with steroid creams. Infestations such as those caused by penetrating insect larvae or flea eggs can be managed by removing the foreign material, as in adult travelers. Pyogenic bacterial skin infections respond to topical mupirocin (applied 3–4 times daily for 5–10 days) or, when extensive, to oral cephalexin (15 mg/kg per dose, three times daily for 10 days).

CONCLUSION

Travel offers a wealth of good experiences for children and their families. With careful pre-travel evaluation of risks and protective interventions, the health risks of travel can be minimized. Managing these risks, health-care providers and families can ensure that foreign experiences during childhood are memorable and positive.

REFERENCES

1. Fischer PR. Travel with infants and children. *Infect Dis Clin North Am* 1998; **12**(2):355–368.
2. Knirsch CA. Travel medicine and health issues for families traveling with children. *Adv Pediatr Infect Dis* 1999; **14**:163–189.
3. Lanigan C, Wheeler M. *Lonely Planet Travel with Children*, 4th edn. London: Lonely Planet; 2002.
4. Wilson-Howarth J, Ellis M. *Your Child's Health Abroad: A Manual for Travelling Parents*. Bucks, UK: Bradt Publications; 1998.
5. Hostetter MK. Epidemiology of travel-related morbidity and mortality in children. *Pediatr Rev* 1999; **20**(7):228–233.
6. Bull MJ, Sheese J. Update for the pediatrician on child passenger safety: five principles for safer travel. *Pediatrics* 2000; **106**(5):1113–1116.
7. Biagioli F. Proper use of child safety seats. *Am Fam Physician* 2002; **65**(10):2085–2090.
8. Orlowski JP. Szpilman D. Drowning: rescue, resuscitation, and reanimation. *Pediatr Clin North Am* 2001; **48**(3):627–646.
9. Hargarten SW, Grenfell RD. Travel-related injuries (motor vehicle crashes, falls, drownings): epidemiology and prevention. In: DuPont HL, Steffen R, eds. *Textbook of Travel Medicine and Health*, 2nd edn. London: BC Decker; 2002:371–375.
10. Hebert RL, King GE, Bent JP. Tympanostomy tubes and water exposure: a practical model. *Arch Otolaryngol Head Neck Surg* 1998; **124**(10):1118–1121.
11. Ackerman MJ, Tester DJ, Porter CJ. Swimming, a gene-specific arrhythmogenic trigger for inherited long QT syndrome. *Mayo Clin Proc* 1999; **74**(11):1088–1094.
12. Committee on Sports Medicine and Fitness. Medical conditions affecting sports participation. *American Academy of Pediatrics* 2001; **107**(5):1205–1209.
13. Center for Diseases Control and Prevention. Health Information for International Travel 1999–2000, DHHS. *Atlanta* 1999; **212**
14. Parkins KJ, Poets CF, O'Brien LM, *et al*. Effect of exposure to 15% oxygen on breathing patterns and oxygen saturation in infants: interventional study. *BMJ* 1998; **316**:887–894.
15. Committee on Injury and Poison Prevention. Restraint use on aircraft. *Pediatrics* 2001; **108**(5):1218–1222.
16. Csortan E, Jones J, Haan M, *et al*. Efficacy of pseudoephedrine for the prevention of barotrauma during air travel. *Ann Emerg Med* 1994; **23**:1324–1327.
17. Buchanan BJ, Hoagland J, Fischer PR. Pseudoephedrine and air travel-associated ear pain in children. *Arch Pediatr Adolesc Med* 1999; **153**:466–468.
18. Gloster HM, Brodland DG. The epidemiology of skin cancer. *Derm Surg* 1996; **22**:217–226.
19. Kim HJ, Ghali FE, Tunnessen WW. Here comes the sun. *Contemp Pediatr* 1997; **14**:41–69.
20. Coogan PF, Geller A, Adams M, *et al*. Sun protection practices in preadolescents and adolescents: a school-based survey of almost 25,000 Connecticut school children. *J Am Acad Derm* 2001; **44**:512–519.
21. Diffey BL. When should sunscreen be reapplied? *J Am Acad Derm* 2001; **45**(6):882–885.
22. Durmowicz AG. Recognizing high-altitude illnesses in children. *J Resp Dis Pediatr* 2002; **4**(1):34–40.
23. Theis MK, Honigman B, Yip R, *et al*. Acute mountain sickness in children at 2835 meters. *Am J Dis Child* 1993; **147**:143–145.
24. Yaron M, Waldman N, Niermeyer S, *et al*. The diagnosis of acute mountain sickness in preverbal children. *Arch Pediatr Adol Med* 1998; **152**:683–687.
25. Pollard AJ, Niermeyer S, Barry P, *et al*. Children at high altitude: an international consensus statement by an ad hoc committee of the International Society for Mountain Medicine, 12 March, 2001. *High Alt Med Biol* 2001; **2**(3):389–403.
26. West JB. Consensus statement on children at high altitude. *High Alt Med Biol* 2001; **2**(3):322–323.
27. Gamponia MJ, Babaali H. Yugar F, *et al*. Reference values for pulse oximetry at high altitude. *Arch Dis Child* 1998; **78**:461–465.
28. DeMeer K, Heymans HS, Zijlstra WG. Physical adaptation of children to life at high altitude. *Eur J Pediatr* 1995; **154**(4):263–272.
29. Sui GJ, Liu YH, Cheng XS, *et al*. Subacute infantile mountain sickness. *J Pathol* 1988; **155**(2):161–170.
30. Khoury GH, Hawes DR. Primary pulmonary hypertension in children living at high altitude. *J Pediatr* 1963; **62**:177–185.
31. Sime F, Banchero N. Penaloza, *et al*. Pulmonary hypertension in children born and living at high altitudes. *Am J Cardiol* 1963; **11**:143–149.
32. Getts AG, Hill HF. Sudden infant death syndrome: incidence at various altitudes. *Dev Med Child Neurol* 1982; **24**(1):61–68.
33. Brouillette RT, Nixon G. Risk factors for SIDS as targets for public health campaigns. *J Pediatr* 2001; **139**(6):759–761.
34. Arguin PM, Krebs JW, Mandel E, *et al*. Survey of rabies preexposure and postexposure prophylaxis among missionary personnel stationed outside the United States. *J Travel Med* 2000; **7**:10–14.
35. Haley RW, Fischer RP. Commercial tattooing as a potentially important source of hepatitis C infection. Clinical epidemiology of 626 consecutive patients unaware of their hepatitis C serologic status. *Medicine (Baltimore)* 2001; **80**(2):134–151.
36. American Academy of Pediatrics. Report of the Committee on Infectious Disease, 25th edn. In: Pickering LK, ed. *2000 Red Book*. Elk Grove Village, IL: American Academy of Pediatrics; 2000.
37. American Academy of Pediatrics. Recommended childhood immunization schedule – United States, 2002. *Pediatrics* 2002; **109**(1):162.
38. Fischer PR, Bialek R. Prevention of malaria in children. *Clin Infect Dis* 2002; **34**:493–498.
39. Fradin MS. Mosquitoes and mosquito repellents: a clinician's guide. *Ann Intern Med* 1998; **128**:931–940.
40. Qui H, Jun HW, McCall JW. Pharmacokinetics, formulation, and safety of insect repellent N,N-diethyl-3-methylbenzamide (DEET): a review. *J Am Mosq Control Assoc* 1998; **14**:12–27.
41. Fradin MS, Day JF. Comparative efficacy of insect repellents against mosquito bites. *New Engl J Med* 2002; **347**:13–18.
42. Fischer PR, Christenson JC, Concentrated DEET. Safe - and sometimes necessary. *Contemp Pediatr* 1998; **15**(25):28.
43. US Environmental Protection Agency. EPA promotes safer use of insect repellent DEET (press release 24 April). Washington, DC: US Environmental Protection Agency; 1998.
44. Weil WB. New information leads to changes in DEET recommendations. *AAP News* 2001; **Aug**:52–53.
45. Wilson ME. Prevention of tick-borne diseases. *Med Clin North Am* 2002; **86**(2):219–238.
46. Poland GA. Prevention of Lyme disease: a review of the evidence. *Mayo Clin Proc* 2001; **76**:713–724.

47. Stauffer WM, Konop RJ, Kamat D. Traveling with infants and young children. Part III: travelers' diarrhea. *J Travel Med* 2002; **9**:141–150.

48. Pitzinger B, Steffen R, Tschopp A. Incidence and clinical features of traveler's diarrhea in infants and children. *Pediatr Infect Dis J* 1991; **10**(10): 719–723.

49. Provisional Committee on Quality Improvement. Practice parameter: the management of acute gastroenteritis in young children. *Pediatrics* 1996; **97**(3):424–433.

50. Duggan C, Nurko S. 'Feeding the gut': the scientific basis for continued enteral nutrition during acute diarrhea. *J Pediatr* 1997; **131**:801–808.

51. Bowie MD, Hill ID, Mann MD. Loperamide for treatment of acute diarrhoea in infants and young children. A double-blind placebo-controlled trial. *S Afr Med J* 1995; **85**:885–887.

52. Kaplan MA, Prior MJ, McKonly KI, *et al.* A multicenter randomized controlled trial of a liquid loperamide product versus placebo in the treatment of acute diarrhea in children. *Clin Pediatr (Phila)* 1999; **38**(10):579–591.

53. Markowitz JE, Bengmark S. Probiotics in health and disease in the pediatric patient. *Ped Clin North Am* 2002; **49**(1):127–141.

54. Wong CS, Jelacic S, Habeeb RL, *et al.* The risk of the hemolytic-uremic syndrome after antibiotic treatment of Escherichia coli O157: H7 infections. *N Engl J Med* 2000; **342**(26):1930–1936.

55. Jick S. Ciprofloxacin safety in a pediatric population. *Pediatr Infect Dis J* 1997; **16**:130–134.

56. Fischer PR, Christenson JC, Pavia AT. Pediatric problems during and after international travel. In: Bia FJ, ed. *Travel Medicine Advisor.* Atlanta: American Health Consultants; 1998:TC2, 9–18.

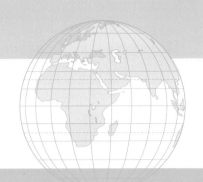

CHAPTER 22 The Elderly Traveler

Kathryn N. Suh

KEYPOINTS

- Cardiovascular disease and accidental trauma are the leading causes of death among older travelers

- Older travelers should plan their trip, have their fitness for travel assessed, and seek proper travel health advice well ahead of travel

- All older travelers – regardless of their health – should have adequate health insurance to cover medical and repatriation costs while abroad

- Recommended vaccines may be less immunogenic in the elderly, and the protective efficacy of many travel vaccines is unknown in this population

INTRODUCTION

Advancing age is less of a barrier to international travel than at any time in the past. The elderly account for an increasing number of the estimated 500 million travelers who cross international boundaries each year, and as the proportion of elderly in the population continues to increase, so too will the number of older travelers. The conveniences of modern day travel and the increased accessibility of formerly remote or exotic destinations may inspire older travelers to venture farther than they previously thought possible.

Age alone should not be considered a contraindication to travel. However, older travelers need to know that they are at increased risk of illness, injury, or death while traveling, even in the absence of pre-existing medical problems. The healthy elderly will often have greater difficulty acclimatizing during travel; they may take longer to adjust to extremes in temperature or humidity and changes in altitude, and may be more prone to motion sickness, jet lag, insomnia, and constipation.

With advancing age comes a greater likelihood of underlying medical conditions. Underlying disease may make the older traveler more vulnerable to acquiring travel-related infections, and may increase the severity of these illnesses. Specific travel recommendations (e.g., malaria chemoprophylaxis; vaccines) may also be affected by the traveler's medical condition and age.

While pre-travel assessments tend to focus on the prevention of travel-related infections, it is important to realize that only 1–3% of deaths in travelers are attributable to infectious diseases. The majority are due to natural causes – mostly cardiovascular disease – or trauma.[1,2] Evaluation of an individual's overall fitness for travel should be performed by the individual's own physician prior to travel. This is

particularly true for the older traveler, especially if the agenda includes a marked increase in physical activity. General advice regarding easily overlooked details, including preparation for travel, personal safety measures, insurance, and medical services during travel may be invaluable (Table 22.1). The pre-travel visit provides an opportunity to address these issues, and to offer practical advice that can minimize the chance of illness and injury and contribute to an enjoyable travel experience.

GENERAL ADVICE

Choosing a trip

Planning a trip well ahead of time is especially important for the older traveler. Knowledge of the travel destination(s) and nature of the trip is key if appropriate advice is to be provided. It may take longer to optimize the pre-travel condition of the older individual.

For some older travelers, all-inclusive resorts, organized tours, or cruises may be attractive alternatives to individually planned trips. They are usually well organized and feature a predetermined itinerary, choices in activities, leisurely travel with adequate opportunity for rest, reliable accommodations, assistance with luggage, and access (if necessary) to reliable medical care.

Fitness to travel

A general check-up is an excellent starting point for the elderly traveler, but does not replace the need for specific travel advice. A complete medical history and physical examination should be performed to assess fitness for travel. Ideally, this encounter should take place far enough in advance to allow for investigation and treatment of any undiagnosed conditions that might otherwise preclude (or delay) travel. There are few absolute contraindications to air travel: pneumothorax or pneumomediastinum; acute coronary syndromes, congestive heart failure, or significant dysrhythmias within 4 weeks of travel; thoracic, cardiac, abdominal, or middle-ear surgery within 3 weeks; cerebrovascular accidents within 2 weeks; and some infectious diseases during the period of communicability (e.g., chicken pox, measles, SARS, tuberculosis).[3] Respiratory tract infections and other pulmonary disorders, anemia, and most communicable diseases, are relative contraindications to air travel; with time and appropriate therapy, most will improve sufficiently to permit travel. It is essential that underlying medical conditions be taken into account prior to recommending *any* pharmacologic agents, including malaria chemoprophylaxis, immunizations, and over-the-counter remedies for common illnesses. Advice for travelers with underlying medical conditions is reviewed in other chapters and will not be discussed here (see Chapters 23–26).

Table 22.1	General advice for the older traveler

Plan your trip well ahead of time. Decide what kind of trip you want to take, and where. Make sure the destination is safe and that no travel advisories have been issued.

When booking travel, make sure that any special requests can be adequately accommodated, and ask about supplemental health insurance (if required) and cancellation insurance. Be certain to clarify limitations and exclusions prior to purchase.

Verify the extent of your current health insurance. Does it cover out-of-country expenses and repatriation costs?

Consider purchasing a medical bracelet if you have underlying medical conditions or medication allergies.

See your personal physician for a general physical examination prior to travel.

If medical services will be required during travel, ask your doctor if these can be arranged ahead of time, before you leave.

If required, consult a travel medicine specialist at least 4 weeks prior to departure (to allow adequate time for immunizations). Be sure that you understand the advice provided, and how to use medications that are prescribed.

Start a conditioning program 1 to 2 months prior to travel, if appropriate.

Take a first-aid kit containing commonly used items.

Carry any prescription medications with you (do not pack them in checked baggage). Bring extra medications and prescriptions for each. Check to ensure that all medications can be brought into the country or countries you are visiting.

Carry your personal physician's phone number and any relevant medical records with you.

Bring extra batteries for hearing aids or mechanical devices, and extra eyeglasses. A small repair kit may also come in handy.

Acclimatize gradually to heat, cold, and altitude. Drink adequate fluids, and drink alcohol judiciously.

Use common sense during travel to avoid accident and injury.

Seek medical attention if you develop a fever or other health problems during your trip or after your return home. Inform your doctor of your recent travels and the details of your trip.

If a significant increase in activity is anticipated during travel, a fitness or conditioning program started 1 or 2 months before can identify potential problems and improve both cardiovascular condition and muscular strength. Exercise stress testing is not routinely recommended during a pre-travel assessment, but may be considered for travelers who will be starting vigorous exercise as part of their trip or who are anticipating lengthy or remote treks – particularly men over 40 years of age, women over 50 years, and those with a history of coronary artery disease, or two or more risk factors for coronary disease.[4]

Making travel arrangements

Specific needs of individual travelers, both during travel and at the travel destination(s), should be discussed with the travel agent at the time of booking to ensure that they can be accommodated. When making travel reservations, aisle or bulkhead seats, both of which have increased legroom compared with standard seats, may be requested; aside from being more comfortable, legs can be stretched without having to stand. On flights where smoking is still permitted, seating in the non-smoking section should be requested if desired. Travelers requiring or preferring special diets for medical or personal reasons should request them 48 h prior to travel; most carriers have a reasonable selection to choose from, but cannot reliably accommodate last minute requests. Other special needs during travel – for example, the need for a wheelchair or motorized transportation at the terminal – should be requested and arranged with the individual carrier at least 48 h in advance.

Travelers should confirm their travel schedules prior to departure. Adequate time should be allowed for travel to the terminal and for check-in. If the departure gate is a considerable distance from the check-in desk or the security checkpoint, a motorized cart can be requested from the airline at check-in. While porters are available to assist with luggage in many terminals, this is not always the case; wheeled suitcases with extendable handles may be easier for the older traveler to negotiate through crowded areas.

Health insurance

More than most other travelers, the elderly should pay particular attention to ensuring that their health insurance is adequate for their intended travel. Government funded health insurance plans do not usually cover out-of-country medical expenses. Private insurance plans may, but the limitations of benefits while abroad should be carefully reviewed and clarified with the insurance provider. If required, supplemental travel insurance may be purchased through several providers, including most insurance and credit card companies and through travel agencies, as well as from travel insurance firms. Insurance must be purchased in the country of residence, prior to departure. Some companies will sell travel insurance on a fixed term basis (e.g., for a 12-month period), suitable for frequent travelers. For any supplemental insurance policy, options, restrictions, and conditions regarding coverage should be clarified with the provider. Most travelers will only purchase what they need (i.e., coverage from the day of departure to the intended day of return), but it may be wise to pay for a few extra days' of coverage in case return is delayed. Ensure that the policy will cover repatriation costs, and clarify under what conditions these can be claimed. In foreign countries, payment for medical services may be requested or required 'up front'; an itemized invoice or receipt for medical care or prescription medications will be required for subsequent reimbursement.

Travelers should carry details of any insurance policies with them, including policy numbers. Family or friends at home should also know how to contact the insurance carrier.

Medications and medical supplies

Commonly used medications and medical supplies may be useful to bring on any trip and are no different for the elderly, with the exception of laxatives, as constipation is more common in this age group. Denture wearers should be aware that denture adhesive may be difficult to find in some countries, and should carry a sufficient supply for the entire trip. First aid medications are not to be used indiscriminately in the elderly, as they can cause uncomfortable and potentially serious side-effects. If possible, older travelers should try to include medications that they have tolerated without incident in the past. Regardless, their use should be reviewed with the traveler prior to departure.

It is important to renew prescriptions for medications that might run out or expire during the trip. Prescription medications should be carried with the traveler at all times, to minimize the chance of loss or theft. Travelers should bring enough medications to last the duration of the trip, plus an extra several days' worth. Duplicate medications, and a prescription for each, should also be carried with the traveler and in some instances can be critical. Medications should be kept in their original bottles, each labeled with the medication name. Some medications and medical supplies – including but not limited to opiate analgesics, narcotics, and needles and syringes – may pose problems for importation across borders; a legitimate prescription can help to overcome this, as can an official (letterhead) letter from the traveler's personal physician. If prescriptions do need to be filled while away from home, it is preferable to obtain the identical medication from the same manufacturer, as differences do exist between different brands of the same medications. Although some medications may be cheaper in developing countries, the increasing problem of counterfeit medications should be used to dissuade travelers from purchasing medications while abroad. Travelers should contact the embassy or consulate of each country they intend to visit to find out if there are any restrictions in bringing medications into or out of the country.

Travelers should also carry the name and phone number of their physician and personal contacts in the event of an emergency, as well as a summary of their medical record, a complete list of current medications, and a copy of the most recent electrocardiogram if appropriate.

Medical services abroad

Health-care standards vary greatly throughout the world, and may differ significantly from those in the country of residence. Any acute illness, which alone can be traumatic in the elderly, is made even more stressful by an unfamiliar environment and language barriers.

A list of medical services available abroad can be obtained prior to travel through several sources, including the International Association for Medical Assistance to Travelers (IAMAT) (www.iamat.org). WorldMed.MD/Executive Physicians Worldwide, (www.executive-physicians.net), will arrange medical appointments ahead of time with English speaking physicians (including specialists) in the travel destination(s). International SOS provides global emergency assistance and medical services including, in many countries, the availability of overseas international clinics geared to the care of travelers (www.internationalsos.com).

Tips during air travel

Extended periods in a cramped environment can make travel to and from any destination unpleasant. The elderly traveler should take measures to ensure that travel comfort and safety are optimized.

Wear comfortable clothing. Intestinal gas expands with altitude and can cause abdominal discomfort, although this is rarely of any medical significance. Avoid foods that cause bloating (e.g., apple juice, carbonated beverages, sorbitol-containing sugarless gum). Alcohol and caffeinated beverages are both diuretics and should be avoided during flight. Dehydration can worsen jet lag and add to fatigue, and may contribute to the development of deep venous thrombosis. Regular contraction of leg muscles while seated, and short walks if safe to do so, may reduce the risk of thrombosis.

Travel safety

All travelers are advised to ensure that no travel advisories have been issued for their intended destination(s). Most federal governments (e.g., the US State Department, the Department of Foreign Affairs and International Trade in Canada, and the Foreign and Commonwealth Office in the UK) will provide regularly updated travel advisories by individual country.

A significant proportion of deaths in older travelers is due to accident or injury, many of which are preventable. Common safety precautions should always be taken. Slowed reaction times, auditory or visual impairment, and medication side effects may make the older traveler more vulnerable to accidents and crime.

MEDICAL CONDITIONS ARISING DURING TRAVEL

Motion sickness

Adults over 50 years of age and very young children are less susceptible to motion sickness, the former possibly related to an age-related decline in vestibular function.

Non-pharmacologic methods that may reduce motion sickness include closing eyes or fixing the gaze on the horizon, limiting head and neck movements, lying down (versus standing or sitting), and avoiding reading while in transit. In-flight turbulence may elicit symptoms, and seating over or near the wings may reduce its nauseagenic effects (possibly at the risk of having to open the window exits in an emergency, however). On cruise ships, the effect of the location of the passenger cabin on motion sickness is controversial, but in general, the rocking motion of a ship is less the closer a person is to its centre. Requesting a cabin with a window instead of an inner cabin may also reduce motion sickness.

Commonly used pharmacologic measures to combat motion sickness include dimenhydrinate, diphenhydramine and related antihistamines, and the anticholinergic agent scopolamine (hyoscine). Scopolamine can be administered orally, transdermally or intranasally; orally, it is the most effective drug for use in motion sickness, but the risk of side effects (drowsiness, dry mouth, blurry vision) is greater than with other agents. Its anticholinergic actions may also precipitate serious conditions including narrow-angle glaucoma, urinary retention (particularly in older men with prostatic hypertrophy) and intestinal ileus. Inhibition of sweating with scopolamine can contribute to heatstroke, especially when used in warmer climates. Dimenhydrinate and diphenhydramine are generally safer for use but may also lead to drowsiness, confusion, or ataxia, which may be exaggerated or prolonged in the elderly.

In-flight emergencies

The majority of medical emergencies in air travelers occur while still on the ground.[5] A wide variety of in-flight emergencies can occur, however, and may be related to the stress of travel, the cabin environment (turbulence, barometric pressure changes), or accident or injury. Unrelated medical emergencies also arise, and although less common, they are likely to be the most serious and may require diversion of the flight. Serious medical conditions most commonly reported during flight include cardiac events, syncope, bronchospasm, and seizures. It is estimated that as many as one in 10 000 air travelers will suffer from some in-flight medical emergency. Death during flight is relatively rare, with 21 to 90 reported each year in the US.[6] Most are sudden cardiac deaths, occurring in middle-aged men with no prior history of coronary disease.[7] The increasing use of automated external defibrillators on board may improve survival in some individuals.[8]

Cramped quarters and the limited medical equipment on board can complicate management of in-flight emergencies. All commercial air carriers have a basic medical kit, but the contents may vary. Flight attendants are trained in basic first aid, but commercial airlines are not responsible for delivery of medical care during flight. Flight crews will call ahead and arrange for medical personnel to meet the aircraft on arrival, if necessary.

Thromboembolic disease

An increased incidence of venous thromboembolic disease (VTED) in travelers, also called traveler's thrombosis or 'economy class syndrome', was first suggested in the 1950s. The exact incidence of VTED in travelers is unknown. Traveler's thrombosis appears to affect younger age groups and has a high incidence of symptomatic pulmonary embolism.[9] In one 3-year study of 104 deaths in long-distance travelers arriving at Heathrow Airport, 12% of all deaths and 18% of those occurring in-flight were attributed to pulmonary embolism.[10] Several case series suggest a causal association between long-haul flights and thrombosis, but prospective data to confirm this are lacking.

Ferrari et al.,[11] in a small case-control study, found travelers to have a four-fold increased risk of idiopathic VTED; 72% of the 39 cases had a history of recent automobile travel, whereas only 23% had traveled by air. Most travelers who develop VTED do so in the presence of known risk factors: a past history of VTED, malignancy, recent lower extremity trauma, recent major surgery, hyperestrogenic states, past or family history of thrombophilia, or prolonged immobilization. In the absence of predisposing risk factors and regardless of age, air travelers do not appear to have an increased risk of thrombosis.[9]

Adequate hydration and frequent leg stretching during travel (or short walks, if safe to do so) are recommended. Compression stockings may reduce the incidence of thrombosis during travel[12] and, in addition to aspirin or low molecular weight heparin, should be considered for use in high-risk travelers. For the majority of older travelers, however, these are not indicated. Most cases of VTED become clinically apparent within 96 h of flight.[9] Travelers should be educated about signs and symptoms of VTED, and advised to seek medical attention if one or more develops.

Jet lag

Jet lag, a mismatch between the body's circadian rhythm and the external environment due to travel across multiple time zones, is characterized by fatigue, sleep disturbance, and impaired overall function. The syndrome is more pronounced as the number of time zones crossed increases, and with eastbound travel. Normally lasting up to 7 days, it is more common and may be more severe or prolonged in the elderly.

Adequate rest prior to travel and proper hydration during may improve overall well-being independent of any effect on jet lag. Dividing long trips into segments (with multiple stopovers) can reduce jet lag, but often with additional inconvenience. Adapting one's daily routine to the current time of day upon reaching the destination can minimize jet lag. Exposure to bright outdoor light may help readjust the circadian rhythm. Other interventions such as exercise and diet are unproven in reducing jet lag.

Benzodiazepines provide some relief from sleep disturbances, but can result in daytime sleepiness as well as general drowsiness, impaired memory, and fatigue. These effects may be more pronounced in older travelers, especially those unaccustomed to taking these medications. Zolpidem (Ambien®), a short-acting imidazopyridine hypnotic that is used for short-term treatment of insomnia, has been shown to be more effective in the treatment of jet lag than melatonin.[13] Elimination half-life and adverse effects of zolpidem such as confusion, ataxia and falls, and gastrointestinal side effects (cramps, nausea, vomiting, diarrhea) are increased in the elderly; the initial dosage should be halved (5 mg before bedtime) in the older individual. Clinical trials examining the use of melatonin have reported conflicting results[14,15] although a recent meta-analysis supports its use.[16] In one dose finding study, the 5 mg fast-release formulation was most effective in combating jet lag, although lower doses (0.5 mg) were also effective; however, no sub-jects older than 65 years of age were included.[17] Melatonin is not currently licensed as a drug but is widely available as a nutritional supplement. The long-term safety of melatonin is unknown. Detailed information on jet lag is provided in Chapter 42.

Hyperthermia and hypothermia

The elderly are more susceptible to the effects of heat and cold. Proper clothing is essential in both extremes of temperature. Acclimatization to heat or cold may take several days. The older traveler should limit outdoor activity if weather conditions are extreme, or at least gradually adapt to the climate over several days.

Heat

Peripheral vasodilation is impaired with advanced age and perspiration is diminished, reducing the body's cooling mechanisms in hot climates. The thirst response may also be diminished in the elderly, leading to dehydration. The risk of overheating and heatstroke may be further increased by medications that impair thermoregulation, including antihistamines, anticholinergics, beta and calcium channel blockers, diuretics, tricyclic antidepressants, and antiparkinsonian medications. Older travelers need to use caution in hot weather and drink adequate fluid, avoiding caffeine and alcohol, which will worsen dehydration. Travelers with renal disease and those on diuretics are especially prone to volume and electrolyte abnormalities if they develop dehydration or heatstroke.

Cold

The elderly are also more susceptible to the cold. Heat generating mechanisms (i.e., shivering) are diminished in older individuals. Appropriate clothing (layered) is essential, and damp clothes should be changed immediately. Alcohol and cigarette smoking can increase the risk of cold-related illnesses (hypothermia and frostbite). Proper hydration is as important in cold climates as it is in the heat.

Altitude sickness

Altitude sickness refers to several different clinical syndromes, the most common of which is acute mountain sickness (AMS). Interestingly, the elderly are at lower risk for AMS than younger travelers.[18] With a 5-day acclimatization period, the healthy elderly can tolerate altitudes of 2500 m well; hypoxemia, sympathetic activation, pulmonary hypertension, and reduced plasma volume do contribute to reduced exercise capacity, however.[19] Those with underlying cardiopulmonary disease or anemia may have more severe hypoxemia or cardiac ischemia at higher altitudes. Beta-blockers can reduce the expected compensatory tachycardia and give rise to dyspnea. A reasonable level of fitness and adequate acclimatization will minimize the risk of AMS in the elderly.

Accidents and injury

Trauma is a significant cause of morbidity and mortality in the traveler. Injury accounted for 25% of deaths in US travelers between

1975 and 1984,[1] and 38% in Canadians in 1995.[2] Trauma-related deaths in travelers are more common in males, and in the young and elderly.[1] The elderly may be at higher risk of injury or accident due to slowed reaction times, auditory and visual impairment, and medication side effects. Motor vehicle accidents are by far the most common accidental cause of death, with the victim often a passenger. Other causes include drowning and diving mishaps, falls, maulings, and natural disasters. Homicide is an unusual cause of death while abroad. Most (80%) travelers who die from trauma do so before reaching a hospital; even if transport to a hospital occurs, evacuation is often required because of inadequate medical facilities.

TRAVEL-RELATED INFECTIONS IN THE ELDERLY

Malaria

Prevention of malaria is essential for any traveler venturing to a malarious area, regardless of age. Older travelers might be considered less likely to acquire malaria because the activities they pursue may place them at lower risk, but this assumption can lead to fatal outcomes. Illness may be more severe in the elderly, and mortality from malaria increases with age. Assessment of malaria risk cannot be ignored in the elderly.

There is no increased toxicity from N,N-diethyl-3-methylbenzamide (DEET) in the elderly. Chemoprophylaxis is always indicated; it can be safely administered in the elderly and may be better tolerated than in younger age groups, but caution must be exercised in certain settings. Chloroquine can rarely cause irreversible retinal damage if used in the presence of known retinal disease, and hearing loss has been reported in those with auditory impairment. Mefloquine should not be used in the presence of cardiac conduction defects or neuropsychiatric disorders but is otherwise safe to use in the elderly. Beta or calcium blocker use does not preclude the use of mefloquine. Atovaquone-proguanil is generally well tolerated when used for prophylaxis, but only small numbers of travelers aged 65 years and older have been included in studies performed to date.

Travelers' diarrhea

Young adults are more likely to acquire travelers' diarrhea (TD) than other travelers: they eat more (and more adventurously), and may be less immune to TD pathogens. In theory, older travelers should be more susceptible to TD because decreased gastric acidity – due to achlorhydria, H_2 blocker or proton pump inhibitor use, or prior gastrectomy – lowers the bacterial inoculum required to produce disease, but this has not been proven in epidemiologic studies. Complications of TD including dehydration and electrolyte imbalance are more poorly tolerated in the elderly, however, especially in those with underlying cardiac, renal, or gastrointestinal disease, the immunosuppressed, and those on diuretics.

Preventive measures emphasizing safe eating and drinking, supportive therapy, and self-treatment should be discussed. Antimicrobial chemoprophylaxis is not recommended for most travelers, but may be considered in the elderly, for reasons noted above; however, evidence of any benefit is lacking. A daily dose of a fluoroquinolone would be recommended, beginning one day prior to departure and continuing until 2 days after the last exposure, for a maximum of 3 weeks. Arguments against antimicrobial prophylaxis include the availability of highly effective (even single dose) antimicrobial therapy, adverse effects, development of antimicrobial resistance, and the false sense of security provided.

Antimotility agents (loperamide, diphenoxylate hydrochloride-atropine) can be used for symptomatic relief of TD in the absence of bloody diarrhea, but may cause constipation, paralytic ileus, and central nervous system depression (especially with diphenoxylate, which is a narcotic). Anticholinergic side effects can also contribute to hyperthermia. Older fluoroquinolones (ciprofloxacin, norfloxacin, ofloxacin) remain the antimicrobial agents of choice for treating TD; dose adjustment is required for reduced creatinine clearance.

VACCINE PREVENTABLE INFECTIONS

The pre-travel visit provides an opportunity to update routine immunizations (influenza, measles, tetanus, polio, and pneumococcal vaccine), as well as to administer appropriate travel immunizations. Vaccine-induced antibody responses can take longer in the elderly, and vaccines should therefore be given well ahead of travel. Data regarding the immunogenicity and efficacy of many vaccines in the elderly are scarce. Recommendations for travel immunizations are the same as those for younger adults.

Routine immunizations

Influenza

Influenza vaccine is recommended annually for all adults over age 65 (over age 50 in the USA). The effectiveness of the vaccine depends on the age and immune status of the recipient, as well as the similarity between vaccine and circulating viruses. The vaccine is at least 70% effective in preventing illness in adults less than 65 years of age. Vaccine induced antibody titers are lower in those over age 65, in whom vaccine effectiveness falls to as low as 30%. Despite this, immunization of the elderly does reduce influenza-attributable mortality and the need for hospitalization.

Measles

Measles continues to be a public health problem in many parts of the world. Older travelers should be immune and do not require measles vaccine. Only those born after 1957 in the USA (after 1970 in Canada), who have not received two doses of measles vaccine or have not had natural infection are at risk of contracting measles.

Pneumococcal vaccine

Pneumococcal polysaccharide vaccine is recommended for adults over 65 years of age. Over 80% of young healthy adults develop antibody responses to immunization, but both the frequency and magnitude of response fall in the elderly population. Overall vaccine efficacy in the elderly is around 60%. Antibody titers and possibly vaccine efficacy fall with increasing time since immunization, but protection lasts at least 5 years and re-immunization is recommended only in select circumstances.

Poliovirus

Seroprevalence studies demonstrate high rates of poliovirus seropositivity in adults of all ages, including the elderly. Unimmunized or inadequately immunized adults who are traveling to areas where polio still occurs should receive or complete their primary series (three doses at 0, 1–2, and 6–12 months) with inactivated vaccine. The need for booster doses in immune adults is unknown.

Tetanus

Tetanus seropositivity declines with age, but deaths from tetanus are exceedingly rare in those who have completed their primary series, suggesting that protection is probably long lasting in this group. Nonetheless, a decennial tetanus toxoid booster (combined with diphtheria toxoid, or given alone) is still recommended. A single booster dose will induce protective immunity of at least one year's duration in over 80% of elderly individuals who have inadequate levels of tetanus antibody.[20]

Travel vaccines

Cholera

Since 1992, no country has required a certificate of vaccination against cholera. Most travelers are at low risk of acquiring cholera and immunization is not routinely recommended. The live inactivated oral vaccine (CVD103HgR) is currently the vaccine of choice, with 82–100% overall protection but only 62–67% against the *El Tor* biotype. There are no efficacy data specifically for elderly populations, however. The new oral B sub-unit whole cell cholera vaccine has not been tested in the elderly.

Hepatitis A

Hepatitis A is the most common vaccine-preventable infection among travelers. Both severity of illness and mortality increase with age (2–7% mortality over age 50). Older travelers who have lived or traveled in endemic regions, or who have a prior history of jaundice, have a higher prevalence of hepatitis A antibody; screening prior to immunization may be cost-effective in this population.

Non-immune older travelers should receive inactivated hepatitis A vaccine, which is well tolerated in most recipients regardless of age. Few studies have examined age-related responses to hepatitis A vaccine, and none has included subjects over age 65.[21] Overall sero-conversion rates in adults are highest (85–95%) in those less than age 40 and fall to 60–84% beyond this age, regardless of the vaccine preparation used. The response to immunization is also slower, and antibody titer lower, in older recipients. For the older traveler, this means they should be immunized at least 4 weeks before travel, and that immunization may be less effective (no data). While vaccine-induced immunity is expected to be long lasting, the lower antibody titer seen in older individuals could translate into a shorter duration of protection, although this is currently unknown. Immunoglobulin remains an alternative to active immunization.

Hepatitis B

Immunization against hepatitis B should be considered for non-immune travelers to highly endemic regions and those who are likely to be exposed to blood or sexual contacts.

Pre-immunization serologic evaluation is appropriate in those who are likely to have had prior infection. Seroconversion rates and antibody titer after 3 doses of vaccine are lower, and the response to immunization slower, with advancing age.[22] Over 90% of adults less than 40 years of age will develop protective levels of antibody, but only 70% of those aged 50 to 59 and 50% of those aged 60 and over will respond. Antibody titer declines with time since immunization, and persistence of hepatitis B surface antibody is dependent on the peak titer obtained. However, protection against infection persists even if antibody titer becomes undetectable. Overall vaccine effectiveness is approximately 95%. Protection lasts at least 15 years and probably for life; booster doses are not currently recommended.

Japanese encephalitis

Travelers to Asia are extremely unlikely to acquire Japanese encephalitis; few cases have been reported in travelers to date. Most infections are subclinical. Encephalitis occurs in less than 1% of infections but has a high mortality rate, and poor neurologic recovery in survivors. The incidence and severity of infection, and the risk of death, increase with advancing age. Immunization of adult travelers

to epidemic zones and those who will spend more than 1 month in endemic areas is recommended.

The currently available formalin inactivated vaccine, administered as a three dose series, produces antibody titers of >1:10 in over 90% of young, non-immune adults (i.e., those not residing in endemic areas). Antibody persists for at least 3 years in this population. The exact relationship between titer and immunity is unclear however. Protective efficacy has not been studied in travelers. Studies have not been conducted in older, non-immune populations, and the immunogenicity, efficacy, and duration of protection in this age group is unknown. Local and systemic side-effects occur in approximately 20% and 10% of recipients, respectively. Rarely, encephalitis and hypersensitivity reactions may occur. It is unknown whether the incidence and severity of adverse events are increased in the elderly.

Meningococcal vaccine

Meningococcal vaccine is recommended for travelers to areas with a high incidence of meningococcal disease, particularly those planning a prolonged (≥3 weeks) stay. Meningococcal disease affects mainly children and young adults, and vaccine efficacy studies have focused on these groups. A single dose of quadrivalent polysaccharide vaccine (serogroups A, C, Y, W-135) results in 90–95% protection against disease. The exact duration of immunity is unknown but is probably at least 5 years. There are no data regarding immunogenicity, efficacy, and safety in the elderly.

Rabies

The risk of contracting rabies is low in most travelers; immunization is advised only for those planning extended stays in remote, high-risk areas or in whom occupational exposures are likely. Two doses of human diploid cell vaccine produce protective levels of antibody in almost all healthy recipients, with intramuscular administration producing higher titers than the intradermal route. Adults over age 60 do respond adequately to immunization, but peak titers are lower in this age group.[23] Antibody duration is generally 1.5 to 2 years, but it is unclear whether lower peak titers in the elderly correlate with a shorter duration of protection. The incidence and severity of adverse effects do not appear to be age-related.

Typhoid fever

Typhoid fever is relatively rare in travelers, but vaccine should be offered to older travelers to endemic areas, particularly those intending to have prolonged (≥3 weeks) stays. Severity of illness and mortality from typhoid fever increase with age.

Two vaccines are available: purified Vi polysaccharide vaccine, and a live attenuated oral vaccine. The polysaccharide vaccine is easily administered and relatively well tolerated, but adverse events (fever, headache, local reactions) are more common than with the oral vaccine. In polysaccharide vaccine trials, a fourfold rise in antibody titer was noted in over 90% of subjects. Most efficacy trials have been performed in children and young adults living in endemic areas; protective efficacy is comparable for both vaccine preparations, between 60 and 70%. Additional doses are recommended every 3 years for the parenteral vaccine and every 5 years for the oral vaccine, if ongoing or renewed exposure is anticipated. In some countries, health officials recommend booster doses annually as long as exposure occurs. No studies using either vaccine preparation have specifically examined seroconversion rates or protective efficacy in the elderly, and studies of vaccine efficacy in travelers are also lacking.

Varicella

Most (90%) adults from temperate climates have been infected with varicella during childhood. Severity of illness and mortality both increase with age. Both humoral and cell-mediated immune responses occur following natural infection and both decline with age.

Adult travelers without a history of varicella can be tested for the presence of antibodies and, if seronegative, offered the live attenuated vaccine. Seroconversion rates following a single vaccine dose are age-related, and are lower in adults than in children (75 versus >95%, respectively); with a second dose in adults, this rises to >95%. The overall effectiveness of varicella vaccine is approximately 90%, but is lower in adults. Breakthrough infection can occur despite immunization; severity is inversely related to antibody titer, but in general the disease is milder than natural infection, with fewer skin lesions and a lower complication rate. Local reactions and fever are the most common vaccine side effects; injection site or generalized varicella-like lesions occur in ~5% of immunized adults. There are no immunogenicity or adverse event data specifically pertaining to the elderly. The duration of protection and the need for booster doses are unknown. Immunization of the elderly also enhances cell-mediated immunity which may protect against herpes zoster (shingles), although the vaccine is not currently licensed for this indication.

Yellow fever

Yellow fever is rare in travelers. Adults over age 50 are at higher risk for severe disease and death from yellow fever. Certain countries in endemic areas require immunization for entry; others require it for those arriving from an endemic area.

Although antibody is assumed to correlate with protection against disease, efficacy studies have not been performed. In young adults, practically all vaccine recipients will seroconvert by 4 weeks, and immunity is expected to last at least 10 years; however, there are no such data for the elderly. Up to 40% of recipients will develop mild local or systemic reactions. Anaphylaxis occurs in 1:131 000 doses; meningoencephalitis is an extremely rare adverse event in adults. The risk of serious side-effects, hospitalization, and death following immunization appear to be more common in the elderly. Retrospective analysis of passively reported adverse events suggests that the relative risk of a serious systemic adverse event is 3.7 for those aged 65–74 years and 11.6 for those over 75 years of age, compared with those aged 25–44 years.[24] Approximately 1:50 000 vaccinees over age 65 is at risk of severe adverse reaction to the primary dose of vaccine. In practical terms, these data suggest that it would be prudent not to immunize elderly travelers who are at no risk for yellow fever, even if the vaccine is required by international regulations, e.g., travelers aboard cruise ships stopping at ports along the coast of South America, but not traveling inland where yellow fever is a risk. A medical certificate indicating that the vaccine is 'contraindicated for medical reasons' is a reasonable alternative.

CONCLUSION

The number of older travelers will only continue to increase in the future. While some limitations and restrictions to travel may be necessary for health reasons, there is little reason why the elderly cannot travel to a broad range of destinations. With adequate preparation and appropriate advice, the elderly traveler can enjoy good health during travel.

REFERENCES

1. Hargarten SW, Baker TD, Guptill K. Overseas fatalities of United States citizen travelers: an analysis of deaths related to international travel. *Ann Emerg Med* 1991; **20**:622–626.
2. MacPherson DW, Guerillot F, Streiner DL, et al. Death and dying abroad: the Canadian experience. *J Travel Med* 2000; **7**:227–233.
3. Jong EC, Benson EA. Travel with chronic medical conditions. In: Jong EC, McMullen R, eds. *The Travel and Tropical Medicine Manual*, 2nd edn. Philadelphia: WB Saunders; 1997:142–150.
4. Backer H. Medical limitations to wilderness travel. *Emerg Med Clin North Am* 1997; **15**:17–41.
5. Cummins RO, Schubach JA. Frequency and types of medical emergencies among commercial air travelers. *JAMA* 1989; **261**:1295–1299.
6. Rodenberg H. Medical emergencies aboard commercial aircraft. *Ann Emerg Med* 1987; **16**:1373–1377.
7. Cummins RO, Chapman PJC, Chamberlain DA, et al. In-flight deaths during commercial air travel. *JAMA* 1988; **259**:1983–1988.
8. Page RL, Joglar JA, Kowal RC, et al. Use of automated external defibrillators by a U.S. airline. *N Engl J Med* 2000; **343**:1210–1216.
9. Kesteven PJL, Robinson BJ. Clinical risk factors for venous thrombosis associated with air travel. *Aviat Space Environ Med* 2001; **72**:125–128.
10. Sarvesvaran R. Sudden natural deaths associated with commercial air travel. *Med Sci Law* 1986; **1**:35–38.
11. Ferrari E, Chevallier T, Chapelier A, et al. Travel as a risk factor for venous thromboembolic disease. A case-control study. *Chest* 1999; **115**:440–444.
12. Scurr JH, Machin SJ, Bailey-King S, et al. Frequency and prevention of symptomless deep-vein thrombosis in long-haul flights: a randomised trial. *Lancet* 2001; **357**:1485–1489.
13. Suhner A, Schlagenhauf P, Hofer I, et al. Effectiveness and tolerability of melatonin and zolpidem for the alleviation of jet lag. *Aviat Space Environ Med* 2001; **72**:638–646.
14. Petrie K, Conaglen JV, Thompson L, et al. Effect of melatonin on jet lag after long haul flights. *BMJ* 1989; **298**:705–707.
15. Spitzer RL, Terman M, Williams JBW, et al. Jet lag: clinical features, validation of a new syndrome-specific scale, and lack of response to melatonin in a randomized, double-blind trial. *Am J Psychiatry* 1999; **156**:1392–1396.
16. Herxheimer A, Petrie KJ. Melatonin for preventing and treating jet lag. *Cochrane Database Syst Rev* 2001; **1**:CD001520.
17. Suhner A, Schlagenhauf P, Johnson R, et al. Comparative study to determine the optimal melatonin dosage form for the alleviation of jet lag. *Chronobiol Int* 1998; **15**:655–666.
18. Roach RC, Houston CS, Honigman B, et al. How well do older persons tolerate moderate altitude? *West J Med* 1995; **162**:32–36.
19. Levine BD, Zuckerman JH. deFilippi CR. Effect of high-altitude exposure in the elderly. The Tenth Mountain Division study. *Circulation* 1997; **96**:1224–1232.
20. Alagappan K, Rennie W, Lin D, et al. Immunologic response to tetanus toxoid in the elderly: one-year follow-up. *Ann Emerg Med* 1998; **32**:155–160.
21. Leder K, Weller PF, Wilson ME. Travel vaccines and elderly persons: review of vaccines available in the United States. *Clin Infect Dis* 2001; **33**:1553–1566.
22. Andre FE. Summary of safety and efficacy data on a yeast-derived hepatitis B vaccine. *Am J Med* 1989; **87**(**suppl 3A**):14S–20S.
23. Mastroeni I, Vescia N, Pompa MG, et al. Immune response of the elderly to rabies vaccines. *Vaccine* 1994; **12**:518–520.
24. Martin M, Weld LH, Tsai TF, et al. Advanced age as a risk factor for illness temporally associated with yellow fever vaccination. *Emerg Infect Dis* 2001; **7**:945–951.

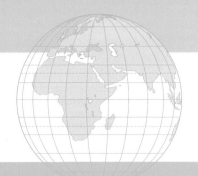

CHAPTER 23   The Disabled Traveler

Kathryn N. Suh

INTRODUCTION

In the USA alone, an estimated 49 million people live with disabilities, of whom over 70% are able to travel. Physical or cognitive disability, similar to advancing age, pose less of a hurdle to international travel today than ever before. Travel companies and carriers have become more aware of the growing number of disabled travelers. Furthermore, legislation has been enacted to protect the traveler with special needs against unfair treatment. The Air Carrier Access Act[1] in the United States and the Canada Transportation Act[2] in Canada were enacted to allow disabled travelers to travel safely and without discrimination on commercial aircraft. A draft of the Code of Practice for Access to Air Travel for Disabled People[3] serves a similar purpose in the UK, and the European Commission has started proceedings to legislate air carrier contracts and passengers' rights within the European Union.[4] Legislation also exists to ensure that disabled travelers have improved accessibility to rail and ferry transport.

Physical or cognitive limitations should not prevent most affected individuals from traveling. Advance planning can reduce or eliminate many of the hassles of travel for the disabled individual and contribute to a positive experience.

GENERAL ADVICE

General advice for the physically disabled or impaired traveler is similar to that recommended for older travelers. Issues relevant to specific disabilities will be discussed below. One excellent source of travel information for the disabled is the Society for Accessible Travel and Hospitality website (www.sath.org), which provides an extensive list of resources for the disabled traveler. Other resources for the disabled traveler are listed in Table 23.1.

An assessment by the traveler's personal physician should precede any trip, in order to determine overall fitness to travel, to determine whether the specific disability will impose certain travel restrictions (e.g., on the mode of transportation, or the need for specific accommodations or accompaniment), and to identify other health issues that could pose problems during the trip. Specific travel advice about safe eating and drinking, prevention and self-treatment of traveler's diarrhea and malaria, and immunizations should be sought from a travel medicine specialist.

Careful attention should be paid to health and cancellation insurance; purchase of a supplemental health insurance policy may be prudent. Travelers requiring medical equipment including mobility devices (such as wheelchairs, walkers, prostheses), and hearing and visual aids, should check if their insurance policy covers theft, loss, or damage of these devices. Finally, if medical attention will be required while abroad, an appointment(s) arranged prior to departure (with specialists if required) can relieve the stress of finding appropriate medical attention in a foreign country.

CHOOSING A TRIP AND MAKING TRAVEL ARRANGEMENTS

The nature and severity of one's disability, and the need for physical assistance, special accommodations, or mobility devices obviously have some bearing on the type of trip that the disabled traveler can enjoy. Some travel agencies have expertise in arranging trips for the disabled, and some organizations specialize in providing group tours or cruises for individuals with particular needs (e.g., dialysis cruises, group travel for the developmentally disabled or for wheelchair users, etc.). These trips, offered to a variety of destinations, provide the traveler with a pre-determined itinerary at a suitable pace, companionship, professional supervision, and medical services where necessary. Some organizations offering these services are listed in Table 23.1.

Specific needs of disabled travelers that are likely to arise during travel and at the destination(s) should be discussed with a travel agent, and their availability confirmed prior to booking travel. These arrangements should be verified again at least 48 hours prior to departure, and at check-in. Written confirmation of arrangements for special services may also be useful. Because pre-boarding and de-planing assistance are often required, disabled travelers are usually the first on and last off aircraft. This should be taken into account when booking connecting flights, and adequate time should be allowed between flights. The airline should provide help for the disabled traveler to reach connecting flights. Individuals traveling with a wheelchair, scooter, or other assistive device should inform the carrier and ask how these can be transported. Special seating requests should also be made at the time of booking – for example, aisle or bulkhead seats may facilitate wheelchair transfers, and seats closer to

Table 23.1 **Resources for disabled travelers**

General information: organizations

Access-Able Travel Source
www.access-able.com
e-mail: access-able@webaccess.net
PO Box 1796
Wheat Ridge CO 80034 USA
Tel: (303) 232-2979

Society for Accessible Travel and Hospitality
www.sath.org
e-mail: sathtravel@aol.com
347 Fifth Avenue
Suite 610
New York NY 10016 USA
Tel: (212) 447-0027

Canadian Transportation Agency
www.cta-otc.gc.ca
e-mail: cta.comment@cta-otc.gc.ca
Ottawa, Ontario K1A 0N9
Tel: (888) 222-2592
TTY: (800) 669-5575

United States Department of Transportation
Federal Aviation Agency Office of Civil Rights
www.faa.gov/acr/dat.htm
e-mail: dot.comments@ost.dot.gov
400 Seventh Street SW
Washington DC 20590 USA
Tel: (202) 366-4000

General Information: Books

Rosen F. *How to Travel: A Guidebook for Persons with a Disability*
Manchester, MO:
Science and Humanities Press, 1997.
website: http://banis-associates.com

Physically Disabled Travelers

Mobility International USA
www.miusa.org
e-mail: development@miusa.org
PO Box 10767
Eugene OR 97740 USA
Tel: (541) 343-1284

Royal Association for Disability and Rehabilitation
www.radar.org.uk
e-mail: radar@radar.org.uk
12 City Forum
250 City Road
London EC1V 8AF
Tel: 020 7250 3222

Disabled Persons Transport Advisory Committee
(DTPAC) Working Group
www.dptac.gov.uk
e-mail: dptac@dtlr.gov.uk
c/o Secretariat
Great Minster House
76 Marsham Street
London SW1P 4DR
Tel: 020 7944 3238

www.holidaycare.org
e-mail: holiday.care@virgin.net
2nd Floor Imperial Buildings
Victoria Road
Horley
Surrey RH6 7PZ
Tel: (0) 1293 774535

Accessible Cruises and Tours
www.medicaltravel.org
e-mail: ada@medicaltravel.org
5184 Majorca Club Drive
Boca Raton FL 33486 USA
Tel: (800) 778-7953

Accessible Journeys
www.disabilitytravel.com
e-mail: sales@disabilitytravel.com
35 West Sellers Avenue
Ridley Park PA 19078 USA
Tel: (800) 846-4537

The Guided Tour Inc.
www.guidedtour.com
e-mail: gtour400@aol.com
7900 Old York Road
Suite 114-B
Elkins Park PA 19027-2339 USA
Tel: (800) 783-5841 or (215) 782-1370
Also arranges tours for developmentally
disabled travelers.

Hearing Impaired Travelers

Canadian Association of the Deaf
www.cad.ca
e-mail: cad@cad.ca
203-251 Bank Street
Ottawa ON K2P 1X3 Canada
Tel: (613) 565-2882
TTY/TDD: (613) 565-8882

Royal National Institute for Deaf People
www.rnid.org.uk
19-23 Featherstone Street
London EC1Y 8SL
Tel: 020 7296 8000

National Association of the Deaf
www.nad.org
e-mail: nadinfo@nad.org
814 Thayer Avenue
Silver Spring MD 20910-4500 USA
Tel: (301) 587-1788
TTY/TDD: (301) 587-1789

World Federation of the Deaf
www.wfdnews.org
e-mail: info@wfdnews.org
PO Box 65
00401 Helsinki Finland
TTY: +358 9 580 3573

Table 23.1   Resources for disabled travelers—cont'd

Deaf Dude Travel
http: //members.aol.com/deafdude6/travel
e-mail: beasleyinc@aol.com

Beasley Travel
154 Ridge Road NW
Largo FL 33770 USA
Tel: (727) 584-5266
Arranges tours for the deaf and hearing impaired.

Visually Impaired Travelers
  American Council of the Blind
  www.acb.org
  e-mail: info@acb.org
  1155 15th Street NW
  Suite 1004
  Washington DC 20005 USA
  Tel: (800) 424-8666 or (202) 467-5081

  Canadian National Institute for the Blind
  www.cnib.ca
  1929 Bayview Avenue
  Toronto ON M4G 3E8 Canada
  Tel: (416) 486-2500

  The Campanian Society, Inc.
  www.campanian.org
  e-mail: campania@one.net
  PO Box 167
  Oxford, OH 45056 USA
  Tel: (513) 524-484
  Specializes in travel programs for the blind and
    visually impaired.

  National Federation of the Blind
  www.nfb.org
  e-mail: nfb@nfb.org
  1800 Johnson Street
  Baltimore, MD 21230
  (410) 659-9314

  Royal National Institute for the Blind
  www.rnib.org.uk
  224 Great Portland Street
  London W1N 6AA
  Tel: 020 7388 1266

Developmentally Disabled Travelers
  The Guided Tour Inc. (see under Physically Disabled
    Travelers)

  Sprout
  http://users.rcn.com/sprout.interport
  e-mail: sprout@interport.net
  893 Amsterdam Avenue
  New York NY 10025 USA
  Tel: (888) 222-9575 or (212) 222-9575
  Specializes in tours for the developmentally
    disabled and mentally challenged.

Note: Reference to or listing of selected organizations does not necessarily signify endorsement by the author.
All websites, addresses, and phone numbers were verified at the time of writing.

the washroom may be more convenient for the mobility impaired. The airline may not be able to guarantee such requests, but should be able to tell the traveler which seats are most accessible. Airline attendants should assist with managing carry-on baggage, transferring to and from a wheelchair, getting to the washroom (unless lifting or carrying the individual is required), and opening food packages and identifying food. Although flight attendants may help with eating, they are not required to do so, nor are they required to help with administering medications or to provide assistance in washrooms.

Passenger trains, buses, and ferries in developed countries can usually accommodate the needs of most disabled travelers, but these standards may not be the same in other countries. The transportation company should be notified and any special services requested well in advance. Travelers (or their travel agents) should ensure that hotels, restaurants, and attractions of interest can accommodate their needs. Inquiries about accessible ground transportation to the departure terminal and at the destination(s) (if required) should be made in advance, and reserved well ahead of time if possible.

The travel schedule should be confirmed prior to departure. Ample time must be allowed for transportation to the terminal, taking into account the time required for any transfers. Adequate time should also be allowed at the terminal for check-in and for transportation to the departure gate. Any physical assistance, assistive devices required at the terminal (e.g., wheelchairs, or motorized transportation within the terminal), or help with boarding or disembarking should be requested at the time of booking travel and again at check-in.

TRAVELING WITH AN ATTENDANT

Some disabled individuals may prefer or need to travel with a companion who can assist the traveler. The level of assistance required by the traveler should be discussed with the carrier at the time of booking. If the carrier is unable to provide the degree of assistance that it feels the traveler requires, it may request that the individual travel with an attendant.

Circumstances in which the safety of the traveler or fellow passengers can be jeopardized may prevent a disabled individual from traveling unaccompanied. Examples include cognitive or developmental impairment, severe physical disability impairing mobility, or combined visual and hearing impairments, any of which may prevent the traveler from understanding instructions or taking appropriate action in the event of an emergency.

Although a carrier may require an attendant to accompany a disabled traveler, it is not responsible for finding or providing this attendant. Occasionally an off-duty employee traveling on the same flight or a kind-hearted fellow traveler will assume this role. Airlines and other carriers may offer significant discounts for a medically necessary travel companion; proof of disability (medical documents) may be required for this discount to apply.

THE PHYSICALLY DISABLED TRAVELER

Physically disabled travelers may require assistance with boarding and disembarking, and this can be requested at the time of booking and check-in. Most airline carriers will announce pre-boarding and deplaning assistance for those who require it.

Air travel with wheelchairs and scooters

Tips for the wheelchair or scooter traveler are listed in Table 23.2. Wheelchair or scooter rental may be an option for some travelers, particularly short-term travelers or those who depend on these devices only for distance travel. Airlines will transport wheelchairs and scooters at no extra cost to the traveler. Those traveling with a wheelchair or scooter should notify the carrier at the time of making reservations, and should specify whether the device is manual or electric; this should be confirmed with the airline at least 48 h prior to departure. A smaller or lightweight manual wheelchair may be preferable for travel, being easier to transport and less prone to damage. If airport or overnight layovers are scheduled, the traveler can request that the wheelchair or scooter be returned to him or her; this will not only be more convenient for the individual, but will also minimize the risk of loss or damage to the device.

The traveler should verify whether or not the wheelchair or scooter is covered by (or can be added to) an existing insurance policy. Prior to departure, proper functioning of the device should be ensured, and consideration given to having it serviced if this has not been done recently. This might prevent unforeseen mechanical problems that could result in wasted time during the trip. Locating a wheelchair or scooter service agency in the destination may prove useful, just in case. Electric wheelchairs or scooters will require occasional recharging – an appropriate voltage adaptor should be brought along if necessary! The device and any removable parts should be labeled with proper identification prior to travel. Finally, a small repair kit should be carried, including tire repair equipment for pneumatic tires.

Manual wheelchairs may be stored in the aircraft cabin, depending on their size and the cabin space available. Some smaller aircraft may not allow these items to be stored in the cabin, but the carrier should inform the passenger of this. Most larger, modern aircraft can accommodate one wheelchair in the cabin, usually on a first-come, first-served basis; early arrival at the terminal can reduce the chances of wheelchair and traveler going separate ways. If a wheelchair cannot be brought on board, or if a scooter is used, it can be gate-checked and a baggage claim check obtained for the item; this will allow the traveler to use the device within the terminal and up to the aircraft door. Removable parts (seat cushions, baskets, etc.) should be removed before checking the item. The traveler may need to transfer to a smaller 'aisle' wheelchair to board the aircraft. The airline should supply this, especially for boarding smaller aircraft. In cases where a ramp to the aircraft door cannot be used, the traveler may need to board the plane by a mechanical lift. The traveler's device will then be placed in the baggage hold. For battery-powered equipment, use of dry cell (non-spillable) batteries is preferable; wet cells (spillable), which contain battery acid, must be removed and packed separately in special containers (another item to lose). Note that some wheelchairs may need to be disassembled in order to fit into the baggage compartment of certain aircraft, and attaching instructions for disassembly and disconnection of batteries (and reassembly and reconnection) may be helpful for airline personnel. Mobility aids should be returned to the traveler, fully assembled, either at the aircraft door or at the baggage claim area, as specified by the traveler.

Washrooms in older aircraft may be unable to accommodate even aisle wheelchairs, whereas those in newer or remodeled aircraft generally can. If an aisle wheelchair will be required on board (e.g., on long flights where a trip to the washroom may be necessary), it should be requested ahead of time. In addition, travelers should be aware that washrooms are often too small to allow an assistant to accompany the traveler into the washroom. The carrier should provide details about washroom space if this information is requested.

The carrier is responsible for the intact transportation of any mobility aid to the traveler's destination, including proper disassembly and reassembly. Damage to (or loss of) wheelchairs, scooters, and batteries does occur during transport, especially in baggage compartments. Damage during flight is the airline's responsibility, and the carrier is obliged to provide a suitable replacement at no cost to the traveler until the damaged item is repaired or replaced. Coverage for loss may depend on federal policies in the country of travel; for example, loss of a device by a Canadian carrier within Canada

Table 23.2	Practical tips for the wheelchair (or scooter) traveler
Request any special services well in advance, including accessible ground transportation if necessary.	
Consider insuring the wheelchair or scooter.	
Have the wheelchair serviced prior to travel.	
For electric wheelchairs, bring a voltage adapter if necessary; for battery-operated chairs, try to use dry cell batteries (they do not have to be removed).	
Label the wheelchair and all removable parts with your name and address.	
Attach instructions for disassembly and reassembly of your chair, and for disconnection and reconnection of batteries if necessary.	
Arrive early at the terminal.	
Use your chair within the terminal, then check it at the gate. Remove any removable parts and take them with you before checking it.	
Make sure the carrier is clear about where the wheelchair is to be returned to you.	
Bring a repair kit, including tire repair equipment.	

requires the carrier to replace it with an identical unit or reimburse the replacement cost, whereas a maximum liability of US $2500 is provided for travelers in the USA.

Cruising with a wheelchair or scooter

Cruising is an attractive and convenient form of travel for many disabled individuals. Newer cruise ships are more user-friendly for the disabled, with features such as wheelchair-accessible washrooms and roll-in showers. In addition, some cruise lines offer cruises specifically for the disabled and are accustomed to the needs of wheelchair travelers.

An appealing feature of most cruises, apart from the all-inclusive nature of travel, is the opportunity to visit many countries by disembarking at several ports of call. Ships can dock if the pier is large enough and in sufficiently deep water to allow this. For wheelchair and scooter travelers, disembarking onto a pier may mean that they and their device have to be carried separately onto the pier; alternatively, the traveler may be seated in the wheelchair or scooter and be 'walked' onto the pier by means of a specialized mechanical contraption which transports both together.

If water is too shallow to permit the ship to dock at shore, the ship will anchor a short distance from land and, weather permitting, passengers must transfer to a smaller ship in order to come ashore – a process known as tendering. Most cruise lines will provide physical assistance to allow the wheelchair traveler to tender.

Ports of call may have many sights to visit in a relatively short period of time. Disabled travelers can usually access these by taxi or other tour company. It may be helpful to inquire about special excursions or services that are available at the different ports when booking the cruise.

Canes, crutches, walkers, and other medical devices

Travelers requiring canes, crutches, walkers, and other medical devices can also travel with these at no extra charge. These devices can generally be stored in the aircraft cabin. The airline's policy regarding replacement of a device in the event of damage or loss should be the same as that for wheelchairs and scooters.

THE HEARING IMPAIRED TRAVELER

Deaf and hearing-impaired travelers may encounter difficulty with many aspects of travel that others take for granted, such as hearing announcements and using telephones. Hearing impairment may also subject the traveler to potential safety risks, particularly in emergency settings where verbal or overhead instructions are provided, or where alarms are sounded. If a travel attendant is required, a companion discount may be available. Travelers who use hearing aids should bring extra batteries.

Reservations should be made ahead of time whenever possible; the travel agent, tour company, transportation carriers, and hotels should be informed about hearing difficulties ahead of time. A written confirmation of travel arrangements and a written agenda can help to ensure that travel plans are correct. Travelers should inform the agents at check-in, at the boarding gate, and on the carrier of their impairment. Since information on overhead announcements may go unheard, travelers should request that this information be given to them individually.

Hotel staff must be made aware of a traveler's hearing impairment. Some hotels will provide visual aids for the hearing impaired so that they can be alerted to alarms or phonecalls. If these are unavailable, knowledge that a traveler is hearing impaired is essential in the event of an emergency. Teletypewriter (TTY) telephones may also be available and should be requested when making reservations.

THE VISUALLY IMPAIRED TRAVELER

Travelers needing eyeglasses should travel with an extra pair, as well as a repair kit and a copy of the most recent prescription. Contact lens wearers should take all required equipment with them and avoid using solutions prepared with iodine-disinfected water, as this can permanently stain lenses. Daily disposable contact lenses offer a convenient and reasonably priced alternative to conventional lenses and eliminate the need to bring solutions.

As for the hearing impaired, visually impaired travelers should make advance reservations when possible, arranging any special services ahead of time. They should alert their travel agent, transportation carriers, and hotel staff of their disability. Agents should be informed at the time of making reservations, and again at check-in and at the boarding gate. Written directions and specific addresses are helpful, especially if the traveler will rely on public transportation or taxis. Carrying a white cane will make others aware of the individual's visual impairment.

Some blind travelers may prefer to travel with an escort. Special discounts may be available for travel companions; inquiries about special rates should be made prior to booking travel. Traveling with guide dogs is discussed below.

SERVICE ANIMALS

Service animals, most commonly dogs, are specifically trained to help an individual with a disability. Less often, other animals may also work as service animals; for the purpose of this section, service animals are assumed to be dogs.

While service dogs are most commonly used by the visually impaired, they may also act as guides for the hearing impaired and those with other disabilities. Certification of service dogs is provided by some agencies, but is not necessary in order for them to work as such; however, proof of certification will be required in some circumstances and may be valuable in others. Service dogs are working animals and not pets, and should not be barred entry to areas where pets are disallowed. The Americans with Disabilities Act[5] in the USA stipulates that service animals be permitted to accompany their owners in all areas where the public is allowed, including taxis, public buses, airplanes, restaurants, hotels, and other public facilities. Restrictions may apply, however, where safety concerns take precedence. For example, an individual and his service dog may be prohibited from sitting in an aisle seat or at an emergency exit in an airplane, where the animal may block passage or hinder access to the exit; or a service dog may be barred if its behavior poses a safety risk to others.

Advance preparation can make traveling with a service animal easier (Table 23.3). The appropriate individuals and organizations should be aware of the traveler's need for a guide dog, and special arrangements made ahead of time. Some countries may quarantine imported animals; restrictions or requirements for transporting a service dog both into and out of a given country can be clarified by contacting the embassy or consulate of that country. Travelers should also remember to make sure the dog will be allowed to re-enter the home country after travel, and ask what restrictions might apply on return. Prior to travel, a veterinarian should examine the dog and ensure that any required immunizations or routine treatments are up to date. A certificate of health and a record of immunizations for the dog should be obtained; some countries will require these documents to be certified.

Table 23.3	Traveling with a service animal
Contact the embassy or consulate of each country you intend to visit and determine what rules or regulations may apply for entering and leaving the country.	
Have your vet examine the animal prior to travel. Make sure immunizations are up to date and obtain a record of the animal's health and immunizations.	
Have the animal officially certified as a service animal.	
Consider buying travel health insurance for the animal.	
Make sure the animal has a sturdy (non-metallic) collar; attach proper identification and date of the most recent rabies immunization to the collar.	
Bring a harness or vest that will identify your animal as a service animal.	
Immediately prior to boarding, make sure the animal has exercised and voided.	
Do not feed or sedate the animal immediately prior to travel.	
Check with your country of residence to find out what procedures must be followed in order to bring your animal back home after travel.	

A vest or harness that identifies the dog as a service animal can make others aware that the dog is working and is not a pet. A secure collar with tags identifying the name of the owner, address and phone number, and date of the most recent rabies immunization can be crucial if for some reason animal and owner are separated. A non-metallic collar and harness are preferable, as they will not set off security alarms. The dog should not be fed immediately before travel and should not be sedated, but should be exercised and have voided prior to boarding. Maintenance and feeding of the animal during the trip are the responsibility of the owner. The traveler should remember to pack whatever essentials the dog might need while away from home. Finally, the traveler may consider purchasing health insurance for the service animal prior to travel. Some policies will include or offer coverage for veterinary services required during travel, but conditions and limitations should be clarified prior to purchase.

THE DEVELOPMENTALLY OR COGNITIVELY IMPAIRED TRAVELER

Developmental disabilities should not prevent travel. Some organizations specialize in excursions exclusively for developmentally challenged travelers (Table 23.1). General advice given to other travelers also applies to those with developmental or cognitive impairment. These travelers should carry an identification card with the address of their destination, in case they get lost. Any special services required should be arranged when booking travel, and requested again at the time of check-in. Provided that the individual is relatively inde-pendent and can understand and follow instructions (e.g., in the event of an emergency), there is no need for accompaniment; if the disability is severe enough to jeopardize the safety of the traveler or fellow travelers, an escort may be required.

CONCLUSION

Most disabled individuals are able to travel. Severe limitations may restrict or even preclude travel, but many physical and cognitive disabilities do not present barriers to traveling. Although some aspects of a trip may be limited depending on a traveler's specific impairment, proper advance planning can ensure that disabled or impaired individuals have a fulfilling, enjoyable, and healthy travel experience.

REFERENCES

1. United States Department of Transportation. *Air Carrier Access Act.* Available online at: www.dot.gov/airconsumer/horizons.htm
2. Canadian Transportation Agency. *Air Travel Accessibility Regulations.* Available online at: www.cta-otc.gc.ca/access/regs/air_e.html
3. United Kingdom Department for Transport. *Consultation Draft, Code of Practice, Access to Air Travel for Disabled People.* Available online at: www.mobility-unit.dft.gov.uk/consult/aviation/access/index.htm
4. European Commission. *Airlines' Contracts with Passengers.* Available online at http://europa.eu.int/comm/transport/air/contrat-cons_en.pdf
5. United States Department of Justice. *Americans with Disabilities Act of 1990.* Available online at www.usdoj.gov/crt/ada/pubs/ada.txt

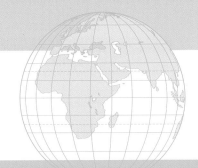

CHAPTER 24 Travelers with Pre-existing Disease

Anne E. McCarthy

KEYPOINTS

- Prior to travel, early pre-travel health consultation is important, and adequate health insurance, including evacuation insurance, should be arranged

- Copies of prescription medications and medications in original containers should be carried in hand luggage

- When indicated, an assessment of safety to fly or to travel should be arranged especially for those with recent surgery or known cardiorespiratory disease

- Renal and diabetes patients and those with gastrointestinal disease should maintain adequate hydration and consider antibiotic prophylaxis for the prevention of travelers' diarrhea during short trips

- For individuals with diabetes, on insulin therapy, a pre-travel consultation with a diabetes educator may be appropriate

GENERAL PRINCIPLES

Medical advances in the twenty-first century allow many people with historically debilitating diseases to live full active lives that include exotic travel. Travel, like life, entails risks which can be minimized with the proper precautions to ensure that the risk does not outweigh the benefits of the travel experience.[1,2] It is imperative for travelers to understand the true risk of their travel, taking into account their particular state of health and their planned itinerary. At times, where choice exists, it may be worthwhile to make a small change in itinerary to minimize health risk without detracting from the benefit of travel.

This chapter will address travel medicine considerations for individuals with pre-existing medical conditions, specifically cardiovascular disease, respiratory disease, renal disease, diabetes, gastrointestinal disease (including chronic liver disease) and severe or life-threatening allergies. Considerations for travelers with underlying conditions such as pregnancy (see Chapter 20) and immunodeficiency (see Chapters 25 and 26) are presented in other chapters of this text.

BEFORE YOU GO

Travelers with underlying medical conditions should seek pre-travel care as soon as an international trip is planned and at a minimum 4–6 weeks before departure. This time is required not only to carry out the pre-travel consultation and administer needed vaccines, but also to provide time to stabilize or optimize underlying disease and to establish a health management plan for the destination country.[3,4] This health management plan should include prevention strategies and self-treatment instructions for anticipated complications, arrangements for any required routine treatments (such as dialysis), and instructions for where to seek help in the event of particular medical complications. Consideration should be given to the provision of a 24-h medical contact in the event of an unexpected or severe complication (such as an on-call number or e-mail address).

Adequate health insurance is a must for travelers with underlying medical conditions. These travelers should ensure that they have a clear understanding of the coverage provided. In particular, they need to know the options for medical evacuation and medical treatment. Many health insurance or medical evacuation plans will transfer a patient based on the medical indications for the transfer rather than patient preferences for the geographic location of their medical care.

Travelers should carry all medication with them in their hand luggage. This includes medications that are routinely taken and any drugs that are taken on an as needed basis (such as sublingual nitroglycerine), with enough supply for the duration of the journey with extra in case of delays. They should also carry along with their passport and immunization record, an official copy of all prescriptions with generic names of all medications (most pharmacies are computerized and can provide a printed copy of all medications and instructions for use). It is advisable to have the medication expiry date clearly visible on each prescription label and to carry each medication in the original container (if a smaller container is required then the traveler should visit their pharmacist who can re-package the medication in a smaller container with a new label). Border guards are understandably suspicious about home-packaged medications. Each traveler should be encouraged to discuss with his or her pharmacist the planned journey and ask for storage tips, keeping in mind that 'room temperature' in the planned destination may far exceed temperatures experienced at home. It is prudent to consider providing the traveler with a supply of medications for anticipated complications of their underlying disease (e.g., urinary tract infection) in addition to the routine travel related medications, with strict instructions as to whether or not medical supervision is required for their use. Table 24.1 summarizes practical tips concerning medication and travel.

Drugs used for prevention (e.g., malaria chemoprophylaxis) or treatment (e.g., antibiotics for travelers' diarrhea) of travel-related illness may interfere with the routine medication used to control the underlying disease. Therefore, all potential interactions should be considered before finalizing the choice of medication for prevention and treatment of travel-related illnesses.

Travelers should be warned that in many countries, a large number of drugs, including antibiotics and oral corticosteroids, are available over-the-counter. However the 'buyer beware' policy should apply when purchasing these products, since the medication received may

Table 24.1	Sample medical disclaimer – Health Canada's Travel Medicine Program (adapted)

Date: _____

Certificate of authorization

_____ (Traveler's name) is carrying in his/her personal possession a medical kit, prescription medications and disposable needles and syringes to be used by a physician for safe administration of medication, if required, while overseas. These items are recommended for this person's individual use and to prevent the accidental transmission of disease through a contaminated needle. They are not for re-sale.

_____ (Name, Address, Signature of physician)

The US rule governing persons visiting the country or passing through *en route* to another country states: 'Those entering the U.S. with syringes should declare them to U.S. Customs and be in possession of a valid medical prescription or authorization. U.S. Federal law prohibits importation of 'drug paraphernalia' (U.S. Code, Title 21, Section 857). Whether hypodermic syringes constitute drug paraphernalia depends on the facts and attendant circumstances of each case. Additionally, many of the States also have laws prohibiting possession of drug paraphernalia similar to that of New York. Travelers should therefore be advised that hypodermic syringes and needles must be medically prescribed or authorized, and must be declared to U.S. Customs.'

be inappropriate, dangerous (for example a drug no longer licensed at home due to safety concerns), or may not be produced using good manufacturing practices, leading to under or over dosing of the medication.

MedicAlert® bracelets are designed to give important medical history when the wearer is incapable of providing details. They can save lives particularly in the event of an acute reversible, but disabling event such as hypoglycemia or allergy. It is important to remember that the information may not be written in the native tongue of the health-care provider in the destination country, and may not be universally recognized. There is an emergency phone number on the back of each medallion, where health-care providers can receive details of the medical history. MedicAlert® has a program specifically designed for travelers, called the Travel Plus℠ program. More information is available at www.medicalert.org.

The International Association for Medical Assistance to Travelers (IAMAT) is a non-profit foundation that provides written information for travelers about health risks, geographical distribution of diseases and immunization requirements for all countries. It also provides a list of western-trained doctors from around the world who speak English in addition to their mother tongue and have agreed to see travelers. Further information is available at www.iamat.org.

The International Air Transport Association (IATA) is made up of a group of experts, including senior airline medical professionals and World Health Organization representatives, who provide guidelines to airlines to improve the awareness of health risk factors associated with air travel and to increase passenger comfort before and during flights. More information is available at www.iata.org/inflight.

There are many support groups and organizations that work to afford maximum life benefit for those with specific underlying disease, such as the American Diabetes Association (www.diabetes.org). Most of these are easily accessible by phone or through the Web. For any traveler with underlying health concerns, the Society for Accessible Travel and Hospitality www.sath.org is a valuable resource.

Although vaccines for travel are discussed in detail elsewhere in this text, some vaccines may be contraindicated or less effective due to underlying disease. In addition, certain vaccines may be recommended specifically because of the underlying disease, such as pneumococcal and influenza vaccine.

Health-care providers should supply an official medical disclaimer letter for any traveler with underlying medical concerns even though it may not be a guarantee for smooth border crossings. An example

from Health Canada's Travel Medicine Program website (www.travel-health.gc.ca), Table 24.1, emphasizes that any needles, syringes or medication carried by the traveler are for legitimate medical purposes and intended only for use by the individual traveler or a medical provider.

Table 24.2 provides a summary of essential health related items for the traveler with an underlying medical condition.

THE VOYAGE

Air travel, particularly over long distances and multiple time zones, exposes passengers to a number of different factors that may have adverse effects on individuals with underlying medical conditions.[5–18] The health risks associated with flight can be minimized in these travelers with careful planning and precautions to reduce the risk.

Airport terminals are often poorly laid out and provide a physical challenge, because they require significant commuting between gates. This exertion may exacerbate angina in those susceptible and may necessitate a wheelchair for transit through the airport. Wheelchair ground transportation can be arranged through the airlines at the time of reservations – the traveler will have to be prepared to supply details of any limitations as the company may want to ensure that the individual is fit to fly. In-flight special needs such as a stretcher can be arranged through the individual airline. Such special arrangements often require a travel companion or caregiver and may require additional cost – all of which should be worked out with the airline far in advance.

The cabins of commercial aircraft are pressurized, but only to 6500–8000 ft (2000–2400 m) above sea level. The result is a reduction in available oxygen and expansion of gases within body cavities. The subsequent mild hypoxia in healthy individuals is inconsequential,

Table 24.2	Essential items to be carried by travelers with underlying medical conditions

All required medications
MedicAlert® bracelet
Health insurance
Medical contact in destination country
Emergency medical contact at home

but may lead to significant compromise in someone with borderline cardiac or respiratory function or with severe anemia. Gas expansion associated with ascent can cause discomfort in some, but may lead to significant problems in those who have recently undergone gastrointestinal surgery. Those with ear, nose and sinus infections should avoid flying because pain or injury may result from the inability to equalize pressure effectively. Aircraft cabin humidity is low (10–20%). This may result in mild symptoms, such as dry eyes, nose and mouth, that can be minimized by maintaining fluids preflight and during flight. Occasionally, this dryness may lead to respiratory irritation and an exacerbation of underlying reactive airways diseases.

The need for in-flight supplemental oxygen should be evaluated in those with underlying cardiac or respiratory disease (see the Respiratory Disease section, below). If required, in-flight oxygen may be arranged with commercial carriers, but requires at least 48 h advanced notice. Passengers should note that they cannot use their own oxygen in flight and that they are responsible for arranging oxygen supply at the departure and arrival terminals.

Motion sickness is not usually a significant problem in air flights, but may be significant when traveling by sea. Obviously, nausea and vomiting could have adverse consequences for the traveler with diabetes. In an aircraft, symptoms can be minimized by utilizing anti-nausea drugs, and choosing a seat over the wing.

Prolonged immobilization associated with air travel leads to venous pooling in the lower extremities. Most travelers suffer little consequence other than mild peripheral edema. However, long flights have been causally associated with deep venous thrombosis or even pulmonary embolus in some travelers.[19–31] As a result of recent scientific and lay press interest, many airlines have provided instructions for in-flight exercises to minimize these effects. A recent review by Hirsh and colleagues[19] categorizes travelers according to their risk of venous thromboembolism:

- Travelers at low risk of thromboembolism are those under 75 years of age; women taking oral contraceptive pills (OCPs); pregnant women; and those less than 45 who are carriers of genetic traits for hypercoagulability. Preventive strategies include regular exercise and maintenance of hydration.
- Moderate risk travelers include those over 75 years of age; women older than 45 who take estrogen containing hormone replacement therapy; and those with traits for hypercoagulability who are taking OCPs. Preventive strategies include below knee graduated compression stockings or ASA.
- High-risk travelers include those with a history of venous thromboembolism; active malignancy; gross obesity; marked restriction in mobility due to muscular or cardiovascular disease; large varicose veins; and those older than 75 years with cardiac and pulmonary disease. Preventive strategies include the use of graduated compression stockings, the addition of ASA, or, if stockings are not used, low molecular weight heparin.

Health risks associated with air travel can be minimized if the traveler plans carefully and takes some precautions before, during and after the flight (Table 24.3).[32,33] A simple and useful test to assess whether an individual is fit for air travel is to determine whether he or she can walk 50 metres (150 feet) or climb one flight of stairs without severe dyspnea or angina.[34] If there is concern about an individual's fitness to fly the health-care provider should contact the airline's physician for medical clearance which is provided on a case by case basis. Commercial airlines do have the right to refuse passengers who are medically unfit to travel. Contraindications for flying include those summarized in Table 24.3. For individuals with a history of epilepsy many airlines recommend dose modification of anti-seizure medications, but this is controversial. For those with an unstable seizure disorder it is advisable to carry preventive and treatment medications

Table 24.3	**Medical contraindications for air flight***

Patient sick enough to have a low probability of surviving flight

Any serious and acute contagious disease

Cardiovascular disease:
  Unstable angina or chest pain at rest
  Recent myocardial infarction – uncomplicated within past 2 weeks, complicated within the past 6 weeks (time period depending on severity of MI and duration of travel)
  Coronary artery bypass graft within the past two weeks
  Decompensated heart failure
  Uncontrolled arrhythmia
  Uncontrolled hypertension with systolic BP >200 mmHg

Respiratory diseases:
  Baseline PaO_2 <70 mmHg at sea level without supplemental O_2.
  Pneumothorax within the past three weeks
  Large pleural effusion
  Exacerbation or severe chronic obstructive respiratory disease
  Breathlessness at rest

Neurologic disease:
  Cerebral vascular accident (stroke) within the past 2 weeks
  Uncontrolled seizures

Recent surgery or injury where trapped air or gas may be present, such as abdominal trauma, gastrointestinal surgery, craniofacial and ocular surgery.

Adapted from *International Travel and Health 2002* (WHO)[12] the International Air Transport Association and others.[32,33]
*Check with individual airlines for specific restrictions

in their carry-on luggage. In addition, it may be prudent to forewarn the airline and aircrew, and provide written instructions for seizure management.

The incidence of in-flight medical events aboard international flights is increasing and is estimated to be between 1 in 10 000 to 40 000 passengers, with 1 in 150 000 of these incidents requiring the use of in-flight medical equipment or drugs.[17,34] Most in-flight medical events are not serious and many involve vaso-vagal episodes or gastrointestinal problems. Serious events, such as cardiac, neurological or respiratory problems lead to the majority of aircraft diversions for medical treatment.[35] In-flight deaths are much less common and most are attributed to cardiac events (56%) or to predisposing medical conditions (19%).[17] Although the US FAA is requiring enhanced medical support in-flight, items such as a well stocked first aid kit and automated external defibrillators may not be reliably available worldwide.[13]

IN COUNTRY

While in country, travelers have to adjust to heat, exertion, a novel diet and possibly altitude. With prior arrangements made through the destination resorts, cruise lines or hotels, special meals can be made available for those with dietary restrictions. It is important for the traveler to realize that available medical resources may be limited. Deaths abroad among travelers are mainly due to pre-existing heart disease and accidents. Many of the accidental deaths are preventable.[36–39] One study determined that 80% of deaths due to injury occurred before the traveler could reach a medical facility, and that infectious diseases (other than pneumonia) accounted for less than 1% of all overseas deaths.

AFTER THE TRIP

After return, travelers should seek prompt attention, particularly for any febrile illness, and inform the attending physician about their recent travel history. A differential diagnosis should include possible travel-related illnesses, since they may be life-threatening if not diagnosed and treated appropriately.

Specific medical problems

Cardiac disease

Travelers with underlying cardiac disease should undergo a pre-travel examination to optimize cardiovascular status and define preventive measures, including any in-flight oxygen requirements. Travel entails exertion in airport terminals, during the flight and at the destination.[3] Cardiac events are one of the most common causes of death among adult travelers. Cardiovascular events are also the second most frequent reason for medical evacuation, and cause over 50% of deaths recorded during commercial air travel. Most of these adverse cardiac events result from underlying coronary artery disease destabilized by stress and fatigue associated with travel. During the flight there are multiple stressors, including altitude-related hypoxia, pressurization, and cramped seating. Acute exposure to high altitude produces hypoxia-associated stimulation of the sympathetic nervous system resulting in increased heart rate and blood pressure. Cardiovascular contraindications to air travel include recent myocardial infarction (MI) (uncomplicated MI within last 2 weeks; complicated MI within the last 6 weeks), unstable angina, and poorly controlled CHF, arrhythmia or hypertension.[12,32]

Travelers with a history of myocardial infarction or significant heart disease should carry a recent electrocardiogram (EKG) tracing to assist an overseas treating physician in the event that chest pain occurs during the journey. As well, those with pacemakers should carry their pacemaker card along with a recent EKG. Flying is generally safe for those with pacemakers, however people with the older style unipolar pacemakers may be susceptible to electronic interference during flight or during security checks. Those with bipolar pacemakers should not be affected. Implantable automatic defibrillators may be interfered with by hand held security screening devices. Such travelers should carry a physician's letter of explanation with their passport.

Prior to departure the traveler should obtain names of specialist physicians in the cities to be visited in case complications arise. Some drugs that prevent or treat malaria may interfere with cardiac medications or may be contraindicated due to an underlying medical condition. The current medication profile and the specific underlying cardiac disease should be reviewed in detail prior to prescribing any preventive or treatment medication for travel.

Respiratory disease

There are many published recommendations for patients with chronic respiratory disease considering air travel.[12,40–52] In-flight supplemental oxygen is a recognized airline service, but requires planning, a physician's prescription, and possible expense.[53] Many types of pulmonary function tests have been utilized to determine the need for in-flight supplemental oxygen.[3,41,42,46] A simple method recommends the use of in-flight oxygen for all with a PaO_2 of less than 70 mmHg at sea level. A more sophisticated test is the Hypoxia Inhalation Test (HIT), which involves a simulation of the hypoxia experienced at altitude to predict an individual's response to air travel.[47] Arrangements for in-flight oxygen can be made through contact with the individual airline. A physician's prescription is required for in-flight oxygen and should state flight duration, intermittent or continuous use, and flow rate at 8000 feet (2400 m), with an additional 30–60 min to account for flight delays. In general, a flow rate of 2 L/min is provided to those likely to become hypoxic, with an increase in flow by 1 to 3 L/min for those on supplemental oxygen at sea level. Travelers are prohibited from using their personal oxygen devices on board an aircraft. In-flight oxygen, when necessary, is always supplied by the airline. It is up to the traveler to arrange any supplemental oxygen requirements for transfer points and lay overs, as well as at the final destination. For those routinely on home oxygen, the regular vendor can assist with these arrangements. Pulmonary contraindications to air travel include dyspnea at rest, cyanosis, active bronchospasm, pneumonia, and pulmonary hypertension. The British Lung Foundation publishes a free booklet entitled 'Going on holiday with a lung condition', available free of charge at www.lung.uk. It contains extensive recommendations for all types of travel for individuals with pulmonary disease. Other useful websites include those of the National Home Oxygen Patient Association http://www.oxygen4travel.com/tips_air.html and the Pulmonary Hypertension Association http://www.phassociation.org/learn/flightadvice.html.

Renal disease

Travelers with end stage renal disease (ESRD) need a prevention and management plan for diarrheal illness; particular emphasis must be placed on fluid management since dehydration may worsen renal failure. Empiric treatment for travelers' diarrhea, with dosage adjustments based on creatinine clearance, should be provided, along with strict instructions, on when to seek medical help. With sufficient notice, dietary restrictions for individuals with renal disease can often be accommodated with the assistance of airlines, hotels and tour operators.

Any arrangements for dialysis should be made well in advance. Peritoneal dialysis is relatively easy to accomplish except for transport of supplies, which are often extremely cumbersome. Also, reliable transport must be organized to ensure that all necessary supplies arrive safely at the destination. Hemodialysis (HD) is available worldwide, but requires several months notice to implement. Arrangements may be made through the local social worker and/or local branches of the Kidney Foundation (www.kidney.org), or through Global Dialysis (www.globaldialysis.com). The Society for Accessible Travel and Hospitality (www.sath.org) provides information on travel and cruise companies that offer trips specifically tailored for dialysis patients.

Arrangements for dialysis must include specific dialysis orders. Some dialysis units require HBV, HCV, and HIV testing, and may refuse anyone who is an HBsAg carrier. Careful scrutiny of any possible HD site is essential due to the potential for spread of blood-borne pathogens. Plans for travel provide an ideal opportunity to ensure that the traveler is immune to hepatitis B. If the dialysis patient is not yet immune to HBV, vaccination using the high dose series and documentation of protective antibodies should be carried out prior to travel.

ESRD on dialysis does not affect the metabolism of mefloquine[3]; however, the data on most other antimalarials are not readily available. Proguanil, excreted by the kidney, can accumulate and dose reduction may be required after four weeks of therapy. This may be a problem for those on prolonged atovaquone/proguanil (Malarone®) chemoprophylaxis. According to the manufacturer, this dug combination is contraindicated for those with a creatinine clearance less than 25mL/min. Folic acid supplementation should be considered for those with ESRD on proguanil.

Diabetes

Although those with diabetes may face special challenges while traveling, they can usually anticipate or avoid serious problems by thinking things through in advance.[54–59] Travelers with diabetes need a thorough understanding of their disease and a full medical evaluation prior to departure including special instructions on the management of diarrhea, nausea and vomiting. It is unwise for these travelers to rely on foreign purchased medications; therefore, they should carry an adequate supply of everything required for diabetes care (and any other medical conditions) with an additional 50% supply in case of unforeseen transportation delays.

Travel results in unaccustomed exertions and interruptions in routines and meals.[2] During the pre-travel evaluation, realistic goals of diabetes control during the voyage should be established recognizing that tight control runs the risk of hypoglycemic episodes while crossing multiple time zones. It may be safer to accept higher than normal glucose readings during travel. As well, a management plan should be in place for any diabetes complications that may arise during the trip (such as diabetes foot ulcer or urinary tract infection). It should include appropriate self-medications and instructions on when to use them and when to seek medical attention. A physician's letter should be carried with the passport outlining the diagnosis, treatment requirements and the need to carry medication, needles and syringes. In addition to travel-related vaccines, pneumococcal and influenza vaccines should be updated. Because of the risk of accessing healthcare abroad, it would be prudent to vaccinate against hepatitis B. If traveling with a companion, he or she should be educated about the signs, symptoms and management of hypoglycemia. If traveling alone, the flight attendant or tour guide should be given the same information, ideally with written instructions for management.

For all travelers with diabetes, frequent monitoring of blood glucose is essential, particularly while *en route* and crossing multiple time zones. Travelers on oral hypoglycemic medication do not require additional dosages and should take their medication according to the local time. For those on insulin therapy, there are many formulae for adjusting insulin dosing during travel.[3,4,54,56,60] Since each travel situation is unique for each person traveling with diabetes, the best option may be individualized advice from the expert diabetes educator in the diabetes clinic.

The following is one suggested regimen for insulin adjustment during travel:

- If crossing five or less time zones routine insulin dosage should be taken. Frequent blood glucose monitoring should be carried out (every 6 h) and the traveler should anticipate the need for extra insulin and an additional meal or snack.
- Westward travel across six or more time zones leads to a lengthened day. On the day of departure the routine morning insulin dose is taken and, if appropriate, the evening dose is taken 10–12 h later. Blood sugar should be measured 18 h after the morning dose. If blood sugar is >13 mmol/L, the traveler should take one-third of the morning dose and a meal or snack. On the first day at the destination, the usual insulin dose(s) is/are taken according to local time.
- Eastward travel across six or more time zones leads to a shortened day. On the day of departure the usual insulin dose(s) should be taken, with the evening dose taken 10–12 h after the morning dose. On the day of arrival at the destination, two-thirds of the usual morning dose should be taken with blood sugar determination 10 h later. If routinely on a single dose schedule and blood sugar is >13mmol/L then the remaining one-third of the morning dose is required. If routinely on a two dose schedule and the blood sugar is >13 mmol/L, the routine evening dose plus the remaining one-third of the morning dose should be taken. If the blood glucose is <13 mmol/L, the routine evening dose alone should be taken. On the second day at the destination, the routine insulin dose(s) is/are taken.

Another approach for insulin adjustment calls for a two to four percent adjustment in insulin dosage for each time zone crossed.[56] For example, a traveler going west over seven time zones would have a lengthened day, necessitating a 20% increase in the long-acting insulin dose.

Ideally, insulin should be stored in the refrigerator; however, it is stable at room temperature for up to one month.[61] Extremely hot temperatures should be avoided. All medication should be carried in hand luggage since insulin may freeze in the aircraft luggage compartment. While *en route*, the traveler should attempt to maintain treatment schedules based on elapsed time rather than time zone changes. The traveler with diabetes should anticipate long delays and avoid hypoglycemia by bringing extra food, meals, and glucagon (if appropriate). Special diabetic meals are not standardized from airline to airline, especially with foreign airline carriers. It may be wiser to order a regular meal and choose the appropriate food.

Advances in diabetes care, with the use of prefilled syringes and cartridges, provides ease of insulin administration, storage and convenience for travel. It may be worthwhile to consider the use of rapidly acting insulin (insulin lispro/Humalog®) which may be injected at the onset of a meal, instead of regular insulin, which needs to be taken 30–45 min before eating. The rapidly acting insulin can provide safer glycemic control if schedule changes occurred with no notice (a common scenario when traveling). A personal laser-lancing device for glucose monitoring eliminates the need for sharps and is less traumatic. The traveler should note that altitude may alter glucometer and insulin pump performance. Those using insulin pumps may have problems at airport security and need to ensure that they have a physician letter for ease of transit. There have been reports of mechanical malfunction at altitude,[62] therefore the traveler should check with the particular manufacturer about safety with air travel. They should also consider carrying an alternate insulin source in case of pump malfunction.

Those requiring insulin must remember that there is increased insulin absorption in hot climates and should not underestimate the need for a period of adjustment as a result of jet lag.

For the traveler with diabetes, prevention strategies are paramount to decrease the risk of food and water-borne diseases. Foot injury, with resultant diabetic ulcer and possible secondary infection, are a real concern for the traveler with diabetes. Extensive instructions prior to travel should include the need for frequent sock changes, avoidance of new shoes, diligent foot examinations each night, and careful instructions for foot care and management of ulcers. A prescription should be provided for appropriate antibiotics to be used in event of infection, with strict instructions about when to seek medical attention. Urinary tract infections are frequent among females with diabetes; due to an increased risk for upper tract involvement, short course antibiotic treatment regimens should be avoided. Travelers with diabetic retinopathy may experience transient worsening due to hypoxic retinal ischemia after prolonged air travel.

Traveling with diabetes supplies has become a little more complicated since the FAA implemented stepped-up security measures at the nation's airports in response to the tragic events of September 11th, 2001. Some of the new security measures may affect airline passengers with diabetes. Travelers should check the ADA website (www.diabetes.org) and the airline carrier (at least one day in advance of his or her scheduled flight) to confirm the airline's policy with regard to diabetes medication and supplies. In brief:

- Passengers may board with syringes or insulin delivery systems once it is determined that he or she has a documented medical need that can be verified by supplying the insulin with a professional, pharmaceutical pre-printed label on the original box.
- Passengers who must test their blood glucose levels can board with their lancets as long as the lancets are capped and accompanied by the glucose meter that has the manufacturer's name embossed on it. (i.e., One Touch meters say 'One Touch,' Accu-Chek meters say 'Accu-Chek').

■ Glucagon must be in the pre-printed labeled plastic container or box.

■ Due to forgery concerns, prescriptions and letters of medical necessity will not be accepted.

These FAA security measures apply to travel within the 50 United States. Passengers are advised to consult their individual air carrier for both domestic (US) and International travel regulations.

Travel plans may be an excellent stimulus for joining a support association such as the ADA (www.diabetes.org), which can provide educational material and other support for travelers with diabetes. The ADA provides services such as patient monographs on pertinent subjects such as eating out, and a buyers guide for diabetes supplies at home and abroad. It would be worthwhile for travelers with diabetes and their traveling companions to know how to tell someone, in the local language, that they have diabetes and how to request sugar or orange juice in the event of an episode of hypoglycemia. A diabetes alert card, available in several languages from the ADA, should be carried, and a MedicAlert® bracelet should be worn. The ADA and other groups have valuable resources for travelers with diabetes, including the Diabetes Monitor, which contains an edition entitled: 'Traveling with Diabetes', available at www.diabetesmonitor.com. The International Diabetes Federation provides a list of regional and country e-mail addresses should one require specialist care abroad (www.idf.org).

Allergies

People with food allergies may order special meals at the time of the airline ticket reservation. However, these travelers should keep in mind that such measures are not infallible, and that they should observe the same rigorous precautions that they follow whenever they are eating out. Those with life-threatening food allergies should learn how to say what they are allergic to in all the countries that they will transit. As well, they should carry pictures of the ingredient or food to be avoided.

Management of allergic symptoms may be different from that at home, since it is unlikely that '911' services will be available. Since an EpiPen™ may be insufficient treatment if medical care is not readily available, it may be worthwhile to carry multiple EpiPens or to learn how to use an Anakit®, which supplies up to three doses of epinephrine (the latter requires subcutaneous injection). The traveler's medical kit should include antihistamines and possibly a short course of corticosteroids for management of a severe allergic reaction.

Gastrointestinal disease

Travelers with decreased gastric acid due to surgery or medications (H_2 blockers and proton pump inhibitors) have lost an important defense against food and water-borne illness. They are more susceptible to illness since a smaller inoculum of pathogens is more likely to cause disease. For this reason, it is worth considering prophylactic antibiotic therapy for travelers' diarrhea. This should be done with caution since it may predispose to a false sense of security and elicit more risk-taking behavior. For most individuals, it is best to offer antibiotics for self-treatment that should be commenced at the onset of symptoms. Typhoid vaccine should also be considered. In rare cases, it may be worthwhile to consider cholera vaccine. A traveler with a recent ulcer or GI bleed may have problems with intestinal gas expansion at altitude.[8]

Travelers with underlying inflammatory bowel disease (IBD) may experience problems if they acquire food-borne or water-borne infections. Enteric infections may lead to an exacerbation of their underlying disease or cause confusion about the etiology of the symptoms and lead to incorrect management.[63–65] In those with underlying IBD, it may be worthwhile to consider antibiotic prophylaxis for travelers'

diarrhea in conjunction with education about the need for strict food and water precautions. They should also carry contact information for medical assistance in the destination country as well as a contact at home for assistance if symptoms progress. Medication for the treatment of IBD and instructions for use with and without medical consultation should be carried in the carry-on luggage. Individuals with IBD may benefit from information provided by their national organizations such as the UK National Association for Colitis and Crohn's Disease (www.nacc.org.uk) or the Australian Crohn's and Colitis Association (www.acca.net.au). Such organizations provide information on many resources for those living with IBD, including lists of international IBD associations.

Individuals with irritable bowel syndrome may experience worsening of their underlying bowel symptoms. They may require particular vigilance in the prevention of travelers' diarrhea and a specific management plan. Travelers with colostomies have little problems with air transport but should use a large colostomy bag in case gas expansion leads to increased output.

Individuals with cirrhosis or chronic alcohol abuse should avoid raw seafood due to the risk of overwhelming sepsis with *Vibrio vulnificus*.[3] and superinfection with hepatitis A. Also, in this risk group, dehydration may lead to severe consequences such as decompensation of underlying liver disease. Therefore, empiric antibiotic treatment for travelers' diarrhea should be provided as well as strict instructions for its avoidance and management. Cirrhotic patients should avoid mefloquine for the prevention and treatment of malaria since it undergoes hepatic metabolism and biliary excretion.

CONCLUSION

Those with underlying health problems should, with appropriate pre-travel planning and behavioral modification during travel, be able to minimize the health risks associated with travel. However, they must have realistic expectations concerning health maintenance and travel restrictions. These individuals at special risk have the option of making use of numerous resources[66] that are now available to make travel an enjoyable and rewarding experience.

REFERENCES

1. Virk A. Medical advice for international travelers. *Mayo Clin Proc* 2001; **76**:831–840.
2. Thomas RE. Preparing patients to travel abroad safely. Part 1: Taking a travel history and identifying special risks. *Can Fam Physician* 2000; **46**:132–138.
3. Mileno MD, Bia FJ. The compromised traveler. *Infect Dis Clin North Am* 1998; **12**:369–412.
4. Bia FJ, Barry M. Special health considerations for travelers. *Med Clin North Am* 1992; **76**:1295–1312.
5. Skjenna OW, Evans JF, Moore MS, Thibeault C, Tucker AG. Helping patients travel by air. *Cmaj* 1991; **144**:287–293.
6. Shesser R. Medical aspects of commercial air travel. *Am J Emerg Med* 1989; **7**:216–226.
7. Woods DP. Am I fit to fly? *Practitioner* 1998; **242**:384–387.
8. Wooldridge WE. Medical complications of air travel. Who is at risk? *Postgrad Med* 1990; **87**:75–77.
9. Rodenberg H. Prevention of medical emergencies during air travel. *Am Fam Physician* 1988; **37**:263–271.
10. Aerospace Medical Association. Medical guidelines for air travel, Air Transport Medicine Committee, Alexandria, VA. *Aviat Space Environ Med* 1996; **67**:B1–B16.
11. Anon. Advising patients about air travel. *Drug Ther Bull* 1996; **34**:30–32.
12. Anon. Travel by air: health considerations. *International Travel and Health.* 2002:12–22.
13. Bettes TN, McKenas DK. Medical advice for commercial air travelers. *Am Fam Physician* 1999; **810**:801–808, 810.
14. Brundrett G. Comfort and health in commercial aircraft: a literature review. *J R Soc Health* 2001; **121**:29–37.

15. Cottrell JJ. Altitude exposures during aircraft flight. Flying higher. *Chest* 1988; **93**:81–84.
16. Davies J. Health risks of air travel. *J R Soc Health* 1999; **119**:75.
17. Jagoda A, Pietrza M. Medical Emergencies in Commercial Air Travel. *Emerg Med Clin North Am* 1997; **15**:251–260.
18. Low JA, Chan DK. Air travel in older people. *Age Ageing* 2002; **31**:17–22.
19. Hirsh J, O'Donnell M, Kearon C. Indications for DVT prophylaxis with air travel. *Patient Care Can* 2002; **13**:80–85.
20. Dimberg LA, Mundt KA, Sulsky SI, Liese BH. Deep venous thrombosis associated with corporate air travel. *J Travel Med* 2001; **8**:127–132.
21. Davis RM. Air travel and risk of venous thromboembolism. Pulmonary embolism after air travel may occur by chance alone. *BMJ* 2001; **322**:1184.
22. Cesarone MR, Belcaro G, Nicolaides AN, *et al.* Venous thrombosis from air travel: the LONFLIT3 study – prevention with aspirin vs. low-molecular-weight heparin (LMWH) in high-risk subjects: a randomized trial. *Angiology* 2002; **53**:1–6.
23. Bihari I, Sandor T. Thromboembolism in travelers. *Orv Hetil* 2001; **142**:2469–2473.
24. Benoit R. Traveller's thromboembolic disease. The economy-class syndrome. *J Mal Vasc* 1992; **17**:84–87.
25. Belcaro G, Geroulakos G, Nicolaides AN, Myers KA, Winford M. Venous thromboembolism from air travel: the LONFLIT study. *Angiology* 2001; **52**:369–374.
26. Barczyk A, Pierzchala W. Risk factors of venous thromboembolism. *Wiad Lek* 2001; **54**:311–324.
27. Bagshaw M. Traveller's thrombosis: a review of deep vein thrombosis associated with travel. The Air Transport Medicine Committee. *Aviat Space Environ Med* 2001; **72**:848–851.
28. Badrinath P. Air travel and venous thromboembolism – the jury is still out. *Cmaj* 2002; **166**:885–886.
29. Ansell JE. Air travel and venous thromboembolism – is the evidence in? *N Engl J Med* 2001; **345**:828–829.
30. Arfvidsson B. Risk factors for venous thromboembolism following prolonged air travel: a prospective study. *Cardiovasc Surg* 2001; **9**:158–159.
31. Arfvidsson B, Eklof B, Kistner RL, *et al.* Risk factors for venous thromboembolism following prolonged air travel. Coach class thrombosis. *Hematol Oncol Clin North Am* 2000; **14**:391–400.
32. Allemann Y, Saner H, Meier B. High altitude stay and air travel in coronary heart disease. *Schweiz Med Wochenschr* 1998; **128**:671–678.
33. Giangrande PL. Air travel and thrombosis. *Int J Clin Pr* 2001; **55**:690–693.
34. Gendreau MA, DeJohn DO. Responding to medical events during commercial airline flights. *N Engl J Med* 2002; **346**:1067–1073.
35. Touze JE, Fourcade L, Heno P, *et al.* Cardiovascular risk for the traveler. *Med Trop (Mars)* 1997; **57**:461–464.
36. Baker TD, Hargarten SW, Guptill KS. The uncounted dead – American civilians dying overseas. *Public Health Rep* 1992; **107**:155–159.
37. Guptill KS, Hargarten SW, Baker TD. American travel deaths in Mexico: causes and prevention strategies. *West J Med* 1991; **154**:169–171.
38. Hargarten SW, Baker TD, Guptill KS. Overseas fatalities of United States citizen travelers: an analysis of deaths related to international travel. *Ann Emerg Med* 1991; **20**:622–626.
39. MacPherson DW, Gueriollot F. Steiner Dl, Ahmed K, Gushulak BD, Pardy G. Death and dying abroad: the Canadian experience. *J Travel Med* 2000; **7**:227–233.
40. Berg BW, Dillard TA, Rajagopal KR, Mehm WJ. Oxygen supplementation during air travel in patients with chronic obstructive lung disease. *Chest* 1992; **101**:638–641.
41. Gong H. Jr. Air travel and patients with chronic obstructive pulmonary disease. *Ann Intern Med* 1984; **100**:595–597.
42. Celli BR. ATS standards for the optimal management of chronic obstructive pulmonary disease. *Respirology* 1997; **2**:S1–S4.
43. Celli BR. Standards for the optimal management of COPD: a summary. *Chest* 1998; **113**:283S–287S.
44. Dillard TA, Beninati WA, Berg BW. Air travel in patients with chronic obstructive pulmonary disease. *Arch Intern Med* 1991; **151**:1793–795.
45. Coker RK, Partridge MR. Assessing the risk of hypoxia in flight: the need for more rational guidelines. *Eur Respir J* 2000; **15**:128–130.
46. Lien D, Turner M. Recommendations for patients with chronic respiratory disease considering air travel: a statement from the Canadian Thoracic Society. *Can Respir J* 1998; **5**:95–100.
47. Robson AG, Hartung TK, Innes JA. Laboratory assessment of fitness to fly in patients with lung disease: a practical approach. *Eur Respir J* 2000; **16**:214–219.
48. Stoller JK. Oxygen and air travel. *Respir Care* 2000; **221**(45):214–212.
49. Sullivan P, Geddes D. Advising the traveller with lung disease. *Practitioner* 1998; **242**:379–383.
50. Vijayan VK. Air travel and chronic respiratory diseases. *Indian J Chest Dis Allied Sci* 1999; **41**:131–133.
51. Vohra KP, Klocke RA. Detection and correction of hypoxemia associated with air travel. *Am Rev Respir Dis* 1993; **148**:1215–1219.
52. Dillard TA, Berg BW, Rajagopal KR, Dooley JW, Mehm WJ. Hypoxemia during air travel in patients with chronic obstructive pulmonary disease. *Ann Intern Med* 1989; **111**:362–367.
53. Stoller JK, Hoisington E, Auger G. A comparative analysis of arranging in-flight oxygen aboard commercial air carriers. *Chest* 1999; **115**:991–995.
54. Dewey CM, Riley WJ. Have diabetes, will travel. *Postgrad Med* 1999; **105**:111–113, 117–118, 124–126.
55. Driessen SO, Cobelens FG, Ligthelm RJ. Travel-related morbidity in travelers with insulin-dependent diabetes mellitus. *J Travel Med* 1999; **6**:12–15.
56. Sane T, Koivisto VA, Nikkanen P, Pelkonen R. Adjustment of insulin doses of diabetic patients during long distance flights. *BMJ* 1990; **301**:421–422.
57. Perlstein R. Diabetes. Sweet journeys. *Community Outlook* 1990; July:11–13.
58. Cradock S. Nurse – I'm going on holiday. Considerations for people with diabetes. *Prof Nurse* 1990; **5**:600–602, 604.
59. Dunning D. Diabetes now – safe travel tips for the diabetic patient (continuing education credit). *RN* 1989; **52**:51–55.
60. Patterson JE, Patterson TF, Bia FJ, Barry M. Assuring safe travel for today's elderly. *Geriatrics* 1989; **49**(53):44–46, 49–53, 57.
61. Pollard AJ, Murdoch DR. *Travel Medicine*. Oxford, UK: Health Press Limited; 2001.
62. Giordano BP, Thrash W, Hollenbaugh L. Performance of seven blood glucose testing systems at high altitude. *Diabetes Educ* 1998; **15**:444–448.
63. Yanai-Kopelman D, Paz A, Rippel D, Potasman I. Inflammatory bowel disease in returning travelers. *J Travel Med* 2000; **7**:333–335.
64. Schumacher G, Kollberg B, Ljungh A. Inflammatory bowel disease presenting as travellers' diarrhoea. *Lancet* 1993; **341**:241–242.
65. Schumacher G. First attack of inflammatory bowel disease and infectious colitis. A clinical, histological and microbiological study with special reference to early diagnosis. *Scand J Gastroenterol Suppl* 1993; **198**:1–24.
66. Keystone JS, Kozarsky PE, Freedman DO. Internet and Computer-Based Resources for Travel Medicine Practitioners. *CID* 2001; **32**:757–765.

CHAPTER 25 # Preparation of Immunocompromised Travelers

Maria D. Mileno

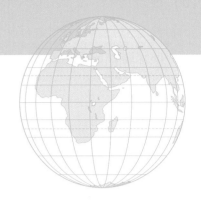

KEYPOINTS

- Live vaccines are contraindicated for most immunocompromised travelers and should be avoided for at least 3 months after completion of cancer chemotherapy

- Asplenic travelers have increased susceptibility to encapsulated bacteria, *Babesia* species and some enteric bacteria and respond poorly to polysaccharide vaccines

- After bone marrow transplantation, the highest risk period for acquisition of an infectious disease is in the first 3 months suggesting that high-risk travel should be avoided during that period

INTRODUCTION

The complex and unique characteristics of travelers with compromised immunity warrant special consideration. Additional patient education is often required when advising about the risks of their particular journey. They should know how infectious risks might be avoided, such as advice about acquiring safe drinking water, and they should be instructed about when and how to seek help. There are few absolute contraindications to travel for those who are immunocompromised, however each person should be assessed on an individual basis. Medical providers should carefully review the medical needs and risks of their potentially traveling compromised patients and have frank discussions with them on the wisdom of travel.

Other chapters in this book are dedicated to the standard approach offered to all travelers, as well as to immunocompromised groups such as pregnant travelers, travelers with diabetes, and HIV-infected travelers. Here, we address the approach to persons with other forms of severe immunosuppression which can result from asplenia, solid organ and bone marrow transplantation, cancer chemotherapy, and high dose corticosteroid use. Health-care workers with special underlying conditions (Table 25.1) have additional risks, which must be discussed, such as avoidance of HIV exposure and initiation of highly active antiretroviral postexposure prophylaxis. This is fully addressed in detail elsewhere.[1] Family members and household contacts of severely immunocompromised travelers should receive counseling and be vaccinated with live virus vaccines to protect the compromised individual. Precautions for malaria including choice of chemoprophylaxis and discussion of prevention of food and water-borne disease and other vector-borne diseases generally do not differ from those for immunocompetent travelers.

ASPLENIC TRAVELERS

Once considered a nonessential organ, it is now known that the spleen plays a central immunologic role. It actively facilitates phagocytosis, removing blood-borne bacteria, intraerythrocytic parasites and immune complexes. It also serves as a site for the initiation of both humoral and cellular immunity. Defensive host factors such as cytokine synthesis, natural killer cell function, and complement activation may all be diminished after splenectomy.

Splenectomy has been estimated to carry a lifetime risk of overwhelming sepsis of up to 5%, with the highest risk occurring within the first two years after splenectomy.[2] The lifetime risk for children who have had a splenectomy reaches up to 8.1%. Death rates from overwhelming infections, (OPSI) are thought to be up to 600 times greater than in the general population.[3] Most of the risk relates to an increased susceptibility to pneumococcal infection although other encapsulated bacteria such as *Haemophilus influenzae*, and *Neisseria meningitidis* are also important risks.

Whether functionally or anatomically impaired, splenic dysfunction is a risk for travelers. Functional asplenia occurs in association with a number of conditions including sickle cell anemia, hemoglobin SC disease, splenic atrophy or congenital asplenia and even in such varied diseases as systemic amyloidosis, lupus erythematosus, or rheumatoid arthritis. Common indications for splenectomy in children relate to malignancies such as Hodgkin's lymphoma and other hematological disorders, while adults more often require splenectomy because of trauma or hypersplenism. The various reasons for splenectomy may affect the subsequent risk of sepsis in any given individual. Patients who undergo splenectomy for hematological disease may be at greater risk of infection than those who have splenectomy following trauma.[4] There is no evidence that splenic tissue left in the peritoneal cavity following trauma surgery provides any useful splenic function. However, patients undergoing splenectomy for hematological and reticuloendothelial diseases, or for portal hypertension, have been shown to have a higher incidence of subsequent sepsis than those undergoing splenectomy for trauma.[3] Moreover, increased mortality occurs in those with underlying reticuloendothelial disease and in patients treated with chemotherapy or radiation. Lifetime incidence rates of up to 25% reported after child-hood splenectomy for hematological disorders warrants vigilance in the education and evaluation of all persons without a spleen who anticipate travel, not only in the first 2 years after splenectomy but for a lifetime.

Table 25.1	Immunization of health-care workers with special conditions				
Vaccine	Severe[a] Immuno-suppression	Asplenia	Renal failure	Diabetes	Alcoholism and alcoholic cirrhosis
BCG	C	UI	UI	UI	UI
Hepatitis A	UI	UI	UI	UI	R
Hepatitis B	R	R	R	R	R
Influenza	R	R	R	R	R
Measles, Mumps, Rubella	C	R	R	R	R
Meningococcal	UI	R	UI	UI	UI
Poliovirus vaccine, inactivated (IPV)	UI	UI	UI	UI	UI
Pneumococcal	R	R	R	R	R
Rabies	UI	UI	UI	UI	UI
Tetanus/Diphtheria	R	R	R	R	R
Typhoid Vi	UI	UI	UI	UI	UI
Typhoid, Ty21a	C	UI	UI	UI	UI
Varicella	C	R	R	R	R
Vaccinia	C	UI	UI	UI	UI

R, Recommended; C, Contraindicated; UI, Use if indicated.
[a]Severe immunosuppression can be caused by congenital immunodeficiency, leukemia, lymphoma, generalized malignancy or therapy with alkylating agents, antimetabolites, ionizing radiation, or large amounts of corticosteroids.

There is no evidence that live vaccines pose any risk to asplenic individuals.[4] Although asplenic individuals respond poorly to polysaccharide vaccines, with resulting low antibody titers that wane unpredictably,[5] a serious attempt should be made to immunize asplenic travelers. Ideally, such travelers would have been previously immunized with the pneumococcal vaccine 2 weeks prior to splenectomy. A one time only pneumococcal booster after 5 years is recommended, and meningococcal immunization, along with all other routine travel immunizations.

Recently, 7-valent pneumococcal conjugate vaccines have been produced by linking polysaccharide to protein carrier molecules, thus stimulating T and B cells in a concerted fashion. Such conjugation results in increased immunogenicity and the ability to prime for a booster response. This vaccine is currently indicated for infants at birth and for children up to 59 months of age. It has been shown to be immunogenic in very young infants, and may have a role in the asplenic individual.[5]

Amoxicillin for asplenic travelers is often provided, should they become ill when abroad. However, the worldwide emergence of drug-resistant *S. pneumoniae* and the continued observation of severe invasive pneumococcal infections,[5,6] raise significant concerns. This problem has been recognized not only in the USA and Canada, but also in Latin America, the Asia-Pacific region, Europe and South Africa. The possibility of complicated skin infections may also occur in asplenic travelers. Asplenic individuals with fever are advised to seek medical help using the suggested resources in the chapter on healthcare abroad. Additional extended-spectrum quinolone agents that have excellent activity against resistant *S. pneumoniae*, *H. influenzae*, and *Moraxella catarrhalis* infection are offered to asplenic individuals who may not be able to seek care in a timely fashion.[6]

Levofloxacin has demonstrated activity against gram-positive and gram-negative aerobes implicated in complicated skin infections as well as excellent efficacy for treatment of pneumonia. A higher dose

(750 mg, instead of the customary 500 mg dose) ensures high drug concentrations in skin and soft tissue. Alternatively, azithromycin is a well tolerated broad-spectrum macrolide agent, which can be offered for initiation of urgent treatment of suspected upper respiratory infections.

There are no data to confirm any increased risk of severe malaria in asplenic individuals, although it is theoretically possible.[7] Asplenic individuals are susceptible to overwhelming infection caused by *Babesia* species, the red cell parasite infection that largely occurs along the eastern seaboard of the United States, the West Coast and in some parts of Eastern Europe. There are no case-controlled studies comparing normal hosts and asplenics with regard to parasite clearance times or incidence of clinical reactivation. Malaria prevention should be no different than for other travelers to malarious regions, and must include a rigorous discussion of personal protection measures in addition to chemoprophylaxis. The importance of urgent evaluation of fever in asplenic individuals cannot be overemphasized, along with a thoughtful discussion about avoiding infections - such as malaria.

Other vector-borne diseases may pose risk and warrant prevention. Recently, a case report of a splenectomized individual who developed severe trypanosomiasis with central nervous system involvement indicated no difference in the onset of symptoms, laboratory studies or disease progression than in persons who have a spleen. The patient was treated successfully with suramin and melarsoprol. Further observation is necessary to ultimately define the role of the spleen in trypanosomiasis and other possible parasite exposures.[8]

TRANSPLANT RECIPIENTS

Immunosuppressive agents, particularly cyclosporin and tacrolimus used to prevent graft rejection in transplant recipients, have profound effects on T-cell function. Azathioprine and corticosteroids may also be part of an immunosuppressive regimen and further impair neutrophil function. Intracellular pathogens pose the greatest risk to these individuals. Persons who have undergone allogeneic bone marrow transplantation (e.g., for leukemia) are more severely immunosuppressed than are solid organ recipients, and are considered functionally asplenic.

Infections which pose most risk for persons who have undergone hematologic transplantation are ubiquitous pathogens. Cytomegalovirus (CMV disease) remains in the spotlight of post-transplantation complications and HHV-6 and HHV-7 seem to exacerbate CMV infections in these patients.[9,10] Adenoviruses are increasingly recognized pathogens that affect blood and marrow transplant recipients (often within the first 100 days of transplant), with highest mortality among those who develop pneumonia and disseminated disease. The intensity of immunosuppressive therapy has an independent contribution to the risk of dissemination.[11] Invasive mold infections (most commonly *Aspergillus*) are usually late in presentation among allogeneic bone marrow transplant patients, and overall prognosis is poor despite antifungal therapy.[12] Timing travel plans beyond the period during which these infections are more likely to occur may be the most important factor in avoiding illness while abroad. Patients who have had bone marrow transplantation are presumed to be immunocompetent if they are at least 24 months post-transplant, are not receiving immunosuppressives, and do not have graft versus host disease. Strategies for safe living after transplantation have been published, particularly for those who have undergone hematopoietic stem cell transplantation (HSCT).[13] Surrounding the time of transplantation and for the first 100 days after oral prophylaxis is given for early prevention of CMV disease (ganciclovir), herpes simplex (acyclovir), Candidiasis (fluconazole) and *Pneumocystis-carinii* pneumonia (trimethoprim-sulfamethoxazole). HSCT-transplanted patients should subsequently continue to adhere to strict food precautions. They should not eat any raw or undercooked meat, (to avoid in particular risk of *E. coli* 0157: H7 and other gram negative enteric organisms) including beef, poultry, pork, lamb, and venison or other wild game. Also, they should avoid combination dishes containing raw or undercooked meats or sweetbreads from these animals, such as sausages (risks of parasitic infection such as toxoplasmosis, trichinellosis, tapeworm and neurocysticercosis) or casseroles which may not allow meats to cook well. Primary infection of toxoplasmosis is more severe than usual for an immunocompromised host. In addition, transplant persons should not consume raw or undercooked eggs or foods that may contain them (e.g., some preparations of Hollandaise sauce, Caesar and other salad dressings, homemade mayonnaise, and homemade eggnog) because of risk of infection with *Salmonella enteritidis*. Outbreaks of listeriosis have been traced to turkey products as well as soft cheeses. To prevent viral gastroenteritis and exposure to *Vibrio* species and *Cryptosporidium parvum,* HSCT patients should not consume raw or undercooked seafood, such as oysters or clams mostly to avoid risk of severe hepatitis A. In situations where the HSCT patient or his or her caretaker does not have direct control over food preparation (e.g., in restaurants), HSCT patients and candidates should consume only meat that is cooked until well done.[13] In the United States, campylobacter is quite high on the list of common food-borne illnesses. Poultry is a usual source and should be thoroughly cooked every time it is served.

In general, live virus vaccines should be avoided since there is a risk that disease associated with a vaccine strain of yellow fever or polio might emerge. Overall, transplant recipients have weaker and less durable antibody responses than normal individuals (Table 25.2). Responses of heart transplant recipients to pneumococcal vaccine antigens were suppressed in one study.[14] Fortunately, there is no evidence to suggest that immunizations lead to a greater risk of graft rejection, although there have been anecdotal reports of rejection asso-

ciated with influenza vaccine.[15] Another study concluded that influenza vaccine can be safely administered to heart transplant recipients.[16]

Some evidence shows that the hepatitis A vaccine is both safe and immunogenic in liver and renal transplant recipients.[17] A smaller study showed suboptimal protection in patients with advanced liver disease or transplanted livers. Given the safety of this vaccine and the high prevalence of hepatitis A infection, we advocate its use in all transplanted persons. Ideally, if used for liver transplant candidates it should be administered to patients early in the course of liver disease.[18] Inactivated polio vaccine can be used when necessary, but travelers to countries requiring yellow fever vaccination should be provided with a waiver letter to the embassy of the country to be visited.

Guidelines recommend giving three doses of DPT or Td, inactivated polio, *H. influenzae,* and hepatitis B vaccines to solid organ transplant patients at 12, 14, and 24 months post-transplant (Table 25.3).[15] The MMR vaccine, which is a live-virus vaccine, is contraindicated within the first 2 years after transplant. Administration of MMR vaccine is recommended at 24 months or later post-transplant if the patient is presumed immunocompetent. It is recommended that lifelong seasonal administration of influenza vaccine should be given beginning before transplant and resuming ≥6 months post-transplant. In addition, 23-valent pneumococcal vaccine is recommended for HSCT patients at 12 and 24 months post-transplant. MMR vaccine viruses are not transmitted to contacts of vaccine recipients and varicella vaccine virus transmission is rare. Family, close contacts, and health-care providers of transplant patients should be vaccinated against measles and varicella if indicated and annually against influenza.[13]

Increased risk of bacteremia during episodes of gastroenteritis caused by *Salmonella* or *Campylobacter* spp. warrants empiric treatment of diarrheal episodes for all transplant recipients with a quinolone antibiotic or its equivalent.

Malaria advice need not be different from usual, although the effects of antimalarials such as chloroquine or mefloquine upon levels of immunosuppressive medications are not fully known. Documenting such levels during antimalarial prophylaxis would be prudent prior to travel.

Also, transplant recipients have an increased risk of skin cancers and this risk may be increased by excessive exposure to sunlight. Specific advice concerning hats and sunblocking agents with UVA and UVB protection is warranted.

CANCER CHEMOTHERAPY

While hematological malignancies lead to immunosuppression beyond that caused by chemotherapeutic regimens used to treat them, solid organ tumors may lead to more subtle immune defects. There was a steady increase in mortality from 1980–1997 due to aspergillosis associated with malignancy, although mortality rates from endemic mycoses (i.e., histoplasmosis, and coccidioidomycosis) remained unchanged.[19] Cryptococcosis is rare in patients with cancer but it can be confused with lung or brain metastases. Yet, if suspected, there is good diagnostic yield from serology, CSF culture and usually an excellent therapeutic outcome.[20]

Patients respond less well than do normal hosts to immunizations after cancer chemotherapy, with the poorest responses occurring in those with primary hematological malignancies[21] (Table 25.3).[15] Live virus vaccines should be avoided until at least 3 months following completion of chemotherapy. It is likely that responses to the other travel immunizations will also be poor. Persons with chronic lymphocytic leukemia or myeloma are functionally antibody deficient and will not produce useful responses to most immunizations (Table 25.4). It is better to provide these patients with empiric

Table 25.2 Recommended vaccinations for hematopoietic stem cell transplant (HSCT) recipients, including both allogeneic and autologous recipients

	Time after HSCT		
	12 months	14 months	24 months
Inactivated vaccine or toxoid Diphtheria, tetanus, acellular pertussis: children aged <7 years	Diphtheria toxoid-tetanus toxoid-acellular pertussis vaccine (DTaP) or diphtheria toxoid (DT)	DTaP or DT	DTaP or DT
Diphtheria, tetanus, acellular pertussis: children aged ≥7 years	Tetanus-diphtheria toxoid (Td)	Td	Td
Haemophilus influenzae type b (Hib) conjugate	Hib conjugate	Hib conjugate	Hib conjugate
Hepatitis (Hep B)	Hep B	Hep B	Hep B
23-valent pneumococcal polysaccharide (PPV)	PPV	–	PPV
Hepatitis A	Routine administration not indicated.		
Influenza	Lifelong, seasonal administration, beginning before HSCT and resuming at >6 months after HSCT.		
Meningococcal	Routine administration not indicated.		
Inactivated polio (IPV)	IPV	IPV	IPV
Rabies	Routine administration not indicated.		
Lyme disease	Routine administration not indicated; limited data regarding safety, efficacy, or immunogenicity among HSCT recipients.		
Live-attenuated vaccine Measles-mumps-rubella (MMR) Varicella vaccine Rotavirus vaccine	– Contraindicated for HSCT recipients. Not recommended for any person in the USA.	–	MMR

For these guidelines, HSCT recipients are presumed immunocompetent at ≥24 months after HSCT if they are not on immunosuppressive therapy and do not have graft-versus-host disease (GVHD)

antibiotics for use if they become febrile while abroad. In addition, standard malaria advice is indicated.

DENGUE FEVER IN PERSONS WITH CHRONIC THROMBOCYTOPENIA

Two recent case reports of dengue fever occurring in persons with underlying thrombocytopenia illustrate the importance of identifying dengue infection in such patients. Dengue may possibly enhance the risk of hemorrhage and may lead to an unnecessary workup because of the profound and possibly misleading decrease in the platelet count.[22]

Classic dengue fever (DF) may induce marked thrombocytopenia[22] in up to 50% of healthy subjects, with platelet counts sometimes as low as 10 000 platelets/mm³. Dengue hemorrhagic fever (DHF) diagnosis requires evidence not only of fever, bleeding and thrombocytopenia, but also of plasma leakage (serous effusions, hypoalbuminemia, hypoproteinemia, or a 20% increase in hematocrit level caused by hemoconcentration). See Table 25.5. Neither case represented DHF; however, the excessive bleeding complications seen in the first case seemed to result from a lack of knowledge regarding the scope of the clinical features asso-ciated with dengue fever.[22]

CORTICOSTEROID USAGE AND NEWER AGENTS

Increasing numbers of travelers are using high dose corticosteroids or other agents such as methotrexate and cyclophosphamide for connective tissue diseases and other immune-mediated disorders. Other persons with rheumatoid arthritis or Crohn's disease may be using newer agents that neutralize the activity of tumor necrosis factor-alfa (TNF-α): infliximab (Remicade®), etanercept (Enbrel®) and adalimumab (Humira®). If a patient on these agents develops a serious infection, these drugs should be stopped while treating the infectious process. Warnings are strongest for TB or invasive fungal infections. Infliximab was linked to 70 cases of TB in US patients between 1998 and May 2001.[23] Should travel medicine practitioners warn these patients about risk of TB from prolonged intimate exposure to high risk populations? What about risks from kicking up dirt horseback riding in the desert southwestern USA?

Table 25.3 **Recommendations for administration of childhood vaccines before and after solid organ transplant**

Vaccine	Recommended for use after transplantation	Re-immunization required after transplantation[a]	Assessment of immunity required after vaccination
Live attenuated			
Varicella	No	No	Yes
Measles	No	No	Yes
Mumps	No	No	No
Rubella	No	No	Yes[b]
Rotavirus	No	No	No
BCG	No	No	Yes
Inactivated			
Polio	IPV only	Yes	No
Acellular pertussis	Yes	Yes	No
Diphtheria	Yes	Yes	No
Tetanus	Yes	Yes	No
Hepatitis B	Yes	Yes[c]	Yes
Neisseria meningitis	Yes[d]	Yes	No
Rabies	Yes[e]	Yes	No
Hepatitis A	Yes	Yes[c]	Yes
Influenza	Yes	Yes	No
Streptococcus pneumoniae	Yes	Yes	No

Note: IPV, all inactivated polio vaccine.
[a]Immunization schedule should be re-instituted once immunosuppression is decreased (typically 6 months to 1 year after transplantation). Once resumed, immunizations should follow the recommended schedule.
[b]Documentation of immunity recommended for women of childbearing age.
[c]Decision to re-immunize should be based on assessment of serological response to the vaccine.
[d]Recommended for college-age students and others at risk.
[e]Recommended for those at risk due to avocation or vocation.

Table 25.4 **Immune suppression and immunization**

Type of immune suppression	Cautions	Suggestions
Travelers with solid organ transplants	Avoid traveling <1 year post-transplant	Pneumococcal, meningococcal, and *H. influenzae* type B vaccines. Hepatitis B and influenza vaccines pre-transplant.
Travelers with hematological malignancies	No live virus vaccines <3 months after last therapy	Pneumococcal and *H. influenzae* type B vaccines, ideally 2 weeks before suppressive therapy. DTaP, Td, influenza, IPV as indicated. MMR and varicella if not severely immunosuppressed.
Congenital immune disorders	No live vaccines.	Intravenous immunoglobulin is used in the management of a number of these disorders but the benefit only lasts for 2–3 weeks.
Drug-induced immunosuppression	No live vaccines if taking >20 mg/day steroids for >2 weeks.	Vaccinate 1 month after last dose of steroid therapy.
Other immunosuppressive drugs/therapy[a]	No live vaccines. Suppression may last up to 3 months from last dose. Can use double dose for hepatitis B vaccine.	Vaccinate >1 month after last dose. If vaccinated while receiving immunosuppressive therapy or in the 2 weeks preceding therapy, revaccinate ≥ 3 months after therapy is discontinued.
Autoimmune disorders: Multiple sclerosis		Immunize as normal.
Chronic diseases and drugs associated with immune defects	No live vaccines with significant immunosuppression	Pneumococcal, influenza, *H. influenzae* type B, hepatitis B vaccines
Hyposplenism		Pneumococcal, meningococcal, *H. influenzae* type B, and influenza vaccines. Prophylactic Penicillin V

[a]Immunosuppressive agents and procedures: alkylating agents; cyclophosphamide; tnf blocking drugs (infliximab, etanercept); plasma exchange; methotrexate (including low dose), 6-MP + azathioprine; cyclosporin and tacrolimus; total lymphoid irradiation; antilymphocyte globulin

---

Table 25.5 **Example cases of dengue fever (DF) in persons with chronic thrombocytopenia**

Case 1
A 32-year-old West Indian man with idiopathic thrombocytopenic purpura and chronic refractory thrombocytopenia and splenectomy developed an acute, febrile, painful illness during an epidemic of dengue fever (DF) due to DEN-2 virus. He presented with extensive superficial bleeding, confusion and nuchal rigidity. The patient had not taken aspirin. On day 2, despite negative blood cultures, and a platelet count of 12 000/mm³ (his baseline ranged from 14 000–50 000 cells/mm³) lumbar puncture was performed and bacterial meningitis was excluded. Within four days of onset of DF the bleeding worsened, and the platelet count decreased to 1000/mm³. Low back pain, impotence, sacral dermatomal anesthesia and sphincteric disturbance ensued. An intradermal hematoma of the conus medullaris was documented. The hematocrit remained within normal limits. Treatment with IVIG and high-dose steroids had no effect. Platelet transfusions produced transient increases to 40 000 cells/mm³ and stopped the bleeding. Clinical diagnosis of DF was confirmed by positive results of an IgM antibody capture assay and by virus culture of blood that yielded a DEN-2 stain. The patient recovered from DF within 6 days and from neurologic impairment within 1 month. Continued follow-up over 4 years showed no other bleeding episodes, despite persistently low platelet counts (10 000 to 20 000/mm³).

Case 2
A 27-year-old West Indian woman with systemic lupus erythematosus, treated with prednisone 20 mg/day, presented with fever, rash and diffuse pain during an epidemic of DF due to DEN-2 and DEN-4. On day 5, the patient's platelet count decreased to 3000/mm³ (baseline 30 000/mm³) and extensive purpura developed, although hemoglobin and hematocrit levels remained within normal range. High dose corticosteroids were given for 3 days. Within 1 week the patient had a complete recovery and a platelet count of 32 000/mm³. IgM serologic tests confirmed the presence of DF infection. No other episodes of acute severe thrombocytopenia occurred during the following 3 years.

Infection risk varies greatly depending on concomitant therapies and the underlying immune disorder. Studies in patients with SLE and other autoimmune disorders have demonstrated that prednisone doses in excess of 20 mg/day (~ 0.3 mg/kg of body weight) can lead to an increased risk of serious infections, with up to eight-fold increased risk in persons receiving doses above 40 mg/day.

Most experts agree that corticosteroid therapy also is not a contraindication to live virus vaccines when it is short-term (i.e. <2 weeks); long-term, alternate-day treatment with short-acting preparations; replacement therapy (i.e., physiologic doses) or doses administered topically (skin and eyes) or by intraarticular bursal or tendon injection. Infections with atypical or opportunistic organisms are seen more than 40 times more often in patients given corticosteroids than in those not given them.[21] Several studies, however, have failed to confirm a significant increased risk of reactivation of tuberculosis in some groups of corticosteroid users. One report, for example, found a reactivation rate of only 3%, which could have been in part due to the underlying diseases. Despite these results, conventional wisdom suggests that any patient with a positive PPD skin test, a suggestive chest radiograph, or a strong family history of tuberculosis should receive antituberculosis prophylaxis prior to starting corticosteroid therapy.

Defects in cell-mediated immunity in these individuals result in weakened responses to immunizations.[24] As with recipients of solid organ transplants, live vaccines should be avoided and a standby course of antibiotics should be given in case such individuals develop fever (Table 25.4). Corticosteroid therapy does not appear to block the antibody response to influenza vaccine and this should be given.

Persons with impaired humoral immunity (e.g., hypogammaglobulinemia or dysgammaglobulinemia) should be vaccinated.

A discussion on strongyloides prevention must occur for the traveler with cancer and for persons on corticosteroids, or individuals who have underlying HTLV-1 infection. Overwhelming strongyloidiasis and septic shock are higher risks for these groups. Avoidance of barefoot walking particularly in damp or muddy areas must be emphasized. Persons who report such exposure should be further evaluated upon return from travel, with an eosinophil count and, if elevated, strongyloides serology. Infected persons can be treated to avoid severe complications of strongyloidiasis.

POSTEXPOSURE RABIES PROPHYLAXIS IN A PERSON WITH LYMPHOMA

Lastly but importantly, what about postexposure rabies prophylaxis in immunocompromised individuals? Although data are limited, a case report of a patient with lymphoma who was bitten by a rabid animal illustrates this issue.[25] The Advisory Committee of Immunization Practices (ACIP) guidelines recommend postponing preexposure vaccination if possible in immunocompromised patients and refraining from immunosuppressive agents, if possible, during post-exposure rabies prophylaxis.

The important case (Table 25.6) suggests that post-exposure rabies treatment schedule in immunocompromised individuals might include doubling the dose, monitoring antirabies antibody titers daily for at least one year and postponing chemotherapy whenever possible until a protective antibody titer is achieved.[25]

Table 25.6 **Example case of post-exposure rabies prophylaxis in a person with lymphoma**

A 55-year-old man newly diagnosed with Stage IV lymphocytic B cell lymphoma was attacked by a jackal, experiencing multiple bites on his right index finger, hand, forearm, elbow and abdomen. He received a standard course of post-exposure rabies vaccine with human rabies immunoglobulin (HRIG) and refrained from beginning chemotherapy. Two days after the fifth (and final) dose, his antirabies antibody titer was low (0.2 IU/mL – protective level is 0.5 IU/mL). A second course of rabies vaccine was administered using a double-dose vaccine and single HRIG intramuscularly. The patient's antirabies antibody titer rose to 2.73 IU/mL, 2 days before the fourth double dose. Chemotherapy was initiated after the fifth double dose and his antibody titer was followed every 3 months. Four months after beginning chemotherapy the titer was acceptable (1.93 IU/mL), but fell to 0.15 IU/mL, 3 months later. The antibody level remained nonprotective after three standard doses given over 7 days, but increased to 3.84 IU/mL after a series of three double doses. The patient had no signs of rabies and his lymphoma was in remission 2 years later.

CONCLUSION

In summary, advice tailored to immune-compromised travelers can help to facilitate safe travel for those who seek destinations with a variety of health risks.

REFERENCES

1. Mileno MD. Occupational HIV Exposure. *Med Health R I* 2000; **83**(7):207–210.
2. O'Neal BJ, McDonald JC. The risk of sepsis in the asplenic adult. *Ann Surg* 1981; **194**(6):775–778.
3. Lynch AM, Kapila R. Overwhelming postsplenectomy infection. *Infect Dis Clin North Am* 1996; **10**(4):693–707.
4. Conlon CP. Travel and the immunocompromised host. *Hosp Med* 2000; **61**:167–170.
5. Kobel DE, Friedel A, Cerny T, *et al*. Pneumococcal vaccine in patients with absent or dysfunctional spleen. *Mayo Clinic Proceedings* 2000; 75.
6. Hoban DJ, Doern GV, Fluit AC, *et al*. Worldwide prevalence of antimicrobial resistance in Streptococcus pneumoniae, Haemophilus influenze, and Moraxella catarrhalis in the SENTRY antimicrobial surveillance program, 1997–1999. *Clin Inf Dis* 2001; **32**(suppl 2):S81–S93.
7. Styrt BA. Risks of infection and protective strategies for the asplenic patient. *Infect Dis Clin Pract* 1996; **5**:94–100.
8. Malesker MA, Boken D, Ruma TA, *et al*. Rhodesian trypanosomiasis in a splenectomized patient. *Am J Trop Med Hyg* 1999; **61**(3):428–430.
9. Nguyen O, Estey E, Ruad I, *et al*. Cytomegalovirus pneumonia in adults with leukemia: an emerging problem. *Clin Inf Dis* 2001; **32**(4):539–545.
10. Paya CV. Prevention of cytomegalovirus disease in recipients of solid-organ transplants. *CID* 2001; **32**(4):596–603.
11. LaRosa AM, Champlin RE, Mirza N, *et al*. Adenovirus infections in adult recipients of blood and marrow transplants. *Clin Inf Dis* 2001; **32**(11):871–876.
12. Baddley JW, Stroud TP, Salzman D, *et al*. Invasive mold infections in allogenic bone marrow transplant recipients. *Clin Inf Dis* 2001; **32**(9):1319–1324.
13. Dykewicz CA. Summary of the guidelines for preventing opportunistic infections among hematopoietic stem cell transplant recipients. *Clin Inf Dis* 2001; **33**(2):139–144.
14. Blumberg EA, Brozena SC, Stutman P, *et al*. Immunogenicity of pneumococcal vaccine in heart transplant recipients. *Clin Inf Dis* 2001; **32**(2):307–310.
15. Burroughs M, Moscona A. Immunization of pediatric solid organ transplant candidates and recipients. *Clin Inf Dis* 2000; **30**(6):857–869.
16. Blumberg EA, Fitzpatrick J, Stutman PC, *et al*. Safety of influenza vaccine in heart transplant recipients. *J Heart Lung Transplant* 1998; **17**(11):1075–1080.
17. Stark K, Gunther M, Neuhaus R, *et al*. Immunogenicity and safety of hepatitis A vaccine in liver and renal transplant recipients. *J Infect Dis* 1999; **180**(6):2014–2017.
18. Avery RK, Dumot J. Hepatitis A vaccine in liver transplant recipients [Correspondence]. *Clin Inf Dis* 2001; **32**(11):1656–1657.
19. McNeil MM, Nash SL, Hajjeh RA, *et al*. Trends in mortality due to invasive mycotic diseases in the United States, 1980–1997. *Clin Inf Dis* 2001; **33**(5):641–647.
20. Kontoyiannis DP, Peitsch WK, Reddy BT, *et al*. Cryptotoccosis in patients with cancer. *Clin Inf Dis* 2001; **32**(11):45–50.
21. Atkinson WL, Pickering LK, Schwartz B, *et al*. General Recommendations on Immunization. Recommendations of the Advisory Committee on Immunization Practice (ACIP) and the American Academy of Family Physicians (AAFP). *Morbidity and Mortality Weekly Report* 2002; **51**(RR-2):1–36.
22. Strobel M, Muller P, Lamaury I, *et al*. Dengue Fever: A harmful disease in patients with thrombocytopenia. *Clin Inf Dis* 2001; **33**(4):580–581.
23. Keane J, Gershon S, Wise RP, *et al*. Tuberculosis associated with Infliximab, a tumor necrosis factor α-neutralizing agent. *N Engl J Med* 2001; **345**(15):1098–1104.
24. McDonald E, Jarrell MP, Schiffman G, *et al*. Persistence of pneumococcal antibodies after immunization in patients with systemic lupus erythematosus. *J Rheumatol* 1984; **11**:306–308.
25. Hay E, Derazon H, Bukish N, *et al*. Rabies prophylaxis in a patient with lymphoma. *JAMA* 2001; **285**(2):166–167.

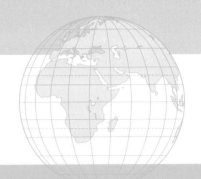

CHAPTER 26 The Traveler with HIV

Francesco Castelli and Cecilia Pizzocolo

KEYPOINTS

■ Immunizations may be less efficacious and have more adverse effects (live vaccines contraindicated in most cases) depending on the host's immune response

■ Increased potential for serious infectious disease and therefore need for greater health precautions

■ Drug interactions with anti-retroviral agents must be considered

■ Restrictions on international border crossings may be problematic for long-stay travelers

INTRODUCTION

As for any sexually transmitted disease the relationship between HIV infection and travel is complex and multifactorial in nature. HIV has spread following human mobility since the beginning of the epidemic. Many aspects may be considered for discussion:

■ May the HIV-infected subject travel safely?
■ How does HIV infection influence pre-travel advice for the HIV-infected subject?
■ What is the risk of HIV acquisition in the host country?
■ What is the potential for HIV spreading in the host country?

The availability of new potent antiretroviral drugs active against Human Immunodeficiency Virus (HIV) has dramatically improved the natural history of HIV-infected subjects in those countries where HAART (Highly Active Anti-Retroviral Therapy) has become the standard of care since 1996. In these countries, the mortality and hospitalization rates have decreased steadily and HIV infection has become a chronic condition, manageable on a long-term basis. Many HIV patients in western countries return to their active social life and to their work. It is then no surprise that many of them are willing to travel overseas, including to tropical destinations, as part of their leisure or as an essential component of their professional life. Recent reports suggest that as many as 20% of HIV infected subjects from North America travel each year to foreign destinations.[1,2]

The travel medicine professional is then challenged by the reportedly higher infectious risk that immunocompromised HIV-infected travelers are likely to face during a stay in developing countries where circulation of infectious agents is substantially higher than in industrialized countries.

On the other hand, casual sex abroad may transmit HIV infection. It has been estimated that as many as 35.7% of heterosexually acquired HIV infections reported in the Netherlands in the period 1997–99 were probably linked to a stay abroad.[3] This is also true when the migrant population is considered. Difficult socioeconomic condi-

tions often leading to promiscuous sex, poor access to health services, and low literacy rates are factors that increase risk of the migrant acquiring sexually transmitted diseases including HIV infection. Recent data in migrant populations settled in industrialized countries also underline the risk of acquiring HIV while visiting friends and relatives in their country of origin.

Meanwhile, the spread of HIV infection in the developing world continues unopposed, due to the lack of infrastructure and economic resources needed to implement HAART. Travel, among other socio-behavioral factors, is one of the main factors influencing the spread of HIV in the developing world and particularly in Africa where over 28 million HIV-infected subjects are estimated to live at the end of 2001.[4]

While excellent reviews on immunocompromised travelers have already been published,[5] this chapter will mainly focus on the special precautions that the travel medicine specialist should consider when advising HIV-infected subjects traveling from western countries to tropical areas.

PRE-TRAVEL ADVICE

The travel-related risk in the HIV-infected traveler depends on the immune status of the subject. As a general rule, travelers with a peripheral CD4+ lymphocytic count over 500 cell/µL may travel safely to any destination and may undergo chemoprophylaxis or vaccination as would any immunocompetent traveler, with the notable exception of BCG vaccine that is always contraindicated. On the other hand, special attention and skills are needed to balance infectious risk, medication requirements, and preventive measures in HIV-infected subjects whose CD4+ peripheral count is low. Whenever possible, an expert center with adequate experience and resources for the management of HIV-related complications should be identified in advance in the destination country and this information should be provided to the traveler.

The most important elements to be taken into account to provide adequate advice to HIV-infected travelers are reviewed below.

Behavioral modification

High priority should be given to the provision of counseling to ensure that the traveler avoids risky sexual practices while abroad, in order to prevent the spread of HIV infection in the host country as well as to prevent the traveler from acquiring other sexually transmitted diseases or additional HIV variants. It has been proven that other sexually transmitted infections may increase the genital shedding of HIV and may then facilitate transmission of HIV infection. Furthermore, the possible acquisition of HIV variants other than the original one may make the therapeutical success of antiretroviral therapy more difficult to achieve. Specific and detailed counseling on adequate food and water precautions is mandatory, not only to prevent travelers' diarrhea, but also to avoid the ingestion of possible opportunistic agents that may cause significant illnesses in the subsequent course of the HIV infection. Among those opportunistic infections, *Toxoplasma gondii*, *Isospora belli*, *Salmonella spp* and *Cryptosporidium parvum* are particularly relevant from a clinical standpoint. Raw vegetables and foods are to be avoided, as well as tap water and fruit juices from street vendors.

It has also been reported that bathing in pools or rivers may increase the risk of skin mycotic, bacterial or helmintic infections. Prolonged sun exposure should be avoided to prevent photosensitivity reactions which are frequently associated with drug therapy.

Vaccination

The safety and efficacy of the various vaccinations in HIV-infected persons have been the subject of many debates. Excellent reviews on this topic are available.[6] The travel health professional should carefully evaluate four key elements in order to make a risk-benefit assessment of a specific vaccine.[7] A summary of the present knowledge on vaccination in HIV-infected persons is found in Table 26.1.

Risk and severity of vaccine-preventable diseases in the HIV-infected traveler

As for non-HIV-infected subjects, an assessment of the risk of acquiring a specific infection should be made for any destination. Many infectious diseases are reported to be either more frequent and severe in immunocompromised subjects. Among those, *Salmonella* spp., pneumococcal and meningococcal infections deserve particular attention. The high susceptibility of HIV-positive patients to invasive *Salmonella* spp. disease is well described. The yearly incidence of invasive pneumococcal disease may be as high as 1% in the HIV infected population in the USA, 100 times higher than in the general population.[8]

Viral hepatitis is particularly dangerous in HIV-infected patients because hepatitis B and C are more likely to be chronic and progress faster than in HIV-negative subjects. Hepatitis A infection, highly prevalent in developing countries, has a more severe course in patients with chronic liver disease. Since hepatitis B and C are transmitted in the same way as HIV, many HIV patients, especially drug addicts and homosexuals, are also co-infected with one or both hepatitis viruses. On the other hand, the prevalence of HAV immunity in travelers is decreasing and only a minority of young travelers from western countries have detectable HAV antibodies. Therefore, hepatitis B vaccination should be considered in previously unexposed HIV-infected individuals, and hepatitis A vaccination should be considered in all HIV-infected travelers to medium to high risk areas.

There is no evidence that influenza occurs more frequently in HIV-infected subjects, but the incidence of complications has been reported to be higher. To date, no information is available on the incidence and/or severity of other vaccine-preventable infections, such as tetanus, diphtheria or typhoid, in the HIV-infected traveler.

Nature of the vaccine

As for any other clinical situation in which immunosuppression is an issue, live vaccines should be avoided as a general rule, especially when the immune status of the patient is severely compromised (CD4+ peripheral cell count below 200/μL). The risk of live vaccines in HAART-treated patients with satisfactory CD4+ response, but whose CD4+ peripheral count nadir is below 200 cells/μL is still controversial. It has been suggested that at least 3–6 months are required after the initiation of HAART therapy before lymphocytes recover full functionality. Nevertheless, some live vaccines (yellow fever, measles) may

be used safely in HIV infected patients whose CD4+ peripheral cell count are stable and consistently exceed 200 cells/μL.[9] A fatal case of measles pneumonia was reported following MMR vaccination in an immunocompromised HIV-infected patient with a CD4+ peripheral count below 200 cells/μL. Yellow fever and measles vaccinations should be limited to situations where a substantial risk of contracting the diseases exists. Inactivated Salk polio vaccine should be used instead of the Sabin live polio vaccine in HIV travelers. Also, inactivated vaccines should nevertheless be used instead of live ones against typhoid and cholera, if indicated. BCG vaccine is always to be avoided. Polysaccharide vaccines, such as vaccines against *Streptococcus pneumoniae* and *Neisseria meningitidis* appear to elicit a CD4+ independent immune response, as demonstrated by the adequate immune titers obtained in immunocompromised hosts. Despite this consideration, clinical protection against pneumococcal disease is impaired in vaccinees whose CD4+ cell count is below 200/μL regardless of the elicited antibody serotiter. The protective efficacy of the 23-valent pneumococcal polysaccharide vaccine to prevent invasive pneumococcal disease in HIV-infected persons was not confirmed in a recent trial in Ugandan adults. After 3 years, invasive disease was reported in 15/697 (2.1%) of vaccinated subjects and in 10/695 (1.4%) of unvaccinated persons, without significant differences.[10] Inactivated, subunit or polysaccharidic vaccines may be administered safely without any risk for the HIV-infected vaccinee, preferably in the early stage of HIV infection (CD4+ peripheral cell count above 300 cells/μL) to ensure adequate immune response.

Immune status of the traveler

The most reliable and simple marker to quantify the immune status of the HIV-infected traveler is the peripheral count of CD4+ lymphocytes. This marker has important prognostic and surrogate value since it predicts the individual risk to develop clinical signs of opportunistic infections and permits one to monitor the success of antiretroviral therapy. Also, it may provide important clues to the prediction of the immune response to specific vaccinations, since most vaccines have a CD4+-dependent antibody response. Such a CD4+-dependent antibody response (the lower the peripheral CD4+ value, the lower the antibody response) has been demonstrated for influenza vaccine, hepatitis A vaccine and hepatitis B vaccine, but it may be true for others for which no evidence has so far been published. For these vaccines, an impaired immune response is to be expected when the CD4+ peripheral cell count is below 300/μL. Vaccination is usually not recommended when the CD4+ peripheral cell count is below 100 cells/μL. Interestingly enough, however, children undergoing antiretroviral treatment have been reported to develop a significantly higher anti-measles antibody response in comparison to untreated children, regardless of the baseline CD4+ peripheral cell count.[11]

Most HIV patients under (HAART) therapy have experienced a dramatic increase in their absolute peripheral CD4+ cell counts. Nevertheless, since regenerated lymphocytes may recover function only after several months, it is safer to consider the above mentioned thresholds for immunization after at least 3–6 months in those patients under HAART whose CD4+ cell count had previously fallen below those limits.

Risk of virological rebound as a consequence of vaccination

The observation that most vaccinations induce a discrete increase in plasma HIV viral load as a result of the activation of the immune system has raised concerns about the appropriateness of vaccination practices among HIV-infected persons. The bulk of the most recent published evidence now shows that the plasma HIV-RNA increase following vaccination is transient, usually returning to pre-vaccination

Table 26.1   Vaccinations in HIV infected travelers[7]

Vaccine	Severity of vaccine preventable diseases in HIV+ subjects	Safety and immunogenicity of vaccine	Recommendation
Cholera	No data available	Potential risk of vaccine-induced disease for live oral vaccine No data on immune response in HIV+ subjects	Live oral vaccine is contraindicated. Use killed (oral or parenteral) vaccine, if substantial risk exists
Diphtheria	No data available	Safe No data on immune response in HIV+ subjects	Use whenever indicated
Influenza	Possible higher incidence of complication	Safe, but temporary HIV-RNA increase CD4+ dependent immune response. Do not vaccinate if CD4+ count is below 100 cells/μL	Recommended in HIV+ subjects
H. influenzae type B	Higher incidence and severity in HIV-infected subjects	Safe, no data on possible HIV-RNA increase Low response if CD4+ count below 100/μL	Early vaccination is recommended in HIV+ subjects
Hepatitis A	Clinical course of hepatitis A is accelerated in patients with chronic hepatitis	Safe, but temporary HIV-RNA increase Reduced response if low CD4+ count	Vaccination is recommended for travelers to HAV endemic areas
Hepatitis B	Progression of hepatitis B is accelerated in HIV+ subjects	Safe, but temporary HIV-RNA increase High rate of non responders. Double-strength dose or additional dose may be required	Early vaccination is recommended in HIV+ subjects. Check antibody titer
Japanese encephalitis	No data available	Safe (inactivated vaccine) No data on immune response in HIV+ subjects	Use if substantial risk exists
Measles	Clinical course of measles is more severe in HIV+ subjects	Vaccination in patients with low CD4+ count may be dangerous Reduced response if low CD4+ count	Avoid vaccination unless high risk of exposure. Avoid vaccination if CD4+ count is below 200/μL
N. meningitidis	Clinical course of meningitis is more severe in HIV+ subjects	Safe Immune response to C serotype may be reduced in HIV+ patients	Use when indicated, particularly in splenectomized subjects traveling to meningitis belt, Umrah, Hadj
Poliomyelitis	No data available	Potential risk of vaccine-induced disease for live oral vaccine (OPV) Reduced response if low CD4+ count	Live oral vaccine (OPV) is contraindicated (also in close contacts). Use killed parenteral (eIPV) vaccine, if substantial risk exists
Str. pneumoniae	Higher incidence and severity in HIV-infected subjects	Safe, but temporary HIV-RNA increase Possible reduced protection if CD4+ count below 200/μL	Usually recommended in HIV+ subjects, but recent reports question its effectiveness
Rabies	No data available	Safe (inactivated vaccine) No data on immune response in HIV+ subjects	Use if substantial risk exists
Tetanus	No data available	Safe, but temporary HIV-RNA increase Reduced response if low CD4+ count	Use whenever indicated
Tick-borne encephalitis	No data available	Safe (inactivated vaccine) No data on immune response in HIV+ subjects	Use if substantial risk exists
Tuberculosis	Incidence of disease is significantly higher in HIV+ subjects	Live attenuated vaccine (BCG): risk of vaccine-induced diseases	The use of BCG is contraindicated in HIV+ subjects
Typhoid fever	Incidence and severity of salmonellosis are higher in HIV+ subjects	Potential risk of vaccine-induced disease for live oral vaccine No data on immune response in HIV+ subjects	Live oral vaccine is contraindicated. Use Vi parenteral vaccine if exposure is likely
Yellow fever	No data available	Potential risk of vaccine-induced disease in patients with CD4+ below 200/μL No data on immune response in HIV+ subjects	Vaccination may be considered only for HIV+ travelers with CD4 count above 200/μL who are exposed to substantial risk

Adapted from Castelli F. and Patroni A,[7] with permission.

baseline values after 4–6 weeks, and even sooner if the patient is under effective antiretroviral treatment, without any substantial risk of HIV disease progression. On the other hand, it has been suggested that there may be a risk of HIV disease progression following the natural occurrence of many vaccine-preventable diseases.

In conclusion, most HIV-infected travelers to tropical destinations will benefit from travel-related immunizations, whenever indicated from a risk-benefit assessment.

Principles regarding the immunization of HIV-infected travelers:

- Inactivated vaccines should be used instead of live vaccines
- HIV-infected persons should be vaccinated as early as possible in the course of HIV infection to ensure an adequate immune response to all vaccines
- CD4+ cell count is a useful marker to predict the response to vaccination; vaccination is not likely to be effective in those with CD4 counts below 100 cells/µL
- In patients receiving HAART, at least 3–6 months must elapse before regenerated CD4+ cells may be considered fully functional and predict antibody response. It is preferable to wait until an effective immune response is possible.

Many antiretroviral drugs are metabolized in the liver via the Cytochrome P450 pathway. It has been suggested that some vaccines, notably influenza vaccine, may impair the function of this metabolic system, resulting in altered drug metabolism and disposition. However, published data do not support this hypothesis.

Chemoprophylaxis

Antimalarial chemoprophylaxis

The interactions between HIV infection and malaria infection have been studied extensively, with conflicting results. Recently, however, many reports have strongly suggested that HIV infection is a predisposing factor for higher parasitemias and a more severe infection, at least in the semi-immune population.[12] Chloroquine treatment for uncomplicated malaria was also less effective in HIV-infected Ugandan children when compared with HIV-negative controls.[13] On the other hand, acute *Plasmodium falciparum* infection has been demonstrated to induce higher HIV proviral loads and to stimulate plasma HIV replication thus possibly accelerating HIV progression in untreated HIV patients. Although no data are currently available on the non-immune HIV population undergoing antiretroviral therapy, such as the HIV-infected traveler from industrialized countries to the tropics, one would expect that HIV-malaria interactions should be even more dramatic, making malaria prevention mandatory. The use of personal protection measures such as mosquito repellents, impregnated bednets, and protective clothing is to be strongly promoted as first line protection. As a general rule, chemoprophylaxis in the HIV-infected traveler should follow national guidelines as for HIV-negative individuals. Interestingly, recent *in-vitro* data have demonstrated an antiviral effect of chloroquine, exerted against both HIV-1 and HIV-2 by a novel antiviral mechanism.[14]

The consideration that many antimalarial drugs and antiretroviral drugs, namely the protease inhibitors, share common hepatic metabolic pathway (Cytochrome P450) has raised concerns, about possible pharmacokinetic interactions. A recent study of healthy volunteers suggested that concomitant mefloquine and ritonavir administration may result in decreased plasma levels of ritonavir.[15] On the other hand, no significant influence of concomitant mefloquine administration on indinavir nor nelfinavir plasma levels was detected in two HIV-infected travelers.[16] To the authors' knowledge, no information is currently available for proguanil and chloroquine, while doxycycline is probably safe.

Chemoprophylaxis of travelers' diarrhea

No data are currently available on the incidence of travelers' diarrhea among HIV-infected travelers. However, it is probably higher than in the general population among those whose peripheral CD4+ cell count is below 200 cells/µL. For these patients, chemoprophylaxis rather than self-treatment may be indicated. HIV-infected patients with CD4+ cell counts below 200 cells/µL are often administered co-trimoxazole as prophylaxis for *P. carinii* pneumonia; this regimen may also prove useful in preventing travelers' diarrhea, even if in some areas of the developing world, resistant enteropathogens may be encountered. However, HIV-infected patients are at higher risk of experiencing drug-related hypersensitivity reactions to co-trimoxazole. Fluoroquinolones have proven effective and safe for gastrointestinal illness prevention and treatment in the HIV-infected population.

Drug interactions

Antiretroviral drugs

- *Nucleoside Reverse Transcriptase Inhibitors (NRTI):* Zidovudine (AZT), Didanosine (ddI), Zalcitabine (ddC), Stavudine (d4T), Lamivudine (3TC), Abacavir (ABV)
- *Nucleotide Reverse Transcriptase Inhibitors* (NtRTI): Tenofovir
- Non-Nucleoside Reverse Transcriptase Inhibitors (NNRTI): Nevirapine (NVP), Delavirdine (DLV), Efavirenz (EFV)
- *Protease Inhibitors (PI):* Saquinavir (SQV), Indinavir (IDV), Ritonavir (RTV), Nelfinavir (NFV), Amprenavir (APV), Lopinavir (LPV)
- *Fusion Inhibitors (FI):* T2O

As noted above, many of these drugs, namely protease inhibitors, have a complex metabolic pathway in the liver utilizing Cytochrome P450. The possible interactions between these drugs and other commonly prescribed drugs are numerous and potentially clinically important, resulting in sub-optimal or conversely toxic plasma concentrations of the antiretroviral or the companion drug.

Table 26.2 provides a short summary of the potential pharmacokinetic interactions between various drugs and antiretroviral drugs belonging to the NNRTI and PI classes, drugs belonging to the NRTI class having less potential for pharmacokinetic interactions. It should be stressed that reliable information is not currently available on the potential interactions of antiretrovirals with most of other pharmacoactive substances, including herbal remedies. Therefore, the HIV-infected traveler under antiretroviral treatment should avoid taking other non-prescription medications that could lead to potentially serious toxic drug interactions.

HEALTH RISK TO THE TRAVELERS AND HEALTH CARE ABROAD

Even if there is general agreement that immunocompromised HIV-infected travelers are at higher risk to develop travel-related infectious health problems, only very few and small studies have assessed the incidence of travel-related health problems in HIV-infected subjects. In the pre-HAART era, health disturbances were reported by as many as 43% (15/35) of HIV-infected travelers,[17] including potentially life-threatening infections (coccidioidomycosis, cryptococcosis, PCP and bacterial pneumonia). In another questionnaire-based survey,[2] the most frequent health problems reported by HIV-infected travelers were diarrhea (32% incidence over the 3-week median period of travel) and skin disorders, reported by 28% of respondents, with high consultancy rates both abroad (5% of respondents) and after return (28% of respondents). According to other reports, respiratory symptoms were reported to be the most frequent health disturbance in HIV travelers.[17]

Table 26.2 Drugs that should not be used with antiretrovirals because of pharmacokinetic interactions[7]

Drug category	Indinavir	Ritonavir	Saquinavir	Nelfinavir	Amprenavir*	Nevirapine	Delavirdine*	Efavirenz
Ca++ channel blockers	None	Bepridil	Ca++ channel blockers	None	Bepridil	None	None	None
Cardiac	None	Amiodarone Encainide Flecainide Propafenone Quinidine	None	Amiodarone Quinidine	None	None	None	None
Lipid lowering agents	Simvastatin Lovastatin	Simvastatin Lovastatin	Simvastatin Lovastatin	Simvastatin Lovastatin	Simvastatin Lovastatin	None	Simvastatin Lovastatin	None
Anti-mycobacterial	Rifampin	Rifabutin	Rifampin Rifabutin	Rifampin	Rifampin	Rifampin Rifabutin	Rifampin	None
Anti-histamine	Astemizole Terfenadine	Astemizole Terfenadine	Astemizole Terfenadine	Astemizole Terfenadine	Astemizole Terfenadine	None	Astemizole Terfenadine	Astemizole Terfenadine
Gastrointestinal drugs	Cisapride	Cisapride	Cisapride	Cisapride	Cisapride	None	Cisapride H2 blockers Proton pump inhibitors	Cisapride
Neuroleptic	None	Clozapine Pimozide	None	None	Pimozide	None	None	None
Psychotropic	Midazolam Triazolam Alprazolam	Midazolam Triazolam Diazepam Zolpidem Clorazepam Estazolam Fluoroazepam Alprazolam	Midazolam Triazolam	Midazolam Triazolam	Midazolam Triazolam Diazepam Fluoroazepam	None	Midazolam Triazolam	Midazolam Triazolam
Ergot Alkaloids	Dihydroergotamine Ergotamine	Dihydroergotamine Ergotamine	Dihydroergotamine Ergotamine	Dihydroergotamine Ergotamine	Dihydroergotamine Ergotamine	None	Dihydroergotamine Ergotamine	Dihydroergotamine Ergotamine
Analgesics	None	Meperidine Piroxicam Propoxyphene	None	None	None	None	None	None
Other	St John's Wart	Bupropion	Phenytoin Phenobarbital Carbamazepine	St John's Wart Phenytoin Phenobarbital Carbamazepine	St John's Wart	Ketoconazole		Clarithromycin

*It is advisable to check the Package insert before prescribing any medication to HIV-infected persons. Adapted from Castelli F. Patroni A[7], with permission.

No sizable study on the incidence of health problems among HIV-infected travelers has been carried out since HAART has become the standard of care in the industrialized world. In our experience, as many as 31.6% of the traveling HIV population have peripheral CD4+ cell counts below 400 cells/μL. The level of immunosuppression is directly related to the risk of malaria parasitemia, with rates of 140, 93 and 57 cases per 1000 person-year in the <200 CD4+/μL, 200–499 CD4+/μL and >500 CD4+/μL groups of Ugandan HIV-infected adults, respectively.[18] The immune restoration induced by antiretroviral drugs is marked by a dramatic increase in peripheral CD4+ cell count even to normal values, which is in turn due both to the expansion of the memory cell compartment and to the *ex novo* production of naïve cells. It is expected that HAART will substantially reduce the risk of infection in the HAART-treated HIV-infected traveler by increasing the peripheral CD4+ pool. Nevertheless, as previously noted, a 3–6 months period is needed for CD4+ lymphocytes to recover full function and this time lag should be considered when planning prophylactic measures in the HIV-infected traveler.

Travel to tropical destinations may be an opportunity for the HIV-infected traveled to encounter new opportunistic pathogens: *Toxoplasma gondii*, *Cryptosporidium parvum*, *Cyclosporacayetanensis* and *Isospora belli* may be ingested from raw vegetables, and untreated water. *Mycobacterium tuberculosis* is a particular risk factor among those who have prolonged close contact with the indigenous population. Salmonella infections are more severe in immunocompromised individuals. Therefore, it is particularly important for HIV-infected travelers to strictly adhere to food and beverage precautions in developing countries.

Apart from the infectious risk, the HAART-treated HIV-infected person should be aware of many other potential problems that may arise during travel[19]:

- Antiretroviral drugs should be carried in hand-baggage to avoid loss while abroad, since antiretroviral drugs are not available everywhere in the world
- Most drug-related adverse events occur within several weeks after initiation of therapy; it is preferable to avoid travel immediately after antiretroviral therapy has been changed
- Drug-related food and liquid intake (i.e., hydration during indinavir therapy) may need adjustment in hot climates where excess fluid loss due to sweating may occur
- Pharmacokinetic interactions with other drugs which may be of potential use during travel (Table 26.2) should be taken into account

Access to specialized health care abroad may be sometimes difficult to achieve for HIV-infected travelers in need. In any case, the HIV-infected traveler should always try to identify in advance a reference center for treatment of HIV patients in the destination country should the need arise. The Directory of the International Society of Travel Medicine may help the travel medicine professional to identify such expertise abroad before departure. A health insurance policy covering repatriation costs and flight cancellation insurance should also be purchased in advance.

CROSSING INTERNATIONAL BORDERS

There is no evidence that border restrictions for HIV-infected individuals limit the spread of HIV infection in any given country. The World Health Organization has always advised against such restrictions which are considered to be useless from the perspective of disease transmission.

However, in spite of this clear-cut position of the scientific international community, many countries have put in place a variety of entry requirements in an attempt to prevent further spread of the AIDS epidemic locally.

These restrictions usually apply to those travelers requesting a long stay permit for work or educational purposes, but may sometimes apply to tourists or other short-term travelers

Table 26.3[20] reports the list of travel restrictions as proposed by the German AIDS Federation DAH which is available on the internet (http://www.aidsnet.ch/immigration/).

However, this list changes very frequently and therefore, country-specific border requirements should be checked by HIV-infected travelers before leaving their country of origin.

It has long been debated whether migration from HIV-endemic areas in developing countries to western countries is regarded as a risk to the host country. On the other hand, many factors contribute to increase the risk of acquisition of HIV infection in migrants in the host country, mainly via the sexual route: social isolation and single status, poverty and psychological distress may be considered independent risk factors for any sexually transmitted infection including HIV. The impact of migration on HIV spread outside migrant communities has never been demonstrated in western countries, even where prostitution in HIV-endemic areas is highly prevalent.

From an epidemiological standpoint, the impact of immigration on the HIV epidemic in the host country and on the possible circulation of genetically different strains is still debated. In the Netherlands, over 50% of heterosexually acquired HIV infections have been reported to come from a foreign country.[3] The introduction of non-B subtype HIV strains following migration (migrants, military personnel, tourists, expatriates, etc.) has been demonstrated[21] with possible implications for therapeutic strategies and the design of preventive vaccines. In Italy, the proportion of notified AIDS cases in migrants from endemic areas has been increasing during the last 10 years, from 3% in the period 1983–93 to 14.4 % in 2001. However, since antiretrovirals are now available free of charge even to illegal immigrants past comparisons are unreliable.

CONCLUSION

The number of HIV-infected travelers from western countries to the tropics will probably increase in the future as a result of the clinical benefits of new Highly Active AntiRetroviral (HAART) regimens that have dramatically improved survival rates and quality of life of HIV-infected persons.

The impact of travel on HIV infection has not been studied extensively. Most studies refer to the theoretical increased infectious risk in the immunocompromised person before the HAART era, while little is known about the real risk in HIV travelers with HAART-restored CD4+ peripheral cell counts. Most data suggest that these HIV patients may travel safely to any destination, provided that adequate prophylactic measures are taken (Tables 26.4 and 26.5).

A particular area of research that needs further investigation concerns the many pharmacokinetic interactions between antiretroviral drugs and antimalarial drugs, since antimalarial chemoprophylaxis is required for most tropical destinations.

Despite strong advice to the contrary by the World Health Organization, many countries still deny entry to HIV-infected travelers requesting long-stay visas.

The impact of migration on the HIV epidemic in the host country has for the most part been reported to be negligible, but the introduction on HIV non-B subtypes may be of concern in some western countries. The provision of adequate access to health care may be the most potent tool to prevent further spread of HIV infection and other sexually transmitted infections among migrants.

Table 26.3 **Country-specific entry restrictions for HIV-infected travelers**

Country	Entry and stay restriction
Argentina	Foreigners requesting a permit of stay longer than 3 months are submitted to a medical exam with HIV test.
Armenia	HIV positive persons are denied entry to the country.
Aruba	HIV test is required for long-term immigrants.
Australia	HIV test is usually required by foreigners older than 15 years requesting permit of stay. Permit may be denied if test is positive. HIV test may be requested in case of clinical suspicion in any situation requiring medical evaluation.
Bahrain	Negative HIV test is required to obtain permit of stay. Diplomats exempted.
Bangladesh	HIV positive persons may be expelled from Bangladesh.
Belgium	A negative HIV test and a clinical examination is necessary for foreign citizens requesting a permit of stay, a work permit or for reasons of study. Exceptions: citizens of the European Community.
Benin	Negative HIV test is required to obtain permit of stay.
Belize	A recent (<2 months) negative HIV test is required to obtain permit of stay. Diplomats exempted.
Bolivia	Negative HIV test is required to obtain permit of stay >3 months.
Bosnia-Herzegovina	Negative HIV test is required to obtain permanent permit of stay.
Botswana	Negative HIV test is required to foreign students.
Byelorussia	Negative HIV test is required to obtain permit of stay longer than 3 months
Brunei	Persons HIV positive could be denied entry to the country. Negative HIV test is required for foreign citizens to obtain permit of stay. Expulsion for persons with a positive HIV test.
Bulgaria	Negative HIV test is required for foreign citizens between 14 and 70 years old (especially students and workers) requesting permit of stay longer than 30 days; as well as for the Bulgarian citizens coming back from a stay abroad longer than 30 days and for any candidate wishing to get married in Bulgaria. Tests are to be performed in a hospital or laboratory within 72 h of arrival. Expulsion for persons with a positive HIV test. Diplomats exempted.
Canada	Short-term visitors will not be tested for HIV and normally will not be excluded from entering Canada if known to be HIV. Migrants requesting permit of stay longer than 6 months, must undergo HIV testing. If test is positive, permit of stay will be denied.
Chile	Negative HIV test is required for foreign workers and students.
China	All travelers requesting a permit of stay in China longer than 1 year should undergo an HIV test (the certificates of any foreign public hospital will be accepted if executed within the last 6 months and approved by a Chinese diplomatic representative). Diplomats exempted. Tourists are requested at the border to fill in an AIDS questionnaire. Chinese citizens after an over 1 year stay abroad are requested to undergo an HIV test. An HIV test is not necessary to enter or stay in Hong-Kong.
Colombia	Foreigners that request a permit of stay in the country have to present a negative HIV test as well as tests confirming the absence of other communicable diseases. Foreign certificates are accepted. The person suspected of being HIV positive will not be allowed to enter the country.
Costa Rica	A negative HIV test is necessary for those persons requesting a permit of stay, study or work.
Cyprus	A negative HIV test is necessary for foreign candidates in order to be employed or to obtain student status.
Cuba	HIV test required for the persons requesting a permit of stay longer than 3 months. HIV positive persons are repatriated. Medical controls for Cuba citizens coming back from 'endemic' zones and for students.
Dominican Republic	A negative HIV test is necessary for persons requesting a permit of stay.
Egypt	A negative HIV test is necessary for persons requesting a permit of stay longer than 3 months. Exception: married with a person of Egyptian nationality.
El Salvador	A negative HIV test is necessary for persons over 15 years of age to obtain a permit of stay.
Estonia	A negative HIV test is necessary for persons, including students, requesting a permit of stay or a work permit.
Georgia	HIV test is necessary for persons requesting a permit of stay longer than 1 month.
Germany	Bavaria only: HIV test necessary to obtain a permit of stay for more than 6 months. Exceptions: European Union and Swiss citizens.
Jordan	HIV test is necessary for persons requesting a permit of stay >1 month. Diplomats exempted.
Greece	HIV test required for foreigners to obtain a permit of stay >3 months and to work in entertainment centers.
Guatemala	A negative HIV test is necessary for foreigners to obtain a permit of stay.
Guyana	HIV test is necessary for persons requesting a permit of stay longer than 3 months.
Hong Kong	HIV test is required for immigrants.
Hungary	Test necessary for immigrants and foreigners requesting a permit of stay >1 year. Employers can ask their employees to undergo an HIV test.

Table 26.3 **Country-specific entry restrictions for HIV-infected travelers—cont'd**

Country	Entry and stay restriction
India	Test requested for: all foreign students (>18 years old) accepted by a university, foreigners that request a permit of stay for more than 1 year as well as the adult members of their families. Blood test is to be undertaken within one month from arrival. Those with a positive HIV test as well as those who refuse to undergo the test are not allowed to stay in the country. Exceptions: diplomatic personnel, United Nations personnel, accredited journalists, ecclesiastical persons, foreigners younger than 18 years and older than 70 years, persons possessing a negative HIV test done within the last month.
Iran	A negative HIV test is necessary for persons requesting a permit of stay or work. Exception: diplomatic personnel under service, tourists and businessmen staying in the country less than 3 months.
Iraq	A recent negative HIV test is necessary to enter Iraq; test may be made at the border Exceptions: diplomatic personnel, persons aged more than 65 years or less than 12 years.
Israel	HIV test is required to obtain permits of stay longer than 3 months.
Kazakhstan	HIV test is necessary for persons requesting a work permit or of stay >3 months.
Kirghizistan	HIV test is required to obtain permit of stay longer than 1 month. Diplomats exempted.
Kuwait	Negative HIV test is required to obtain permit of stay or a permit of work. Diplomats exempted.
Latvia	Negative HIV test is required to obtain permit of stay or work permit. Test is necessary for persons (>15 years old) requesting permit of stay >90 days.
Lebanon	HIV test is required to obtain a permit of stay or a work permit. Diplomats exempted.
Libya	Negative HIV test is required to obtain a permit of stay or a work permit. Diplomats exempted. 'All the foreigners with AIDS are to be deported and cannot return to the country any more'. (Decision no. 92 of 1987, General Secretary of Health).
Lithuania	Negative HIV test is required to obtain a permit of stay or a work permit.
Malaysia	HIV test is required to obtain a work permit as an unskilled laborer.
Maldives	HIV test is required to obtain permit of stay for a long period.
Marshall Islands	HIV test is required to stay in the country for longer than 30 days or to obtain a permit of stay or a work permit.
Maurice Islands	Negative HIV test is required to obtain permit of stay or work permit.
Micronesia	HIV test is required to obtain permit of stay for more than 90 days or work permit.
Moldova	Negative HIV test is required to obtain permit of stay for more than 90 days; students and spouses of Moldovan citizens.
Mongolia	Obligatory test for foreign citizens without a recent negative test or to obtain permit to stay >3 months. Test should be repeated after some months.
Montserrat	Negative HIV test is required for foreign students.
Namibia	HIV test could be required to obtain permit of stay.
Nicaragua	HIV test is required to obtain permit of stay >3 months.
Norvegia	Free HIV and tuberculosis screening is offered to persons who stay more than 3 months.
New Zealand	Negative HIV test is required to obtain permit of stay for more than 3 months (students who ask to stay more than 2 years and refugees).
Oman	Negative HIV test is required to obtain work permits in private sector or to renew permit of work.
Pakistan	Negative HIV test is required for foreigner citizens to obtain permit of long-term stay, to refugees and to returning Pakistan citizens.
Panama	HIV test is required to obtain a work permit for women working in leisure sector and for foreigners requesting the renewal of permit of stay >1 year
Papua New Guinea	Negative HIV test is required to obtain permit of stay or work permit.
Paraguay	Negative HIV test is required to obtain a temporary or permanent permit of stay.
Philippines	Applicants seeking permanent residence visa must submit to a medical exam, which includes HIV test.
Poland	HIV test is required to obtain permit of stay
Qatar	Negative HIV test (executed within the last 6 months) is required to obtain permit of stay or work permit. Diplomats exempted. Expulsion for persons with HIV positive test.
Russia	Negative HIV test is required to obtain permit of stay for more than 3 months and for all Russians returning to Russia after 1 month stay abroad. Expulsion for persons with positive HIV test. Diplomats, consulates and accredited media representatives exempted.
Saudi Arabia	Negative HIV test is required to obtain or prolong permit of stay or work permits. Expulsion for persons with HIV positive test.
Seychelles	Negative HIV test is required to obtain a work permit.
Singapore	HIV test is required for a person with a monthly income below $1250 and to obtain permit of stay >6 months or work permit. Expulsion for persons with positive HIV test.

Table 26.3   Country-specific entry restrictions for HIV-infected travelers—cont'd

Country	Entry and stay restriction
Slovakia	Negative HIV test is required to obtain permit of stay for more than 3 months.
Slovenia	Negative HIV test is required to obtain permit of stay for more than 3 months.
South Africa	HIV test is required for foreign mine workers.
South Korea	HIV test is required only for artist travelers (dancers, singers etc.) working without their wife/husband to obtain permits of stay >3 months.
Spain	A medical test including HIV test can be required for persons asking for permit of stay, work or permit for students.
Sri Lanka	Persons suspected to be HIV positive could be denied entry to the country.
St Christophe and Nevis	HIV test requested for workers, students and foreign residents.
St Vincent and Grenadines	Negative HIV test is required to obtain permanent or temporary permit to stay.
Syria	HIV test is required (allowed Institutions: Blood Bank, Damaskas; Direction of Hygiene, Alep; Direction of Hygiene, Lattakla) for: – all the foreigners of 15–50 years old who want to stay in the country for longer than 15 days – Syrian students studying abroad after their return to Syria – foreigners marrying a Syrian citizen – Exceptions: diplomats, consulates, international organization members.
Sudan	Visa could be denied to HIV positive persons.
Suriname	HIV test requested for workers and immigrants.
Taiwan	HIV test is necessary at arrival for foreigners to obtain a permit of stay for more than 3 months, a work permit or a permit of residence. Expulsion in the case of a positive test result or refusal.
Tadjikistan	HIV test requested for foreigners to obtain a permit of stay for more than 90 days.
Thailand	HIV test could be required for renewal of visa.
Trinidad et Tobago	Foreigners that request a permit of stay or a work permit are obligated to undergo a medical exam.
Tunisia	HIV test requested for prolonged permit of stay.
Turkmenistan	Persons HIV positive could be denied entry to the country. HIV test is obligatory if seropositivity suspected.
Turks and Caicos Islands	Foreigners requesting a work permit or permit of stay need to undergo a medical exam including HIV test.
United Arab Emirates	HIV test obligatory for foreigners older than 18 years to obtain a permit of stay or a work permit. Test to be executed in the country. Test positive - denied permit. Exception: diplomats.
United States of America (USA)	All non-citizens with HIV may be restricted (including tourists) but in practice tests are required only for those seeking permanent residency. Entry is not allowed for persons with a positive test or AIDS (exceptions possible for persons infected going for meetings, to visit families, to undergo therapies, coming for business, who may obtain 1 month visa).
Ukraine	Visitors who want to stay in the country for more than 6 months or 3 months.
Uruguay	Foreigners need to undergo medical exam including HIV test to obtain a permit of stay.
Venezuela	According to the law, permission to enter Venezuela could be denied to persons suffering from various illness; this could apply to HIV/AIDS.
Virgin Islands	A negative HIV test is needed to obtain a permanent permit of stay or to obtain a contract of employment.
Yemen	HIV test requested for foreigners to obtain a permit of stay >2 months. Diplomats exempted.

Situation may change over time. It is necessary to check border requirements before leaving the country of origin.
Available on the Internet at http: //www.aidsnet.ch/immigration/. Date accessed: 21 February, 2003.

Table 26.4	Check list for HIV-infected travelers

Assess CD4 count, viral load and anti-retroviral therapy

Consider vaccine efficacy and contraindications, and potential drug interactions

Assess travel risks (especially those with CD4 counts <200 cells/µL) and counsel on infectious disease and risk reduction (consider prophylaxis for travelers' diarrhea for trips <3 weeks)

Encourage traveler to carry current medical history including medications, and if possible, name of an HIV-knowledgeable physician at destination

Advise traveler to determine *anonymously* any travel restrictions for HIV-infected persons at an intended destination.

Adapted from Mileno MD, Bia FJ,[5] with permission.

Table 26.5	Prevention of selected infectious disease risks among HIV-infected travelers

Disease	Location	Preventive measure
Toxoplasmosis	global	Food and water precautions; avoid raw meat; avoid cats
Coccidiosis		
Isosporosis	global	Food and water precautions
Cryptosporidiosis	global	Food and water precautions
Cyclosporiasis	global	Food and water precautions
Salmonellosis	global	Food and water precautions
Histoplasmosis (H. capsulatum)	C. and S. America	Avoid bat caves
Tuberculosis	global	Avoid close, prolonged contact with indigenous population
Chagas' disease	C. and S. America	Avoid sleeping in adobe or thatched roofed huts
Visceral leishmaniasis	C. and S. America, Middle East, Africa	Precautions against sandfly bites

REFERENCES

1. Kemper CA, Linett A, Kane C, Deresinsky SC. Frequency of travel of adults infected with HIV. *J Travel Med* 1995; 2:85–88.
2. Simons FM, Cobelens FG, Danner SA. Common health problems in HIV-infected travelers to the sub-tropics. *J Travel Med* 1999; 6:71–75.
3. Op Coul ELN de, Coutinho RA, Doornum GJJ van, et al. The impact of immigration on env HIV-1 subtype distribution among heterosexuals in the Netherlands: influx of subtype B and non-B strains. *AIDS* 2001; 15:2277–2286.
4. WHO. Global situation of the HIV/AIDS pandemic. *WER* 2001; 76:381–388.
5. Mileno MD, Bia FJ. The compromised traveler. *Infect Dis Clin North Am* 1998; 12:369–410.
6. Rousseau MC, Moreau J. Delmont J. Vaccination and HIV: a review of the literature. *Vaccine* 2000; 18:825–831.
7. Castelli F. Patroni A. The Human Immunodeficiency Virus-infected traveler. *Clin Inf Dis* 2000; 31:1403–1408.
8. Moore D, Nelson M, Henderson D. Pneumococcal vaccination and HIV infection. *Int J STD AIDS* 1998; 9:1–7.
9. Goujon C, Tohr M, Feuillie V, et al. Good tolerance and efficacy of yellow fever vaccine among carriers of human immunodeficiency virus. *J Travel Med* 1995; 2:145.
10. French N, Nakiyingi J, Carpenter LM, et al. 23-valent pneumococcal polysaccharide vaccine in HIV-1-infected Ugandan adults: double-blind, randomized and placebo-controlled trial. *Lancet* 2000; 355:2106–2111.
11. Berkelhamer S, Borock E, Elsen C, et al. Effect of Highly Active Antiretroviral Therapy on the serological response to additional measles vaccinations in Human Immunodeficiency Virus-infected children. *Clin Inf Dis* 2001; 32:1090–1094.
12. Whitworth J, Morgan D, Quigley M, et al. Effect of HIV-1 and increasing immunosuppression on malaria parasitaemia and clinical episodes in adults in rural Uganda: a cohort study. *Lancet* 2000; 356:1051–1056.
13. Kamya MR, Kigonya CN, McFarland W. HIV infection may adversely affect clinical response to chloroquine therapy for uncomplicated malaria in children. *AIDS* 2001; 15:1187–1188.
14. Savarino A, Gennero L, Chu Hen H, et al. Anti-HIV effects of chloroquine: mechanisms of inhibition and spectrum of activity. *AIDS* 2001; 15:2221–2229.
15. Khaliq Y, Gallicano K, Cameron DW, et al. Mefloquine decreases ritonavir exposure in healthy volunteers. *Program and abstracts* of the 7th Conference on Retroviruses and Opportunistic Infections, San Francisco, 2000: abstract no. 92.
16. Schippers EF, Hugen PWH, Hartigh MW, et al. No drug-drug interaction between nelfinavir or indinavir and mefloquine in HIV-1 infected patients. *AIDS* 2000; 14:2794–2795.
17. Kemper CA, Linett A, Kane C, et al. Travels with HIV: the compliance and health of HIV-infected adults who travel. *Int J STD AIDS* 1997; 8:44–49.
18. French N, Nakiyingi J, Lugada E, et al. Increasing rate of malaria fever with deteriorating immune status in HIV-infected Ugandan adults. *AIDS* 2001; 15:899–906.
19. Colebunders R, Nachega J, Gompel A Van. Antiretroviral treatment and travel to developing countries. *J Travel Med* 1999; 6:27–31.
20. German AIDS Federation DAH. http://www.aidsnet.ch/immigration/.
21. Thomson MM, Nàjera R. Travel and the Introduction of Human Immunodeficiency Virus Type 1 Non-B Subtype Genetic Forms into Western countries. *Clin Inf Dis* 2001; 32:1732–1737.

CHAPTER 27 The Corporate Traveler

John Piacentino, Cloe Murray, Edith R. Lederman and Stephan Mann

KEYPOINTS

- Corporate responsibility is essential to ensure that employees are adequately screened, prepared, and cared for in the event of illness or injury during overseas travel

- The business traveler has a responsibility to the corporation to ensure compliance with health and safety recommendations in order to ensure a successful trip

- An effective travel medical consultation should anticipate the health and safety concerns of the corporate traveler and provide customized prevention interventions and counseling

- Infectious threats can be prevented through appropriate vaccination, prompt medical attention and chemoprophylaxis

- Routine immunizations should be up-to-date and special immunizations should be actively anticipated in order to prepare for last-minute travel plans

- Travel medication kits, the contents of which range from antibiotics for travelers' diarrhea to jet lag remedies, improve traveler comfort, and may intervene in illness progression, thereby maintaining readiness and promoting mission accomplishment

- Non-infectious causes of illness and injury must be screened and counseled for, including personal safety and security, alcoholism and deep venous thrombosis

INTRODUCTION

The health and safety of the corporate traveler is critically important not only to the individual traveler, but also to the success of the business trip. Considerable resources, both human and financial, are expended each time a representative of the company embarks on travel related business. Consequently, the medical practitioner must treat the corporate traveler as a work athlete, whose peak performance will be necessary in order to successfully complete the task at hand.

Similar to the recreational traveler, the focus of the corporate travel physical examination is on prevention. Maintenance of travel health and safety during corporate travel will be more easily accomplished if appropriate pre-travel preparation has occurred. Proper vaccinations, prevention of food and water-borne illness, insect precautions, and leisure activity risks must be considered. Standard travel medical kits are also recommended. However, the mutual responsibilities of employer and employee, and the financial motivation of business travel, require special consideration from the advising practitioner. For example, recreational travelers do not require medical clearance

from a health care provider prior to departure and may not even seek travel advice. In contrast, the business traveler has a personal and corporate responsibility to follow pre-travel recommendations and may even be medically deferred, pending resolution of a medical condition. Similarly, documentation is essential. The corporation and employee should maintain copies of all travel documents and itineraries. Use of a traveler checklist is helpful. A post-travel consultation may also be necessary for the corporate traveler for both medical and liability purposes.

In short, the business traveler, corporation, and medical practitioner have a shared responsibility to ensure the health and safety of the corporate traveler and as a result, the successful completion of the business trip. The most effective way to manage this responsibility is through the use of medical practitioners with an expertise in both occupational and travel medicine.

BEFORE TRAVEL

The initial travel consultation is the beginning of the relationship between medical practitioner and corporate traveler and should assess both the patient's fitness for travel and provide any necessary anticipatory guidance or preventive measures.

Chronic diseases

The determination of medical fitness is one of the initial decisions that the medical practitioner will make during the travel consult. This determination is especially important because it affects not only the traveler, but the corporation as well. When considering travel medical fitness, the practitioner should be guided by the patient's medical history, physical condition, employee/employer medical confidentiality, and the Americans with Disabilities Act.

Medically, special attention should be given to those conditions that have the potential to decompensate during travel (e.g., cardiovascular illnesses, chronic obstructive pulmonary disease, diabetes and immunodeficiency). Additionally, chronic medical conditions that may not receive adequate care in the developing world should be carefully considered before granting medical clearance. Employees with decompensated disease, who frequent emergency departments in their country, may find themselves in imminent danger in the developing world. Patients with HIV may not be able to receive the appropriate vaccinations because of their immune suppression (e.g., yellow fever) nor will they likely be able to replace any lost medication. Travelers with predisposition to psychiatric illness, including depression, should be carefully evaluated. Adequate preparation, which may include formal classroom instruction and role-playing, will ensure smooth business transactions as well as the prevention 'culture shock.'[1] A World Bank study reviewing post-travel insurance claims revealed that men who traveled overseas two or more times per year had a relative risk that was three times greater than their non-traveling counterparts of placing a claim for a psychiatric condition.[2] Corporate managers who remain abroad for long periods of time have been observed to suffer from 'reverse culture shock' as they become re-acquainted with their own culture (see Chapter 37).[3]

Legally, if a traveler is deemed not medically fit for travel, the medical practitioner must convey this information to the employer without divulging non-work related, medical details. Communication of chronic disease diagnoses or other medical conditions to the employer is a violation of patient confidentiality. Additionally, when declaring an employee as not medically fit for travel, the practitioner must adequately define the health or safety risk. Failure to do so could lead to a violation of the Americans with Disabilities Act (ADA). The ADA protects employees with pre-existing medical conditions from employ-ment discrimination and limits medical consideration to the essential function of the job. Consequently, a history of cardio-vascular disease would not suffice for denial of medical clearance, but documented unstable angina or frequent high-grade ventricular ectopy would be more helpful in ascertaining whether the condition represents a valid medical risk.

Infection prevention

Preventing infection among business travelers is one of the key areas of the travel consult. Prevention methods include timely vaccination, food and water safety, insect precautions and tuberculosis screening. Standardizing company recommendations emphasizes the corporation's foresight and investment in employee health.

Vaccination

Perhaps no other area of infection prevention is as well recognized as proper vaccination. Establishing company policy on maintaining up-to-date vaccination status for employees who engage in international travel will eliminate last minute scrambles for vaccinations (which may take considerable time to become effective) and take advantage of the most effective medical treatment – prevention.

In addition to tetanus vaccination, there are others that should be considered routine. For example the influenza vaccine is highly effective, especially in young, healthy adults, and should be utilized whenever possible. Other routine immunizations to update might include inactivated polio virus (IPV) and measles, mumps and rubella (MMR). The morbidity of primary varicella-zoster infection is greater in adults and an effort to screen adults serologically without a history is reasonable. HIV testing prior to administration of varicella vaccination is recommended. Opportunities to vaccinate for Hepatitis B should be actively sought as the potential for emergent blood transfusion and/or intimate contact with locals increases with each out-of-country excursion.

The spontaneity of business trips calls for foresight and planning where 'immediate' protection is a requirement. Any employee who potentially might travel to a developing country should be prophy-lactically vaccinated for Hepatitis A and typhoid fever. A bout of Hepatitis A, which is vaccine-preventable, may waylay a corporate traveler for over a month.[4] The immunity that the Hepatitis A vaccine provides is effective and long-lasting. While the typhoid vaccine may be protective only 70% of the time, it is still a good investment as it may prevent an acute febrile illness in addition to life threatening complications such as intestinal perforation.

Anticipating the need for more exotic vaccinations such as yellow fever or Japanese Encephalitis B Virus (JE-V) that require lead-time may prevent disastrous delays either prior to travel, or worse yet, at the destination airport. For example, all active duty US Navy person-

nel must maintain their yellow fever vaccination status to prevent delays in emergency deployment; these vaccines are usually administered twice a month (pay day) to efficiently utilize the multi-dose vials that have a very short half-life. Newer, single-dose preparations have increased administration convenience but are more costly. Additionally, if it were to become the company policy to maintain yellow fever vaccination status, HIV testing would be necessary, creating other legal and ethical issues. Although HIV testing is voluntary in the private sector, it would be prudent to perform the test prior to yellow fever vaccination. JE-V vaccination requires a window of over a month to safely administer the series and avoid the potential for anaphylaxis during travel.

Potential animal contact should be assessed and rabies counseling and/or vaccination should be provided accordingly. Travel limited to cities only does not exclude the need for rabies vaccination. An employee who frequents Bangkok, where the prevalence of infection in stray dogs exceeds 5%, should likely receive this vaccine, especially if he or she is a jogger or cyclist. Risk assessment for other routine travel-associated vaccines like the meningococcal vaccine will need to be determined for each individual case.

In accurately assessing the need for vaccinations, the provider should not forget to inquire about intentions for side trips during leisure time. Often these destinations are more rural, and knowledge of these additional travel plans may not only alter your vaccination recommendations but also highlight the need for malaria prophylaxis.

Food and water safety

Business travelers may be particularly susceptible to food and water-borne illnesses due to the nature of their stay. Unlike the recreational traveler, the corporate traveler may not have control over the agenda of the day, including meals. Meals are frequently planned for both sustenance and as business activities. This may range from five star hotel buffets to food from street vendors whose carts are situated over open sewer systems. Refusal of meals and food items may not be culturally acceptable and could result in the ingestion of some local fair that otherwise might have been avoided. Basic food and water precautions like avoiding ice-containing drinks and local seafood delicacies (e.g., ceviche) can prevent unnecessary illnesses.[5] However, inspite of good pre-travel counseling, more than 10% of corporate travelers from one company reported ingesting raw meat or seafood while more than 50% ate from cold salad bars and drank tap water during their travel abroad.[6] Other more active methods for prevention include hepatitis A vaccination, self-medication with ciprofloxacin or loperamide, and water purification using tablets or filters. In critical business situations where the health of the short-term traveler is paramount, and where food and water may be particularly risky, daily antibiotic prophylaxis or post-exposure prophylaxis (the 'evening after' antibiotic pill) might be considered.

Insect precautions

Malaria remains one of the most frequently reported infectious diseases in the world and can be a significant source of medical risk and lost opportunity for the business traveler and the corporation. A thorough evaluation for the risk of malaria at least 2 weeks in advance is highly recommended as antimalarials that are poorly tolerated will likely lead to noncompliance. Advanced planning by both the company and the traveler will allow for adjustments to the medication regimen to one with more tolerable side effects. Malaria prophylaxis regimens need to be tailored to the specific travel destinations and medication resistance patterns. Newer prophylaxis regimens that do not require month-long post-exposure therapy such as atovaquone/proguanil or primaquine are gaining in popularity. The administration of primaquine requires an evaluation for G-6PD deficiency to prevent significant hemolysis in those who are deficient in this enzyme. In addition to chemoprophylaxis, insect precautions should include wearing protective clothing, avoiding outdoor exposure at dusk, use of insect repellants (e.g., DEET) and use of permethrin-impregnated bednets. It is worthwhile informing the corporate traveler that although malaria is primarily a rural disease in most parts of the world, dengue fever, from a day-biting mosquito, is found primarily in urban centers. Dengue fever is a particular risk for business travelers because it is transmitted by an urban day-biting mosquito. Insect precautions in the early morning and late afternoon are critical to dengue prevention.

Tuberculosis screening

There are little data regarding the risk of acquiring tuberculosis through work-related travel. However, one recent study has demonstrated that people who travel from countries where tuberculosis has a low background rate to countries with high rates of tuberculosis are at risk of infection (as manifested as tuberculin skin test conversion).[7] Ultimately, long-stay travelers to high endemic areas of tuberculosis will develop the infection at the rate found in the indigenous population. Rates of infection have been shown to be even higher among those engaged in the provision of health care.

Although latent tuberculosis infection may not have an immediate impact on the success of the business trip, it does have an impact on both the traveler and the company. Work related tuberculosis infection could be claimed under the company's workers' compensation plan and more importantly employees with tuberculosis need to be identified and treated for personal and public safety. Prior to prolonged or repeated travel to highly endemic areas, corporate travelers should be screened for tuberculosis. Additionally, upon return, the long-stay or frequent corporate traveler should be re-screened (ideally 3 months after return, or annually) and monitored for any symptoms consistent with tuberculosis infection.

Risk behavior counseling

Although the corporate traveler will be engaged in business, leisure activities and their risks should also be addressed. Screening for alcoholism is important as it may accompany and exacerbate depression. Trends toward alcohol abuse may be fueled by social isolation, as well as easy access to inexpensive liquor. Alcohol use may also be encouraged as a socio-cultural activity during business travel. Recommendations for those with a potential for alcohol abuse may include: avoidance of settings that feature alcohol, substitution of alcohol with non-alcoholic beverages, and pre-travel discussions with the company concerning this issue. Illicit substances such as marijuana and opioids may also be easily accessible. In addition, the medical practitioner should review safe sex practices and consider hepatitis B vaccination for those who are likely to engage in casual sex outside of a monogamous relationship. In a recent study of travelers to South America, 12.2% reported having sex with a new partner during their stay. Risk factors for sexual behavior included being male, unmarried, length of stay greater than 30 days, and traveling alone or with friends.[8]

In order to minimize culture shock, the company should provide the employee with basic guidelines on local customs and practices. This will help the employee establish cultural competency and may help defray any anxiety or depressive symptoms. With access to the internet, companies and travelers alike can utilize government web-sites for travel related information, including travel advisories, political assessments, and location of embassies and consulates abroad.

Basic medical supplies

Medical kits for corporate travelers are highly recommended. Basic components include the following: anti-diarrheal agent and/or laxative, analgesics/antipyretics, standard 'cold' preparations/decongestants, an antibiotic for self-treatment of travelers' diarrhea (first-line therapy will depend upon the travel destination), a set of sterile needles and intravenous sets, first aid dressings, insect repellant, and oral rehydration salts. Optional components may include short acting benzodiazepines for that much desired but often eluded airplane slumber, a portable water purifier to provide potable water, and acetazolamide for altitude sickness. Corporate travelers, especially those traveling for prolonged periods, might wish to carry a broad spectrum, multi-purpose antibiotic such as levofloxacin or azithromycin, which may be used to treat travelers' diarrhea, urinary tract, respiratory, and skin infections. In a World Bank study, male international travelers were significantly more likely (RR >2) than non-travelers to report skin/soft tissue infections, back pain, asthma, conjunctivitis, venous disorders (including DVT), and psychological/stress disorders.[4] Given these results, one might also consider including a beta-agonist metered dose inhaler and erythromycin eye ointment in a travel medical kit.

Providing one standard medical travel kit may be impractical. Not all travelers will need all the components of a standard medical travel kit, and the cost of supplying each travel kit may not be easily absorbed by smaller companies. One solution would be to develop several types of kits that are destination dependent, containing such basic items as insect repellants, a water purification system, and appropriate over-the-counter medications (Table 27.1).

Health and safety administrative activities

Both the employer and the employee have a responsibility to ensure that all administrative steps have been taken to either prevent health and safety incidents, or provide a mechanism for effectively dealing with any incidents that might arise during the course of travel. The health-care provider should use the travel consult to remind the traveler to check with his/her company regarding health insurance coverage abroad, pertinent corporate contacts in the event of an emergency, and location of medical facilities. In addition, the traveler should be reminded to pack enough medications for the duration of the trip, as some medications may not be available abroad. These medications should be placed in clearly labeled bottles and packed in the traveler's carry-on luggage. Travelers with pre-existing medical problems may want to keep a list of medications in their wallet or purse. Some employees may choose to identify a co-worker who could administer an epinephrine pen in case of a severe allergic reaction.

Documentation is another key element of preparedness for potential health and safety-related incidents. The corporation should maintain copies of all travel documents and exact itineraries. In addition, the employee may want to give similar documents to a reachable family member or trusted co-worker. All business travelers should carry extra passport photos in the event that a new passport is needed. A traveler checklist and medical practitioner checklist are often helpful to ensure that all preventive measures have been taken prior to leaving for business travel (Fig. 27.1 and Table 27.2).

DURING TRAVEL

As discussed above, maintenance of travel health and safety during corporate travel will be more easily accomplished if appropriate pre-travel planning and preparation has occurred. Corporate travelers should strive to arrive at their destination in good health and adequately rested in order to be at peak performance.

Table 27.1	The medical travel kit

The medical travel kit may include a variety of items depending on the needs of the individual and the location and duration of travel. The following is a partial list of types of medical travel kits. Not all items need be included in each kit.

Insect travel kit
  Insect repellant (DEET-containing), bed netting, permethrin, tweezers, plastic bags for saving insects, wound dressings, antimalarial prophylaxis.

Injury and illness travel kit
  Ace wrap, finger splints, ice pack, antibiotic ointment, wound dressings (gauze, band aids, tape), gloves, thermometer, ibuprofen and/or acetaminophen.

Food and water travel kit
  Ciprofloxacin (travelers' diarrhea), loperamide (anti-diarrheal), laxative or stool softener, antacids, chemical water treatment (iodine, chlorine or silver tablets), filter water treatment

Surgical travel kit
  Iodine or alcohol preps, sterile instruments (hemostat, pick-ups, scissors, suture material), wound dressings (gauze, band aids, tape), gloves, antibiotic ointment, biohazard bag.

Pharmacy travel kit
  Ibuprofen and/or acetaminophen, pseudoephedrine (decongestant), diphenhydramine (antihistamine), laxative or stool softener, loperamide (anti-diarrheal), fluconazole (vaginal yeast infections) and terbinafine or ketoconazole (fungal skin infections), steroid cream, cough syrup and lozenges, antacids, nicotine replacement, sun screen, levofloxacin or azithromycin (skin, urinary tract, respiratory or GI infections).

In addition to the above medical travel kits, individuals should remember to bring enough of their usual pre-travel medications, in properly labeled bottles, for the duration of their trip along with extra amounts in case of delayed return.

Comfort, safety and travel-related medical disorders

Prolonged international flights are fraught with the potential for medical misadventures. This can be of a minor, inconveniencing nature (e.g., ear pain, nicotine cravings, muscle cramps, jet lag), or a potentially life threatening disorder (e.g., deep vein thrombosis and pulmonary embolism). Carry-on luggage should include medications for treatment of minor symptoms, as well as all essential prescription medications. Medications or medical supplies packed in checked luggage must be considered 'expendable' due to the frequency of lost or delayed luggage. Smokers should obtain and use nicotine patches to avoid uncomfortable cravings on overseas non-smoking flights.

Personal health will also be aided by proper attention to physical comfort during the flight. Choosing an aisle seat will facilitate stretching and make movement within the aircraft easier in order to avoid muscles cramps and pooling of blood in the leg veins. Pooling of blood in the dependent vessels could lead to the development of a deep venous thrombosis (DVT) and ultimately, a pulmonary embolism (PE). Unfortunately, the current medical literature on quantifying the risk of developing DVT and PE during air travel is conflicting and especially incomplete when limiting consideration to the corporate traveler.[9,10] Given that prolonged inactivity may lead to blood pooling, it seems reasonable to encourage business travelers to stretch during long flights, particularly those with additional risk factors for development of DVT (dehydration, smoking, prior history of DVT, heart disease, diabetes and birth control pills).

Dehydration is a possibility on longer flights due to inadequate fluid intake and low cabin humidity. In-flight beverage service is often delayed, so corporate travelers may want to include a supply of drinking water in their carry on luggage. A supply of easily packed snack foods may also be a prudent addition to the carry-on luggage, since in-flight dining service is not known for large portions (and recently for dieters only!). Avoidance of uncooked vegetables, drinks that are not commercially bottled, and ice cubes might be considered when flying on air carriers from developing countries.

Acute ear pain (barotitis media or ear squeeze) from air pressure differences between the middle ear and the outside environment may occur during the aircraft's descent. In the normal ear, the Eustachian tube which connects the middle ear and the throat will open up to equalize these pressures. Certain medical conditions such as upper respiratory infections ("colds"), and chronic sinus or ear conditions can lead to malfunction of the Eustachian tube, leading to a painful pressure build up within the middle ear. Severe cases can lead to rupture of the tympanic membrane (ear drum). Similar painful sinus pressure conditions can also occur. Travelers with acute upper respiratory infections should consider decongestant medications for symptom control and prevention. If acute ear pain occurs during aircraft descent, the traveler can try to open the Eustachian tube by pinching the nostrils closed and gently blowing through the closed nose. Most cases of acute ear or sinus pain resolve within hours, but severe or prolonged pain may require medical care.

Many corporate travelers find themselves at less then peak effectiveness during the first day or two after arrival at their destination due to the effects of jet lag. Jet lag is essentially a failure of the internal clock to reset to local time. This can lead to sleepiness, fatigue, irritability, and difficulty concentrating – not exactly conducive to peak performance! Adequate sleep prior to travel, avoidance of dehydration, and avoidance of alcohol can help decrease symptoms. Many travelers on long flights ask their physician for a prescription sleep aid to ensure some sleep during the flight. If necessary take a brief nap on arrival at the destination, but avoid prolonged daytime sleep the day of arrival to ease adaptation to local sleep times. (See chapter 42 on Jet Lag).

Health maintenance abroad and safety incidents

Upon arrival at the destination, corporate travelers should proceed directly to the hotel to secure their luggage. Unmarked cabs, and

Figure 27.1 Practitioner travel consult worksheet.

Appendix Table two. Practitioner Travel Consultant Worksheet

Name.................................Birth date.....................Date...................
Travel Destination..................................Dates of travel....................

Chronic or current medical conditions
Cardiovascular Pulmonary Gastrointestinal Immune system Neurologic Rheumatologic Skin Urogenital Gynecologic/Pregnancy Psychiatric

Medications	Vaccination history	
	DT MMR Tetanus Hepatitis A Hepatitis B Varicella	Influenza Yellow Fever JEV Typhoid Meningitis Rabies

Allergies (Foods/Medications)	Alcohol, Cigarette and drug use
Diphenhydramine or Epinephrine needed?	

Tuberculosis History (including last ppd)

Councelling	
Food and water safety Hepatitis A vaccination, ciprofloxacin, loperamide, Water treatment **Risk councelling** Alcohol, Drug, Mental health, Safe sex, Motor vehicle **Insect precautions** Malaria Prophylaxis, DEET, Permethrin, Bednet, Person protection methods	**Basic medical supplies** Travel medical kit Chronic medication kit Over-the-counter medications **Administrative** Health insurance abroad, Corporate contacts, International vaccine card, Location of medical facilities, Medical alert bracelet

unknown persons offering guide assistance should be avoided. Once at the hotel, all valuables and essential medications should be kept in the hotel safe. Other prudent measures to ensure personal safety include the avoidance of flashy clothing and jewelry, displaying large amounts of cash, and travel away from crowds or to poorly lit areas. The traveler should try to be nondescript. Carrying a personal alarm device is suggested, but beware of local laws regarding other protective equipment such as pepper spray and stun devices. The traveler should know the location and phone number for local law enforcement agencies, and carry a functioning cell phone for emergency use.

Avoidance of excessive alcohol and illicit drug use will help reduce the risk of compromising situations such as blackmail and kid-napping. As mentioned in the preceding section, awareness of local social customs and cultural differences should be part of pre-travel planning to avoid embarrassing and potentially dangerous situations. Sexual encounters are to be discouraged due to the high prevalence of sexually transmitted diseases (including HIV) in many countries. The use of condoms and safe sex practices are mandatory if sexual contact does occur.

Despite the best travel preparations, health and safety incidents abroad do occur. A preliminary investigation of World Bank workers showed that rates of medical insurance claims were 80% higher for men and 18% higher for women than their non-traveling counterparts.[11] These claims were mostly associated with psychological illnesses. However, other studies have documented an

Table 27.2	Corporate traveler health and safety checklist	
Medical consultation	Travel medicine consult to address vaccines and travel health and safety Personal physician consultation for ongoing medical conditions	
Pre-travel medications	Enough for length of stay, individually labeled and in carry-on luggage	
Over-the-counter medications	Acetaminophen Antacids Cough syrups and lozenges Decongestants (cold tablets)	Ibuprofen Miconazole Nicotine replacement Sun screen
Allergy precautions	Diphenhydramine Self-injectable epinephrine	Steroid cream (hydrocortisone)
Food and water precautions	Antacids Ciprofloxacin (traveler's diarrhea) Loperamide (anti-diarrheal),	Laxative or stool softener, Chemical treatment or other water purifier
Insect precautions	Antimalarials, insect repellant (DEET), bednet	
Medical supplies	Medical travel kit, condoms, birth control, routine personal hygiene items, levofloxacin or erythromycin (broad spectrum antibiotic)	
Medical information	International immunization record (photocopies) Medication list in wallet Medical alert bracelet	
Documents	Passport, visa and photocopies Additional photo identification	
Important contacts		
Emergency corporate Embassy/Consulate Local hospital Health insurance Family		

increase in a variety of complaints including, gastrointestinal complaints, minor injuries, insomnia and skin disorders.[12]

Any visit to medical care facilities in a foreign country is fraught with potential dangers due to language barriers and differences in hygiene practices. This is most pronounced in developing countries where medical instruments are often not adequately sterilized between uses, and proper screening of blood products for infectious agents such as HIV may not occur. Corporate travelers should thus try to self-treat minor medical conditions utilizing over the counter and prescription medications in their travel medical kit. If medical treatment is necessary, the traveler should insist on the use of the sterile medical supplies and avoid any blood draws, injections and transfusions if at all possible. The corporation should have a medical evacuation plan for traveling employees needing to return to home for treatment.

Health maintenance abroad and avoidance of safety incidents is dependent upon good pre-travel preparation, consistent personal behaviors and corporate responsibility. The travel consultant should emphasize that once abroad, the employee should continue maintenance health activities (e.g., taking pre-travel medications and basic safety precautions such as limiting alcohol consumption). The medical practitioner should also help the corporation define its responsibilities, such as arranging for non-alcoholic beverages at work functions, providing safe transport and company contacts in the event of an emergency. If a health or safety incident does occur, the corporation should function as the point of contact for the employee and facilitate any care necessary.

The travel medicine practitioner should review these mutual responsibilities of employee and employer with both parties, prior to travel.

AFTER TRAVEL

Post-travel medical consultation is useful for both the short-term and long-term business traveler. Lapses in preventive behavior can make short term and long term business travelers equally susceptible to infectious and non-infectious hazards. Consequently, the re-entry physical can serve as an opportunity for the medical practitioner to assess the overall health of the traveler as well as address any concerns of the employee.

Re-entry physicals and counseling

Depending on the length of travel or the corporate traveler's experiences, a re-entry physical exam with counseling may be offered. A recent study showed that 76% of international business travelers reported travel-related health problems. These problems included jet lag, travelers' diarrhea and gastrointestinal complaints, climate adaptation problems, and accidents and minor injuries.[12] This is a good opportunity to readdress safe sex practices and identify the need for further sexually transmitted disease testing and counseling with the patient's primary care physician. The practitioner can also screen for signs of anxiety, depression, culture shock and decompensation of chronic medical illnesses. It is important for the health-care provider to convey to the corporation that the medical assessment of the returned employee can help distinguish between travel related and non-travel related illnesses. In addition, post-travel physical examinations help to maintain the overall health of the individual and may help minimize lost time from work. This is especially important for the frequent traveler.

Continuance of care and symptom follow-up

Emphasis on the continuation of malaria prophylaxis after return, will help to ensure the full benefit of chemoprophylaxis. Similarly, it is important to see to it that vaccination schedules have been completed to ensure that individuals are fully immunized in anticipation of future travel. Re-assessment of tuberculin skin test status should be performed on all travelers coming from high endemic regions for tuberculosis. Finally, it is important for the practitioner to remember that not all symptoms will present immediately upon return. Health-care providers, business travelers and corporate officials need to be educated about the fact that symptoms developing many weeks or even months after travel may be related to a previous business trip.

CONCLUSION

The business traveler, corporation, and medical practitioner have mutual responsibilities to ensure the health and safety of the traveler and consequently the success of the trip. The most effective way to manage this responsibility is through the use of medical practitioners with an expertise in both occupational and travel medicine. An effective travel consult should identify opportunities for prevention and provide the appropriate anticipatory guidance to the individual traveling. In addition, the travel consult should also address the potential health and safety liabilities to the company when clearing personnel for business-related travel.

In spite of the best efforts at prevention, lapses in human behavior are guaranteed to occur. The corporate traveler and employer must have an effective plan for medical emergencies prior to the traveler's departure. Upon return, long-term corporate travelers should have re-entry physicals and health debriefings. Finally, in order to maximize preventive efforts, particularly in relation to future travel, business travelers should complete vaccination series that were begun prior to travel.

REFERENCES

1. Stewart L, Leggat PA. Culture shock and travelers. *J Travel Med* 1998; **5**:84–88.
2. Liese B, Mundt KA, Dell LD, *et al.* Medical insurance claims associated with international business travel. *Occup Environ Med* 1997; **54**:499–503.
3. Guzzo RA, Noonan KA, Elron E. Expatriate managers and the psychological contract. *J Appl Psychol* 1994; **79**:617–626.
4. Perry GF. Occupational medicine forum. *Occup Environ Med* 1996; **38**(4):339–341.
5. Dinman BD. Responsibilities of corporate medical directors for health management in developing countries. *J Occup Med* 1983; **25**(10):757–759.
6. Kemmerer TP, Cetron M, Harper L, *et al.* Health problems of corporate travelers: risk factors and management. *J Travel Med* 1998; **5**:184–187.
7. Cobelens FG, Deutekom H van, Draayer-Jansen IW, *et al.* Risk of infection with Mycobacterium tuberculosis in travelers to areas of high tuberculosis endemicity. *Lancet* 2000; **356**:461–465.
8. Cabada MM, Echevarria JI, Seas CR, *et al.* Sexual behavior of international travelers visiting Peru. *Sex Transm Dis* 2002; **9**:510–513.
9. Gallus AS, Goghlan DC. Travel and venous thrombosis. *Curr Opin Pulm Med* 2002; **5**:372–378.
10. Dimberg LA, Mundt KA, Sulsky SI, *et al.* Deep venous thrombosis associated with corporate air travel. *J Travel Med* 2001; **3**:127–132.
11. Liese B, Mundt KA, Dell LD, *et al.* Medical insurance claims associated with international business travel. *Occup Environ Med* 1997; **7**:499–503.
12. Roger HL, Reilly SM. A survey of the health experiences of international business travelers. *AAOHN J* 2002; **10**:449–459.

CHAPTER 28 International Adoption

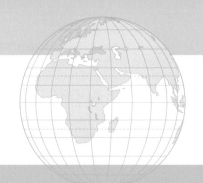

Jean Francois Chicoine and Dominique Tessier

KEYPOINTS

- Counseling for international adoption includes: (1) pre-travel health advice for the parents, (2) issues concerning travel with a young child, (3) infectious disease risks to parents from contact with the adoptee, and (4) acute and chronic health problems of the adopted child

- Before travel, parents should learn as much as possible about the adoptee's living conditions, culture and health problems, preferably from an international adoption center

- Pre-travel health advice for adoptive parents includes, in addition to the usual recommendations, greater emphasis on hepatitis B immunization

- Adoptees from developing countries, especially those who have been institutionalized or neglected, frequently suffer from infectious diseases, malnutrition, cognitive and physical developmental delays, problems with socialization, and behavioral disorders

INTRODUCTION

Your patient is virtual. Has never been in your country, let alone in your office. The information you can gather on the child's health status is scarce and full of uncertainties. You know the sex but the age is approximate. You cannot immunize the patient before travel. Yet, you have already spent more than an hour in consultation and so many questions are unanswered. Welcome to international adoption counseling!

The practice of adoption has existed in most civilized nations. In several African tribes, the Maori in Polynesia, as well as the Inuit in Canada, the child is a jewel shared by a widened family. Other countries will be unaware of adoption, without necessarily forbidding it: such is the case of Chad and Mongolia. Algeria, Mauritania, Pakistan, Morocco and several Islamic countries have always prohibited adoption. In the twentieth century, many children born out of wedlock were offered to adoptive families, initially within their own country and eventually in foreign countries. For example, between 1950 in 1970, hundreds of Canadian-born children of single mothers, the 'children of sin' as it was said, were adopted in the USA, Puerto Rico, Venezuela and France. These were the early days of 'international adoption'. The Vietnam and Korean Wars, and famine in developing countries turned international adoption into a universal reality. The increasing problem of infertility, the regulation of births, and the recognition of civil rights of illegitimate children are factors that contributed to the need for families to seek children in other countries. The liberalization of international trade in China, the fall of the Ceaucescu system, the institutionalization of orphans in Eastern European countries, Perestroika, and the globalization of poverty, will continue to bring more abandoned children available for adoption. In several African countries, 15% of the children are AIDS orphans. In the world of tomorrow, abandonment and adoption are likely to rise exponentially.

If one counts the travel of adopting parents and of the adopted children, those of international adoption agencies and international conferences on the rights of children, one realizes that each year, the practice of international adoption generates hundreds of thousands of trips around the world, and potentially a large number of consultations with travel medicine experts before departure or on return. The adopting parents must realize that a demographic boom and the facilitation of the international passage of children by governments are not absolute guarantees the health and security for themselves or for the child they are about to welcome. Health-care professionals in travel medicine are ideally placed to support the process before, during, and after international adoption.

Every year, approximately 16 000 international adoptions take place in the USA, about 4000 in France, 3000 in Sweden and 2000 in Canada. At this rate, by the year 2020, more than 200 000 adopted children will have emigrated to the USA. Great Britain and Germany on the other hand have a comparatively small number of international adoptions, with only 258 for Great Britain in 1998. In North America, most of the adopted children come from China, Korea, Russia, India, Haiti, Romania, Guatemala, Vietnam and Colombia. Recently, Madagascar, Ethiopia, Brazil and Oceanic countries were added to the list of sources of adoptees by Western Europeans. While in France, males account for more than 50% of adoptions, three-quarters of internationally adopted children in Canada are girls. Half of these children are less than 1 year old when adopted, but a quarter of them are over the age of 3. In fact, the tendency to adopt older children is increasing in North America.

The Convention of The Hague concerning international adoption stipulates that states should make it a priority to take measures to insure that every child be maintained in his or her biological family, or if not possible, that a proper family be found for him/her in the country of birth. This statement is clear: international adoption should be considered a last resort. Several years ago, Paraguay closed its doors to international adoption to constrain a highly corrupted system. Recently, Russia closed and then reopened adoption to the USA, while Vietnam did the same for France. In Canada, the province of Québec broke with the Guatemalan government because DNA testing performed by Canadian authorities to validate the maternity of pregnant mothers had not been enough to control local networks of baby conception 'a la carte', strictly for adoption purposes; this problem has been magnified by the commerce of children on the Web! The corruption and criminality associated with international adoptions has driven organizations such as UNICEF to withhold unconditional support for the process.

THE PRE-ADOPTION EVALUATION

The request of parents for pre-adoption medical consultations is rising. Additional information on the health of orphans in their countries of origin would go a long way to predict future challenges for families that come to consult health-care providers concerning international adoption, i.e., the relative risk of AIDS in Cambodia, fetal alcoholism syndrome in Russia, and malnutrition in Romania.[1–3] The question of health risks of the adoptee are often addressed to the travel health adviser. Unfortunately, the actual medical condition according to written medical documentation, photographs or videos, may turn out to be highly inaccurate. It would be ideal for this evaluation concerning potential health risks be done at an expert center in international adoption, of which there are ~30 in North America.

THE PARENT'S MEDICAL PREPARATION

Except for adoptions from Korea and Taiwan, the majority of parents will have to travel in order to have their initial encounter with their child, and will thus benefit from a travel medicine consultation. Many parents will have never traveled to a foreign country before. Some countries like Bulgaria or Vietnam demand trips from adopting parents. Others, like Bolivia, require extended stays of over a month before parents can proceed to adopt the child. Some trips can be made in luxurious conditions, while others may require parents to live in very modest, somewhat precarious conditions, at the orphanage or in a local pension in a rural area. When both parents cannot travel together, a grandparent or a friend will often be part of the expedition. These individuals should be prepared health-wise in the same way.

Recommendations from the travel medicine expert need to be tailored in each case. The usual immunizations according to destination are recommended, but special attention should be given to hepatitis B immunization. The child to be adopted may be a chronic carrier, often HBe antibody positive, and therefore highly contagious. Acute hepatitis B infection among adopting parents is well described. Travel counseling should address all preventive measures: care related to food and water, vector borne diseases including malaria and dengue, and sun and environmental protection. The specific characteristics of the adoption generally confine parents to their hotel rooms in large cities. Malaria chemoprophylaxis is rarely necessary except for Haiti, Madagascar and India. In those highly endemic areas for malaria, chemoprophylaxis is usually recommended even for very short stays. Atovaquone/proguanil or primaquine are very good options since they need to be initiated the day before arrival and continued for only 7 days after exposure. In considering the choice of chemoprophylaxis for malaria, one must keep in mind the possibility that the mother might become pregnant. There is some evidence that the fertile adopting mother has increased potential for becoming pregnant soon after the adoption. Also, transmission of cytomegalovirus from the adopted child to the pregnant mother is a consideration. Mothers should be advised to be careful and frequently wash their hands and/or use a disinfectant. The prescription of a presumptive treatment for diarrhea, such as ciprofloxacin or azithromycin should not be forgotten, as our already vulnerable parent in charge of a child will be under considerable stress.

The dynamics of group travel can be difficult. International adoption delegations usually have very tight schedules and precise tasks to accomplish in a limited time, often dealing with bureaucratic red tape they are not used to. Whenever possible, it is preferable to organize a group information session regarding major risks and recommended prevention measures. This usually avoids confusion when travelers from the same location compare prescriptions or vaccines they received from different health-care providers. This also helps the medical provider to determine whether each traveler should carry his/her own first-aid kit or if a single group-kit would be more appropriate. In international adoption, the latter is often preferable since most parents would like to bring the equivalent of an entire pharmacy in case they might need it (Table 28.1). If possible, it is advisable to identify within a delegation preparing for international adoption an individual, preferably someone in the health-care field, who will be in charge of the first-aid kit, and ensure that this person understands clearly how to use its contents.

Planning meals, with a baby to feed and take care of, may be more difficult than expected. Parents with medical conditions that could be affected by irregular meals, like diabetes, need to be well prepared. On long flights, citrus fruits are easy to carry and useful in maintaining hydration. Energy or granola bars, dried fruits, and nuts should be packed in carry-on luggage. For long flights, recommendations should be given regarding the prevention of deep vein thrombosis and counseling to help the child travel safely.

Health and repatriation insurance should be purchased before departure. On arrival, adoptive parents should register with their embassy or consulate, especially in a country where the socio-political situation is unstable. They should also be prepared to improvise when facing unexpected hazards. Inexperienced travelers with a baby in their arms may be more prone to forget their luggage, money, etc. Carrying the baby in a front pack during stressful periods, such as check-in at the airport, can help free ones hands while keeping the baby in sight. Security issues need to be reviewed carefully. Simple measures can be the most useful; for example, always carrying the hotel address written in the country's language, renting a cell phone and pre-programming important numbers when possible, having tips ready to avoid rummaging in a deep purse or diaper bag, keeping the number and the size of luggage bags to a minimum in order to be more self-sufficient, and wearing sensible shoes to provide more stability when carrying a baby. Finally, the risk of rabies should also be carefully addressed. Any bite in developing countries should be considered a rabies risk. Parents should be taught about preventative measures and post-exposure prophylaxis.

Table 28.1	Suggestions for first aid kit for international adoption
Milk substitute without lactose (soy or lactose free)
Hand cleaner (70% ethyl alcohol)
Hydration cream (glaxal base)
Topical antibiotic (2% mupirocin)
Sulfacetamide
Topical steroid cream (1% hydrocortisone)
Physiological nasal spray
Azithromycin or clarithromycin
Scabicide
Multivitamin and iron supplements
Essential fat supplement (carthamus oil)
Diaper (nappy) rash cream (zinc oxide)
Antipyretic, liquid or pediatric strength
Rehydration preparation

As time remains an uncontrollable dimension, jet lag is a common but serious problem for adopting parents. The adult's natural body clock does not take kindly to rapid changes across time zones. Children tend to adapt faster, but the anxiety of parents and their fear of letting the baby cry, may open the door for unsuitable sleeping patterns and habits. Adults should try to spend time out-of-doors to be exposed to natural sunlight. If this is not suitable for security reasons, a short-acting hypnotic for the first 2–3 days in each direction is a safe solution to be considered. If no-one else can take charge of the baby during the night, parents should take turns using a sedative. Avoidance of caffeine, excessive alcohol, and food too close to bedtime, are common sense precautions that often need to be reinforced.

THE ADOPTEE 'PRE-TRAVEL' CONSULTATION

The pre-travel consultation for the adoptee has the very unusual characteristic that it is being done for a traveler about whom there is often little information except possibly for a brief technical report, photograph, or video. The child waiting at the other end of the world will nevertheless require clothing, food, and other basic necessities that parents often desperately try to identify before their departure. These requirements are often discussed with travel medicine professionals, challenging their pediatric knowledge. Adoptive parents should try to address their questions and share answers with other parents, especially those who have successfully completed an international adoption, the adoption agency, associations of adopting parents, and their family doctor or future pediatrician.

Parents should not be too concerned with food allergies and should feed the child as soon as possible. It is essential for parents to be prepared for the fact that the child might be severely malnourished. Most children will never have been in diapers, and could very well know how to use the potty as early as 9 months of age. It is easy to understand why so many children suffer from constipation. Parents should know about basic medical care and signs that would warrant a consultation with a health-care provider. Respiratory infections are common, as are diarrhea and skin problems. A first-aid kit as described in Table 28.1 is well adapted to the specific needs of adoptive parents. Many prescription drugs are included and should be provided. Scabies is extremely common and will usually leave scars for many weeks. Parent should be instructed on the appropriate use of scabicides and warned that symptoms (pruritus) may not resolve for several weeks after successful treatment. The scabies lesions may be secondarily infected and a topical antibiotic may be needed. Other skin conditions such as dermatophytosis and other non-specific rashes are not uncommon, but can wait to be treated at home.[4–7]

The transition from the orphanage to a loving family is likely to be a tremendous relief for the child who is used to lying on his/her back under physical constraints, to hunger, to the paucity of human contact, and to the incessant noise of institutional life. Even under these adverse circumstances the instantaneous attachment of the child for the parents and of the parents for the child is more myth than reality. The child will need days, perhaps even months or years, to deepen the links with the adopting parents. Profoundly deprived children will require a considerable amount of time before being able to find the neurophysiological mechanism that allows for bonding. If taken from the arms of a loving nurse or foster parent with whom the child has slept, he/she may cry immediately when put down, an unexpected event for the new inexperienced parents. The new parents will also need to adjust, preferably sharing their worries with other adopting parents. The confidence in oneself can be further shaken if the child focuses attention on only one of the adopting parents. The other parent should not be concerned or alarmed. When more than one child from the same family is adopted, the task is further complicated.

HEALTH PROBLEMS ENCOUNTERED DURING TRAVEL

Parents should receive the same advice and medications as any other traveler to the country visited. Detailed written instructions on how to use each medication are advisable since parents may not pay enough attention during the pre-travel consultation to advice concerning their own potential medical problems. They should be able to properly use rehydration fluids and self-treatment for diarrhea. Personal hygiene measures should be reviewed as well as standard food, water, and insect precautions.

Close contact with their new child should not be limited unless there is a very serious risk of infection; scabies should not be included in this category. Scabies is such a common parasitic infection in developing countries that parents should be mentally prepared to be confronted by the infection – and even be infected themselves. Although unappealing intellectually, the infection can easily be controlled with appropriate medication without complication. Infested children should still be hugged and embraced to promote bonding.

The usual items contained in the first aid kit adapted for international adoption should be sufficient to treat common problems while away. All parents should have a thermometer and know how to use and read it. The criteria for fever should be known and first step interventions well understood. A medication chart, indicating approximate doses to be given according to weight, should be provided. If possible, an overseas doctor should be identified by the embassy, the adoption agency, or an association such as the International Association for Medical Assistance to Travellers (IAMAT), should the need arise for interventions in emergency situations.

It is not rare for parents to discover that their adopted child is trisomic, hydrocephalic, mentally challenged, or suffering from acute meningitis. In extreme situations, parents may return home without a child or with a child requiring special, prolonged care. In some countries, e.g., China, parents will be offered another child. Such exchanges are often very traumatic.

POST-ADOPTION MEDICAL CONSULTATION

Several authors have indicated that the clinical examination after adoption is essential and should include hematological, biochemical, and serological screening.[7] Unsuspected medical conditions have been identified in more than half of the adopted children from foreign countries.[6–9] A medical evaluation done on arrival is important in order to assess nutritional state, identify transmissible infections and possible psychoaffective disturbances, and to listen to the concerns of the adopting family. The infectious disease screening should be tailored to the infectious disease epidemiology of the country of origin: malaria in Africa, syphilis in Ethiopia or Russia, HIV/AIDS in Thailand, Cambodia, Romania and Haiti. The ethnic and geographic origin of the child may mandate other tests such as a hemoglobin electrophoresis, to search for hemoglobinopathy such as thalassemia. Child development should be carefully evaluated. The usual assessment done at Sainte-Justine Hospital in Montreal is indicated in Table 28.2.[7,9,10]

THE NUTRITIONAL STATUS

The nutritional status of evaluation starts with a thorough clinical exam followed by an anthropometric evaluation.[11] Weight, height, and cranial parameters are noted and charted on percentile charts to follow the child's progress. Chinese, Vietnamese, and Colombian growth charts have been developed. For the majority of undernourished children, the North American Nelhaus, the National

Table 28.2	Screening tests for newly-arrived international adoptees

Routine
  CBC
  Hepatitis B[a] (HsAg,HbsAb,anti-core antibody)
  Hepatitis C[a]
  HIV (Elisa, PCR)[a]
  Syphilis screening (VDRL or RPR)
  Stool O&P (1–3)
  Tuberculin skin test[a]
  Newborns screen: phenylketonuria, thyroid, etc.
  Dental evaluation
  Bone age (girls older than 4 years)
  Urinalysis

Optional, depending on nutritional status:
  Liver function tests, ,calcium, phosphate,
  Albumin, creatinine, serum iron, zinc etc.
  Serial bone age

Optional, depending on a suspected infection:
  Chest X-ray
  Thick and thin films for malaria
  Anti-HCV (RIBA)
  HIV viral load
  Syphilis
  Rubella, toxoplasmosis serology etc.
  H. pylori

Optional, depending on developmental assessment:
  Ergotherapist evaluation
  Psychological evaluation
  Speech therapist evaluation
  Hearing and vision screens

Optional, depending on the geographic country of birth:
  Hemoglobin electrophoresis, G6PD screening
  Lead blood level

[a]Repeat at 3–6 months depending on circumstances

Center for Health Statistics (NCHS), or the European Sempe and Pedron growth charts are recommended as reference tools.[12,13] Culturally adapted growth charts such as the one for East Indian or Korean children can also be used. Microcephaly, a common finding among institutionalized children, can be so severe as to alter the interpretation of age.

In Quebec, 808 Chinese girls (average age 11.5 months) were examined consecutively in the month following their arrival.[14] One quarter of them suffered from wasting and more than half of the group suffered from stunting to various degrees. In China, as in Eastern Europe, chronic malnutrition reaches the highest severity after the age of 1 year. UNICEF reported that up to 75% of children institutionalized 13–24 months in Romania suffered from chronic malnutrition.[6,15,16] Low birth weight, an extended period of malnutrition, and slow cranial growth carry the risk of permanent damage affecting the psychomotor development of the child.[16–18] Vitamin and mineral deficiencies are common and are associated with iron deficiency anemia, rickets, and vitamin A visual disturbance. Rickets is particularly common in China and Eastern Europe. Iron and other mineral supplements should be administered and hematological follow-up be carried out until the child is fully recovered. Contributing factors such as folic acid deficiency, thalassemia, lead intoxication, and intestinal parasitosis such as hookworm infection, should be evaluated.

Growth delay will affect newly adopted children more than any other medical problem.[19] Height under the fifth percentile has been described for nearly one child out of two on his/her first medical evaluation. Genetic, ethnic, environmental and medical causes should be considered in all cases. Children from Haiti, Somalia, or northern China are generally taller than those from Southeast Asia or the Chinese provinces of Guangdong or Hunan. Dwarfism caused by a deficit in growth hormone will often improve considerably after adoption. More disturbing is the high prevalence of microcephaly in institutionalized children. Improvement in time may be significant but this is not always the case. These factors will all contribute to the great difficulty in evaluating the true age of the child. Also, it is important to take into consideration the possibility of precocious puberty in girls adopted after the age of 4 years.[20,21]

THE INFECTIOUS ASPECTS

According to the authors, between 2 and 5% of adoptive children will be hepatitis B carriers having contracted the virus from their biological mother by vertical transmission in China, Vietnam, Thailand or Cambodia, or by horizontal transmission via syringes or contaminated products in Romania, Ukraine or Russia. Also, transmission of hepatitis B is well documented to occur between children, especially siblings under the age of 5 years, by direct transmission of secretions and excretions. Other risk factors for infection include those children who were transfused when premature, those who were hospitalized for lengthy periods, or those who were institutionalized in their country of origin. At particular high risk were those who received vitamins, parenteral sedatives and other 'therapeutic' injections.[18,22–25] Cases of hepatitis C were reported to occur in less than one percent of children from China, Russia and Moldavia Republic; however, this finding was often due to transplacental transmission of antibodies to children less than one year old and not a true infection. Fewer than 1% of overseas adopted children had syphilis *in utero* or at birth. In general, children with congenital syphilis do not have any detectable clinical abnormality and therefore require serological screening.

The prevalence of parasitic infections is high among adoptive children, except for babies coming from Korea for whom age and the pre-adoption living conditions do not usually predispose to infection. In several studies, 4–51% of stool samples of adopted children revealed the presence of protozoa, and nematodes or more rarely, cestodes.[8,10,26] These infections may contribute to malnutrition, anemia, and psychomotor delays. Hookworm infections and strongyloidiasis are common. Adopted children usually come from countries where the prevalence of tuberculosis is 10–20 times greater than that in Western Europe or in North America. It is not surprising, therefore, to note that the authors found 2–19% of adopted children had latent tuberculosis on the basis of a positive tuberculin skin test.[27] HIV-infected children were adopted in Haiti as well as Romania, where the number of seropositive institutionalized children exceeded 10%.[28] The discovery of infection in the newcomer is rare thanks in part to the testing of potential candidates for adoption in the countries of origin before the decision to adopt is made.

IMMUNIZATION CONSIDERATIONS

Both the World Health Organization and the Centers for Disease Control and Prevention consider that immunizations administered to children in developing countries can be trusted and that these adoptees should be considered to be effectively protected provided that there is adequate documentation.[29,30] However, recent data suggest that this may not be true for children from many orphanages around the world. There are many possible explanations for the low levels of protective antibodies noted in some series: breakage of the cold chain, falsification of immunization records, and inappropriate vaccine dosage and use. Almost all children will be appropriately immunized against tuberculosis, diphtheria, tetanus, polio and pertussis, and children older than 9 months old, against measles. Hepatitis B vaccination is usually administered in Thailand, Romania and Colombia. Haemophilus influenza vaccination is offered in Korea, Colombia and Guatemala, and Japanese encephalitis in China and Vietnam. In some African countries, yellow fever immunization will also be offered. Immunizations against mumps, rubella, chicken pox and hepatitis A are rarely included.

CHILD DEVELOPMENT

It has been reported that 70% of children upon arrival in the host country suffer from global motor delays. As noted in several series of adoptees from Eastern Europe, delays were more frequent and more severe in the presence of malnutrition and when the stay in the orphanage was prolonged. The majority of children will improve within a few months of parental care. The deplorable living conditions, mostly because of malnutrition and maltreatment, may also harm the cognitive growth of many orphans. An adoption carried out before 6 months of age with good conditions at the orphanage or qualified foster home, as is done in Vietnam or in Colombia, will allow for normal cognitive development both in the short and long term. Persistent language delay could hide a global delay, or a communication or hearing disorder that requires an audiogram evaluation and future multidisciplinary care. Close follow-up is necessary to monitor for the development of autism, emotional problems, and neuropsychological disorders such as attachment disorders and neurocognitive disorders, the latter associated with fetal alcohol syndrome.[31-34]

THE SOCIAL IMPACT OF ADOPTION

Several Scandinavian and American studies indicate that the majority of overseas adopted children will enjoy a balanced adolescence on a socio-emotional level, both from the family and educational point of view. On the other hand, a significant study from the Netherlands on 2118 youths from age 10 to 15 years who had been adopted abroad in early childhood, showed a high prevalence of behavioral disorders such as delinquency, aggressiveness, and depression, especially among the boys. The younger the child was at adoption, the lower was the risk of socio-emotional maladaptation and neuropsychological problems during the teenage years. Some retrospective studies note that the prevalence of attention deficit disorders in children adopted abroad may be associated with a history of small birth weight or prolonged severe malnutrition.

Central to a successful social adaptation is an identity search. The box containing the child's garments at the time of adoption, the plane tickets, and the photographs and videos of the trip, will facilitate the development of identity. A lack of self-esteem, a major disability, and experiences of racism, may result in the failure of certain children to solve their personal search and consequently their social adequacy.

In spite of their importance, developmental delays, attachment problems, and autistic-like behavior observed on the arrival of the child should give rise to supportive care rather than to hasty diagnoses and irrevocable labels by adoptive parents or the medical care team. Some children more than others will have the capacity to rebound; their strength often lies in their empathy, capacity to organize, autonomy, and even in their sense of humor. Good interpersonal relationships before adoption and an early adoption by loving and qualified family are factors that make it possible to ensure the establishment of permanent family bonds and reduce the impact of childhood abandonment. From adversity and in abandonment, international adoption brings new challenges and rewards for both the adopted child and new parents. But most of all, it enables all members to travel a new pathway towards growth and evolution as a family.

REFERENCES

1. Jenista JA. Preadoption review of medical records. *Pediatr Ann* 2000; **29**:212–215.
2. Jenista JA. Preadoption medical review and revolutionary process. *Adoptive Families* 1999; **322**:14–18.
3. Albers LH, Johnson DE, Hostetter MK, Iverson S, Miller LL. Health of children adopted from the former Soviet Union and Eastern Europe: comparison with preadoptive medical records. *JAMA* 1997; **278**:922–924.
4. Mitchell MAS, Jenista JA. Health care of the internationally adopted child. *J Pediatr Health Care* 1997; **11**:51–60.
5. Hostetter M, Iverson S, Doles K, Johnson D. Unsuspected infectious diseases and other medical diagnoses in the evaluation of internationally adopted children. *Pediatrics* 1989; **83**:559–564.
6. Johnson DE, et al. The health of children adopted from Romania. *JAMA* 1992; **268**:3446–3451.
7. Aronson J. Medical evaluation and infectious considerations on arrival. *Pediatr Ann* 2000; **29**:218–223.
8. Hostetter M. Infectious diseases in internationally adopted children: Findings in children from China, Russia and Eastern Europe. *Adv Pediatr Infect Dis* 1999; **14**:147–161.
9. Hostetter MR, et al. Medical evaluation of internationally adopted children. *N Eng J Med* 1991; **325**:479–485.
10. Miller L. Caring for internationally adopted children. *NEJM* 1999; **34**:1539–1540.
11. Miller L. Initial assessment of growth, development and the effects of institutionalization in internationally adopted children. *Pediatr Ann* 2000; **29**:224–231.
12. Nelhaus G. Head circumference from birth to eighteen years. Practical composite international and interracial graphs. *Pediatrics* 1968; **41**:106–114.
13. Hamill PVV, Drizd TA, Johnson CL, et al. Physical growth: National Center for Health Statistics Percentiles. *Am J Clin Nutr* 1979; **32**:607–629.
14. Cichoine JF, Blancquaert I, Chicoine L, Raynault MF. *Bilan de santé de 808 chinoises nouvellement adoptées au Quebec.* Tours, France: Résumé XXXIIe congrès de l'association des pediatres de langue française; 1999.
15. Benoit TC, Jocelyn IJ, Moddemann DE, et al. Romanian adoption: the Manitoba experience. *Arch Pediatr Adolesc Med* 1996; **150**:1278–1282.
16. Kaler SR, Freeman BJ. Analysis of environmental deprivation: congnitive and social development in Romanian orphans. *J Child Psychol Psychiatr* 1994; **35**:769–781.
17. Johnson D. Long-term medical issues in international adoptees. *Pediatr Ann* 2000; **29**:234–241.
18. Miller LL, Kiernan MT, Mathers MI, Klein-Gitelman M. Developmental and nutritional status of internationally adopted children. *Arch Pediatr Adolesc Med* 1995; **149**:40–44.
19. Proos LA, Hofvander V, Wennquist K, Tuvernot B. A longitudinal study on anthropometric and clinical development of Indian children adopted in Sweden 1. Clinical and anthropometric condition at arrival. *Upsala J Med Sci* 1997; **97**:79–92.
20. Bourguignon JP, Gerard A, Alvarez-Gonzales ML, Fawe L, Franchinout P. Effects of changes in nutritional conditions on timing of puberty: clinical evidence from adopted children and experimental studies in the male rate. *Horm Res* 1992; **38(suppl 1)**:97–105.
21. Virdis R, Street M, Zampolli M, et al. Precocious puberty in girls adopted from developing countries. *Arch Dis Child* 1998; **78**:152–154.
22. Christenson B. Epidemiological aspects of the transmission of hepatitis B by BVHSAg-positive adopted children. *Scand J Infect Dis* 1986; **18**:105–109.
23. Davis LC, Weber DJ, Lemon SM. Horizontal transmission of hepatitis B virus. *Lancet* 1993; **889**(893)
24. Darmany JM. HIV infection and hepatitis B in adopted Romanian children. *BMJ* 1991; **302**:1604.
25. Jenista JA, Chapman DD. Medical problems of foreign-born adopted children. *AJDC* 1987; **141**:298–302.
26. Hostetter MR. Infectious diseases in internationally adopted children: Findings in children from China, Russia and Eastern Europe. *Adv Pediatr Infect Dis* 1999; **14**:147–161.
27. Lange WR, Warnock-Eckhart E, Beam ME. Mycobacterium tuberculosis infection in foreign born adoptees. *Pediatr Infect Dis J* 1989; **8**:625–629.
28. Hersh BS, Popouici F, Jerzek Z, et al. Risk factors for HIV infection among abandoned Romanian children. *AIDS* 1993; **7**:1617–1624.
29. Hostetter MK, Johnson DE. Immunization status of adoptees from China, Russia and Eastern Europe. *Pediatr Res* 1998; **43**:147A.

30. Miller LC. Internationally adopted children: immunization status. *Pediatrics* 1999; **103**(1078)

31. Verhulst F, Althaus M, Versluis-Den Bieman HJM. Damaging backgrounds: Later adjustment of international adoptees. *J Am Acad Child Adolesc Psychiatry* 1992; **29**:420–428.

32. Verhulst F, Althaus M, Versluis-Den Bieman HJM, *et al.* Problem behavior in international adoptees III. Diagnosis of child psychiatric disorders. *J Am Acad Child Adolesc Psychiatry* 1990; **29**:94–103.

33. Faber S. Behavioral sequelae of orphanage life. *Pediatr Ann* 2000; **29**:242–248.

34. Verhulst F, Althaus M, Versluis-Den Bieman HJM. Problem behavior in international adoptees: I. An epidemiological study. *J Am Acad Child Adolesc Psychiatry* 1990; **29**:94–103.

CHAPTER 29 # Visiting Friends and Relatives

Ronald H. Behrens

KEYPOINTS

- VFRs make up a substantial proportion of international travelers

- VFRs are at increased risk of a variety of infections associated with travel

- Children of VFRs born in industrialized countries, young VFRs and those from the higher socio-economic strata of society may be at greater risk of Hepatitis A

- VFRs travelling to certain countries are at increased risk of typhoid fever, malaria, STDs and possibly tuberculosis

- VFRs are less likely to seek pre-travel health advice and often travel in high-risk environments that expose them to particular infectious diseases

INTRODUCTION

The definition of those who visit friends and relatives (VFRs) has not been standardized but the term is used to cover ethnic travelers who have immigrated at some period in the past and maintain family links in their country of origin. Because of the differences in definition across studies and publications, varied terminology is used to describe ethnic travelers, and these may not be describing equivalent groups. The terms migrant, immigrants, semi-immune and foreign (born) are used to indicate citizens and immigrants born abroad and of different ethnic and cultural background to the natives of a country. Studies have also used a number of terms to describe the natives or major group of the host country including European, non-migrants, nationals and non-immunes. This failure of a common definition makes it difficult to make direct comparisons between groups and to adequately identify their reasons for traveling. The VFR may be third or fourth generation from the original migrant, but has both social and cultural attachments with their country of origin, or they may be immigrants who have settled for 10 years or longer in a new country and travel back to their country of origin. A 'VFR' is culturally and racially distinct from the natives of the country in which they now reside. Refugees and displaced persons, are often temporary residents in a host country and their health problems often relate to exposures they had in their countries of origin as well as those that occurred during their migration.

The reason for travel can influence the pattern of morbidity during and after travel. Both the health of the individual and the public health of the country to which he/she returns may be affected by travel. There are a number of factors, which may impact on a VFR's risk of illness. Health beliefs held by the traveler will influence the use of pre-travel advice and prophylaxis. [1] Many VFRs believe they will not suffer from infections such as malaria because they consider themselves to be immune, and may feel it unnecessary to seek advice on disease prevention. Many asylum seekers and new immigrants on social support, have problems accessing health services. Pre-travel health advice services are clinic based and the majority charge for their services. To realize the benefit of these services, travelers must recognize the risks associated with travel and benefits of pre-travel advice and prophylaxis. Travelers must have confidence in the service and rapport with the health personnel. Finally, the cost benefit of the advice and prophylaxis needs to be appreciated. Language barriers, bureaucracy in the health system, anxiety over immigration status, and ignorance of rights to health services are some of the non-economic reasons why this population may fail to use a travel health service when planning to travel. Pre-travel health services are customized to deal with the leisure and business traveler and focus on the language and culture of the predominant community requirements. It is often difficult to adjust for the many diverse and small ethnic groups within a community. This unequal access to services has also led to delays in the treatment of ill returned travelers and can contribute to more severe pathology in this group.

EPIDEMIOLOGY OF TRAVEL BY VFRs

In the UK, ethnic groups make up 6.7% of the total population, however as can be seen from the graph, they make up a total of 20% (6.5 million) of all visits made abroad. There are around half a million citizens whose country of origin is Africa. In the year 2000, around 2 million visits were made from the UK to Africa, of which 40% were made by VFRs. In the USA in the year 2000, VFRs constituted around 27% of total overseas journeys made by US citizens abroad, around 7.2 m travelers that year. [2] Although this group makes up a smaller proportion of journeys to disease endemic areas than other travelers, VFRs appear to suffer the greatest proportion of illness of all groups of travelers. Data and research exist on the epidemiology of imported hepatitis A, typhoid, malaria, tuberculosis and HIV. Comparing the trends and differences between groups of travelers helps define important and relevant risk factors for travelers.

Hepatitis A

Hepatitis A Virus (HAV) is responsible for roughly 50% of acute hepatitis cases in the USA. In the USA and the UK, travel is identified as a risk factor in around 10–20% of all reported cases. Transmission of this RNA picornavirus is by fecal contamination of water or food. In developing countries, most children by the age of 5 years have developed antibodies to HAV. This pattern is not complete and there are high socio-economic strata of society where, because exposure to infection is limited, children remain susceptible to infection.[3] In the developed countries of Europe, North America (except for the Arctic), Japan, and Australia, exposure to HAV does not occur and the majority of the adult population are antibody negative and therefore susceptible to infection. Populations born after 1945 have an HAV-antibody prevalence of less than 20% in many industrialized countries. Adult ethnic immigrants born in a developing country are often immune, while their children born in a developed country have no HAV antibodies and are susceptible to HAV infection. Children rarely develop clinical symptoms after exposure to HAV, but adults have symptomatic evidence of infection.[4,5] In a study by Behrens et al.,[6] children under 15 years of age from VFR families traveling to the Indian sub-continent appeared to be twice as likely to develop symptomatic hepatitis A than older travelers. In the same study, ethnic travelers were eight times more likely to develop hepatitis A than tourists or other travelers. The study revealed that the majority of travel associated cases of hepatitis A (60%) into the UK were contracted on the Indian sub-continent. The finding that young travelers developed clinical hepatitis A was unexpected. One interpretation of this finding is that non-immune children may be exposed to a high inoculum of virus when living in a less sterile environment with their relatives during their visit. Notifications of hepatitis A from the Netherlands between 1995–1997[7] report a striking seasonal fluctuation in incidence of HAV. In the autumn, there was a significant increase in the number of pediatric notifications of HAV in Moroccan and Turkish children. This was due to infection occurring during their summer holiday when visiting relatives in their country of origin. This pattern was seen annually over a 5-year period. Following this seasonal increase, the authors reported a temporal increase in notifications of HAV in adult Dutch citizens in the Netherlands. The authors suggest this is a result of secondary infection from the imported primary pediatric cases. The ethnic child is vulnerable to hepatitis A for three likely reasons: the child does not receive pre-travel counseling and immunization; the living environment which they visit is different from that encountered by tourist and business travelers, and the contact they make with the local population is more direct and sustained, therefore exposing the visitor to infectious pathogens.

Typhoid fever

Most reports of typhoid fever in North America and Europe are associated with travel. The Indian sub-continent (ISC) including Pakistan, India, and Bangladesh result in around 37–91% of travel associated typhoid.[8,9] The risk to American travelers of typhoid, during travel to the Indian sub-continent, is 18 times that to other regions of the world and as a foreign-born-US citizen, the risk is increased by a further 25%.[10] All the typhoid cases in a 2-year study in north-west England were travel associated and all but one were from the ISC. In contrast to the previous citing of secondary transmission of hepatitis A, there were no secondary cases of typhoid reported. In Nottingham,[9] all cases of enteric fever were in travelers who had visited the ISC, and were VFRs. In the 1980s, 70% of typhoid fever cases in England and Wales were contracted during visits to the ISC and 90% of paratyphoid A were similarly acquired. In all the studies, the proportion of cases that had received pre-travel immunization was very low. A similar proportion (77%) of reported cases of typhoid fever imported into the USA were in VFRs.[11]

Malaria

Malaria is one of the most important infectious diseases acquired by ethnic travelers. Sub-Saharan Africa is the region where the highest risk of falciparum malaria exists and the risk of transmission to a

visitor has been estimated to range from around 0.1% per visit to Zimbabwe to as high as 1.7% per visit to Nigeria.[12] In Europe, the surveillance network TropNetEurop has described the pattern of malaria imported into Europe. Over a 2-year period, they describe 48% of the falciparum cases in semi-immune immigrant travelers and 54% in travelers who were visiting friends and 63% of all cases reported were contracted in West Africa.[13] Over the decade 1990–2000, 10 227 cases of *Plasmodium falciparum* infections from sub-Saharan Africa were reported to the Malaria Reference Laboratory in the UK. A total of 69% were from West Africa, 18% from east Africa, 10% from South and 3% from Central Africa. Of these, 55% of *P. falciparum* and 48% of *P. ovale* were in VFRs. Recent analysis of *P. falciparum* imported into the UK reveals that two-thirds of cases are reported from London and that 71% occurs in travelers of African descent and 64% of non-falciparum malaria is in travelers of S. Asian descent. The relative risk of *P. falciparum* occurring in a London citizen of African descent is a staggering 139-fold that of a Londoner of Caucasian descent (David Bradley, personal communication, 2002).

Interestingly, incidence in visitors to the UK from endemic countries, was as high as that of tourists.[14] For visits to the Indian sub-continent where *P. vivax* is the strain most commonly acquired, the risk is 0.15% per visit made.[15] Data from reported cases by region, and ethnic travel are shown in Figure 29.1 and Table 29.1. These confirm West Africa as the region of highest transmission risk for *P. falciparum* and that over half the visits made to this region are by ethnic travelers, many of whom are also traveling for business. The risk in East Africa where the proportion of ethnic travelers was much lower at 21% of visits, appears to have a similar risk of developing malaria to that of tourists visiting this region (Fig. 29.1).

Immigrant and ethnic workers in Italy have a growing prevalence of malaria. The reporting is regional, however the pattern is similar from different parts of the country. National statistics from Romi[16] and colleagues describe 44% of malaria cases in ethnic travelers, the majority of whom are VFRs. Calleri[17] and colleagues describe that the proportion of ethnic travelers who developed malaria in and around Turin increased from 0% in 1983 to 54% in 1992. In Bressica[18] the infectious disease clinic reports that 80% of imported *P. falciparum* cases are in ethnic travelers with the proportion of migrants to resident increasing from equal in 1990 to six-fold higher by 1998. In Lombardy, in the North of the country, 54% of analyzable cases were in migrants, of whom 87% were VFRs.

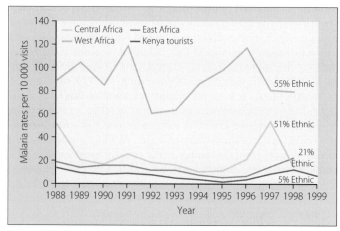

Figure 29.1 The incidence of malaria in UK residents visiting sub Saharan Africa by regions. The incidence in Kenya of tourists is also shown. The figure shows the proportion of visits made by VFRs to the regions. The data is provided courtesy of the Malaria Reference Laboratory and the International Passenger Survey.

Table 29.1	Average attack rates for all species of malaria in UK residents by reason for travel 1999–2001		
	Attack rates (cases/10 000 visits)		
	VFRs	**Tourist and business travelers**	**Relative risk of VFR versus tourist**
Kenya	13	6	2
Tanzania	16	11	1
Uganda	107	26	4
East Africa	**45**	**14**	**3.2**
Ghana	63	24	3
Nigeria	91	14	6
West Africa	**77**	**19**	**4.1**
India	1.30	0.39	3
Pakistan	3.05	0.17	18
Indian sub-continent	**2.18**	**0.28**	**7.8**

The RR is the relative risk of infection of ethnic travelers compared with tourist and business travelers to the same region. (Surveillance data provided courtesy of the Malaria Reference Laboratory and numbers of travelers is provided by the International Passenger Survey.)

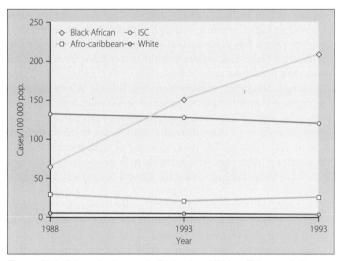

Figure 29.2 Tuberculosis rates in England and Wales. This reveals the dramatic increase in tuberculosis in Black Africans. The data also shows the large difference in rates between the white and non white populations in the UK. (Adapted from ref.[33]).

Children are at a similar risk of malaria infections as adult ethnic travelers. Out of a group of 49 pediatric cases of malaria in Spain, 44 children were from endemic countries (immigrants or adopted children) and five were Spanish-born children who had traveled to tropical areas, where four were sons of immigrants who had also contracted malaria while visiting their families in the tropics. None of the five traveling children had taken correct malaria prophylaxis.[19]

In a review of pediatric malaria in the UK, Brabin and Ganley[20] describe that 15% of all imported malaria cases between 1990–1995 were in children (under 15 years of age). The majority of cases were in VFRs visiting West Africa. Only 50% were taking chemoprophylaxis.

Another major factor influencing VFRs risk of acquiring malaria when traveling to areas of high transmission is inadequate use of chemoprophylaxis only. A total of 28% of ethnic malaria cases admitted using chemoprophylaxis when asked in a study of malaria in returned travelers, which compares poorly with the 75% usage in tourists with malaria.[21] A similarly low proportion (31%) of Canadian residents of south Indian origin travelling to India intended taking chemoprophylaxis, despite many believing themselves to be at risk.[22] Matteelli et al. report that 92.6% of ethnic travelers with malaria in the Lombardy region had not used chemoprophylaxis, while 50% of tourists and business travelers had used a prophylactic drug regimen.[23] In the study from Bressica,[18] the authors reported that only 11% of migrants started chemoprophylaxis, compared with 55% of non migrants. The National Analysis of Italian Malaria Cases supports this dismal picture with 36% of non migrant and 4% of ethnic travelers using regular prophylaxis. In the TropNetEurop surveillance data, 72.4% of ethnic travelers had not used chemoprophylaxis, a proportion which is similar to that of prophylaxis usage in European malaria cases (60%). This finding is somewhat disparate to previous reports where there is a clear difference in use of chemoprophylaxis between ethnic and non ethnic travelers.

The reasons for lack of use of prophylaxis in this high-risk group are unclear, and is likely to be multi-factorial. One factor may be the cost of purchasing chemoprophylactic drugs.

Cost was considered to contribute to the low level of use of malaria chemoprophylaxis by VFRs.[24] A study based in Walsall, UK, which has a large proportion of ethnic residents describes the consequences following the removal of the government subsidy on malaria prophylaxis in 1995 in the UK. There was a dramatic decrease in prescriptions issued for malaria prophylaxis and an equally significant increase in malaria cases compared to the preceding years. There is also some evidence of travelers selecting cheaper but inappropriate drug regimens because of cost after the removal of the same drug subsidy in the UK.[25]

Another contributing factor to low prophylaxis use is lack of knowledge, ignorance or misinformation held by ethnic travelers. This may in part relate to the lack of advice or not seeking advice prior to travel. Of the ethnic travelers studied on departure from Canada, 54% had sought advice and only one-third planned to use chemoprophylaxis.[22] Only 7% had been prescribed an appropriate regimen. French VFRs departing from Paris were twice as likely to be taking unsuitable chemoprophylaxis as tourists taking package holidays.[26]

In a population-based study of knowledge, attitudes and practices of Italian foreign-born citizens, 70% were aware of how malaria was transmitted. Of those who had traveled home to a malarious region, only 18% had sought pre-travel advice; 52% of this group were unaware of the malaria risk at their destination, and a further 40% were ignorant of suitable protective measures against infection. The large majority of those who had traveled had not taken prophylactic measures on their journey.[18]

An interesting feature reported by a number of investigators is that the severity of malaria differs between VFRs or migrant travelers and non-immune western tourists. There appears to be anti-disease immunity persisting in VFRs and migrant travelers, which protects against severe and fatal disease despite the lack of chemoprophylaxis. In Lombardy, severe disease occurred in 9.2% of non-migrant cases with falciparum malaria compared to 1.3% in migrants. In Bressica, the proportion was similar 8.9–1.2%. Fatality reports give a similar picture. In two Italian studies, the case fatality rate for non-immune Italians travelers was 1.6% nationally and 3% in Lombardy. Deaths were rare in the migrants and VFR groups. Data from TropNetEurop shows that all deaths were in Europeans and the clinical complication rate in Europeans (6.3%) was double that of the immigrant semi-immune traveler (3.7%). Of the 91 deaths from malaria reported in the UK between 1990–2000 the case fatality rate was 5.5 times higher in tourists and 16 times higher in business compared to deaths in ethnic travelers. It appears from this evidence that although the ethnic traveler is at significantly higher risk of infection, the risk of dying from malaria is lower than in tourists.

Although falciparum malaria from Sub-Saharan Africa makes up the largest portion of imported malaria, there is still a significant proportion of malaria imported from the Indian sub-continent. Three quarters of imported vivax malaria in the UK are in ethnic travelers to India and Pakistan. The peak reporting of vivax malaria is in the 4th quarter of each year, which correlates closely to the peak period of travel to the Indian sub-continent, around the 2nd and 3rd quarter of the year.

The malaria problem facing ethnic travelers is clear from the published data. They make up the largest group of travelers developing malaria during travel abroad reported from many European countries, and this proportion is increasing. Those from West Africa face a significant risk of infection; many fold higher than tourists to other parts of Africa. They are frequent travelers and their destinations are in rural settings where vector control may not occur. There are some clues to the contributing factors to this high risk – low chemoprophylaxis use. This may be due to ignorance of risk or misinformation in regard to their vulnerability.

Reducing imported malaria in many parts of Europe is unlikely to be achieved until the large problem of malaria among ethnic travelers is resolved. The current most commonly used strategy of improving and introducing new chemoprophylaxis regimens is unlikely to have an impact on the majority of imported malaria. Travel advisors need further information on why ethnic travelers are at high risk and more knowledge about their current behavior, then an appropriate strategy can be rationally implemented. It is almost certain to be a community-based intervention to improve knowledge, attitudes and practice and enhanced use of pre-travel services.

HIV and sexually transmitted diseases

Although the black-African ethnic group make up around 0.4% of the total population of the UK[27] they carry a disproportionate burden of HIV in the UK. In the year 2000, 30% of cases were reported to be in black-Africans, while 70% of all cases were in one of the many minority ethnic groups.[28] De Cock estimated that relative risk of infection in black African adults was 20 times and for children 355 times higher than in non-African equivalent groups living in the UK. There is evidence of similar high incidence rates of gonorrhea in Afro-Caribbean men living in Leeds, UK. They were 54 time more likely to be diagnosed with the sexually transmitted diseases than the white population.[29] The link that these infections are travel associated is unclear. Fenton and colleagues[30] examined travel of black Africans living in London to their home countries in Central Africa, and the acquisition of new sexual partners while abroad; 44.5% had returned to their country of origin within the previous 5 years. A total of 40% of men and 21% of women acquired a new sexual partner abroad. Predictors of new sexual partners while abroad include increased sexual activity with larger number of sexual partners and previous STDs in the UK. In the group, 42% had not used a condom at last intercourse and one-third perceived themselves to be at risk of catching HIV. Over 2% of recently returned travelers were identified as HIV antibody positive in a London hospital. A significant risk factor of infection in this study was again having been born in East, Central or Southern Africa.[31] The role of travel and risk of HIV is therefore an important one for the ethnic traveler. Interventions to address this hazard need to be developed and evaluated and will need to be targeted at each cultural group so as to ensure effectiveness.

Tuberculosis in the ethnic traveler

There is much more data on the prevalence and risk factors of travel associated tuberculosis. As a notifiable disease, this data is collected with much more discipline and detail. Both in the USA and UK, there has been an increase in the proportion of cases of tuberculosis in ethnic (defined as foreign born in the USA) travelers. Between 1986 and 1997 there was a 56% increase in cases among foreign-born persons from 22–39% of the total numbers of cases reported in the USA.[32] In the UK, the TB incidence rose by 20% in residents originating from the Indian sub-continent and 124% in black Africans.[33]

It is predictable that most of the states or cities with higher populations of ethnic residents have higher than national rates of tuberculosis. Persons born in the Indian sub-continent and living in the USA had a tuberculosis incidence/per year of 68/100 000 population,[34] while in the UK in 1998 the incidence for the same group was 121/100 000 population. The black African community has the highest rate of all at 210 cases per 100 000 population per year and as is shown in Figure 29.2, this continues to rise.[33]

The relation of acquisition of tuberculosis and travel is more difficult to identify. However, the data from the UK and USA show that recent arrivals of ethnic migrants in these countries (<5 years) from sub-Saharan Africa have rates of tuberculosis of 3 and 4 times higher than that of residents originating from the same region but who have been resident for longer than 5 years. There are likely to be many other factors which will affect and influence these high rates in ethnic groups, including the numbers of visits made by relatives from highly endemic countries and the targeted screening of ethnic travelers on entry to the USA and Europe. The changing trends of tuberculosis in their country of origin needs to be considered. Developing countries have rates in their general population, which are 5–100 times higher than in the developed regions of the world.[35] Travel to and from these regions of the world and exposure of migrants, business and tourist travelers to such high transmission areas will affect disease and carriage of *M. tuberculosis* as they travel and mix across the world.

CONCLUSION

The ethnic travelers, particularly the VFRs, have the highest morbidity of infectious diseases, including typhoid, Hepatitis A, malaria, tuberculosis and HIV. This is associated with their lifestyle, behavior, culture and beliefs. This pattern of morbidity is only just being recognized and there is a dearth of data on the major contributing factors to the problem. Improvements in travel medicine practice, including the development of new antimalarial drugs and novel vaccines have been of little benefit to this group of travelers as can be seen from the increasing trend of morbidity. Pre-travel services are under utilized by this population and there is little material adapted to the language and cultures of ethnic travelers. A major shift in practice will be necessary to benefit this vulnerable group.

REFERENCES

1. Farquharson L, Noble LM, Barker C, Behrens RH. Health beliefs and communication in the travel clinic consultation as predictors of adherence to malaria chemoprophylaxis. Abstract from the 7th ISTM Conference: 2001; FC02.02.
2. US Department of Commerce ITA Tourism Industries. *Profile of US Resident Travelers Visiting Overseas Destinations.* US Department of Commerce; http://tinet.ita.doc.gov/view/f-2000-101-001/. Accessed 01-07-2001.
3. Mall ML, Rai RR, Philip M, *et al.* Seroepidemiology of Hepatitis A infection in India: changing pattern. *Indian J Gastroenterol* 2001; **20**(4): 132–135.
4. Villarejos VM, Serra J, Anderson-Visona K, Mosley JW. Hepatitis A virus infection in households. *Am J Epidemiol* 1982; **115**(4):577–586.

5. Lednar WM, Lemon SM, Kirkpatrick JW, *et al.* Frequency of illness associated with epidemic Hepatitis A virus infections in adults. *Am J Med* 1985; **122**:226–233.

6. Behrens RH, Collins M, Botto B, Heptonstall J. Risk of British travelers acquiring Hepatitis A [letter]. *BMJ* 1995; **311**:193.

7. Termorshuizen F, van de Laar MJ. The epidemiology of Hepatitis A in the Netherlands, 1957–1998. *Ned Tijdschr Geneeskd* 1998; **142**(43):2364–2368.

8. Caumes E, Belanger F, Brucker G, Danis M, Gentilini M. Diseases observed after return from travels outside Europe. 109 cases. *Presse Med* 1991; **20**(31): 1483–1486.

9. Lighton LL. Follow up in north west England of cases of enteric fever acquired abroad. *Communic Dis Pub Health* 1999; **2**(2):145–146.

10. Mermin JH, Townes JM, Gerber M, *et al.* Typhoid fever in the United States, 1985-1994: changing risks of international travel and increasing antimicrobial resistance. *Arch Intern Med* 1998; **158**(6):633–638.

11. Steinberg E, Frisch A, Rossiter S, McClellan J, Ackers M, Mintz E. *Typhoid Fever in Travelers: Who Should We Vaccinate?* Abstract from the 49th meeting of the American Society of Tropical Medicine and Hygiene: 2000; 60.

12. Muentener P, Schlagenhauf P, Steffen R. Imported malaria (1985–95): trends and perspectives. *Bull World Health Organ* 1999; **77**(7):560–566.

13. Jelinek T, Schulte C, Behrens RH, *et al.* Imported Falciparum Malaria in Europe: Sentinel Surveillance Data from the European Network on Surveillance of Imported Infectious Diseases. *Clin Infect Dis* 2002; **34**(5).

14. Phillips-Howard PA, Bradley DJ, Blaze M, Hurn M. Malaria in Britain: 1977–86. *BMJ* 1988; **296**:245–248.

15. Anonymous. Surveillance of malaria in European Union countries. *Eurosurveillance* 1998; **3**:45–47.

16. Romi R, Sabatinelli G, Majori G. Malaria epidemiological situation in Italy and evaluation of malaria incidence in Italian travelers. *J Travel Med* 2001; **8**(1):6–11.

17. Calleri G, Macor A, Leo G, Caramello P. Imported malaria in Italy: epidemiologic and clinical studies. *J Trav Med* 1994; **1**:231–233.

18. Castelli F, Matteelli A, Caligaris S, *et al.* Malaria in migrants. *Parassitologia* 1999; **41**(1–3):261–265.

19. Huerga H, Lopez-Velez R. Imported malaria in immigrant and travelling children in Madrid. *Eur J Clin Microbiol Infect Dis* 2001; **20**(8):591–593.

20. Brabin BJ, Ganley Y. Imported malaria in children in the UK. *Arch Dis Child* 1997; **77**(1):76–81.

21. Behrens RH, Curtis CF. Malaria in travelers: epidemiology and prevention. In: Behrens RH, McAdam KPWJ, eds. *Travel Medicine.* London: Churchill Livingstone; 1993:363–383.

22. dos Santos CC. Anvar A, Keystone JS, Kain KC. Survey of use of malaria prevention measures by Canadians visiting India. *Can Med Assoc J* 1999; **160**(2):195–200.

23. Matteelli A, Colombini P, Gulletta M, Castelli F, Carosi G. Epidemiological features and case management practices of imported malaria in northern Italy 1991–1995. *Trop Med Int Health* 1999; **4**(10):653–657.

24. Badrinath P, Ejidokun OO, Barnes N, Ramaiah S. Change in NHS regulations may have caused increase in malaria. *BMJ* 1998; **316**(7146):746–747.

25. Evans MR. Patients may start to take cheaper over the counter regimens. *BMJ* 1996; **313**(7071):1554b.

26. Semaille C, Santin A, Prazuck T, *et al.* Malaria chemoprophylaxis of 3,446 French travelers departing from Paris to eight tropical countries. *J Trav Med* 1999; **6**(1):3–6.

27. Office of Population Censuses and Surveys. *The 1991 census.* London: HMSO; 1993.

28. Anonymous. AIDS and HIV infection in the United Kingdom: Monthly report. *Commun Dis Rev Wkly* 2001; **11**(8):11–13.

29. Cock KM De, Low N. HIV and AIDS, other sexually transmitted diseases, and tuberculosis in ethnic minorities in United Kingdom: Is surveillance serving its purpose? *BMJ* 1997; **314**(7096):1747.

30. Fenton KA, Chinouya M, Davidson O, Copas A. HIV transmission risk among sub-Saharan Africans in London travelling to their countries of origin. *AIDS* 2001; **15**(11):1442–1445.

31. Hawkes S, Malin A, Araru T, Mabey DCW. HIV infection among heterosexual travelers attending the Hospital for Tropical Diseases, London. *Genitourin Med* 1992; **68**:309–311.

32. Working Group on Tuberculosis among Foreign-Born Persons. Recommendations for prevention and control of tuberculosis among foreign-born persons. A report from the Working Group on Tuberculosis Among Foreign-Born Persons. *Morb Mortal Wkly Rep* 1998; **47**(RR-16).

33. Rose AM, Watson JM, Graham C, *et al.* Tuberculosis at the end of the 20th century in England and Wales: results of a national survey in 1998. *Thorax* 2001; **56**(3):173–179.

34. McKenna MT, McCray E, Onorato I. The epidemiology of tuberculosis among foreign-born persons in the United States, 1986 to 1993. *N Engl J Med* 1995; **332**(16):1071–1076.

35. World Health Organization. *Global Tuberculosis Control.* WHO/CDS/TB/ 2001.287. Geneva: WHO; 2001.

CHAPTER 30 Expatriates

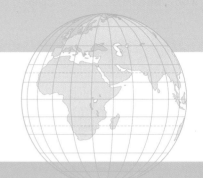

Ken L. Gamble and Deborah M. Lovell-Hawker

KEYPOINTS

- In the pre-departure assessment, attention must be paid to:

  a Health issues that must be managed during the international assignment that are not related to tropical and infectious diseases

  b Psychosocial issues that are associated with long-stay travel

- Counseling must consider low risk infectious diseases and behavior, which demonstrate cumulative risk over prolonged periods

- Cross-cultural training and re-entry issues are a priority

- 'Self-Care' is central to successful care abroad

- Consideration must be given to comprehensive post-travel screening and psychological debriefing

INTRODUCTION

Foyle has defined expatriates as those who take up residence in another country for occupational purposes, returning to their original country when their assignment is completed.[1] Business personnel, diplomats, embassy personnel, aid-workers, missionaries, explorers, geologists, miners, military personnel and professional domestic employees are among those who readily fit those criteria. There is no published census that has delineated the size of this community but it could amount to millions.

The length of stay varies from months to years, long enough to necessitate some form of assimilation into the host culture. Some will emerge fully bicultural, whereas others will choose to fully maintain their identity with those from the sending culture. All will by necessity be forced to adapt to some aspects of the host culture.

As diverse as the backgrounds, are the strategies for preparation, health management and risk reduction. The corps diplomatique are usually carefully selected, professionally trained and skilled for their specific role in the international communities. They tend to be more affluent, enjoy ready access to the best available health facilities that are carefully monitored for quality control, or have ready opportunity to transfer to an alternative location.

In contrast, many aid-workers volunteer for short-term assignments with minimal thought of health implications and may receive minimal preparation and training for their intercultural experience. Many may live in relatively primitive settings with a minimum level of support and must individually determine who their health-care provider will be. Only under extreme circumstance will they have an opportunity for a medical evacuation.

Other variables such as the choice of lifestyle will dramatically influence risk. Less affluent expatriates may be isolated from amenities found in industrialized countries but live a relatively simple lifestyle in a predictable and risk managed environment whereas expatriates with multinational companies may live and work surrounded by modern amenities, buoyed by an intricate support structure, yet embark on risk taking diversions throughout their sojourn, thereby increasing their risk of accidental injury. Occupation and nationality become major factors in some hostile settings, exposing expatriates to risk of harm and death from intentional violence.[2]

The risk of illness among expatriates is influenced by all factors that impact the health of short-term business travelers or tourists including: age, sex, behavior, climate, environmental specific risk factors, accidental injury and infectious diseases. However, the complexity of intercultural assignments has a profound affect on the impact of illness in that setting. Repatriation for health reasons may mean dislocation from employment opportunities, disruption of education and dissolution of social networks. Isolation and limited resources increase the scope of responsibility that must be taken for self-care. Intense and prolonged exposure to the physical, environmental, political and social challenges could have a negative impact on their psychosocial well being.

Frequently the medical and psychological dimensions of an illness are intertwined. The Foreign Service has estimated that 60% of all referrals for medical treatment have a stress-related basis; therefore it is prudent for health-care providers to recognize the relevance of the psychological factors that influence the health status of expatriate personnel when providing expatriate communities preventive or therapeutic care. To that end, both health aspects will be represented in concert as a practical approach to screening, preparation, and care during the international assignment and re-entry is developed throughout this chapter.

UNDERSTANDING THE RISKS

A basic understanding of the epidemiology of illnesses that pertain to expatriates will be useful as the health-care provider focuses on the evaluation and provision of preventive care.

Morbidity

The Peace Corps were the first to develop a formal epidemiological surveillance system, and have monitored health trends in over 5500 volunteers in 1985. Bernard,[3] Banta[4] and Lange[5] have all demonstrated similar trends. The most commonly reported health problems are shown in Table 30.1.

GeoSentinel, a global, provider-based sentinel surveillance system has compiled some useful data from 7116 ill patients who presented to

Table 30.1	The most commonly reported health problems
Event	Frequency (per year)
Diarrheal disease	48/100
Respiratory illnesses	27/100
Injuries	20/100
Skin conditions	19/100
Psychological	4/100

25 different clinics after travel to five regions of the world.[6] With the exception of injuries, which would not commonly present to the clinics involved in the GeoSentinel surveillance system, they demonstrated that the relative frequency of health events on a global scale is similar to that noted by the Peace Corp Volunteers (PCV) with a trend toward regional differences (Table 30.2).

Stress takes its toll on expatriate volunteers and missionaries

Though most describe their time overseas as enjoyable and fulfilling, expatriates as a group encounter a variety of potentially stressful experiences. Anxiety and fatigue accounted for only 4% of the identified events in Banta's analysis of PCV in 1966, comparable to that reported by GeoSentinel; yet, the 'burden of illness' is in fact greater than infectious diseases when the cumulative impact of stress is considered.

In a survey of 390 missionaries, Parshall[7] found that 97% reported experiencing tension, 88% found anger to be a frequent or occasional problem, and 20% had taken tranquilizers since becoming missionaries. In a longitudinal study, Paton and Purvis[8] administered the General Health Questionnaire (GHQ-30) to 18 nurses before they went to work in Romanian orphanages for three months, and again on their return. GHQ-30 scores significantly increased during the time in Romania, indicating an increase in health related problems, which was maintained at one-month follow-up. The nurses were also administered the Impact of Event Scale (IES), and were found to report symptoms of intrusive thoughts and avoidance which resembled those of clinical trauma patients. In addition, 22% reported sleep problems. Paton also found high levels of symptomatology among relief workers in El Salvador, Armenia, Iran and the Philippines.

In another study, overseas aid and development workers representing 62 different organizations completed anonymous questionnaires after returning to their home country. Participants were recruited randomly, and the response rate was 82%, with 145 individuals completing the questionnaires. The mean time spent as expatriates was 51 months, although there was a wide range. Forty-six percent of these respondents reported that they had experienced a psychological illness of clinical severity either while they were away, or on their return home. In 87% of cases the primary diagnosis was depression, with another 7% having been clinically diagnosed as having chronic fatigue syndrome. Four percent of the cases had received a diagnosis of post-traumatic stress disorder PTSD, and 2% had other diagnoses[9] (Table 30.3).

Premature attrition

The profound negative impact of premature attrition was recognized in the late 1800s and continues to be a major factor impacting the cost of international placement. Crude data from a global survey of aid and missionary agencies indicates an attrition rate of 3–8% per year. Some 20–40% of all expatriate managers return home early due to their inability to adjust to the new culture, and/or their poor performance in that culture. Moreover, nearly half of those who do *not* return early function below their normal level of productivity while working as expatriates.[10] The rate may be much higher among expatriates sent to the countries that are culturally the most different from their home country.

Mortality data

A review of published studies demonstrates a considerable variance in the mortality rate of expatriates with estimates ranging from 100% greater among aid and development workers compared with colleagues remaining at home[11] to 40% lower than would be expected in a comparable US population.[12]

Frame and Hargarten[13] observed that motor vehicle accidents were the leading cause of death among missionaries and PCV, respectively. A recent study of deaths among humanitarian workers demonstrated that intentional violence was responsible for most of their deaths (68%) followed by Motor Vehicle Accidents (17%).[14] From 1970 to 1985, the rate of death from infectious diseases approximated that reported in the US; now that HIV exposure has been found to be an occupational risk for aid workers in some parts of the world that may change.[11]

PRE-DEPARTURE ASSESSMENT

The purpose of pre-departure assessments

There are very little data in the literature that provide specific counsel to guide the pre-travel assessment. Much can be extrapolated from literature that pertains to clinical preventive health and travel medicine. Pre-travel consultations may be sought for:

- a baseline health assessment

Table 30.2	Relative frequency of health events on a global scale				
	Africa	S.E. Asia	India	S. America	Central America/Caribbean
Acute diarrhea	18	28.3	37	21	22.4
Chronic diarrhea	4.1	6.2	2.8	10.9	1 1.9
Respiratory infections	8.4	14.8	16.7	5.9	5.2
Skin conditions	8.3	9.2	7.2	7.6	10
Anxiety/fatigue	3.9	4.2	4.4	3.8	3.9

Most frequently occurring diseases in travelers (% of ill travelers by travel destination)[6]

Table 30.3	Difficulties commonly reported include (not rank ordered)
Cross-cultural adjustment	
Loneliness	
Communication problems	
Unpredictable circumstances	
Role ambiguity	
Long working hours	
Little opportunity to relax or socialize	
Overwhelming responsibility	
Ethical dilemmas	
Powerlessness	
Extreme temperatures	
Uncomfortable living and working conditions	
Danger	
Wide-scale poverty	
Injustice	
Suffering	
Despair	
Death	
Limited access to any form of psychological support.	

- risk appraisal
- counsel regarding appropriate immunization and malaria prophylaxis
- third party health appraisal for sending organizations designed to enhance the support services that they can provide and circumvent legal liability

Defining appropriate expectations – the volunteer

Organizations vary widely with respect to their provision of cross-cultural preparation and support of their personnel. People who offer their services as volunteers or missionaries are advised to choose an organization that offers good training, medical, emotional and practical support. In particular, it is worth checking the policies of organizations, and asking whether they adhere to *Best Practice Guidelines* (such as those promoted by the organization 'People in Aid' – www.peopleinaid.org). Organizations that have never heard of such principles and show no interest in considering them may offer insufficient support to their personnel.

See Table 30.4 for the minimum questions to ask before signing up with an organization.

The sending organization – protecting their investment

Legal constraints will influence the purpose, nature and extent of pre-departure assessments. Host countries often impose limited medical prerequisites as part of the visa granting process. If health constraints have a critical bearing on the outcome of an assignment, the sending agency bears responsibility to define health prerequisites, which in many jurisdictions must be posted along with the job description. Increasingly care must be taken to ensure that health prerequisites are judged to be non-discriminatory in nature. At a more pragmatic level, sending organizations should view the pre-departure assessment as an initial step toward the provision of care for their employees, protecting their investment, which may amount to US$500 000 per family.

Therefore, candidates receiving conditional acceptance may be required to have a 'third party assessment' by an 'agent' who is often their personal primary health-care provider or a travel medicine consultant. The sending organization bears the responsibility of defining the purpose of the evaluation for the candidate and agent. The health-care provider is responsible to carefully appraise candidate to determine the status of their current health, personal risk factors as well as their personal resources. Usually the agent's conclusions are recorded on a standardized form or compiled in a formal

Table 30.4	Minimum to ask before signing up with an organization
Do you adhere to any 'Code of Best Practice', or any other standard recognizing the importance of caring for personnel?	
What training or orientation is provided before workers leave?	

Financial arrangements (finances are a major source of stress, especially for volunteers)
    Do volunteers raise their own costs, and if so, how much must be raised?
    Is language training a requirement? Who defrays the costs?
    Is there a 'resettlement payment' after return home? Any pension provision?	

What medical and/or emotional support is provided while workers are away from home?
    Is there a mechanism for feedback and communication?
    How do I make requests for help: elective, urgent and emergent	

What are your policies regarding
    Evacuation
    Compassionate leave
    Schooling for children
        Options available and supported by the organization
        Support for children with special needs and learning styles
        Location of placement and length of contract	

What help is provided for dealing with the return home? (see Ch 37)
    Do you routinely offer debriefing?
    Is longer-term support provided if there are any stress-related problems?	

Can you put me in contact with some of your previous workers, so I can ask them about their experiences?	

report directed to the sending organization. A formal consent for release of confidential information should be obtained prior to release of such documentation. The report delineates salient health risks, appropriate management directives and preventive measures. Care will be enhanced if these conclusions and directives are discussed with the candidate, the one who must take ultimate responsibility for his/her health and personal development.

Transition from one's country of origin to an international setting necessitates a transition from a certain form of dependency on one's personal health-care provider to shared responsibility, requiring a level of reciprocity among the expatriates, health-care professionals and the agency. Frequently, expatriates will need to assume more responsibility for self-care. Health care professionals retained by the sending organization may assume the role of a health coach/consultant and the organization extends care by prudent placement, adherence to appropriate occupational and public health measures, and the provision of logistical support.

When complete, the health assessment should serve to:

- Establish a risk profile for each individual
- Enable appropriate management and deployment (corporate responsibility)
- Encourage the adoption of appropriate preventive measures and preparation (individual and corporate responsibility)
- Empower the individual to effect meaningful self care

Pre-departure medical assessment

There is no perfect assessment that will produce an outcome guaranteeing that an individual will make a successful transition and be interculturally effective; therefore a health assessment that is limited to a verdict stating that a person is fit or not fit is flawed. Less than 1% of candidates will be challenged to reconsider their decision based on new medical data gleaned from the pre-departure medical assessment. It is more appropriate to consider this assessment to be a more in-depth risk appraisal than that required for short-term travelers. The pre-departure assessment serves as an access point, allowing the health management team an opportunity to determine where a candidate is on the health continuum. The collective goal is to provide care and support so as to minimize the expatriate's health risks.

Because of the multinational nature of expatriate task forces it is difficult to establish one standard assessment protocol that can be uniformly applied to all jurisdictions. The minimum standard of care

for pre-departure assessments should ensure that each person has received care in accordance with the national guidelines in the candidate's country of origin. Additional testing, at the discretion of the agency's medical director, may be necessary depending on the nature and location of the assignment and/or government regulations that pertain to visa applications.

A comprehensive history thorough enough to provide a baseline profile of an individual's medical and mental health is the most essential component of the pre-departure health and risk assessment. The physical assessment and laboratory testing should focus on health concerns identified in the history as well as age and gender specific risk factors. Though one is encouraged to follow national guidelines, it is prudent to do so in the context of the location and duration of the proposed assignment. For example, a person may be scheduled for a screening colonoscopy in 2 years but assigned for 4 years to a location where colonoscopy is not available.

A complete report should include everything shown in Table 30.5.

Managing the outcome

If a person is medically stable there are very few conditions that would absolutely contraindicate an intercultural assignment. However, there are many pre-existing health conditions such as cardiac conditions, diabetes mellitus, inflammatory bowel disease and reactive airway disease that could suddenly change or be exacerbated by environmental conditions, geography (high altitude) or infectious diseases. The example in Table 30.6 will illustrate how the medical consultant can work with the agency and candidate to affect the best possible outcome.

Appropriate selective interventions for other target conditions such as diabetes mellitus, coronary artery disease, hypertension, osteoporosis and sexually transmitted diseases should be recommended in accordance to the standard of care in the applicant's country of origin. It is folly to assume that all primary care physicians have already uniformly applied these standards for all of their patients. Furthermore, one must not overlook the significance of an equivocal finding in a client who will be living in a remote setting where follow-up testing is not available.

A mammogram report read 'suspicious lesion in the left breast. Recommend follow-up in 3 months'. Though appropriate counsel in a setting with good access to care, this individual was assigned to a country that did not have mammography equipment. A lumpectomy was done prior to departure, revealing early intraductal cancer. Thus,

Table 30.5 A complete report

Record relevant positive findings
    History
    Positive physical findings (especially blood pressure)
    Dental records

Record abnormal laboratory findings (e.g., ECG)
Identify long-term problems that could jeopardize the well-being of the individual or compromise his capacity to complete the assignment (e.g. congestive cardiac failure)
Identify long-term problems where health management issues impact care or the nature and location of the assignment (e.g., asthma)
Delineate risk factors that should be monitored because of future implications (e.g., diabetes mellitus)   Record blood group and type
Record reaction to skin testing for tuberculosis
Record immunization status and relevant recommendations for geographic risk
Document recommendations for prophylaxis (especially malaria)
Delineate health and safety issues

Table 30.6	Example to illustrate how the medical consultant can work with the agency and candidate to affect the best possible outcome

An aid worker is assigned to a remote region where access to pharmaceuticals is limited and houses are heated with a low-grade coal. The history reveals that he has reactive airway disease, triggered by chemical irritants. Based on this history a more thorough, selective assessment was done to evaluate his reactive airway disease, which included a pulmonary function test. It was determined that the aid worker had moderate persistent asthma according to the National Asthma Education and Prevention Program.

After being apprised of the risks the management team and the applicant may re-evaluate their options: either reconsider this placement based on the information available or opt to proceed. If they opt to proceed the following must be in place:
    The medical consultant should prepare a plan that includes: recognition of early warning signs, guidelines to evaluate severity, how to administer appropriate therapy and when to call for help.

The management team must develop a plan to ensure that the directives can be followed. In this case study, they would ensure that resources are available to monitor the reactive airway disease, provide supplies of necessary medications and formulate an acceptable contingency plan in the event that this individual's condition deteriorates.

the consultation served the applicant by apprising her of a health risk and served the agency by delineating the responsibilities that were appropriate for the context of placement, services and support.

Pre-departure psychological assessment

As noted earlier, the importance of including a psychological assessment might be inferred from the fact that 20–40% of all expatriate managers return home early due to their inability to adjust to the new culture, and/or their poor performance in that culture. Moreover, nearly half of those who do *not* return early function below their normal level of productivity while working as expatriates.[10] These figures do not appear to be restricted to managers, as similar results have been reported for all overseas employees.[15] Personal and family stress is thought to be the primary causes of early repatriation.[16] Therefore, it is recommended that candidates for intercultural assignments have a pre-departure psychological assessment.

A pre-departure psychological assessment will:

■ Indicate how the candidate is likely to be affected by living and working in a different culture
■ Evaluate the spousal relationship and the potential impact on adjustment
■ Evaluate the impact of the family's transition on the children
■ Determine where there is a vulnerability to psychological disorders
■ Determine where coping mechanisms may be inadequate (e.g., alcohol or substance abuse)
■ Foster a model of dialog and open communication
■ Guide personnel managers in their training programs to maximize the probability that the candidate will adjust well
■ Assist in determining the need for and/or type of psychometric testing
■ Guide personnel managers in their selection process and provide support should they conclude that an international placement is not appropriate

Psychological interview

The recommendation is that a psychological assessment should be part of the selection procedure for every assignment. This assessment should take place early enough in the recruitment process to allow it to influence decisions, and should not be left until the day before the person gets on the plane, by which time it is much more difficult to stop the process.

Even if the applicant has worked overseas previously, there should be a re-assessment before every new assignment. One study found that approximately 25% of people who were applying for a new short-term expatriate position, having already worked as expatriates previously, were suffering from depression or another psychological condition.[9] Clinical observation also supports the view that applicants with clinical disorders are sometimes accepted for re-assignments without further psychological screening, to the detriment of them-selves and those who have to support them in their post.

If a couple will be moving overseas together, it is useful to interview them both separately and then together, even if only one of them will be working. One of the predictors of an expatriate's adjustment is the spouse's adjustment.[16] If the couple has children, it is useful to assess the whole family. Concern about the children is a common cause of early return, and potential problems might be identified during the assessment, avoiding much distress later on (Table 30.7).

Psychological interview – when there is no time or expertise

Sending organizations do not all subscribe to a 'Code of Best Practice' and many do not assume responsibility to ensure that appropriate assessments are part of pre-departure preparation. In the event that time is limited or a team of counselors with expertise in this discipline is not readily available, a 'triage' approach could be adopted. All candidates should be privileged with an opportunity to explore the salient issues, which could impact them in a personal way, in the context of their own unique person and psychological makeup. Should any risk factors become apparent, every effort should be made to ensure that those individuals have an opportunity to meet with someone who does have expertise in this field.

An abbreviated psychological interview: salient issues

■ current mental state (e.g., any current symptoms of depression)
■ current stressors, what causes them stress and how they handle it (e.g., illness in family, aging parents, recent bereavements/traumas etc.)
■ history of psychiatric or psychological problems (including depression, eating problems, self-harm, alcohol or drug misuse, psychotic experiences)
■ symptoms of traumatic stress or other anxiety conditions (obsessive-compulsive tendencies, phobias, panic attacks)
■ any psychological treatment, counseling, anti-depressant medication or other psychiatric treatment received

Table 30.7	Topics for a thorough psychological interview (allow for about 90 min)

The candidate's childhood and adolescence

Education and employment up to the current day, including reasons for leaving jobs

Strengths and coping mechanisms

Weaknesses, and areas of vulnerability

What causes them stress and how they handle it

How they deal with anger and frustration

Their motivation for applying for the post

Their expectations about the job and living in a different country

Any previous experience of working in other countries

Traumatic incidents (including abuse)

Interpersonal relationships (how they get on with people)

Their support network

How flexible they are

Alcohol/ drug use

Eating patterns and exercise habits, and how they will feel if these have to change (e.g., unable to exercise as they like to)

History of psychiatric or psychological problems (including depression; obsessive-compulsive tendencies; phobias; panic attacks; symptoms of traumatic stress or other anxiety conditions; eating problems; self-harm; alcohol or drug misuse; psychotic experiences). Any psychological treatment, counseling, anti-depressant medication or other psychiatric treatment received. Current mental state (e.g., any current symptoms of depression)

Family psychiatric history

Psychosexual history, if this is deemed an appropriate topic to consider (e.g., If HIV risk is high in the area of work)

Current adjustment to their singleness, marriage or other relationships

Current stressors (e.g., illness in family; aging parents; recent bereavements/traumas etc.)

■ alcohol/ drug use
■ family psychiatric history

Managing the outcome

A psychological assessment can be used to provide recommendations, which will help to maximize the probability that the candidate will adjust well. Knowledge of vulnerabilities can assist in placement, and highlight any special support which might be beneficial. In some cases it is wise to advise delaying the move until there has been time to engage in language study, cross-cultural training, personal or marital therapy, or address some other issue to ensure that the person goes with the right tools and leaves behind unhelpful 'baggage'. It may also be advisable to recommend a delay if the candidate has suffered from a recent bereavement or relationship breakdown. Moving to a new culture inevitably involves losses, and to add these losses to pre-existing ones can be overwhelming. Moreover, returning home at the end of an assignment can be especially difficult if the candidate left shortly after a bereavement before getting used to 'home' without the loved one.

Candidates who have a past history of psychological difficulties need not be automatically excluded from expatriate positions. Those who have successfully overcome past difficulties and have developed more effective ways of coping may adjust and perform well as expatriates. However, where there is a vulnerability to psychological disorders, either due to personal history or family history, this should be carefully assessed. Foyle et al.,[1] found that affective disorders among expatriates were associated with a past personal history of depressed mood, and a family history of suicide, psychosis, personality disorder or neuroses. They concluded that:

'Those with heavily loaded family and personal psychiatric histories should not be accepted for overseas service unless there is clear evidence that they have remained well for several years, have a good work record in their home country, and have shown a capacity for coping in general, and for maintaining good interpersonal relationships. There must also be good personal and medical support in the locations to which they will go'.

The role of psychometric testing

Some assessors like to use psychometric tests as part of the assessment. These can add useful information when used alongside a clinical interview, but should not replace the interview. One advantage of such tests is that the candidate's score can be compared with standardized scores. Some assessors find it easier to justify a decision on the basis of an objective number than on the basis of a subjective 'intuition' following an interview. Some psychometric tests are effective in terms of time and expense, especially if they can be sent to the candidate and scored relatively quickly, perhaps by computer. On the negative side, tests can provide a false sense of security. Many psychological factors are useful in predicting how an expatriate is likely to adjust and perform overseas, and no one test covers all of these aspects.

Little empirical research has been conducted on the effectiveness of psychological tests for predicting expatriate adjustment. The limited research which has been performed has mainly concerned the use of the Minnesota Multiphasic Personality Inventory (MMPI),[17] which is the most widely used personality test. The MMPI has been effectively used in some areas of personnel selection.[18] It provides a broad range of information about psychological disorders and normal personality traits. Norms exist for people of different backgrounds and cultures.[19] If one perceives that there is a need for psychometric testing it is prudent to select professionals familiar with the use of this instrument in the prediction of expatriate adjustment.[20,21] Though it appears to be self-evident, the fact that many continue to interpret MMPI scores with minimal training make it necessary to reinforce that these tests should be interpreted by someone with expertise, training and an understanding of the inherent deficiencies.[22]

When making a referral to a psychologist, clearly identify the issues that are of greatest concern. Are they being assigned to a hardship post, a leadership role for a field staff that forced the resignation of the last leader or is it a politically sensitive region that makes diplomatic skills an essential prerequisite? Have they recently recovered from an addiction to alcohol? A screening method, which is useful for one type of post, may be of little value for another post. Some tests can help screen out people with psychological disorders, while other tests help to identify strengths and weaknesses, or interests and values. These tests can assist in deciding where an individual will best be placed, in terms of the location and the role that they are best suited to.

PRE-DEPARTURE: PREPARATION

Many expatriates report feeling under-prepared for their international assignment,[23] which can only add to their levels of stress and uncertainty. One cannot assume that guidelines prepared by the sending organizations will be comprehensive and current nor can one assume that personnel have been adequately prepared if they have seen their local health practitioner.[24,25] Personnel managers from 42 leading Non Government Aid Organizations responded to a survey of infection control policies for bloodborne viruses as shown in Table 30.8.[26]

A comprehensive preparation program could help to reduce both psychological and medical problems with the potential benefit of ameliorating the impact of attrition among expatriates. See Fawcett (1999) for further briefing guidelines.[27] When preparing your material ask yourself 3 practical questions:

1 Is it likely to happen?
2 Will your audience recognize the issues when they happen?
3 Is there a meaningful solution or management option if it does happen?

A careful review of the data in section 2 will serve as a guide to that which is relevant based on current literature. In addition, include a discussion on geographic risk factors, occupational health and safety issues, disease specific risks and practical tips on stress management. Most of the guidelines in this book that apply to the short-term traveler will also apply to expatriates. The reader is referred to the other chapters that deal more specifically with these subjects.

Table 30.8	Survey of infection control policies for bloodborne viruses[26]	
		(%)
Health is the sole responsibility of the expatriate themselves		42.3
Health is the sole responsibility of the local staff		56.5
No information was provided regarding bloodborne pathogens		11.5
Did not evaluate hepatitis B vaccine status pre-departure		53.8
Supplied hepatitis B post-exposure prophylaxis		24%
Supplied HIV post-exposure prophylaxis		16%
Did not have a policy regarding HIV post-exposure prophylaxis		72.7

Immunizations

Immunization counsel is thoroughly addressed in Chapter 10. However, there are some issues that are particularly relevant for the expatriate community and will be briefly addressed.

Hepatitis B

Hepatitis B is an established risk for expatriates, primarily but not confined to risks that pertain to occupation and sexual activity. Given the very low potential for adverse outcomes, the efficacy of the vaccine and the relatively low cost, universal immunization for the expatriate task force can readily be justified.[28,29]

Encephalitis

Japanese encephalitis B and tick-borne encephalitis

Expatriates dwelling in urban settings are generally not advised to receive vaccines against encephalitis even if endemic in the rural areas. However, the cumulative risk of exposure may warrant administration of the three dose series.

Rabies

Countries at greatest risk include Asia, Africa and Latin America. Most post exposure treatment is for canine bites though the risk should be considered for most mammalian bites. Post exposure treatment should closely parallel the risk of exposure that is approximately 1 per 1000 volunteers per month among expatriates living in rabies enzootic regions.[30] In Nepal the risk among expatriates was noted to be higher than that noted among tourists. The limited data available suggest that in the majority of cases management is sub-optimal.[31] The risk of children being bitten is conservatively estimated to be four times greater than that of adults. Furthermore, the bites in children are usually higher on the trunk or face and are more severe or, conversely, minimized and neglected.

Specifically, counsel expatriates assigned to rabies enzootic regions and recommend pre-exposure rabies vaccination to the following:

- Families with children
- Families with pets
- Personnel with limited access to care and transportation
- Personnel in countries where access to Human or Purified Equine Rabies Immune Globulin and/or modern tissue culture vaccines is limited
- Personnel who visit or travel into remote regions or explore caves for work or recreation
- Personnel who will be working with animals, e.g. veterinarians

Expatriates should 'street proof' their children to prevent animal bites:

- Never approach an unfamiliar animal
- Remain motionless when approached by an unfamiliar dog
- If knocked over, roll into a ball and lie still
- Stay away from any animal displaying unusual behavior
- Do not pet an animal that is in a cage, crate or pen
- Do not try to separate pets if attacked by other animals
- If bitten, report it immediately to an adult and for treatment details refer to Chapter 46.

Malaria

Risk factors

Malaria (see Chapters 12–15 for details) is the leading cause of death among expatriates who died from infectious diseases and continues to pose a threat in sub-Saharan Africa, PNG and Papua (Irian Jaya) where the rate of malaria is at least 10-fold greater than in other malarious coun-tries.[32] The incidence of malaria in expatriates ranges from 31/1000 per year in Asia to 209/1000 per year in West Africa, a rough estimate because:

- Not all personnel will report their illness
- Self-diagnosis is based on a fever without laboratory testing
- False positive reports from laboratories in developing countries are as high as 75%[33]

Myths and practices among expatriates

Persons who provide pre-departure counsel to expatriates should understand that personnel living in endemic regions often disregard counsel from travel medicine consultants who live in malaria-free countries. Many of the 'experts' are not trained physicians, provide counsel without an understanding of the literature, and may rely completely on their anecdotal experience. For example, a recent survey showed that pyrimethamine is among the most popular regimens in Africa.

Personal protection measures are overlooked. In one study, only 38% of expatriates screened doors and windows, 53% used mosquito netting and less than 20% treat their nets with insecticides. Less than 75% of expatriates will take the recommended regimen and frequently change their medication without seeking appropriate counsel.[34] Many will judge the efficacy of their choice based on their personal experience as well. Those who do not contract malaria will assert that their regimen was effective even if their choice was pyrimethamine whereas others, who have false positive malaria smears or undiagnosed fever will conclude that the mefloquine they were taking, is ineffective. Unfortunately, misdiagnosis has resulted in some personnel switching from an effective to an ineffective prophylactic regimen, a practice directly implicated in the recent death of one Canadian missionary.

Malaria and pregnancy

Pregnant women have to understand that they are the main group of adults at risk for malaria. Susceptibility to malaria increases during the second and third trimesters, reaching its peak during the first 60 days postpartum. *Plasmodium falciparum* infection during pregnancy increases the risk of abortion, maternal anemia, intrauterine growth retardation, prematurity, and stillbirth and is a risk factor for neonatal death. Therefore, it could be argued that the risks that pertain to the use of mefloquine or other commonly accepted regimens are far less than that posed by malaria. Likewise, mosquito repellents including DEET are safe in the context of risk. However, one survey of pregnant expatriates demonstrated that many pregnant expatriates stop their prophylaxis or change to an inferior regimen during pregnancy.

Malaria prevention in children

Children and adolescents are at special risk of malaria, perhaps because of poor compliance or inaccurate calculation of the dose,[33] and they may rapidly become seriously ill. Babies, including breast-fed infants, and children should be well protected against mosquito bites and receive malaria chemoprophylaxis. Children are at greater risk than adults for DEET toxicity though the complications recorded in the literature, which includes seizures among other central nervous system abnormalities, are very rare.

Chemoprophylaxis

Guidelines on the prevention of malaria in expatriates should not deviate significantly from standard guidelines (see Chapter 13). Most experts concede that mefloquine is the preferred antimalarial in regions where chloroquine resistance is well established when convenience, cost and efficacy are the primary considerations. However, in a study that involved 1200 persons from a broad sector of the expatriate community working in sub-Saharan Africa, only 3% continued to use mefloquine primarily because of concerns regarding neuropsychiatric side-effects.

Mefloquine is the least popular among expatriates, primarily because of the fear of neuro-psychiatric side-effects. Many express concern about long-term safety though data to date, primarily from Peace Corp Volunteers, demonstrate improved tolerance over time. Most expatriates can afford it though cost is not usually a consideration.

Expatriates rarely use doxycycline, in part because many are uncomfortable using antibiotics for extended periods of time. Dermatologists have the most safety data, however when prescribed for acne it is provided usually at a lower dose. Compliance is the most significant limitation from a medical perspective.

Atovaquone/Proguanil (Malarone) will have a limited role with expatriates. Personnel who live in malaria-free enclaves but venture overnight for short periods of time into endemic regions are most likely to benefit from this drug because they can start immediately prior to the trip and discontinue it one week later. Cost will be the limiting factor for most if it is approved for long-term prophylaxis.

The chloroquine and proguanil combination is the most popular regimen among expatriates despite spreading chloroquine and proguanil resistance. Though reported adverse events approximate that of mefloquine, the frequency of neuropsychiatric side-effects was lower and probably accounts for the preference for that combination. Mouth ulcers are frequently reported, probably secondary to proguanil.

Primaquine is a second line option, rarely recommended unless other effective alternatives have been exhausted. Efficacy and safety data are limited though it appears to be as effective as doxycycline, and was proven to be safe in personnel who used it up to a year. All personnel who use primaquine should have a G6PD level measured because the drug is a very potent oxidizing agent.

Dapsone and pyrimethamine (Maloprim) and pyrimethamine (Daraprim) alone are also popular, but the use of both of these regimens is discouraged because of widespread resistance. At least one Canadian missionary died while using dapsone and pyrimethamine for prophylaxis.

Self-diagnosis

Self-diagnostic kits have proven to be accurate and reliable in the hands of laboratory workers but less accurate in the hands of travelers.[35] Expatriates are highly motivated, are in settings of risk for longer periods of time, have very limited access to quality laboratory services and are accustomed to assuming responsibility for self-treatment. Therefore, this population may prove to be an appropriate subset of travelers to select for training. Self-diagnosis with reliable kits could prove to be one of the major advances for the management of malaria among expatriates (see Chapter 14).

Self-treatment

Self-treatment (see Chapter 14) implies that access to expert supervision is limited. Though it is an option that many expatriates are comfortable with, there are pitfalls. Many will assert that they can distinguish malaria from other infectious diseases based on the symptoms that they have grown to associate with malaria. Common expatriate practices that could lead to harm include using the same drug for treatment that they were using for prevention, using an effective drug for prevention but an inferior drug for treatment, and administering the dose that has been recommended for semi-immunes rather than that recommended for non-immunes, especially the newer artesunate derivatives and the use of single agents in chloroquine resistant zones.

It is currently estimated that 90% of global episodes of clinical malaria and deaths occur in sub-Saharan Africa; therefore expatriates and team leaders assigned to that region, where widespread chloroquine and multi-drug resistant malaria is a particular threat, should be selected for self-treatment training. Safety, efficacy and drug tolerance must also be considered priorities when selecting medication. The Roll Back Malaria Program advocates the use of fixed combination therapy to improve compliance and efficacy and to reduce errors and the emergence of drug resistance.

Tuberculosis

It is estimated that between the years 2000 and 2020, nearly one billion people will be newly infected and 70 million will die if control is not strengthened. Also of concern is the exponential development of multi-drug resistant tuberculosis.

The risk of latent mycobacterium tuberculosis is about 3% per year for aid workers and missionaries working in refugee camps, in long-term health and development, or in urban health programs. However, none are exempt including children attending public or boarding schools where the risk of latent TB is about 2%.[36]

The European and North American guidelines are distinctly different. In the UK, BCG vaccination is offered to those without contraindications or a previous exposure or immunization, going to a developing country or high-risk location or occupation for more than 1 month. In North America, BCG is not usually recommended for adults; however, many advocate the immunization of children under 5, primarily to prevent disseminated disease. Recent studies suggest that current strains of BCG have been over-attenuated and thus may be less effective than they were during earlier trials.[37]

Diarrheal diseases

Diarrheal diseases related to bacterial infections consistently account for the majority of reported illnesses among expatriates. Expatriates who reside in 'high risk communities' for less than 2 years are likely to experience attack rates similar to that of short-term travelers, though the severity may gradually decrease over time.[38] There is both regional and seasonal variation in the attack rate and etiological agents; therefore expatriate families should be instructed in both self-treatment protocols and should be made familiar with the varied presentations and seasonality to ensure that the most appropriate regimen is applied to their situation.

Preventive measures include: strict adherence to basic hygiene principles, especially hand washing for household food handlers and employees in addition to standard counsel regarding water purification and food precautions (see Chapter 16 for details).

Risk behavior

Excessive alcohol consumption (see Chapter 35) and a high rate of extramarital sexual activity are common among certain groups of expatriates.[39] Peer pressure and expectations, loss of norms, boredom, stress, loneliness, separation from the social support network, spousal separation or avoidance strategies are among reasons cited for these behavioral changes.

Sexually transmitted diseases

Sexually transmitted diseases have historically proven to be a major public health challenge. Travelers and expatriates, reflecting norms in their countries of origin, are no exception. In Great Britain males are more prone to having non-monogamous relationships when compared with their female counterparts; 31.2% of men and 21.4% of women had formed new heterosexual or homosexual partnerships in the past year and in Greater London the mean number of lifetime heterosexual partners is 15.5 and 7.3 for males and females, respectively.[40] A study of approximately 900 Dutch expatriates living in four different geographic regions showed that 41% of males and 31% of females reported having sex with casual or steady local partners. Of concern is the inconsistent use of condoms especially among those who had two or more partners, which in Great Britain peaked at 33% for males, and 24% for females; likewise, in many cases expatriates do not consistently use condoms during sexual activity.[41]

HIV

HIV transmission is primarily related to occupational hazards and sexual activity. The mean occupational risk of HIV was 0.11%/person per year among Dutch medics.[42] HIV transmission is extremely rare in some groups whereas well documented among Belgian advisers and European expatriates working in AIDS endemic areas. Denial appears to be one of the impediments to compliance to prevention guidelines. In Great Britain only 4% of those at increased risk for HIV transmission judged that they were so. The rate among expatriates is expected to increase, given the explosive increase in HIV infection in many parts of the world where expatriates work, increased occupational exposure and behavioral patterns that include inconsistent use of condoms.

Expatriates may need pre-departure HIV testing and counsel:
- for visa applications
- to assess employer liability if personnel return HIV positive after their assignment
- as part of a bloodborne pathogen control program
- for eligibility to join a trusted donor blood group (Walking Blood Bank)

Infection control policies

Guidelines for post-exposure prophylaxis following an occupational health exposure have been carefully developed and are constantly under review (http://www.cdc.gov/ncidod/hip/guide). The guidelines that pertain to sexual assault have been developed based on the same principles though there are no data to support the recommendations (http://www.cdc.gov/hiv/pubs/facts/petfact.htm). Kits are increasingly available, especially where the risk of occupational exposure is high. Recommendations regarding drug combinations will change periodically as new guidelines are established.

Basic principles include:
- sending organizations should develop policies regarding all bloodborne pathogens
- pre-departure training should be provided
- provisions and protocols should be established for rape and/or sexual exposure, and occupational exposure
- protocols should be regularly updated in accordance in International Guidelines

Health briefing – possible structure

Most personnel assigned to an international setting will have at least one private consultation with a travel medicine specialist specifically for vaccines, skin testing for tuberculosis and malaria counsel. However, time constraints will limit the scope of that encounter. Group sessions are often a very manageable and cost-effective approach to the educational component of preparation, especially for personnel assigned through a sending organization that will be deploying others to an international setting. Web based educational modules will prove to be a viable and cost-effective medium for education.

The curriculum should include:

- Vaccine counsel
- Basic hygiene and sanitation: food and water preparation, sewage disposal
- Injury prevention and security
- Self-management of the commonest medical ailments:
  - Diarrhea
  - Respiratory tract infections
  - Malaria
  - Skin diseases
- Sexual health
- General health: sleep, diet, exercise, rest and relaxation, alcohol use
- Personal Medical Supplies and emergency Kits
- How to select health-care providers

Health briefing – 'the extended family'

Many will choose to hire persons to provide 'domestic support' in the international setting and in essence they become part of the 'extended family'. It is prudent to prepare personnel to consider the impact that that could have on the health status of members of the family. Areas of concern include infectious diseases such as tuberculosis, blood borne pathogens, and enteric pathogens as well as public health issues including food and water preparation and sanitation.

Psychological training and preparation

As mentioned earlier it is very important that expatriates learn, before they go overseas, that certain signs of stress and 'culture shock' are normal among expatriates (see Chapter 35). They should be encouraged to accept as normal any mild stress-related symptoms (e.g., sleeping problems, poor concentration, fatigue, tearfulness, irritability, weight changes, indecisiveness etc.). They may experience emotions more intensely than they ever have before, and others around them may be very emotional too. Should they experience such symptoms, they should be 'kind to themselves', taking time to relax and do things they enjoy, and they should talk (or e-mail or write) to someone about their experiences, rather than keeping them to themselves. If they can accept such feelings as normal, given the situation, they are likely to feel better much more quickly than if they think they should not feel that way.

Information and general counsel

As part of the preparation package, expatriates should receive information about where they can go for help should any symptoms of stress persist or become more severe. For mild difficulties, self-help books and information (available over the Internet) may be sufficient. In more severe cases, consultation with a mental health professional should be arranged. Ideally, organizations should obtain information about mental health services in the area, and how they can be accessed, before the expatriate arrives. Professional help should certainly be sought in cases of psychoses, severe depression, suicidal ideation, anorexia nervosa, post-traumatic stress disorder, serious difficulties with a child (including the possibility of abuse), or any mental health problem which appears to be getting much worse. If other people are suffering (e.g., because the individual is acting in violent or unsafe ways, or has a personality disorder that is causing difficulties within the community), outside help should be sought. Many other conditions may also benefit from professional help, and the expatriate should be encouraged to seek such help at an early stage. It is better to err on the side of caution and seek professional help if one is not sure. If appropriate treatment is not available locally, there may be a need for repatriation. A local medical professional may be able to liaise with the organization in such cases. The expatriate should be helped to accept that repatriation because of psychological difficulties

is no more a sign of failure than repatriation due to physical problems i.e. a psychological illness is an illness, and not a character fault (on psychiatric disorders, see Chapter 35).

Preparatory information can be given during a 'stress briefing' (or 'health briefing') session. This can be achieved through independent private consultations or through group sessions that are specifically designed to maximize the chances of maintaining good emotional and physical health while working in another country. Such a briefing is especially important if this will be the first experience of living in a different culture. Two handouts for use in such briefings are shown in Tables 30.9 and 30.10.

Stress briefing – possible structure

- If they have worked in similar situations before, it is useful to start by asking what they found most stressful, what their reactions were, and what helped them.
- Whether or not it is their first cross-cultural placement, it is helpful to discuss what they expect *this* placement will be like. (Unrealistic expectations can be a major cause of stress. The individual should be warned not to expect that this trip will be similar to any previous assignment. Encourage them to exchange unrealistic expectations for realistic ones. Unmet expectations are a common cause of frustration, and modifying them in advance can reduce difficulties later on).
- What do they think might be stressful or difficult this time? Discuss in detail how they are likely to cope. (Change is itself a cause of stress).
- When they are under stress, how does it generally affect them?
- How have they coped with previous stressful experiences? What have they learned that might be helpful this time?
- What will they do to relax?
- What social support network do they have? (If they have few close relationships, how can they build up a stronger network of friends?) Who will they talk to if they feel low or under stress? Who will they contact if they have *significant* problems? (Ensure there is a named person).
- Discuss stress management techniques and help them identify strategies which they might find useful (e.g., exercise, expressing feelings in a diary/letters, reading, listening to music, getting away from their base, talking to others). Will they take anything with them to enable them to do these things (e.g., music tapes)?
- What hours do they expect to work, and how often do they plan to have a day off? Encourage sufficient time to rest and relax – that is essential, not optional when living in a different culture. Excessive working hours contribute to the difficulties, which can cause premature return. If they have a specific plan for taking time off, they are less likely to be 'sucked in' to over-working. (If the expatriate is not going alone, but will be accompanied by partner and/or family, it is especially important that they make time to spend with their partner or family).
- How do they feel about the organization? What support is available?
- What are their views on security arrangements? Are they likely to adhere to guidelines (e.g., if evacuation is recommended)?
- Thinking ahead, encourage them to have a debriefing when they return 'home' at the end of their placement, and sufficient time off before resuming work.

Further preparation

Encourage the candidate to seek further information or training if this will not be provided and you judge that it is likely to be useful. For instance, depending on their experience and the location, it may be appropriate to recommend that they receive additional information about any of the following.

Table 30.9   Handout: 'Before you go'

Before you go

Most expatriate workers report finding life in a different culture enriching, and a positive experience overall. However, that does not mean that working in a foreign country is not problematic, or that it is easy to readjust to life at home afterwards. People who are well prepared before they go often gain the most from living in a different culture.

Preparing to go

1. Think about what difficulties you might encounter, and how you plan to deal with these. Problems can be tackled more easily when you have thought in advance about how you might handle them. With planning, it may be possible to avoid some problems. Talk over your main concerns with someone, particularly someone who has been in a similar situation

2. Try to find out as much as you can about the culture before you go. Different attitudes towards time, decisions, goals, ethics and values may cause frustration. If you are prepared for such differences, you are likely to be able to recognize and accept them more easily. Finding out about local customs will also make it less likely that you will offend people. It is definitely worth learning some basic words in a local language before you go. Remember that everyone makes mistakes.

3. Well in advance of traveling, find out about any health precautions you will need to take, and ensure you stick to these. It's not worth taking risks with dirty water, unprotected sexual activity, neglecting vaccinations or antimalarial precautions etc.

4. Feeling isolated and unsupported increases stress. Before you go, build up a 'support network' - people you will be able to rely on to support you. While you are away from home, keep the network alive by communicating with your family and friends, and letting them know how they can continue to show support (e.g., if there is anything you would like them to send you). If possible, invite close friends or family members to come and visit you while you are abroad, so that they gain a fuller picture of what life is like for you there, and are able to share in some of your rich experiences. Also make time to build up friendships in your new location, whether with local people or other expatriates.

5. Make a list of things you like to do for enjoyment and relaxation. Plan to do as many of these as you can while you are away. Ensure you pack any equipment you will need (e.g., novels to read; favorite music to listen to; sports equipment).

6. Think about the signs you show when you are under stress. (Some people have headaches or back ache; others lose their appetite or 'comfort eat'; some have sleeping difficulties; some become irritable). Become aware of your response to stress, so that you will recognize when you feel stressed and you can take steps to lighten the load and relax a bit more. If you have time and think it will be useful, learn about stress management techniques, or buy a relaxation tape.

Table 30.10   Handout: health & stress management strategies for expats

1. Remember that it takes time to adjust to a new culture. Do not expect to fit in straight away.
2. We are all more vulnerable when we are tired. Ensure that you get enough rest. Take at least 1 day off work each week, and have regular holidays. People who work 'all the hours' are at risk of burnout. Make sure that you fit leisure time into each week. Leisure is not an optional extra, it is a necessary ingredient for health.
3. Moderate exercise (such as walking) is good for both mental health and spiritual health. Make time to be active in ways you enjoy (and are possible and safe in your new location).
4. Avoid too much alcohol, caffeine or nicotine, as these can increase symptoms of stress.
5. Look after your health
    eat a balanced diet; drinking plenty of water
    avoid excessive exposure to sun
    accidents are more likely when you are tired, so
        take enough rest
        take special care when driving
        do not drive at night
        do not 'drink and drive'
    Adhere to the malaria prevention guidelines
        If a change is necessary, seek the wisdom of an expert in that area
6. If you become ill, take enough time off to recuperate, rather than trying to continue working while unwell.
7. If other people have unrealistic expectations of you, discuss the situation with them. Check out any information that seems ambiguous or unclear. Don't be afraid to ask questions.
8. Relationship problems can be especially stressful when you are cut off from your normal circle of family and friends. If a problem arises, try to speak about it objectively with the person concerned, and see if you can resolve it. Try to give encouragement to others when possible.
9. Maintain regular contact with friends at home. This can make life more pleasant while you are away, and ease the transition when you return home.
10. Some people find it helpful to record their thoughts and feelings in a journal or in letters. Research suggests that this can be good for your physical health as well as your emotional well-being! Solutions to problems may emerge as you write.
11. If you are used to being an expert, it can be difficult to suddenly become a newcomer who has to learn new ways of doing things. Acknowledging this frustration and trying to be patient can make it easier to bear.
12. Remember that it is completely normal to experience some signs of stress when living in a different culture. Most expatriates have times when they have problems concentrating or sleeping; become unusually irritable; feel overwhelmed; feel tearful or low; have difficulty making decisions; experience changes in their appetite, etc. If you experience such symptoms, remind yourself that this is a normal part of the adjustment process. Let people know that you are feeling under stress. Recognizing your limitations is a sign of strength, not a sign of weakness. It is best to acknowledge and deal with stress early on, so that it does not escalate.
13. Seek professional help if any symptoms of stress persist for more than a few weeks, or if they start to interfere with your ability to work or to function well. Also seek help if you find that you are drinking excessive amounts of alcohol as a way of coping.
14. Try to maintain your sense of humour, and have some fun!

Culture shock and cultural adaptation

Learning as much as possible about the culture in advance can make the transition easier (and in a few cases, leads candidates to decline the job opportunity, as they realize it would not be appropriate for them) (see Table 30.11).

Security issues and evacuation policies

Many expatriates are at increased risk of experiencing traumatic incidents, perhaps related to terrorist bombing, war situations, evacuations, hostage taking, rape, robbery, riots, violence, traffic accidents, or natural disasters. Training in crisis management is relevant, at least for team leaders. Expatriates report that they were glad that they were prepared for the worst, because if it happened they had already thought through how to deal with it, and if it didn't happen their time overseas was even better than they had expected (Table 30.12).

Interpersonal skills

Interpersonal issues are common causes of frustration and attrition among expatriates. Training in problem solving skills, negotiation techniques and conflict resolution can be effective in reducing stress and attrition and enhancing productivity. Some organizations have also found it beneficial to teach potential expatriates about personality differences or cross-cultural differences, in order to help expatriates understand themselves and others better.[43]

Family dynamics

If children will be included in the move, it is important to help the parents understand how to make the cross-cultural transition successful for their children.

'Solo Expatriates'

Much of what has been written assumes that the expatriate is working through an agency that has a moral and legal obligation to provide minimum logistical support for their international employees. Many embark on such adventures without the benefits of that support struc-ture in place. Though the principles apply, there will not be a formal structure to ensure that the details are cared for. For the 'Solo Expat', Table 30.13 has recommendations that will ensure adequate support.

CARING FOR EXPATRIATES IN INTERNATIONAL SETTINGS

The health status of this select group of people is likely to be skewed toward the 'healthy' side of the health continuum because of self-selection and to some extent because of the health pre-requisites that were determined by the sending organization. Nevertheless, not all will be in perfect health and obviously not all will remain healthy and some health issues will be exposed in the crucible of the intercultural experience. Sieveking[44] counseled us to remember that, 'Regardless of how valid our selection is, and how thorough our orientation, most any employee will encounter difficulties ... we can never leave even the best employee alone' (pp. 201–202). It has been reported that expatriates who feel very confident in company support, will adjust better than those who feel uncertainty and stress about their future; therefore, it is reasonable to conclude that the care extended to expatriates will contribute to a successful transition.

Models of care

- Self-reliant staff who develop their own network of health-care providers
- Reliance on national health-care providers who have received international training and who are familiar with the culture the home country
- International clinics staffed by persons who are also members of that expatriate community
- Clinics staffed by members of the same organization (mission hospitals)
- Reliance on networks that have been established through the effort of the sending organization's administrative staff or by contacts made by previous members of the expatriate community (e.g., embassy networks for their personnel)

Self-care

The emphasis on a 'continuous flow of care' is ideal, but almost an oxymoron when applied to a globally mobile population with varied options for communication, resources and access to health care systems. One could approximate a flow of care if all that was invested in

---

Table 30.11	Cultural adaptation: stages of adjustment

1. Before you go: Anticipation and anxiety.
2. When you first arrive: A 'honeymoon' period, when everything is new and interesting – it is an adventure.
3. The honeymoon comes to an end: You may miss home, and become depressed, irritable and anxious. Everything may seem too much effort. Remember that these feelings are normal and will pass.
4. Adjustment: The new culture begins to feel like home. You are able to enjoy your experiences again.
5. Leaving: Saying goodbyes can be difficult.
6. Readjustment when you return home: You may experience 'reverse culture shock', feeling that you no longer quite 'fit' back in your own culture. For example, the supermarkets may seem overwhelmingly big; people may appear unfriendly, you may feel isolated or that no-one really understands what your life abroad has been like. You may feel very tired, so try to take sufficient time off work. Feeling low is common and will pass with time – do not tell yourself that you are 'over reacting'.

In each stage you can aim to manage stress through:
- S   Social support (family and friends)
- T   Talk, do not bottle feelings up
- R   Rest and relax
- E   Exercise, and eat sensibly
- S   Sleep enough
- S   Sing, laugh, or do whatever else you enjoy

Table 30.12	Crisis management package

Measures to prevent crises wherever possible:
- being alert to potential danger
- taking precautions to enhance safety
- knowledge of established policies and procedures
- how to access extra resources during a crisis

Stress management skills that train expatriates under duress to:
- stay calm during the crisis
- emphasize the importance of not 'switching off' or abandoning hope during a crisis
- engage in active problem solving
- anticipate, believing that there is some way out (associated with a reduction in negative psychological after-effects)
- make use of 'defusing' (informal support between colleagues) in the hours after the incident
- gain further support if required

the 'screening assessments' was viewed as the foundation upon which management strategies for care were built, rather than isolating the assessment to a bureaucratic process that serves no other purpose than to flag 'high risk candidates'. Pre-departure assessments could have a value added component if we were to view that step to be similar to the work of a 'financial planner'. If the health information gleaned during the assessment was reorganized and transferred back to the 'patient-provider', the 'patient-provider' could be trained to

Table 30.13	Recommendations that will ensure adequate support for the 'Solo Expat'

Research your chosen country and location
- Community available for your spouse (if applicable)
- Educational facilities for children
- Health facilities and access to tertiary care
- Sanitation standards and facilities for water purification
- Communication systems
- Evaluate the job opportunities
- Develop a contingency plan

Schedule an appointment with your primary health-care provider
- Request a health evaluation, projecting your needs for the chosen term
- Request copies of relevant material
- Seek counsel regarding health surveillance while away
- Ensure that you have an adequate supply of medication
- Inquire regarding openness to interaction while away

Seek a referral to a Psychologist aware of intercultural dynamics
- Review salient issues that pertain to personal well-being
- Discuss
  - Spousal relationship
  - Interaction with children
  - Adaptation and re-entry

Have a dental check-up and copies of your dental records

Find adequate health insurance
- Covers pre-existing illnesses
  - Ensure that the 'limit' is adequate
- Evacuation insurance
  - Explore the impact of evacuation on family members
  - Details of evacuation support
  - Contact numbers in event of emergency

Visit a travel medicine specialist
- Immunization
- Malaria counsel
- Schedule a longer visit to discuss specific geographic risk factors

Seek out counsel of other expats who have domiciled in that country
- Identify facilities that can be part of your support network
- Identify support groups such as 'Expat Moms'
After arrival report to your Embassy

become the key resource for the model that puts emphasis on a 'continuous flow of care'. The pre-departure preparation would in essence become part of the training for effective self-care in the international setting.

Disease management consultants in the USA estimate that self-care, defined as diagnosing and managing medical symptoms without a health-care professional, account for at least 80% of the care that is provided. It has been documented that trained 'patient providers' can effectively manage complex medical problems and prove to be invaluable assets in the creation of an affordable health-care team. No formal studies have been done to determine how expatriates compare with their American counterparts, but one can infer from the content of this textbook that most pre-travel counsel is within the grasp of this intelligent and motivated group. It is reasonable to assert that training expatriates to become proficient in key aspects of self-care coupled with ongoing support will be fundamental to the successful provision of excellent primary health care.

Telemedicine and the Internet

By 2010, it is estimated that 50% of all health-care ambulatory services will be delivered in the home, largely through telemedicine. Training and providing ongoing support for 'patient providers' is even more plausible now that most countries of the world have access to web-based products. Chat rooms and bulletin boards with health news could considerably improve the quality of self-care that one can provide.

Web-based services will likely substitute for some telemedicine applications as the cost of IT infrastructure decreases and patient acceptance and security increases. Even in a rudimentary stage of development with all of the problems evident, Callahan reported that the electronic medical record was valuable in 27% of emergencies that occurred during 'Transit risk days' defined as periods when outside of expatriate medical coverage areas. Though the authors expressed disappointment with the outcome, very few interventions have that level of return. Clearly, for expatriates in particular, the potential value of electronic communications compels us to develop this concept further.

Organizational support

Though 'self-care' is necessary, it appears that most do seek help from health-care professionals for more complex medical problems. Organizations could increase the potential for more effective care by fostering a culture that promotes help-seeking behavior.

It can be useful to check that expatriates are not working excessively long hours, and that they are taking days off regularly. They should be informed about how they can provide feedback, make requests or ask for help (practical or emotional) at any time should they require it. Adequate supervision should be provided. Inviting their suggestions for changes and improvements can foster job satisfaction. Chronic stress problems are less likely to materialize in an environment where people feel free to acknowledge difficulties and request help at an early stage.

Repatriation and medical evacuation

For a minority of problems, medical evacuation may be necessary, either because appropriate treatment is not available locally or if for various reasons the care was not considered acceptable. In 1996 the medical evacuation reported among PCV was 7.7/100. The major causes for medical evacuations in a recently published retrospective descriptive study of UNHCR employees were: infectious diseases (17%), accidents (15%) and obstetrical/gynecological conditions (15%).[2] AIDS, malaria and hepatitis accounted for the majority of those with infectious disease. The majority of events occurred in Africa (60%) where only one-third of the task force was working at the time.

Organizations should have clear policies on evacuation, abuse, and hostage situations that expatriates are asked to adhere to as a condition of their contract. If they have consented to a policy before going overseas, they are more likely to adhere to it later. During periods of political unrest it is not uncommon for expatriates to lack the capacity to exercise sound judgment – perhaps because they do not perceive danger, or because they are reluctant to abandon their local friends. Critical Incident Stress Debriefing should be offered to all who are evacuated in times of crisis. Training in CISD should be offered to suitable members of a task force if a number are working in the same vicinity. It is also wise to ensure that they have adequate time to rest, and follow-up support should be offered.

HEALTH SCREENING AND CARE ON RETURN

In-depth attention to post-travel screening is found in Chapter 51. Churchill[45] noted that some would 'seek medical help because of specific symptoms, while others who are asymptomatic will request screening investigations to reveal latent infections which might give rise to symptoms later in life. A third group will ask for help with retrospective diagnosis of illnesses suffered while abroad. People from all three groups may express concern about the risk of passing on infections to close contacts or may be worried about their fitness to return to the tropics. The precise value of screening for tropical illness is hard to quantify, as the chance of finding an important treatable illness in any one individual will depend on the level of risk of infection to which that individual has been exposed.

Post-travel screening for expatriates must move beyond the limited screening judged to be prudent when the risk of infectious diseases is the sole consideration. Many expatriates will have minimal to no exposure to tropical and parasitic diseases, yet there are compelling reasons to reassess expatriates upon their return. For this subset of travelers, the post-travel health assessment could be considered an access point for health-care professionals to become involved in the 'continuous flow of care'. Based on the model alluded to earlier in this document, the post-travel assessment would review the data based on previous assessments and in addition would serve as a combination of case finding, screening and health debriefing. Patients' perceptions should be explored from the context of the challenges that they expe-rienced which may have had a perceptible impact on their health. It is also appropriate to explore

their understanding of some of the basic prevention principles for it is not unusual for expatriates to absorb colloquial and anecdotal perspectives that weaken the utility of the self-care model. Many will have somatic concerns that are directly related to the psychosocial challenges that they have encountered. It is important for health-care professionals to recognize that they can more effectively address the health concerns of expatriates when they function as a team.

The context

Missionaries/volunteers and Non-Government Organizations (NGOs) – Social and Psychological Impact

Missionaries, volunteers and aid and development workers may face particular challenges. For some people, the belief that they are doing something worthwhile sustains them in difficult times. Others become disillusioned when they see few results from their work, and begin to feel that their efforts were 'a drop in the ocean'. Working for charities can lead to financial pressures, and charities may be unable to provide funding for projects with which the workers would like to assist. Lack of resources may lead to workers feeling unsupported themselves, and there may be no funds available for holiday breaks, or training, or counseling.

Some feel guilty about taking time off when the needs are great, while others state that there was little to do in their environment apart from work. In one study of 200 aid workers, 50% claimed they regularly worked more than 60 h/week. One respondent said that in retrospect, 'more breaks and less work would have been more efficient, as we were all burnt out'. Missionaries and humanitarian workers appear to be at increased risk of developing chronic fatigue syndrome, and this is probably related to excessive work demands and other stressors.[46]

Expatriates who reported that they had experienced psychological problems were found to have spent significantly longer overseas than those who did not report such problems. In the same study, participants were asked what the worst part of their expatriate experience had been. The question was open-ended, and their responses were subsequently categorized as shown in Table 30.14.

Several respondents who had been shot at or shelled, or witnessed deaths, or lived in conditions of poverty, stated that the worst part of the experience had been relationship problems, or the internal politics of the sending organization. This highlights the importance of good cross-cultural preparation, and adequate support while they are away, as well as choosing an organization which one is likely to find satisfactory.

Table 30.14	Worst part of the expatriate experience[9]
	(%)
Cultural difficulties and frustrations	21.4
Relationship problems	17.9
Dissatisfaction with the agency or the work	17.2
Missing home, or problems at home	11.7
Traumatic incidents	7.6
Living conditions/health	6.2
Isolation	4.8
Returning home	4.8
Everything/no response	8.3

Much of the above information about volunteers and missionaries also applies to people who are employed by NGOs. NGO staff often experience or witness distressing experiences. Many are involved with traffic accidents or illness epidemics, or have their offices or homes broken into. Some encounter the effects of war, both first hand or meeting survivors afterwards and hearing about the violent deaths of adults and children, and seeing evidence of mass destruction. Some experience death threats or are taken hostage or raped. Others live in fear of such experiences although they do not happen.

Research has indicated that about 25% of NGO workers report clinically significant symptoms of intrusive thoughts and avoidance (related to post-traumatic stress disorder) several months after returning from a placement abroad.[47]

Medical problems and infectious diseases

This continues to generate a great deal of debate. There have been few papers written on the value of screening longer-term travelers, or indeed of the major health problems they suffer while abroad. Carroll[48] studied a mixed group of travelers including diplomats, long-term volunteers and trekkers and concluded that screening was useful but could be largely done through structured history taking and relevant laboratory tests: specialist examination added little. Jones and Wintour[49] reviewed the records of 613 adults and children who presented to the Elphinstone International Health Centre over a decade. One cannot assume that the assessments were strictly for the purpose of screening but it is important to note that the range of illnesses diagnosed included a significant number that were non-tropical in nature. One-third required secondary or tertiary care, primarily in the fields of gastroenterology, cardiology and nephrology/urology.

Peppiatt and Byass[50] looked at the health of 212 persons who served in 27 countries for 488 person years. All were members of one mission society evaluated over a period of 3 years and therefore 212 may come close to being a denominator for that particular group. Self-reporting from overseas showed malaria, diarrhea and giardia were the most common perceived illnesses, but psychiatric illness accounted for nearly 110 episodes per 1000 person years.

Brouwer et al (1999) looked at 282 check-ups of children, the majority of whom had lived in sub-Saharan Africa and ranged in age from 3 months to 16 years with stays ranging from 3 months to 13 years. One hundred and fifty-six diagnoses of travel-related infectious and parasitic illnesses were found: 23% of check-ups showed asymptomatic giardiasis, 10% eosinophilia and 8% schistosomiasis. If infectious diseases were the only consideration one could question the value and cost effectiveness of screening asymptomatic children. However, based on the model proposed, the broader picture including parental concern, development and adjustment issues could well be the most important elements of the assessment and may be overlooked by persons who are not familiar with the impact of adjustment to an intercultural lifestyle and the impact of the re-entry transition.

Selective assessments

HIV
Aid workers may qualify for counsel and screening because of:
- occupational exposure
- lifestyle risk
- re-entry Visa requirements

TB surveillance
TB is the most important infection from a public health perspective and latent TB, as noted earlier, could impact as many as 3% per year in countries where TB is widespread. Standard screening involves tuberculin tests with Purified Protein Derivative (PPD) before and at least 3 months after possible exposure to TB. In Europe PPD is often administered as a Heaf Test whereas in North America the standard protocol is based on the Mantoux skin test with 5 tuberculin units of PPD administered intradermally.

Tuberculin skin testing has many practical drawbacks. It is generally not convenient for it means at least two visits. Also, if the 2-step mantoux is used as a standard an additional two visits are required. Many are unfamiliar with the interpretation of the test and thus may under or over report and although one is advised to disregard the impact of a previous BCG vaccination, in some instances it is likely a contributor to a positive test. Furthermore, false positives may arise due to exposure to nontuberculous mycobacteria.

This variability and subjectivity has prompted research for a more sensitive and noninvasive test. Blood tests to detect infection with tuberculosis have been developed. Though further validation is required, initial research is promising and authorities anticipate that it will replace skin testing with PPD.[51]

Debriefing

Some organizations routinely offer critical incident debriefing to all staff who have been working in conflict zones, or have been exposed to any kind of traumatic incident. Some reports have suggested that critical incident debriefing may be ineffective for people who have experienced one-off traumas, but the studies on which this is based had methodological problems.[52]

The critical incident debriefing process can be modified to allow discussion of stressful experiences over a period of time, and not simply individual incidents. Research suggests that debriefing in this manner is beneficial for people who have worked overseas (e.g., as aid workers or missionaries) and experienced a number of stressful incidents over a period of time. For example, one study found that 25% of aid workers who did not receive personal debriefing reported clinical levels of symptoms of intrusion and avoidance (related to post-traumatic stress) several months after returning to their home country. Among a group who received a session of personal debriefing (which lasted approximately two hours), only 7% reported clinical levels of these symptoms.

REPORTING

If a report is to be sent to the agency, the same principles outlined for the pre-departure assessments apply. In that case, the health care practitioner serves as an agent and as for the pre-departure assessment, the sending organization should clearly articulate the purpose of the assessment, and that request should be accompanied by a signed release of information document.

If one considers this interaction to be a part of the 'continuous flow of care', the report should be formatted to summarizing health problems, list testing done, provide copies of all relevant investigations and develop a detailed action plan for the expatriate to follow if returning to an international assignment (Table 30.15).

CONCLUSION

For those counseling personnel in preparation for an international assignment, remember the following:
- During the pre-departure assessment pay particular attention to: health issues that must be managed during the international assignment that are not related to tropical and infectious diseases and psychosocial issues that are associated with long-stay travel (Table 30.16)

Table 30.15	Checklist for pre-return assessment

Update the immunizations

Evaluate the prophylaxis regimen for persons in malaria endemic regions
    Record adverse reactions if they limit use of specific medications
    Evaluate compliance regimen
    Review personal protection measures

Record relevant history and positive physical findings

Record abnormal laboratory findings
    provide a management plan for new problems
    report on long-term problems that were identified
    review health issues that impact placement
    outline management responsibilities for sending organization

Table 30.16	Pre-travel checklist expatriate

Medical evaluation
  Pre-travel risk appraisal and counsel
    Discuss cumulative risks
    Complete recommended vaccines
    Choose appropriate prophylaxis (malaria)
  Routine health assessment
    Ensure assessment includes all age and sex specific screening tests
    e.g.: mammogram, PSA etc.
  Summary of health profile
    Current health issues
    Risk factors
      e.g., allergies
    Copies of relevant investigations
      e.g., CBC, lipid profile, ECG, Blood group and type
    List of current medications
    Immunization record
    Eyeglass prescription
  Personal psychosocial health appraisal
  Dental Assessment and pre-departure care

Medical Kit (see Chapter 8)
  Ample supply of prescription medication
  Extra pair of glasses
  Safety and first aid supplies
  Gloves

Medical training
  Prevention
    Food and water safety
      Screened kitchens
      Adequate refrigeration
      Water purifiers
    Training servants
      Basic health
      Sanitation and hygiene
      Food preparation
    Risk reduction
      Activities
      Behavior
  Self-management of common problems
    Diarrhea   Respiratory illnesses   Fever
    Malaria   Common skin problems

Health care abroad
  Prepare a living will
  Appoint medical proxy
  Obtain adequate health insurance
    Evacuation insurance
  Obtain a list of references from other expatriates
    Physicians
    Facilities
    Services
  Join a list serve
    Expat-Moms.com

Table 30.16	Pre-travel checklist expatriate–cont'd

Sending Organization Check List
  Risk appraisal of assignment:
    Occupational
    Geographic/climate
    Personal
  Health and psychosocial assessment
  Factored health risks into placement priorities
  Logistical support for known health priorities
  Facilitated opportunities for training
    Health and safety
    Management of exposure to blood and body fluids
    Transition issues
      Culture shock
      Re-entry
      TCK (Third-Culture Kid)

Provision of adequate insurance

- Counseling must consider low risk infectious diseases and behavior, which demonstrate cumulative risk over prolonged periods
- Cross-cultural training concerning the international assignment and re-entry issues is a priority
- Preparation should include contingency plans for evacuation and repatriation
- 'Self-care' is central to successful care abroad
- Consideration must be given to comprehensive post-travel screening and psychological debriefing

REFERENCES

1. Foyle MF, Beer MD, Watson JP. Expatriate mental health. *Acta Psychiatr Scand* 1998; **97**:278–283.
2. Peytremann I, Baduraux M, O'Donovan S, *et al*. Medical Evacuations and Fatalities of United Nations High Commissioner for Refugees Field Employee. *J Travel Med* 2001; **8**:117–121.
3. Bernard KW, Graitcer PL, Vlugt T van der, *et al*. Epidemiological surveillance in Peace Corps Volunteers: A model for monitoring health in temporary residents of developing countries. *Int J Epidemiol* 1989; **18**:220–226.
4. Banta JE, Jungblut, E. Health problems encountered by the Peace Corps overseas. *Am J Public Health* 1966; **56**:2121–2129.
5. Lange WR, Frankenfield DL, Frame JD. Morbidity among Refugee Relief Workers. *J Travel Med* 1994; **1**:111–112.
6. Pechersky R, Weld L, Kozarsky P, *et al*. *Geosentinel: Disease Profiles of Travelers. Abstract FC10.01*. 7th Conference of the International Society of Travel Medicine, May 2001.
7. Parshall P. How spiritual are missionaries? In: O'Donnell KS and O'Donnell ML, eds. *Helping Missionaries Grow: Readings in Mental Health and Missions*. Pasadena, California: William Carey Library; 1988:75–82.
8. Paton D, Purvis C. Nursing in the aftermath of disaster: Orphanage relief work in Romania. *Disaster Prev Manage* 1995; **4**:45–54.
9. Lovell DM. Psychological adjustment among returned overseas aid workers. Unpublished D Clin Psy Thesis, University of Wales, Bangor, 1997.
10. Deshpande SP, Viswesvaran C. Is cross-cultural training of expatriate managers effective: A meta analysis. *Int J Intercultural Relat* 1992; **16**:295–310.
11. Schouten EJ, Borgdorff MW. Increased mortality among Dutch development workers. *BMJ* 1995; **311**:1343–1344.
12. Frame JD, Lange WR, Frankenfield DL. Mortality Trends of American Missionaries in Africa, 1945–1985. *Am Soc Trop Med Hygiene* 1992; **46**:686–690.
13. Hargarten SW, Baker SP. Fatalities in the Peace Corps. A retrospective study: 1962 through 1983. *JAMA* 1985; **254**:1326–1329.
14. Sheik M, Gutierrez MI, Burnham G. Death Among Humanitarian Workers. *BMJ* 2000; **321**:166–168.
15. Tucker MF, Benson PG, Blanchard F. The development and longitudinal validation of the navy overseas assignment inventory. *Task Order 77/95/D*. US Navy Contract; 1978.
16. Stroh LK, Dennis LE, Cramer TC. Predictors of expatriate adjustment. *Int J Organ Anal* 1994; **2**:176–192.

17. Hathaway SR, McKinley JC. Minnesota Multiphasic Personality Inventory-2. Minneapolis, Minn.: University of Minnesota Press; 1989:

18. Westefeld JS, Maples M. The MMPI-2 and vocational assessment: A brief report. *J Career Assess* 1998; **6**:107–113.

19. Butcher JN. *International Adaptations of the MMP1-2*. Minneapolis, MN: University of Minnesota Press; 1996.

20. Schnurr PP, Friedman MD, Rosenberg SD. Premilitary MMPI scores as predictors of combat-related PTSD symptoms. *Am J Psychiatry* 1993; **150**:479–483.

21. Schubert E, Ganter K. The MMPI as a predictive tool for missionary candidates. *J Psychol Theology* 1996; **24**:124–132.

22. Helmes E, Redden JR. A perspective on developments in assessing psychopathology: A critical review of the MMPI and MMPI-2. *Psychol Bull* 1993; **113**:453–471.

23. Dunbar E, Ehrlich MH. Preparation of the international employee: Career and consultation needs. *Consult Psychol J* 1993; **45**:18–24.

24. Dwelle TL. Inadequate basic preventive health measures: Survey of missionary children in sub-Saharan Africa. *Pediatrics* 1995; **95**:733–737.

25. Lange WR, Kreider SD, Kaczaniuk MA, Snyder FR. Missionary health: the great omission. *Am J Prev Med* 1987; **6**:332–338.

26. Ghent M, Boyle J, Zuckerman J. *Overseas Aid Non-Governmental Organizations – Infection Control Policies for Bloodborne Viruses. Abstract PC106.02.* 7th Conference of the International Society of Travel Medicine, May 2001.

27. Ad-Mission FG. *The briefing and debriefing of teams of missionaries and aid workers.* Harpenden, England: self-published; 1999.

28. Lange WR, Frame JD. High incidence of viral hepatitis among American missionaries in Africa. *Am J Trop Med Hygiene* 1990; **43**:527–533.

29. Smalligan RD, Lange WR, Frame JD, et al. The risk of viral hepatitis A, B, C, and E among North American missionaries. *Am J Trop Med Hygiene* 1995; **3**:233–236.

30. Arguin PM, Krebs JW, Mandel E, Guzi T, Childs JE. Survey of Rabies Preexposure and Postexposure Prophylaxis among Missionary Personnel Stationed Outside the United States. *J Travel Med* 2000; **7**:10–14.

31. Pandey P, Shlim DR, Cave W, Springer MF. Risk of Possible Exposure to Rabies among Tourists and Foreign Residents in Nepal. *J Travel Med* 2002; **9**(3):127–131.

32. Adera T, Wolfe MS, McGuire Rugh K, Calhoun N, Marum L. Risk factors for malaria among expatriates living in Kampala, Uganda: The need for adherence to chemoprophylactic regimens American. *J Trop Med* 1995; **52**:207–212.

33. Lobel HO, Varma JK, Miani M, et al. Monitoring for mefloquine-resistant Plasmodium falciparum in Africa: Implications for travelers' health. *Am J Trop Med Hygiene* 1998; **59**:129–132.

34. Schneider G. MSc Thesis, London School of Hygiene and TM, London.

35. Funk M, Schlagenhauf P, Tschopp A, Steffen R. MalaQuick versus ParaSight F as a diagnostic aid in travelers' malaria. *Trans R Soc Trop Med Hygiene* 1999; **93**(3):268–272.

36. Cobelens FG, Deutekom H van, Draayer-Jansen IW, et al. Association of tuberculin sensitivity in Dutch adults with history of travel to areas of with a high incidence of tuberculosis. *Clin Infect Dis* 2001; **33**(3):300–304.

37. Behr MA, Small PM. Has BCG Attenuated to Impotence? *Nature* 1997; **389**:133–134.

38. Shlim DR, Hoge CW, Rajah R, et al. Persistent high risk of diarrhea among foreigners in Nepal during the first 2 years of residence. *Clin Infect Dis* 1999; **29**:613–616.

39. Graaf R De, Zessen G van, Houweling H. Underlying reasons for sexual conduct and condom use among expatriates posted in AIDS endemic areas. *AIDS Care* 1998; **10**:661–665.

40. Johnson AM, Mercer CH, Erens B, et al. Sexual Behavior in Britain: Partnerships, practices and HIV Risk Behaviours. *Lancet* 2001; **358**:1835–1842.

41. Moore J, Beeker C, Harrison JS, et al. HIV risk behavior among Peace Corps Volunteers. *AIDS* 1995; **9**(7):795–799.

42. Houweling H, Coutinho RA. Risk of HIV infection among Dutch expatriates in sub-Saharan Africa. *Int J STD AIDS* 1991; **4**:252–257.

43. Lingenfelter SG. Mayers MK. *Ministering Cross-Culturally*. Grand Rapids, Michigan: Baker Book House; 1986.

44. Sieveking N, Anchor K, Marston RC. Selecting and preparing expatriate employees. *Pers J* 1981; **60**:197–202.

45. Churchill DR, Chiodini PL, McAdam KP. Screening the returned traveler. *Br Med Bull* 1993; **49**:465–474.

46. Lovell DM. Chronic fatigue syndrome among overseas development workers: A qualitative study. *J Travel Med* 1999; **6**:16–23.

47. Eriksson CB, Vande Kemp H, Gorsuch R, et al. Trauma exposure and PTSD symptoms in international relief and development personnel. *J Traumatic Stress* 2001; **14**:205–212.

48. Carroll B, Dow C, Snashall D, Marshall T, et al. Post-tropical screening: how useful is it? *BMJ* 1993; **307**(541).

49. Wintour K, Jones ME. Routine medical evaluation of expatriate volunteers-retrospective analysis of 613 patients. *Abstracts from the 7th Conference of the International Society of Travel Medicine*, May 2001; Abstract No. FC09.03.

50. Peppiatt R, Byass P. A survey of the health of British missionaries. *Br J Gen Pr* 1991; **41**:159–162.

51. Mazurek GH, LoBue PA, Daley CL, et al. Comparison of a whole-blood interferon gamma assay with tuberculin skin testing for detecting latent Mycobacterium tuberculosis infection. *JAMA* 2001; **286**(14):1740–1747.

52. Lovell-Hawker DM. *Effective Debriefing Handbook*. London: People in Aid.

CHAPTER 31 Expedition Medicine

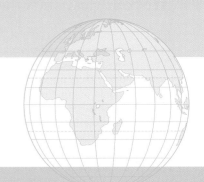

Eric L. Weiss and Trish L. Batchelor

KEYPOINTS

- The expedition physician must first assess his/her expertise and responsibility to determine whether the role is appropriate

- Pre-travel preparation includes a risk assessment analysis, risk management strategies including the development of a first aid kit

- Potential medical problems are most often determined by the health of the group, the nature of the activities and the environment in which they are carried out

- Meticulous preparation, medical expertise, communication and problem solving skills, creativity and improvisation are qualities that make for a successful expedition physician

INTRODUCTION

In the early 1900s, expeditions were the reserve of the privileged few who could devote months or even years of their lives to the pursuit of discovery. The heroic exploits of the early Antarctic explorers such as Scott and Shackleton define our concept of 'expedition'. What, now, a century later, is an expedition? The Collins English Dictionary defines an expedition as 'an organised journey or voyage, esp. for exploration or for a scientific or military purpose'.[1] The range of expeditions undertaken today is enormous. In the UK alone, it is estimated that the 'expedition market' involves between 12 000 and 15 000 travelers annually.[2] At one end of the scale are those who one would consider the 'purists' – the Scott's and Shackleton's of our era. These are the individuals who impose a stratagem of 'arbitrary self-limitation'[3] to overcome the lack of 'blank places' on our earth. These individuals will often travel alone or in very small groups with little or no support, for example Goran Kropp, a Swede who rode his bicycle from Sweden to the base of Mt. Everest and then climbed to the summit entirely unsupported. For the majority of people, however, an expedition is a group exercise. This may be a group of friends or colleagues, a university or school group, a commercial climbing trip, an ecological group or perhaps a charity support group. A uniting theme is that expeditions will usually visit areas of climatic extremes – mountains, polar regions, desert, the tropical jungle or the ocean and that they will undertake some kind of activity, whether this be scientific research or an adventure activity such as climbing, kayaking, rafting, diving, caving or sailing.

Expedition doctors are rarely paid to accompany such a group, often they are invited by friends or have an interest in the particular activity being undertaken. In fact, many expeditions leave with no physician or other medical provider – here another opportunity for travel medicine outreach and education. The aim of the expedition doctor is to minimize risk by taking sensible precautions – advising on the correct pre-travel preparation, managing potential environmental risks and being as prepared as possible to manage emergencies that may arise. Risk cannot be eliminated, and neither should it be – part of the appeal of undertaking an expedition is an element of risk. However, as in all aspects of travel medicine wise pre-planning can only contribute to a successful journey.

Many of the topics relevant to expedition doctors are covered in more detail in other chapters of this text – particularly high altitude medicine, diving, remote destinations, psychological disorders, diarrhea, and food and water issues. This chapter attempts to give some guidance on deciding whether being an expedition doctor is right for you; how to prepare yourself and your group for the expedition; how to put together an appropriate first aid kit; an awareness of common problems that may occur in various climatic conditions or undertaking particular activities, and how to deal with some of the more difficult situations you may be faced with on your journey.

'To solve a problem which has long resisted the skill and persistence of others is an irresistible magnet in every sphere of human activity ...' (Sir John Hunt, expedition leader of the first successful ascent of Everest)

QUESTIONS TO ASK

The opportunity to be a trip physician may come as an unexpected phone call or e-mail or at other times, the expedition physician may be a founding member of the expeditionary team. Either way, there are important questions to ask, both of yourself, as well as of the organizing group, to ensure a good match of expectation, ability, and responsibility.

Perhaps the overriding consideration for the expedition physician to be is a careful evaluation of the expedition team. Strong communication abilities, interpersonal skills, and sensitivity are all vital components for all members of the expedition leadership – physician included. Be honest with yourself regarding your personality, your skills, and your overall suitability for this exciting, but often demanding role. For more challenging expeditions to austere environments, strong interpersonal skills are obviously important for all team members. However, for more commercially organized, group expeditions, or trips, the expedition physician will likely be a member of the staff and it is essential that he or she be willing and able to work as a team player.

The converse is also true – the organizing group also needs to be willing to grant medical authority to the physician. Everyone's respective roles and responsibilities need to be clearly defined long before the first medical issues arise far from the peaceful comforts of the meeting room. Even then, medical action (once the patient has been medically stabilized) should take place in a coordinated fashion with all team members aware of and agreeing on the plan. For this to all work smoothly, there are questions that every potential expedition physician should put on the table. Before, during, and after the trip, what are the physician's responsibilities to the program? Will he or she be responsible for pre-travel medical screening? Will a health questionnaire be administered and who will write the questions? Who has final say regarding passenger participation in borderline cases? And who will provide 'pre-travel' education and information to leadership and participants alike? The authors feel strongly that these responsibilities fall clearly in the expedition physician's domain. Less clear is the role of the physician on the trip regarding non-medical issues, so this should also be discussed. Some programs simply want a physician available should a medical situation arise, others view the physician as an integral member of the leadership team. The more challenging the expedition the more important it is to be a member of the team.

Other issues that need to be considered include the provision or requirement of travel health/repatriation insurance. Many companies allow this to be an optional addition for their participants setting the stage for difficult situations and/or decision making later on. Be aware that the traditional limits on payment (often US$50 000 in the US) or on pre-existing illness with standard policies are insufficient for even the most vanilla of expeditions. The expedition physician is in a position to lobby for appropriate attention to be paid to this often-neglected issue.

Responsibility for the expedition medical kit is another very important issue for discussion. Smaller expeditions may expect the physician to be completely responsible for the medical kit, other programs may have an established kit built at the corporate office. The latter can be perfectly acceptable, but it is essential that the trip physician be very familiar with the kit contents, both in name as well as location. Taking the kit apart and putting it back together several times before departure is an excellent idea!

Not to be forgotten in the pre-adventure enthusiasm are the issues of compensation, and unfortunately, liability. The latter, more an issue for physicians where the ratio of legal to medical professionals is higher, will be discussed separately below. The former should be put simply on the table before the significant responsibility of providing on-trip medical care is agreed and assumed.

Depending on the size, nature, duration, destination(s), of the expedition, simply being included may be sufficient reward. For more commercially oriented trips, the trip physician is typically not charged the fee that his or her fellow passengers may have to pay. Some companies may only reduce the fee, rather than eliminate it all together. The expectant expedition physician should be wisely counseled that the trip at hand may include a significant amount of work. Clearly, many factors are at play here. Young healthy travelers going on a short rafting expedition are less likely to need significant medical intervention than a group of elderly travelers on a 4-week trip around the world (see quote by Iain McIntosh, below). For programs where the need for medical care can be expected to be high it is not unreasonable to ask for payment for services rendered.

'One should avoid at all costs accompanying the elderly devotees on tours specially designed for them, with a suicidal urge to embark on a holiday of a lifetime to the end of the earth. These old-timers carry their chronic disorders with them and are always accompanied by suitcases full of medicaments. Grounded by gout and arthritis, deterred by dyspnoea and congestion, few are fit enough to view the sights of global travel and seek recompense by monopolizing the attention of the captive tour-doctor to his/her great discomfort…the holiday spirit, can, however, be experienced to excess in younger groups where over-indulgence in cheap, potent, local libations brings

maudlin merriment, self-inflicted injury, drunken coma and resultant inconvenience to the harassed group medic.

It is well to eschew well-publicized jaunts to conquer K4 or climb to some inaccessible summit in Bhutan. The 'tigers' of the high tops frequently peel off the mountain at a moment of maximal discomfort for the expedition doctor and rendering first aid, where exposure is both vertical and climatic, is not without hazard. Simple school trips to Gwent or Tangier must also be viewed with misgiving for youngsters start vomiting the moment the boat leaves the harbour, if not before, and a series of bruises, breaks and blood-letting will exasperate the medical companion.

Better by far to choose a group of the middle-aged in robust health, long separated from the boisterous over activity of youth, devoid of desire to climb impossible peaks and seeking only their creature comforts and a modicum of culture in a distant sunny clime. They never wander very far from life's simpler pleasures such as hot baths, flushing loos and good cuisine.' (Iain McIntosh, 1992)[4]

In sum, there are many issues to be considered before signing up for the exciting, but often challenging role, as expedition physician. Be sure you are comfortable with expected roles and responsibility, do not underestimate the amount of work involved, and be satisfied with the compensation offered, even if it is simply the opportunity to participate in an adventure that will hopefully broaden your horizons forever.

RISK ASSESSMENT AND PREPARATION

After positively answering the question: 'Am I right for this expedition' (and is it right for me?) it is now time to prepare. A risk assessment analysis should be prepared. All the potential aspects of the trip that could potentially cause a problem should be reviewed, and work on ways to minimize the risk should be thought through. It is prudent to reduce the risk to acceptable levels as ultimately it is the expedition physician who will have to deal with the medical problems that will arise.

Personal preparation

The expedition physician will need to learn as much as possible about the group members, the environment they are traveling to, and the activity/ies the group will be undertaking.

A medical questionnaire (see Table 31.1) is designed to (a) identify group members who may be unsuitable for the trip and (b) identify members with pre-existing conditions.

Having to say 'no' to a potential participant is one of the more difficult tasks you may be faced with – this is more likely to happen on a commercial expedition. It is possible that the individual concerned will dispute the decision, therefore asking for a second opinion from another physician with a reputation as an expert in the relevant field is recommended. This may not be necessary if a positive relationship is established with the individual's personal physician. This is a relatively uncommon scenario. More common is that some trip members will have pre-existing conditions that do not warrant exclusion from the trip, but require extra preparation. Most pre-existing conditions can be successfully controlled as long as the group member is honest about his/her condition, the appropriate pre-trip preparation has been undertaken, and you as the physician are prepared to manage any exacerbations that may occur as a result of the conditions of the trip. A report from the group member's regular physician including laboratory work, X-ray and EKG interpretation, and contact information (including e-mail), is a wise precaution.

Clinically, it is important that the physician is prepared to handle almost any emergency that may occur. A background combining

Table 31.1	Sample medical questionnaire for group members

Personal details
 Name
 D.O.B.
 Address
 Phone contacts
 E-mail address

Next of kin to be contacted in an emergency
 Name
 Address
 Phone contacts: Home
   Work
   Mobile
 E-mail address

Regular doctor
 Name
 Address
 Contact phone numbers: Surgery
   Emergency
 E-mail address

When did you last see your regular doctor and why?
 Do you have any current medical problems? If so please provide details.
 Have you ever had any medical or psychological problems in the past? If so, please provide details.
 Have you ever had any surgery?
 Have you been hospitalized in the past 2 years, and if so, why?
 Do you take any prescribed medications?
 Do you take any over the counter or herbal medications?
 Do you have any allergies including drugs, foods, stings, Band-Aids etc.?
 What is your blood group?
 Do you drink alcohol? If so how many per day of: Wine
   Beer
   Spirits
 Have you traveled to less developed countries before? If so, when and did you have any problems while you were away?
 Activity, as relevant, e.g. what is the highest altitude you have climbed/trekked to? How deep was your deepest dive? etc.
 Environmentally specific questions as relevant, e.g. have you suffered from altitude sickness before? Have you suffered from the bends before? If so, provide details.
 We have provided a list of recommended immunizations – please mark below the date you received them. List as appropriate.
 What was your most recent blood pressure reading and when was this taken?
 Do you have any particular medical concerns regarding this trip?

Primary Care, Emergency Medicine and Tropical or Travel Medicine would be ideal. Apart from the management of common travel-related illness, such as diarrhea and problems specific to the environment to be visited, the following are some suggestions of pre-requisite skills necessary to ensure the physician is adequately equipped before the expedition is undertaken:

- Basic resuscitation skills on an Emergency Life Support (ELS), Advanced Cardiac Life Support (ACLS) or Acute Trauma Life Support (ATLS) course should be renewed/taken up.
- Management of chronic disease exacerbation (CHF, CAD, Asthma, Diabetes) should be reviewed.
- To be comfortable with SAM splint (or equivalent) to improvise immobilization for common orthopedic conditions including fractures.
- To be familiar with shoulder, ankle, and elbow dislocation management.
- To be comfortable with the use of sports tape to treat common sprains and strains.
- To have some basic dental skills, e.g., using cavit for temporary fillings.

- To manage epistaxis.
- Proficiency with wound care, including lacerations, burns, and foreign bodies.
- To be comfortable with dealing with minor ophthalmological problems, such as corneal foreign body, corneal abrasions, etc.
- To be comfortable with the use of basic transportation and evacuation systems.

The other major contributors to potential medical problems are the environment to be visited and the activities the group is undertaking. Learn as much as possible about the environment to be visited. Environmental extremes of heat, cold, humidity, altitude, depth, UV exposure, or motion all have their consequent medical problems. Table 31.2 'risk assessment' gives some examples to consider. Learn about the endemic diseases of the country – some will be preventable with immunizations or medications, but many will rely on behavior modification, such as insect avoidance and hygiene. Will you be able to diagnose and possibly manage these conditions without sophisticated lab support? There may be concerns about specific forms of wildlife, particularly venomous reptiles. The expedition physician can learn about the environment to be visited, by reading (the bibliography at the end of this section is a good starting point), speaking with doctors or group members who have been to similar environments before, or undertaking one of the increasing number of courses available which focus on specific environmental hazards and activities.

You will also need to be prepared for the health risks specific to the activity you are undertaking, e.g., the risk of dislocated shoulders in kayakers, decompression illness in divers and so forth.

In preparing for a potential 'worst case scenario' an evacuation plan should be in place (Fig. 31.1). You should have made contact with your assistance company and learned as much as possible about any local health-care facilities that may be available. In a very few parts of the world there are well organized rescue facilities in place, e.g., the Himalayan Rescue Association in Nepal, however in most areas for expedition, there will be a dearth of reliable local medical facilities.

Safety and security issues are paramount. In one of the few studies looking at the incidence of health problems on expeditions, the Royal Geographic Society of Britain recorded only two deaths out of 2381 participants in 19 000 expedition days. These were two Indonesian members of a trip to Irian jaya who were kidnapped by West Papuan Independence fighters. In particular, many of the world's highest mountains are in countries with unstable political situations (India, Nepal, Tibet and most recently Pakistan), while piracy on the ocean is a real threat to long-term ocean goers. The local Department of Foreign Affairs website provides updated information (see Table 31.4).

Preparing your group members is vitally important – you should be the one to provide them with specific pre-travel health recommendations including appropriate immunizations, malaria prophylaxis (if relevant) and general health advice. If you run a travel medicine clinic this can be a 'marketing' opportunity for you, otherwise you should refer your members to a well-run specialized travel medicine clinic. For remote expeditions where the rabies risk is high, you should think about ensuring all of your members are pre-immunized against rabies – in many parts of the world obtaining human rabies immunoglobulin is a virtually impossible task. Travel medicine advice is notoriously inconsistent if supplied by different providers – ensuring consistency also gives a sense of confidence to group members. Whilst you will be bringing your own extensive medical kit it is sensible to ensure that each member of the group also carries a basic kit themselves – you do not want to be a 'day and night pharmacy' for basic over-the-counter medications. The only exception to this may be if you are traveling with a group of students under the age of 18 and you prefer to keep a very close eye on them. Your group members

Table 31.2	Risk assessment – an example of some potential risks
Aspect of trip	**Potential risk**
The team	
Pre-existing medical conditions	Deterioration in extreme or remote conditions resulting in medical emergency/death
Fitness of members	Lack of fitness leading to increased risk of injury or illness
Adequate pre travel preparation	Lack of adequate preparation leading to risk of preventable diseases, e.g., Hep A, malaria
Experience and training of members	Less experience and training will lead to increased risk of mishap
Attitudes	Willingness to follow guidelines will decrease risk
Equipment	Poorly maintained equipment adds risk
Team dynamics	A harmonious team is less risky
The environment	
Mountains	Altitude sickness, serious injuries, frostbite, snow blindness, UV damage, hypothermia
Desert	Heat exhaustion, dehydration, UV damage
Tropics/jungle	Heat exhaustion, dehydration, skin infections, wildlife
Ocean	UV damage, sea sickness, decompression illness, CAGE, dehydration, venomous stingers, coral cuts
All less developed countries	Poor food and water hygiene leading to enteric diseases
Specific endemic diseases	Insect-borne diseases, e.g. malaria, dengue, JBE, trypanosomiasis, myiasis, etc
Wildlife	Bites, envenomation, stings, injuries
Transport/road conditions	Motor vehicle accidents/plane accidents leading to serious injury or death.
The activity	
Mountaineering	AMS, serious injuries from falls, hypothermia, frostbite, snow blindness, UV damage
Trekking	AMS, UV damage, minor injuries
Kayaking	Drowning, shoulder dislocations
Diving	Decompression illness, CAGE, coral cuts
Sailing	Drowning, injuries, motion sickness
Caving	Drowning, suffocation
Local population	
Political climate	Risk of kidnapping, terrorist activities, piracy
Attitudes to foreigners	Risk of theft, injury, rape
Hygiene standards	Enteric disease
Medical facilities	Nosocomial infection in local medical facilities (esp. Hep B, HIV)

should receive clear written information about the environmental conditions they are going to face so that they can be mentally and physically prepared. You may even consider giving advice on pre-travel fitness training if appropriate.

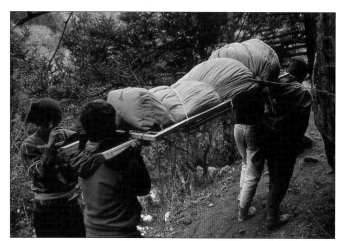

Figure 31.1 Litter evacuation. Nightmare in Nepal – be prepared, do your homework and do not forget evacuation insurance. Photo courtesy of Eric Weiss.

One often-ignored element of group preparation is ensuring that there are other members who can perform first aid in a remote setting. It would be unwise to be the only person in the group capable of managing common problems. There are an increasing number of first aid courses with an emphasis on the wilderness setting being run for lay people. Consider asking other members of the expedition leadership (or other interested parties) to take this, or similar, courses.

A group meeting, if possible, is the ideal environment in which to give a medical briefing to your group – this can be an excellent opportunity to dispel any myths and resolve any conflicting advice that people will have invariably received.

FIRST AID KITS

Nowhere does the adage 'the right tool for the job' ring more true than when trying to deal with a brisk nosebleed or case of urinary obstruction while away from your local emergency department. The expedition physician must be creative and innovative when it comes to caring for those in his or her charge, and this includes the ability to improvise with materials at hand if the first aid kit is not. That being said, duct tape or safety pins are usually no substitute for the 'right tool', so careful consideration of your first aid kit's contents is an essential component of pre-trip planning.

Contents

Expedition participants play several important roles as it relates to the trip first aid kit. Certainly everyone should be advised to travel with their own personal kit, including the simple remedies that many use on a regular basis. Having travelers consider any medication or first aid oriented product that they have used in the past year is a good trigger for what ought to come along. The expedition physician should also carefully review the health status of each participant, and be certain to anticipate potential medical conditions or exacerbations while designing the kit. In addition to being participant specific, the kit should also be itinerary specific: consider the environmental risks as well such as altitude, cold, or heat illness. It is useful to divide the kit contents into categories (wound care, ears/nose/throat, antibiotics, dental, etc.) while planning contents (see Table 31.4). Pack items that can be creatively used for several purposes – for example, a Foley catheter can also be used to control epistaxis, or as a tourniquet. Lastly, the participants themselves unknowingly provide some degree of buffer for the physician as often, should he or she need a medication that is not in the medical kit, a participant may have it in his/her personal stash. This is obviously truer in a larger, commercial group.

Design

In addition to contents, the actual kit design is an important feature. The expedition physician needs to be very familiar with both contents as well as location. Having to struggle to find the epinephrine or nitroglycerine is not wise. To have all of the 'emergency' drugs/interventions in a separate pull away pouch can be very helpful. For trips where the group will be away from packs or baggage for day excursions, the physician should pack a 'day pack', which includes not only the emergency pouch above, but also the commonly used agents, such as acetaminophen, loperamide, and bandaging materials.

Supplies

Before departure, another consideration is drug and supply availability on the road. If the expedition needs to be truly self-sufficient, careful consideration needs to be paid to both first aid kit components and amount. If there is ability to re-stock while on the road, be certain to have a system of tracking first aid kit use. For kits that will be re-used, a careful post trip inventory check is obviously critical.

A final consideration is also perhaps the most difficult. Where will you, as expedition physician, draw the line? Will you include intravenous supplies? What about airway equipment, such as laryngoscopes and endotracheal tubes? Weight and size of the first aid kit are obviously important considerations, but so too are issues of 'what then?'. If your patient requires respiratory support in the middle of nowhere, how long can you reasonably sustain such efforts? 'Triage' becomes even more important, as well as more difficult, when far from home.

LIABILITY

In the USA, the issue of medical legal exposure arises quickly in any environment where a health-care provider is involved with caring for patients. Over time, this issue is unfortunately being exported around the world. However, medical legal sensitivity does not mean that fear of a lawsuit needs to drive all decision making, or even be front of mind. Providing quality patient care and providing documentation that serves as a good communication tool should be your guiding principals. That being said, the expedition physician would be wise to consider malpractice insurance because there is in fact some liability assumed.

The simplest way to do this, if you are currently covered through your practice, is to approach your insurance provider and ask that a 'rider' be added to the existing policy. Often this can be accomplished at no additional expense, or perhaps a one-time fee will be involved.

Table 31.3	Useful websites
Subject area	**URL**
Mountaineering	
International Society of Mountain Medicine	www.ismmed.org
High Altitude medicine Guide	www.high-altitude-medicine.com
The British Mountaineering Council UIAA Mountain Medicine Centre	www.thebmc.co.uk/world/mm/mm0.htm
The International Porter Protection Group	www.ippg.net
Kayaking and rafting	
America Canoe Association	www.acanet.org
The American White Water Affiliation	www.americanwhitewater.org
Canadian Recreational Canoeing Association	www.crca.ca/CRCACore.cfm
British Canoe Union	www.bcu.org.uk
Scuba diving	
South Pacific Underwater Medical Society	www.spums.org.au
Divers Alert Network	www.diversalertnetwork.org
Undersea and Hyperbaric Medicine Society	www.uhms.org
Safety & security	
US Dept of State	www.travel.state.gov/travel_warnings.html
UK Foreign and Commonwealth Office	www.fco.gov.uk/travel/
Canada Dept of Foreign Affairs	www.voyage.dfait-maeci.gc.ca/destinations/menu.e.htm
Australian Department of Foreign Affairs and Trade	www.dfat.gov.au/consular/advice/advices_mnu.html
New Zealand Dept of Foreign Affairs	www.mft.govt.nz/travel/index.html
German Foreign Office	www.auswaertiges-amt.de/www/de/laenderinfos
The Anti-Piracy Center in Kuala Lumpur	www.icwbo.org/ccs/menu_imb_piracy.asb

Table 31.4	Example of physician level first aid kit

Category

Emergency
    Epinephrine 1:1000 (1 mg/mL)
    Nitroglycerin spray, metered dose inhaler
    Oral glucose gel
    Pocket mask (e.g., by layerdal)
    Diphenhydramine 50 mg/mL injectable via
    Albuterol metered dose inhaler
    No. 11 scalpel
    No. 10 scalpel
    5.0 endotracheal tube, cuffed
    1 cc pre-packaged syringe (27 gauge needle)
    3 cc pre-packaged syringe (21 gauge needle)
    Oral airways (assorted sizes)
    Laryngoscope with machintosh 3 blade
    Mcgill forceps
    Nasal trumpet (30 french)
    Foley catheter (16 french)
    Sawyer snake bite extractor
    Morphine sulfate
    Diazepam

Other injectables
    Promethazine
    Furosemide
    Dexamethasone

Wound care / preparation
    0.25% bupivacaine
    0.25% bupivacaine w/epinephrine
    20 cc irrigating syringe
    Povidone iodine solution
    Povidone iodine swab stick
    Needle driver
    Mosquito clam
    Iris scissors
    Toothed forceps
    3 cc syringe (25 gauge needle)
    5 cc syringe (25 gauge needle)
    Alcohol wipes

Wound closure
    Dermabond tissue glue
    Disposable skin stapler
    6.0 Surgilene suture
    5.0 Surgilene suture
    4.0 Surgilene suture
    4.0 Dexon suture
    Steri-Strips (3 mm, 5mm)
    Tincture of benzoin swabs

Wound dressings
    Band-Aids (assorted sizes)
    2 x 2 gauze
    4 x 4 gauze
    2 inch Kling gauze
    Polysporin ointment
    One inch cloth tape
    1/2 inch pink tape
    Xeroform gauze
    Q-tips   Mole skin
    Sam splint
    Ace wrap
    Duct tape

Eyes, ears, nose and throat
    Sterile eyewash
    Tetracaine drops
    Mydriacyl drops
    Sulamyd drops
    Ciprofloxacin drops
    Erythromycin ointment
    Fluorescein strips
    Ophthalmoscope/otoscope

Table 31.4	Example of physician level first aid kit—cont'd

Category

    Alligator forceps
    Earwick
    Cortisporin otic suspension
    Rhinoguard epistaxis device
    Lidocaine 2% jelly
    Ear speculum
    Afrin nasal spray
    Sucrets (oral anesthetic)

Dental
    'tempadent' (dental filling)
    Oil of clove

Dermatologic
    Topical steroid (sample size)
    Clotrimazole cream (sample size)
    Topical 'sting relief'
    Sunscreen (UVA & UVB blocker)

Oral medications
    Pain / sedation
        Acetaminophen
        Ibuprofen
        Acetaminophen / hydrocodone
        Diazepam
        Haloperidol

Antibiotics
    Ciprofloxacin
    Azithromycin
    Penicillin VK

Gastrointestinal
    Imodium AD
    Docusate sodium (stool softener)
    Oral rehydration salt packets
    Ranitidine

Cough / cold
    Sudafed decongestant
    Echinacea herbal supplement
    Zinc tablets

Altitude
    Acetazolamide 125 mg
    Dexamethasone 4 mg
    Nifedipine 10 mg

Other
    Diphenhydramine
    Prednisone
    Caffeine (nodose)

Miscellaneous

21 and 25 gauge butterfly needles

Small ziplock plastic bags w/labels

Small breakout emergency medical bag

One liter normal saline

Trauma scissors

Latex gloves

Small flashlight

Electronic thermometer

Eye protection

Stethoscope

Bp cuff

Safety pins

Lighter

Small notepad

Table 31.4	Example of physician level first aid kit—cont'd
Category	
Pen or other writing instrument	
Pregnancy test	
Urine dip stick test	
Pocket pharmacopoeia reference	
Pocket emergency medicine reference	

The other terms of your insurance will remain the same. Detailed discussion of 'occurrence' versus 'claims made' insurance, with a 'tail', are beyond the scope of this discussion, but if these terms are unfamiliar, it would be wise to familiarize yourself with them. Simply stated, occurrence coverage will cover any event that occurs within the timeframe of the policy – if a trip participant chooses to bring a lawsuit several years later, you would still be provided for. In contrast, is the 'claims made' insurance, where you are only covered against malpractice claims during the time you are paying premiums. Legal action years later may find you unprotected, unless a 'tail' to your policy is purchased. The 'tail' extends the policy for a fixed period of time, for a fixed price.

If you are providing medical services on behalf of a larger travel organization, it is possible to be covered under the auspices of the parent company. This practice, however, is rare – most travel companies looking for a 'trip physician' will require the physician to provide his/her own malpractice insurance. Do not overlook this issue during your discussions with such a company. The expedition physician assumes liability even if not formally paid. Simply receiving a trip discount brings responsibility and potential exposure. So-called 'Good Samaritan' laws do not apply here.

If you currently have no malpractice insurance, and the expedition itself is unable or unwilling to provide this, it is wise to explore insurance options simply for the duration of the trip. That being said, this sort of coverage is increasingly difficult to obtain. One physician, having exhausted the local options, actually turned to Lloyds of London to craft a customized insurance product.

In sum, medical legal exposure is one of the unfortunate realities of providing medical care in almost any situation. Signing up as the expedition physician will ensure adventure, but also brings added responsibility. Generally practicing 'good medicine' is the best advice, but having a good malpractice policy will provide an additional layer of comfort.

ON THE ROAD

As expedition medical officer, the responsibility will be that of caring for the group members should they become unwell; managing any medical emergencies that may occur and organizing evacuations and repatriations should they be necessary. In the field of Wilderness Medicine, the following attributes have been suggested as desirable for a 'wilderness physician' and they translate well into selection criteria for an expedition doctor: 'forethought, preparation, experience, confidence in your knowledge and abilities, the ability to step into a "wilderness" mindset, and especially, the ability to take a thorough history, do a meticulous and accurate physical examination, and draw the proper conclusions from your findings …'.[5] All this has to be accomplished in potentially hostile environmental conditions, with no back up and limited communications.

It is important to remember that the group will probably include local staff – their health on the expedition is also the expedition physician's area of responsibility. There is a popular misconception that porters in the developing world are made of 'tougher stuff' than Westerners. Recently, the health of porters, particularly in the Himalayas and Andes has been studied, and it has been found that even on commercial high altitude treks, porters are just as likely as Western trekkers to become ill or injured at altitude.[6] Concerned individuals have established an organization known as the International Porter Protection Group (IPPG) to educate trekking and climbing groups of their responsibilities toward their local staff (www.ippg.net).

It is wise to lay down the ground rules at the beginning of your trip – you should set aside a specific time each day for 'clinic'. All non-urgent problems should be dealt with at this time, including problems of the local staff. Treating the local population is a contentious issue,[7] and will be discussed later in the chapter.

This section will look briefly at the more common types of expedition and the conditions the expedition physician should be prepared for. Some aspects will be covered in more detail in other chapters, and specific texts should be consulted for more detailed information.

There has been little published research on the actual incidence of medical problems on expeditions. Physicians will have a 'feel' for the emergencies they should be prepared for, but how does this correlate with what actually happens in the field?

The Expedition Advisory Center of the Royal Geographic Society in London has established a 'medical cell' that is studying the incidence of medical problems during expeditions. Data published by them in the year 2000 examine expeditions that were in the field between 1995 and 1997.[1] The data are based on the voluntary submission of questionnaires from expedition leaders. The study authors recorded information from 36% of the expeditions registered with the Society over this time period.

Their data examine 2381 participants in 246 expeditions who visited 105 different countries for a total of 130 000 'man-days' in the field. Of these expeditions, 41% visited the mountains, 33% the tropics and the remaining groups visited variously polar regions, desert or marine environments. Group sizes ranged from 1–90 members, with a mean of nine. The average length of trip was 8 weeks with a range of 2 weeks to more than 3 months. The main purposes were scientific study (45%), adventure (39%), community work (2%) and a mix of science and adventure (14%).

Most notably, only 13% of expeditions had any medical provider accompanying them. Some 65% relied on a trained 'first aider', 6% on a registered nurse and 4% on a paramedic. A total of 13% had no-one with any medical training accompanying them. This is a marked improvement on data collected in 1983, which showed that 52% of 95 expeditions had no individual with even basic first aid training accompanying them.[8] Despite this, nearly three-quarters of the groups reported medical problems. A total of 181 groups reported a total of 835 incidents resulting in an incident rate of 6.4/1000 'man-days' in the field. Some 78% of incidents were classified as mild (the person could return to their activity after treatment); 17% were intermediate (the person was unable to return to activity but did not require evacuation) and 5% were serious (resulting in death, evacuation or hospitalization). Repatriation back to the UK was required by only 0.3% of expeditioners.

Not surprisingly, the most common problem affecting expedition members was gastrointestinal illness, particularly diarrhea – this accounted for 33% of problems recorded. Similar figures were reported by the British 1992 winter expedition to Mt. Everest[9] and reflect the rate of GI illness in travelers to less developed countries in general (see Table 31.5). What may be a nuisance for the leisure traveler can be a devastating illness that risks the success of an expedition.[16] Chapters 16–19 in this volume cover this topic in detail. The expedi-

Table 31.5	Conditions treated on British Mt. Everest winter expedition
Category	**Number of cases**
GIT	
Gastroenteritis	43 (30%)
Upper GI bleed	1
Dyspepsia	2
Persistent vomiting	1
Hemorrhoids	3
TRAUMA	
# Tibia	1
STI incl. lacerations	10
RESP	
Sore throat	14
High altitude cough	18
Cough induced intercostal myalgia	2
Respiratory tract infection	5
Persistent nasal congestion	2
ENVIRONMENTAL	
Hypothermia	2
Sunburn	5
AMS mild	24
AMS severe	2
Frostbite	6
GENERAL MEDICAL	
Ileofemoral venous thrombosis	1
Insomnia	5
Macular hemorrhage	1
Presumed retinal ischaemia	1
DENTAL	
Abscess	2
Lost crown	2

Adapted from[10].
The team consisted of 18 climbers, 15 trekkers, two base camp staff, 10 Sherpas and 10 porters. A total of 28% of complaints in porters and Sherpas; the remainder in members and trekkers.

tion physician should ensure that the incidence of any specific pathogens that could be of concern during the trip has been researched, e.g., are you visiting Nepal at the end of the monsoon when Cyclospora is still a problem? Ensure that your method of water purification and armament of antibiotics reflects the pathogens to which your group will be exposed. Anecdotally, it appears that individuals who are suffering from an intercurrent illness such as diarrhea are more susceptible to altitude sickness.[10] In an expedition situation any illness should be treated at an early stage.

'General medical conditions' accounted for 21% of problems recorded by the RGS expeditioners, and these included chest, ear and skin infections, typhoid fever, 23 cases of confirmed or suspected malaria, seven cases of dengue fever and 16 disabling drug side-effects. Interestingly, mefloquine was felt to be the offending drug in 75% of these cases.

A total of 17% of problems were classified as 'orthopedic'. These were predominantly falls on rough terrain, burns, lacerations, bruises, and concussion. Only 11 people were involved in motor vehicle accidents and one in an avalanche. Fourteen percent of problems were 'environmental' – 50% of these being altitude related, with sunstroke and heat exhaustion making up 35%. Eight percent were unwell as a result of arthropod, or other wildlife bites – particularly scorpions, snakes and jellyfish. Surgical disorders were rare and accounted for only 3% of complaints including two cases of appendicitis, 10 minor dental problems and 13 cases of minor ophthalmic trauma.

Of the serious disorders, altitude sickness accounted for 27% of cases, 'general medical' (predominantly malaria) for 27%, and serious fractures or dislocations in the mountains for 23%. Only two deaths were recorded and these were both as a result of kidnapping. The authors of the paper suggest that 'participation in a well-planned expedition is comparatively safe, with a medical incident rate of 6.4 per 1000 man-days and a death rate of 1 per 12 000 participants'.[1] They compare this to the risk of a medical incident at other events that young people participate in: 10 per 1000 at a scout camp; 17 per 1000 at a rock concert, and 28 per 1000 running a marathon.[11]

There is no doubt that the level of risk varies according to the style of expedition that one is undertaking. As only 13% of the studied expeditions took a medical officer with them it is tempting to suggest that many of them would be considered relatively low risk by the organizers and participants. High altitude mountaineering is known to be a very dangerous past time, with a death rate of 2.9% quoted by Shlim and colleagues.[12] An analysis of British mountaineering deaths on peaks of over 7000 m from 1968 to 1987 gave a mortality rate of 4.3 per 100 mountaineers. A total of 70% of deaths were due to falls, avalanches, or crevasse accidents.[13]

'The next phase of the expedition is ambitious: climb Rakaposhi, a huge mountain reaching into sky and cloud. But ambition has left, replaced by unshakeable illness in us all. A combination of dysentery and dehydration flattens me, and I end up back in Karambad, in the hospital for a day, and I'm prostrate for a week. It was a small thing that entered our guts, bacterial in dimension, but devastating out of all proportion to its size. Our conversation dwells on it. Bowels and intestines...'[14]

Although acute psychiatric problems appear to be rare on expeditions, they are without doubt one of the more difficult problems to manage in a remote area. Expeditions will invariably involve significant levels of stress, discomfort and interpersonal conflict. Most individuals will cope under these circumstances, however there is a small chance an individual may decompensate, resulting in a psychiatric crisis. Pre-travel screening is crucial in trying to avoid such potential problems. There are no hard and fast rules, but some issues to consider include:

- Past behavior. Find out what your team members have done in the past and speak to people who have traveled with them – how have they coped under difficult circumstances previously? Past behavior is a better predictor of future behavior than words and intentions.
- Enthusiasm of the individual for not only the trip but for life in general. What are the persons' motivators? Negative reasons for joining a trip (such as getting over a major life crisis) are not necessarily a contraindication to joining the group, but these issues should be explored prior to departure.
- Past mental health history. Very serious thought should be given before considering someone with a past history of hospitalization for a psychiatric illness.

A good team leader will be working on keeping open and effective communication throughout the team, and a good team physician should be unobtrusively monitoring the mental health of his or her group.

Acute psychosis is a diagnosis feared by the team doctor. In the case of travel, most cases of acute psychosis occur in individuals with no past history of mental illness. The exact diagnosis under these circumstances has not been systematically studied, however it has been suggested that acute situational psychosis is the most common diagnosis in this situation.[15] Team doctors should have an injectable antipsychotic in their medical kit, and follow-up medication as required. Repatriation is often very difficult in these situations, as the patient needs to be stabilized before boarding a passenger aircraft and he/she will often need a medical (Dr or RN) escort home. A lack of familiar medical facilities and personnel in developing countries can further exacerbate the situation.

Other less dramatic problems include dealing with 'difficult' patients such as the hypochondriac, or potentially more dangerously, the stoic. Those who have never traveled to a less developed country before may find the whole experience overwhelming and can develop symptoms such as anxiety, fear, depression, being over anxious about their health, insomnia and withdrawal. Some doctors have coined the term PUTA – Psychologically Unfit to Travel in Asia, to describe this condition.[16] This can, of course, occur at any destination away from the individuals' home.

Post-traumatic stress disorder is a serious consideration in anyone who has been involved in a major trauma while traveling. It is important that the trip physician remains involved with such individuals and ensures appropriate follow-up on their return home.

'The most insidious danger on any expedition where men have to rub shoulders for weeks is a mental sickness which might be called 'expedition fever' – a psychological condition which makes even the most peaceful person irritable, angry, furious, absolutely desperate because his perceptive capacity gradually shrinks until he sees only his companions faults while their good qualities are no longer recorded by his grey matter'.[17]

Polar environments

Travel to polar regions has increased enormously over recent years. In 1998, there were 37 winter stations run by 18 nations located south of the 60th parallel, and over 10 000 tourists and adventurers visited Antarctica during the summer season.[18] Virtually all published data on polar medicine have come from individuals working in these research stations.[18–20] While these stations do have medical facilities and usually one physician, conditions are extreme and emergencies can be very difficult to manage.[21]

Analysis of problems on Antarctic bases shows that the most common cause of medical consultation is injury or poisoning (42% of cases). Other frequent problems are categorized as respiratory (9.7%); skin and subcutaneous tissue (9.6%); CNS (7.5%); GIT (7.4%); infections and parasitic diseases (7.3%); musculoskeletal and connective tissue (7.1%), and psychiatric disorders (2.3%). According to the researchers 'high rates of dental problems and skin diseases contrasted with low rates of disease related to the environment (e.g., cold injury, sunburn, snow blindness) and psychiatric problems'.[19] British investigators have reported similar results. In a retrospective study of medical records compiled by the British Antarctic Survey from 1986–1995, only 2.5% of medical consultations were for cold injury. A total of 95% of these cases were frostbite (Fig. 31.2); in three-quarters of cases this was superficial, and most commonly affecting the face. Trench foot and hypothermia accounted for only a very small number of cases. The majority of the cases occurred as a result of recreational skiing or snowmobile driving. The most significant factor associated with the development of frostbite was previous cold injury. The authors conclude that 'cold injury is uncommon on Antarctica. Despite this, it warrants a continued high profile as under most circumstances it may be regarded as an entirely preventable occurrence.'[20] This pattern is in contrast to what one might expect of small group expeditions to these regions who do not have access to the climate-controlled facilities of a scientific base.

Mountaineering

Mountaineering expeditions are increasingly becoming high profile public events. Books such as *Into Thin Air* chronicling the tragic

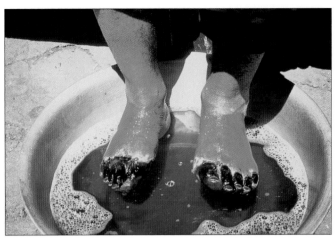

Figure 31.2 Frostbite in a Himalayan porter. With permission from Dr Urs Hefti.

events of 1996 on Mt. Everest have highlighted the danger inherent in high altitude climbing. Those who have survived the 1970s and 1980s climbing scene are the exceptions rather than the norm (Figs 31.3 and 31.4). Many classics of mountaineering literature are based on stories of serious falls and miraculous survivals.[22,23] Technical climbing, even at moderate altitudes, has a significant death rate. Analysis of death

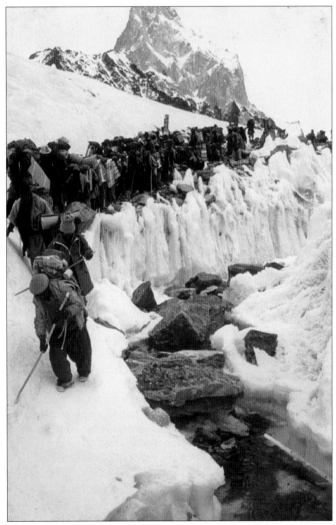

Figure 31.3 Porters approaching K2 base camp. With permission Dr Jim Duff.

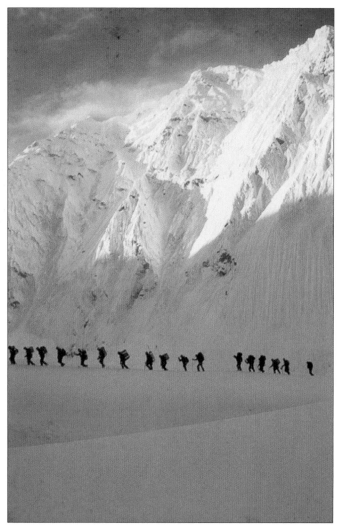

Figure 31.4 High altitude porters climbing on Mt Everest. With permission Dr Jim Duff.

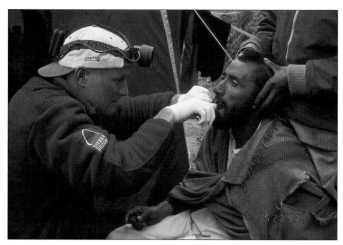

Figure 31.5 Dental extraction.

data in the New Zealand Alps (Mt. Cook is the highest mountain at just over 3000 m), showed that the risk of death in the more technically difficult areas of the park was 6.5/1000 days – a similar rate to that reported for high altitude climbing.[24] The world's two highest mountains, Everest and K2 have significant mortality rates.[25]

As many of the world's highest and most challenging mountains are located in countries known to have high rates of enteric disease (Nepal, Pakistan, India, Tibet, Peru, Bolivia, Kazakhstan, etc.) it is not surprising that diarrhea ranks highest on the list of likely problems encountered on a mountaineering expedition. Meticulous attention to hygiene standards on arrival in the host country, on the walk in, and at base camp are necessary to try and minimize this risk – often a huge challenge. Early treatment is recommended to limit the debilitation that can be caused by a bout of bacterial diarrhea.

Respiratory problems are also frequent – particularly the ubiquitous high altitude cough – known as the Khumbu cough in the Everest region of Nepal. 'Sore throat, chronic cough, and bronchitis are nearly universal in persons who spend more than two weeks at an extreme altitude (over 5500 m or 16500 f)'.[26] Of note is that these symptoms are not usually accompanied by the traditional signs of infection such as fever, myalgias or lymphadenopathy. The disorder is considered to be the result of a combination of obligate mouth breathing due to exertion, the cold dry air, and the addition of vasomotor rhinitis.

Acute mountain sickness, frostbite, hypothermia, UV keratitis, and sunburn are the most common environmental problems for which one must be prepared. Dental problems often pose a significant challenge for doctors in remote areas – it would be wise to gain some basic dental skills before going on a major expedition (Fig. 31.5). Replacing lost fillings and managing dental abcesses appear to be the most common issues.

Major trauma is the major fear of the mountaineering expedition doctor. Falls are likely to be serious and to result in major injuries. Larger expeditions will carry commercial splinting and traction systems to stabilize such patients.[10] If traveling with a smaller expedition one should familiarize oneself with possible methods of improvised splinting and traction systems. An excellent review of this topic can be found by Weiss and Donner in *Wilderness Medicine*.[27] Blood and fluid loss can present a potentially life threatening situation. Intravenous isotonic crystalloids or perhaps colloids should be carried. Cross transfusion between group members is potentially an option. This can be done by creating a donor-recipient chart after checking each group member for blood group antibodies and blood-borne infection. There are also commercial cross match kits available for use in the field but these do not provide any information about infectivity. Field blood transfusion would obviously be an enormous medical and logistical challenge.

Many doctors involved in climbing expeditions are experienced climbers themselves. There is also a more formal qualification known as the International Diploma of Mountain Medicine. These European-based courses are intensive, with over 100 h of course work, and require a certain level of mountaineering skill. There are two parts to the course – the common thread and then a choice of one of the specialty courses studying mountain rescue or expedition and wilderness medicine.[28]

Dr Jim Duff shares his experience as team doctor on this daring, small group climb of the North face of Everest by four Australians in 1988. Two of the team summitted on a route that is still considered one of the most difficult on the mountain.

'*After several weeks of hard and unsupported effort a team of four climbers set off from their high camp in a bid for the summit. Taking a purist approach, no fixed rope or supplemental oxygen was used on this summit push. The climbers accepted that they were essentially soloing on the mountain as each person had little in reserve to help the others.*

On a 100-meter steep mixed section one of the climbers discovered he had a broken crampon. He was in a precarious position and the crampon required repair. In order to achieve this he had to remove all of his gloves apart from the lowest layer, a pair of thinsulate gloves. The climber's hands became increasingly frostbitten as he continued up to the top of the west ridge and he was within 50 vertical meters of the summit when his friends returned from the summit and he accompanied them back down to their top camp in the dark. On return to top camp radio contact was established. This was our only means of communication for diagnosis and treatment over the next 40 hours, before the climber reached the foot of the mountain face. He was met at the base of the face and treated with oxygen, but no rewarming was attempted until his return to base camp when we could ensure that no refreezing would occur. This climber ultimately lost all of his fingers down to the PCP joint and required ongoing physical and emotional support until surgery was performed some months later, and beyond.'

This case demonstrates some of the unique aspects of providing care in such extreme circumstances – equipment failure is a potent source of injury or death; the treating physician may be remote from the victim and may need to treat by proxy; victims of severe injuries such as this one need long term support. As the initial emotional shock wears off depression is common.

Useful websites are listed in Table 31.4.

Desert environments

Desert environments are characterized by high daytime temperatures, low nighttime temperatures and potentially huge temperature variations over a single 24-h period – up to 45 °F.[29] Additionally, there is little surface water, minimal vegetation, clear sunny skies, potentially strong winds and sparse human habitation. Planning ahead in such an unforgiving environment is essential – 'in deserts, travelers have the potential to kill themselves quite easily through bad planning, and this is a wasteful way to go'.[30]

Clearly, the major health risks in desert environments result from the heat and UV exposure. Humans do have some ability to adapt to heat (as opposed to cold), however this takes at least 7–10 days.[31] There should be adequate time for acclimatization before starting the expedition and activities should be designed to reduce the risk of heat exhaustion or, more seriously, heat stroke. Activity should be avoided during the hottest part of the day (usually 10 a.m. until 3 p.m.), and appropriate clothing should be worn. As little skin as possible should be exposed to the sun. Broad brimmed or legionnaires-style hats are a necessity, as are sunglasses. Shoes should balance the need for protection against the harsh surface and comfort in order to avoid blisters. Awareness of the symptoms of heat exhaustion and dehydration among group members is paramount, and they should ensure they are keeping an eye on each other. Important warning signs include headache, nausea, dizziness, vomiting and anorexia. Recent work on hikers in the Grand Canyon has highlighted the risk of exercise-induced hyponatremia that can occur as a result of over hydration in individuals exercising in conditions of extreme heat.[32] The authors note 'heat exhaustion is difficult to distinguish from mild hyponatremia; we did not find statistically significant differences in symptoms or signs until clinically apparent alterations in mental status appeared.' They found that hyponatremia was the most common cause of serious illness related to exercising in the heat, and that altered mental status, convulsions (in the absence of hypoglycemia and extreme hyperpyrexia), and the development or progression of symptoms after the cessation of exercise were suggestive of hyponatremia. The remarkably simple prevention for this serious problem is the regular ingestion of sodium-containing foods.

Heat exhaustion may also progress to heat stroke – a true medical emergency. Before 1950, the mortality rate for heat stroke was between 40 and 75%,[31] and without the benefits of a hospital emergency room,

this statistic is likely to hold true in the field. The obvious answer is to avoid the problem in the first place through behavior modification, however the expedition physician needs to be familiar with the clinical spectrum of heat illness and its management in the field.

Jungle/tropical environments

Heat is also the main threat in tropical jungle environments, however it is the accompanying humidity that particularly characterizes these areas, and significantly increases the risk of heat related illness (See quote Redmond O'Hanlon).

First time visitors to such regions may waste an enormous amount of time trying to stay dry – when in reality this is a futile effort. It is however worth putting in an effort to stay dry at night, and to have dry clothes to change into at the end of the day. Skin is particularly vulnerable to the constant 'wetness' of jungle travel with fungal infections, maceration, cuts that refuse to heal and prickly heat all potential problems. As with all hot environments careful attention to fluid and electrolyte replacement is essential to avoid heat exhaustion, hyponatremia and heat stroke. Water is generally abundant in these environments, but will usually require purification to avoid enteric disease.

Malaria and other vector-borne disease are likely to be a significant risk in most tropical jungle areas of the world. These important topics are covered elsewhere in this text.

Other arthropods such as ants, chiggers, botfly, sandflies, wasps, bees, spiders and scorpions may also be prevalent in your patch of the jungle. Mammals such as bats are a rabies risk, snakes and fish such as candiru, piranha, eels and stingrays have fearsome reputations. Research your destination thoroughly so you are aware of the potential hazards you may encounter.

'The heat seemed insufferable, a very different heat from the dazzling sunlight of the river-side, an all-enclosing airless clamminess that radiated from the damp leaves, the slippery humus, the great boles of the trees…my shirt was as wet as if I had worn it for a swim in the river…with a humidity of 98% there is nowhere for sweat to evaporate, no relief by cooling, just an added body-stocking of salt, slime, smell and moisture'. (Redmond O'Hanlon: Into the Heart of Borneo)

Kayaking and rafting

White water enthusiasts are now traveling to increasingly remote destinations in their aim to run 'first descents'. The Himalayas – particularly Nepal, Bhutan and Tibet are renowned for their difficult rivers.

Rivers are graded from Class I to Class VI – class VI describing runs that 'exemplify the extremes of difficulty, unpredictability and danger. The consequences of error are very severe, and rescue may be impossible.'[33] A recent well-publicized white water kayak trip to the Tsangpo River in Tibet exemplifies the exploratory and dangerous nature of some kayak expeditions.[34]

Health risks of particular relevance to white water kayak and raft trips include:

- Ingestion or immersion in contaminated water. Apart from the obvious risk of contracting enteric disease from swallowing water, diseases such as leptospirosis and schistosomiasis have been contracted by groups undertaking trips on rivers in countries such as Costa Rica, Thailand and Ethiopia[35–37]
- Dehydration – despite proximity to water, heat and strenuous activity may result in inadequate fluid replacement
- Drowning and near-drowning. Almost all fatalities on rivers are as a result of submersion.[38] Wearing a PFD (personal flotation

device, or life jacket) may reduce the risk of drowning; however, on extreme rivers entrapment may be inescapable

■ Trauma. One of the injuries commonly associated with kayaking is anterior shoulder dislocation. If you are accompanying a kayak trip you should feel comfortable with relocation techniques. One analysis of white water injuries showed that shoulder dislocation accounted for 16% of injuries. Other common injuries included fractures (17%), leg injuries (13%), near drowning (13%), and lacerations (10%).[38] Ankle injuries commonly occur as a result of portaging (carrying the raft or kayak overland in areas where the river is not navigable), or while scouting ahead. Head injuries in a remote area can be disastrous: always wear a helmet and a PFD in white water

■ Blisters from paddles, and other abrasions, can be slow to heal in the constantly wet environment

■ Burns are a significant risk as a result of campfires lit at evening riverside camps

■ UV damage from sun exposure, exacerbated by almost 100% reflection of UV by the water

Doctors accompanying kayaking or rafting expeditions should be particularly versed with managing trauma.

Useful websites are listed in Table 31.4.

Scuba diving expeditions

Scuba diving is covered in detail in Chapter 39. Doctors accompanying dive trips should have undertaken extra training in hyperbaric medicine. Participants should be carefully screened. They should have a recent and thorough diving medical and should be screened for past diving related problems, particularly DCI (Decompression Illness). A contingency plan for the management of DCI, including the location of the closest hyperbaric chamber and a plan for how to get there, should be made in advance. An update on basic skills and emergency responses for all members of the group is wise – a common cause of dive accidents is a failure to respond rapidly to an emergency. Equipment failure poses a real risk in scuba diving, so thorough attention to maintenance of equipment is essential.

While some dive expeditions will be undertaken in cold environments (there are many commercial dive trips to the Antarctic), most dive locations are in the warmer tropical areas of the world. In particular, the expedition physician should ensure the group has appropriate antimalarial prophylaxis if relevant, e.g. many authorities still recommend avoiding mefloquine in divers. The availability of Malarone (atovaquone/proguanil combination) has made the choice of antimalarial medication for divers easier. Other vector-borne diseases are also likely to be prevalent. The expedition physician should ensure that the group is insured specifically for diving – many policies will actively exclude cover for treatment in a recompression chamber, or evacuation to such a facility. Groups such as DAN (Divers Alert Network) offer specialized insurance packages for diving, including phone support with a doctor trained in hyperbaric medicine, and cover for evacuation to the nearest recompression chamber. There are little data on the exact risk of diving expeditions, however data on recreational divers show that the most common cause of hospitalization is decompression illness. One Australian study looking at hospital admissions in tourists to the state of Queensland found that in a 3-year period, there were 296 overseas visitors admitted for water related injuries. A total of 55% of these admissions were to treat decompression illness, 15% were for fractures or dislocations (predominantly as a result of rafting and kayaking) and 15% for drowning and non-fatal submersion.[39]

Specific problems to address with pre-planning yet still be prepared to manage include:

■ Coral cuts. These are notorious for developing secondary infection. Divers should wear protective clothing to minimize the risk of coral cuts.

■ 'Swimmers ear'

■ Venomous sea creatures, such as sea snakes, jelly fish etc. Ensure the area to be visited has been thoroughly researched in order to be aware of specific risks, e.g., box jellyfish.

■ Penetrating injury (sea urchin spines)

■ Marine acquired wound infection (*Vibrio species*)

■ Ciguatera poisoning if catching your own fish.[40] Commercial kits are available for detection of this toxin and may be useful.

■ Decompression illness

■ Barotrauma of any gas filled space

■ Arterial gas embolism

■ Motion sickness

■ Severe sunburn

Useful websites are listed in Table 31.4.

The luxury expedition

Rather than the rigors of the outback or Spartan existence of base camp, the expedition physician may find him/herself surrounded by relative luxury during the 'expedition'. A variety of factors have contributed to a new breed of upscale adventure travelers. As our population has aged, a lucky few have found themselves with an abundance of time, money, and desire to travel the world. Many travel companies provide 'high end' adventure travel, from safaris, to large private jets. The clientele are often older, and arguably sicker, than the average traveler. They have also paid for a very expensive trip and may have a different set of expectations regarding their medical care. This being said, these travelers are also often sophisticated, fun loving, well-read, world-traveled, and wonderful expedition companions.

Advice for the physician joining such a group would include extra attention to pre-travel health screening and considerations that the medical kit needs to be able to accommodate the potentially special needs of the group. Although still rigorous, such an expedition opens the door to a different set of travelers: chronic, hopefully stable, illness is common, and the expedition physician has an important role in the overall program. 'Clinic hours' before dinner, or on the jet, provide both a sense of service as well as help manage the physician's time. Lastly, having a supply of alternative remedies such as zinc tablets or echinacia will help keep the peace during the invariable outbreak of cough and cold.

LOCAL HEALTH CARE

Although serious emergencies on expedition are rare, they will provide you with the greatest level of stress. You should establish an evacuation plan and find out as much as you can about any local medical facilities that may be available.

The most logical way to prepare for any serious medical situation is to make contact with an evacuation assistance company in the middle to late planning stages of the expedition. In general, insurance companies contract assistance companies to undertake communication with the expedition doctor/local medical facility should an emergency occur, and to organize repatriation to the nearest relevant medical facility. It is also possible to have a corporate subscription directly with an evacuation company. Assistance companies have an extensive network of local care providers, and generally have practical knowledge of the quality of care that is available in a given location.

Contacting the assistance provider allows the company to be aware of your activities and location and therefore are forewarned of any potential problems. It is far better that the provider is aware there is a group of 20 paddlers in a remote area of Tibet, rather than being contacted for the first time in the middle of an emergency. If the company feels the risk is warranted it will set up a contingency network. Making this contact ensures that financial issues are also taken care of, as larger companies will have provisional guarantees pre-organized with local care providers.

Nepal, among the countries popular for expeditions, is unique in that it has a very comprehensive rescue network, with multiple helicopter companies offering their services. In this situation, access to a satellite phone will allow easy access to a helicopter rescue company. Limitations on rescue are imposed by weather and altitude/location, rather than access to facilities. This is one country where the involvement of an assistance company may not be required until repatriation back to Katmandu. One should still however be aware of the local facilities with which the assistance company has arrangements – this will facilitate further management, whether it be hospitalization, repatriation to Bangkok, or repatriation home. Nepal is also unusual in that there are two well-respected private medical clinics run by Western-trained physicians and usually staffed by a number of Western doctors. In most countries, finding reliable local medical care is far more difficult. Ideas for trying to find local facilities include contacting doctors who have previously visited the area in question, contacting local members of the ISTM, and contacting members of IAMAT. If the expedition physician is able to locate the closest reasonable facility prior to the expedition, it would be valuable to visit the facility and meet the treating physicians there, so that the level of care avail-able can be fully assessed. This will assist enormously when communicating with the assistance company should an evacuation be required. One important challenge is when to decide to turn over the care of your patient to another provider or medical team. Although the expedition physician has an obvious duty to care for his/her patient, the physician also has a duty to be available to care for the other members of the expedition, who may well be pressed, for a variety of reasons, to move on. This highlights the importance of having other members of the group trained in first aid, so that you are not entirely indispen-sable! An evacuation will be an enormously stressful situation – pre-planning for the eventuality can only be helpful.

DIFFICULT SITUATIONS

Above and beyond the obvious challenges of group medical care in an austere environment, there are several other situations that may or may not arise to challenge you in your role as expedition physician. Some depend on the nature of your expedition (trekking to Everest base camp or beyond versus an organized tour of the Galapagos), some on your destination (Middle East versus Northern Europe), and some simply on circumstance.

Medical care of others

It is not uncommon for expeditions, even to relatively remote parts of the globe, to cross paths with other expeditions. This can be an opportunity for cultural exchange, learning from groups who are returning from your destination, and even occasionally shifting the load of food or equipment. There may, however, be an expectation of sharing the expedition physician and medical supplies. This can be acutely problematic in the setting of another group that is not medically prepared and/or has an acute medical problem. Obviously, for urgent or life threatening cases, medical concerns come first. But, non-urgent requests can strain the time and resources of the medical team. Plenty of expedition physicians have awoken to a line outside the tent of porters or climbers seeking medical attention. The expedi-

tion physician and other members of the team should be prepared for this eventuality. Again, preparation is key: will there be other groups at your destination? Is it appropriate to contact them in advance of the trip? Should extra medical supplies be packed, and if so, how much? Discussing this situation in advance and deciding on a party line will help when the situation arises.

More difficult is the issue of providing medical care to the local population. This will be less of an issue for the average commercial trip, but can be a challenging situation for expeditions traveling through local villages. Locals may go out of their way to pursue medical assistance or advice from a traveling physician. As with caring for other expeditions, this issue needs to be thought through and prepared for, in advance.

Safety and security

Although technically not the responsibility of the expedition physician, as a member of the expedition team, it is not uncommon for the physician to get involved in issues of safety and security for the group. Obviously, if there is a threat of injury or harm, the medical concerns can quickly become paramount. As with many of the other issues touched on in this chapter, preparation is extremely important. The expedition leadership should do their homework on their destination. US State department, or equivalent, information should be sought out and read. Friends or colleagues who have traveled recently to your destination can provide invaluable inside advice. Be familiar with the local cultural and political situation, and have at hand emergency contact information both for local police as well as appropriate embassies or consulates. A substantial supply of local currency can be invaluable.

If you have the budget, technology allows for excellent communication fixes in the way of international cellular telephones. Even satellite-based phones can be taken – with many vendors offering 'emergency only' subscription services which are worth looking into.

Useful websites are listed in Table 31.4.

REPATRIATION

Despite best efforts at screening trip participants and at keeping them well on trip, the situation may arise where one of the group becomes sufficiently injured or ill to warrant emergency evacuation to a site where more sophisticated medical care can be provided. Here the expedition physician's role can become quite challenging.

The first issue will be simply one of communication. Does the group have the means of calling for help? Even an investment in a satellite phone does not ensure success in all parts of the world, and one might need to rely on a porter or other messenger to deliver word by foot. In this case, it will have been extremely important to have set up a plan in advance. For example, in Nepal, a private, or even military helicopter can be requested to evacuate an ill or injured trekker, but only if that trek is registered in advance with the appropriate authorities. More commonly, phone communication is available, but the issue of advance planning is just as important.

There are many excellent companies dedicated to the medical repatriation of sick or injured travelers. The arrival of a sophisticated medical team, ready to swoop the patient off in a dedicated jet air ambulance is a relief for both patient and physician alike. But this moment comes at a price, and that price can be steep if the team is unprepared.

Aeromedical evacuation, with a physician-based team, can easily cost over US$100 000. This raises several very important points. It is essential that on any international expedition where there is a risk of significant illness or injury, each participant carry insurance to cover medical repatriation. In addition, pay particular attention to the 'cap' on the policy: less expensive policies may only cover up to US$50 000 leaving the patient with significant financial liability. Also, pre-existing illness clauses should be looked for and addressed if appropriate. The notion of paying out of pocket and then submitting receipts to your insurance company once back home is simply not practical for anything but the most minor of medical problems.

Note also that the first stop for such an evacuation may not be 'back home', but rather to a relatively local center where appropriate medical interventions can be provided. This may cause some fear or frustration for the ill passenger. Setting expectations, but also working closely with the medical repatriation company (and at times lobbying on behalf of the patient or family) are important roles for the expedition physician.

Lastly, the expedition physician caring for a patient who needs to be hospitalized or repatriated is faced with a difficult decision. When does he or she leave the patient to re-join the group for which he or she continues to have overall medical responsibility? This is a complicated question depending on many variables, and should be discussed with expedition leadership as soon as possible.

DEATH OVERSEAS

There can be no more challenging a situation for the expedition physician than to have one of the team die under his or her watch. The circumstances here can vary, ranging from an accident taking the life of a young and healthy climber to the sad, but not entirely unexpected death of a chronically ill elderly traveler on their last tour of the Caribbean. In any case, the issues for the trip physician are many.

For the patient suffering from a life-threatening illness or injury, there is the issue of coordinating local care and/or repatriation. Transporting an infirm victim from a remote location can be difficult, but even at the local hospital there are a number of obvious challenging issues such as language, finances, and physician or equipment availability. Less obvious can be issues of gender (male expedition physician and female patient, or vice versa), hours of operation (hospital pharmacy is closed overnight), to medical culture. Western physicians may be surprised to find a system where medications and supplies need to be purchased (cash only) at a pharmacy and then provided to the local doctors for use. Also, friends or family may be expected to provide nursing care, such as bathing the patient, simple wound care, and providing meals. It is important for the expedition physician to be aware of these potential issues when coordinating local medical care for the group.

Emotionally, having one of the team die while under your care is very difficult. The fact that other physicians or health professionals may have been involved may actually make the situation more complicated. It is difficult to be in a situation where you do not speak the language, do not know the system, and are left with a nagging feeling that you should have done more. Other members of your team will have the same feeling and a 'post incident' debriefing session is very important.

Practically, there are a number of issues that need to be handled in the event of a death overseas. Foremost is the need for communication. The victim's next of kin should be advised of injury, illness, or death as soon as possible. Also, communicating with the expedition's parent company or organization is very important. They may be able to coordinate communication and other efforts back home. Local burial or cremation may be available, depending on the desires of the victim's family. Repatriation of remains is usually arranged by the appropriate local embassy or consulate. Regulations may require that the deceased be embalmed prior to transport. Regardless, repatriation of remains can be an expensive proposition, and payment will need

to be provided before any action will be taken. Early involvement of the local embassy or consulate is advantageous, but do not overestimate their ability to intervene and problem solve on your behalf.

BACK HOME

On your return home, the expedition physician's obligations will depend upon the style of trip undertaken.

If you have been employed by a company, you should write a trip report outlining the medical problems you encountered, how they may be better prevented next time, comments on your experience with the evacuation company (if relevant) and any improvements you could recommend to the group and individual medical kits. If the company plans to employ a physician for their next trip, it is wise to make contact so the next trip doctor can be informed of any relevant issues.

If you had any dealings with local care givers, a letter of thanks and information on the outcome of the patient they cared for will be greatly appreciated, and will undoubtedly pave the way for even better relations should another injured or ill expedition member come their way in the future.

Finally, it is important to consider the health of the group in the post-travel period. It is wise to give them a list of symptoms and signs to be aware of over the ensuing weeks, based on the incubation times of common endemic diseases in the area visited. If there were any exposures that require screening for at a later stage, e.g., for schistosomiasis after 3 months, they should be given an appropriate protocol to follow with their local physician. Additionally, the group members should have your contact details so they can get in touch if they are concerned or need their regular physician to discuss any issues with you. You should keep in contact with anyone who has had a significant injury that will require extensive post travel treatment, e.g., frostbite. And of course, anyone who has been involved in a significant trauma or rescue situation should be counseled regarding post-traumatic stress disorder and advised to seek care should they develop symptoms.

Post travel illness is covered in detail in Chapters 52–57.

CONCLUSION

The role of the expedition physician has come a long way in the past century, coinciding in part with the sense of the world becoming ever smaller while our need for exploration and self-discovery ever larger. Such a personal expedition is no longer restricted to the extremely wealthy and privileged, although to a lesser degree this continues to be true. More and more, groups of travelers are organizing to explore the vastness of nature, the richness of other cultures, or the depths of their own spirits. The field of travel medicine has matured along with this change in travel patterns and as such even so called 'adventure travelers' are paying more attention to their health and more liberally involving physicians and other travel medicine professionals in the medical aspects of their planning.

The expedition physician, whether occupying the team to the summit, or simply advising the group from the office, has an increasingly complex role to play. The job begins long before departure with assessing the health of the party, educating participants, building a quality medical kit, doing destination homework, and working closely with other members of the expedition leadership. Once on the road the job responsibilities become more obvious, but there are many hidden pitfalls, including difficult patients, challenges to time and resources, and perhaps having to deal with significant injury, illness or death in an environment that is extremely remote both physically and culturally.

On the other hand, there are numerous rewards, not the least of which is traveling to an interesting or physically challenging corner of the globe. There is satisfaction to be had from providing quality health care with little besides a medical kit and personal creativity, improvising solutions while actually finding time to enjoy the expedition itself. It is hoped that, for your next expedition, this chapter will be one of the essential tools in your 'pre-travel' medical kit.

REFERENCES

1. McLeod WT, ed. *The New Collins Concise Dictionary of the English Language*. London: Collins; 1986.
2. Anderson SR, Johnson CJ. Expedition health and safety: a risk assessment. *J R Soc Med* 2000; **93**:557–562.
3. Roberts D, ed. *Points Unknown: A Century of Great Exploration*. New York: WW Norton & Co.; 2000.
4. McIntosh I. Trials and tribulations of an expedition doctor. *Trav Med Int* 1992; 72–77.
5. Bowman WD. Perspectives on being a wilderness physician: is wilderness medicine more than a special body of knowledge? *Wild Env Med* 2001; **12**:165–167.
6. Basnyat B, Litch JA. Medical problems of porters and trekkers in the Nepal Himalaya. *Wild Env Med* 1997; **8**:78–81.
7. Bishop RA, Litch JA. Medical Tourism can do Harm. *BMJ* 2000; **320**:1017.
8. Johnson CJH. Expedition medicine, a survey of 95 expeditions. *Travel Med Int* 1984; **2**:239–242.
9. A'Court CHD, Stables RH, Travis J. How to do it: Doctor on a mountaineering expedition. *BMJ* 1995; **310**:1248–1252.
10. Prativa Pandey. Personal communication from Dr Prativa Pandey MD. Medical Director, the CIWEC Clinic Kathmandu, Nepal.
11. Hodgetts TJ, Cooke MW. The Largest Mass Gathering. *BMJ* 1999; **318**:957.
12. Shlim DR, Houston C. Helicopter rescues and deaths among trekkers in Nepal. *JAMA* 1989; **261**(7):1017–1019.
13. Pollard A, Clarke C. Deaths during mountaineering at extreme altitudes. *Lancet* 1988; **1**(1277).
14. Child G. *Mixed Emotions*. Seattle: The Mountaineers; 1997.
15. Shlim DR. Psychological aspects of adventure travel. *Wild Med Lett* 2001; **18**(1).
16. Duff J, Gormly P. *First Aid and Survival in Mountain and Remote Areas*. Katmandu: Dr Jim Duff; 2000:158.
17. Taylor A. *Antarctic Psychology*. Wellington: DSIR Science Information Publishing Centre; 1987.
18. Lugg DJ. Antarctic medicine. *JAMA* 2000; **283**(16):2082–2084.
19. Sullivan P, Gormly PJ, Lugg DJ. Watts DJ. The Australian Antarctic Research Expeditions Health Register: three years of operation. In: Postl B, Gilbert P, Goodwill J, *et al.*, eds. *Circumpolar Health 90*. Winnipeg: University of Manitoba Press; 1991.
20. Cattermole TJ. The epidemiology of cold injury in Antarctica. *Aviat Space Environ Med* 1999; **70**:135–140.
21. Priddy RE. An 'acute abdomen' in Antarctica. *MJA* 1985; **143**:108–111.
22. Plowright RK. Crevasse fall in the Antarctic: a patients perspective'. *MJA* 2000; **173**:583–584.
23. Lamberth PG. Death in Antarctica. *MJA* 2001; **175**:583–4.
24. Malcolm M. Mountaineering fatalities in Mt Cook National Park. *NZ Med J* 2001; **114**(1127):78–80.
25. Huey RB, Eguskitsa X. Supplemental oxygen and mountaineer death rates on K2 and Everest. *JAMA* 2000; **284**(2):181.
26. Hackett PH, Roach RC. High altitude medicine. In: Auerbach PS, ed. *Wilderness Medicine*. St Louis, Mosby; 2001:2–43.
27. Weiss EA, Donner HJ. Wilderness improvisation. In: Auerbach PS, ed. *Wilderness Medicine*. St Louis, Mosby; 2001:466–494.
28. Peters P. Practical aspects in mountain medicine education. *Wild Environ Med* 2000; **11**:262–268.
29. Otten EJ. Desert survival. *Wild Med Lett* 2000; **17**(2).
30. Dryden M. Tropical and desert expeditions. In: Warrell D and Anderson S, eds. *The Royal Geographical Society Expedition Medicine*. London: Profile Books; 1998.
31. Gaffin SL, Moran DS. Pathophysiology of Heat-Related Illness. In: Auerbach PS, ed. *Wilderness Medicine*, St Louis, Mosby; 2001:240–289.
32. Backer HD, Shopes E, Collins SL, Barken H. Exertional heat illness and hyponatremia in Hikers. *Am Jour Emerg Med* 1999; **17**(6):532–538.
33. American Whitewater Affiliation. *Safety Code of the American Whitewater Affiliation*. New York: Phoenicia; 1989.
34. Balf T. *The Last River. The Tragic Race for Shangrila*. New York: Crown; 2000.
35. Centres for Disease Control and Prevention. Outbreak of Leptospirosis among white-water rafters – Costa Rica 1996. *Morb Mortal Wkly Rep* 1997; **46**:577–579.
36. Pinner R. Update on Emerging Infections: Outbreak of Acute Febrile Illness Among Athletes participating in Eco-Challenge - Sabah 2000 - Borneo, Malaysia 2000. *Ann Emerg Med* 2001; **38**(1):83–86.
37. Istre GR. Acute Schistosomiasis among Americans rafting the Omo River, Ethiopia. *JAMA* 1984; **251**(508).
38. Weiss EA. Whitewater medicine and rescue. In: Auerbach PS, ed. *Wilderness Medicine*. St Louis, MO: Mosby; 1995:1238.
39. Wilks J, Coory M. Overseas visitors admitted to Queensland hospitals for water-related injuries. *MJA* 2000; **173**(5):244–246.
40. Farstad DJ, Chow T. A brief case report and review of Ciguatera poisoning. *Wild Envir med* 2001; **12**:263–269.

CHAPTER 32   Remote Destinations

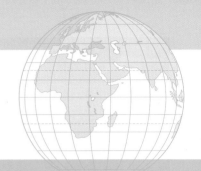

Michael V. Callahan and Davidson H. Hamer

INTRODUCTION

Travelers to remote destinations include employees of petroleum, mining and construction companies, scientists, members of the armed service and intelligence communities, adventure travelers, and expedition teams. In recent years, there has also been an increase in middle-aged travelers to remote destinations and among certain adventure activities such as moderate altitude mountaineering.[1] The rising popularity of adventure travel among this group has increased both the likelihood and complexity of medical problems occurring in remote, rural regions of both developed and developing countries.

One important feature of remote destination travel is that part of the itinerary places the traveler beyond the reach of adequate health facilities, air evacuation (medevac) services, and the support services of embassies. Travel in rural areas also places expatriates beyond the protective reach of centralized, typically urban, law enforcement agencies. Back-country travelers are more likely to run afoul of criminal or anti-government factions. When these travelers become sick, injured or victimized by the ill-intentioned, assistance may be delayed many hours, or even days. When immediate medical care is required, local health clinics are likely to be primitive, and physicians, when available, often lack resources to manage complicated or multi-casualty emergencies. A growing awareness about these dangers has prompted many travel advice resources to recommend that remote destination travelers obtain air evacuation insurance in the belief that commercial medevac operations can be reliably deployed to remote international locations. In reality, international medevac services often lack the required authorization, in-country staff, and appropriate airships necessary to extricate patients from rural regions of developing countries. For this reason, reliance upon medevac companies to provide emergency extraction from remote regions is ill advised. The distinction is made here between evacuation from rural regions, which remains problematic, and air medical evacuation from the capital cities of developing countries, which is common. In recent years, the quality of aeromedical services and training of providers has improved secondary to competition between quality providers and the expectations of the receiving hospital or physician.

PRE-TRAVEL SCREENING

The above considerations emphasize the point that remote destination travelers require a more comprehensive approach to pre-travel screening, immunization, personal security and health education. Pre-travel consultation to this group involves more than routine services, immunizations and health education. In the case of extreme and solo travelers, the risks to health and personal security are sufficiently great as to warrant the addition of protective measures to ensure autonomy and self-reliance. Examples of such measures include prearranged *in-country* legal, personal security and emergency medical services, and equipping disaster response teams, expeditions and small groups with handheld satellite phones and advanced medical kits.

Aggressive pre-travel health screening has been shown to reduce both the number of in-country medical emergencies and the number of air medical evacuations among a group of 1770 expatriates living in rural regions of several developing countries.[2] Routine health screening, which is covered by health maintenance plans, is usually insufficient for the subset of travelers that spend significant time in remote environments. Most travel medicine practitioners agree that unrecognized medical or psychiatric conditions are often unmasked by the stresses associated with prolonged placement in austere international settings. This observation is important as medical facilities in developing countries often lack resources to manage complex illnesses associated with western lifestyles such as chronic diseases imported by middle-aged petroleum management, business consultants or missionaries. In particular, exacerbations of chronic obstructive pulmonary disease (COPD), cardiac disease, neurological emergencies, and complications resulting from alcohol excess or withdrawal are the cause of considerable morbidity. Medical emergencies resulting from these conditions tend to do worse as medical resources become less advanced (Fig. 32.1). As a consequence, comprehensive medical exams are critical steps in the preparation of long-term travelers to remote destinations. It should be noted that routine health screening guidelines in western countries are based on probable age-adjusted health risks and the expectation that emergency medical care may be accessed in a reasonable amount of time.

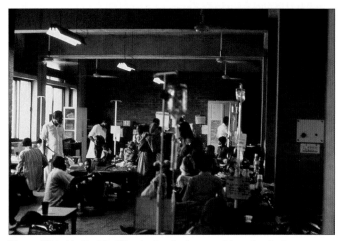

Figure 32.1 Medical facilities in developing countries often lack resources and experience treating chronic illnesses imported with western expatriates. The comprehensive medical exam is a critical component in reducing the likelihood of exacerbations of cardiac or pulmonary disease.

Table 32.1	Screening test for travelers to remote destinations

Highly recommended
Detailed review of the individual's medical history
Evaluation for risk factors for acute medical or psychiatric disease (e.g., family history, history of alcohol or drug abuse, sexually transmitted diseases, and psychiatric illness)
Complete physical examination
Dental examination
Screening for previously unrecognized psychiatric illnesses
Screening laboratory studies (e.g., complete blood count, fasting glucose, lipid profile, serum creatinine, transaminases)
Chest X-ray
12-lead electrocardiogram

Additional tests to be considered
Urinalysis
Glucose tolerance test
HIV testing
Pregnancy for women of child-bearing age
Pap smears
PPD
Maximum expiratory peak flow
Cardiac stress testing
Colonoscopy
Mammography

The value of thoughtful pre-travel screening is dramatically illustrated when the travel medicine practitioner is called upon to assist in the management of overseas medical or trauma emergencies involving patients they have seen in the travel clinic. During these emergencies, medical decisions must often be based in part on dubious data, circumspect laboratory findings, and the bedside assessment of foreign clinicians with uncertain qualifications. In these situations, it is comforting to have access to the results of a comprehensive pre-travel workup. Access to the patient's pre-travel record allows the travel medicine practitioner to refine the differential diagnosis, identify a likely etiology, and select the best treatment plan from the available options. For these reasons the pre-travel consultation for the remote-destination traveler will likely exceed the recommended tests and reimbursement for a patient of a given gender and age. The pre-travel consultation for this group of travelers should also include two frequently overlooked areas: dental examinations and screening for cryptic psychiatric illness such as depression.

The components of a pre-travel consultation for the remote destination traveler include an in-depth review of the individual's medical history, a complete physical examination, and screening laboratory studies appropriate for the patient's age, health, individual risk and the destination environment (Table 32.1). The intent of the studies is to identify previously unrecognized medical disorders. Careful evaluation of certain risk factors (e.g., family history, history of alcohol or drug abuse, sexually transmitted diseases, and psychiatric illness) will guide the selection of additional tests – many of which would not have otherwise been considered. It is not uncommon for these comprehensive work-ups to uncover evidence of psychological problems, inflammatory bowel conditions, malignancies, or deteriorating cardiac or pulmonary reserves. Routine tests for this special group of travelers should include a chest X-ray and a 12-lead electrocardiogram. More in-depth testing includes maximum expiratory peak flow, glucose tolerance tests, cardiac stress testing, serum creatinine, urinalysis, viral serologies, colonoscopy, and for women, pregnancy tests, Pap smears and careful mammography. The importance of identifying drug and alcohol dependency, and quiescent depression or other psychiatric illnesses cannot be overemphasized as these conditions are likely to be unmasked during stressful situations and unfamiliar surroundings.

Any abnormalities encountered during the pre-travel evaluation must be carefully addressed and treated prior to travel. In certain cases, new medical or psychiatric conditions identified during screening may preclude travel or long-term international placement. The traveler's insistence that the overseas health clinic, or on-scene medical provider, is capable of managing any medical complications that arise, will need to be verified. Careful consideration should also be given to travelers with certain chronic diseases that are uncommon in many developing countries. Stent-stabilized coronary artery disease, cardiac dysarrhythmias, brittle diabetes and exacerbation of COPD are particularly difficult to manage in rural regions of developing countries. Physicians in many developing regions often lack experience and resources necessary for managing these routine but dangerous medical problems.

Dental emergencies are an under appreciated cause of trip interruption and a leading reason why travelers access local medical care.[3] The primitive conditions of dental facilities may exceed that of rural medical clinics. In one study, dental problems affecting corporate management accounted for up to 8% of medical problems implicated in business interruption at several overseas jobsites.[2] Pre-travel dental examinations should be performed for any patient with oral discomfort, those with history of odontological disease and any patient who has not been evaluated in the last year. The dentist who performs the exam should be informed that the traveler may not have access to dental care for an extended period. The dental consultant should be encouraged to perform the exam in a manner that will identify dental problems, which will evolve over the next 6–12 months.

Long-term travelers, disaster assistance personnel, medical providers, and expatriates are likely to have prolonged contact with the local population, which often increases the risk of tuberculosis. Even short-term travelers to certain parts of the world (Africa, Central America, Southeast Asia, and the Indian sub-continent) are at risk for exposure to and acquisition of tuberculosis, especially if they are involved in some type of health-care work.[4] The increased risk underscores the need for tuberculin skin testing prior to and after travel.

Special considerations

Western travelers receiving treatment in foreign hospitals may also experience complications resulting from adverse drug interactions. It is not uncommon for the adverse reaction to result from interaction between the patient's prescription medications and a foreign produced pharmaceutical. One of the more dangerous potential adverse events is dysarrhythmias resulting from interaction between halofantrine, used to treat malaria, and the patient's class IA antiarrhythmics, or amiodarone. A common feature to these cases is that the complication often results from interactions between new generation medications prescribed to the traveler and an overseas pharmaceutical that is unavailable in the traveler's home country. There are several risk-reduction strategies that may be used to reduce drug–drug interactions in the traveler who is taking prescription medications prone to dangerous drug interactions. One practical approach is education regarding adverse interactions between the patient's prescription drugs and foreign pharmaceuticals. The value of focused drug education is limited, as it requires that the travelers have some understanding of medical care, and that he or she is conscious and able to comprehend the treatment plan in the foreign hospital. An alternative is to change the traveler's medication to a drug with fewer interactions. The decisions to swap medications should be made with input from the patient's prescribing sub-specialists, in particular, the cardiologists, endocrinologists and HIV specialist. In cases where treatment in overseas medical clinics is likely, or when the traveler is uncertain about drug allergies, the travel medicine practitioner should consider hypersensitivity drug testing, with particular attention to sulfa-, phenol- and penicillin-based medications.

IMMUNIZATIONS AND EDUCATION

Pre-travel consultation provides an excellent opportunity to update adult immunizations, while providing more specialized vaccines for the prevention of meningococcal meningitis, rabies, and Japanese encephalitis. Hepatitis B should be provided to all travelers but especially to those at increased risk of trauma, emergency surgery and others at risk for blood transfusions, medical relief personnel, or expatriates with prolonged placement. In certain circumstances, the traveler's activities or unique risks may require administration of restricted and specialty vaccines, such as the tick-borne encephalitis, plague, and anthrax vaccines (see Chapter 10).

All travelers should receive standard pre-travel advice about food and water safety, self-treatment of travelers' diarrhea, anti-vector measures, and safe sexual practices. However, in the case of the remote destination traveler, pre-travel education needs to be more extensive and expanded to include unique risks for a given natural ecotone, region, season, political climate and travel activity. For example, emphasizing that the traveler should drink only bottled or boiled water is useless if the traveler will be in areas where bottled water is unavailable, or boiling is impossible. In these cases, education should focus on field viable methods of water purification, such as improvised flocculation-halogenation using 4% hypochlorite, and recommendations regarding selection of a durable water purification filter. The value of tailoring pre-travel education to the traveler's medical condition and itinerary cannot be overemphasized. Special issues, such as avoidance of contact with fresh water for travelers to candiru or schistosomiasis-endemic areas, prevention of altitude illness for trekkers, and hypobaric illness for divers who use aircraft to travel between dive sites, should all be reviewed and practical risk reduction strategies recommended.

TRAVEL MEDICAL KIT

After the completion of the detailed medical and dental evaluations, the remote destination traveler should be provided with a first aid kit. The kit should be simple, compact, and contain a minimum number of prescription medications (Table 32.2). The traveler (and travel

Table 32.2 Remote travel emergency kit
Individual traveler (low to moderate risk activities)
Identification Knife multi-tool Compass/GPS Map Flashlight (LED, low power consumption) Whistle (plastic) Adhesive compresses Lighter, or 'strike anywhere' matches (dipped in candle wax to waterproof) Magnesium fire starters Bandana (silk) Cord Coins for telephone Radio/Satellite phone Personal first-aid material Prescription medication, labeled (in plastic or waterproof aluminum box) Medications for specific prior illness (e.g., insulin, glucose test strips, and buccally absorbed glucose for diabetics; bronchodilators for asthmatics; injectable epinephrine for insect-sting allergy; transdermal scopolamine for motion sickness Permethrin/DEET Spare sunglasses Sunscreen Signal mirror Aluminum foil Cagoule (e.g., Ikokatat®)
Two or more travelers: All items above plus the following: Pencil and paper (waterproof paper preferred) Accident report forms (waterproof) Spare bulb, batteries Closed-cell foam pads (1 × 1 foot sections, 3 oz) 'Space' blanket (1 oz) Surveyor's trail tape (50 ft, 1 oz) Nylon utility cord (2 oz) Heat source (candle; fuel tabs, 2 oz) Cagoule bivouac poncho (10 oz)
Polar/alpine traveler(s): All items listed under 'Individual traveler' plus the following additional items: Shovel (metal for avalanche or snow cave, 16–32 oz) Altimeter (2 oz) Road flare (5 min, 3 oz) Emergency shelter Thermometer, outdoor (0.5 oz) Aluminum adhesive tape (gutter tape Glue (JB Weld) Spare bale and screws Climbing skins (11–16 oz) 'P-tex' ski base stick Spare crampon wrench

medicine practitioner) should be reminded that the medical kit is no substitute for poor planning or bad judgment, and should not impart a false sense of security for either party. The traveler should be carefully counseled about the limitations of the kit's resources and medications. The kit should contain a laminated card that contains reminder recommendations, international assistance numbers and a basic decision-making algorithm written in lay terminology.

Long-term travelers must carry a supply of prescription medications that will comfortably exceed the duration of their stay. Medication must be professionally labeled with the patient's name in order to reduce unpleasant encounters with foreign customs officials or police. If the traveler requires narcotic-based analgesics, a minimum number of tablets should be carried and packaging should be well organized in order to reduce the likelihood of detainment or incarceration. In one small study of expatriate imprisonment in four developing countries, five (13%) of 39 incarcerations involved possession of allegedly illegal drugs.[5] In these cases, release of the expatriate was secured only after 'fines' were extorted from the employee's company or travel companions. The above case underscores the need for clear documentation. Patients or medical personnel carrying narcotics, sterile syringes, and in some countries, antiretroviral medications, should also carry a physician's note. Whenever possible, the traveler should also be provided with a 24-h physician contact number. All critical medications should be separated into multi-day aliquots and one supply should be carried with the traveler at all times. Many medications, such as long acting nitrates and first generation hypoglycemics, oxidize after exposure to air. Other medications contain anhydrous additives and gel-coverings, which degrade under warm, humid conditions. Warm temperatures also cause clumping of tablets, resulting in tearing of acid-protective coatings when tablets are manually separated. Problems with labile medications and degradation of gel coats may be reduced by repackaging tablets in blister packs or sealing small quantities of tablets in airtight poly bottles (e.g., Nalgene®).

Travel medical kits should be tailored for each client, based on trip itinerary, the patient's risk factors, and the types of health problems encountered in the destination environment. For example, nonsedating antihistamines to prevent 'hyperbaric squeezes', and meclizine, to reduce motion sickness, are usual additions to the recreation diver's medical kit. Conversely, a high altitude or polar trekker's kit should include analgesic lozenges for tracheal chapping and topical ointment and acrylamide skin glue to treat cuticles split by dry, cold, low torr conditions. A recommended list of routine and supplemental medications for different types of activities is provided in Table 32.2.

SELF-TREATMENT

The benefits of self-treatment of diarrheal diseases are well established,[6,7] and many clinics regularly provide travelers with antidiarrheal regimens. A growing number of travel medicine services are expanding self-treatment to include stand-by therapy for acute respiratory infections, hypersensitivity reactions, and the repair of dental amalgams. In recent years, rapid finger-stick blood tests have improved the ability to diagnose malaria in rural settings, but not without problems regarding interpretation of results or improper performance of the test.[8] While self-treatment seems to be reasonable for diarrheal illness, and most likely, malaria, it raises questions when more esoteric medical conditions are considered or when the therapy is associated with dangerous side-effects (Fig. 32.2). Examples of therapies that should not be included in travel medical kits include antivenin immunotherapy, which requires i.v. administration and protection against dangerous allergic reactions, and i.v. dexamethasone for treating neurotrauma and high altitude cerebral edema. In both cases, pre-travel education that emphasizes risk-avoidance strategies will do far more to prevent these dangerous events than will access to a dangerous therapy.

Providing instruction to go along with the medications does not insure that the traveler, or the traveler's companion will use the medication correctly.

Depending on the medical skills of the traveler, trip duration, number of travelers, trip activities and hazards endemic to the destination environment, additional diagnostic and therapeutic resources may be considered. Recommended basic medical kits for common adventure travel activities are provided in Table 32.3.

ADVENTURE TRAVEL GROUPS

Groups traveling to remote destinations are likely to include wilderness adventure charters, expeditions, scientific and disaster response teams, and small military deployments. Among these, guided adven-

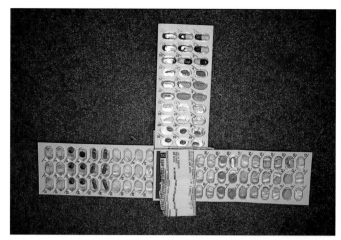

Figure 32.2 Travelers that spend extended time in remote locations should be instructed in stand-by treatment. Medication provided to these patients should be correctly labeled and packaged to resist environmental degradation. The medical packs depicted here provide standby therapies for 17 severe medical illnesses affecting expatiates living in remote areas.

ture travel groups are most likely to seek pre-travel advice, immunizations, and appropriate provisioning. However, in recent years, the popularity of *casual expeditions*, involving paying clients and moderately difficult wilderness travel, has increased the number of adventurers seeking more sophisticated pre-travel health services. Consultation for this group includes all the elements of the comprehensive pre-travel exam, education and screening discussed above, as well as questioning about the charter company. Many travel companies prioritize profit margins and client enrollment over emergency preplanning and preparedness. Medical responsibility is often deferred completely to the travel medicine practitioner. By necessity, consultation for these travelers should include in-depth questioning about the charter company's own pre-travel preparation, the level of medical and disaster training of the travel guides, and formal arrangements with medical evacuation organizations. The shared experience of air evacuation providers indicates that a disquieting number of adventure travel companies respond ineffectually to emergencies among clients. Medical problems tend to reflect inadequate screening of the middle-aged or elderly, inadequate stewardship of clients, lack of adequate medical training for group leaders and poor judgment following the onset of potentially severe events such as chest pain, dyspnea, absence seizures, and syncope. Adventure travel companies that provide inappropriate pre-travel recommendations should be approached and provided with a list of reasonable recommendations. Working with, rather than against these companies can lead to better screening of the adventure-minded traveler and may enrich the referral network.

EXPEDITIONS

Few remote location travelers will be as great a pre-travel consult challenge as the expedition team. In contrast to the wilderness adventure charters and casual expeditions described above, expeditions are more likely to undertake high-risk activities in environments that are both extreme and remote (Fig. 32.3). The challenge of providing pre-travel services for expedition team members is mitigated in part by advantages derived from standardizing pre-travel evaluations among the team and the probability that safe travel behavior will be reinforced between team members. For select cases the travel medicine practitioner may consider augmenting team resources to increase the

Table 32.3   Remote destination group medical kit (expedition 4–8 team members)

Item/type/purpose	Description and approximate weight
Povidone-iodine	1% 6–12 swabs (1 oz)
Soap (liquid)	Biodegradable (1 oz)
Adhesive bandages	10–15, 1' (1 oz)
Gauze compress	Telfa, 2–8, 4 × 4 (2 oz)
Trauma compress	2–4, 8 × 8 (2 oz)
Tape (cloth)	1–2, 1' wide (2 oz)
Rolled gauze	Kling®, 4 rolls, 4' × 5 yards (2 oz)
Triangular bandage	(2 oz)
Elastic bandage	3–6' width (2–4 oz)
Aluminum finger splint	e.g., SAM® (0.5 oz)
Tongue depressors	(1 oz)
Sanitary napkins	Plastic wrapped (3 oz)
Poly bags	2 mm; 40 gallon (13 oz)
Traction splint	Kendrick® femur device (19 oz)
Skin closures	SteriStrip® (1 oz)
Splinting material	SAM®, 4 oz, or wire/ladder (2 oz)
Airways, nasal	Tygon® (1 oz)
Scissors, bandage	EMT scissor (heavy duty)(4 oz)
Tweezers	(1 oz)
Thermometer (hypothermia rates)	Low reading (to 75 °F)
Safety pins	Large (for splint and airway)
Lighter	(1 oz)
Blood pressure cuff	Adult cuff used for tourniquet, tamponade and BP determination. Obtain Helistat model for cold environments
Stethoscope Lightweight	(5 oz)

Topical medications	
Type	Description
Antibiotic irrigation	Povidone-iodine 10% solution (diluted to 1%)
Antibiotic ointment	Bacitracin–polymixin B
Antibiotic/Anti-inflammatory, OTIC	Acetic acid 2% plus hydrocortisone 1%
Antifungal	Ketoconazole 2% cream
Corticosteroid cream	Lidex 0.05%
Decongestant spray, nasal	Oxymetazoline; phenylephrine
Dental filling, temporary	Acrylamide base (Cavit®)

Oral medications	
Acute mountain sickness	acetazolamide; adult prevention: 125–250 mg Q 12 h; Treatment: 250 mg Q 6–12 h and/or dexamethasone, 2 mg Q 6 h
Analgesic/anti-inflammatory	Non-steroidal anti-inflammatory agent, e.g., naproxen sodium or ibuprofen
Analgesic	Acetaminophen-codeine (Tylenol # 3) ibuprofen-hydrocodone (Vicoprofen®)
Antacid	Antacid tablets with simethicone; Mylanta II
Antibiotic	Ciprofloxacin 500 or 750 mg; doxycycline 100 mg; amoxicillin 500 mg/clavulanate 125 mg (may substitute Augmentin® 875 mg tablets)
Antiemetic/antinausea (rectal)	Promethazine 25 mg suppository
Antihistamine	Diphenhydramine 25 mg capsules
Corticosteroid	Medrol Dosepak
Decongestant	Pseudoephedrine 30 mg tablets
Sedative	Haloperidol, long-acting benzodiazepines (Valium®)

High risk travel (expeditions and disaster response teams)
  Airway, nasopharyngeal (impaired mental status; resuscitation)
  Cricothyrotomy cannula or catheter (e.g., Abelson cannula)
  Chest tube set (chest trauma; empyema – practical only on major expeditions)
  Glucose-testing strips and buccally absorbed glucose preparation (strips must be protected from freezing)
  Handheld ophthalmoscope with high nm blue filter and fluorescein strips to stain corneal lesions (retinal hemorrhages; anterior eye exam – practical only on expeditions)
  Oxygen (hypoxemia; shock; cerebral/pulmonary edema; impaired mental status)
  Sphygmomanometer (aneroid, plastic housing – practical only on expeditions)
  Stethoscope (lightweight, noise-reducing)
  Suction device (mechanical) (clearing oral cavity; chest tube drainage – practical only on expeditions)
  Surgical tools (practical only on remote expeditions)

General use
  Intravenous solutions (isotonic) and tubing (for hydration; route for i.v. medications)
  Needles and syringes (for i.m. and i.v. medication)
  Antibiotic, i.m. (practical only for expeditions) (e.g., ceftriaxone)
  Beta agonist metered-dose inhaler (for asthma; anaphylactic reaction)

Table 32.3	Remote destination group medical kit (expedition 4–8 team members) —cont'd

Item/type/purpose

Dextrose 50% injection (hypoglycemia; non-traumatic coma; hyperthermia)
Epinephrine injection (1:1000 multidose vials)
Nitroglycerin tablets (Dx and treatment of chest pain syndromes, e.g. angina pectoris)
Ophthalmic anesthetic (e.g., proparacaine or tetracaine 0.5%) (to facilitate eye examination and to provide short-term analgesia only)

High risk of trauma
  Nalbuphine (Nubain) or butorphanol (Stadol) injectable (for pain; pulmonary edema) and include naloxone (Narcan) to antagonize narcotic-induced respiratory depression or hypotension
  Diazepam (or lorazepam; Ativan) injectable (for major sedation; seizures)
  High risk of altitude illness
  Corticosteroid injection (e.g., dexamethasone) (cerebral/pulmonary edema; severe allergic reaction; asthma)
  Furosemide injection (cerebral/pulmonary edema)

High risk of snowblindness
  Ophthalmic cycloplegic (e.g., cyclopentolate 1%) (for pain due to snow blindness)
  Ophthalmic corticosteroid/antibiotic combination (e.g., Maxitrol) (recommended for short-term use in snow blindness *only* if blue filter ophthalmoscopic exam using fluorescein stain rules out herpetic keratitis)

Total weight approximately 56 oz (4.25 lb; 10 x 6 x 4 in). Equipment is based on Wilderness EMT Training (reproduced with permission, from Rescue Medicine, Inc.)

---

capability for self-treatment of health problems and self-evacuation from dangerous environments. Identifying quality training resources for self-evacuation and wilderness medical decision-making is difficult. One reliable resource for peer-reviewed remote medical care training resources is the Wilderness Medical Society (www.wms.org).

The ability of an expedition to care for team members varies markedly with travel environment, medical skill of team members, and the type and amount of equipment carried. For example, blue water sailing and river rafting expeditions allow more medical resources to be transported compared to mountain and polar expeditions. The ability of certain groups to transport an increased number of emergency medical supplies is no assurance that the equipment or medication will be used correctly. In expeditions that do not have a qualified medical officer, potent medications may be used incorrectly, or extended to individuals beyond the original screened group. For this reason, travel medicine practitioners should be wary about providing advanced medical kits and dangerous pharmaceuticals to groups, even when all team members are evaluated at the same travel clinic.

A different scenario involves travel groups with medical providers among the team members. An appropriately skilled medical provider coupled with a well-configured medical kit can play an important role in maintaining team health and responding to life-threatening medical problems (Table 32.4). An important concept in the design of the team's medical capability is matching medical resources, in particular drugs and emergency invasive technologies, to the skill level of the provider (Fig. 32.4).

Medical providers should not be placed in the position of having to attempt dangerous interventions for the first time, especially during the chaotic setting of a wilderness medical emergency. This situation can be avoided by increasing the medical skill level of the team, or by limiting the level of intervention supported by the medical kit. It should be pointed out that selection of medical personnel should not be based on convenience and availability, but rather upon legitimate

Figure 32.3 Medical evacuation of a critically injured climber from the 14 000 foot high altitude research station on Denali.[5]

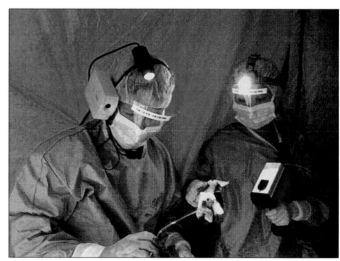

Figure 32.4 Portable OR for emergency surgery in remote locations. This portable, self-contained surgical theatre allows field medical officers in Nigeria to provide emergency surgical care to a gun shot victim, assisted by video link to Rescue Medicine surgeons in the United States.[5]

Table 32.4   Medical training for expeditions

Pre-hospital provider	Training required (h)	Certification body, contact organizations and comments
First Responder	40	National standard. American Red Cross DOT course, www.redcross.org
Wilderness First Responder	60+	No national standard. Highly variable quality of training. Established programs include the National Outdoor Leadership School, nols.edu; SOLO, stonehearth.com; Wilderness Medical Associates, wilmed.com
Search & Rescue Medical Responder	60+	Oriented to the disaster team member. Strengths include medical decision making regarding medical evacuation. National Association for Search and Rescue, www.nasar.org
Emergency Medical Technician (EMT)	120	State and federal standards and certification. Skills include CPR, BTLS, splinting and standing orders for certain therapeutics. National resource is National Association for Emergency Medical Technicians, naemt.org; Highly appropriate for remote destination travelers
EMT-Wilderness	120+	Expanded scope of training with a focus on wilderness medical problems such as insect stings, hypothermia and patient packaging for medevac. Contact organizations same as wilderness first responder
Paramedic	1800+	Urban pre-hospital programs, which provide excellent field experience. Paramedics are skilled in i.v. access, pre-hospital emergency airways and patient assessment. Several programs offer extended wilderness modules appropriate for expedition medical officers

clinical skill as evidenced by prior field experience and formal medical training (Fig. 32.5).

Unfortunately, medical personnel are often selected based on their ability to provide costly medical kits, rather than upon wilderness and emergency medical skill level. One overlooked point regarding the medical skill level of the remote destination team medical provider: effective field medical care is often achieved by experienced pre-hospital medical care providers with ALS training. One reason for this groups' improved performance reflects their familiarity with delivering care with minimal resources, minimal assistance and beyond the walls of the emergency department. Table 32.4 describes the levels of pre-hospital skills for select levels of pre-hospital medical providers.

PERSONAL SECURITY

Many adventure travel destinations are found in regions of political instability or relative lawlessness. Travelers to these areas are more likely to be victimized by armed robbers, corrupt law enforcement officials, or by political factions opposing the central government. While travelers tend to be aware of criminal and terrorist activity in

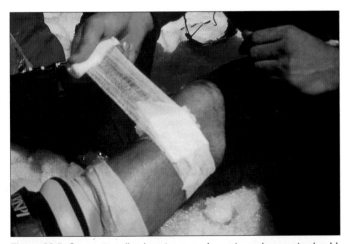

Figure 32.5 Groups traveling in extreme and remote environments should prepare be able to treat local risks and probable injuries. Here, an expedition physician treats a laceration to the patellar tendon during the 10 week 1995 Trans Greenland Ski Expedition.[5]

foreign cities, they are often naïve about risks to personal safety in rural regions.

Travel advisories published by consular offices and the US State Department are often too generalized, and rarely reflect current conditions in remote destinations. The often-cited advisories produced by British, US, German, Australian and Israeli governments are based in part on embassy figures for kidnappings, and homicides, all of which have reporting biased for cities and popular tourist attractions. For these and other reasons, criminal activity against remote-region travelers and expatriates working in the back-country, are often under-reported.

Quality information on the current 'scam du jour', political unrest, police corruption and terrorist activity in rural regions can often be obtained by contacting the safety officers of non-governmental relief agencies that are active in the region of interest. The remote destination traveler should also be encouraged to seek current information in the capital city prior to departing for back-country locations. In-country sources for travel intelligence include newspapers, and places where adventure travelers congregate such as cyber cafes, youth hostels, tourist areas and consular offices. In recent years, escalation of anti-western sentiments in many regions has resulted in specific targeting of western travelers and expatriates.

Significant embassy resources and thousands of personnel hours are expended annually, addressing incidents of kidnapping for ransom, fraudulent imprisonment, and other crimes against western travelers. In some regions, the financial costs of 'fines' undermine the morale of expatriate workers and impact corporate profits. Educating travelers about current risks to personal security are a necessary component of a thorough pre-travel consultation, and should not be overshadowed by reimbursed procedures, such as immunization. In many cases, travel medicine practitioners will need to first educate themselves about up-to-date risks in a specific region of the destination country and then communicate this information to the traveler. Recommendations regarding personal security should be specific for the traveler's itinerary and intended activities. Consultation should identify viable risk-avoidance measures, contingency plans, and default communication links. It should be noted here, that international communication kiosks such as Internet cafes and the business centers of hotels frequented by Westerners are often staked-out by groups that target Westerners. Individuals traveling beyond the reach of centralized law enforcement should be encouraged to set up regularly scheduled communication links with a responsible person back at home. In countries such as Indonesia and the Democratic Republic of the Congo, rural law enforcement authorities may be the most common risk to personal security and steps should be taken to avoid this group if possible. It should be noted here that many international travel support services lack factual experience and in-country resources to address the needs of clients who were victimized, imprisoned, or detained far from major cities. Several additional resources that have proven to be helpful in the determination of security risks for specific countries are provided in Table 32.5. More generalized resources for determining risks to personal security are provided in Chapter 50.

MEDEVAC

Air evacuation services are designed to transport patients from the hospital bed of a capital city to the patient's home country (See Chapter 49). The economic realities of the international medical evacuation business guide usage and availability of jet aircraft. These constraints mean that evacuation services are either unavailable or markedly delayed in less traveled regions. In many developing regions, communist countries, and areas under non-governmental control,

medevac companies often lack appropriate authorization, aircraft resources, and appropriately skilled aero-medical personnel. In these cases, the medical evacuation provider will often subcontract third party services to provide aircraft services locally. In these circumstances, the quality of medical care is more likely to be marginal, the evacuation improvised, and medical outcome unsatisfactory.

CONCLUSIONS

The dramatic increase in remote destination travel, adventure travel and expeditions to extreme environments present the travel medicine practitioner with new dilemmas in pre-travel screening, health and safety education, and medical provisioning. For this group of travelers, the effectiveness of pre-travel consultation may be limited by the consultant's lack of familiarity with the destination environment and attendant risks. The delivery of quality consult services to this group requires that travel medicine clinicians extend services beyond the routine and reimbursable, to include candid and careful education regarding risk reduction behaviors, and personal provisioning, preparedness and contingency planning.

Table 32.5	Resources for travel health and personal security information
Source	**Comment**
United States Department of State Travel Advisory Updates	Reports are based on incidence, are biased toward security risks in cities and locations where expatriates congregate. Warnings may be overstated to reduce burden on consular resources.
British Consular Affairs	Frequently updated with extensive coverage of many African countries.
Premium service providers	Several credit card companies and Insurance plans develop composite security risk recommendations for clients including e-mailed and satellite transmitted warnings
Corporate websites	Intended for expatriates traveling to overseas jobsites. Highly variable in quality and content, but are often the most accurate source for local risks in remote locations. Many corporations do not require PIN numbers for access and permit use by third parties.
Internet subscription services	Services often derive information from the same source and re-package it. Quality of information varies widely between services. Many providers disappear overnight and comparisons cannot be made. Several providers employ ex-government threat analysts and maintain accurate and up-to-date information.
CD ROM services	Many services are excellent for identifying in-country medical resources but provide outdated information on security risks.
Medical evacuation service providers	Highly variable services. Security information varies with provider, and with type of plan. Information is often provided via a weblink to a dedicated information resource.
Internet chat rooms	Popular among the adventure budget travelers. Information, both factual and mystical, is quickly disseminated. Emerging risks and patterns of corruption are often first reported here and confirmed months later by government agencies. Requires time to research and validate the claims.
Electronic and traditional news	Many websites allow quick evaluation of changing conditions (e.g., political coups, natural disasters, terrorist activity). While up-to-date, stated risks rarely reflect conditions in rural regions of a specific country.

REFERENCES

1. Saito S, Tobe K, Harada N, *et al.* Physical condition among middle altitude trekkers in an aging society. *Am J Emerg Med* 2002; **20**(4):291–294.
2. Callahan MV, Hamer DH, Bailey SA, *et al. Medical Emergencies in Expatriates: Analysis of 1770 cases* (Ab-FC10.04). Seventh Conference of the International Society of Travel Medicine, Innsbruck, Austria, 2001.
3. Kedjarune U, Leggat PA. Dental precautions for travelers. *J Travel Med* 1997; **4**:38–40.
4. Cobelens FG, Deutekom H van, Draayer-Jansen IW, *et al.* Risk of infection with Mycobacterium tuberculosis in travellers to areas of high tuberculosis endemicity. *Lancet* 2000; **356**:461–465.
5. Callahan MV. Expatriate imprisonment. *Analysis of 39 Short-term Incarcerations.* Seventh Conference of the International Society of Travel Medicine, Innsbruck, Austria, 2001.
6. Adachi JA, Ostrosky-Zeichner L, DuPont HL, Ericsson CD. Empirical antimicrobial therapy for traveler's diarrhea. *Clin Infect Dis* 2000; **31**:1079–1083.
7. Wistrom J, Jertborn M, Hedstrom SA, *et al.* Short-term self-treatment of travellers' diarrhoea with norfloxacin: a placebo-controlled study. *J Antimicrob Chemother* 1989; **23**(6):905–913.
8. Jelinek T, Amsler L, Grobusch MP, *et al.* Self-use of rapid tests for malaria diagnosis by tourists. *Lancet* 1999; **354**:1609.

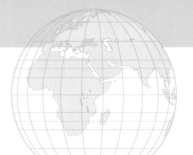

CHAPTER 33 The Health-seeking Traveler

Richard Dawood

KEYPOINTS

- Hazards of spas include bacterial, toxins and radioactive contaminated water

- Travelers on large religious pilgrimages are at particular risk of illness during infectious disease outbreaks

- Hazards of health-care abroad include inadequate medical facilities, as well as language and transcultural problems

- Pre-travel research, planning, and preparation will help to prevent illness among health seeking travelers

INTRODUCTION

Why do we travel? Leisure travelers seek relaxation or a change of scene, hoping to return home feeling re-invigorated, with a sense of well-being, and at ease. For some travelers however, the quest for 'health' is the primary – perhaps the sole – purpose of going abroad. It is one that follows in a long tradition: man has been traveling in search of health for millennia.

Where does this quest take us? Beaches, parks, mountains, open spaces; but also to spas, sanatoria, places to convalesce in a more favorable climate, cruise ships, places perhaps with healing powers, such as shrines and holy places around the world.

SPAS AND HEALTH RESORTS

Staying at a spa for a couple of weeks, relaxing and being pampered, may certainly make the traveler feel rested and at ease. Take away the stress of a hectic job or the daily routine; and add in some exercise and fitness training, a healthy diet, massage, sympathetic company, and above all, a strong sense of taking positive steps to improve one's health: what could be more likely to engender a feeling of health and well-being. But, is there any hard evidence that the health benefits go deeper than this?

The spas of Europe are not like spas and resorts in the USA: the emphasis is on cures and healing, not just fitness and having fun. Claims for cures date back through the ages – to the ancient Greeks, Romans and Biblical times. In Tunbridge Wells, a spa town in England that received royal patronage, a physician in the sixteenth century listed the following among the medical complaints likely to benefit from taking the local waters: 'obstructions, especially of the spleen and liver; dropsy, jaundice, scurvy, the green sickness, defect and excess of female courses, inward inflammations and hot distempers, palsy, apoplexy, rheums, hypochondriacal melancholy, pox, pimples and other external infirmities; the waters scoureth and cleanseth the urinary passages ... and nothing is better against barrenness.' The purgative effect of the waters of Epsom, in Southern England, was discovered in the early seventeenth century, and Epsom flourished as high society flocked there to take the waters; magnesium sulphate was later extracted and identified for its laxative properties, and to this day is sometimes referred to as Epsom Salts.

Here is a more modern list of healing powers from Vichy in France (as published on its website), and typical of many: 'digestive and nutritional problems, such as migraines and headaches caused by digestive or psychogenic problems; the after effects of surgery for gallstones; after effects of viral or drug-induced hepatitis; slow digestion, heartburn, bloating, digestive somnolence, hiatus hernia, non-ulcerative gastritis; digestive allergies, diabetes, hyperuricemia and gout, and obesity. Also, arthritis, rheumatism, and the after effects of injury ...' It is difficult to read a list like this in French without thinking of the so-called physicians in Molière's 'Malade Imaginaire'. Conventional British and American medical practice is not really in tune with this approach.

Skeptics have argued that such ailments belong to the repertoire on which all spa towns grow rich – common conditions, and preferably chronic ones that keep people coming back, but with a real prospect of natural cure or remission, excluding, of course, any serious or acute illnesses, since a clearly visible failure rate would be extremely bad for business.

In some parts of Europe – not Britain, but especially France, Italy, and Germany – spas are very much part of daily life, and health insurance schemes are often prepared to cover costs of treatment. In Eastern European countries, some are even owned by the State. Under former communist regimes, they were used not just for treatment, but also to provide free healthy vacations for the workers. Doctors from spa towns are almost always enthusiastic about the benefits and cite examples from their own practice, but objective evidence of medically proven benefit, as documented by trials and reports in medical journals, is sketchy. Most of the claims that are made still have no conclusively proven scientific basis. Attempts to conduct objective trials – notably in Hungary, which has more than 500 natural springs and probably more rheumatologists *per capita* than anywhere else in the world – have been fraught with problems. Evidence in support of the benefits ought perhaps to be stronger if they are indeed genuine.

On the other hand, many of the claims relate to slowly- or non-progressive long-term conditions for which conventional treatment may have little to offer or has let people down. Doctors, clinics, and health centers at some of the spas are undeniably good at looking after their patients, listening to their problems, and addressing their needs. Different spas have different specialities. The spa waters at Bagnoles-de-l'Orne, (France) are said to have 'filtering, resolving, keratolytic and sedative' actions, and attract many sufferers of lymphedema.[1]

A lymphology unit at the local clinic finishes off a spell at the spa with intensive treatment: postural drainage, massage, bandages, pneumatic pressure, and physical therapy. Regardless of the properties of the waters, the level of focused care for this, a clinical condition that is notoriously difficult to manage, seems very appealing.

There are hazards. A survey of 37 brands of domestic and imported bottled mineral waters found that 24 that contained salts or minerals in concentrations that did not comply with drinking water standards in the USA. Isolated cases of infective contamination have occurred – such as the cases of amebic meningitis in Bath, England, in the 1970s and 1980s[2] – and a number of studies have found bacteria in bottled mineral water. There have been cases of poisoning following excessive inhalation of hydrogen sulfide at spas in Taiwan, where bathing in hot springs is an especially popular recreation.[3]

Hydrotherapy in whirlpools and hot tubs may be associated with transmission of infection – notably Pseudomonas folliculitis,[4] and legion-nellosis[5,6] There is also a need for caution in subjecting people with underlying debilitating illness to undue physical or environmental stress.[7]

Surprisingly, some European spas make much of the radioactivity of their water, or of the local rock or mud. There are examples of bottled mineral waters proudly stating radioactivity content on their labels. Spa radioactivity usually arises from radium or uranium salts, or radon – a radioactive gas that is weakly soluble in water. Staff working at spas in Poland are known to receive excessive doses, though the risk to short-term visitors is probably very small.

Making people feel better is of course a worthy objective in its own right, and in reality, it matters little how that is achieved, or whether or not there may be a psychosomatic component. Many spas have become a focal point for research and expertise in rehabilitation. Heat treatment and hydrotherapy are now used by physical therapists everywhere, and take their origin from the spas of old. The surroundings tend to be beautiful, staff have a positive attitude, and there is a pervasive atmosphere of relaxation and hope. Spa treatment should not be offered in a manner that discourages people from seeking more effective treatment where such treatment can be given, and exposure to radiation should certainly be avoided.

HOLY PLACES

The world's holy places can be a magnet for the ailing, the disabled and the infirm. There may be powerful benefits to well-being and morale, and such visits can restore a sense of purpose and hope for the future; on the negative side, however, there may be additional stresses and risks imposed by a journey that may be long and perhaps arduous. Long-haul air travel and the associated hypoxia may prove to be the final insult, in the terminally ill. Further hazards arise from fasting; from exertion at high altitude (as in pilgrims to the holy mountain lakeside of Gosainkunda, Nepal)[8]; from heat exhaustion and exposure to the elements; and from disease transmission under conditions of overcrowding (such as the periodic outbreaks of meningitis that have occurred in Muslim pilgrims undertaking the Hajj[9]). This catalog of possible ills has led one authority to propose 'pilgrimage medicine' as a new medical specialty. In some parts of the world, local health resources that may be barely adequate for the needs of the indigenous population, may rapidly become overloaded and unable to cope with the demands imposed by an influx of visitors.

'Holy water' also poses a potential hazard:[10] coliforms, staphylococci, yeasts, molds, and unidentified 'little green worms' have all been reported growing in fonts in Irish churches. In holy water from the River Ganges, pilgrims appear unperturbed by the presence of carbonized human remains, but there is also a problem with arsenic and pesticide contamination. In a study of holy water from Thailand,

only nine out of 76 samples met WHO drinking water standards.[11] Holy water brought into hospitals has been the source of outbreaks of infection in western countries.[12] Travelers should know that the basic principles of food and water hygiene apply even in this context.

TRAVELERS SEEKING SPECIFIC MEDICAL TREATMENT

Many of the anticipated health benefits described thus far are intangible ones. The quest for more specific medical treatment, however, is one that motivates millions of travelers all over the world.

Many individuals from countries with limited medical resources may travel to centers of medical excellence in developed countries when they need skilled care. Centers of excellence in Europe and the USA attract substantial numbers: the governments of some Middle Eastern countries, for example, find it more cost-effective to cover the cost of overseas health care, at least in some medical specialties, than to attempt to establish local services from scratch.

Travel for medical treatment is sometimes mandated by legal or social considerations – the quest for termination of pregnancy, for example, motivates thousands of Irish women each year, to travel to the UK.[13] In Germany, restricted access to in-patient treatment with radio-iodine for thyroid disease prompted many to seek treatment elsewhere.[14] Travel from one developed country to another has been proposed as a way of tackling long hospital waiting lists; in the UK, the government is considering sending patients to France, Greece and Germany for surgical care.

Travel from developed to less developed countries for medical treatment – notably elective surgery – is now also a growing phenomenon, though the primary motivation is usually one of cost rather than access. Cosmetic surgery in parts of the world, such as the Far East, Central America and South Africa is a growth industry.[15,16] Favorable exchange rates, availability of surgical expertise, existence of reasonable hospital facilities, plus the option of convalescing 'on safari' or in a holiday environment, in privacy or away, perhaps, from the scrutiny of friends and family who might disapprove, add to the attraction.

Treatment of this kind is not entirely without risk (over and above the risks of the same type of procedure, carried out at home): skills and resources may prove to be inadequate to achieve a good result, or inadequate to cope with rare but life-threatening complications that might supervene – complications that might not pose a particular problem at a center of excellence in the traveler's own home country. Additional hazards may be present, such as a possible increased risk of blood-borne infections such as hepatitis B, HIV or malaria – infections that may have a much higher prevalence in the local population that in the traveler's home. Additional hazards may also arise from the journey itself – immobility, for example, might increase the risk of transport-related problems such as deep vein thrombosis. Surgical complications appearing during a long journey may be almost impossible to treat. Also, other travel-related health risks always loom in the background.

Whatever procedure is being contemplated, travelers undergoing medical treatment outside their accustomed environment are almost always at a disadvantage. Language and cultural differences may hinder both verbal and non-verbal communication. Religious and ethical differences can become almost impossible to resolve, over issues such as heroic efforts to preserve life or limb, perhaps in the terminally ill. Lack of familiarity with the local medical system, limited access to past medical history, unfa-miliar drugs and medicines, and limited options for follow-up after the event, may each be a problem. If complications occur, the insur-ance situation can become difficult to resolve and costs may escalate. And if things go wrong, legal recourse may be fairly limited or diffi-cult to obtain.

Travelers not going abroad specifically for medical care may nonetheless be tempted to 'stock up' on locally produced medicines in order to save money. This can pose a particular risk in parts of the world, where counterfeit medicines or vaccines are common – such as parts of Latin America, Eastern Europe, the Indian sub-continent and Far East, and sub-Saharan Africa.[17] High-cost medicines such as some types of antibiotic, and antimalarials, are common candidates for purchase overseas. Medication hazards arise both from poor efficacy and from potential toxicity. Travelers should always be encouraged to buy all of the medicines they might need whilst still in their home country.

COMPLEMENTARY THERAPIES AND INDIGENOUS MEDICAL AND HEALTH-RELATED PRACTICES

A desire to try out complementary therapies of one kind or another may constitute the primary purpose of a trip; alternatively, the traveler may be drawn to experiment with therapies and practitioners encountered fortuitously while abroad. In either case, the traveler may be healthy but interested in a transcultural experience, or already suffering from symptoms and searching for relief.

Specialist tour operators now offer the opportunity to combine travel with exactly these kinds of therapy – Ayurvedic medicine in the Indian sub-continent, for example. Ayurvedic medicine purports to be based on a 3000-year old tradition; its name means, literally, 'meaning of life.' Enthusiasts claim it to be 'the only system of medicine in the world which has methods to totally rejuvenate the Body and Mind'. Treatments such as oil application, Yoga, special diets and steam baths, 'drain body toxins, re-establish the biochemical balance, and help customers emerge as new, invigorated individuals'.

On the other hand, even within India, the Ayurvedic system has come under heavy attack for irrational and outdated practices. A news report in the Lancet quoted Vaidya Balendu Prakash, chair of the Health Ministry's Central Ayurvedic, Siddha, and Unani Drugs technical advisory board: 'The majority of Ayurvedic formulations available on the market are either spurious, adulterated, or misbranded'.[18]

Such therapies have their following, and may bring comfort, relief and encouragement, particularly to those suffering from chronic conditions such as strokes, paralysis and chronic musculoskeletal problems for whom modern, Western-style medicine, may have disap-

pointingly little to offer. The potential for harm, however, arises when Western medicine really can help, but is shunned in favor of therapies that offer no prospect of benefit. A notable example is the problem of snakebite in Sri Lanka: Ayurvedic medicine has nothing to offer, but has denied many victims the option of effective treatment. A homeopathic antimalarial prophylactic is currently popular among western travelers to Africa, with no conventional scientific evidence of efficacy.

Herbal cures and remedies are more likely to be encountered serendipitously in the course of travel, and all travelers need to be alert to the possible problems. Such remedies may seem harmless enough, but the fact that a substance is herbal or 'natural' does not mean that it has no potential for harm. Many such medicines are adulterated with toxic contaminants, or occasionally 'spiked' with powerful conventional medicines such as steroids.

In a well-documented case in the USA, a Korean man died after drinking herbal tea made with hai ge fen, powdered clam shell, that was heavily contaminated with lead.[19] Hard shell clams, barnacles, oysters, mussels and sea urchins may be used medicinally, but may readily become contaminated with heavy metals. Unfortunately, there is seldom any control over the way in which 'natural' medicines are formulated and prepared.

Also, herbal remedies may interact with conventional medications. A summary of possible side-effects and interactions may be found at: www.asahq.org/publiceducation/list2.htm.

Other therapies that the traveler may come across include: acupuncture, traditional Chinese medicine, homeopathy, reflexology, and a variety of massage and manipulative therapies that may be carried out by practitioners with varying degrees of skill (or sometimes none). Unskilled manipulation may cause obvious complications. Any therapy involving penetration of the skin poses a hazard of blood-borne infection: needle sterility and scrupulous attention to hygiene should be an unfailing rule, and any traveler intending to undergo such treatment should also consider prior immunization against hepatitis B. Hazards may also arise from sensitization and contact dermatitis – now seen increasingly with henna tattoos – a form of body adornment widely practiced in North African and Asian cultures that is very popular with visitors.[20-22]

Some of the ways in which complementary therapies may cause harm are summarized in Table 33.1, and adverse outcomes more generally associated with health-seeking behavior are summarized in Table 33.2.

Table 33.1	Hazards from complementary therapies abroad
Non-efficacy: expected/promised benefits may not appear	
Treatment may be frankly hazardous or harmful	Contamination/adulteration Use by unskilled practitioner Poor hygiene, limited resources
Genuine, underlying problems may fail to be recognized/adequately treated	
Absence of skilled conventional medical resources to cope with complications	
Disadvantages of health care in an unfamiliar environment	Language/cultural issues Communication problems Unfamiliar drugs/medicines Difficulty arranging long term follow-up/continuity of care Limited legal recourse, if or when things go wrong
Instrumentation/skin piercing/lack of sterile supplies Blood-borne infection	HIV Hepatitis B Hepatitis C Syphilis Malaria Chagas disease
Sensitization, allergic reactions, scarring	

Table 33.2   Health-seeking behavior: adverse outcomes and possible precautions

Therapy	Possible adverse outcomes	Preventive measures
Balneotherapy (Spas, mud baths etc.)	Heat associated illness Hypotension Skin infection Ear infection Legionellosis Acanthamoeba Hydrogen sulfide exposure Other chemical toxicity Radiation exposure	Research your spa well Take local advice on possible hazards Moderate your exposure
Pilgrimages, religious healing experiences	Emotional stress Heat-associated illness Altitude illness Food/water-borne infection Meningococcal disease SARS	Planning and preparation Awareness of possible risks Access to local medical facilities Immunization
Voluntary or involuntary medical/surgical tourism	Absence of adequate facilities to achieve desired result/ manage complications Language and transcultural problems Risk of blood-borne infection Other tropical /travel-associated risks/complications	Appropriate medical insurance with clarification of any contentious issues in advance Awareness of safety measures/personal risk reduction Careful research of local medical facilities, where possible Traveling with others rather than alone
Use of local remedies, herbal medicines	Potential for toxicity Non-efficacy Transmission of blood-borne infection (through instrumentation, skin piercing)	Avoidance

REFERENCES

1. Vezard C. The thermal cure at Bagnoles-de-l'Orne, (in French). *Phlebologie* 1982; **35**(2):587–595.
2. Cain AR, Wiley PF, Brownell B, Warhurst DC. Primary amoebic meningoencephalitis. *Arch Dis Child* 1981; **56**(2):140–143.
3. Deng JF, Chang SC. Hydrogen sulfide poisonings in hot-spring reservoir cleaning: two case reports. *Am J Ind Med* 1987; **11**(4):447–451.
4. Ford-Jones L, Clogg D, Delage G, Archambault A. Health spa whirlpools: a source of Pseudomonas folliculitis. *CMAJ* 1981; **125**(9):1005–1006.
5. Martinelli F, Carasi S, Scarcella C, Speziani F. Detection of Legionella pneumophila at thermal spas. *New Microbiol* 2001; **24**(3):259–264.
6. Jernigan DB, Hofmann J, Cetron MS, *et al*. Outbreak of Legionnaires' disease among cruise ship passengers exposed to a contaminated whirlpool spa. *Lancet* 1996; **347**(9000):494–499.
7. Gehrke A, Schnizer W. Rehabilitative treatment measures in coronary heart disease. Value balneology therapy–advantages disadvantages, (in German). *Med Welt* 1983; **34**(16):491–493.
8. Basnyat B. Pilgrimage medicine. *BMJ* 2002; **324**:745.
9. Anonymous. Serogroup W-135 meningococcal disease among travelers returning from Saudi Arabia – United States. *MMWR* 2000; **49**(16):345–346.
10. Payne D. Holy Water not always a blessing. *BMJ* 2001; **322**(7280):190.
11. Phatthararangrong N, Chantratong N, Jitsurong S. Bacteriological quality of holywater from Thai temples in Songkhla Province, southern Thailand. *J Med Assoc Thai* 1998; **81**(7):547–550.
12. Rees JC, Allen KD. Holy Water – a risk factor for hospital-acquired infection. *J Hosp Infect* 1996; **32**(1):51–55.
13. Clarity JF. Irish girl, 13, to abort baby in England. *New York Times* 1997; December 2:**A7**.
14. Schicha H, Scheidhauer K. Radioiodine therapy in Europe – a survey. *Nucl Med* 1993; **32**(6):321–324.
15. Castonguay G, Brown A. 'Plastic surgery tourism' proving a boon for Costa Rica's surgeons. *CMAJ* 1993; **148**(1):74–76.
16. Mydans S. The all-purpose Thai vacation: sun, sea and surgery. *New York Times* 2002; 11 September.
17. Dawood R. Medicines for travel. In: Dawood R, ed. *Travellers' Health: how to stay healthy abroad*, 4th edn. Oxford: Oxford University Press; 2002.
18. Kumar S. Indian herbal remedies come under attack. *Lancet* 1998; **351**(1188).
19. Hill GJ, Hill S. Lead poisoning due to hai ge fen. *JAMA* 1995; **273**(1):24–25.
20. Brancaccio RR, Brown LH, Chang YT, *et al*. Identification and quantification of para-phenylenediamine in a temporary black henna tattoo. *Am J Contact Dermatitis* 2002; **13**(1):15–18.
21. Jappe U, Hausen BM, Petzoldt D. Erythema-multiforme-like eruption and depigmentation following allergic contact dermatitis from a paint-on henna tattoo, due to para-phenylenediamine contact hypersensitivity. *Contact Dermatitis* 2001; **45**(4):249–250.
22. Lewin PK. Temporary henna tattoo with permanent scarification. *Canadian Medical Association Journal* 1999; **160**(3):310.

CHAPTER 34   # Fear of Flying – Aviophobia

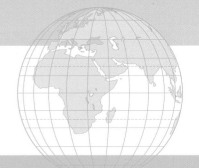

Helmut Müller-Ortstein and Andrea Kropf

KEYPOINTS

- Surveys and estimates reveal that 60% of the population suffers from some degree of anxiety related to air travel

- For a diagnosis of aviophobia to be made, avoidance behaviors must be demonstated

- Causes of aviophobia vary from fear of lack of control ('passenger syndrome') to agoraphobia to fear of death and dying (e.g., airplane crash)

- By examining the different causes of aviophobia it is possible to identify areas in which treatment can be very effectively applied

- Providing information, teaching passengers to practice active strategies and confrontation form the basis of intensive seminars designed to allow aviophobics a chance to overcome their fears

INTRODUCTION

In the civilizations of the industrialized world, time is an ever-scarcer commodity. Most people therefore regard flying as an opportunity for unrestricted mobility. Those unable to take advantage of this freedom because of fear of flying suffer a disadvantage in terms of their quality of life, both private and professional. An aviophobic is often a victim of irrational negative fantasies and may also be aware of this fact.

Fear of flying was already a highly complex phenomenon before 11 September 2001. Since the disaster in America, fear of flying has taken on an additional dimension: the fear of using a means of transport that could be used by terrorists as a weapon. All of us in future will fly with this knowledge. Despite terrorism, bio-terrorism (e.g., anthrax) and many other disasters, it is important that we do not allow ourselves to feel permanently under threat. These days there are many reasons to be afraid, but it is also possible to deal intelligently with these fears.

Given the high incidence of fear of flying, we can assume that doctors and psychologists will be increasingly confronted with the problem. The knowledge that fear of flying is treatable, coupled with information on what treatments are available, should help considerably to encourage patients to take steps to overcome their fear.

Surveys and estimates indicate that only about 40% of airplane passengers feel totally at ease. The other 60% experience anything from slight uneasiness to fear or panic. At least 10% of the population do not fly at all because of their fear.[1] For a diagnosis of aviophobia (Table 34.1) (fear of flying that presents as a mental disturbance), to be made, subjects have to demonstrate, among other things, *avoidance*

Table 34.1   Aviophobia: fear of flying which presents as a mental disturbance

Avoidance behaviors	
Direct	Not flying
Indirect	Reducing fear through alcohol or anxiolytics

behavior; in other words, they will directly avoid the object of their fear, namely flying, by not flying or they will reduce their fear by drinking alcohol or taking tranquillizers (indirect avoidance).

In both cases the fear is real to those affected, but the reasons for the fear are *irrational*, i.e., they cannot tackle the grounds for their fear without help, but they know that their fear is inappropriate measured objectively against the danger of the situation. Most aviophobics are well aware of the statistics that are published time and again in the immediate aftermath of a crash, proving the relative safety of flying compared with travelling by road or rail, for instance, yet they are still unable to control the fear that torments them. To many people, the circumstance of being up in the air in 'empty' space out of contact with the ground still seems to be an act of presumption ('Icarus complex'). The following statement made by an actor at a fear-of-flying seminar (quoted in the *Lufthansa Magazine* of 10/1999) is a good example of this irrationality: 'I feel fulfilled, I have a great family and a glittering career. When the aircraft takes off, I'm afraid that I might be punished for it'.

Fear of flying manifests itself not only in irrational thoughts of impending disaster and avoidance behavior, but also in physiological symptoms such as trembling, sweating, a racing heart, breathing difficulties, dry mouth, dizziness, etc. (Fig. 34.1) We know that these automatic physical changes are part of a human being's inbuilt protective reaction to threat (either real or perceived), designed to trigger a quick response (fight or flight). Locked in an aircraft, a person can no longer use the energy to flee, and the only way he can fight is by displaying aggression to fellow passengers or the flight crew (one phenomenon of 'the unruly passenger'). But, the 'wellbred', controlled passenger remains in his seat, tensely observing his physical reactions, and aggravating his feelings of anxiety to the degree that (out of ignorance) he gauges the physical changes brought about by fear to be dangerous or even threatening.

HOW CAN SUFFERERS CONQUER THEIR PHOBIA?

The first step is to encourage people to spell out their (mostly) diffuse feelings of anxiety and engage intensively with their fear in order to identify the specific conditions and background to the fear, and what

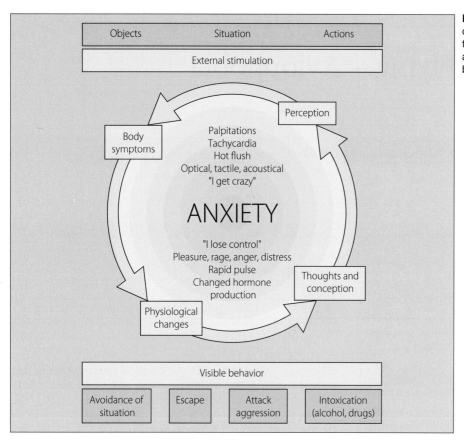

Figure 34.1 Diagnosis of aviophobia. The 'vicious circle' in anxiety attacks. The diagram illustrates the typical 'circulus vitiosus' that occurs during anxiety attacks and is responsible for the rapid build-up of fear (after J. Margraf & S. Schneider).

triggers and intensifies their reactions. Strategies to conquer fear of flying are most effective if they are applied in a targeted fashion once the precise context of the fear has been clarified.

It is therefore necessary to apply differential diagnosis to determine whether fear of flying is linked to 'fear of crashing' (i.e., fear of dying and death) or fears linked in sufferers with how they will react and behave in flight.

In the case of people whose principal fear is that of crashing, we can distinguish two main categories of fear:

- Conditioned fear of flying: where a person has experienced unpleasant events during previous flights such as severe turbulence, nosedives, emergency landings or near-misses that have triggered feelings of anxiety.
- Fear of flying based on a lack of information: where gaps in a person's knowledge and misinformation regarding aircraft technology, aircraft maintenance, control of airspace, pilot training, etc. make them vulnerable to imagining possible disaster.

For many such people, the situation is aggravated by the realization that they are 'condemned' to passivity. In other words, they are forced to put their trust in technology and the people who operate the technology and to surrender themselves to feeling powerless and *helpless* (passenger syndrome). The main problem in the case of those whose fear of flying is centred on themselves is the flight situation, the fact that they cannot get off when they wish to. These are people with *agoraphobic* symptoms in the broadest sense of the term (ICD-10:F 40.00). They anticipate being trapped in their own fear, which they associate in turn with the danger of having a heart attack, losing consciousness such as loss of control (screaming, being sick, fighting, etc.) and associated embarrassment, as well as loss of self-worth. For many passengers, these symptoms are triggered in particular by the feeling of being restricted by the tubular shape of the aircraft and the

discomfort of the seats (claustrophobic symptoms). For others, the altitude at which they are flying is the main cause of their anxiety.

People with agoraphobia-related fear of flying also often experience fear of panic attacks in other situations in which they are unable to make a quick and inconspicuous exit, e.g., elevators, the supermarket, cinema, subway, hairdresser, dentist.

By examining the different aspects of aviophobia as described above, it is possible to identify the areas in which treatment can be effectively applied to control excessive levels of anxiety.

Providing theoretical information

Having some knowledge of the technical aspects of flying and what happens during the course of a flight helps make people feel more confident and calmer.[2] Equally important for sufferers is trusting their own bodies, which means knowing something about the physiological processes triggered by fear in the human body.

Teaching active strategies to overcome fear

These include physical techniques such as progressive muscle relaxation and correct breathing, which are effective on their own in reducing many symptoms of anxiety such as hyperventilation and dizziness.[3] Cognitive approaches are also helpful: examining personal lifestyle is a way of revealing hitherto unrecognized stress factors which can help to lower the fear excitation threshold and therefore the individual's general vulnerability. Calmness has to be rehearsed. Identifying irrational, dysfunctional patterns of thought and restructuring them, thinking through disaster fantasies including the preoccupation with dying and death, and practising positive imagination are effective long-term strategies for controlling flight anxiety.[4]

Confronting the object of fear

According to psychological learning theory, avoiding fear-inducing situations has the long-term effect of increasing the symptoms of anxiety. While any flight from a situation that triggers fear may initially attenuate the fear, this attenuation conditions avoidance tendencies. Only by facing the object of fear and holding their ground in a fear-inducing situation can people learn that they have up to now overestimated their reactions in anticipation, that these reactions are endurable, and that they will eventually wear themselves out. In psychotherapy, various forms of confrontation therapy are applied, including systematic desensitization, gradual confrontation and flooding (in sensu, *in vivo*). The method is selected according to the personality type of the sufferer and also the possibilities offered by the therapeutic setting.

The methods discussed here to overcome fear of flying: providing information, practicing active strategies and confrontation, also form the components of seminars on flying without fear which are held regularly at virtually all major western airports (Table. 34.2).

The intensive seminars, under the guidance of psychologists, involve small groups of 8–12 participants. The courses, held at weekends, last 2 days. An experienced pilot is on hand to answer all technical queries and give a detailed explanation of what goes on during a flight from preparations for take-off through landing. After practicing the relaxation methods and cognitive strategies describe above, participants next listen to an audio-cassette presenting a simulation of all the typical in-flight noises and crew announcements as a mental preparation for flying. In the final part of the seminar, participants take a domestic flight.

The seminars have a very high success rate. The technical information provided personally by a pilot is instrumental in building up the confidence of the sufferers in the 'aircraft' as an object, while learning psychological strategies to handle themselves helps prevent them from exaggerating their anticipated reactions of fear. Another factor explaining the success of the seminars is that in many cases, the seminar will represent the first time that aviophobics deal intensively and in a differentiated fashion with their phobia and discover new, sometimes completely unexpected, aspects. The very fact of verbalizing their feelings of anxiety in a group of people who are plagued by the same or at least similar problems is obviously a relief.

During the course of the 2 days of the seminar, the participants, who come from all walks of life and are of all ages, grow so close to each other and help each other so much that it is rare for anyone not to take part in the final flight. Failure to do so is usually for understandable reasons.

For many of those taking part, the seminar is successful, in that it enables them to stop avoiding flying by using the strategies they have learned to overcome their fear. Nevertheless, the process of reflecting on the circumstances of their lives can highlight problems that it is impossible to resolve given the short duration of the seminar and which may require further therapy.

Fear of flying is such a complex matter that not every individual taking part in a course will see all his or her symptoms cured. But it can make the situation clearer and, under certain circumstances, provide a basis for further treatment by a psychotherapist.[5]

Not everybody is so badly affected by fear of flying that they feel it necessary to take a 2-day seminar. They may feel it is sufficient to do something active themselves such as reading about the subject or working through a self-help scheme.[6,7] Therapy with virtual worlds is also a promising approach.[8]

Those who have to fly only rarely, but who have severe aviophobia may feel that taking a tranquillizer is their best option. In this instance is the responsibility of the doctor to advise the patient to test out the tranquillizers before flying in order to avoid possible paradoxical reactions during the flight. The doctor might also recommend trying herbal remedies. Likewise, the advice to severe aviophobics not to drink coffee before or during a flight is probably best coming from a doctor (Fig. 34.2).

Because of the numbers of plane crashes and emergency landings that have occurred in recent months, doctors and psychologists, who are most likely to be approached for help and advice by those suffering fear of flying, have no easy job to allay people's fears. If we have time, we can encourage patients to start to reflect on aspects such as their feelings of not having lived properly yet, being at the mercy of fate, etc.

Those who look pessimistically into the future and complain that they could not bear, even in their imagination, the actual moment of a crash, could be referred to Saint Exupery's *Wind, Sand and Stars*. The aviator and writer, who crashed many times in his airplane, wrote in 1939: 'One day I was trapped in the cabin of an aircraft sinking underwater and thought I was going to drown. I didn't suffer much. Many times I was convinced that it would soon be all over for me. But it never seemed a very significant event to me. Even in the current adventure (a crash in the Egyptian Sahara), I experienced no torments of fear.'

Humans can withstand threats and dangers that have actually occurred far better than they might previously have imagined they would cope. But how many of us make our lives hell simply by fearing what might happen and imagining disaster instead of taking charge of our life and making the most of it!

Table 34.2	Fear of flying courses
Northwest Airlines: www.fearlessflying.com, info@fearlessflying.com Tel: 1 888 577 4455	
Alaska Airlines: contact Ms Marilyn Moody, Tel: 206 772 1122	
Lufthansa: Individualized Seminars for Relaxed Flying, Agentur Texter Millot GmbH, Hohenstaufenstraße 1, 80801 München, Tel: ++49 (0) 89391739, info@flugangst.de, www.flugangst.de	
British Airways: Aviatours Ltd UK, Tel: 01 250 793 250	
San Francisco Fear of Flying Clinic: www.fofc.com Tel: 650 341 1595	
Stichting Valk, Postbus 110,2300 AC Leiden, Tel: ++31 (0) 71-527 37 33, info@falk.org, www.valk.org	

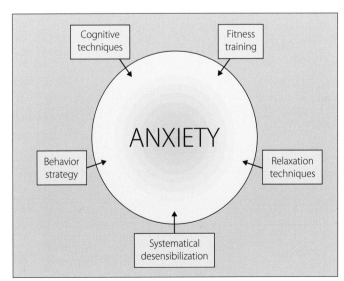

Figure 34.2 How to cope with fear of flying.

REFERENCES

1. Institut für Demoskopie Allensbach (1995) Allensbacher Berichte, Nr. 5: Angst vorm Fliegen.
2. Heermann J (2000) Warum sie oben bleiben, Frankfurt am Main: Insel Verlag
3. Ohm D (1992) Progressive Relaxation, Stuttgart: Trias Verlag.
4. Greco TS (1989) A cognitive-behavioral approach to fear of flying: A practioner's guide. *Phobia Practice and Research* J2 (1): 3-15.
5. Doctor RM (1990) Long-term behavioral treatment effects for the fear of flying. *Phobia Practice and Research* J3 (1): 33-42.
6. Müller-Ortstein H, Baumeirster HP (1997) Mut zum Fliegen, München: Urban & Fischer Verlag.
7. Müller-Ortstein H (2001) Angstfrei fliegen. Das interactive Selbsthilfeprogramm, München Urban & Fischer Verlag.
8. Kuntze Mf, Bullinger AH (2001) Höhenangst und andere spezifische Phobien, Bern: Verlag Hans Huber.

CHAPTER 35

Psychiatric Disorders and Psychiatric Emergencies Overseas

Thomas H. Valk

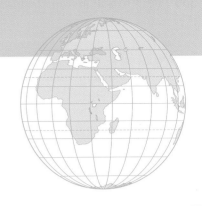

KEYPOINTS

- Traveling and living overseas involves unique stressors and frequent international travel may correlate with increased need for mental health services

- Various classifications of travelers and/or expatriates have been proposed, based upon presumed motivations and more overt reasons for travel. Data is insufficient to determine if any of these systems have clinical relevance

- The international traveler and expatriate population generally suffer from the same range of mental disorders as those seen in clinics or hospitals

- Disorders that are seen frequently, are most likely to qualify as emergencies, or can be especially problematic when they occur overseas, and other problems of special interest are examined. These include certain mood and psychotic disorders, panic attacks, selected substance use disorders and special situations such as the Jerusalem syndrome and psychiatric reactions to mefloquine

- The clinical operating environment overseas provides clinicians with many challenges, given the wide variation from country to country in the availability of culturally compatible clinicians, hospital and laboratory facilities, and medications. Nurse staffing and training varies and difficult cross-cultural situations are frequently encountered. The associated legal environment with respect to commitment and substance abuse also varies widely with consequent impact upon treatment

INTRODUCTION

International travel is a stressful experience. Travelers face separation from family and familiar social supports, and must deal with the impact of foreign cultures and language, jet lag, and bewildering, unfamiliar threats to health and safety. Having to accomplish even the most mundane tasks of everyday living while overseas can become an hours- or days-long challenge leading to a loss of the sense of active mastery over the environment. Under the stress of travel, pre-existing psychiatric disorders can be exacerbated and pre-dispositions towards illness may emerge for the first time. Reflecting these stressors, international business travelers have been found to file insurance claims at higher rates than non-traveling counterparts. This effect was greatest for claims for psychological disorders and increased with the frequency of travel.[1] In a follow-up survey, international travelers reported that one third of those responding reported high to very high levels of stress. Concerns about the impact of travel on family and isolation contributed the most to the stress.[2] Travel across time zones, interestingly, did not seem to correlate to the amount of experienced stress. Streltzer, in his study of psychiatric emergencies in travelers to Hawaii, estimated an incidence of emergencies of 220 per 100 000 population/year for tourists, 2250 per 100 000/year for transient travelers, those who arrived in Hawaii with no immediate plans to leave, versus a rate of 1250/100 000 per year for the non-traveling population.[3] Diagnostically, the problems seen, in order of decreasing frequency, were schizophrenia, alcohol abuse, anxiety reactions, and depression.

Despite the clear stress involved, international travelers generally suffer from the same range of disorders as seen in a clinic or hospital. Rather than deal with all possible psychiatric disorders, this chapter will focus on a select subset: disorders that are seen frequently, are most likely to qualify as emergencies, or can be especially problematic when they occur in the overseas environment. This subset includes certain mood and psychotic disorders, panic attacks, and selected substance use disorders. Special situations of interest such as the Jerusalem syndrome and psychiatric reactions to mefloquine will also be examined.

TYPES OF INTERNATIONAL TRAVELERS

International travelers can be classified in a number of ways and have a variety of conscious and unconscious motivations for their travel. Cohen generated a typology for tourist travelers that focused upon the intrinsic motivation for travel. Although applied to tourist travelers, some of the modes are seen in the non-tourist. His five modes of tourism include: (1) a recreational mode, or travel as entertainment; (2) a diversionary mode, or travel for escape from boredom or routine; (3) an experiential mode when travelers, without a sense of the authenticity in their own life, search for vicarious experiences of authenticity in the lifestyles of others in foreign cultures; (4) an experimental mode, wherein the tourist seeks a sense of authenticity by actually adopting the lifestyles of others; (5) and an existential mode, which is most similar to a religious pilgrimage.[4] Others have pointed to such motivations as seeking adventure, escape from family or other aspects of life, a higher standard of living, a desire to improve a marriage or other family circumstances (the 'geographic cure'), or better education.[5] For some, an extended trip or assignment overseas represents a distinct career opportunity. These various, possible motivations behind travel overseas, although not exhaustive, are summarized in Table 35.1. Another, more prosaic, classification is based upon the overtly stated reason for travel: tourism, study overseas, business and expatriate

Table 35.1	Possible motivations for travel

Modes of tourist travel[4]
  Recreational
  Diversionary
  Experiential
  Experimental
  Existential

Other possible motivations
  Adventure seeking
  Escape from family or other aspects of life
  Increased standard of living
  The 'geographic cure' of family or personal problems
  Better educational opportunities
  Career advancement

travel. Although there is no universally accepted definition of when a business traveler or student becomes an expatriate, certainly a person who takes up residence in a foreign country for one year or more is a reasonable place to separate the two.

The clinical relevance of any system of classification is not clear. Further, it is difficult to put into operational terms unconscious motivations behind travel in order to conduct studies. Epidemiological data on the rates of psychiatric disorders by type of traveler is nonexistent. Anecdotal and clinical evidence point to possible differences, however, but more study is necessary to establish differences in incidence and prevalence rates. One expatriate group studied by the author, for example, rarely seemed to experience anxiety disorders, judging from a clinical population.[6] However, in tourists to Nepal, panic attacks, especially those occurring in individuals for the first time, were not infrequent.[7] Business and expatriate executives are almost certainly less likely to suffer from the more debilitating, chronic mental disorders, such as schizophrenia, if only because such a disorder is incompatible with high office in the workplace and because the disorder usually begins in younger patients. Such would not necessarily be true of the expatriate's family members, however. Within the context of this chapter, the classification by overtly stated reason will be used.

CLINICAL OPERATING ENVIRONMENTS OVERSEAS AND THEIR VICISSITUDES

Although travelers may not present with an unusual range of disorders, the clinician tending to this population will find many challenges in the clinical operating environment overseas. Countries and even cities within countries vary enormously in a number of parameters that impact upon dealing with psychiatric emergencies. Some countries do not have well-developed mental health systems. Hospital facilities for the psychiatric patient may be lacking and culturally compatible clinicians may be rare or non-existent. Nurse staffing, training and practices can differ enormously from country to country. Cross-cultural problems arise, as examined by Fennig et al. in their paper on the Arab nurse and the Jewish psychotic patient.[8] The range of psychotropic medications available locally may be limited and of unknown quality. Laboratory facilities to determine blood levels of frequently used mood stabilizers such as lithium, valproic acid or carbamazepine may not be reliable or available in some settings.

The legal environment within which a clinician practices can also vary widely. This may be especially relevant when facing a patient in imminent danger to self or others. Local commitment laws can vary widely from country to country and some countries may not have any laws dealing with such matters.[9] Laws dealing with illicit substance use vary considerably and can, in some countries, be quite severe.

As a result of these mental health and legal infrastructure differences, which are summarized in Table 35.2, the first decision a clinician frequently will have to make is the strategic one of whether or not a given patient can be managed in place or requires evacuation. Even having decided this key issue, clinicians frequently will have to be quite creative in their management of patients overseas. Problems that normally would require hospitalization, such as the psychotic or suicidal patient, may have to be handled on an outpatient basis, using friends, family and/or private duty nurses to monitor and contain the patient pending medical evacuation. In some countries, psychiatric problems are normally handled on general medical wards, albeit with extra nursing assistance. If hospital facilities are present, but of questionable quality, safety or cultural compatibility, the treating physician will have to balance carefully the relative benefits of containment in hospital versus some more ad hoc arrangement outside. The same balance will have to be made in countries with no or few legal provisions for commitment of the dangerous patient. The physician will need to be familiar with the legal situation and how the laws, if any, are normally carried out, in order to make a good decision to invoke commitment or not.

MOOD DISORDERS

Mania

Although relatively rare, mania is probably one of the most difficult problems to handle overseas. This state usually occurs as part of manic-depressive or bipolar disorder. Patients frequently present with a truly vexatious combination of inflated self-esteem, abundant energy, heightened libido, poor judgment and negligible insight into the nature of their illness. These symptoms can continue for weeks and can lead to ruinous loss of fortune, numerous and indiscreet sexual contacts and even loss of career. In the author's experience, a single manic patient can completely paralyze a sponsoring overseas organization until such time that either the symptoms spontaneously subside, the patient spirals into incoherence allowing hospitalization or other immediate care, or the patient consents to effective treatment or evacuation. To compound the problem, commitment under criteria of imminent danger to self or others is not always possible and the patient's lack of insight can make voluntary consent to treatment difficult to achieve. Frequently, some sort of leverage or pressure from family or sponsoring organization is necessary to obtain the patient's cooperation. Table 35.3 is a clinical vignette, which is illustrative of the presentation and problems encountered in dealing with a person with a manic

Table 35.2	Challenges found in some clinical operating environments overseas

Lack of well-developed mental health system

Inpatient facilities either not available or not culturally compatible

Nursing practices, scope of duty and training vary widely

Culturally compatible mental health clinicians rare or not present

Locally available psychotropic medications limited or of unknown quality

Laboratory facilities for serum levels of psychotropic medications not available or of unknown reliability

Wide variations in the legal environment, effecting commitment and treatment of drug abuse

Table 35.3	Clinical vignette of typical features of a patient with mania overseas

Mr A was a businessman traveling overseas for a temporary posting in a developing nation. His sponsoring company did a pre-travel medical evaluation without any specific screening for mental health problems. As a result, Mr A's first, relatively mild hypomanic episode, occurring some time before his transfer, and for which he did not receive treatment, went unnoticed.

Over the course of a few weeks, Mr A began to display an elevated and expansive mood along with seemingly endless amounts of energy, albeit applied to projects in an uneven, even haphazard manner. Uncharacteristically, he soon required only a few hours of sleep at night. His colleagues noticed increasingly rapid and pressured speech and sometimes had problems following Mr A's train of thought. Even more disturbing, however, was Mr. A's deteriorating business and social judgment. He began talking about and attempting to implement highly questionable business deals and was very easily irritated at any question of his plans. Socially, Mr A at first became the life of every party, but soon began making increasingly bothersome and overt sexual advances towards women. His colleagues finally approached the company's medical division when Mr A started singing loudly in the office, convinced that he was a world class, albeit undiscovered, baritone and talking about the fact that he was receiving direct, divine guidance and that his business schemes could not fail as a result.

Company medical had a consultant physician in country. Fortunately, this physician suspected a manic episode, although substance abuse could not be entirely ruled out. As this was a developing country, however, hospital facilities for psychiatric treatment were poorly staffed and were judged to be potentially worse for Mr A than his disorder. Culturally compatible psychiatric care was also not available. As Mr A had virtually no insight into his condition and would not acknowledge the fact that he was ill, and since he had made no threats to himself or to others, the lack of inpatient facilities and specialists was a moot point as he refused treatment anyway.

There began several weeks of increasingly difficult and embarrassing incidents, damaging both to Mr. A's and the sponsoring company's reputation, as colleagues and finally Mr. A's home country supervisor exerted considerable pressure upon Mr. A to accept medication and a return to his home country for care. The company's business came to a standstill for the duration. Eventually, having been told by the company that he would be summarily dismissed if he did not accept recommend medical care, Mr A accepted haloperidol, the most appropriate medication available on the local market. It was never clear, however, if his acceptance was the result of the gradual diminution of his symptoms with time or the pressure from multiple sources. Lithium carbonate was available, but laboratory facilities for monitoring serum lithium levels were judged to be unreliable. After being sufficiently stabilized to fly, Mr A was flown to his home country with a colleague and a male nurse as escorts. He was not allowed to return to his assignment overseas.

episode overseas. The vignette is a composite of typical features and is not based upon any actual patient.

Incidence, prevalence and etiology

Incidence and prevalence data for this disorder are not available for international travelers. Data from a general population study in the USA found a 6-month prevalence rate of 0.4–0.9%, depending upon gender and location.[10] In the US Foreign Service population studied by the author, manic and hypomanic states accounted for 2.8% of all psychiatric medical evacuations.[11] Hypomanic states are less serious versions of mania that usually do not cause serious social or economic impairment or require hospitalization. The etiology of mania has been extensively studied. Genetic, environmental, and neurotransmitter factors all appear to play a role and the reader is referred to general psychiatric textbooks for review of this interesting subject. With regards to a specific link to travel, some investigators have found a tendency towards more hypomanic or manic symptoms in travelers who had transited time zones in the eastbound direction.[12,13] These studies also found the opposite effect: there were more depressive symptoms associated with westward travel. Methodological limitations preclude a definitive statement, however, and the question of illness causing travel versus travel causing illness is not clearly answered. Nevertheless, sleep deprivation has been thought to have an antidepressant effect and to precipitate elevated moods.[14,15] The question is, then, does the phase advance of the sleep-wake cycle of eastbound travel that crosses time zones particularly induce manic or hypomanic episodes in susceptible individuals in contrast to the general sleep deprivation often associated with any extended travel? Further research is necessary.

Diagnosis and differential

Diagnostic criteria for manic episodes are included in Table 35.4. This set of criteria is from the American Psychiatric Association's Diagnostic and Statistical Manual for Mental Disorders, Fourth Edition, Text Revision (DSM-IV-TR). It is recognized that these criteria are not in use worldwide although they are very widely used in the United States and in a number of other countries. The mixed episode, to which the criteria refer, is when criteria are met for a manic episode and a major depressive episode (see below) nearly every day over at least a week. Most manic episodes will be part of bipolar disorder and it is important to establish if the patient or family has such a history. Occasionally, patients will progress in symptoms to become floridly psychotic with incoherence, delusions and hallucinations. In these instances, the episode may be mistaken for an acute or schizophreniform psychosis that only prior history or subsequent course will clarify. Substance abuse can produce manic symptoms, especially the stimulants such as amphetamines or cocaine. Alcohol use during episodes occurs and may or may not be part of a comorbid alcohol abuse or dependence disorder. Thus, prior or current drug use is important to establish. In addition, there are a number of medical conditions and medications that can produce manic symptoms. Medical conditions include various brain lesions, infections producing encephalitis, hyperthyroidism and Cushing's disease. In practice, these are not frequently encountered although they can be catastrophic if missed. Medications of particular note include virtually any antidepressant. The reader is referred to any general psychiatric textbook for a more complete list. For the present purposes, practitioners should be alert for any signs or symptoms of delirium, which would suggest an organic etiology. A general medical examination

Table 35.4	Criteria for manic episode

A. A distinct period of abnormally and persistently elevated, expansive, or irritable mood, lasting at least 1 week (or any duration if hospitalization is necessary).

B. During the period of mood disturbance, three (or more) of the following symptoms have persisted (four if the mood is only irritable) and have been present to a significant degree.
  (1) inflated self-esteem or grandiosity
  (2) decreased need for sleep (e.g., feels rested after only 3 hours of sleep)
  (3) more talkative than usual or pressure to keep talking
  (4) flight of ideas or subjective experience that thoughts are racing
  (5) distractibility (i.e., attention too easily drawn to unimportant or irrelevant external stimuli)
  (6) increase in goal-directed activity (either socially, at work or school, or sexually) or psychomotor agitation
  (7) excessive involvement in pleasurable activities that have a high potential for painful consequences (e.g., engaging in unrestrained buying sprees, sexual indiscretions, or foolish business investments)

C. The symptoms do not meet criteria for a mixed episode.

D. The mood disturbance is sufficiently severe to cause marked impairment in occupational functioning or in usual social activities or relationships with others, or to necessitate hospitalization to prevent harm to self or others, or there are psychotic features.

E. The symptoms are not due to the direct physiological effects of a substance (e.g., a drug of abuse, a medication, or other treatment) or a general medical condition (e.g., hyperthyroidism).

Note: Manic-like episodes that are clearly caused by somatic antidepressant treatment (e.g., medication, electroconvulsive therapy, light therapy) should not count toward a diagnosis of Bipolar 1 Disorder.

should be conducted at the first opportunity and should include testing for substance abuse.

Treatment

As discussed earlier, management of manic episodes can be very difficult even in those situations overseas where there is an adequate, culturally compatible mental health system. Treatment in the overseas environment is frequently aimed at either hospitalization, if such is possible, or stabilization pending medical evacuation. Use of a potent antipsychotic medication is frequently the first step in order to gain some control of the situation in the least amount of time. In fact, in the absence of laboratory facilities to monitor blood levels of the various mood stabilizers, such medication may be the practitioner's only choice. Haloperidol, an older, typical antipsychotic is often available, is effective and can be used in doses between 2–10 mg/d.[16] Higher doses up to 20 mg/d may occasionally be necessary as will use of the i.m. form. Side-effects are fairly common, however, and include extrapyramidal symptoms that can mimic Parkinson's disease with bradykinesia, tremor and muscular rigidity. These may be treated with anticholinergic agents such as benztropine or trihexyphenidyl and/or reduction in dose. Akathisia also occurs, can be quite uncomfortable, and can easily be mistaken for an increase in agitation. It is experienced as a continuous restlessness and may lead to an inability to sit down and pacing. This side-effect may respond to a beta-blocker, such as propranolol and/or dose reduction. Acute dystonias occur, sometimes with the first dose, and can be treated with diphenhydramine 25–50 mg i.m. If available, olanzapine, a newer, atypical antipsychotic, in doses of 5–20 mg/d may be used instead of haloperidol and may be as effective.[16,17] Extrapyramidal side-effects are much less common with olanzapine and it is generally better tolerated than haloperidol. Further, its sedative side-effect may be of particular use in this setting. If adequate laboratory facilities exist, patients should also be started on a mood stabilizer. Lithium continues to be the prin-

cipal drug for this purpose. Starting doses of 300 mg t.i.d. are reasonable and blood levels should be established between 0.8–1.2 mEq/L.[16] In the long term, patients with mania frequently lack the insight, at least initially, to comply with treatment. This tendency and the natural history of the disorder suggests that further travel or residence overseas is not in the patient's best interests until the pattern of recurrence is known and until they achieve a good degree of insight into their illness accompanied with a high level of compliance with treatment.

Major depression

The other mood disorder of particular note for the overseas clinician is that of major depression. Of all the types of depression, this one is the most serious and can result in the most impairment or even mortality. Since it can take a matter of weeks to develop, the disorder itself is not the proximate cause of a psychiatric emergency. Unlike the manic patient, patients with major depression are relatively inactive, anergic and unmotivated. The emergent problem associated with such depressions is the risk of suicide and/or psychotic symptoms, if present. Table 35.5 is a clinical vignette, which is illustrative of the presentation and problems encountered in dealing with a person with a major depressive episode overseas. The vignette is a composite of typical features and is not based upon any actual patient.

Incidence, prevalence and etiology

As with other disorders in the population of international travelers, incidence and prevalence data are lacking. Data from a general population study in the USA found a 6-month prevalence rate of 1.3–4.6%, depending upon gender and location, with women being more likely to have the problem than men.[10] In the US Foreign Service population, depression of all sorts, to include major depression, accounted for 20% of all psychiatric medical evacuations from overseas, second only to alcoholism.[11] In an overseas, clinical population of US Foreign Service personnel and dependents living overseas, 9.5% of patients suffered from major depression.[18]

As with mania, the etiological causes of major depression have been studied extensively. Genetics, environmental and neurotransmitter factors have all been explored and the reader is referred to a general textbook of psychiatry for a review of this interesting subject. As noted, there appears to be some association between westbound travel across time zones and depressive symptoms, although more study is necessary.[12,13] The stressors of international travel or overseas residence, the isolation from family and familiar social supports, reactions to a foreign culture and language, all likely contribute to depression, major or otherwise, at least in the susceptible individual.

Diagnosis and differential

Table 35.6 presents diagnostic criteria for a major depressive episode, according to the DSM-IV-TR. The mixed episode, to which the criteria refer, is when criteria are met for a manic episode and a major depressive episode nearly every day over at least a week. Major depression can occur as a single episode, as recurrent episodes, or as part of bipolar or manic-depressive disorder. A number of medical conditions can cause depression of this sort, including pancreatic cancer, hypothyroidism, sleep apnea, and a number of infectious and inflammatory diseases, to name a few. Some medications have been associated with major depression, such as reserpine, methyldopa and propranolol. The reader is referred to a textbook of general psychiatry for a complete listing. A general medical evaluation is recommended. A personal or family history of prior episodes or of bipolar illness may help clarify the diagnosis. Substance abuse does occur with major depression, and patients with a primary diagnosis of alcohol depend-

Table 35.5	Clinical vignette of typical features of a patient with major depression overseas

Mrs B was the wife of an expatriate employee, in her early thirties and posted overseas to a developing country. Over the course of several months, her fellow expatriate spouses noted increasing withdrawal from the usual active expatriate social life. At home, over the course of weeks, her husband noted an unrelentingly depressed outlook and mood, worse in the mornings, frequent crying spells, a complete disinterest in sexual relations, and unremitting fatigue. She began to be unable to keep up with managing the household and staff, spending much of her time either in bed or walking aimlessly around the house in her pajamas. Mrs. B also began to show little interest in personal care and dress and was consistently waking up in the early hours of the morning, unable to return to sleep. Her appetite fell off and she lost some fifteen pounds, which was over 10% of her initial body weight.

Mrs. B's husband brought his wife to the company approved, host country physician shortly after she began to talk openly of having suicidal thoughts, albeit, without specific plans or apparent intent. On evaluation, she was noted to be disheveled and dressed in a bathrobe and pajamas. She complained of being depressed, and had nothing good to say about herself or her situation in life. The future looked bleak to her and her affect was noted to be invariant and depressed in nature. Although she was oriented in all spheres, her speech was noticeably slowed as were all her motor movements. She was unable to concentrate. She admitted on direct questioning to having daily, frequent suicidal thoughts of a fleeting nature, but denied current plans or intent. She denied any hallucinations or delusions, and none were evident. There was no history or evidence of substance abuse. She had no prior history of psychiatric disorder, much less suicide attempts, although there was a family history of depression. There was no significant medical history and no particular findings on physical exam except those related to weight loss and her slowed motor movements.

The physician suspected a major depression, first episode. There were no adequate or culturally compatible psychiatric in-patient facilities or specialists available. Also, many of the newer antidepressants were not available on the local market. Because of the suicidal ideation, which was judged to be serious, if not of immediate danger over the next several days, it was arranged for Mrs. B to fly to her home country the next day with her husband and a female nurse as escorts. Although Mrs. B did not believe she could be helped, she reacted passively and did not resist these arrangements. Immediate psychiatric evaluation was arranged upon their arrival and she was hospitalized for several weeks, during which she responded rapidly to antidepressant medications. Extended outpatient follow up over the next month found continued improvement to the point of remission of symptoms. Working with her psychiatrist, the company's medical department and the host country consulting physician, a plan was devised for her return to her husband's overseas posting. The psychiatrist was willing to maintain telephone contact both with the consulting physician and with Mrs. B and her husband on a regular basis. Both Mrs. B and her husband were agreeable to regular follow up visits to the consultant physician and to a follow up visit to the psychiatrist in several months. Arrangements were made to ship Mrs. B's medication to her overseas post. In all, it was felt that a return was safe. In making this judgment, multiple factors were considered: (1) Mrs. B suicidal ideation had never progressed to a point of imminent danger and she had no history of prior attempts; (2) her symptoms evolved over a matter of months allowing for timely intervention in the event of recurrence; (3) she displayed good insight into and acceptance of the fact that she had had a major depression; (4) her husband was both understanding and supportive of her; (5) she responded quickly to medication and was both motivated in treatment and compliant; (6) she did not have any psychotic symptoms; and (7) this had been her first episode and there was no personal or family history to suggest bipolar disorder.

ence can often appear severely depressed. Patients may also use alcohol, stimulants or marijuana concurrently with major depression, either to alleviate symptoms or because of concurrent substance abuse disorders. Certainly evaluation should include a substance use history in some detail. Major depressive episodes can also occur with psychotic features such as delusions or hallucinations. The presence of psychotic features can mean that the patient will be more difficult to treat and certainly makes the situation emergent.

Assessment of suicide risk

Suicidal ideation is frequently present with major depression and suicide risk is the usual reason that major depression becomes an emergency overseas. One estimate of the risk of suicide in an individual hospitalized for severe major depressive disorder is 15%.[19] Careful assessment of this risk in a forthright manner is imperative. Assessment should include the following elements:

- frequency and persistence of suicidal ideation (SI); frequent SI with ruminative quality indicates higher risk;
- ascertainment of any plans for suicide attempt; presence of plans, especially realistic, non-contingent ones indicate higher risk;

- access to lethal means for an attempt; assess access to firearms, medications, knives, tall buildings, etc.
- assessment of intent; how serious or 'close' to attempting suicide is the patient?
- family history of suicide or suicide attempts;
- personal history of suicide attempts and their exact nature; e.g., if prior attempts, were they conducted in a lethal manner with low chance of discovery? Such would indicate higher risk;
- presence of psychotic features and/or any substance use or abuse greatly increases risk;
- presence of any major adverse life events or their anniversaries, such as the death of a spouse, parent or significant other.

Although the above points represent a reasonable first assessment, the reader is referred to any general psychiatric text for a more complete discussion of all known risk factors and associations with age, gender, race, and other diagnoses.

The risk of suicide should always be taken seriously and if there is doubt as to the degree of risk, it is best to proceed with an abundance of caution. Should the risk appear to be substantial, immediate hospitalization is best, if available. If not available, then evacuation to the

Table 35.6	Diagnostic criteria for major depressive disorder, single episode

1. Presence of a single major depressive episode.
2. The major depressive episode is not better accounted for by schizoaffective disorder and is not superimposed on schizophrenia, schizophreniform disorder, delusional disorder, or psychotic disorder not otherwise specified.
3. There has never been a manic episode, a mixed episode, or a hypomanic episode.

Note: This exclusion does not apply if all of the manic-like, mixed-like, or hypomanic-like episodes are substance or treatment induced or are due to the direct physiological effects of a general medical condition.

If the full criteria are currently met for a major depressive episode, *specify* its current clinical status and/or features:

   Mild, moderate, severe without psychotic features/severe with psychotic features
   Chronic
   With catatonic features
   With melancholic features
   With atypical features
   With postpartum onset

If the full criteria are not currently met for a major depressive episode, *specify* the current clinical status of the major depressive disorder or features of the most recent episode:

   In partial remission, in full remission
   Chronic
   With catatonic features
   With melancholic features
   With atypical features
   With postpartum onset

nearest adequate facility is the next best option. While waiting for evacuation, the clinician should do the utmost to implement appropriate suicide prevention steps as can be done under the circumstances. These may include arranging for a 24 h continuous watch of the patient by family, private duty nurses, or others, removal of any obvious means of suicide, such as firearms, medications, knives, ropes, razors, etc., and frequent checks on the patient's status. If the patient has been actively using substances, access should be removed, if at all possible, and careful watch kept for withdrawal symptoms.

Treatment

Treatment in serious cases of major depression, especially those with high risk of suicide, should be aimed at preventing suicide prior to evacuation or hospitalization. If psychotic features are present, these should be treated aggressively with antipsychotic medications. Which antipsychotic to use depends upon availability, of course. Haloperidol can certainly be used in a similar dose range as for manic episodes. However, if available, newer, atypical antipsychotics, such as risperidone, olanzapine, quetiapine, and others, can be preferable because of their better side-effect profiles. If the patient has had particular difficulty sleeping, use of a sedative-hypnotic may be of use. Benzodiazepines can be used although they may worsen depression. Trazodone is frequently helpful in these instances in doses of from 50 to 200 mg p.o. at bedtime.

The patient should be started on an antidepressant. Given the fact that virtually any antidepressant has a delayed response effect on the order of weeks, such may not be of immediate benefit. However, in the seriously ill patient, time is of the essence. Choice of antidepressant depends upon local availability, of course. Certainly, if the patient has had prior episodes and has responded to a particular antidepressant, then that is the drug of choice. In general, the newer antidepressants are preferable over either the older tricyclics or the MAO inhibitors because of their better side-effect profiles and safety in overdose situations. A reasonable place to start would be the specific serotonin re-uptake inhibitors (SSRI) such as fluoxetine, sertraline, paroxetine, fluvoxamine or citalopram.

PSYCHOTIC DISORDERS

Psychosis is a state that can occur in many different psychiatric disorders, including mania, depression and a number of substance use disorders. A psychotic state is a serious break with reality and can be characterized by delusions, hallucinations (often auditory; visual, tactile and olfactory hallucinations are suggestive of an organic etiology) and thought disorder. Thought disorder is a disruption of the normal train of thought such that sequential ideas are not connected. It can be mild to severe in nature, such as in word salad where the patient is seemingly stringing words together without any connection at all. The presence of psychosis, especially in a patient who is not chronically, mentally ill, or who has never had prior episodes, represents a psychiatric emergency, regardless of its causation. The following section reviews two types of disorders, brief psychotic disorder and schizophrenia. Both are characterized by psychosis and that are frequently seen overseas. The following section reviews two types of disorders, brief psychotic disorder and schizophrenia.

Brief psychotic disorder

Diagnostic criteria for brief psychotic disorder are found in Table 35.7. It is important to note the duration criteria (Criterion B) and the fact that individuals with this disorder should return to full functioning. Equally important are the differential criteria, Criterion C. As psychotic states can occur as a result of depression or mania, substance use disorders, schizophrenia, general medical conditions, or medications, these must be excluded in order to make the diagnosis. In the international travel arena, one must consider cerebral manifestations of malaria and use of mefloquine in this differential.

Psychotic states are frequently cited in the literature as being associated with travel and some of these may fulfill the criteria of brief psychotic disorder. The author found that 6.2% of psychiatric evacuations within the US Foreign Service involved a psychotic state, exclusive of mania or hypomania.[11] In an outpatient population of US Foreign Service personnel and dependents living overseas, brief psychosis accounted for 1.6% of adult patients.[18] Episodes of acute situational psychosis have been reported in tourists to Nepal and in American expatriates in South Vietnam.[20,21] Flinn and Singh have commented upon transient psychotic reactions associated with long travel. Flinn in particular cited isolation of long distance travel, increased alcohol intake, irregular food and fluid intake and insomnia as contributing factors.[22,23] Bar-el *et al.* identified a type of Jerusalem Syndrome (see below) that may meet the criteria for brief psychotic disorder.[24] Acute psychotic reactions have been reported in Japanese honeymooners traveling to Honolulu. These cases appeared to occur with greater frequency among honeymooners than among non-honeymoon Japanese tourists and the authors speculated that arranged marriages and other cultural factors might be at play.[25] In many of these reported situations, the psychotic state evolved rapidly, there was no prior history of such problems, and symptoms resolved quickly with treatment. Given all the various stressors from international travel, and the fact that brief psychotic disorder is recognized to be associated with significant life stresses, this presentation may be one of the psychiatric disorders truly related to travel in all its vicissitudes.

Table 35.7   Diagnostic criteria for 298.8 Brief psychotic disorder

A. Presence of one (or more) of the following symptoms:
  (1) delusions
  (2) hallucinations
  (3) disorganized speech (e.g., frequent derailment or incoherence)
  (4) grossly disorganized or catatonic behavior

Note: Do not include a symptom if it is a culturally sanctioned response pattern.

B. Duration of an episode of the disturbance is at least 1 day but less than 1 month, with eventual full return to premorbid level of functioning.

C. The disturbance is not better accounted for by a mood disorder with psychotic features, schizoaffective disorder, or schizophrenia and is not due to the direct physiological effects of a substance (e.g., a drug of abuse, a medication) or a general medical condition.

Specify if:
  With marked stressor(s) (brief reactive psychosis): if symptoms occur shortly after and apparently in response to events that, singly or together, would be markedly stressful to almost anyone in similar circumstances in the person's culture
  Without marked stressor(s): if psychotic symptoms do not occur shortly after, or are not apparently in response to events that, singly or together, would be markedly stressful to almost anyone in similar circumstances in the person's culture
  With postpartum onset: if onset within 4 weeks postpartum

Treatment

Treatment depends upon accurate diagnosis, with due regard to differential diagnosis. Organic causes of psychosis, to include cerebral malaria, intoxication with stimulants or hallucinogens, alcohol withdrawal, use of mefloquine and a number of other medications and general medical conditions such as brain tumors need to be ruled out. Certainly a general medical evaluation is indicated and should include appropriate laboratory tests for detection of substance abuse. Due attention to any suicidal ideation is important. The use of antipsychotic medications, such as haloperidol, fluphenazine, olanzapine, risperidone, or quetiapine, often in relatively low doses, may be all that is required. The former two medications are older, typical antipsychotics and have the side-effect profile outlined for haloperidol in the section above on mania. The latter two medications are relatively new, may not be as available in all overseas environments, and are atypical antipsychotics that have generally better tolerated side-effect profiles, a fact that is true for most atypicals as a class. If hospitalization is not available, then the clinician should use a safe, contained environment allowing for frequent monitoring. Rapid response to treatment, within hours or a few days are consistent with brief psychotic disorder. Evacuation may not be necessary, although it is prudent for the patient to break travel and return home.

Schizophrenia

Schizophrenia is a chronic, debilitating mental illness that often begins in the teens or early adulthood and can last for a number of years. Fifty percent of individuals with schizophrenia will experience onset before the age of 25.[16] It is characterized by psychotic symptoms that can wax and wane over time and, with treatment, may be absent for extended periods. Diagnostic criteria for schizophrenia are presented in Table 35.8. There are a number of recognized subtypes. All are dependent upon satisfying the criteria for schizophrenia, and each emphasizes a specific set of symptoms. Subtypes include paranoid, disorganized, catatonic and undifferentiated. The residual type is where the symptoms of psychosis (delusions, hallucinations, disor-

ganized speech) are not prominent and negative symptoms such as flat affect, lack of motivation, and poverty of speech are still in evidence.

Relation to international travel

It is abundantly clear that individuals with schizophrenia travel internationally. Numerous authors have found this disorder in travelers at international airports, in Hawaii, and as travelers to Jerusalem.[3,13,26,27] In the author's experience, and that of a number of US Consular Officers, individuals that probably meet the criteria for schizophrenia are known to wander about internationally, occasionally showing up at Embassies for some form of assistance, and may constitute an international form of chronically mentally ill homeless persons. The prevalence of this disorder in the internationally traveling population is not known. Lifetime prevalence is from 1 to 1.5%.[16] As mentioned in the introduction, given the nature of schizophrenia, it is less likely to be seen in some types of international travelers, such as the business traveler or the expatriate employee. Given the chronic nature of the illness and the relatively early age of onset, it is unlikely that travel in itself can be considered a causative factor. Etiology has, as with other disorders, been extensively studied for many years. Suffice it to say that the illness can run in families, can arise without a family history, and likely has no single, predominant etiology. Readers with a particular interest are referred to any general psychiatric text for a review of current theories.

Treatment

Individuals with schizophrenia can and do abuse substances of all types and can have co-existing substance use disorders. Substance abuse can complicate treatment considerably. In assessing patients, it is important to obtain as clear a history of substance use as possible. Appropriate laboratory tests, if available, are warranted. Since some of these patients have been wandering internationally for periods of time, a general medical examination is also advisable. Treatment depends primarily upon the patient's status upon first contact. If the patient is compliant with medication and there are few prominent psychotic symptoms, hospitalization may not be necessary. Psychotic symptoms, however, should be treated with antipsychotic medications, such as haloperidol, fluphenazine, olanzapine, risperidone, or quetiapine, to name a few. Frequently, the patient can tell the physician which medications have been of most benefit in the past, and if available, these should be re-instituted. Due attention to substance abuse, to include intoxication and withdrawal states may be necessary. The presence of suicidal ideation should be assessed and a risk assessment, similar to that outlined in the discussion of major depression above, should be carried out. If there are hallucinations present, part of this assessment should address whether or not they are auditory and command in nature. Command auditory hallucinations can urge the individual to commit suicide, which clearly increases risk. Individuals at high risk of suicide should be hospitalized, if possible, or contained as outlined in the section on major depression. Given stabilization, individuals should be sent home to family or their country of origin although they may not comply and may continue traveling despite admonition.

SUBSTANCE USE DISORDERS

Virtually any mind altering, intoxicating or addicting substance, has a corresponding substance use disorder diagnosis. A complete account of all possible substances is beyond the scope of this chapter and the reader is referred to general psychiatric textbooks or specific works on addictions for a full review. Rather, in this section, some specific problems related to substance use that are likely to culminate in emergencies are discussed along with more general information

Table 35.8	Diagnostic criteria for schizophrenia

A. *Characteristic symptoms:* Two (or more) of the following, each present for a significant portion of time during a 1-month period (or less if successfully treated):
  (1) delusions
  (2) hallucinations
  (3) disorganized speech (e.g., frequent derailment or incoherence)
  (4) grossly disorganized or catatonic behavior
  (5) negative symptoms, i.e., affective flattening, alogia, or avolition

Note: Only one criterion A symptom is required if delusions are bizarre or hallucinations consist of a voice keeping up a running commentary on the person's behavior or thoughts, or two or more voices conversing with each other.

B. *Social/occupational dysfunction:* For a significant portion of the time since the onset of the disturbance, one or more major areas of functioning such as work, interpersonal relations, or self-care are markedly below the level achieved prior to the onset (or when the onset is in childhood or adolescence, failure to achieve expected level of interpersonal, academic, or occupational achievement).

C. *Duration:* Continuous signs of the disturbance persist for at least 6 months. This 6-month period must include at least 1 month of symptoms (or less if successfully treated) that meet Criterion A (i.e., active-phase symptoms) and may include periods of prodromal or residual symptoms. During these prodromal or residual periods, the signs of the disturbance may be manifested by only negative symptoms or two or more symptoms listed in Criterion A present in an attenuated form (e.g., odd beliefs, unusual perceptual experiences).

D. *Schizoaffective and mood disorder exlusion:* Schizoaffective disorder and mood disorder with psychotic features have been ruled out because either (1) no major depressive, manic, or mixed episodes have occurred concurrently with the active-phase symptoms; or (2) if mood episodes have occurred during active-phase symptoms, their total duration has been brief relative to the duration of the active and residual periods.

E. *Substance/general medical condition exclusion:* The disturbance is not due to the direct physiological effects of a substance (e.g., a drug of abuse, a medication) or a general medical condition.

F. *Relationship to a pervasive developmental disorder:* If there is a history of autistic disorder or another pervasive developmental disorder, the addition diagnosis of Schizophrenia is made only if prominent delusions or hallucinations are also present for at least a month (or less if successfully treated).

Classification of longitudinal course: (can be applied only after at least 1 year has elapsed since the initial onset of active-phase symptoms):

  Episodic with interepisode residual symptoms (episodes are defined by the reemergence of prominent psychotic symptoms); *also specify if: with prominent negative symptoms*
  Episodic with no interepisodes residual symptoms
  Continuous (prominent psychotic symptoms are present throughout the period of observation); *also specify if: with prominent negative symptoms*
  Single episode in partial remission; also specify if: with prominent negative symptoms
  Single episode in full remission
  Other or unspecified pattern

concerning substance use disorders and their appearance and consequences overseas.

Most substances of abuse have both a dependence and an abuse diagnostic category. Essentially, for either category, the affected individual continues to use the substance despite repeated and serious problems associated with its use. For abuse, these problems do not include either the development of tolerance or withdrawal symptoms. Rather, the emphasis is upon continued use despite substance related social, family, work or legal problems and repeated use in hazardous situations (e.g., driving while intoxicated). Dependence includes the possibility of the development of either tolerance or withdrawal for many substances, along with a range of cognitive and behavioral symptoms. These include consumption of the substance in larger amounts than anticipated, attempts or a desire to cut down on use, continued use despite adverse medical or psychiatric consequences and a loss of social or other activities due to continued use.[28]

Relation to international travel, etiology

Virtually any substance of abuse is encountered in the international traveler population. In the US Foreign Service population, substance use disorders of any type were the leading cause of psychiatric medical evacuation, accounting for 28% of the total. Alcohol abuse or dependence accounted for the majority of these evacuations and for 22.9% of the total.[11] Similarly, in a clinical population of US Foreign Service personnel and dependents living overseas, 12.5% of patients were alcohol dependent and 1.6% had cannabis abuse.[18] Heavy alcohol use or dependence among international travelers have also been reported by a number of authors in a variety of settings.[3,5,13,21,22,26] For a number of travel oriented clinicians, and quite a few expatriates, it is axiomatic that the expatriate population has a high rate of alcohol abuse and dependence. However, actual prevalence data in this or any other type of international traveler is not available either for alcohol or any other substance of abuse.

The etiologies of substance use disorders have been studied extensively. As with other psychiatric disorders, genetic, environmental and neurobiological factors have been found, without any single cause predominant. With regards to travel, given the number of years it takes to develop alcohol dependence (some 3 to 15 years in one longitudinal study), travel itself is unlikely to be a key determinant.[29] Anecdotally, however, for those alcoholics in remission, international travel and/or expatriation with their inherent stressors can threaten sobriety. Being in new and sometimes exotic places, freed from the family and social restraints of home, and having access to cheap substances of all sorts would certainly be a situation ripe for abuse. In some countries, minor tranquilizers and even stimulants are readily available on the open market, are legal, and can be purchased without prescription. Such is an open invitation to self-medication, which certainly does occur and can lead to abuse and dependence.

When does substance abuse or dependence become a psychiatric emergency? Usually, alcohol intoxication by itself does not become a psychiatric emergency, unless the patient becomes violent or suicidal. The vast majority of cases of alcohol intoxication never come to medical attention. However, intoxication with hallucinogens, stimulants, inhalants, cannabis, and phencyclidine can result in psychotic states that can present as a psychiatric emergency.[28] In general, treatment of these psychotic states should include careful observation for possible overdose, and evaluation for concomitant use of other substances or medical conditions, to include laboratory tests for the detection of substances of abuse.[16]

Treatment of intoxication states

Severe agitation associated with amphetamine, other sympathomimetics, or amphetamine-like substance intoxication, may be treated with diazepam i.m. or p.o. from 5 to 10 mg every 3 h, as needed. The addition of vitamin C 0.5 g p.o. q.i.d. may increase excretion of these substances by acidifying the urine. Delusions and hallucinations associated with intoxication states may be treated with haloperidol i.m. or p.o. from 1–5 mg every 2–6 h as necessary. Phenothiazines should not be used in the treatment of intoxication with hallucinogens (except LSD) and PCP or PCP like substances. Tachyarrhythmias encountered with amphetamines and other sympathomimetics and in the anti-cholinergic toxic psychosis may be treated with propranolol 10 to 20 mg p.o. every 4 h as necessary. The antidote for anticholinergic psychosis is physostigmine 2 mg i.v. every 20 min with no more than 1 mg/min being administered at any given time. For opioid intoxication when overdose is apparent, the airway should be kept open, O_2 should be used and reversal may be accomplished with naloxone 0.4 mg i.m. every 20 min for three doses.[16]

Given the complexity of treating these states of intoxication, hospitalization or at least treatment in an emergency room over the course of hours is the preferred route. The immediate goal is to support the patient as necessary, deal with acute agitation and psychotic symptoms, and prevent injury, morbidity or mortality from overdose. As with the other disorders discussed previously, if hospitalization is not available or adequate, the physician may need to set up treatment in a contained and controlled environment with 24-h monitoring using private duty nurses or other personnel as available. After the acute phase is dealt with, considerations of longer-term treatment for substance abuse or dependence that generally rely upon abstinence will frequently be necessary. Obtaining such treatment may involve return to the patient's country of origin. In this regard, clinicians and patients should be mindful that laws in some countries are quite severe regarding illicit drug use and that relapse risk is generally felt to be higher if long-term treatment of those with substance abuse or dependence is not undertaken.

Alcohol withdrawal

Withdrawal states seen in patients that are substance dependent can also present as psychiatric emergencies. Alcohol, opioid, and sedative, hypnotic, and anxiolytic withdrawals can lead to hallucinations, delusions, agitation and delirium that may prompt psychiatric attention. Of these substances, alcohol is probably the most likely culprit in the overseas travel oriented environment. For the specifics of management of opioid and sedative, hypnotic and anxiolytic withdrawal states, the reader is referred to a general textbook of psychiatry or addiction medicine. The diagnostic criteria for alcohol withdrawal are presented in Table 35.9.

As with the other substance use disorders, patients presenting with alcohol withdrawal should be evaluated for concurrent medical conditions and for concurrent use of other substances that might complicate management or diagnosis. Medical conditions to be especially looked for are those associated with prolonged alcohol intake, such as cirrhosis, gastritis, GI bleeding, pneumonia, subdural hematomas, and dehydration. Thus, a thorough medical evaluation is quite important. Development of a state of delirium, with altered consciousness, disorientation, memory and concentration difficulties, is significant because somewhere between 4% and 20% of these patients die.[30,31] History should include any prior episodes of withdrawal and the signs and symptoms thereof.

Treatment of medically complicated cases or those with significant amounts of agitation or hallucinations is best carried out in a hospital, should that option be available. If not, individuals will need to be in a well-lighted environment with minimal stimulation and frequent monitoring. Concurrent medical problems will need to be treated. Suicidal ideation should be assessed and dealt with appropriately. Although there are many methods used to withdraw patients, probably the most utilized is with the benzodiazepines, which are cross-tolerant with alcohol. A loading procedure can be used in those patients with significant withdrawal symptoms. Oral or i.v. doses of diazepam 10–20 mg or chlordiazepoxide at 50–100 mg are delivered and repeated every hour until the patient is sedated, has signs of intoxication or there is a significant reduction in withdrawal signs and symptoms. Obviously, close observation during the loading period is necessary to titrate the cumulative dose correctly. After this period, either only occasional or no further doses are necessary.[32] Should the circumstances not permit the kind of close monitoring necessary for a loading procedure, lesser amounts of diazepam in the 5 to 10 mg range, i.m. or p.o., can be given every 3 h on a PRN basis based upon assessment of the severity of withdrawal. i.m. vitamin B complex should be given.[16]

Any patient with alcohol withdrawal disorder is virtually certain to be alcohol dependent. Thus, after withdrawal is completed, patients

---

Table 35.9 Diagnostic criteria for 291.81 alcohol withdrawal

A. Cessation of (or reduction in) alcohol use that has been heavy and prolonged.
B. Two (or more) of the following, developing within several hours to a few days after Criterion A:
   (1) autonomic hyperactivity (e.g., sweating or pulse rate greater than 100)
   (2) increased hand tremor
   (3) insomnia
   (4) nausea or vomiting
   (5) transient visual, tactile, or auditory hallucinations or illusions
   (6) psychomotor agitation
   (7) anxiety
   (8) grand mal seizures

C. The symptoms in Criterion B cause clinically significant distress or impairment in social, occupational, or other important areas of functioning.
D. The symptoms are not due to a general medical condition and are not better accounted for by another mental disorder.

Specify if:
With perceptual disturbances

should undergo longer-term treatment aimed at abstinence on either an inpatient or outpatient basis. Travel to undertake such treatment may well be necessary and careful thought should be given following successful treatment as to the possible impact upon sobriety of a return to international travel or posting overseas.

PANIC ATTACKS

The criteria for diagnosing a panic attack are presented in Table 35.10. These attacks can occur on an occasional basis, can be part of a panic disorder with recurrent attacks, and can occur as a result of substance abuse, such as during cannabis intoxication or during alcohol withdrawal. In the general US population, panic disorder has a 6-month prevalence of between 0.3–1.2%.[10] Panic attacks as seen in the fear of flying syndrome and their treatment are discussed in Chapter 34.

Relation to international travel

Anxiety intense enough to lead to an emergency room visit has been noted in some 18% of psychiatric emergencies in tourists traveling to Hawaii. Curiously, in transients traveling to Hawaii, those who arrived without any immediate plans to return, anxiety reactions accounted for only 1.6%.[3] Among tourists to Nepal, panic attacks were noted to be common. For the most part, these were first time episodes in persons who appeared to be adjusting well. Reassurance and the offer of a benzodiazepine appeared to be all that was needed to prevent recurrences. Altitude did not appear to be a factor in most cases.[7] In the US Foreign Service expatriate population studied by the author, however, panic attacks, and in fact, anxiety disorders in general, were relatively infrequent. Anxiety disorders of any sort accounted for less than 3% of psychiatric medical evacuations and in a clinical population overseas, only 1.6% of patients had a panic disorder and only 3.2% had any sort of anxiety disorder. This rate was much less than would be expected in a clinic population in the US.[6,11]

The apparent disparity between the general population and that of expatriates is an interesting phenomenon, which may be mirrored in the similar disparity between the percentage of anxiety reactions between tourists and transients traveling to Hawaii. One hypothesis is that persons with established panic disorder simply do not travel. That is, there is an element of self-selection. The panic attacks seen in

tourists to Nepal were, for the most part, first episodes, which is at least consistent with this hypothesis. Further studies, comparing rates of panic attacks and panic disorders, between selected traveling populations versus populations that do not travel internationally would be helpful. Table 35.11 is a clinical vignette, which is illustrative of the presentation and problems encountered in dealing with a person with a panic attack overseas. The vignette is a composite of typical features and is not based upon any actual patient.

Treatment

For the most part, panic attacks do not constitute a psychiatric emergency in the sense that they involve immanent danger to the patient or others. To the person having a first episode, however, it certainly feels like an emergency and frequently results in a trip to the emergency room where work-ups for various medical conditions such as coronary artery disease, pulmonary embolus and even pheochromocytoma may be undertaken. Certainly, medical evaluation in those having a first time attack is warranted to rule out organic pathology

Table 35.10	Criteria for panic attack

Note: A panic attack is not a codable disorder. Code the specific diagnosis in which the Panic Attack occurs (e.g., Panic Disorder With Agoraphobia).

A discrete period of intense fear or discomfort, in which four (or more) of the following symptoms developed abruptly and reached a peak within 10 min:

(1) palpitations, pounding heart, or accelerated heart rate
(2) sweating
(3) trembling or shaking
(4) sensations of shortness of breath or smothering
(5) feeling of choking
(6) chest pain or discomfort
(7) nausea or abdominal distress
(8) feeling dizzy, unsteady, lightheaded, or faint
(9) derealization (feelings of unreality) or depersonalization (being detached from oneself)
(10) fear of losing control or going crazy
(11) fear of dying
(12) paresthesias (numbness or tingling sensations)
(13) chills or hot flushes

Table 35.11	Clinical vignette of typical features of a patient with a panic attack overseas

Mr C was a young, healthy adventure-seeking tourist, traveling to a developing country for the first time. Although his trip was going well and in the absence of any particularly dangerous situation or even vigorous exertion, Mr C experienced the sudden onset of the most profound anxiety and panic, accompanied by an equally awful dread that he was about to die. His hands trembled, he felt short of breath, began sweating profusely and felt his heart pounding within his chest. His symptoms swelled over the course of minutes and ended as abruptly as they had started, leaving Mr C feeling limp and exhausted.

Fearful of what these symptoms could mean and thinking that he had some terrible cardiac condition, Mr C. sought medical attention as swiftly as he could. Although laboratory, radiological and cardiovascular studies were limited, what was available, plus the complete absence of findings upon physical along with negative medical, psychiatric and substance abuse histories, all pointed towards Mr C's experience as having been a panic attack, his very first.

The evaluating physician, having some knowledge of panic attacks, and since there were no culturally compatible psychiatrists available, undertook to educate and reassure Mr C. Although not all possible medical tests could be performed, Mr C's history, the rapid onset and equally rapid termination of symptoms, without residual, the absence of findings or history, all made panic attack a high probability if not a medical certainty. Mr C was told that panic attacks are not unusual but that they were virtually never fatal and did not represent some grave medical illness. Fortunately, Mr C was reassured. Given the fact that he had no prior psychiatric history or history of panic attacks, no specific treatment was undertaken although a follow-up visit with his personal physician was recommended upon his return home some weeks hence.

or substance abuse. The list of possible medical and neurological causes of anxiety or panic attacks is long and the reader is referred to any general psychiatric textbook for review. However, when such evaluations are negative or non-contributory, then treatment should be aimed at education about the fact that panic attacks are a well-known psychophysiological phenomenon and are rarely, if ever, life-threatening. The patient can be given a benzodiazepine to help in any future attacks, although given the abrupt onset and relatively short duration of attacks, its use is probably not going to be terribly helpful physiologically. It can be reassuring, however. For those patients having recurrent panic attacks, especially those that fulfill the criteria of panic disorder and having frequent attacks several times per week, regular benzodiazepine use is a reasonable immediate treatment. Longer acting benzodiazepines such as diazepam or clonazepam are preferable so that blood levels do not fluctuate rapidly. Long-term treatment of panic disorder, however, should begin with the use of an SSRI antidepressant, such as fluoxetine, paroxetine, sertraline, or citalopram in standard dosages. Once these have been established at sufficient dosage for four to six weeks, the patient should be slowly withdrawn from benzodiazepines over a matter of weeks. Withdrawal is important since the benzodiazepines are addictive.

SPECIAL SITUATIONS OF NOTE

The following section deals with two particular situations of interest to the travel medicine practitioner but which do not represent specific disorders. These are the Jerusalem Syndrome and the psychiatric side-effects of mefloquine.

Jerusalem syndrome

Jerusalem syndrome refers to acute, frequently psychotic reactions that occur during travel to Jerusalem or to other locations that have powerful religious or spiritual significance. The hypothesis is that the powerful religious symbolism of Jerusalem when coupled with 'the messianic, redemptive yearnings of Jews and Christians' provides a stimulus that is overwhelming for some individuals.[33]

In their work on Jerusalem syndrome, Bar-el, *et al.* looked at the 1200 tourists to Jerusalem between the years of 1980 and 1993 that were referred for psychiatric evaluation due to symptoms or behavior that came to attention after their arrival.[24] They noted that the number of such cases averaged 100/year, of which 40 required hospitalization. Three types of patients with Jerusalem syndrome were identified. Type I included individuals with pre-existing psychosis that came to Jerusalem due to their condition along with a sometimes delusional idea that they had to undertake a religious mission. These persons usually traveled alone and had a history of schizophrenia or bipolar illness. Type II were people who usually traveled in groups and who had obsessive or fixed, non-delusional but idiosyncratic ideas concerning Jerusalem and their purpose for traveling there. These individuals were not psychotic and did not often come to psychiatric attention. Type III consisted of only 42 individuals during the course of the study. The authors postulated three diagnostic criteria for these individuals:
1. No prior history of psychiatric episodes
2. Individuals travel to Jerusalem as tourists without any particular mission
3. Upon arrival, these persons have an acute psychotic reaction.

In the authors' experience, there was also a characteristic progression towards psychosis characterized by seven stages including initial agitation followed by a desire to split away from traveling companions, a need to be clean and pure and preparation of a toga-like gown that was always white. Subsequent steps included a need to shout or sing verses from the Bible followed by a procession to a holy place in

Jerusalem and finally the delivery of a sermon at a holy place. The sermon was usually confused.

Of note was the fact that hallucinations were usually not present and that afflicted individuals returned to normal within 5–7 days. Treatment consisted of removing patients from holy sites and Jerusalem and the use of minor tranquilizers or melatonin. On recovery, patients had full recall of their behaviors and experienced shame, rarely being willing to talk about their episode. Of the 42 cases, 40 were Christian and one was Jewish.

A syndrome similar to the Type I variant of the Jerusalem syndrome has been called the Stendhal syndrome. In this syndrome, art-loving persons visiting Florence, Italy have acute psychotic reactions upon or related to viewing the many works of art there. The author indicated that most had some form of latent psychiatric problem.[34]

Kalian and Witztum have pointed out the infrequency of Jerusalem syndrome, about 50 patients per year among almost 2 million tourists and have disagreed with the notion that Jerusalem is a pathogenic factor. Rather, in their opinion, the syndrome should be viewed as an exacerbation of pre-existing, chronic mental illness, although it could be seen also as a unique phenomenon of a cultural nature.[35,36]

In fact, Type I Jerusalem syndrome variant would appear to be cases in which pre-existing, serious mental illness was exacerbated concurrent with travel to Jerusalem. The question unanswered is whether or not travel was the result of the exacerbation or the other way around. Subtle prodromal symptoms of decompensation in the chronically mentally ill can take place over weeks' time and could easily be missed on evaluation in Jerusalem. On the other hand, the Type III variant of Jerusalem syndrome does not appear to be related to prior mental illness, although thorough study of these few individuals was hampered by their reluctance to talk about their experience and the fact that detailed psychological evaluation was not done. Further, it is unclear what diagnosis would be appropriate for these individuals.

In summary, it is probably fair to say that for some tourists with pre-existing mental illness, the intense religious symbolism of Jerusalem either results in a decompensation in conjunction with the other stressors of travel or that with an impending decompensation, the symbolism becomes imbedded in the pathology resulting in travel. For a very small number of tourists, only 42 over 13 years, there appears to be a de novo decompensation without any apparent antecedent mental illness. This group may represent the true Jerusalem syndrome: hospitalization after arrival in Jerusalem; no preceding mental illness; psychotic symptoms; and quick recovery with minimal pharmacological intervention. However, further information on this small group of individuals, such as diagnosis, a recounting of their experience after recovery and psychological testing would be in order.

For travel clinicians who may encounter some form of Jerusalem syndrome, most patients would require treatments as outlined under the section in this chapter for brief psychotic disorders. Details concerning the very small group of Type III variant of Jerusalem syndrome are too few to formulate a treatment regimen save to note that benzodiazepines seemed to suffice for many.

Psychiatric reactions to mefloquine

As detailed in Chapter 13, mefloquine is an effective antimalarial agent used both for prophylaxis and treatment of chloroquine-resistant malaria. Its use in either manner has been associated with a number of psychiatric symptoms including depression, psychosis with hallucinations or paranoia, anxiety, and agitation. Its use is contraindicated, according to the manufacturer's package insert, for prophylaxis in individuals with active depression or a history of psychosis. An estimate of incidence rate for moderate to serious neuropsychiatric reactions, based upon figures from several different databases and several assumptions, is 1 in 215 for those taking therapeutic doses and 1 in 13 000 for prophylaxis.[37]

In one study undertaken in Germany, 12 patients with neuropsychiatric reactions to mefloquine were identified through contact with 12 infectious disease units in German hospitals. Of the 12 patients, four were on prophylaxis, the rest on therapy, and none had pre-existing psychiatric illness. Symptoms started 1–2 days after therapeutic doses and in one patient on prophylaxis, symptoms began after the first dose. Reactions lasted from 2–10 days and no patient had manifestations of cerebral malaria. Eight patients had psychiatric manifestations to include psychosis with hallucinations and/or delusions, depression, agitation or anxiety. The rest had primarily neurological or medical symptoms, such as seizures, abnormal coordination, vertigo, or nausea. Of the eight with psychiatric manifestations, only two had what might be considered purely psychiatric presentations. Both had psychotic symptoms. One was on a therapeutic dose and the other on prophylaxis. All the other individuals with psychiatric symptoms had either concurrent neurological symptoms or had suggestions of organicity with confusion or disturbed consciousness.[37] Another report of a single case of apparent reaction involved a 45-year-old woman on prophylaxis for 7 weeks. She was admitted to a psychiatric ward four days after her last dose with acute depression and confusion that improved without medical treatment. She had no prior history of psychiatric difficulties and no recurrence in 6 months of follow-up.[38]

For the travel medicine clinician, it is important to keep in mind that mefloquine should be in the differential for any psychotic presentation or depression. Based upon the cases reviewed, prior history of psychiatric illness is lacking and for most some concurrent neurological symptom and/or confusion or alteration of consciousness is likely to be present. Differential should also include, given the circumstances, malaria infection to include cerebral malaria. Treatment would consist of stopping the mefloquine and appropriate containment and monitoring in the hospital or, if a hospital is not available, appropriate containment as discussed above. Symptomatic treatment may be undertaken with use of antipsychotic medication for psychotic symptoms and benzodiazepines for anxiety and sleep. It appears that the duration of symptoms is a matter of days.

REFERENCES

1. Liese B, Mundt KA, Dell LD, *et al.* Medical insurance claims associated with international business travel. *Occup Environ Med* 1997; **54**:499–503.
2. Striker J, Luippold RS, Nagy L, *et al.* Risk factors for psychological stress among international business travellers. *Occup Environ Med* 1999; **56**:245–252.
3. Streltzer J. Psychiatric emergencies in travelers to Hawaii. *Compr Psychiatry* 1979; **20**(5):463–468.
4. Cohen E. A phenomenology of tourist experiences. *Sociology* 1979; **13**:179–201.
5. Heltberg J, Steffen R. *Psychiatric and psychological problems in travellers.* Paper presented to the First Scandinavian Symposium on Travel Medicine and Health, Uppsala, 21–22 May 1992.
6. Valk TH. Psychiatric practice in the Foreign Service. *Foreign Serv Med Bull* 1990; **280**:6–11.
7. Shlim DR. Personal communication. **10** *January* 2002.
8. Fennig S, Tevesess I, Gaber K, *et al.* The Arab nurse and the Jewish psychotic patient in the closed psychiatric ward. *Int J Soc Psychiatry* 1992; **38**(3):228–234.
9. Rodgers TA. *Involuntary commitment of the mentally ill: The overseas experience.* Paper delivered to the psychiatrists of the US Department of State, New York City, May 1990.
10. Meyers JK, Weissman MM, Tischler GL, *et al.* Six-month prevalence of psychiatric disorders in three communities. *Arch Gen Psychiatry* 1984; **41**:959–967.
11. Valk TH. Psychiatric medical evacuations within the Foreign Service. *Foreign Serv Med Bull* 1988; **268**:9–11.
12. Young DM. Psychiatric morbidity in travelers to Honolulu, Hawaii. *Compr Psychiatry* 1995; **36**(3):224–228.
13. Jauhar P, Weller MPI. Psychiatric morbidity and time zone changes: a study of patients from Heathrow Airport. *Brit J Psychiatry* 1982; **140**:213–235.
14. Wehr TA. Improvement of depression and triggering of mania by sleep deprivation. *JAMA* 1992; **267**(4):548–551.
15. Wehr T, Goodwin F, Wirz-Justice A, *et al.* 48-hour sleep-wake cycles in manic-depressive illness: naturalistic observations and sleep deprivation experiments. *Arch Gen Psychiatry* 1982; **39**:559–565.
16. Sadock BJ, Sadock VA. *Kaplan & Sadock's Pocket Handbook of Clinical Psychiatry.* 3rd edn. Philadelphia, PA: Lippincott Williams & Wilkins; 2001.
17. Bhana N. Perry CM. Olanzapine: a review of its use in the treatment of bipolar I disorder. *CNS Drugs* 2001; **15**(11):871–904.
18. Valk TH. Psychiatric practice in the Foreign Service. *Foreign Serv Med Bull* 1990; **280**:6–11.
19. Coryell WR, Clancy J. Excess mortality in panic disorder: A comparison with primary unipolar depression. *Arch Gen Psychiatry* 1982; **39**:701–703.
20. Shlim DR. Personal communication, 11 January 2002.
21. Talbot JA. The American expatriate in South Vietnam. *Am J Psychiatry* 1969; **126**(4):555–560.
22. Flinn DE. Transient psychotic reactions during travel. *Am J Psychiatry* 1962; **119**:173–174.
23. Singh HA. A case of psychosis precipitated by confinement in long distance travel by train. *Am J Psychiatry* 1961; **117**:936–937.
24. Bar-el Y. Durst R, Katz G, *et al.* Jerusalem syndrome. *Br J Psychiatry* 2000; **176**:86–90.
25. Langen D, Streltzer J, Kai M. 'Honeymoon psychosis' in Japanese tourists to Hawaii. *Cultural Diversity and Mental Health* 1997; **3**(3):171–174.
26. Shapiro S. A study of psychiatric syndromes manifested at an international airport. *Compr Psychiatry* 1976; **17**:453–456.
27. Bar-el T. Witztum E, Kalian M, *et al.* Psychiatric hospitalizations of tourists in Jerusalem. *Compr Psychiatry* 1991; **32**(3):238–244.
28. APA. *Diagnostic and Statistical Manual of Mental Disorders*, 4th edn. Text Revision Washington, DC: American Psychiatric Association; 2000.
29. Vaillant GE. *The Natural History of Alcoholism.* Cambridge, MA: Harvard University Press; 1983.
30. Slaby AE. *Handbook of Psychiatric Emergencies*, 4th edn. Norwalk. Stamford, CN: Appleton and Lange; 1994.
31. Giannini AJ, Slaby AE. *Handbook of Overdose and Detoxification Emergencies.* New York: Medical Examination Publishing Co.; 1983.
32. Sellers EM, Narango CA, Harrison M, *et al.* Diazepam loading: Simplified treatment for alcohol withdrawal. *Clin Pharm Ther* 1983; **6**:822–827.
33. Bar-el T, Witztum E, Kalian M, *et al.* Psychiatric hospitalizations of tourists in Jerusalem. *Compr Psychiatry* 1991; **23**(3):238–244.
34. Magherini G. *Syndrome di Stendhal.* Milan: Fettrinelli; 1992.
35. Kalian M, Witztum E. Comments on Jerusalem syndrome. *Br J Psychiatry* 2000; **176**(492).
36. Kalian M, Witztum E. Jerusalem syndrome or paranoid schizophrenia. *Psychiatr Serv* 2000; **51**(11):1453.
37. Weinke T, Trautmann M, Held T, *et al.* Neuropsychiatric side-effects after the use of mefloquine. *Am J Trop Med Hyg* 1991; **45**(1):86–91.
38. Bjorkman A. Acute psychosis following mefloquine prophylaxis. *Lancet* 1989; **2**(865)

CHAPTER 36 Cultural Adaptation

Deborah M. Lovell-Hawker

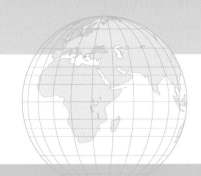

KEYPOINTS

- The process of cultural adaptation often involves four stages: honeymoon, disillusionment, partial adjustment and adjustment

- It is common to experience some stress-related symptoms while adjusting to life in an unfamiliar culture

- Reassurance that adjustment difficulties are normal and will pass facilitates recovery

- Depression is the most common psychological disorder diagnosed among expatriates, and can be effectively treated with cognitive-behavioral therapy and medication

- Cultural adaptation can be made easier by ensuring there is sufficient time to rest, relax, pursue pleasurable activities and interact with supportive people

Table 36.1	Factors associated with easier cultural adaptation
The individual feels it was their choice to come to this culture	
Less 'cultural distance' (i.e., the two cultures being more similar)	
Previous experiencing of traveling or living in different cultures	
Being well-prepared for the cultural transition, and having more knowledge about the culture	
Realistic expectations	
Understanding the language	
Having a clearly defined role	
Helpful employer or supervisor	
Supportive family/friends/colleagues in the new environment (and elsewhere)	
Feeling accepted in the new culture	
Flexibility, resourcefulness and ability to tolerate ambiguity and frustrations	
Good health (physical and psychological)	
No major family problems	
A belief that being in the new culture is worthwhile	

CULTURE SHOCK, AND THE U-CURVE HYPOTHESIS

'Culture shock' is a term which has slipped into common usage since it was coined by Oberg in 1960.[1] Most people understand it to mean the 'shock', anxiety and difficulties commonly experienced by people who have just arrived in an unfamiliar culture.

Cultural adaptation is a complex process, which occurs over time (usually over the course of many months), rather than a sudden 'shock', which strikes when a traveler steps off a plane. People are affected in different ways, and the same person will not necessarily go through the same process every time they enter a different culture. The process of adjustment will vary depending on a number of factors. Some of these factors are listed in Table 36.1.

The motives and expectations of the traveler also have an influence in their adjustment. For example, some business people and military personnel living overseas are happy to stay within the expatriate community and have little desire (or time) to learn about and adapt to the local culture. In contrast, international students, voluntary workers and missionaries may have chosen to travel in order to interact with local people and adjust to a new environment. Migrants and refugees may feel that they have to adapt and make the host culture 'home' because they expect to stay there for the rest of their lives. It is hoped that at least some of this chapter will be relevant to people in each of these groups, although most of the research has been based on aid workers, missionaries, business people and international students.

In 1955 Lysgaard[2] described cultural adjustment as following a typical pattern of a U-shaped curve of well-being plotted against time (Fig. 36.1).

This has become known as the U-curve model of adjustment. It is intended to depict initial optimism on arrival in a new culture, followed by a dip in well-being, before gradually recovering. Over the past 50 years, this model has been widely accepted and used to teach travelers about the reactions they might expect to experience. The pattern has been applied to various groups of long-stay travelers including students, business people, diplomats, aid workers, missionaries, and family members accompanying these people. Different terminology has been used, but the overall pattern has remained the same. Many authors have described a four-stage process[1] (see Table 36.2):

1. The 'honeymoon period': An initial stage of fascination where everything is perceived as new and exciting. The expatriate is a detached observer. This stage may only last for a few days, or it may persist for many weeks.

2. Disillusionment: The expatriate becomes disillusioned with the new culture, as it begins to intrude on their life in unexpected ways. They can no longer remain a spectator, as they have to deal with practical problems. They may feel overwhelmed and inadequate due to difficulties experienced and an inability to function at the level they would like to (e.g., due to language constraints, or because familiar cues are lacking). Feelings of irritability, anxiety, loneliness, frustration, confusion, disorientation, self-blame, depression and hostility towards the new culture are common during this stage. There may be a longing to return home (and home may be idealized).

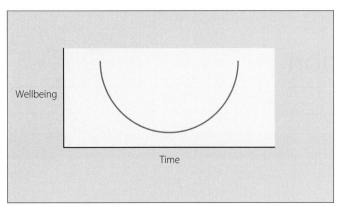

Figure 36.1 The U-curve pattern of adjustment to a new culture.

3. Partial adjustment: They believe that they are developing an understanding of the culture and its cues, and they now feel able to function reasonably well. However, some anxiety about the culture remains.

4. Adjustment: Both cultures are re-evaluated, and good and bad elements can be perceived in each. A more balanced perspective develops. They feel more relaxed (as most of their anxiety has disappeared), and they are able to react warmly towards local people, and to accept their customs. They feel more in control and confident about their ability to live independently in this culture.

The process of cultural adaptation is not always a smooth, linear process as the curve might suggest. Some people never leave the 'honeymoon' stage, especially if their visit is reasonably short. Others miss out on the 'honeymoon', and plunge immediately into feelings of inadequacy and despair. Some leave while still in the second stage, never progressing to adjustment. Others have a more pleasant experience, passing from the 'honeymoon' into adjustment without any noticeable drop in well-being. Some progress towards adjustment, but later return to a stage of despair and a longing to go home. Only rarely do people achieve as high a level of functioning in the new culture as they did at home and feel equally comfortable in both cultures. For this reason, some authors have chosen to use a curve shaped like a backwards J, rather than a U, to illustrate the process.

Research has provided some support for the U-Curve hypothesis,[3,4] although there have been very few well-designed longitudinal studies. Researchers argue about how many stages there are and exactly what format they take. Despite these limitations, the U-curve remains a popular and useful model, as many travelers say that their experience was in line with this basic pattern. If nothing else, the U-curve model can help to prepare travelers for a probable drop in their mood after the initial excitement of arrival in a new land. Such preparation can help them cope with decreased well-being if they do encounter it, and no harm is done if they do not.

'NORMAL' ADJUSTMENT DIFFICULTIES

As suggested by the dip in the U-curve, it is not uncommon to experience a period of low mood while adjusting to an unfamiliar culture. There are several factors which contribute towards low mood, including a sense of loss (of family, friends, possessions, lifestyle and perhaps status in the home culture); confusion about role, values, expectations and identity in the new culture; feelings of inadequacy due to finding it difficult to cope with the new environment; feeling rejected by the new society, or rejecting of it; fatigue and strain due to the effort of having to learn new ways of doing things; and discomfort, anxiety or disgust concerning some cultural differences.[5] If poverty is characteristic of the new culture in comparison with the old one, feelings of guilt and anger may emerge. Where there are major security issues (e.g., in conflict zones), anxiety is common, and people may also feel frustrated because they are not able to move about freely. In some environments there is a high risk of experiencing or witnessing a traumatic event (such as a traffic accident, gunfire, violent attack, theft, or natural disaster), or developing a serious illness.

Even in relatively 'low risk' settings, mild stress-related symptoms are common during the process of acculturation. Table 36.3 lists some of the symptoms that may be experienced.

As Table 36.3 illustrates, symptoms of stress may be physical, emotional, behavioral, cognitive or spiritual/philosophical. Expatriates may seek help from a variety of sources. Many people who travel abroad have a strong spiritual commitment, and may seek help from a religious source. Some find that traveling raises intellectual or philosophical questions, which they want help to resolve. Others seek counseling for interpersonal or occupational difficulties (listed under 'behavioral symptoms' in Table 36.3). Some people are reluctant to acknowledge emotional difficulties, but willing to consult a health professional about somatic complaints. As well as considering physical causes, the possibility of emotional factors contributing to the problem should not be overlooked. For example, anxiety related to concerns about living in the new culture may cause expatriates to over-react to minor physical complaints (such as skin problems or minor pains). It is worth asking directly whether the expatriate is finding any aspect of adjustment (or life in general) difficult. Some people feel that when they consult a health professional they should only mention their physical problems, and they do not know who they can talk to about other difficulties. Many expatriates are willing to disclose their adjustment difficulties if they are asked by someone who appears understanding, non-judgmental, and willing to listen –

Table 36.2	Stages of adjustment	
Stage	**Perception of new culture**	**Feelings of expatriate**
1. Honeymoon	New, exciting	Detached observer, interested
2. Disillusionment	Intrusive, problematic, unfamiliar	Disillusioned, overwhelmed, inadequate, irritated, anxious, isolated, depressed, tired
3. Partial adjustment	Becoming easier to predict and understand	Starting to feel at home
4. Adjustment	Is preferable to the home culture in some ways, although not in others	Comfortable, at home, relaxed, accepting of local people and customs, confident

Table 36.3	Symptoms of stress, which may occur during cultural adaptation

Physical
Tiredness; Difficulty sleeping, or else spending a lot of time in bed; Nightmares; Headaches; Back pain; Inability to relax; Dry mouth and throat; Feeling sick or dizzy; Pounding heart; Sweating and trembling; Stomachache and diarrhea; Loss of appetite, or over-eating; Feeling very hot or cold; Shortness of breath; Shallow, fast breathing; Hyper-vigilance; Irregular menstruation; Frequent need to urinate; Increased risk of ulcers, high blood pressure and coronary heart disease

Emotional
Depression; Tearfulness, or feeling a desire to cry but being unable to; Mood swings; Anger (at self or others); Agitation; Impatience; Guilt and shame; Shock; Feelings of helplessness and inadequacy; Feeling different or isolated from others; Feeling overwhelmed/ unable to cope; Feeling rushed all the time; Anxiety; Panic/phobias; Loss of sense of humour; Boredom; Lowered self-esteem; Loss of confidence; Unrealistic expectations (of self and others); Insecurity; Self-centered/inability to think about others; Feelings of vulnerability; Feeling worthless

Behavioral
Withdraw from others or become dependent on them; Irritability; Critical of self and others; Relationship problems; Lack of self-care; Nail biting; Picking at skin; Speaking in slow monotonous voice, or fast, agitated speech; Taking unnecessary risks (e.g., when driving); Trying to do several things at once; Lack of initiative; Working long hours; Poor productivity; Loss of job satisfaction; Carelessness; Absenteeism; Promiscuity, or loss of interest in sex; Increased smoking or use of alcohol or drugs (including prescription drugs); Excessive spending or other activities to try to take one's mind off the situation; Loss of motivation; Self-harm or suicidal behavior

Cognitive
Concentration and memory difficulties; Indecisiveness; Procrastination; Pessimism; Thinking in 'all or nothing' terms; Very sensitive to criticism; Self-critical thoughts; Loss of interest in previously enjoyed activities; Imagining the worst will happen; Preoccupation with health; Expecting to die young; Less flexible; Confusion and disorientation; Excessive fears (e.g., about being attacked); Trying to avoid thinking about problems; Flashbacks, or intrusive thoughts about difficulties; Hindsight thinking ('If only...' 'why didn't I...'); Negative thoughts about oneself, one's work, family, the future and the world; Time seems to slow down or speed up; Suicidal thoughts

Spiritual/Philosophical
Questioning the meaning of life; Loss of purpose; Loss of hope; Changes in beliefs; Doubts; Giving up faith; Legalism; Rigidity; Cynicism; Loss of sense of community with others; Sense of being abandoned; Submission to excessive control (e.g. may join a religious cult); Spiritual dryness; Unforgivingness; Bitterness; Feeling distant from God; Difficulty praying; Anger at God or at life

especially if they can be assured that their difficulties are not a sign of weakness, but are common among people who have moved to a new culture.

Education and reassurance can be of considerable importance. In particular, it is helpful to provide education about normal adjustment difficulties. Some people experience symptoms of 'culture shock' and accept these as normal, and respond by seeking support (through sharing their feelings with others), and making time to do things that help them to feel better (e.g., making extra time for leisure, relaxation and treats). In such cases, the feelings of discomfort are generally short-lived. Other travelers in contrast, feel that they are over-reacting or 'having a breakdown' when they experience normal symptoms of culture shock. They become depressed about being depressed, as they believe they should be 'able to cope better'. They are likely to try to hide the difficulty, rather than seeking help. Such a reaction tends to maintain and heighten the symptoms. A tendency to invalidate one's feelings (i.e., to conclude 'I should not feel this way') is one of the best predictors of the development of psychological disorders among overseas aid workers.[6] Reassuring travelers that their adjustment difficulties are normal and will pass assists in breaking the cycle.

MORE SEVERE EMOTIONAL DIFFICULTIES

Most expatriates feel homesick from time to time – missing their family and friends, their home and possessions, and their former way of life. Most also feel under stress at times, as they try to learn what is expected of them in the new culture, as well as getting to know the area, meeting people, adapting to a change of climate and different living conditions, and perhaps learning a new role and language. Even good changes are tiring, and symptoms such as fatigue, irritability, tearfulness, and difficulty sleeping and concentrating are natural. In most cases such symptoms can be relieved by doing something enjoyable, or perhaps going away for a weekend.

Reassuring travelers that these reactions are normal is useful in most cases, but not in every case. Health professionals should be alert for symptoms that go beyond normal culture shock. For example, in rare instances expatriates become totally overwhelmed by unhappiness and appear unable to function. They may refuse to make any attempt to integrate into the new culture. For instance, they may stay in the house and show no interest in the culture, not wanting to try new food or learn new customs. They may write frequent e-mails or letters home outlining their distress, or make long phone-calls, and continually talk about home, repeatedly breaking into tears. Self-care and regular duties may be neglected. If such behavior persists, it is wise to consider an early return to the home culture. In cases of severe depression, suicide risk should be assessed, with immediate action being taken if necessary to ensure the safety of the individual. It has been reported that sojourners are at increased risk of committing suicide,[7,8] although there is a lack of satisfactory research in this area.

Cases of uncomplicated clinical depression are often less apparent and go undetected. In one study of overseas aid workers, 7% reported that they had been diagnosed as suffering from depression while they were working overseas although they had never previously suffered from any clinical disorder.[6] Those with a family history (or personal history) of psychiatric disorder are at greater risk of developing an affective disorder themselves when overseas.[9] Most overseas workers who become clinically depressed do not tell their organization about the depression, often fearing that to do so would interfere with future job prospects. Many expatriates prefer to complete their assignment and then return home, rather than returning prematurely due to 'psychological difficulties'. Such an early return is often regarded by the worker (and perhaps by others) as an indication of failure. The best response for these workers may be to provide emotional support and to help them identify the stresses that are contributing to their difficulties, and to help them decide how to cope with these, using a problem-solving approach. On the other hand, workers who do choose to return early can be reassured that such a decision is not uncommon.

Overseas workers generally report that the worst part of their experience was not any traumatic incident (such as warfare, a traffic accident, or a natural disaster), although they may well have been involved with such incidents. In most cases, the worst part of life overseas is reported to be either the cultural difficulties and frustrations; or relationship problems; or else dissatisfaction with their work or the organization they work with.[6] Such on-going, personal problems cause more difficulties than short-lived traumas. In many cases expatriates also feel that there is too much to do. In one study of 200 aid workers, 50% reported that they regularly worked more than 60 h a week, with some stating that as a result they became 'burnt out'.[10] They may overwork because the needs seem great and there are not enough workers to meet them; or because they feel guilty that their standard of living is much higher than that of local people; or because they have little else to do, as they feel isolated and there are few leisure facilities available. Some expatriates are constantly visited by local people, and although this may be enjoyable, it can also become very tiring. Living and working alongside colleagues who are stressed also takes its toll. Many expatriates become exhausted. The best medicine in this situation is to take time off to relax, and to take steps to deal with underlying stresses.

Non-working spouses of overseas workers should not be forgotten as they may have more adjustment problems than their working partners.[3] Their needs should be taken into account, and they should be encouraged to build up a network of friends and to find their own role.

Studies suggest that 15–25% of international students have significant adjustment difficulties, in terms of frequent homesickness, loneliness or depression.[3] Increasing social interaction generally leads to a reduction in these symptoms, and this can be achieved through support groups and social activities. As a lack of motivation and reduced activity are characteristic of depression, it is useful to help depressed students plan activities which will give them a feeling of achievement or pleasure, and to gradually increase their social involvement. In some cases depression may be related to being the target of discrimination, or other external pressures (e.g., financial difficulties or academic problems), and these issues need to be addressed.

Depression is by far the most common psychological disorder reported by expatriates.[6] Cognitive-behavioral therapy (CBT) is an effective treatment for depression, and can be used in combination with medication; medication alone is less effective in the long term than CBT.[11] Depression is not the only disorder which has been identified among expatriates. Excessive alcohol intake is commonly reported among international travelers, and drug abuse may also be a problem[12] (see Chapter 35). This may be a means of trying to cope with feeling homesick, lonely or depressed. Others respond to such feelings by engaging in sexual encounters, which they would not have engaged in at home, including unprotected sex, increasing the risk of HIV infec-tion.[13,14]

Occasionally, adjustment difficulties play a part in the development of problems such as eating disorders. Women who move from a culture which does not place great value on thinness to a culture which highly values thinness may be at increased risk of developing eating disorders, perhaps due to over-idealizing the new culture, or perceiving thinness as a way to help them become accepted. Nasser compared matched samples of female Arab students attending universities in London and Cairo. A total of 12% of the Arabs in London were found to have bulimia nervosa, compared with no cases in the Cairo sample.[15] Nasser also reported a higher incidence of anorexia nervosa among Greek girls living in Munich than among those in Greece.[16]

A higher than expected proportion of development workers appear to develop chronic fatigue syndrome while working overseas.[17] This appears to be related to working excessively; feeling under stress; and failing to rest adequately after developing physical illnesses.

Anxiety disorders (including post-traumatic stress disorder) are sometimes reported among overseas workers, and should be treated with the recognized effective treatments for such disorders (e.g., CBT, in combination with medication if this is indicated).

Psychotic disorders occasionally occur, often where there has been a family history of such problems. The onset of psychotic symptoms may be triggered by the stress of arriving in an unfamiliar culture. When assessing psychiatric symptoms, it is important to ask about the use of any medication (e.g., malaria prophylaxis). Psychiatric disorders are discussed further in Chapter 35. Whenever there is a possibility of psychiatric disorder, it is better to seek help sooner rather than later.

CHILDREN

The American Academy of Child and Adolescent Psychiatry (1999) reports:

> 'Moving to a new community may be one of the most stress-producing experiences a family faces. Frequent moves or even a single move can be especially hard on children and adolescents. Studies show children who move frequently are more likely to have problems at school. Moves are even more difficult if accompanied by other significant change in the child's life, such as ... loss of family income, or a need to change schools'.[18]

Moving from one community to another within the same culture can be stressful; crossing cultures is an even greater challenge. Children who spend a significant part of their developmental years outside their parents' culture have become known as 'Third Culture Kids' (TCKs), because they do not belong fully to either their parents' culture or to the culture in which they are living. They belong to a 'third culture' which is a mixture of these two. Many TCKs move several times during their early years. TCKs may be at increased risk for a number of difficulties, including learning problems and speech disorders (possibly due to language changes), depression, anxiety disorders and behavioral problems. In addition, eating disorders are becoming increasingly prevalent in international schools, which cater for the children of expatriates. This may be related issues of identity, self-esteem, and body dissatisfaction (which may be heightened in cultures in which females are perceived as inferior, or where women have to cover up their bodies). Eating disorders are also more prevalent among high achievers, and many TCKs feel under considerable pressure to achieve academically. Issues of control are also relevant – some TCKs feel that they have no control over most aspects of their life (e.g., over cross-cultural moves; or even issues related to clothing, food, and the freedom to go out on their own). Food and the body may be the only area they feel they have control over, and some TCKs have felt that starving themselves was the only method they could use to persuade their parents to take them back to the home country.

As stated in Table 36.1, cultural adjustment is generally easier if the individual feels it was their choice and they had time to prepare for it (it was predictable). Sometimes a cultural move is voluntary and predictable for the parents in a family, but involuntary and unpredictable for the children. It is important to be aware of such differences. Although TCKs may have little choice in the decision to relocate, it is important to explain why the family is moving, and to seek out their views, and to attempt to prepare them for the move well in advance. Children should be encouraged to ask questions, as this helps to reduce anxiety. Involving them as much as possible in decisions helps them to feel less powerless. They should be asked which clothes and toys they want to take with them. If possible, children should be involved in the choice of schooling (which may be in a local school; at an international day school or a boarding school in the host country; at a day school or boarding school in the home country; or they may be home-schooled, perhaps with the help of satellite schooling or cyber-schooling).

On arrival in the new culture, stressed parents need to remember to make plenty of time to listen to and talk with their children. Otherwise children may feel that they are less important than their parent's job, which can lead to a loss of their self-esteem and self-confidence. Spending time with children and listening to them shows that they are of value, and helps them to understand the reasons for the move, which makes it easier to accept. The presence of the parents also calms children's fears, and so the parents should aim to be with the child as much as possible, at least during the initial weeks. Children should be asked whether there is anything they would like help with, or anything that could make adjustment easier for them. For example, if children are frequently approached by strangers who want to touch their hair, parents can teach them how to deal with this. Parents should also teach their children about appropriate and inappropriate touch. For instance, in certain cultures children are disciplined at school by a teacher touching their (clothed) genitals; while in others, babies are masturbated to send them to sleep. If children are to be looked after by other people, parents should try to ensure that no inappropriate behavior will take place.

Keeping up routines (such as stories at bedtime) helps children feel secure. For most children, 'home' is wherever their parents are, and so they can adapt to relocation, especially if they are able to keep in touch with friends and family. Some TCKs spend a long time observing children in the new culture playing before they feel comfortable about participating. They want to ensure that they have understood what is going on before they attempt to join in. This can be a healthy choice, providing they do take part eventually.

Children may become anxious if they perceive that their parents are anxious. Symptoms of stress vary with age, but common symptoms among children include regressing to behaviors which they had grown out of (e.g., clinging; bed-wetting; thumb sucking); appetite loss; abdominal pain or headaches; sleeping problems and nightmares, and fears. Some children become withdrawn, while others display outbursts of anger. Most children get over such problems relatively quickly as soon as they feel more familiar with the new environment, and parents should remember that all children go through difficult times, with or without a relocation. Reading about normal child development can help parents determine whether or not the patterns displayed by their child are unusual. If they are unusual and no improvement is seen, help should be sought.

It is particularly difficult to adjust to moving to a new culture during the adolescent years, as adolescence brings enough change in itself. It is generally wise to avoid a first cross-cultural move during these years, if possible. If the move is unavoidable, extra support should be offered.

Moving to a new culture can have considerable benefits for children, but also presents a number of challenges. There may be confusion about identity (not knowing which nationality they are or where their loyalties lie); they may feel out of place in both cultures; and moving between two (or more) cultures can make it difficult for them to form close friends or feel settled. Often TCKs have to accept that they live in a highly mobile community, where friends (fellow expatriates) come and go constantly. There may be family separations too, if children are sent to boarding school. This may lead to grief reactions. Some react to this by becoming self-sufficient and deciding never to form deep relationships, as goodbyes seem too painful. This may reduce the pain of parting, but leaves a sense of constant loneliness.

Some TCKs move so often that they conclude that there is no point in planning ahead (as plans have been changed and their hopes disappointed so often). Others decide that it is not worth addressing problems or conflict, because they can move away instead. Consequently, as adults they may decide to move whenever they face problems (e.g., changing college if they decide they do not like their course; seeking divorce rather than attempting to resolve marital conflict, etc.).

Pollock and Van Reken[19] and Knell[20] have provided excellent accounts of the experience of TCKs, and offer many useful suggestions.

FACTORS THAT CAN FACILITATE CULTURAL ADAPTATION

Some writers have suggested that people who choose to leave home and work in another culture often have pre-existing psychological difficulties. In reality, this does not seem to be the case. The majority of expatriates are psychologically healthy and well-equipped to face the challenges of adaptation (although a few slip through the net and go overseas with pre-existing emotional difficulties, perhaps motivated by a desire to escape from problems).[6] Many organizations now include a 'psychological assessment' in their selection procedure, to assist them in selecting psychologically healthy workers.[21] Good psychological briefing and cross-cultural training before departure play an important part in equipping them to adapt well[22] (see Chapter 30). The greater the understanding of the new culture, the better.

As has been explained above, a key factor in preventing the onset of psychological disorders during the adaptation process is understanding that some stress-related symptoms are to be expected. They signal a need to take extra care of oneself. If the new culture appears overwhelming, it may be helpful to withdraw briefly (either by going away for a few days, perhaps to stay at a hotel which feels more familiar; or else by staying inside for a while and doing familiar things – such as watching videos, eating familiar food, or playing games from the home country.) Then the expatriate should reemerge slowly, perhaps only interacting with the new culture for a few hours at a time at first, and gradually building this up. Having a routine can provide a feeling of security and consistency. During this time it is helpful to actively seek out positive aspects of the new culture, to help create a more balanced viewpoint. It is important to have realistic expectations throughout the time in the host culture.

It is generally useful for expatriates to have a mentor to guide them through the adjustment process. This may initially be another expatriate who has already been through a similar process and realizes what is likely to be helpful. Later, it is useful to find a local mentor, who can explain the reasons for customs, and help the newcomer to begin to understand the culture more fully. People are most likely to thrive if they have a good support system, which may include local friends, friendships with other expatriates, and on-going support from friends and family in the home country. E-mail can play a part in keeping long-distance relationships active.

Adjustment takes time. Pressure for productivity adds to the strain felt, and so it is better to allow time for adjustment without having to meet demanding goals during the initial period. (On the other hand setting a few small, achievable goals, and then meeting these, can dissipate feelings of inadequacy, helplessness and frustration. When feeling overwhelmed, it is usually best to start with the easiest tasks, as succeeding in these promotes confidence and leads to further success). The traveler should be encouraged to try to reduce other pressures in their life while they are adjusting to the new culture. If language school is exhausting, they might be advised to drop something else for the time being. Pressure may be reduced by accepting practical help – for example, by employing someone to assist with cleaning, washing clothes and cooking. Some expatriates reject this idea on the principle of being opposed to having 'servants', but local people are generally glad of the job, and it is not seen as demeaning, and should not cause the expatriate to feel guilty.

Expatriates are still something of a novelty in many areas. Local people may stare, call after them, beg from them, or follow them around. Even local colleagues and friends can seem intrusive, as they often find it natural to ask questions that appear very personal to people from elsewhere. For instance, in many cultures people think nothing of asking questions such as, 'How much do you earn?', 'How old are you?', 'Why don't you have children (or more children)', or 'Why are you not married?' This last question may be followed by an offer to arrange a marriage, or simply, 'Will you marry me?' The easiest way to deal with such questions is to think in advance of a suitable response.

Some expatriates (especially those with children) choose to keep one evening each week on which to do things they would do in their home culture. For example, they might dress as they do at home (staying inside if necessary to avoid offending local people), cook what they eat at home, and put on music or videos from their own culture, or go to a hotel to swim or play squash. This can reduce feelings of loss and homesickness, by showing that they are still able to experience home comforts from time to time. Other people find that going to an expatriate club, or simply meeting up with other expatriates, serves a similar purpose. It can be helpful to identify activities which were enjoyed in the home culture, and to consider which can be pursued in the new culture, and also to add new activities which can be enjoyed in the new locality.

Having enough time to rest and relax, doing pleasurable activities, maintaining a sense of humor, and having a supportive network of family and friends all play a part in helping expatriates to enjoy living in a different culture. Basic stress management techniques can help during the more difficult times.[23] Cultural adaptation is a difficult process for some people, but it is not usually a negative experience. It can lead to personal growth and greater self-confidence and self-esteem. Most expatriates rate their overseas experience as a positive one overall, reporting the 'best part' to be the people they met in the new culture (41%) or the work satisfaction (30%).[6] Children who move to a different culture also tend to rate the experience as a positive one, in retrospect. When asked what they gained from it, their most frequent responses are international friendships, independence, language ability, cultural awareness, confidence and the climate![20]

CONCLUSION

Cultural adaptation takes time, and often follows a pattern of initial excitement followed by a dip in mood, and then adjustment to the new culture. Realizing that low mood is a normal part of the process can help expatriates to cope when they do feel low. If emotional difficulties are more severe or prolonged, professional help should be offered. Given support and time, most adults and children can adapt well to a new culture.

REFERENCES

1. Oberg K. Cultural shock: adjustment to new cultural environments. *Pract Anthropol* 1960; **7**:177–182.
2. Lysgaard S. Adjustment in a foreign society: Norwegian Fulbright grantees visiting the United States. *Int Soc Sci Bull* 1955; **7**:45–51.
3. Church AT. Sojourner adjustment. *Psychol Bull* 1982; **91**:540–572.
4. Zapf MK. Remote practice and culture shock: social workers moving to isolated northern regions. *Soc Work* 1993; **38**:694–704.
5. Taft R. Coping with unfamiliar cultures. In: Warren N, ed. *Studies in Cross-cultural Psychology*. Vol. 1. London: Academic Press; 1977:121–153.
6. Lovell DM. Psychological adjustment among returned overseas aid workers. Unpublished D. Clin. Psy. Thesis, University of Wales, Bangor, 1997.
7. Furnham A, Bochner S. *Culture Shock: Psychological Reactions to Unfamiliar Environments*. London: Methuen; 1986.
8. Stack S. The effects of interstate migration on suicide. *Int J Soc Psychiatry* 1980; **26**(1):17–26.
9. Foyle MF, Beer MD, Watson JP. Expatriate mental health. *Acta Psychiatr Scand* 1998; **97**:278–283.
10. Macnair R. *Room for Improvement: The Management and Support of Relief and Development Workers*. London: Overseas development institute; 1995.
11. Williams JMG. *The Psychological Treatment of Depression*. London: Croom Helm; 1984.
12. Lange WR, McCune BA. Substance abuse and international travel. *Adv Alcohol Subst Abuse* 1989; **8**:37–51.
13. Graaf R De, Zessen G Van, Houweling H. Underlying reasons for sexual conduct and condom use among expatriates posted in AIDS endemic areas. *AIDS Care* 1998; **10**:651–665.
14. Moore J, Beeker C, Harrison JS, et al. HIV risk behavior among Peace Corps Volunteers. *AIDS* 1995; **9**(7):795–799.
15. Nasser M. Comparative study of the prevalence of abnormal eating attitudes among Arab female students at both London and Cairo universities. *Psychol Med* 1986; **16**:621–625.
16. Nasser M. Eating disorders: the cultural dimension. *Soc Psychiatry Psychiatr Epidemiol* 1988; **23**:184–187.
17. Lovell DM. Chronic fatigue syndrome among overseas development workers: a qualitative study. *J Travel Med* 1999; **6**:16–23.
18. American Academy of Child and Adolescent Psychiatry. *Children and family moves*. AACAP fact-sheet 14: American Academy of Child and Adolescent Psychiatry; 1999. Available at: http://www.aacap.org/publications/factsfam/fmlymove.htm
19. Pollock DC. Van Reken RE. *The Third Culture Kid Experience: growing up among worlds*. Yarmouth, Maine: Intercultural Press; 1999.
20. Knell M. *Families on the Move*. London: Monarch; 2001.
21. Gamble KL, Lovell D, Lankester T, et al. Aid workers, expatriates and travel. In: Zukerman JN, ed. *Principles and Practice of Travel Medicine*. Chichester, UK: John Wiley & Sons; 2001:447–466.
22. Bhawuk DPS, Brislin RW. Cross-cultural training: a review. *Appl Psychol: An Int Rev* 2000; **49**:162–191.
23. Fontana D. *Managing Stress*. Leicester, UK: British Psychological Society; 1989.

CHAPTER 37

Re-entry after Long-term Travel/Living Abroad

Fredrick J. Summers

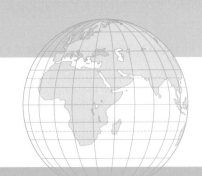

KEYPOINTS

■ Re-entry or reverse culture shock can be just as powerful an experience as moving to an unknown culture

■ Travel physicians and clinics are in an ideal position to assist their patients to develop the balanced lifestyle that will enable them to re-enter successfully

■ Teaching a straightforward model of the hormonal stress reaction gives people a strategy to self-monitor, reduce their distress, and avoid counter-productive behaviors

■ Advice to families should be tailored to the age and developmental stages of the children and the sophistication of the parents, with particular attention to the vulnerabilities of adolescents

■ A well-conceived travel program will offer families and individuals re-entry material at the time of departure and follow up with re-entry strategy several months prior to their return home

INTRODUCTION

Re-entry, Reverse Culture Shock, or simply Coming-Home are names for the phenomenon of returning to one's country and culture after an extended time living away. This transition often presents unexpected challenges to the traveler because the pitfalls are unanticipated. The psychological impact of this return can be just as powerful an experience as that of moving to an unknown culture for the first time. Coping with re-entry is important to individuals and families as well as organizations whose employees are affected by the stress of re-entry. This chapter examines the pitfalls and challenges of re-entry. It presents concepts that travelers can use to develop re-entry tools, gives age and family specific re-entry strategies, and assists the travel medicine specialist in integrating re-entry preparation into his practice.

Three factors contribute to re-entry stress: unrealistic expectations, unrecognized changes in the returnee, and unanticipated changes in the home culture.

Unrealistic expectations

The expatriate often incorrectly assumes that returning successfully from a work or travel experience should be a triumphant time. A subset of returnees think that the expatriate experience makes them special. They feel that living overseas is a life-defining event and that their career, status, or insights are special. They are shocked to learn that some of their countryman may view their overseas life as an aberration to be tolerated as opposed to a sign of great curiosity and mental prowess. The majority are simply indifferent. Finally, travelers leave a novel, stimulating environment in which they often hold a unique or prestigious position to return home to a more mundane lifestyle. Homecoming sometimes means taking out the garbage for the first time in years. This false perception and lack of preparation make the expatriate vulnerable to all the symptoms of cultural shock and stress reactions.

Unrecognized changes in the returnee

Returnees often fail to realize that their foreign experiences have altered their thinking and values in subtle if not dramatic ways. Immersion in an unfamiliar society will change the way the expatriate looks at wealth, family, politics, religion, and values. Even the most ardent patriots are changed forever by their time aboard. In some cases the experience only intensifies the passion of travelers for their home, but for most travelers the first-hand experience of another country and people leaves them with a more refined view of politics, poverty, education, freedom, and so on. The returnees also neglect to accept the unconscious learning from the ubiquitous host culture's eating rituals, queues, driving etiquette, dress and social attitudes, and more. As Mark Twain pointed out travel is the best antidote for ignorance. Travel inexorably works its wonders on us.

Unanticipated changes in the home culture

During the traveler's time away, the home culture has changed. While many of the familiar visual, verbal, and non-verbal cues remain, returnees find themselves strangely out of synch with their compatriots.[1] This cultural evolution can range from superficial changes in fads, popular music, and the time of mail delivery, to a profound rethinking of cultural values such as gun control, abortion, and capital punishment. They take the home coming for granted and can overestimate the protective power of returning to the same job, neighborhood, friends, relatives, schools, commute, consumer goods, road signs, values, popular culture-sports and entertainment. Travel medicine practitioners are in an ideal position to educate and reassure their patients about re-entry and reduce the risk of excessive symptoms and psychiatric syndromes.

While few people would knowingly risk going abroad without evaluating the physical health risks at their destination, evaluating their own health status, providing for routine medications, and updating their inoculations, very few will consider their psychological health or the mental health risks to themselves and their families before packing for a foreign destination. Education about the inevitable stress of relocating to another country is essential for a successful tour and return. Most travelers are unlikely to need their catastrophic health insurance and most travelers are unlikely to need psychiatric services. Nonetheless it makes sense to be prepared.

AVOIDER-ENGAGER CONTINUUM

Ideally, travelers would be advised before the outward bound portion of their trip to begin thinking about re-entry. Doctors would orient their patients to the psychological tasks facing them as part of the overseas preparation. Since the symptoms of culture shock often overlap with the re-entry symptoms the outward bound preparation is valuable for both experiences. They would tell them that there is a range of adaptation from the engager to the avoider and advise them to seek a stable middle ground. Then at the time of their return, travel medicine practitioners would ascertain where their clients fell on a spectrum of adaptation from the avoider to the engager. The patients' coping mechanisms can be easily gauged from a brief interview or one of the many psychological testing instruments.

The avoiders, much like polar bears preparing for winter, insulate themselves from their surroundings. Generally somewhat anxious and without innate curiosity about others, they assume a defensive lifestyle and hermetically seal themselves from their environment trying to create a world identical to the one they left behind. Ineffective tools for this include workaholism, the Internet, shopping exclusively in stores from home, videos, alcohol, and a condescending attitude to the values of the local culture.

At the other extreme are the engagers who immerse themselves in their new home, they adopt wholesale the dress, customs, mannerisms, servants, and culture of their local. Sitting in gallabayas in a Cairo coffeehouse, they absorb the very sands of the Sahara. As defensive as the avoiders who see no virtue in their new country, engagers see no virtue in their homeland. This defensive strategy may allow them to function, but neither extreme has the resiliency and safeguards to survive major stressors in a new environment. Both of these lifestyles invite re-entry problems for neither has dealt honestly with the reality of living as a foreigner in a different land.

Fortunately, the majority of people fall between the extremes; this group while remaining balanced and flexible tends to oscillate successfully from one end of this continuum to the other depending on external conditions. This group becomes competent in the culture without denying its origins and intention to return home. This moderation gives these returnees an honesty and adaptability lacking in the caricature of the extreme positions.

HEALTH CARE PROVIDER'S FOUR TASKS

- After gauging their coping style, the health-care provider must emphasize that individuals are not returning home as the identical people who left. Their world view has changed. Any attempt to recreate an identical lifestyle will produce distress and symptoms. A corollary to this is to accept that most if not all of their former social circles will not understand or be curious about their experiences beyond cursory accounts. This is not a criticism of any group, but simply an acknowledgment that relationships are generally built around shared experiences and not adventures. Foreign experiences will not make anyone special.
- Health-care providers must emphasize the psychological task of leave-taking and preparation for re-entry which are the first tasks for a successful return.
- They can give their patients information about the concept of stress and the related notion of culture shock. This simple structure will allow their clients to understand and accept their reactions more easily and to develop their own problem solving strategies.
- Health-care providers must address the special issues of families and their children. There is evidence that intervention should be directed toward families rather than individuals. The clinician should briefly explain or provide literature that illustrates the develop-

mental tasks of children and how the adaptation to the homeward journey must vary depending on the child's age. Parents should plan accordingly. After all of this, health-care providers can point out that millions of people live abroad and several hundred thousand children attend International Schools; they can say confidently that the majority of families adapt, are enriched by their experiences, integrate their new perceptions of the world, and return home with minimal disruption.

Generally speaking, families that have shown resilience in the past will do so abroad. Those families whose functioning is not based on strong relationships will pack their troubles with them. Travel is not an antidote for pre-existing psychological problems. For people who experience more profound symptoms, the phenomena of re-entry are well known and expert assistance is available. Half will find a niche within three months of returning home, but others will take a year or longer. This is normal.

LEAVE-TAKING

All departures involve sorrow and loss. Most people will not have the opportunity to return and work in the same foreign land. There is often a finality to the departure. The experience of mourning, loss, and separation will be jumbled together and be influenced by the excitement of departure. Mixed emotions are common during this period.

The tasks are to recall and thank the many people who assisted you during your stay. Remember that people will handle this loss in much the same way as they have handled other transitions, e.g., moves, job changes, terminating relationships, or serious illness and death. It is important to think back, recall those events, and anticipate that you will react in a similar way. For those who have experienced intense difficulty in the past separations, anticipation allows them to seek help and develop more effective coping strategies.

The Peace Corps, which has extensive experience returning people to the USA, offers the advice not to postpone any activity in the host country.[2] Bring your experience to closure by visiting the last tourist site, buying the last keepsake, and making the most of the unique opportunity. Advise your patients to make the rounds of vendors, shopkeepers, taxi drivers, guides, and say good-bye and thanks to all the people who assisted them in any way to be comfortable during their visit. Remember what they take with them, a rare and unique experience, is a priceless gift. No matter what their experience, there will be moments of nostalgia and longing.

At work, employees must finish projects, prepare for a successor, and acknowledge all those who assisted them. Particularly in cross-cultural work environments it is critical for those leaving and those staying to acknowledge each other and accept the sometimes profound cultural differences.

Leaving school and shutting down a home require similar preparation: farewells, the sorting of papers and records that will be needed immediately upon re-entry, and preparation for the nuts and bolts of daily living in the home country. All of this must be done while accepting the emotional ups and downs knowing that the impact of traveling home is yet to hit.

STRESS

In the last 20 years of the twentieth century, the West developed a fascination with the concept of stress and its reduction. This rediscovery turned the notion into a cliché and gave the appearance of a totally fresh idea. However, stress is a crucial part of daily life and has existed since the dawn of evolution, and many ideas useful to managing re-entry have evolved from this work.

- Stress is the nonspecific reaction of individuals to demands on them to adapt and change. Re-entry is a powerful stressor. While there are individual styles of managing stress, the emotions and experience of stress is mediated by hormones and neurotransmitters and is common to everyone. Because of our unique psychological makeup, no one can predict with certainty which stressors will impact which person adversely.

- The goal of stress management and successful re-entry is not, and cannot be, the elimination of the common and sometimes uncomfortable pressures of life. People can in fact, learn strategies that can keep their reaction to change in a range which enhances their adaptation. Stress is unavoidable, and the healthy adaptation is a state called *eustress*. Remember that insufficient stimulation leads to boredom and *amotivation*. Properly managed, stress is a tool that can be used to modulate the effects of re-entry.

- Stress is a common final pathway for many stimuli. While the best predictor of one's response to re-entry is to look at past experience, there is no certainty that a similar event will not produce a different reaction next time. One should not become overconfident.

- Everyone has survived a variation of re-entry. Each time people change cultures and return to their original environment they have re-entered. These moves are common and not thought of in the context of re-entry and cultural adaptation, but changing schools, taking a new job, moving across town or to a different part of the country, living with new roommates, are all a variation on culture change.[3] They involve leaving a context where one is comfortable and can perform most tasks unconsciously to a new culture where you do not immediately fit. The normal visual, verbal, and behavioral cues that make people comfortable are gone. Familiar tasks become challenges and social acceptance is crucial. This precipitates the same stress response that one could experience at the time of re-entry. In a sense, everyone is a stress expert.

- Once the acute stress reaction has begun, there is no way to stop the chemical and emotional cascade. One must learn to accept it and shape it. Unfortunately, this fight or flight reaction has not evolved to deal with modern constructs such as the office, airport, and school environment. Therefore we must learn to modulate the response. The effect of acute stress reaction may remain for several hours and is partially dependent on the external conditions, the psychology of the person, and the half-life of the neurotransmitters and hormones involved. For many people if they recall the effects of several strong cups of coffee on their body, and the duration of the phenomenon, they will have a basic idea of the physiology of a stress reaction.

First, stress stimulates the brain. No one who has stepped in front of a moving car or faced a deadline can deny the power of the acute brain stimulation from stress. Reactions range from freezing with fear to split second problem solving.

Second, stress stimulates a wave of hormone release that affects every tissue and function of the body. Neural stimulation of the adrenal glands stimulates release of adrenaline and noradrenaline, which instantaneously drives the emotions of fear and anger and the most obvious symptoms of the 'fight or flight' response.[4] This is thought to be a primitive reaction to help us escape overwhelming danger, but if too intense is not helpful to problem solving in the work, school, or home setting. The symptoms include: increased heart rate, increased blood pressure, cold, sweaty palms, dry mouth, dilated pupils, increased blood flow to the brain and muscles, decreased flow to the digestive tract, scanning behavior.

At the same time, adrenocorticotrophic hormone (ACTH) reaches the adrenal cortex releasing primarily glucocorticosteroids such as cortisol and corticosterone. These hormones initiate the production of glucose thus providing a ready supply of energy for meeting the crisis. They also inhibit immune and inflammatory responses. In the short term, these effects may enhance one's ability to manage crisis, however, when experienced chronically as during re-entry, they can cause symptoms which inhibit the ability to problem solve (Table 37.1).

While the hormonal interactions and neural components are much more complex than what is presented here, people who understand this simple model of the mechanism, symptoms, and consequences of unmanaged stress are much more motivated to self-monitor. These people understand that once the hormonal cascade has started the stress reaction will sustain itself for several hours. Since it cannot be aborted, people can only accept their symptoms and attempt to modulate them. This construct gives them a tool that allows them to gauge their reaction and formulate effective responses.

STRESS RESPONSE PATTERNS

Another useful preventive concept is to consider the effect of stress on decision making.

In the Janis and Mann (1977)[5] concept, there are five basic patterns that people assume when making decisions during stressful times. These are given below.

Unconflicted inertia

The posture takes the passive position of ignoring critical new information and leaving behavior patterns unchanged. Safe in their psychological bunker, the person hopes that re-entry will eventually pass by.

Unconflicted change

In this pattern, change is embraced without any analysis or contingency planning. This returnee will often adopt willy-nilly all coping suggestions and attempt to remain insulated from the feelings and challenges of re-entry.

Table 37.1	Emotional and physical symptoms of long-term stress include

Emotional symptoms
Loss of confidence
Anxiety
Insomnia
Anger
Irritability
Impatience
Depression
Fatigue
Appetite changes – both an increase and a decrease
Poor concentration
Fearfulness
Mood swings
Misperceptions
Depression and related symptoms of sadness, hopelessness, poor self-esteem, pessimism. Withdrawal.

Physical symptoms
All the illnesses that can be influenced by psychological factors. This means nearly every affliction known, however some are particularly pertinent to the re-entry syndrome.
Increased susceptibility to illness from a depressed immune system
Cardiovascular symptoms, e.g., Chest pain, throbbing pulses
Muscle tension and headaches
Gastrointestinal symptoms including diarrhea and cramping as well as constipation.

Defensive avoidance

In this complex, returnees abrogate responsibility for themselves and shift it to supervisors and organizations. The company and its managers are magically empowered with knowledge and responsibility for the individual and are expected to provide an anxiety free re-entry for the employee and his family. This is often seen in large organizations which are thought to provide cradle to grave care.

Hypervigilance

In this state, one sees rapid swings from one poorly planned solution to another. There is constant scanning for new information on which to base new solutions. Consequences are not considered and doing for the sake of doing is stress relieving. This state results in the poorest decision making.

Vigilance

In this mode, the individual collects, discusses, and evaluates material in a rational and timely way. Clearly the clinician wants to encourage patients to develop this coping mechanism. Within families, the healthcare provider should insist that all family members participate in an age-appropriate way in the decision making process. In this state, people are able to develop the ability to self-monitor, and the most effective way to do this is to develop relationships where there can be direct and honest feedback.

PREPARATION FOR RE-ENTRY

Mental health concerns should be given equal time with, and be integrated into, the pre-departure evaluation and preparation within a travel clinic. The physician and the staff should emphasize that even the experienced traveler is at risk of developing a re-entry syndrome. Preparation should be encouraged, which includes at least a basic consideration of coping styles on the engager-avoider continuum. The clients should have a very basic notion of the stress cycle and understand that it is a normal, unavoidable experience, which can enhance re-entry, but when out of control can result in severe symptomatology. Finally, they should know that re-entry stress affects problem solving ability and understand the advantage of the vigilant state for analyzing problems. They should also be aware that each family member may react differently and that there is a time component to the process that cannot be condensed. A normal process can take from 3 months to more than 1 year. Orientations and discussions can be organized for an individual, families, or groups. In many settings, a mental health provider – usually a psychologist – can perform this task. In addition, for clients who are more comfortable with more objective measures, a psychologist could use one of the hundreds of self-report measures, which are easily adaptable to the clinic setting including:

- The Cross-Cultural Adaptability Inventory by Judith Meyers
- State-Trait Anxiety Inventory
- Profile of Mood States
- MMPI -Minnesota Multiphasic Personality Inventory.

PRACTICAL ADVICE

What to do

- The truism that the first step to solving a problem is to acknowledge that it *is* a problem holds for re-entry too.
- Preparation as in any stress reduction program is a life change and involves a daily commitment; it cannot be done the day before the return. For this task the motto of 1 day at a time is appropriate. It also reminds us to divide problems into categories: what can be changed and what cannot, and to know the difference.
- Without a doubt, the one stress reduction technique that works for everyone and in every situation, is exercise. The mechanism by which exercise reduces tension, boosts energy, and lessens negative moods remains unclear but the efficacy is clear. The clinic should build into its physical examination recommendations for an aerobic program. The University of California at Berkeley Wellness Letter, contains a short summary.[6]
- Maintain a balanced life, paying attention to family and recreation as well as work. Many people become too dependent on work to reinforce their self-esteem. This includes maintaining a routine for the daily chores and a healthy lifestyle, which attends to diet, sleep, exercise, recreation, and meditative time.
- The returnee must focus on relationships. While abroad, many friendships may fall by the wayside. They become more difficult to maintain given the aspect of human nature that out of sight is often out of mind. Communication challenges, as well as the major task of adjustment to a new country, take the focus off family and friends. However, many studies demonstrate that the maintenance of strong relationships especially within the family is key to a long, healthy, and well-adjusted life.[7]
- Develop a positive attitude and see return as an opportunity. One of the most powerful discoveries of the twentieth century is that our thoughts can in fact affect our feelings. There is a benefit in seeking an optimistic outlook. Humor and a realistic perspective are effective tools to nourish a positive attitude.
- The power of a positive religious and philosophical underpinning to our life-choices enhances our ability to cope with re-entry. As in most situations, rigid viewpoints do not have the flexibility to accept and appreciate the perspectives of a new culture. Clients should be encouraged to find a community where they can share the comfort of their beliefs.
- People cannot ignore the nitty-gritty of returning. The same checklist they used on departure of banks accounts, address changes, licenses, school and health records, financial papers, wills, and so on needs to be attended to in advance.
- The more that people participate in a decision, the more likely that they will have a successful transition. This applies to families and their children. Clients should be encouraged to involve everyone in the re-entry process and to have frequent and open discussions about the issue.
- People with pre-existing medical and psychiatric conditions may anticipate an exacerbation of symptoms during a major transition. They should be directed to competent follow-up care and be instructed to continue their medication and carry an adequate supply.
- Managing successfully the pressures of re-entry requires a daily commitment and is not a one-time effort.
- Groups have proven an effective way for people to air their worries and to develop problem-solving strategies.

What not to do

Equally important is the notion that there are behaviors that make the transition more difficult.

- Alcohol intake increases with increased stress. This was dramatically illustrated by the increased consumption in New York City after the terrorist attack of September, 2001. Alcohol is a poor anti-anxiety agent and a poor sleeping medication. While it is enjoyable in moderation and may be somewhat protective for coronary disease, it has no place in the management of re-entry.

Clients with short-term insomnia or anxiety reactions should discuss these symptoms with their physician. In some cases, brief therapeutic intervention or short-term use of medications is sufficient.

- An increase in anger and irritability are commonly seen during a stressful time. These negative behaviors have a ripple effect in a family and work environment and are a certain indicator of stress overload. People who employ these mechanisms to reduce short-term stress should consult their doctor and use as many positive coping techniques as possible.
- Besides alcohol, many people self-medicate with other drugs including nicotine, caffeine, marijuana, benzodiazepines and so on. Nicotine and caffeine may well increase anxiety, even in those with tolerance to them. Physicians should monitor prescription medication and inquire about the use of illegal drugs.
- Shopaholism is commonly seen in the re-entry group. Typically, they are seen prowling the sukhs looking for the last perfume jar in Egypt. Acknowledging one's anxiety and remembering the importance of responsible money management usually contain this problem. Nonetheless, many expatriates return home with money problems.
- Re-entry and other stressors often generate rumors and gossip. This behavior is actually stress-inducing; people need to be reminded of the responsibility they have to themselves and others to check their information and speak thoughtfully. Related to this is the temptation to degrade the country that one is leaving. A balanced viewpoint remains best.

For those who may need psychological services outside the scope of the clinic, any major European city and many other major cities worldwide such as Cairo, New Delhi, and Bangkok have Community Service Associations which provide mental health services with expatriate staff. The quality is often uneven, and the health-care provider is advised to evaluate the resources himself. Embassies, Consulates, and major businesses have often researched local medical care, and a call to the Health Unit or the Executive Officer may yield valuable information.

FAMILY UNIT

Typically, expatriates travel as families or couples. Perhaps the most effective and immediate work the travel clinician can perform for re-entry, is to tailor techniques and strategies to the family unit and the special needs of children. The upheaval of changing jobs, schools, environment, and neighborhood should be acknowledged. According to Ruth Useem and Richard Downie, the 'third culture kid' (TCK) does not fully belong to any culture.[8]

An unpublished study from the Ackerman Institute in New York City notes that generally, children and families adjust well to multiple moves, including re-entry. Healthy, communicative families generally adjust well to moves.[9] This is a way of saying that people take their problems with them. Families struggling with marital discord or other psychological issues will not be cured by the move. There is also a sub-group of children who have significant problems. It is often thought that in a healthy family, all children will adjust similarly. This is a serious misconception; every child is unique and has his own coping style and needs. Within any family, different children may have starkly different reactions to re-entry. Parents need to be reminded to be attentive to each child. Other factors that play a role for children returning are age, sex, temperament, intelligence, as well as the complex relationships of siblings and parents.

Strategies for managing re-entry have to be focused on the age of the child.

Infants

The world of infants and younger toddlers is essentially restricted to their family and its environment. Overseas, there may also be a hired, local caregiver who plays a significant role in the child's life. For some children who are left almost solely in the care of a maid, this loss may be the most important aspect of the move home. The problem of adequate child care abroad and its impact on children is a critical issue. Families should actively monitor the quality of child care and not minimize the disruption to the family at the time of re-entry. Children of this age will, within the range of their temperament, react to the emotions of their family. If the primary caregiver tolerates the move well, then this will be communicated verbally and non-verbally to the child in the daily tasks of feeding, toileting, play, and dressing. Parents of children in this age group are encouraged to prepare themselves well for the transition and continue providing for the child as consistently as possible. Because of the child's exquisite sensitivity to the child–caretaker relationship, parents encountering difficulty with the return should consult their physician early to minimize the negative effect on the child. Symptoms requiring intervention in this age group are serious regressive behavior, sleep and eating changes, and a non-specific irritability. After eliminating possible physical causes, these symptoms in the child are most likely a reaction to a change in routine and stress symptoms in the caregivers.

Pre-school

Partly from an increased mobility and partly from a more developed sense of place and time, preschool children already have a much broader sense of the world than infants. With a clearer sense of their surroundings, these children will be well aware of external changes, e.g., packing their bedrooms, changing neighborhoods, and leaving favorite playgrounds and shops. They are very likely to need help in saying goodbye to playmates and their parents. Leave taking for these children requires straightforward discussions, inquiry as to their preferences for departure and arrival, and the opportunities for social good-byes at departure and introductions at arrival. These children will also be aware of their relationships with relatives: grandparents, uncles, aunts, and any disruption that the move brings to their interactions with them. Many expatriate families now have relatives in the host country. All of this needs to be woven into the departure and arrival planning. These children are especially fond of the 'why' question and parents must be prepared to give simple, yet honest explanations for the move. Parents can state without great detail that the move is a challenge for everyone and ask the children to assist the family in age appropriate ways. For all ages the television should be used sparingly to manage emotions and communication. Good television habits should be established and maintained. Worldwide, there are sensitive programs, which model good social interaction and problem solving techniques, rather than showing gratuitous violence.

When to seek help

Parents know their children best, and they should consult the physician concerning any major change in the child's behavior such as a cooperative girl becoming defiant. Other worrisome symptoms include: change in sleep habits, regression in eating or toilet training, an upsurge in temper tantrums, excessive crying or anxiety, separation problems, or withdrawal and sadness beyond the child's normal range of affect. Parents need to be well aware of their own conflicted feelings about moving and the guilt that it engenders in them when moving disrupts a child's life. This can generate secondary conflicts and manipulations. While moving may be difficult, the message must be that it is a necessary part of the family's life and in the long-term best for everyone. Parents must reaffirm their love and support for the child and reassure the child of their support in the family's new life. Regular family meetings should be instituted at this age and maintained until children leave for college as a forum for questions, problem solving, and discussing emotions.

Elementary school

By elementary school age, children have greatly expanded their range of behaviors, have a more sophisticated view of the world, and participate in a more complex social network. These children are likely to be involved in sports, in pursuit of hobbies such as a musical instrument, and in after school activities. Remembering that a child's temperament is a major factor in re-entry, parents must observe if their child is out-going or an introvert, intellectual or hands-on, self-oriented or already emphatic, a leader or a follower, and so on. Generally a child's typical behavior will only intensify under the pressure of re-entry, and parents must plan accordingly, e.g., the introverted child will need more support and introductions to become comfortable socially. Throughout this period, parents can encourage their child to become independent, to experience the move as an opportunity for developing more adaptive traits, and to learn from failures. At the same time, the engaged parent recognizes that each child's needs are unique and that the child needs protection from becoming overwhelmed.

In addition to the strategies for the younger children, more time will be needed for children in this age group to separate from their more complex social network. Questions will be more complicated and require thoughtful answers. They may more openly express their fears. Children should be told that the move is a parental decision and not a reaction to anything they have done. At this age, children may have many useful insights in how to answer their own questions and solve their own re-entry problems. Attention to academic performance and any special needs must be integrated into the plans for re-entry. Members of this age group can understand the explanation that the move is a major undertaking for the family and that they can make an important contribution to their family during it.

When to seek help

The general guidelines for younger children apply. In addition, children in this age group may show signs of depression more often seen in adults – lethargy, withdrawal, poor self-esteem, and social isolation. Older children in this group may develop self-destructive behaviors along with eating disorders and weight change. Aggression is often a symptom of stressors such as re-entry. Extraordinary disobedience and defiance can mark a shift in the child's world and indicate the need for professional help. Academic performance is exquisitely sensitive to a child's worldview and should be tracked. Teacher, peers, and the peer's parents often have insight into a child's reactions that are difficult for parents to see. Again preparation, involvement, and empowerment of the child during re-entry ease the process. Family meetings should address the issues of re-entry, i.e., what each member of the family will miss in the host country, what they anticipate positive and negative in their homeland, and the changes that family members note in each other. At the same time, the child needs the reassurance of clear, firm, predictable guidelines and the consequences for not meeting the family's expectations.

Adolescents

Teenagers are the most problematic group to relocate. At this age, peers have often replaced parents – at least temporarily – as the most powerful relationships. According to Armand Nicholi, this is

occurring at a much earlier age than a generation ago.[10] Their sense of independence and the ability to articulate opposing viewpoints combine to make teenagers comfortable in expressing their view of re-entry. Indeed, depending on their resiliency and temperament, this may be one of the most difficult challenges of their life. For many, returning home is not a reward for giving up a comfortable social structure and a school where they feel accepted and often special. While often overseas schools have all the problems of a school at home – drugs, intense peer pressures, and weak administration – the students often feel special and worldly. They realize from their visits home that they will lose the prestige of their international status. There are many situations that require special thought, e.g., moving during the senior year, during a sports season, taking a child from an intense love relationship, leaving during a 2 year International Baccalaureate program and in the midst of college applications.

This is a period of intense change and psychological struggle. Incidents of depression and suicidal thoughts increase dramatically in the teenage years. Many other disorders manifest themselves during this time. Physicians need to insist that families plan well in advance to include teenagers in the move. With encouragement, a teenager can often verbalize his concerns and needs. For many families, major moves demand that they weigh the needs of a career against the emotional needs of the family. This is not an easy decision. Many schools and overseas communities run re-entry programs for teenagers, and they should be encouraged to participate. In this age group the phenomenon of Third Culture Kids or Global Nomads is seen. These young adults may have formed an attachment to an expatriate lifestyle, which emphasizes international issues and overseas living in preference to returning home.

When to seek help

- Withdrawal and signs of depression. Any comments about hopelessness or suicide
- Increase in aggression or destructiveness to property
- Eating disorders: anorexia and bulimia
- A morbid fascination with the occult or bizarre metaphysical beliefs
- Anxiety and sleep problems
- Any significant change from the adolescent's baseline behavior
- Truancy
- Running away
- Alcohol and other drug abuse
- A fascination with weapons

Physicians should ask the parents to bring the teenager into the office for a confidential interview. Remember in many cases the best way to find out what is wrong is to ask. For serious symptoms, the physician should refer the family to a child psychiatrist.

Adults

After teenagers, this is the most problematic group for re-entry. Adults are often the most naïve when it comes to the impact of returning home. They often do not recognize that adult life has developmental changes and phases, which affect their coping ability. In addition, adults often lack the direct feedback about their stress responses that teenagers and children give and receive so easily. When travel physicians help their clients look at the list of tasks in the re-entry process, they are better able to understand the inevitable consequences of the upheaval. Adults and their families must in short order, pack, find housing, change jobs and schools, say goodbye to friends, travel to their home country, create a new social network, set up a new household, and attend to the innumerable, nitty-gritty tasks. This is a daunting challenge. Most of the strategies in this chapter apply to adults. Most adults and most families manage this transition without outside

Table 37.2   Additional strategies

1	Return home at least once a year. On these visits, they should visit their neighbors and the children must see their friends. If children attend camp, they should return to the same one every year.
2	If there is no home base, create one.
3	Use the Internet and telephone to keep up with developments in home community, changes in the company, and news of friends and relatives.
4	Use the Internet to read national newspapers to stay current with national news and attuned to changes in the home culture.
5	Return children to the same school and neighborhood. Be prepared to be an advocate for them in classroom assignment and in transferring credits from overseas schools.
6	Some expatriates don't experience identity loss for 2–3 years. Stay alert to changes in behaviors and nurture a social network that will confront and support you.
7	While there are many sources of survival techniques, all people are unique and must find their own recipe.

intervention, but with awareness and planning. Table 37.2 shows additional strategies suggested by those who have survived, these involve ongoing activities throughout the overseas experience. Many adults join support groups of expatriates to ease the transition, but all adults should seek help for:

- symptoms of depression: especially weight changes, insomnia, lethargy, profound sadness and hopelessness, lack of enjoyment, and suicidal ideation
- an increase in any of the negative behaviors listed under stress management
- feedback from friends and colleagues that they are not themselves.

ORGANIZATIONS

- Global Nomads International: www.globalnomads.association.com
- Transition Dynamics: www.transition-dynamics.com
- Electronic Magazine of Multicultural Education: www.eastern.edu/publications/emmi/

CONCLUSION

The effective travel clinic will integrate mental health into a comprehensive program for their clients. The psychological risks for families and individuals are as great as the risks for physical illness. Education has a critical role in the prevention of mental health symptoms. In the outward-bound portion of the journey, clients should be given an orientation to stress reactions and cross cultural issues. They should be encouraged to understand their own coping mechanisms and to understand that the re-entry syndrome will affect them. Awareness and anticipation will allow them to minimize the conflicts and utilize the re-entry as an opportunity. One to three months prior to re-entry is an optimal time for the clinic to contact its clients to reinforce the coping strategies.

REFERENCES

1. Valk T. *Shoreland's Travel Medicine Monthly* 1998; **2**(12).
2. Peace Corps. *The Voyage Home*. Washington: Office of Domestic Programs; 1997:7–11.
3. Dickstein L. Other additional conditions. In: Sadock, B, Sadock, V, eds. *Comprehensive Textbook of Psychiatry*, 7th edn. Philadelphia: Lippincott, Williams, Wilkins; 2000:1920–1921.
4. Cannon WB. *The Wisdom of the Body*. New York: Norton; 1932.
5. Janis I. Decision Making under Stress. In: Goldberger L, Breznitz S, eds. Handbook of Stress. NYC: The Free Press; 1993:56–74.
6. The Energizer. University of California at Berkeley *Wellness Newsletter* 1995; **11**(11).
7. Jansson DP. Return to Society: Problematic Features of the Re-entry Process. *Perspect Psychiatr Care* 1975; **13**:136–142.
8. Unseem R, Downie R. Third Culture Kids. In: McCloskey K, ed. *Notes from A Traveling Childhood*. Washington: Foreign Service Youth Foundation; 1994:65–71.
9. Steinglass P, Edwards M. *Family Relocation Study*. NYC: Ackerman Institute for Family Therapy; 1993.
10. Nicholi A. The adolescent. In: Nicholi A, ed. *Harvard Guide to Psychiatry*. Cambridge, MA: Belknap Press; 1999:611–635.
11. Austin C, ed. *Cross Cultural Re-entry: A Book of Readings*. Abilene, Texas: Abilene Christian University; 1996.
12. Kohls L. *Survival Kit for Overseas Living*. 2nd edn. Yarmouth, Maine: International Press; 1984.
13. Meyers J. *The Cross-Cultural Adaptability Inventory*. MN: National Computer Systems; 1992.

CHAPTER 38 Altitude

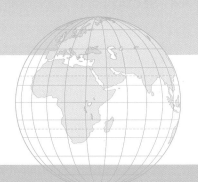

Thomas E. Dietz and Peter H. Hackett

KEYPOINTS

- Most individuals, even those with mild chronic illness, can enjoy traveling to altitude as long as they are properly advised and are careful to acclimatize

- Hypoxia, lower temperatures, UV radiation, and dehydration are the common challenges one faces while at altitude

- Acute mountain sickness is common and affects up to 40% of individuals even at moderate altitudes (2000–3500 m) at popular ski resorts

- Management of acute mountain sickness includes: no further ascent until symptoms resolve, descent to a lower altitude if there is no improvement, and descent if there are any signs of cerebral edema or pulmonary edema

- There are a variety of medications available for the prevention and/or treatment of high-altitude illness, including acetazolamide, dexamethasone, and nifedipine; some data suggest the benefit of ginkgo biloba

INTRODUCTION

The increasing popularity and accessibility of adventure travel trips to high-altitude locations makes it more important than ever for travel clinic physicians to understand the medical problems associated with high altitude. This chapter discusses the unique aspects of the high-altitude environment, acclimatization, the high-altitude illnesses, the impact of high-altitude on pre-existing medical conditions, and whether a pre-existing condition might adversely affect acclimatization to high altitude. A list of online resources is included in Table 38.1 for a more detailed recent review, consult Hackett and Roach.[1]

The high-altitude environment

The high-altitude environment usually refers to elevations over 1500 m (4900 ft). Moderate altitude includes the elevations of most mountain and ski resorts, 2000–3500 m (6600–11 500 ft). Arterial oxygen saturation is well maintained at these altitudes, but mild tissue hypoxia results from low arterial PO_2, and altitude illness is common. Very high altitude refers to altitudes of 3500–5500 m (18 000 ft). In this range, arterial oxygen saturation is not maintained, and extreme hypoxemia can occur during sleep, exercise and illness. High-altitude pulmonary and cerebral edema are most common in this range. Extreme altitude is over 5500 m (18 000 ft). Above this altitude, successful long-term acclimatization is impossible and deterioration ensues; no long-term

human habitations exist above 5500 m. Individuals must progressively acclimatize to intermediate altitudes to reach extreme altitude.

Hypoxia is the primary physiological insult on ascent to high altitude. The fraction of oxygen in the atmosphere remains constant (0.21), but as barometric pressure decreases on ascent to altitude, so does the partial pressure of oxygen (Fig. 38.1). More importantly, the inspired partial pressure of oxygen (P_iO_2) is lower than atmospheric oxygen partial pressure because of water vapor pressure in the airways. At the altitude of Denver, Colorado (1600 m), P_iO_2 is 18% lower than at sea level (122 versus 149 mmHg); in Breckenridge, Colorado (2860 m) it is 105 mmHg; while at La Paz, Bolivia (4000 m), P_iO_2 is only 86.4 mmHg, which is equivalent to breathing a gas mixture of 12% oxygen at sea level. Thus, the high-altitude environment produces significant alveolar and consequent arterial hypoxemia.

The high-altitude environment creates a number of stresses in addition to hypoxia. Temperature decreases with ascent to altitude, on the order of 6.5 °C per 1000 m (3280 ft); the effects of hypoxia and cold can be additive in terms of predisposing to problems such as frostbite and high-altitude pulmonary edema. Ultraviolet radiation increases by 4% per 300 m (1000 ft) gain in altitude, due to less water vapor and particulate matter in the high-altitude atmosphere; this predisposes to sunburn, UV keratoconjunctivitis, and cataracts. Dehydration is common because of increased insensible water loss from the airways and skin.

ACCLIMATIZATION

The body's response to hypoxia depends on both the degree of hypoxia and rate of onset of hypoxia. Acute hypoxia causes feelings of unreality, dizziness, dim vision and rapid unconsciousness given sufficient hypoxic stress; for example, sudden exposure to an altitude equivalent to the summit of Mt. Everest (8848 m; P_iO_2 43 mmHg) will result in unconsciousness within 2 minutes. However, individuals developing the same degree of hypoxia over days to weeks are able to function relatively well. This process of adjusting to hypoxia, termed acclimatization, is a series of compensatory changes in multiple organ systems over differing time courses from days to weeks, and even years. While the fundamental process occurs in the metabolic machinery of the cell, acute physiologic responses are essential, while allowing the cells time to adjust.

The most important and immediate response of the body to hypoxia is an increase in minute ventilation, triggered by oxygen sensing cells in the carotid body. First with an increase in tidal volume and then respiratory frequency, increased ventilation produces a higher alveolar PO_2, thereby reducing hypoxic stress. Concomitantly, a lower alveolar CO_2 produces a respiratory alkalosis, which acts as a brake on the brain respiratory center and limits the increase in ventilation. Only after renal compensation (excretion of bicarbonate ion) does

Table 38.1	Online information resources on altitude illness

International Society for Mountain Medicine: www.ismmed.org
    Detailed practical information on altitude illness available for both physicians and non-physicians.
    Includes diagnostic criteria for AMS, HACE, and HAPE, as well as AMS scoring tools for adults
    and children. An 'ask the experts' section is available for difficult cases.

The High Altitude Medicine Guide: www.high-altitude-medicine.com
    Information on altitude illness and other health issues for travelers and their physicians. Has a
    practical tutorial on field hyperbaric treatment, and comparisons of the various portable hyperbaric
    bags.

EMedicine: www.emedicine.com/emerg/environmental.htm
    Written in a brief, easy-to-review format; targeted at physicians. The cerebral and pulmonary
    syndromes of altitude illness are covered in separate 'chapters'.

Web MD: www.webmd.com
    Has separate consumer and physician sections, and extensive medical info for consumers. Online
    chat rooms cover various topics including altitude illness and travel medicine.

ICAR-MEDCOM: www.mountainmedicine.org/mmed/icarmedcom/papers.html
    A collection of articles on medical management of mountaineering emergencies, including a suggested
    alpine medical kit. Presented by the International Commission for Mountain Emergency Medicine.

Wilderness Medical Society: www.wms.org
    Complete archives of Wilderness and Environmental Medicine and the prior *Journal of Wilderness*
    Medicine. Archives are open, but the current issue is only accessible to subscribers and WMS
    members.

Bibliography of High Altitude Medicine: annie.cv.nrao.edu/habibqbe.htm
    A searchable bibliography of important work in high altitude medicine.

the blood pH return to normal levels does the full increase in ventilation take place. This process, termed ventilatory acclimatization, requires approximately 4 days at a given altitude, and is greatly enhanced by acetazolamide. Patients with insufficient carotid body response (genetic or acquired), or pulmonary or renal disease may have an inadequate ventilatory response and therefore do not adapt well to high altitude.

Just as the ventilatory pump increases in order to supply more oxygen to the blood, the circulatory pump increases to provide more circulating oxygen to the tissues. Ascent to high altitude, through sympathetic activation, initially increases resting heart rate and cardiac output, and mildly increases blood pressure. The healthy heart tolerates extreme hypoxia well; even with arterial PO_2 less than 30 mmHg, ECG and echocardiogram evaluation in experimental

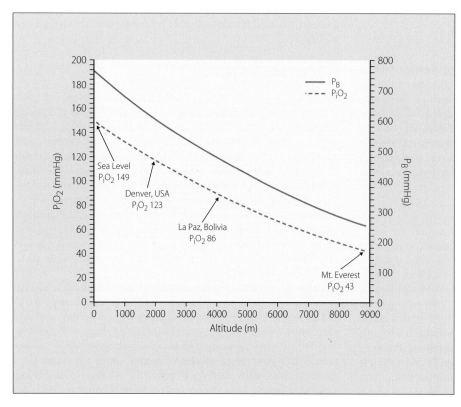

Figure 38.1 Barometric pressure and P_iO_2 at altitude. Barometric pressure (P_B) decreases exponentially with increasing altitude; PO_2 is a constant 21% of P_B, but the partial pressure of inspired air (P_iO_2) is decreased because of water vapor added as the air is warmed and humidified in the respiratory tree.

subjects showed no evidence of ischemia, no wall motion abnormalities, and no depressed contractility.[2,3]

The pulmonary circulation reacts to hypoxia with vasoconstriction, due to smooth muscle activation in the vessel walls. This response is arguably beneficial, somewhat improving ventilation/perfusion matching and gas exchange. The resulting pulmonary hypertension, however, can lead to a number of pathological syndromes at high altitude, including high-altitude pulmonary edema and altitude-related right heart failure.

Cerebral blood flow increases immediately on ascent to high altitude, and then returns toward normal over the first week of acclimatization. This response is variable, but the average increase is 24% at 3810 m, and more at higher altitude. Whether this increased flow relates to the headache of acute mountain sickness is unclear.

Hemoglobin concentration increases on ascent to high altitude, thereby enhancing the oxygen-carrying capacity of the blood. In the first few days, it increases secondary to the reduction in plasma volume; (i.e., hemoconcentration). Over weeks to months, hemoglobin concentration increases due to augmented red cell production stimulated by erythropoietin.

The oxyhemoglobin dissociation curve in vivo remains unchanged until the marked alkalosis of extreme altitude shifts it to the left, thus facilitating loading of the hemoglobin with oxygen in the pulmonary capillary. Reinforcing the notion that a left-shifted hemoglobin is an advantage at high altitude, individuals with a rare naturally occurring left-shifted hemoglobin have exceptional performance at altitude. Whether those with a right-shifted hemoglobin dissociation curve are at a disadvantage at altitude is unknown.

Effects of high altitude on exercise

High-altitude hypoxia dramatically impacts aerobic but not anaerobic exercise performance. Maximum oxygen consumption (VO_2 max) decreases approximately 10% for every 1000 m of altitude, starting at 1500 m. As a result, a person exercising at altitude to the same degree as at sea level will be operating at a higher percentage of VO_2 max, will become more easily fatigued and will reach anaerobic threshold earlier. Also, because of the large increase in exercise ventilation, breathlessness becomes a limiting factor. The result is that persons exercising at high altitude must exercise less intensely to avoid exhaustion, and rest more frequently. Endurance time (minutes to exhaustion at 75% of altitude-specific VO_2 max) does improve, as much as 40% after 12 days.[4]

Sleep at high altitude

Sleep architecture is altered at high altitude, and results in a slight change in sleep stages, frequent arousals, and nearly universal subjective report of disturbed or unsatisfactory sleep. After 3–4 nights at a given altitude, this generally improves, though periodic breathing during sleep (Cheyne-Stokes) is 'normal' at altitudes above 2700 m.

HIGH-ALTITUDE SYNDROMES

Altitude illness refers to a group of syndromes that result from hypoxia; the target organs are the brain and the lung. Acute mountain sickness (AMS) and high-altitude cerebral edema (HACE) reflect the brain pathophysiology, and high-altitude pulmonary edema (HAPE) reflects that of the lung. These illnesses generally occur at altitudes above 2500 m, though particularly sensitive individuals can become ill as low as 1800 m. Everyone traveling to altitude is at risk, regardless of the level of physical fitness or previous altitude experience.

ACUTE MOUNTAIN SICKNESS AND HIGH-ALTITUDE CEREBRAL EDEMA

Epidemiology

The incidence of acute mountain sickness varies, depending on the rate of ascent and the highest altitude reached. In moderate altitude (2000–3500 m) ski resorts, the incidence ranges from 10–40%. In those who hike above 4000 m, 25–50% will suffer from AMS. Travelers flying to a high-altitude destination such as Lhasa, Tibet (3810 m) or La Paz, Bolivia (4000 m) can expect an incidence of 25–35%.

Susceptibility to AMS demonstrates great individual variability because of genetic differences. Individual susceptibility is reproducible: a past history of AMS is the best predictor. Men, women, and children are at equal risk, though risk is slightly decreased after age 50. Physical fitness provides no protection from AMS.

Pathophysiology of AMS/HACE

The exact pathophysiology of AMS/HACE is unknown. The current hypothesis is that hypoxia elicits hemodynamic and neurohumoral responses in both the brain and lung that ultimately result in capillary leakage from microvascular beds and edema (Fig. 38.2).

Whether mild AMS or headache alone is actually due to brain edema remains an open question. Recent magnetic resonance imaging (MRI) studies demonstrated that the brain swells on ascent to altitude in both those with and without AMS, presumably from vasodilatation. True edema, however, was not detected, except with severe AMS and HACE.[5-7] Factors that might contribute to a hydrostatic brain edema are multiple and include sustained cerebral vasodilatation, impaired cerebral autoregulation, elevated cerebral capillary pressure as well as alterations in the permeability of the blood-brain barrier through cytokine activation.

Clinical presentation and diagnosis

Acute mountain sickness is a syndrome of non-specific symptoms and a broad spectrum of severity. Diagnostic criteria and scoring tools for altitude illness for both adults and children are available online (Table 38.1). AMS occurs in non-acclimatized persons in the first 48 h after ascent to altitudes above 2500 m, especially after rapid ascent (one day or less). Symptoms usually begin a few hours after arrival at the new altitude, but may arise a day later (often after the first night's sleep). The cardinal symptom is headache, typically bi-frontal and throbbing. Gastrointestinal symptoms (anorexia, nausea or vomiting), and constitutional symptoms (weakness, lightheadedness or lassitude) are common. AMS is thus similar to an alcohol hangover, or to a nonspecific viral infection, but without fever and myalgia. Fluid retention is characteristic of AMS and victims often report reduced urination, in contrast to the spontaneous diuresis observed with successful acclimatization. As AMS progresses, the headache worsens, and vomiting, oliguria and increased lassitude develop. Ataxia and altered level of consciousness herald the onset of clinical high-altitude cerebral edema (Fig. 38.3).

Patients with AMS appear ill but lack characteristic physical findings. Heart rate and blood pressure are variable, and nondiagnostic. Unless HACE is present, neurological examination is normal. Fundoscopic examination may reveal retinal hemorrhages, but these are not specific to AMS. Pulmonary crackles may be present but oxygen saturation will be normal or at most slightly lower than acclimatized persons at the same elevation. Peripheral and facial edema may be present, particularly in women.

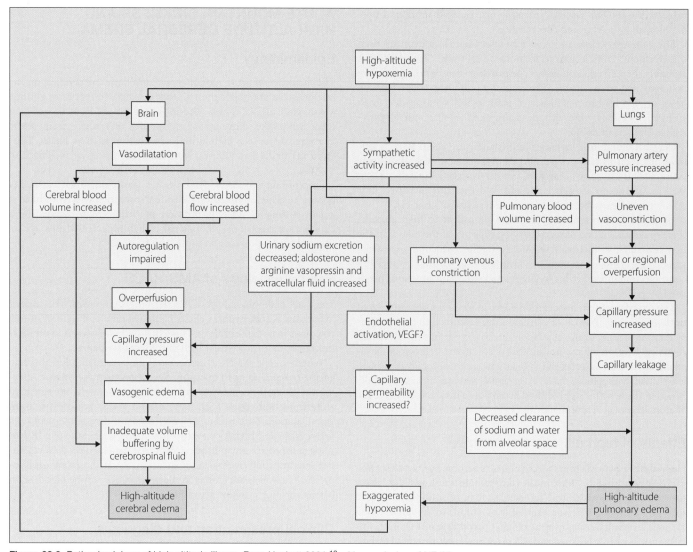

Figure 38.2 Pathophysiology of high-altitude illness. From Hackett 2001,[12] with permission of NEJM.

Most conditions similar to AMS can be excluded by history and physical examination. Onset of symptoms more than three days after ascent, lack of headache, or failure to improve with descent, oxygen, or dexamethasone suggest another diagnosis. Dehydration is commonly confused with AMS, as it can cause headache, weakness, nausea, and decreased urine output.

The natural history of AMS varies with altitude, ascent rate, and other factors. In general, symptoms improve slowly, with complete resolution in one to two days. AMS symptom duration ranged from 6–94 h with a mean of 15 h in one study at 3000 m.[8] A small percentage (<10%) of persons with AMS will go on to develop HACE, especially with continued ascent in the presence of AMS symptoms.

Untreated, HACE may progress to stupor and coma over hours to days, and death is due to brain herniation. Ataxia commonly persists for days to weeks after descent, but persistent mental status changes or the presence of focal neurological deficits should prompt a complete neurological evaluation. Brain tumors that suddenly become symptomatic at altitude,[9] Guillain-Barré syndrome, and cortical blindness have all been misdiagnosed as HACE. Patients who survive typically have full recovery after descending, but reports of persistent neurological sequelae exist.

Treatment

Management of AMS follows three axioms: (1) no further ascent until symptoms resolve; (2) descend to a lower altitude if no improvement with medical therapy; and (3) at the first sign of HACE descend immediately. It is not possible to predict the eventual severity from the initial clinical presentation, and patients must be watched closely for progression of illness.

Suggested medications for high-altitude travelers are listed in Table 38.2. Table 38.3 provides a variety of common clinical scenarios and suggests management options. Descent to an altitude below which symptoms started is always effective treatment, but may not be practical given the topography, or possible given the patient's ultimate trekking or climbing goals or group resources. Thus, a descent of 500–1000 m is usually sufficient. Acetazolamide speeds acclimatization and thus hastens resolution of the illness, but this requires 12–24 h. Dexamethasone rapidly reverses symptoms (2–4 hours), but does not improve acclimatization. Therefore, it is logical to use both agents if the victim does not descend. Also, acetazolamide can be taken episodically without fear of rebound symptoms when it is discontinued. Oxygen is extremely effective, but availability may be

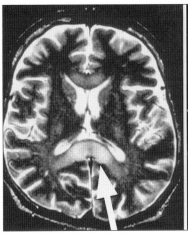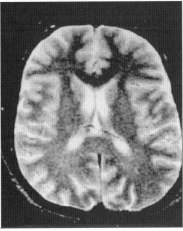

Figure 38.3 Magnetic Resonance Image (MRI) of a patient with high-altitude cerebral edema. Left, axial T₂-weighted magnetic resonance image demonstrating high signal in the splenium of the corpus callosum (arrow) and mildly increased signal in the centrum semiovale. Right, axial T₂-weighted magnetic resonance image of the same patient 11 months later, showing complete resolution. After Hackett 2001,[7] with permission of *JAMA*.

limited. Dexamethasone should be continued for 1–2 days after descent in persons with uncomplicated HACE, or until the mental status clears in cases of severe HACE.

Portable hyperbaric chambers made of coated fabric (e.g., Gamow Bag, CERTEC, and PAC) are now widely available among adventure travel groups, on expeditions, and in high-altitude clinics (Fig. 38.4). The patient is placed completely within the bag, which is sealed shut and inflated with a manually operated pump, pressurizing the inside to 105–220 mmHg above ambient atmospheric pressure.

Coca leaf tea is widely recommended in South America and in the popular press as a cure for altitude illness; however, there are no studies to support this claim. Coca leaf tea may act as a mild stimulant and improve well-being at altitude, which may be its primary effect. Garlic has also been advocated for prophylaxis and treatment of altitude illness. Animal studies show efficacy in preventing hypoxic pulmonary hypertension, but studies in humans are lacking and its use cannot be recommended at this time. Treatments shown to have no benefit include naproxen, calcium channel blockers, phenytoin and antacids. Alcohol and other respiratory depressants should be avoided in someone with AMS due to the risk of exaggerated hypoxemia.

Prevention

Recommendations on staged ascents are generally adequate for the average person, but some persons will still become ill despite a slow, staged ascent. Persons traveling to high altitude should allow adequate time for acclimatization, and pay careful attention to symptoms. Helpful guidelines to avoid altitude illness are included in Table 38.4.

Many travelers wonder how long acclimatization lasts after a sojourn to high altitude. Some value in preventing AMS will persist for a week or more, but only a few days at sea level can render one susceptible to HAPE. Improved exercise ability will last for weeks.

Acetazolamide (Table 38.2) effectively prevents AMS[10]; it accelerates acclimatization by inducing a bicarbonate diuresis, stimulating ventilation and improving sleep-breathing patterns. It does not mask symptoms of AMS. Since it is also useful for treatment,[11] acetazolamide should be in the high-altitude traveler's medical kit, along with written instructions. A recent survey concluded that trekkers carrying acetazolamide did not know how to use it properly. Dexamethasone also effectively prevents AMS, but does not improve acclimatization.[10] Due to the concern of rebound symptoms and the side effect profile, this medication cannot be routinely recommended for prophylaxis.

Several recent controlled trials have shown Ginkgo biloba extract effective in preventing AMS, both with gradual and rapid ascents.[12] It is available in a standardized preparation in Europe, but in North America varies in terms of potency. Preliminary data suggest that acetazolamide is superior to ginkgo for prevention of AMS.

HIGH-ALTITUDE PULMONARY EDEMA

Epidemiology

The reported incidence of HAPE varies from 0.01% to 15%, depending on the altitude, ascent rate, and the population at risk.[1] Individual susceptibility based on genetic factors is perhaps the greatest risk factor, with male gender also being suggested as a risk factor. There is no clear association with age. Pre-existing medical conditions associated with pulmonary hypertension or a restricted pulmonary vascular bed will greatly increase susceptibility to HAPE. Exercise increases risk of HAPE since it increases cardiac output and pulmonary artery pressure at altitude.

Pathophysiology

HAPE is a non-cardiogenic, hydrostatic pulmonary edema, characterized by pulmonary hypertension and increased capillary pressure (Fig. 38.2). Left ventricular function in HAPE is normal. Although increased pulmonary artery pressure due to hypoxic pulmonary vasoconstriction occurs in all who ascend to high altitude, it is exaggerated in those susceptible to HAPE, again primarily a genetically determined susceptibility.[13]

Clinical presentation and diagnosis

HAPE occurs 2–4 days after ascent to high altitude, often worsening at night. Decreased exercise performance is the earliest symptom, usually associated with a dry cough. The early course is subtle; as the illness progresses, the cough worsens and becomes productive; dyspnea can be severe, tachycardia and tachypnea develop, and drowsiness or other CNS symptoms may develop. Patchy unilateral or bilateral fluffy infiltrates, and a normal cardiac silhouette on chest X-ray are characteristic of HAPE (Fig. 38.5). The presence of a low-grade fever has led to misdiagnosis (as pneumonia) and to subsequent deaths.

HAPE varies in severity from mild to immediately life-threatening. It can be fatal within a few hours, and is the most common cause of

Table 38.2	Medications for travelers to high altitude			
Agent	**Indication**	**Dose**	**Adverse effects**	**Comments**
Acetazolamide	Prevention of AMS	125–250 mg orally twice a day beginning 24 h before ascent and continuing during ascent and to at least 48 h after arrival at highest altitude	COMMON: Paresthesias; polyuria; alters taste of carbonated beverages PRECAUTIONS: Sulfonamide reactions possible; avoided in breast-feeding; can decrease therapeutic levels of lithium	Can be taken episodically for symptoms; no rebound effect; pregnancy category C
	Treatment of AMS	250 mg orally every 8–12 h		
	Pediatric AMS	5 mg/kg body weight/day, given orally in divided doses every 8–12 h		
	Periodic breathing	125 mg orally 1 h before bed		
Dexamethasone	Treatment of AMS	4 mg every 6 h orally, i.m. or i.v. for 2 doses	Mood changes; hyperglycemia; dyspepsia	Rapidly improves AMS symptoms; can be lifesaving in HACE; may improve HACE enough to facilitate descent; no value in HAPE; pregnancy category C but preferably avoided by women who are pregnant or breast-feeding
	HACE	8 mg initially, then 4 mg every 6 h orally, i.m. or i.v.		
	Pediatric HACE	1–2 mg/kg body weight initially, then 0.25–0.5 mg/kg every 6 h orally, i.m. or i.v., not to exceed 16 mg/d		
Ginkgo biloba	Prevention of AMS	80–120 mg orally twice daily starting 5 days before ascent and continuing to highest altitude	Occasional headache; rare reports of bleeding	Requires further study; preparations vary; may be used by women who are pregnant or breast-feeding
Nifedipine	Prevention of HAPE	20–30 mg of extended-release formulation orally every 12 h	Reflex tachycardia; hypotension (uncommon)	No value in AMS or HACE; not necessary if supplemental oxygen available; pregnancy category C
	Treatment of HAPE	10 mg orally initially, then 20–30 mg of extended release formulation orally every 12 h		
Promethazine	Symptomatic treatment of nausea and vomiting	25–50 mg orally, i.m. or i.v., or rectally every 6 h	Causes sedation; lowers seizure threshold, caution with history of seizures; extrapyramidal reactions may occur with high doses	Pregnancy category C
Hydrocodone	Symptomatic treatment of high-altitude cough	5–10 mg orally every 4 h	Causes sedation Contraindicated with HACE	May also be helpful for pain of intercostal muscle strain associated with cough
Temazepam	Insomnia	15–30 mg orally at bedtime	Confusion, drowsiness; respiratory sedation	Appears safe for well persons, but should be avoided in those with AMS due to concerns of increased hypoxemia during sleep
Zolpidem	Insomnia	10 mg orally	Rare, short-acting	Does not depress ventilation at high altitude; pregnancy category B

AMS, acute mountain sickness; HACE, high-altitude cerebral edema; HAPE, high-altitude pulmonary edema; i.v., intravenous; i.m., intramuscular
Pregnancy category B: No evidence of risk in humans. Adequate, well-controlled studies in pregnant women have not shown increased risk of fetal abnormalities despite adverse findings in animals, or in the absence of adequate human studies, animal studies show no fetal risk. The chance of fetal harm is remote, but remains a possibility.
Pregnancy category C: Risk cannot be ruled out. Adequate, well-controlled human studies are lacking, and animal studies have shown risk or are lacking as well. Use only if potential benefits outweigh the potential risks.
After Hackett 2001,[12] with permission of *NEJM*.

death related to high altitude. Differential diagnosis is sometimes problematic, but improves dramatically with descent or oxygen, whereas other diagnoses do not and should be pursued in patients who do not fit this pattern.

Treatment

The mainstay of treatment (see Tables 38.2 and 38.3), is descent. Oxygen, if available, is life-saving. Nifedipine should be used if descent or oxygen is not available. Hyperbaric treatment can be given in one-hour increments, and generally three to six hours will be required,

depending on the severity of illness. Dexamethasone should be used only if neurological symptoms or signs are present.

As with HACE, prognosis is excellent for survivors, with rapid clearing of the edema fluid and no long-term sequelae. Patients may need from 3 days to 2 weeks to recover completely; after all symptoms have resolved, cautious re-ascent is acceptable.

Prevention

See AMS prevention; the same staged-ascent recommendations are useful for HAPE prevention.

Table 38.3	Options for management of high-altitude illness
Clinical presentation	**Management**
Mild Acute Mountain Sickness Mild to moderate headache with nausea, dizziness or fatigue within first 24 h of ascent to high altitude (>2500 m).	Stop ascent, rest, and acclimatize Descend 500 m or more Speed acclimatization with acetazolamide (125–250 mg orally twice daily) Treat symptoms with mild analgesics and antiemetics or, use a combination of these approaches.
Moderate Acute Mountain Sickness Moderate to severe headache with marked nausea or vomiting, weakness, dizziness, lassitude, and peripheral edema 12–24 h after rapid ascent to high altitude.	Stop ascent, rest, treat medically Descend 500 m or more Give acetazolamide (250 mg orally twice daily), or dexamethasone (4 mg orally or intramuscularly every 6 h), or both Administer low-flow oxygen (1–2 L/min) or use a portable hyperbaric chamber Treat symptoms or, use a combination of these approaches.
High-Altitude Cerebral Edema Confusion, lassitude, and ataxia 48 h after ascent to high altitude; complained of a headache the day before onset of the confusion.	Start immediate descent or evacuation If descent is delayed or not possible, use a portable hyperbaric chamber and/or administer oxygen (2–4 L/min) Administer dexamethasone 8 mg intramuscularly, intravenously, or orally initially, then 4 mg every 6 h)
High-Altitude Pulmonary Edema Cough, weakness, dyspnea, chest congestion 60 h after arrival at a ski resort at 2750 m.	Administer oxygen (2–4 L/min, to keep SaO_2 >90%) Start immediate descent, minimizing exertion and cold stress If descent is delayed or not possible, or if oxygen is not available, use a portable hyperbaric chamber If descent/oxygen unavailable, administer nifedipine (10 mg orally initially, then 30 mg extended release formulation every 12 h)

The indication for chemoprophylaxis of HAPE is repeated episodes. Whether one previous episode should encourage prophylaxis is arguable, but demonstrated susceptibility certainly requires caution. Often a slower ascent is the only preventive method required. Effective agents for prevention of HAPE include nifedipine (Table 38.2) and salmeterol.[13] Those with a history of HAPE should carry nifedipine to use either prophylactically or with the first signs of HAPE. Salmeterol reduced HAPE by 50% in susceptible persons, appears safe, and should be considered for treatment as well, though it has not yet been studied for this indication.

OTHER ALTITUDE-RELATED CONDITIONS

Syncope within the first 24 h at high altitude is a well-recognized entity, and termed 'high-altitude syncope'.[14] This form of neurocardiogenic syncope[15] does not imply an underlying condition; a complete evaluation is generally unnecessary unless a second episode occurs.

The occurrence of focal neurological deficits, such as transient ischemic attacks in supposedly otherwise healthy individuals, has been noted at high altitude.[1] They are not part of the altitude illness spectrum, and require further evaluation. Patients with previously undiagnosed arteriovenous malformation (AVM), cerebral aneurysm and brain tumors have all become symptomatic on ascent to high altitude,[9] and both ischemic and hemorrhagic stroke have also been reported.

High-altitude retinal hemorrhage (HARH) is common and usually asymptomatic. The incidence of HARH varies from 4% at 4243 m to more than 50% in one study at 5360 m.[16,17] For those who develop visual changes, evacuation to a lower altitude is recommended.[17] No reports claim that such visual changes are progressive in persons who remain at altitude. HARH resolves completely within a few weeks after descent.

Peripheral edema is common at high altitude, especially in women.[1] It is not necessarily associated with altitude illness, but anyone with edema must be evaluated for AMS. Edema will resolve with decent. Diuretics work well; however, one must be cautious to avoid dehydration.

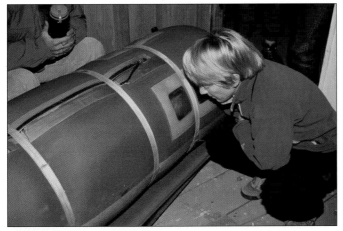

Figure 38.4 The Gamow Bag® portable hyperbaric chamber. Clinic staff talks with a patient undergoing hyperbaric treatment for high-altitude pulmonary edema at 4250 m in Nepal. Courtesy of T. Dietz.[36]

Table 38.4	Practical advice for travelers to altitude

Go slowly
   Avoid overexertion
   Avoid abrupt ascent to sleeping elevations over 3000 m
   Spend one to two nights at an intermediate elevation (2500–3000 m) before further ascent
   Above 3000 m, sleeping elevations should not increase by more than 300–400 m per night
   When topography or village locations dictate more rapid ascent, or after every 1000 m gained, spend
      a second night at the same elevation
Day hikes to higher elevations, with return to lower sleeping elevations help to improve acclimatization
Avoid alcohol consumption in the first 2 days at a new, higher elevation
Memorize the Golden Rules of Altitude

The Golden Rules of Altitude
   If you feel unwell at altitude, it is altitude illness until proven otherwise
   If you have symptoms of AMS, go no higher
   If your symptoms are worsening (or with HACE or HAPE), you must go down immediately

Note: Thanks to Dr David Shlim who originally popularized *The Golden Rules of Altitude*

High-altitude cough increases with elevation, and is a significant cause of morbidity among extreme-altitude climbers. The cough is paroxysmal, and sometimes sufficiently forceful to fracture ribs. Sputum is frequently purulent but fever is absent. Normal exercise performance, lack of dyspnea at rest, and absence of râles or cyanosis help distinguish high-altitude cough from HAPE. A concurrent sore throat is common, without any abnormal findings on exam.

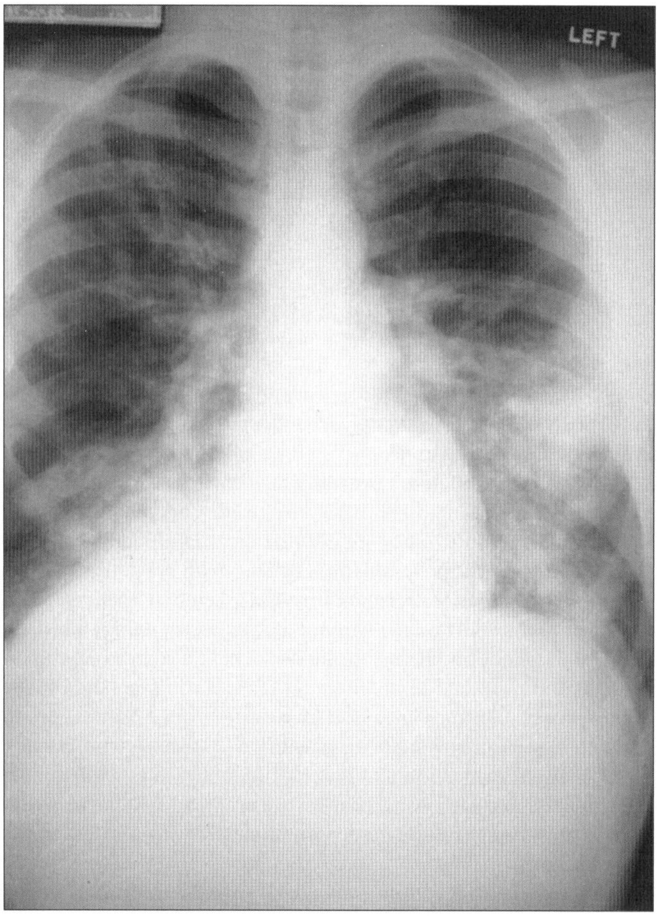

Figure 38.5 Chest radiograph of a patient with high-altitude pulmonary edema. Note the normal heart size and extensive bilateral infiltrates, consistent with high-altitude pulmonary edema. Courtesy of P. Hackett.[7]

The cause of high-altitude cough is unknown, but probably multi-factorial, including mucosal injury from hyperventilation of cold, dry air, airway inflammation, hypoxic bronchoconstriction, and alteration in the cough threshold. Treatment is symptomatic.

The intense UV light at high altitude when reflected off snow can easily cause damage to the unprotected eye, resulting in UV keratitis, also known as 'snow blindness.' Although it can be intensely painful and debilitating, it is self-limited and without sequelae, resolving in 24–48 h. Treatment consists of antibiotic ointment, analgesics and perhaps eye patching. This injury is entirely preventable by proper use of sunglasses with good UV absorbing characteristics. If sunglasses are not available, any material can be placed across the orbits, such as tape or cloth, with horizontal slits to provide essential vision.

EFFECT OF ALTITUDE ON COMMON MEDICAL CONDITIONS

Some pre-existing medical conditions may be exacerbated by high altitude, or affect one's ability to acclimatize or one's susceptibility to altitude illness. Though data are scant, case reports, and a growing number of controlled studies support some reasonable recommendations.[18] Table 38.5 lists common medical conditions in terms of risk stratification for moderate altitude, up to 3500 m; above this altitude data are very scarce.

Pulmonary and cardiac problems

Since the body increases ventilation in response to altitude exposure, any condition that impacts this response might be expected to impact high-altitude tolerance. Persons who have had carotid artery surgery or neck irradiation lose carotid body function and are therefore more hypoxic at high altitude and perhaps more susceptible to altitude illness.[19]

Patients with sleep disordered breathing (SDB) are often hypoxemic at low altitude, and might be much more hypoxemic at high altitude. Supplemental nocturnal oxygen may be advisable, at least for those who are hypoxic at low altitude. In addition, patients on Bi-PAP or CPAP need to make sure that their machine has pressure compensating features; machines without this can be off by as much as 10 cm H_2O pressure at 2500–3000 m.

Patients with hypoxemic lung disease are physiologically at a higher altitude (they have a decreased arterial PO_2) than healthy persons. On ascent to altitude, they might develop altitude illness at relatively lower altitudes, and their exaggerated hypoxemia would likely have other

Table 38.5	Advisability of ascent to high altitude (up to 3000 m)	
Minimal risk	Some documented risk – consider medical monitoring, availability of oxygen	Substantial risk – ascent not advised
Children and elderly Physically fit and unfit Obesity Chronic obstructive pulmonary disease (COPD), mild Asthma Hypertension, controlled Coronary artery bypass grafting, angioplasty, or stenting (without angina) Anemia, stable Migraine Seizure disorder, on medication Diabetes mellitus LASIK, PRK Oral contraceptives Pregnancy, low-risk Psychiatric disorders Neoplastic diseases Inflammatory conditions	Carotid surgery or irradiation Sleep-disordered breathing and apnea COPD, moderate Cystic fibrosis Hypertension, poorly controlled Coronary artery disease, with stable angina Arrhythmias, high-grade Congestive heart failure (CHF), compensated Sickle cell trait Cerebrovascular disorders Seizure disorder, not on medication Radial keratotomy Diabetic retinopathy	COPD, severe Coronary artery disease, with poorly controlled angina CHF, uncompensated Congenital heart disease ASD, PDA, Down's syndrome Pulmonary hypertension Pulmonary vascular abnormalities Sickle cell anemia (with history of crises) Pregnancy, high-risk

consequences as well. Surprisingly, only one field study has addressed the issue of COPD and altitude, and that was at the modest altitude of 1920 m.[20] Minor symptoms occurred, but patients did acclimatize in a similar period of time to otherwise healthy persons. Nonetheless, oxygen prescriptions should be provided to these travelers to be used if necessary. Mobile oxygen services are widely available in mountain resorts and communities, especially in developed countries. For those with COPD who are on oxygen at low altitude, the F_iO_2 needs to be increased by the ratio of the old barometric pressure over the new barometric pressure. Some experts have suggested that the arterial PO_2 at high altitude can be predicted from sea level hypoxic gas breathing, but testing is not generally available in travel clinics, and the correlation between altitude PaO_2 and symptoms is weak.

Patients with cystic fibrosis should be monitored at high altitude and might require oxygen therapy. Patients with cor pulmonale or pulmonary hypertension from any cause must be very cautious regarding altitude exposure both because of exacerbation of their disease and the risk of developing high-altitude pulmonary edema. Patients with pulmonary hypertension, if they do go to a high altitude, should be on supplemental oxygen and avoid exertion.

A number of studies have demonstrated that patients with allergic asthma do better at high altitude, because of decreased allergens and pollution, and decreased air density.[21] Exercise-induced bronchospasm (EIB) was not exacerbated at 1500 m,[22] but this needs to be studied at higher altitudes. Anecdotally, patients with EIB do well at high altitude, but as do all asthmatics, they need to be prepared in the event of an asthma attack. These patients should always have their inhalers on their person, not in a bag or pack from which they can be separated, and they should have a course of steroids to use as necessary. Asthma is not a contraindication to high-altitude exposure.

In high altitude permanent dwellers, blood pressure is lower compared to their low altitude counterparts.[23] Persons with hypertension who move to high altitude also benefit because of a slowing of progression and even regression of the disease after months to years in residence.[24] In contrast, acute induction to high altitude is associated with a slight increase in blood pressure in normotensives (5–10 mmHg in both systolic and diastolic pressure). In those with hypertension, the increase is on average similar as normotensives, but individual variation is great.[25] In terms of advising patients with hypertension traveling to high altitude, the first goal is to optimize blood pressure and medical regimen at low altitude. Because certain individuals with hypertension may have a significant increase in blood pressure on ascent to altitude, and since this abnormal response cannot be predicted, hypertensives should monitor their blood pressure, and consider taking with them additional medication. Calcium channel blockers may be superior to beta-blockers[26] and ACE inhibitors are not helpful.[27]

Limited available data do not suggest an increased risk of sudden cardiac death in travelers to high altitude locations.[28] Most often, individuals doing exercise at high altitude are accustomed to exercise at low altitude and are reasonably fit. However, exercise and hypoxia together seem to be more stressful than either alone (especially in someone who has not been exercising), and any male older than 40 contemplating a trip to high-altitude involving exercise should be conditioned to exercise prior to departing the lowlands.[29]

The slight increase of heart rate and systolic BP on ascent to altitude causes a small increase in myocardial work. As a result, patients with angina may have onset of ischemia at slightly lower workloads than at low altitude.[30] Patients with angina, then, should stay on their medications, reduce their activities somewhat during the first three days at altitude, and perhaps transiently increase their anti-anginal medication if they are more symptomatic than usual.

Patients with previous coronary artery bypass surgery, coronary artery angioplasty or stenting can be stratified into risk categories on the basis of symptoms and exercise treadmill test, as suggested by Hultgren.[31] These patients are considered at a high risk for an acute coronary event only if they have a positive exercise treadmill test. Alexander has proposed other criteria for high risk during altitude exposure: ejection fraction less than 35%, a fall in exercise systolic blood pressure, ST segment depression more than 2 mm at peak heart rate, and high-grade ventricular ectopy.[32]

Perhaps the most common scenario regarding CAD and altitude exposure in the setting of a travel medicine practice is how to assess risk in a male older than 50 years of age without known CAD but who has risk factors for CAD. The same risk stratification should be done as if the client were starting an exercise program at low altitude. For those with no symptoms, no evidence of CAD on ECG and no risk factors, an exercise treadmill test (ETT) is optional. For those without symptoms or evidence of CAD but one or more risk factors, a negative ETT assigns the person to the low risk category, and a positive ETT requires further evaluation. For males younger than 50 years of age with normal ECG and either none or one risk factor, ETT is not indicated.[31]

Limited data and anecdotal observations suggest that patients with active heart failure decompensate at high altitude, and should probably avoid altitude, whereas those with CAD without active CHF may tolerate moderate altitudes without difficulty.[33] Supplemental oxygen should be considered.

Children (and adults) with shunts such as atrial septal defect, patent ductus arteriosus, and those with Down's Syndrome with various defects have developed severe HAPE at modest altitudes of 2500 to 3000 m.[34] Children with a heart murmur that is not clearly benign should be evaluated prior to altitude exposure of more than one-day duration. Those with cyanotic congenital heart disease should avoid high altitude unless using supplemental oxygen.

Pulmonary hypertension (PHT) of any etiology is aggravated by altitude exposure. Unless the PHT is mild, ascent without oxygen should generally be avoided. Persons with other congenital or acquired abnormalities of the pulmonary circulation (e.g., congenital agenesis of a pulmonary artery, thromboembolic pulmonary vascular disease) are also at high risk of HAPE and should not go to a high altitude unless using supplemental oxygen.

Hematologic disorders

Sickle cell anemia, with a history of crises, is a contraindication to high altitude travel, unless with supplemental oxygen. Even the cabin pressure of commercial jets (1500–2500 m equivalent altitude) will precipitate crises in 20% of those with hemoglobin SS, SC and sickle-thalassemia. Persons with sickle cell trait are at small risk of splenic infarction or vaso-occlusive crisis at high altitude, although the exact risk is difficult to quantitate. Left upper quadrant pain at high altitude should raise the suspicion of splenic infarction because of the sickle cell trait, even in phenotypic Caucasians. Persons with low hemoglobin concentration seem to tolerate high altitude surprisingly well; they are not prone to altitude illness, although severe dyspnea and weakness may develop.

Neurologic disorders

Whether ascent to high altitude will increase the frequency or severity of headaches in lowlanders with migraine is not clear, but ascent can certainly trigger migraine in some persons, regardless of prior history of migraine at sea level. Observations have included new focal defects (visual and other) with migraine at altitude.[35,36] Migraine must be included in the differential diagnosis of AMS at altitude. Triptan medication (sumatriptan), often effective for migraine, has had mixed success with altitude headache, suggesting some overlap of mechanism between migraine and high altitude headache.

Some studies in the military have noted an increased incidence of ischemic stroke at high altitude and similar data need to be collected in tourists. Predisposing factors that may particularly contribute to cerebrovascular thrombosis at high altitude include dehydration, polycythemia and episodes of forced inactivity. Because of the significant cerebral vasodilatation on ascent to altitude, persons with cere-brovascular structural abnormalities, such as arteriovenous malformation or aneurysm, may be at risk for an untoward event. The experiences of one of the authors (PH) in the field suggest that it is crucial to advise patients with known cerebrovascular disorders to be very cautious at altitude, report any symptoms, and to perhaps avoid altitudes >3000 m.

Anecdotal reports indicate that ascent to high altitude may lower the seizure threshold. For those with new onset seizure, subsequent evaluation often reveals a previously unknown seizure focus. Persons with well-controlled seizure disorder at low altitude seem to be at no increased risk at altitude if they continue their medication. Individuals with a previous history of seizure but currently not on medication should consider anticonvulsant medication when traveling to high altitude, especially for extended trips to sleeping altitudes above 2500 m.

Diabetes

Some diabetics have more problems at high altitude. First episodes of diabetic ketoacidosis, and death, have been observed in fit trekkers at high altitude (Shlim, personal communication, 2002). None, however, had been monitoring their blood glucose. Expeditions that have included diabetics have had both positive and negative feedback regarding the health of these individuals.[37,38] Some of the problems encountered have included poorly functioning glucometers, possibly related to the cold, confusion between AMS and hypoglycemia, ketoacidosis secondary to nausea and vomiting of AMS, and remoteness of medical care. Taking extra time to acclimatize, keeping glucometers in special bags next to the skin, and active monitoring of glucose, fluid and carbohydrate intake can make a high altitude journey successful.

Ophthalmologic conditions

Since the cornea and the retina are the eye structures most affected by altitude, patients with corneal and retinal conditions may be at increased risk on ascent to high altitude. Persons who have had radial keratotomy no longer have structurally normal corneas, and on ascent to altitude, the typical altitude-related swelling of the cornea is not uniform. Central flattening and peripheral expansion can result in a significant hyperopic shift, up to three diopters. The problem is also likely to become worse with decreasing accommodation as one ages. In contrast, photorefractive keratotomy (PRK) is a laser technique that shaves the anterior cornea uniformly, without incisions, and does not produce significant visual change at altitude. There are no definitive data regarding altitude responses to laser in situ keratomileusis (LASIK) surgery. Those with a history of RK can correct their vision by bringing with them glasses of increasing plus power. No information exists as to whether high altitude may contribute to or aggravate the retinal microangiopathy of hypertension, diabetes, or other diseases. Patients with retinopathy should probably avoid very high sleeping altitudes, over 3500 m.

Contact lenses are used successfully at high altitude, though a few precautions are worth mentioning. Lenses when in a case with liquid should not be allowed to freeze. Good hygiene can be difficult and requires forethought. The contact wearer should bring backup glasses. Rewetting solution and fluoroquinolone drops should be in the person's kit, and should also be kept from freezing.

Obstetrics/gynecology

There are no data to suggest that women who use oral contraceptives at altitude have a greater risk of thrombosis than at sea level. Anecdotal evidence shared by those working at the high-altitude clinics in Nepal has substantiated this. Nonetheless, women on mountaineering expeditions might constitute a special case, because of prolonged exposure to extreme altitude and the attendant problems of dehydration, polycythemia, and immobility. Many expedition doctors recommend an aspirin a day for extreme altitude climbers, and especially for women using oral contraceptives.

There are no data to suggest an increase in pregnancy complications in lowland women who travel transiently to high altitude. Pregnancy of high-altitude dwellers is associated with complications such as pregnancy-associated hypertension, pre-eclampsia and infants small for gestational age, and it is reasonable to wonder whether this fact has any relevance for altitude sojourners. So far, for altitudes up to 2500 m, study results are reassuring. In addition, laboratory data in humans and animals have shown that fetuses with normal circulation tolerate levels of acute hypoxia far exceeding moderate altitude exposure. However, these studies also concluded that a compromised placental-fetal circulation could be unmasked at high altitude. Therefore, when advising a pregnant person contemplating travel to altitude, it seems prudent to make sure the pregnancy is normal. Remoteness from medical care, the quality of available medical care, the risks of trauma and other issues related to wilderness or developing world travel are probably more important than the issue of moderate hypoxia.

Psychiatric conditions

There are no data to help the physician advise persons with psychiatric illness about risks of altitude exposure. Studies demonstrating effects of hypoxia on mood and personality in normal subjects suggest that some changes take place starting at about 4000 m. An interview might help determine if the individual has realistic expectations of the trip and whether the particular trip is suitable for them. A frequent question is whether common psychiatric medications, such as lithium and selective serotonin reuptake inhibitors (SSRIs) are a problem at high altitude. Lithium excretion has been studied, and is normal at high altitude, but little else is known. This is an important area for further study. We advise patients on psychotropic medications to stay on them, to be careful to avoid altitude illness, and to descend if problematic symptoms develop. Again, what may be of greater concern than risk of altitude-related problems may be the remoteness of the environment for those who may suffer from anxiety or depression.

REFERENCES

1. Hackett PH, Roach RC. High-altitude medicine. In: Auerbach PA, ed. *Wilderness Medicine.* St. Louis, MO: Mosby; 2001:2–43.
2. Reeves JT, Groves BM, Sutton JR, *et al.* Operation Everest II: Preservation of cardiac function at extreme altitude. *J Appl Physiol* 1987; **63**:531–539.
3. Suarez J, Alexander JK, Houston CS. Enhanced left ventricular systolic performance at high altitude during Operation Everest II. *Am J Cardiol* 1987; **60**:137–142.
4. Maher JT, Jones LG, Hartley LH. Effects of high altitude exposure on submaximal endurance capacity of men. *J Appl Physiol* 1974; **37**:895–898.
5. Icenogle M, Kilgore D, Sanders J, Caprihan A, Roach RC. Cranial CSF volume (cCSF) is reduced by altitude exposure but is not related to early acute mountain sickness (AMS) (Abstract). In: Roach RC, Wagner PD, Hackett PH, eds. *Hypoxia: Into the Next Millennium.* New York: Plenum/ Kluwer Academic Publishing; 1999:392.
6. Sanchez Rio M del, Moskowitz MA. High altitude headache. In: Roach RC, Wagner PD, Hackett PH, eds. *Hypoxia: Into the Next Millennium.* New York: Plenum/Kluwer Academic Publishing; 1999:145–153.
7. Hackett PH, Yarnell PR, Hill R, *et al.* High-altitude cerebral edema evaluated with magnetic resonance imaging: clinical correlation and pathophysiology. *JAMA* 1998; **280**(22):1920–1925.
8. Dean AG, Yip R, Horrmann RE. High incidence of mild acute mountain sickness in conference attendees at 10 000 foot altitude. *J Wilderness Med* 1990; **1**:86–92.
9. Shlim DR, Meijer HJ. Suddenly symptomatic brain tumors at altitude. *Ann Emerg Med* 1991; **20**:315–316.
10. Reid L, Carter K, Ellsworth A. Acetazolamide or dexamethasone for prevention of acute mountain sickness: a meta-analysis. *J Wild Med* 1994; **5**(1):34–48.
11. Grissom CK, Roach RC, Sarnquist FH, Hackett PH. Acetazolamide in the treatment of acute mountain sickness: clinical efficacy and effect on gas exchange. *Ann Intern Med* 1992; **116**(6):461–465.
12. Hackett P. Roach RC. High-altitude illness. *N Engl J Med* 2001; **345**:107–114.
13. Sartori C, Allemann Y, Duplain H, et al. Salmeterol for the prevention of high-altitude pulmonary edema. *NEJM* 2002; **346**(21):1631–1636.
14. Nicholas RA, O'Meara PD. High-altitude syncope: History repeats itself. *JAMA* 1993; **269**:587.
15. Freitas J, Costa O, Carvalho MJ, Falcao Freitas A de. High altitude-related neurocardiogenic syncope. *Am J Cardiol* 1996; **77**:1021.
16. McFadden DM, Houston CS, Sutton JR, et al. High altitude retinopathy. *JAMA* 1981; **245**:581–586.
17. Butler FK, Harris DJ, Reynold RD. Altitude retinopathy on Mount Everest, 1989. *Ophthalmology* 1992; **99**(5):739–746.
18. Hackett P. High altitude and common medical conditions. In: Hornbein T, Schoene R, eds. *High Altitude: An Exploration of Human Adaptation.* NY, NY: Dekker; 2001:839–886.
19. Basnyat B, Litch J. Another patient with neck irradiation and increased susceptibility to acute mountain sickness (Letter). *Wilderness Environ Med* 1997; **8**:176.
20. Graham WG, Houston CS. Short-term adaptation to moderate altitude. Patients with chronic obstructive pulmonary disease. *JAMA* 1978; **240**:1491–1494.
21. Boner A, Comis A, Schiassi M, Venge P, Piacentini G. Bronchial reactivity in asthmatic children at high and low altitude. Effect of budesonide. *Amer J Resp Crit Care* 1995; **151**:1194–1200.
22. Matsuda S, Onda T, Iikura Y. Bronchial responses of asthmatic patients in an atmosphere-changing chamber. *Inter Arch Allergy Immunol* 1995; **107**:402–405.
23. Hultgren HN. Reduction of systemic arterial blood pressure at high altitude. *Adv Cardiol* 1979; **5**:49–55.
24. Mirrakhimov M, Winslow R. The cardiovascular system at high altitude. In: Fregly M, Blatteis C, eds. *Section 4: Environmental Physiology.* Oxford: Oxford University Press (American Physiological Society); 1996:1241–1257.
25. Savonitto S, Giovanni C, Doveri G, et al. Effects of acute exposure to altitude (3,460 m) on blood pressure response to dynamic and isometric exercise in men with systemic hypertension. *Am J Cardiol* 1992; **70**:1493–1497.
26. Deuber HJ. Treatment of hypertension and coronary heart disease during stays at high altitude (Abstract). *Aviat Space Environ Med* 1989; **60**:119.
27. Hultgren HN. Effects of altitude upon cardiovascular diseases. *J Wild Med* 1992; **3**:301–308.
28. Shlim DR, Gallie J. The causes of death among trekkers in Nepal. *Int J Sports Med* 1992; **13**(1):S74–S76.
29. Burtscher M, Philadelphy M, Likar R. Sudden cardiac death during mountain hiking and downhill skiing. *N Engl J Med* 1993; **329**:1738–1739.
30. Levine BD, Zuckerman JH. deFilippi CR. Effect of high-altitude exposure in the elderly: the Tenth Mountain Division study. *Circulation* 1997; **96**(4): 1224–1232.
31. Hultgren H. Coronary heart disease and trekking. *J Wild Med* 1990; **1**:154–161.
32. Alexander JK. Coronary heart disease at altitude. *Tex Heart Inst J* 1994; **21**:261–266.
33. Erdmann J, Sun KT, Masar P, Niederhauser H. Effects of exposure to altitude on men with coronary artery disease and impaired left ventricular function. *Am J Cardiol* 1998; **81**:266–270.
34. Durmowicz A. Pulmonary edema in 6 children with Down syndrome during travel to moderate altitude. *Pediatrics* 2001; **108**(2):443–447.
35. Murdoch DR. Focal neurological deficits and migraine at high altitude (Letter). *J Neurol Neurosurg Psychiatr* 1995; **58**:637.
36. Dietz TE, McKiel VH. Transient high altitude expressive aphasia. *High Alt Med Biol* 2000; **1**:207–211.
37. Moore K, Thompson C, Hayes R. Diabetes and extreme altitude mountaineering. *Br J Sports Med* 2001; **35**:83.
38. Admetlla J, Leal C, Ricart A. Management of diabetes at high altitude. *Br J Sports Med* 2001; **35**:282–283.

CHAPTER 39 Diving and Marine Medicine

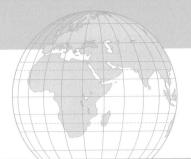

Alan M. Spira

KEYPOINTS

- The hazards of diving and the sophistication of advising travelers with regard to safety in diving are under appreciated by the travel medicine community

- Many with underlying chronic illnesses or with disabilities may dive as long as their medical problems are stable prior to diving and they have taken appropriate measures to ensure their safety

- Dysbarism is a term used to describe the pathology from the altered pressure during diving; the two forms are barotrauma that results from the uncontrolled expansion of gas within body compartments, and decompression sickness resulting from too rapid a return to atmospheric pressure

- Arterial gas embolism ranks second only to drowning as a cause of death in divers

- There are now many legitimate organizations and resources for travelers to contact in order to learn about diving, take lessons, and ask questions about risks of diving and their management

INTRODUCTION

In the past half-century, scuba (Self-Contained Underwater Breathing Apparatus) diving and cruising have become some of the fastest growing activities within the travel industry.[1] As travel health-care professionals, we need to understand the health hazards that accompany this sport. The underwater environment is not a forgiving one: decompression sickness, air emboli, trauma, oxygen toxicity, and other risks face those who enter this world. There are large numbers of people insufficiently trained in scuba and in poor physical condition, and has led to a rise in diving illnesses and injuries. Diving is a high-risk sport. Three to 9 deaths per 100 000 occur annually just in the USA alone, and diving morbidity survivors far exceed this.[2] The most common cause of death in divers is drowning (60%), followed by barometric-related illnesses. The type of gas under pressure and where the gas is in the body may lead to the development of barotrauma, decompression illness, narcosis and specific gas toxicity. Furthermore, there are underwater creatures that can harm or kill by any one of a number of means.

FITNESS/SAFETY TO DIVE

There are numerous factors that affect whether a traveler should dive including age, sex, training, concurrent medical illness or medications and certainly level of fitness; a few will be discussed in detail. See Table 39.1.[2–37]

Age

Elderly

Exercise capacity and strength diminish at around 30 years of age as does optimum oxygen utilization. Reflexes slow down, and endurance drops. Cardiovascular tone gradually diminishes with a resulting decreased maximum heart rate and maximum oxygen uptake; peripheral vascular resistance rises. Older divers need to have a more realistic appraisal of their abilities and not go beyond them. Age-related diseases such as cardiac disease, arthritis, diabetes mellitus, hypertension, and others can be relative or absolute contraindications to diving. Generally those older than 45 years of age, or having underlying chronic illness, should undergo a thorough physical examination that includes a stress EKG, and begin a comprehensive conditioning program before learning to dive.

Youth

The age normally allowed for diving certification is 12 years, although sport diving has no formal age restrictions. Among the prime considerations in allowing children to dive are the levels of physical and emotional maturity, proper eustachian tube function; strength to handle equipment, and equipment fit. Younger children do not have mature sinuses, pulmonary systems or eustachian tube function, all of which are essential to diving safely. Dental braces are not a contraindication to diving. There are insufficient data on the effect of diving on epiphyseal growth plates, so some authorities conservatively recommend waiting until long bone growth is nearly complete.[3]

Women divers and diving during pregnancy

Although there is no clear relationship between female sex and decompression sickness (DCS) risk, possible risk factors include higher body fat levels (on average 10% more than males), use of birth control pills, and menses.[4,5] At present, the incidence rate of DCS in women varies between 0 and 3 times that of men.[4] Menstrual patterns and ovulation do not seem to be affected by recreational diving. Also, there is no evidence that diving during menses increases the risk of shark attack. Menses can induce migraines however, and are themselves a relative contraindication to diving.

Pregnancy is a contraindication to diving.

Training

Proper training courses take several weeks of class work, pool training, and open-water work. Weekend-long certifying courses offered by tourist resorts are usually inadequate, creating divers with insufficient training and a false sense of ability.

Table 39.1	Contraindications to diving

ABSOLUTE CONTRAINDICATIONS

Medical condition	Comments
Seizure disorders	Exclusions include childhood febrile seizures, or those due to medication.[27] EEG may be done if indicated, particularly following head trauma[27]
Cardiovascular problems	Heart disease accounts for up to 25% scuba deaths;[26] myocardial infarction within previous year, symptomatic coronary artery disease, arrthymia, congestive heart failure, atrial septal defect,[28] history of cerebrovascular accident, uncontrolled hypertension[26, 30]
Psychological	Depression, schizophrenia, anxiety/panic disorder,[2, 36] history of psychosis or suicide attempts;[27] children with hyperactivity disorder require evaluation[3]
Sickle cell disease	Homozygous sicklers; risk to heterozygotes as well[3, 31]
Unexplained syncope	
Vertigo	
Inability to equalize middle ear pressures	Temporary contraindication if due to temporary condition
Chronic lung disease Previous POPS	Bullous, emphasematous lung disease, history of spontaneous pneumothorax
Tympanic membrane perforation	Unless healed or surgically repaired

RELATIVE CONTRAINDICATIONS

Asthma	Absolute contraindication for commercial and military; regulations vary country to country; controversial topic – control of illness, medications, maturity of diver[9-19]
Diabetes mellitus[19-25]	Depends on control and whether episodes of hypoglycemia occur
Cardiovascular problems	Those with mitral valve prolapse should have evaluation to make sure no concurrent problems[25]
Migraine headaches	Symptoms can be confused with those of DCS
Limited visual acuity	Contact lenses are safe;[33] post radial keratotomy patients should probably wait 2-5 months (mask squeeze prior to complete healing can be harmful);[34] no problem for those with previously repaired retinal detachments or controlled glaucoma[27, 35]
Post-operative patients	Usually safe to dive when asymptomatic; ostomies fine; those with airtight Kock pouches should not dive; those with breast implants may have higher risk of bubble formation, though appears tissue damage minimal[32]
Hernias	Inguinal or abdominal hernias must be repaired prior to diving
Disabilities	Depends on nature of disability; many who undergo proper training after screening do extremely well[37]
Infectious diseases	Active upper and lower respiratory infections are a temporary contraindication
Pregnancy	Controversial; most do not recommend.[5] May be higher incidence of DCS II;[4, 6, 7] no data to suggest greater risk of spontaneous abortion,[8] though fetal death in utero has been associated with diving[7]
Orthopedic injuries	Contraindicated until healed
Migraine headaches	Diving contraindicated during active headaches

Concurrent illnesses

There are several pathological conditions that can pose a risk when diving. Asthma, cardiovascular conditions, anatomical defects, respiratory conditions are among the most serious of these. General comments and advice are found in Table 39.1, but each case must be examined individually.

Often overlooked is the use of medications, which can have significant effects on a diver's health. Some medications cross the blood–brain barrier under hyperbaric conditions.[38] The short- or long-term use of certain medications may preclude diving, beta-agonists for acute asthma exacerbations, for example, or suppressive seizure therapy or anti-psychotics. For the majority of medications, whether a diver's safety and health would become compromised while taking medications, remains unclear.[39] It is recommended that any traveler or diver to test a medication prior to traveling to see whether they suffer any adverse effects, and if so, change to a different formulation (Table 39.2).[6,20,27,29,37,39–44]

Medical evaluation for diving

Certain levels of physical and psychological fitness are necessary in order to dive safely. Medical evaluation should be undertaken for *all* those who desire to scuba dive. Evaluation for the sport scuba diver should focus on the ears, sinuses, chest/lungs and heart as well as the psychological status. Because divers dive in pairs, a physically or mentally unstable person in the water will endanger two lives.

DIVING DISEASES

Barotrauma

Dysbarism is a general term used to describe the pathophysiology that develops from altered environmental pressure; it has two main forms: barotrauma from the uncontrolled expansion of gas within gas-filled body compartments and decompression sickness from nitrogen bubbles after breathing air under increased pressures.

Barotrauma is the damage or injury from a pressure gradient between the environment and air-containing body cavities distorting tissues. More than 90% of the human body is either water or bone, both of which are incompressible; thus the areas directly affected by pressure changes are those that are filled with air or gas. These sites include the middle-ear, the eustachian tube, the sinuses, the thorax and the gastrointestinal tract (Fig. 39.1). A mechanical problem arises when the pressures are not equal. This gradient may be positive during descent underwater with increasing pressure, or it may be negative during ascent towards the surface when the pressure within the body cavities is greater than the surrounding environment. It can occur in as little as 4 feet of depth without equalization (90 mmHg pressure gradient).

Otic

The middle ear is the most common body part affected by barotrauma, occurring in up to 30–60% of divers.[45] While the inner ear is fluid-filled, the middle and outer ear canal are air-filled. The middle ear is separated from the outer ear by the tympanic membrane; the only way air pressure can be equalized in the middle-ear is via the eustachian tube into the oropharynx (with an intact tympanic membrane).

Middle-ear squeeze occurs during descent (usually in the first 10 m) when the surrounding water pressure exceeds the air pressure in the middle-ear, deforming the tympanic membrane, and is dependent upon rate of descent and the state of eustachian tube function.

Table 39.2 Medications and diving

Medication or Medication Class	Comments
Sedatives/ Analgesics	Narcotics contraindicated;[6, 29] Nonsteroidal anti-inflammatory drugs safe[20] Acetominophen safe
Cardiovascular agents	Beta-blockers relatively contraindicated[29, 39, 40] ACE inhibitors, vasodilators use with caution Cardiac glycosides (digoxin) safe[20]
Birth control pills	Little data; appear safe[37]
Insulin	Insulin requirements may change; Lower levels of glucose/glucagon measured while diving in some diabetics
Antipsychotics	Contraindicated[20]
Anticonvulsants	Contraindicated[27]
Antimicrobial agents	Appear safe, unless underlying acute illness for which there is a contraindication[39]
Antimalarials	Mefloquine may induce adverse events confused with decompression sickness.[41] Test doses may be taken prior to diving to make sure tolerated.[39] Atovaquone-proguanil or doxycycline may be better choices depending upon the circumstances
Antihistamines/ decongestants	Depends on medication and underlying cause for its administration; pseudoephedrine may decrease risk and severity of otic barotraumas[42, 43]
Anti-motion sickness agents	Some may cause sedation; scopolamine has been used safely[44]

Equalizing the pressure is accomplished by opening the eustachian tubes via valsalvae maneuvers, so that pressurized air from the scuba tank present in the mouth can enter the middle-ear space. If middle-ear space air pressure does not rise to balance the pressure on the opposite side of the tympanic membrane, then vascular congestion, hemorrhage, pain and membrane rupture may follow. If the tympanic membrane ruptures and cold water rushes into the middle-ear, the vestibular system is disrupted and vertigo, nausea and vomiting may ensue. Underwater, this may be fatal. Hearing loss and tinnitus may also occur. Common causes for eustachian tube dysfunction are inability to equalize as rapidly as the pressure changes; acute or chronic inflammation; allergy; anatomical deformities; scarring of the tympanic membrane from otitis media during childhood; prolonged use of nasal drops; frequent or acute upper respiratory infection, nasal allergies, nasal obstruction, or ear disease; and excessive smoking. Underwater, if equalization is not successful, the diver must ascend until the level when equalization does occur and then re-descend slowly.

A reverse squeeze is a situation where the air pressure in the middle-ear exceeds that of the ambient water pressure; this may occur due to cerumen, stenosis, atresia, or tight-fitting hoods. Air in the middle-ear will expand (Boyle's Law) as one rises to the surface; if not relieved by opening the eustachian tube, the tympanic membrane will bulge outward as the water pressure decreases closer to the surface. This can also occur when a diver has taken decongestants, which wear off while underwater and edema returns to the eustachian tube and middle-ear before ascending. External ear squeeze occurs if the external auditory canal is obstructed, usually by cerumen, tight-fitting hoods or ear plugs. It may occur on ascent or upon descent. Pain, hemorrhage, and possible tympanic membrane rupture may occur.

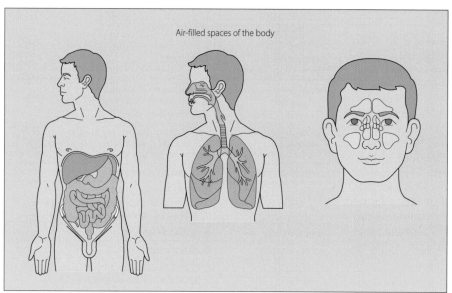

Figure 39.1 Air-filled spaces of the body. (From LifeArt, TechPool Industries, Cleveland OH)

Alternobaric vertigo is asymmetric, middle-ear barotrauma during ascent, where middle-ear air on either side cannot exit on ascent, leading to vertiginous symptoms. Vertigo may be stopped by halting the ascent or by descending again.

Inner-ear barotrauma can have severe consequences, from round or oval window rupture with possible perilymph fistulae, to cochlear hemorrhage with sensorineural hearing loss and vestibular dysfunction. Round window rupture from excessively negative middle-ear pressure is more likely with overly forceful valsalvae maneuvers that raise CSF and inner ear pressures. The round window is located between the middle and inner ears, and rupture often leads to tinnitus and decreased or loss of hearing. This should be suspected when tinnitus and vertigo are severe, or when associated with nerve deafness. It can mimic inner-ear DCS and recompression therapy may be necessary.[46]

Divers who develop otic barotrauma must be able to clear their ears before continuing a dive; if unable to do so, the dive must be aborted. If symptoms do not improve upon surfacing, referral to a otorhinolaryngologist is recommended.

Sinuses

The sinuses are the second most common sites of barotrauma. The ostia draining mucous from the various sinuses into the nasal cavity can easily clog with minimal inflammation, and if the pressure between the sinuses and the surrounding water does not balance, barotrauma results. During descent, when most sinus barotrauma occurs, the negative pressure in the sinus cavity can tear mucous membranes from the sinus walls, which may be both painful and bloody. During ascent, the membranes are compressed and the thin skeletal walls may deform.

Upper respiratory infections, sinusitis, nasal polyps, allergies, nasal spray overusage, cigarette smoking and anatomic abnormalities such as deviated septum can all predispose to sinus barotrauma.

Gastrointestinal

When a diver swallows air during ascent underwater, it will expand and stretch the intestines. This barotrauma of ascent may range from uncomfortable to painful, and may be associated with increased eructation and flatulence post-dive. This is most common in novice divers and those who drink carbonated beverages or eat heavily before diving. It also occurs with steep head-down angles during descent. Rarely, a hollow viscus over-distended by air, such as the stomach, may rupture from barotrauma.[47]

Dental

Barontalgia is also called Tooth Squeeze. It can arise from caries, defective caps or crowns, temporary fillings, root canal therapy, periodontal abscesses, maxillary sinus congestion or dental lesions.[48] By the gas laws, such teeth may actually implode during descent or explode upon ascent. The affected tooth is often sensitive, if not painful, and pain may be referred to the sinuses. The reverse is also possible; many cases of dental pain originating after flying or diving are actually sinus in origin. All divers should have good dental care and those with temporary crowns should not dive.

Mask

A mask squeeze develops as a result of not enough air pressure within the mask during descent. Because of lower pressure, facial tissue is pulled into the mask, and causes subconjunctival hemorrhage, periorbital petechiae or ecchymoses. Although it may appear frightening, it is not serious, and resolves spontaneously within days. Prevention involves exhaling slightly through the nose into the mask during descent.

Pulmonary over-pressurization syndrome

Pulmonary Over-Pressurization Syndrome (POPS) is a dysbaric illness that consists of four clinically important entities: arterial gas embolism, pneumomediastinum, pneumothorax and subcutaneous emphysema. It is due to pulmonary barotrauma (PBT) and is also called 'burst lung'. All may arise during ascent from gas expansion that exceeds the lung's elastic ability, resulting in alveolar tissue rupture.

In healthy lungs, POPS is most likely due to breath-holding during ascent or shooting to the surface too rapidly for adequate exhalation to be able to compensate for the degree of gas expansion. There are several pathological conditions as well, and may predispose patients to pulmonary barotrauma: chronic obstructive pulmonary disease; acute and chronic bronchitis; asthma with mucous plugging and bronchoconstriction; pulmonary blebs with spontaneous pneumothorax; pulmonary abscesses and restrictive lung diseases.

Arterial Gas Embolism (AGE) is the most important and feared form of POPS, ranking second only to drowning as a cause of death in divers.[49] Bubbles of expanding gas rupture from over-distended alveoli into the blood stream and become emboli, lodging in arterioles and capillaries where they produce damage. This condition becomes apparent rapidly (though presentation is occasionally delayed), usually within 10 minutes of surfacing, and often presents with bloody froth at the mouth or chest pain. Cardiovascular collapse may occur. Emboli lodge anywhere. The brain is the primary organ affected by AGE, the bubbles causing unconsciousness, vertigo, paraesthesias, convulsions, paralysis or paresis, nausea, visual disturbances, headache, confusion or even personality disorders, cerebrovascular accidents and seizures or death. In the heart, they may occlude coronary vessels leading to myocardial infarction; in the spinal cord paralysis and numbness may develop. Underwater, arterial gas embolism is often fatal. Dyspnea may or may not be present. AGE may occur in very shallow dives (a matter of feet or a meter) or very brief dives (lasting several seconds).[50] The laws of physics state that the risk of air embolism is actually greatest near the surface: a diver who inhales from a tank at a mere four feet underwater and holds his breath to the surface has enough of a pressure gradient developed to force air across the alveolar membrane into the blood. Therapy requires immediate recompression in a diving chamber. It can be difficult to find a chamber in remote or exotic locations. Divers should always check ahead of time with the dive resort or dive boat to see if one is readily accessible during their trip.

Decompression sickness, or 'the bends'

Air is 21% oxygen, the rest being primarily metabolically inert nitrogen, which is not metabolized and can accumulate in body tissues. The air a scuba diver inhales under pressure increases the amount of nitrogen absorbed into tissues. When this pressure is released, as during ascent from a scuba dive, nitrogen comes out of solution, and if it does so too rapidly, it forms bubbles in extravascular or intravascular tissues. Unlike air emboli, decompression sickness does not occur in shallow water and bubbles are primarily venous. Factors that lead to decompression sickness include too rapid an ascent rate, diving for too long or at too great a depth beyond the limits of no-decompression diving; dehydration; age; obesity; previous injury; alcohol; and cold. The pathophysiology of decompression sickness is very complicated, and includes gas uptake by tissues, gas elimination, and other poorly predictable factors that contribute to bubble formation.[51] Bubbles may cause vascular obstruction, distortion of tissues, denature proteins, aggregate red blood cells and platelets and activate the coagulation cascade with resulting disseminated intravascular coagulation. There are several tables that serve as guidelines for safe depth and time exposures to avoid decompression illness. These are not infallible, however, and one can stay within the limits of the United States Navy Dive Tables, even dive computers, and still develop decompression sickness (DCS).

Divers should make their deepest dives first. After a dive one does not unload all the gas; some remains in the tissues and one can thus enter the next dive with a gas handicap. Deepest dives first reduce the risk of DCS.

DCS syndromes include pain syndromes, spinal cord syndrome, cerebral syndrome, peripheral nerve syndrome and dysbaric osteonecrosis. Generally, the sooner the onset of symptoms after a dive, the more severe the case and often the more rapid the progression (Table 39.3).

DCS is a continuum of bubble-induced injury. For convenience it is often divided into the milder DCS I and the more serious DCS II, although both may occur concurrently. DCS I is defined as having

Table 39.3	Frequency of combined decompression sickness and arterial gas embolism in dive accidents[26,34]		
Symptoms		**Occurrence as first symptom (%)**	**Total occurrence (%)**
Neurologic			
Severe			
	Unconsciousness	2.1	4.2
	Paralysis	0.7	5.7
	Visual disturbance	0.0	6.4
	Difficulty walking	0.5	10.6
	Semiconscious	0.5	3.4
	Bowel control problem	0.0	1.6
	Speech disturbance	0.4	2.8
	Bladder control problem	0.0	3.0
	Convulsion	0.2	0.4
Mild/ambiguous			
	Numbness	21.7	83.4
	Dizziness	8.3	23.7
	Decreased skin sensation	0.5	10.8
	Personality change	0.2	3.2
	Reflex change	0.0	1.2
	Weakness	5.5	25.8
Neurologic total		40.6	81.3
Cardiorespiratory		1.8	4.1
Pain/skin/nonspecific symptoms			
	Pain	33.9	78.4
	Extreme fatigue	5.5	20.8
	Headache	8.1	22.6
	Nausea	3.4	15.9
	Pruritus	2.7	8.3
	Rash	0.7	4.4
	Restlessness	0.4	4.1
	Muscles twitch	0.4	3.5
	Hemoptysis	0.4	0.7
Pain/skin/nonspecific total		55.3	12.7
Ambiguous (Also possibly due to barotrauma)			
	Hearing loss	0.0	1.1
	Tinnitus	0.2	3.4
Other		2.4	6.2

skin rash or muscle and joint pains only. Dermatologic findings usually include pruritus and diffusely mottled erythematous patchy rashes, lividity, marbling, formication or local pitting edema. Musculoskeletal symptoms are the most common feature of decompression sickness. The pain is often vague and diffuse, ranging from superficial to deep and is often near a synovial joint. It is typically asymmetrical, and may shift in both character and temporal pattern. The upper extremities (shoulders followed by elbows and arms) are the most commonly affected. The pain is dull and difficult to localize. Erythema, swelling, tenderness and, increased pain with movement are not typical of DCS. However, inflating a blood pressure cuff over the affected area will often reduce pain when due to bubbles, but not when due to old sport or traumatic injuries.

Any neurological, cardiopulmonary or vestibular findings place the disease into 'type II'. Cases involving the brain, spinal cord, heart or lungs are medical emergencies, requiring urgent recompression. Type II DCS may be considered a diffuse, multifocal central nervous system disease. This can include paraesthesia, hypoesthesia, paresis, paraplegia, hemiplegia, urinary retention, impaired consciousness or ataxia, seizures, coma and death. Among the visual disturbances that occur from decompression sickness are blurred vision, scotomata, visual field defects and blindness, which can be confused with cerebral arterial gas embolism. Chest pain and cough may also occur with intrathoracic intravascular bubbling ('the chokes'). It has been suggested that repeated subclinical DCS from cerebral bubbles may also lead to a condition analogous to multi-infarct dementia.[53]

Spinal cord involvement is the site of the most frequent neurological DCS involvement, and symptoms often include lower back pain, abdominal pain, lower extremity weakness or paraesthesias; signs include paralysis and urinary retention. Symptoms tend to progressively wax and wane, and there may be residual symptoms even after recompression therapy.

Inner Ear DCS is also called vestibular decompression sickness (the 'staggers') and presents with vertigo, tinnitus, hearing loss, or nausea. If these symptoms occur upon descent then it is actually due to inner ear barotrauma and the dive must be aborted; oval and round window ruptures must be included in the differential diagnosis.

Those predisposed to symptomatic decompression illness include divers with a patent foramen ovale (PFO). Approximately 20% of the population have PFO while nearly 40% of DCS cases have PFO.[53] The lungs filter most of the small nitrogen bubbles formed in the venous system during a dive, and in turn limits tissue damage. However, if blood passes from right atrium to left atrium bypassing lung filtration then bubbles may enter the arterial system where they can do great damage as emboli.

The psychological profile of a diver may also contribute to the morbidity of DCS *vis-à-vis* delaying treatment. Denial is the most common factor, with others including anxiety, panic, embarrassment and depression, which prevent divers from presenting for therapy. Rationalization is also a common denominator in postponing evaluation; other divers perversely view being 'bent' as a measure of their experience or machismo. Many such divers refuse to seek medical care or if do, refuse recompression. They may return to diving prematurely, which can lead to further decompression illness or permanent disability.

Flying after diving

As discussed, barometric pressure plays a great role in the development of decompression illness. Modern aircraft keep cabin pressures to about 2400 meters (8000 feet), not sea level. If a diver were to board an aircraft right after ascending from a dive, that diver would be at risk for DCS from further decreasing atmospheric pressure (Boyle's Law: gas bubbles expand as pressure decreases). The probability of DCS drops asymptotically with time after diving; thus, authorities, such as the US Navy, the US Air Force and Divers Alert Network advise intervals of 12–24 h between one's last dive and flying.[53,54]

Returning to diving following diving trauma or illness

To return to diving, there should be no increased risk of recurrence or worsening of tissue damage.

Otic barotrauma
After middle-ear barotrauma, one may return to diving when the hearing is normal and the eustachian tubes can function. If one has suffered with some inner ear damage, however, then specialized evaluation and treatment is recommended before returning to diving.[50]

Pulmonary barotrauma
In the past, anyone who had suffered an AGE was proscribed from ever diving again because of the possibility of an undetected local air trapping in the lungs.[55] Theoretically, one should be able to dive again without a problem occuring, but one requires evaluation for

possible underlying pulmonary pathology.[56] The US Navy dive manual recommends not diving for at least 4 weeks after arterial gas emboli, assuming there has been complete resolution.[55]

Decompression sickness
The risk factors for DCS must be explored and, whether behavioral or anatomical/physiological. One may return to diving after 48 h following complete resolution with simple recompression if only joint pain occurred. If further recompression was required, return to diving should not be for at least 7 days after complete resolution. If there was any neurological involvement, one must wait a minimum of 4–6 weeks after complete resolution.[53]

OTHER PATHOLOGICAL DIVING CONDITIONS

Nitrogen narcosis

Nitrogen under pressure acts as a narcotic. N_2 has a high affinity for lipid, as with gaseous anesthetics. Its effect is related to depth and rapidity of descent, and tolerance develops with repeated deep dives. Jacques Cousteau called it the 'rapture of the deep'. Martini's Law of diving equates the effect of nitrogen as being equal to a single martini for every 50 feet of depth. Symptoms increase with exercise, cold, alcohol, and fear. Symptoms disappear upon ascent.

Hypoxemia and Hyperoxemia

Both hypoxemia and hyperoxemia are dangerous. Over exposure to pure oxygen can result in seizures at depths greater than 33 ft/10 m³, and short exposures of elevated pressure can induce other CNS effects such as abnormal vision, auditory changes such as tinnitus, irritability, dizziness and nausea. The first sign of oxygen toxicity underwater may be a seizure, with possible drowning or aspiration.

CO and CO_2 poisoning

Carbon monoxide (CO) and carbon dioxide (CO_2) may rarely contaminate scuba tanks. CO may enter a tank if using a compressor that pulls in air contaminated with exhaust fumes, oil vapors or hydrocarbon buildup. CO binds hemoglobin 230 times more effectively than does oxygen, rendering red blood cells incapable of tissue oxygen delivery. CO poisoning may present with headache, nausea, vomiting, arrhythmias, loss of consciousness or death. While at sea level the concentration of CO may be tolerable, under pressure it can easily become toxic.

Excessive CO_2 can also develop with breath-holding, defective compressors, or too large a dead space in the mouthpiece. The spectrum of illness includes depression, headache, dizziness, nausea, air-hunger and diminished vision at low levels, stupor and unconsciousness at intermediate levels, and muscle spasms, tetany and death at increased levels of CO_2 poisoning.

Marine trauma

There are several other important hazards to divers in the underwater world. Near-drowning, hypothermia, bite, wounds, and envenomations are also hazards of diving. These are discussed in other chapters in this text.

Diving Resources

There are several professional and recreational international diving and hyperbaric medicine diving organizations. These are listed in Table 39.4.

Table 39.4   Recreational and professional scuba diving organizations and resources

American Canadian Underwater Certification Inc. (ACUC)
1264 Osprey Drive, Ancaster, Ontario L9G 3L2 Canada
Tel: 905 648 5500
Fax: 905 648 5440
www.acuc.es

American Nitrox Divers International (ANDI)
74 Woodcleft Avenue, Freeport, NY 11520 USA
Tel: 516 546 2026
Fax: 516 5446 6010
www.andihq.com

British Sub-Aqua Club (BSAC)
16 Upper Woburn Place, London WC1 0QW, UK
or, Telford's Quay, Ellesmere Port, South Wirral,
Cheshire L65 4FY, UK
Tel: 44 0151 350 6200
Fax: 44 0151 350 6215
www.bsac.com/

The Canadian Association for Underwater Science
P.O. Box 13, Station C
St. John's NF A1C5H5 CANADA
www.caus.ca/

CMAS – Confed. Mondiale Des Activites Subaquatique
Viale Tiziana, 74 Rome, Italy
Tel: 011 39 6 36858480
Fax: 011 39 6 36858490
www.cmas2000.org

Defense and Civil Institute of Environmental Medicine (DCIEM)/Defence
    R&D Canada (DRDC Toronto)
1133 Sheppard Ave. West, Toronto, ON M3M 3B9 Canada
Tel: 1 416 635 2000
Fax: 1 416 635 2104
www.drdc-rddc.dnd.ca/success/diving_e.html

Divers Alert Network
The Peter Bennett Center
6W Colony Pl, Durham, NC 27705-9815 USA
Tel: 919 684 2948
www.diversalertnetwork.org
This organization is an international diving medicine network, which has
    taken a high profile lead in promoting dive medicine and dive safety.

Handicapped Scuba Association
1104 El Prado, San Clemente, CA 92672-4637
Tel./Fax: 714 498 6128
www.hsascuba.com/

International Association of Nitrox & Technical Divers (IANTD)
9628 NE 2nd, Suite D, Miami Shores FL 33138 USA
Tel: 305 751 4873
Fax: 305 751 3958
www.iantd.com/

Japan Underwater Leaders & Instructors Assoc.
Let's Bld 1F 2-18-5, Kohama-Nishi Suminoe-Ku,
Osaka, 559, Japan
Tel: 011 816 6751228
Fax: 011 816 6751229
www.julia.ne.jp/

Korea Underwater Association
Rm. 149, #2 Gymnasium, Oryun-dong, Songpa-ku, Seoul, 138-151, Korea
Tel: 011 822 4204293
www.kua.or.kr

International Diving Educators Association (IDEA)
P.O. Box 8427, Jacksonville, FL 32239 USA
Tel: 904 744 5554
Fax: 904 743 5425
www.idea-scubadiving.com/

MDEA - Multinational Diving Educators Assoc.
Box 3162, 200 22 Malmö, Sweden
Tel: +46 40 290240
Fax: +46 40 290240
www.mdeaeurope.com/

National Association of Underwater Instructors (NAUI)
P.O. Box 14650 Montclair, CA 91763 USA
Tel: 909 621 5801
Fax: 909 621 6405
www.naui.org

Professional Association of Diving Instructors (PADI)
1251 East Dyer Road, #100 Santa Ana, CA 92705
Tel: 714 540 7234
Fax: 714 540 2609
www.padi.com

Scuba Schools International (SSI)
2619 Canton Ct., Fort Collins, CO 80525 USA
Tel: 970 482 0883
Fax: 970 482 6157
www.ssiusa.com/

Sub-Aqua Association (SAA)
19 Harrier Drive, Canford Marina, Wimborne, Dorset BH21 1XG UK
Tel: 0151 287 1001
Fax: 0151 287 1026
www.saa.org.uk

South Pacific Undersea Medical Society (SPUMS)
c/o Australian and New Zealand College of Anaesthetists
630 St Kilda Road, Melbourne, Victoria 3004, Australia
www.spums.org.au/index.html

Surf Life Saving Australia
Locked Bag 2, Bondi Beach, NSW, 2026, Australia
Tel: 02 9130 7370
Fax: 02 9130 8312
www.slsa.asn.au/

Undersea and Hyperbaric Medical Society
10531 Metropolitan Ave, Kensington, MD 20895
Tel: 301 942 2980
Fax: 301 942 7804
www.uhms.org

YMCA National Scuba Program
5825-2A Oakbrook Parkway, Norcross GA 30093
Tel: 404 662 5172
Fax: 404 242 9059
www.ymcascuba.org/

REFERENCES

1. Travel Industry Association of America. Annual Statistics. Washington D.C.: Travel Industry Association of America; 1997.
2. Morgan WP. Anxiety and panic in recreational scuba divers. *Sports Med* 1995; **20**(6):398–421.
3. Dembert ML, Keith JF. Evaluating the potential pediatric scuba diver. *Am J Dis Child* 1986; **140**(11):1135–1141.
4. Robertson AG. Decompression sickness risk in women. *Undersea Biomed Res* 1992; **19**(3):216–217.
5. Cresswell JE, St Leger-Dowse M. Women and scuba diving. *BMJ* 1991; **302**(6972):1590–1591.
6. Taylor M. Women in Diving. In: Bove AA, Davis JC, ed. *Diving Medicine*, 3 edn. Philadelphia, PA: WB Saunders; 1997:89–107.
7. Ducasse JL, Izard P. Medical specificities of diving for women and children. In: Oriani G, Marroni A, Wattel F, eds. *Handbook of Hyperbaric Medicine*. Berlin: Springer; 1996:207–215.
8. St Leger Dowse M, Bryson P, Gunby A, Fife W. Men and women in diving: a retrospective survey: rates of decompression illness in males and females: Data from 142 dived pregnancies. *Undersea Hyperbaric Med* 1995; **22**(suppl):54.
9. Weiss LD Van, Meter KW. Cerebral air embolism in asthmatic scuba divers in a swimming pool. *Chest* 1995; **107**(6):1653–1654.
10. Neumann TS, Bove AA, O'Connor RD. Kelsen SG. Asthma and diving. *Ann Allergy* 1994; **73**(4):344–350.

11. Farrell PJ, Glanvill P. Diving practices of scuba divers with asthma. *BMJ* 1990; **300**(6718):166.

12. Anonymous. *Pressure.* The Undersea & Hyperbaric Medical Society 1995; **24**:5.

13. Curson KS, Dovenbarger JA, Moon RE, Hodder S, Bennett PB. Risk assessment of asthma for decompression illness. *Undersea Biomed Res* 1991; **18**(**suppl**):16.

14. National Institutes of Health. *Global Initiative for Asthma.* Global strategy for asthma management and prevention-NHLBI/WHO workshop report; publication number 95-3659. Bethesda: National Institutes of Health; 1996.

15. Nat Asthma Educ Prog. *Executive Summary; Guidelines for the diagnosis and management of asthma, Publication No. 91-3042A.* Washington D.C.: US Dept of Health and Human Services; 1991.

16. Bove AA. Observations on asthma in the recreation diving population. *So Pac Underwater Med Soc Jour* 1995; **25**(4):222–225.

17. Farrell PJ. Asthmatic divers in the UK. *So Pac Underwater Med Soc Jour* 1995; **25**(1):22.

18. Wilmshurst P. Medical standards with the British Sub Aqua Club for those suffering from various disorders. *So Pac Underwater Med Soc J* 1994; **18**(4): 153–156.

19. Bove AA. Medical aspects of sport diving. *Med Sci Sports Exer* 1996; **28**(5): 591–595.

20. Kindwall EP. The use of drugs under pressure. In: Kindwall EP, ed. *Hyperbaric Medicine Practice.* Best Publishing: Flagstaff; 1995:247–259.

21. Mebane C. The Aging Diver. Alert Diver. Durham, N.C: *Divers Alert Network*; 1993: 6-7.

22. Edge CJ. Medical aspects of scuba diving: Standards for diabetic divers are workable. *BMJ* 1994; **309**(6950):340.

23. Edge CJ, Grieve AP, Gibbons N, O'Sullivan F, Bryson P. Control of blood glucose in a group of diabetic scuba divers. *Undersea Hyperbaric Med* 1997; **24**(3):201–207.

24. Kruger DF, Owen SK, Whitehouse FW. Scuba diving and diabetes. Practical guidelines. *Diabetes Care* 1995; **18**(7):1074.

25. Lerch M, Thurm U. Beyond the frontier – IDDM and Scuba diving – a field study. *Undersea Hyperbaric Med* 1996; **23**(**suppl**):15–16.

26. Schwartz K. Age and Diving. Alert Diver. Durham, N.C: Divers Alert Network; September/October 1996: 36-39.

27. Davis JC. Medical Examination of Scuba Divers, 2 edn., *Medical Seminars Inc.* Medical Seminars: San Antonio; 1986.

28. Bove AA. Diving by the elderly and the young. In: Bove AA, Davis JC, eds. *Diving Medicine*, 3 edn. Philadelphia, PA: WB Saunders; 1997:108–113.

29. Harrison LJ. Drugs and diving. *J Fla Med Assoc* 1992; **79**(3):165–167.

30. Klaus D. Management of hypertension in actively exercising patients. Implications for drug selection. *Drugs* 1989; **37**(2):212–218.

31. Lowbeer L. Complications of sickle cell trait. *JAMA* 1983; **250**:360–361.

32. Vann RD, Riefkohl R, Georgiade GS, Georgiade NG. Mammary implants, diving and altitude exposure. *Plast Recon Surg* 1988; **81**(2):200–203.

33. Brown MS, Siegel IM. Cornea-contact lens interaction in the aquatic environment. *CLAO J* 1997; **23**(4):237–242.

34. Uguccioni D. Diving after Radial Keratotomy. Alert Diver. Durham, N.C: *Divers Alert Network*; March/April 1996:24-25.

35. Kalthoff H, John S, Scholz V. Problems of intraocular pressure in scuba diving. *Klin Mon Augenheilkd* 1975; **166**(4):488–493.

36. McAniff JJ. *US Underwater Diving Fatality Statistics.* Rhode Island: National Underwater Accident Data Center, University of Rhode Island; 1990.

37. Williamson JA, McDonald FW, Galligan EA, *et al.* Selection and training of disabled persons for scuba-diving. Medical and psychological aspects. *Med J Aust* 1984; **141**(7):414–418.

38. Chryssanthou C, Graber B, Mendelson S, Goldstein G. Increased blood–brain barrier permeability to tetracycline in rabbits under dysbaric condi-tions. *Undersea Biomed Res* 1979; **6**(4):319–328.

39. Edmonds C. Drugs and Diving. In: Edmonds C, McKenzie B, Thomas R, eds. *Diving Medicine for Scuba Divers.* Locust Valley, N.Y.: Aquaquest Publi-cations; 1992:414–422.

40. Arnold RW, Nadel ER. The effect of peripheral vasodilators on the human diving response. *Alaska Med J* 1993; **35**(2):204–208.

41. Wright D. Mefloquine and scuba diving. *N Z Med J* 1995; **108**(1013):514.

42. Brown M, Jones J, Krohmer J. Pseudoephedrine for the prevention of barotitis media: a controlled clinical trial in underwater divers. *Ann Emerg Med* 1992; **21**(7):849–852.

43. Sipenen SA, Kulvik M, Leinio M, *et al.* Neuropyschologic and cardiovas-cular effects of clemastine fumarate under pressure. *Undersea Hyperbaric Med* 1995; **22**(4):401–406.

44. Williams TH, Wilkinson AR, Davis FM, Frampton CMA. Effects of transcu-taneous scopolamine and depth on diver performance. *Undersea Biomed Res* 1988; **15**(2):89–98.

45. Koriwchak MJ, Werkhaven JA. Middle-ear barotrauma in scuba divers. *J Wilderness Med* 1994; **5**:389–398.

46. National Oceanic and Atmospheric Administration (NOAA). Diving Manual, Ch. 5. Silver Spring: US Department of Commerce; October 1991.

47. Nachum Z, Shupak A, Spitzer O, *et al.* Inner ear decompression sickness in sport compressed-air diving. *Laryngoscope* 2001; **111**:851–856.

48. Cramer FS, Heimbach RD. Stomach rupture as a result of gastrointestinal barotrauma in a scuba diver. *J Trauma* 1982; **22**(3):238–240.

49. Neblett LM. Otolaryngology and sport scuba diving. Update and guidelines. *Ann Otol Rhinol Laryngol Suppl* 1985; **115**:1–12.

50. Neumann TS. Pulmonary Barotrauma. In: Bove AA, ed. *Bove & Davis's Diving Medicine*, 3 ed. Philadelphia, PA: WB Saunders; 1997:176–183.

51. Huss JH. Medical aspects of skin and scuba diving. *J Sch Health* 1972; **42**(4):238–242.

52. Alexander J. *Hyperbaric Oxygen Therapy Training Course Manual.* Los Angeles: Department of Hyperbaric Medicine, Northridge Hospital Medical Center; 1993.

53. Wilmshurst P. Brain Damage in Divers. *BMJ* 1997; **314**(7082):689–690.

54. Flagstaff, AZ. *U.S. Navy Divers Handbook.* Flagstaff: Best Publishing; 1996:80.

55. Furry DE, Reeves E, Beckman E. Relationship of scuba diving to the devel-opment of aviators' decompression sickness. *Aerosp Med* 1967; **38**(8):825–828.

56. Davis JC. Definitive treatment of decompression sickness and arterial gas embolism. *Hyperbaric and Undersea Medicine.* San Antonio: Medical Seminars Inc.; 1981.

57. Davis JC, ed. *The Return to active diving after decompression sickness or arterial gas embolism*; Publication number 41 (RW) 11-13-80. Bethesda: The Undersea & Hyperbaric Medicine Society; 1980:13–80.

CHAPTER 40   Extremes of Temperature and Hydration

Yoram Epstein and Daniel S. Moran

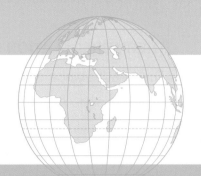

KEYPOINTS

- Heat stress is determined not only by the ambient temperature, but also by the level of solar radiation and humidity

- Heat adaptation, or acclimatization, can be achieved within a few weeks of exposure; men typically acclimatize better to hot, dry conditions while women to hot, wet conditions

- The time it takes for cold adaptation has not yet been well defined; behavioral adaptation, including modification of shelter, clothing, caloric and fluid intake, is more significant in reducing the hazards of cold

- Prevention of exertional heatstroke requires the following of a variety of guidelines; treatment is complex, but most survive

- Intensive treatment of deep hypothermia can be life-threatening in and of itself; definitive treatment should be commenced at a medical center equipped with intensive care facilities

INTRODUCTION

The basic concept of homeostasis requires stability of the 'inner environment'. Body temperature and water are among the main factors that must be constantly controlled to achieve this stability. The human body, being homeothermic, maintains a fairly constant internal temperature regardless of environmental temperature by adjusting the rate of heat loss to the environment to the rate of heat generated by metabolic processes. The volume of total body fluids is also regulated within very narrow limits.

Maintaining constant body temperature requires the involvement of several thermoregulatory mechanisms. The most important is the vasomotor regulatory system, through which blood flow to the skin is regulated. When vasomotor activity alone cannot regulate body temperature, other physiological systems are recruited, such as shivering, when body temperature is reduced, as well as sweating, when body temperature is elevated.

'Normal' body temperature

The phrase 'normal' body temperature, although commonly used, is a misnomer. Body temperature is dependent on various factors such as site of measurement, metabolic state, time of the day, age, and for women, the period during the ovulatory cycle. At rest, body-core temperature ranges from 36–37.5°C. The limits for body temperature to maintain efficient thermoregulation are 35–40°C. Frequently, outdoor activities in a warm climate under high solar radiation may result in hyperthermia. During exhaustive exercise, body-core temperature may increase to 40°C without exhibiting any adverse effects. Likewise, exposure to cold environments may cause body temperature to equilibrate at the lower end of the acceptable limit.[1]

Monitoring body-core temperature

Overall, the status of the thermoregulatory system can be determined by measuring body-core temperature. This requires an accurate measuring instrument and the measuring site should reflect actual body-core temperature.

Measuring instruments

The mercury-in-glass and liquid crystal thermometers, commonly in use, have a number of disadvantages, including a long equilibrium time, a tendency to break, loss of accuracy over time, reading of maximal temperatures, and unsuitability for monitoring extreme hyperthermia or even mild hypothermia because of their upper, and especially lower, limits. 'Tympanic' infrared thermometers respond very quickly but they usually do not accurately reflect body-core temperature because they measure aural canal temperature, which is influenced by environmental conditions, and not direct tympanic temperature. Digital clinical thermometers are simple, available commodities and may be used with relatively high precision (± 0.1°C) in the range of 32–42°C. At extreme temperatures, however, especially at the lower range, measurements tend to be inaccurate and should be regarded as such. The advantages of electronic thermometers are that they contain an easily read digital display, which reduces operator error. They also tend to have shorter equilibration times than mercury-in-glass thermometers. Electronic thermometers, which use either thermistors or thermocouples as sensors, have the requisite degree of wide range accuracy, are very flexible, and are easily applied.

Measurement sites

Non-invasive measurement sites, including the axilla, oral cavity and forehead reflect surface temperatures and are highly influenced by the environment. Minimally invasive sites including rectal, esophageal, and tympanic temperatures, accurately reflect body-core temperature; however, tympanic and esophageal temperatures are less convenient to obtain.

Under emergency conditions (heatstroke, hypothermia), which require continuous accurate monitoring of body-core temperature, it is advisable to measure rectal temperature (at around 10 cm beyond the anal sphincter) by an electronic thermometer.

THERMOREGULATION

The heat balance equation

The delicate balance between heat accumulation in the body and its dissipation can be depicted in a simplified version of the second law of thermodynamics, as follows:

$$\Delta S = M_{net} \pm (R + C) - E$$

where: ΔS = changes in the body's heat content; M_{net} = metabolic heat production; (R+C) = dry heat exchange; E = evaporative heat loss.

Ambient conditions (dry air temperature, mean radiant temperature, and water vapor pressure, as well as clothing) affect the heat flux to and from the body by their influence on dry (sensible) heat exchange and wet (insensible) heat loss.

Metabolic heat production

Metabolic heat production is the fraction of energy from the total body metabolism, which is turned into heat. Since work efficiency is 20–30%, the fraction of energy that is produced as heat ranges from 70–80% of total metabolism.

Heat production at rest is about 1 Met (~50 kcal/m² body surface area/h). Moderate work intensity results in double this heat production level, whereas hard work intensity triples it (Table 40.1). The sustainable 'voluntary hard work' level is about 5 Met (425 kcal/h; 500 W).

Dry heat exchange

Conduction

Conduction is heat exchange between two surfaces in direct contact. Since the contact areas are usually small (e.g., feet contact with the ground), heat exchange by conduction is relatively low. It becomes significant when one lies uninsulated on cold ground, especially if under the influence of vasodilating drugs or alcohol.

Convection

Convection refers to heat transferred from a surface to a gas or liquid. The rate of heat exchange by convection depends on many variables (i.e., density of the medium of air versus water). During cold-water immersion, heat loss occurs at a faster rate than standing nude in cold air because of the much higher heat capacity (1000 versus 0.29 cal/L/°C) and the higher thermal conductivity ($1.4 \cdot 10^{-3}$ versus $5.7 \cdot 10^{-5}$ cal/cm per °C) of water as opposed to air.

Radiation

Radiation refers to the transfer of heat by electromagnetic waves (at the spectrum of infrared wavelength). Radiant heat transfer is very much dependent on the insulation from the environment. A major source of heat gain in hot climates is solar load (up to 250 kcal/h), which can be significantly reduced (by more than 50%) by wearing light clothing.

Collectively, dry heat exchange is directly related to the effective skin area and temperature gradient between the environment and the skin, and inversely related to the thermal insulation of clothing (total insulation of clothing and trapped air layers), corrected for air and body movements.

For an average adult wearing light clothing under mild air movements, a 1°C change in ambient temperature above or below 31°C measured in the shade or 36°C measured in the sun will result in a respective change in body heat content of ±15 kcal/h, respectively.

Evaporative heat exchange

In a thermally neutral environment, sweating does not occur and evaporation accounts for only 15% of total heat loss. Of this, approximately half is due to evaporation from the respiratory tract. When the body is unable to maintain thermal equilibrium by dry heat exchange, however, and body-core temperature thus rises, sweating permits heat loss by vaporization of water.

Evaporation of sweat is the major means of dissipating excessive heat accumulated in the body (evaporation requires 580 kcal/L) but, evaporation is limited by environmental conditions (mainly by the vapor pressure gradient between the skin and the environment). Ambient air, humidity, clothing vapor resistance, and wind velocity determine the maximal evaporative capacity of the environment. In practice, under the same ambient temperature, the lower the humidity, the higher the evaporation; the higher the clothing permeability, the higher the evaporative capacity.

Although it is unusual, the term E in the heat balance equation can become positive (heat is absorbed by the body). This occurs during airway rewarming of hypothermic patients, when water saturated oxygen is inhaled at 43°C; in this situation, water vapors condense and deliver 580 kcal/L of water that is formed.

Environmental conditions assessment

The ability to work in a hostile environment is inversely related to the prevailing environmental climatic stress; the greater the environmental stress, the shorter the tolerance time and the greater the risk for injury. Therefore, safety regulations concerning work intensity, duration, and work-rest cycles in a hostile climate depend on proper assess-ment of the environmental stress.

Heat stress

Ambient temperature by itself does not provide enough information about the prevailing climatic stress. This is better determined by a combination of temperature, solar radiation, and humidity.

The most common index to determine environmental heat load is the Wet Bulb Globe Temperature (WBGT), which combines ambient temperature, wet-bulb temperature (i.e., the temperature of an aspirated thermometer covered with a wet sleeve). The recorded temperature refers to the lowest temperature to which it can be cooled by evaporating water. This measurement is compared with that read by the 'dry thermometer', to estimate the ambient humidity, and black globe temperature, the temperature inside a blackened hollow sphere of thin copper with a given diameter that is used to estimate total heat exchange by radiation and convection. This is quite cumbersome and is rarely used. A comparable index is the Discomfort Index (DI), which is easier to calculate and combines only ambient temperature and wet-bulb temperature. Based on these indices, safety guide-

Table 40.1	Metabolic heat production		
	kcal/h	Watt	Met
Sleeping	70	85	0.8
Rest	90	105	1.0
Sitting	110	125	1.2
Light work[a]	145	170	1.6
Walking[a]	360	420	4.0
Running[a]	900	1050	10.0

[a]Average values

lines have been issued regarding the risk encountered while working in the heat (Fig. 40.1).[2, 3]

Cold stress

Determination of cold stress is much more difficult than assessment of heat stress. Ambient temperature, wind velocity, and precipitation are variables in this respect. The Wind Chill Index (WCI), which estimates the convective cooling power of the environment, is used to assess cold intensity. The calculated 'equivalent temperature', which reflects the lowering effect of wind on ambient temperature, is the link to the perception of cold (Fig. 40.2). Levels of cold intensity may vary according to adaptation and acquaintance with the hazards of cold. Wind chill warnings will, therefore, be given in milder conditions to people who are less accustomed to the cold than to those who are more adapted to the cold.[4, 5]

Acclimatization

Adaptive changes, which occur when an individual undergoes prolonged exposure to a stressful environment (heat, cold, or altitude), and reduce the physiological strain produced by such environment, are regarded as 'acclimatization'. (The term 'acclimation' is used if such physiological adaptations have been achieved in a controlled laboratory setting). The specific adaptive habituations result in an increasing tolerance to the stressful environment and reduce the dangers to health.

Heat adaptation

Acclimatization to heat is specific to the climatic conditions to which a person is exposed, and can be achieved within a few weeks of exposure. (Acclimation to heat can, under controlled laboratory conditions, be attained within 5–10 days by a 2 h daily exposure to an exercise-heat stress). There are some differences in the dynamics of acclimatization to hot/wet and hot/dry climates. While in hot, dry climates, sweating is the predominant effector mechanism, in hot, wet climates, it is the cardiovascular system. There are also gender differ-

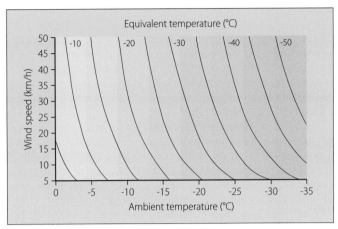

Figure 40.2 The wind chill index chart. The chilling effect of the wind in combination with a low temperature is expressed as the 'equivalent temperature'. Health concern is related to habituation to cold, accordingly thresholds are defined as follows:

	Habituated	Non-habituated
Low	−10 °C	−5 °C
Moderate	−25 °C	−10 °C
High	−45 °C	−25 °C
Extreme	−60 °C	−35 °C

ences in the ability to acclimate to these conditions: while males tend to acclimate better to hot/dry conditions and females acclimate better to hot/wet climatic conditions. The traditional hallmarks of heat acclimatization are lower thermal and cardiovascular strain, manifested primarily by reduced body-core temperature and heart rate, and an increase in sweating following exercise-heat stress. Acclimatization to heat has been found to be very effective in alleviating symptoms related to heat stress. To prevent excessive heat stress and guard against heat injuries, the non-acclimated individual should remember:[6, 7]

- Acclimatization to heat is time-dependent. Working in the heat should be graded in terms of duration and intensity.
- During the first days, a sense of fatigue, headaches, and lassitude will be present. These are 'warning signs'. Rest periods should be lengthened and fluid consumption should be enhanced.
- Within a few days, subjective feeling is improved and more physical work can be done.
- Depending on physical fitness and age, acclimatization to heat at a level that enables adequate performance will take 5–10 days.
- Acclimatization to hot/wet climate takes longer than that to hot, dry climate.

Cold adaptation

The most common observation in regard to adaptation to cold is the great drop in body-core temperature before the onset of shivering. In addition, a metabolic cold adaptation has been suggested, which results in increased heat production, possibly by a shift from shivering to non-shivering thermogenesis. Nevertheless, the time course to achieve cold adaptation has not yet been defined and may prove to be long. The practical advantages provided by these adaptations in terms of conservation of body heat are questionable. In this sense, behavioral adaptation (e.g., seeking shelter, proper clothing, adjusting caloric and fluid intake, and building fires) is much more significant in reducing the hazards of cold.[8]

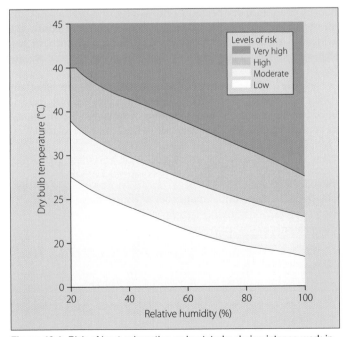

Figure 40.1 Risk of heat exhaustion or heatstroke during intense work in the heat. (Adjusted to the ACSM Position Stand: the prevention of thermal injuries during distance running[2]).

Fever

Normally, body temperature is determined by the delicate balance between heat gain and heat loss, described in thermodynamic terms by the heat balance equation. Under these conditions, heat flux does not affect the 'central integrator'. Fever, in contrast, represents a state in which the body temperature 'set point' has been reset from its base value of 37 °C to a higher value.

The effect of pathogens on regulated temperature occurs through the interaction of components within the immune system. This interaction stimulates the production of pyrogenic cytokines, which in turn induce the release of prostaglandin E_2, leading to an increase in the body's 'set point' temperature. As a result, the body responds by elevating metabolic heat production (shivering).

Antipyretics block fever by inhibiting prostaglandin synthesis. This in turn shifts the 'set point' temperature to the left, back to its natural value, and the body responds by enhancing heat dissipation (sweating). Therefore, antipyretic therapy, which may prove to be effective in febrile conditions, is totally ineffective in reducing body-core temperature that results from a thermodynamic imbalance. Furthermore, heatstroke, when the liver becomes extremely vulnerable, treatment with antipyretic drugs (e.g., paracetamol) is dangerous and life threatening.[1]

Steam baths and saunas

Steam baths and saunas are traditional forms of public bathing recognized for over 2000 years. They have become very popular in the modern era at leisure-time facilities and among travelers visiting those areas where this is still considered part of the traditional way of life.

The common belief that sauna bathing has a therapeutic application, besides being a short-term muscle relaxation, has not been established. On the contrary, the severe heat stress in the sauna (~100 °C; ~40% relative humidity) and the steam bath (~50 °C; ~100% relative humidity) results in a significant physiological strain, especially of the cardiovascular system. This is exhibited by an increase in heart rate, stroke volume, and blood pressure. In addition, a steep increase in body core temperature is evident and the excessive sweating enhances the danger of dehydration.

For most people, sauna bathing, as well as steam baths, is safe, unless misused or abused. Those who wish to bathe in a sauna or in a steam bath should be aware of the potential risk involved. Cardiac patients, hypertensive patients, pregnant women and children are especially vulnerable. Others should:

- Limit the exposure to less than 15 min
- Drink water to reduce dehydration
- Not bathe immediately after physical exertion
- Not consume alcohol during bathing (alcohol increases the risk of arrhythmia and hypotension).

HEAT RELATED ILLNESSES

Heatstroke

Heatstroke is the most serious of the syndromes associated with excess body heat. It is defined as a condition in which body temperature is elevated to such levels that it becomes a noxious agent, causing damage to the body's tissues and giving rise to a characteristic multi-organ clinical and pathological syndrome. The severity of the illness depends on the degree of hyperthermia and its duration. Heatstroke is an extreme medical emergency that can be fatal if not diagnosed and treated promptly.

The literature differentiates between two entities of heatstroke: exertional heatstroke (EHS) and classical heatstroke. EHS occurs when excess heat, generated by muscular exercise, exceeds the body's ability to dissipate it. Patients are typically young and very active physically. Its occurrence is sporadic. Classical heatstroke, which will not be discussed in this chapter, is a common disorder of the elderly during heat waves and occurs in the form of an epidemic.[3, 6, 7]

Pathophysiology

Heatstroke usually occurs when extreme heat stress leads to marked hyperthermia after thermoregulation is subordinated to circulatory and metabolic demands. Collapse occurs because of central nervous system and other secondary non-cardiovascular effects of severe hyperthermia. The latter, such as erythrocyte sphering and disseminated intravascular coagulation (DIC), results in microthrombosis and coagulative necrosis, causing diffuse neurological and other damage leading to death.

Diagnosis

Prolonged exertion, warm climate, very high body-core temperature (above 40.6 °C), and dry skin, and are typically linked with EHS, are misleading yardsticks.

The performance of strenuous physical exercise in the heat has been notorious as a cause for heatstroke. In many instances, however, EHS occurs within the first 2 h of exercise and not necessarily at high ambient temperature.

Body-core temperature of 40.6°C, as a critical temperature to define heatstroke, is arbitrary. In many instances, lower temperatures are recorded because the first measurements are delayed, performed by untrained individuals, or measured incorrectly.

At the stage of collapse, profuse sweating is still likely to be present, unless heatstroke develops in an *a-priori* anhidrotic subject. Dry skin might be evident either in situations where the climate is very dry and sweat evaporates very easily, or when heatstroke coincides with a severe degree of dehydration.

Early presentation

The presentation of EHS is usually acute. Dizziness, weakness, nausea, confusion, disorientation, drowsiness, and irrational behavior are prodromal symptoms, lasting from minutes to hours, and evident in about 25% of all casualties. Failure to recognize the first signs of disability might lead to misassessment of the true physiological status.

The early clinical signs of heatstroke are nonspecific; therefore, any systemic disease or condition (Table 40.2) that presents with increase in body temperature and manifestations of brain dysfunction should be considered only after the diagnosis of heatstroke is excluded.

Table 40.2	Differential diagnosis of heatstroke
Dehydration	
Encephalitis, meningitis	
Coagulopathies	
Cerebrovascular accidents (e.g., hypothalamic hemorrhage)	
Seizures	
Hypoglycemia	
Drug intoxication	
Animal poisoning (snakes, bees)	

Clinical picture

The clinical manifestation of heatstroke usually follow a very distinct pattern of events.

- *The hyperthermic phase*: Central nervous system disturbances are present in all cases of heatstroke, as the brain is extremely sensitive to hyperthermia. Signs of depression in the central nervous system often appear simultaneously in the form of coma, stupor, or delirium, irritability and aggressiveness. Seizures occur in approximately 60–70% of the cases.
- *The hematological and enzymatic phase*: Hematological and enzymatic disorders peak usually 24–48 h after the collapse. Typical, although not pathognomonic, is a marked elevation in plasma CPK activity, which resembles rhabdomyolysis.
- *Renal and hepatic phase*: Manifests 3–5 days after collapse and is characterized by serious disturbances in renal (acute renal failure) and hepatic functions (fulminant hepatitis).

Treatment

Treatment of heatstroke victims is symptomatic (Table 40.3). Cooling should be initiated vigorously immediately upon collapse and only minimally delayed for vital resuscitation measures. Any time-consuming examinations should be postponed until body temperature is controlled.

The most practical and efficient method of cooling is the use of large quantities of tap water, which is readily available and does not require any complicated logistic arrangements. It eliminates the hazard of cold-induced vasoconstriction that reduces the efficiency of heat dissipation. The victim should be placed in the shade and any restrictive clothing must be removed. The patient's skin must be kept wet and the body should be continually fanned. Cooling should be continued until body temperature reaches 38°C. This should not, however, delay the rapid evacuation of the patient to the nearest medical facility, which is of the utmost importance.

No drug is effective in reducing body temperature. Dantrolene is not effective, since in EHS there is no involvement of the calcium channels as there is in the mechanism in malignant hyperthermia. Antipyretics are also ineffective since the thermoregulatory 'set point' is not affected in heatstroke. Antipyretics might be harmful, since they cannot be metabological in the heat affected liver.

To confirm the diagnosis and afterwards the effectiveness of cooling, rectal temperature, not oral temperature, must be measured. Blood pressure and pulse must be checked, a quick clinical examination performed, and if possible, urine and blood should be obtained for examination prior to infusion of fluids.

Usually, not more than 2 L of Ringer's lactate or saline should be infused in the first hour, after which fluids should be administered in accordance with the state of hydration. Overhydration might result in hyponatremia and brain edema.

Some of the clinical manifestations of heatstroke may develop during the 2nd or 3rd day after collapse. Therefore, it is imperative that any suspected case of heatstroke be followed for at least 48 h. During this period, and at 12 h intervals, laboratory and clinical evaluations should be carried out (Table 40.4).

Prognosis

Survival rate from EHS is 95% if diagnosed and treated properly. The noxious effect on the tissues caused by heatstroke is directly and closely correlated with the duration of the high temperature phase. Therefore, misdiagnosis, early inefficient treatment, and delay in evacuation are the major causes for deterioration in the patient's condition. Predictors of poor prognosis include prolonged body temperature above 42°C, prolonged coma, hyperkalemia, oliguric renal failure, and continuous hepatic dysfunction. The vast majority of cases of heatstroke recover with no lasting sequelae.

Neurological deficits may persist in some patients, usually for only a limited period, in the form of cerebellar deficits, hemiparesis, aphasia, and mental deficiency. In rare cases, neurological impairment may be chronic and last for years.

Prevention

Most heatstroke patients are motivated but relatively untrained subjects who exert themselves beyond their physiological capacity. Therefore, frequently EHS occurs during relatively short exertions. Early collapse during exercise may point to the possibility that, besides over-motivation, other underlying factors compromise the individual's thermoregulation. For the young, healthy population, four factors are of relevance: poor physical fitness, lack of heat acclimatization, acute febrile disease, and dehydration.

Following some simple guidelines and providing proper health education can easily prevent EHS.

- Only healthy, fit subjects should participate in strenuous physical activity. Exercise should agree with the participant's capacity.
- Rest periods should be incorporated during long periods of activity (proper night rest is also imperative).
- Physical exertions should avoid the hottest hours of the day.
- Adequate hydration is essential. Water should be readily available and used freely during activity (Fig. 40.4). Proper education for fluid replacement will eliminate dehydration.

Table 40.3	Treatment for exertional heatstroke
Cooling	Tap water (large quantities) Antipyretics are ineffective and dangerous
Seizures	Diazepam (titration I.V. 10 mg) until seizure cease
Rehydration	2L/1st h, then after according to water deficit
Oliguria	Mannitol (0.25 mg/kg) Furosemide (1 mg/kg)
Clotting	Fresh frozen plasma Cryoprecipitate Platelet concentrate
Brain edema	Dexamethasone
Acid-base balance, electrolytes, and glucose levels usually correct spontaneously after cooling and rehydration	

Table 40.4	On admission, and at 12 h intervals, the following should be checked
ECG	
Muscle enzymes	
Transaminases and liver function	
Renal function	
Coagulation indices	
Acid-base balance	
Electrolytes	
Glucose	

Other heat-related concerns

Several other conditions that are associated with exertion outdoors in the heat warrant attention. They are not considered as medical emergencies and can easily be prevented.[4]

Heat exhaustion

Heat exhaustion lies on a continuum with heatstroke. The term 'heat exhaustion' is used to describe the inability to continue exercising in situations of heat stress. Symptoms are milder than those expected for heatstroke and include: dizziness, confusion, nausea, muscle cramps, and mild elevation in body-core temperature. Major neurologic impairment is absent.

Treatment is similar to that applied in heat stroke, and include removal of the patient to a shaded area, cooling with copious amounts of water, and continuously monitoring body-core temperature. Fluid replace-ment by drinking or by infusion should be according to the patient's clinical condition and hydration status.

Heat cramps

The term 'heat cramps' is a misnomer because heat itself does not cause them; rather, they occur in muscles subjected to intense activity and fatigue. Heat cramps are described as painful spasms of skeletal muscles that usually involve the arms, legs, or abdominal muscles. Because heat cramps tend to occur more in physically conditioned subjects, it is difficult to differentiate them from other muscle pains related to physical activity. The etiology is not fully clear but is prob-ably related to sodium depletion. Sodium replacement in diet is effec-tive in prevention of this syndrome.

Heat syncope

This condition 'Orthostatic hypotension' is an orthostatic syncopial episode or dizziness that occurs from prolonged standing in the heat or a sudden change in postural position from lying to standing. It occurs because of the massive peripheral vasodilatation, and reduces venous return and, consequently, inadequate cardiac output. Treat-ment consists of placing the patient in a supine position with legs elevated.

Heat edema

A mild edema occasionally seen during the early stages of heat exposure, especially in the unconditioned subject. It results from plasma volume that expands to compensate for the increased need for thermoregulatory blood flow. This condition has no clinical signifi-cance and will resolve itself spontaneously. Diuretic therapy is not necessary.

COLD INJURIES

Cold injuries occur when the body is unable to protect itself from the environment and heat loss from the body exceeds heat gain. Cold injuries are subdivided into peripheral injuries (chilblains, trench foot, and frostbite) and systemic injury (hypothermia). Cold injuries result mainly because of inappropriate behavior (Table 40.5), and can be significantly reduced by following simple guidelines (Table 40.6).

Hypothermia

Clinically, hypothermia is defined as a body-core temperature of less than 35°C. It occurs when massive body heat is lost to the environ-ment and exceeds the metabolic heat production. Scientific literature differentiates between 'urban hypothermia' and 'accidental hypother-

Table 40.5	Factors that increase the risk for cold injuries
Hypothermia	
Low ambient temperatures (high cold intensity)	
Improper clothing and equipment	
Wet clothing	
Fatigue, exhaustion	
Dehydration	
Poor food intake	
Inactivity	
Lack of knowledge or inappropriate risk taking	
Alcohol intake	
Peripheral injuries	
Improper, constricting, and wet clothing	
Cold intensity	
Immobilization	
Smoking	
Hypothermia	
Vasoconstrictive drugs	

mia'. This classification is based on the etiology and population at risk. 'Urban hypothermia', which is not the focus of this chapter, is characteristic of the elderly population suffering from poor health and poor nutrition, alcoholics and drug users. Young children from lower socio-economic strata are also at risk. The population at risk for 'accidental hypothermia' is usually the young and active popu-lation, e.g. winter sport participants, hikers, travelers, military per-sonnel, and adventurers.[10–12]

Diagnosis

The diagnosis of hypothermia is dependent solely on body-core tem-perature. Accordingly, it is classified as mild, moderate, or severe. All organ systems are affected by hypothermia. This should be kept in mind during rewarming. During the hypothermic stage, however, the central nervous system and the cardiovascular system are the most sensitive.

- *Mild hypothermia*: Body temperature falls in the range of 35–32°C. The patient may be slightly cool and pale, but is usually shiver-ing and conscious. Central nervous system reactions are slowed. Cardiovascular changes include initial tachycardia, which is sec-ondary to catecholamine release, followed by bradycardia. Common in this stage are shivering, confusion, disorientation and dysarthria.

- *Moderate hypothermia*: Body temperature falls in the range of 32–28°C. Shivering ceases, and the patient becomes unconscious to varying degrees. Myocardial irritability is evident by the appear-ance of atrial fibrillation and changes in the ECG complex. A characteristic, although not pathognomonic, deflection at the junction of the QRS complex and ST segment, known as J-wave (Osborn wave) appears.

Table 40.6	Cold injuries are preventable by following simple guidelines
Staying in shelters that protect from wind and rain/snow	
Matching outdoor activities with cold intensity	
Wearing multi-layer, unrestrictive dry clothing	
Performing light-moderate work to prevent sweating	
Adjusting layers of clothing to work rate in order to eliminate wearing wet items	
Eating high caloric diets and eliminating alcohol consumption	

■ *Severe hypothermia*: Body temperature below 28°C. In this condition, arrhythmias in the form of ventricular fibrillation are common. Deep unconsciousness, waxy pale skin, the absence of corneal reflexes, and undetectable breathing, pulse rate, and blood pressure often mislead into thinking that the patient is dead.

In the diagnosis of hypothermia, the working hypothesis should always be *'no patient is dead until warm and dead.'* Asystole usually is seen at body temperature of 18°C. The lowest known survival temperature for adults is 16°C, and for infants, 15°C.

Treatment

Hypothermia is a condition that can also be life threatening during the treatment stage. Therefore, intensive treatment should be commenced at a medical center equipped with ICU facilities.

■ *In the field*: During all stages of hypothermia, the patient should be evacuated to a dry shelter and all wet clothing removed. Passive external heating, by covering the patient with dry blankets, sleeping bags, etc. is the safest first-aid treatment until evacuation to the hospital is possible. The low metabolic rate associated with hypothermia actually has a protective effect on the body's vital organs and function. Therefore, individuals, especially children, have been successfully resuscitated after prolonged severe hypothermia when treated properly.

■ *In the hospital*: Active rewarming should be initiated, concomitant with continuous monitoring of body-core temperature by an electronic thermometer. Aggressive, active rewarming can be accomplished by several means, e.g., warm water bottles, radiant heat, hot-water immersion (42–43°C), warm inhalation (43°C), gastrointestinal irrigation or peritoneal dialysis with warm fluids (42–43°C), and cardiopulmonary bypass (37°C); the last is probably the safest and most effective treatment. Mild hypothermia will resolve itself regardless of the rewarming technique. For moderate and severe hypothermia, aggressive rewarming should be initiated. The rewarming stage, however, might be associated with severe complications, especially for the moderate and severe cases of hypothermia.

Advanced life support protocols, especially defibrillation, may be ineffective when body-core temperature is low (moderate and severe hypothermia). Defibrillation should be tried and medications given only when body temperature is higher than 32°C.

Complications associated with rewarming

The associated complications from rewarming result from abrupt changes in the metabolic rate and effective blood volume.

■ *After-drop*: Despite rewarming, body temperature continues to fall. This phenomenon is related to the return of cold blood from the periphery to the central circulation. After-drop may be significant if rewarming is not sufficiently aggressive. Immersion in hot water and cardiopulmonary bypass result in the lowest after-drop.

■ *Rewarming shock*: During aggressive rewarming, effective peripheral circulation increases, unadjusted to cardiac capabilities. This results in low cardiac output and a state of shock.

■ *Arrhythmias*: The cardiac muscle is extremely sensitive. During rewarming, as cold blood returns from the periphery to the central circulation, arrhythmias may develop. Atrial fibrillations may spontaneously be converted to sinus rhythm. Ventricular fibrillations are resistant and do not respond to conventional medications. Bretylium tosylate may be helpful.

■ *Hypoglycemia*: Rewarming abruptly increases metabolic rate. This requires the recruitment of any available energy source, which, in turn, will cause hypoglycemia. A continuous infusion of 5% dextrose in isotonic sodium chloride solution should be the treatment of choice.

Frostbite

Frostbite is the most serious peripheral cold injury. It occurs when unprotected tissue is exposed to sub-zero cold environments, even for relatively short periods. The tissues in the affected area freeze, and ice crystals form within the cells causing them to rupture.

Frostbite is divided into four levels, depending on the severity of the injury, which can be ascertained only retrospectively (i.e., cold burns).

■ *Level I (frostnip)*: When only the skin surface freezes. It begins with itching and pain. Then, when blood supply to the skin decreases because of extensive vasoconstriction, feeling is lost and the area becomes numb. Because only the top skin layers are affected, healing is short, usually without subsequent problems.

■ *Level II*: In this case, the skin becomes frozen, but deeper tissues are spared and remain soft. Several days after the injury has occurred, hard blisters will form. They often appear black in color, and look worse than they actually are. With proper treatment, healing can be expected within 4–12 weeks. Cold sensitivity may occur afterwards.

■ *Levels III–IV*: These stages of frostbite resemble deep tissue injuries. The muscles, tendons, blood vessels, and nerves of the affected area are frozen. The area feels hard, woody, and numb. The affected area looks red, deep purple, or blackened with blisters usually filled with blood. Often it takes months to determine the extent of the damage. Amputation of extremities is usually required, but is delayed until it is ascertained which tissues cannot be revived (Fig. 40.3).

Treatment

Treatment should be commenced only at a medical installation under conditions that ensure that the affected area will not re-freeze. The proper way to treat trench foot and frostbite is to rewarm the affected area in warm water (40–42°C), usually for 15-30 min. This should be done 3–4 times a day until thawing is complete.[5, 8, 11, 13] In addition:

■ The patient should be kept in a warm environment.
■ The affected area should be kept dry and clean under sterile sheets and should not be dressed.
■ Blisters should not be opened or manipulated.
■ Analgesia (morphine or meperidine) should be administered intravenously or intramuscularly, as indicated.
■ Penicillin G or another broad spectrum antibiotic should be administered parenterally.

'Trench foot' (immersion foot)

The name of this condition is derived from the cold injury that prevailed in soldiers living in the trenches during World War I. It occurs when a part of the body, usually the feet, is exposed to non-freezing cold and wet environments for prolonged periods (>10 h). The feet are especially vulnerable since boots restrict proper blood flow to the feet, thus worsening the condition. The affected area is pale, cold, swollen, and painful. Serous blisters that appear are deep.[5, 8, 12]

Treatment

The treatment of trench foot is similar to that of frostbite.

Chilblains

These are the most common cold injuries. Chilblains tend to occur when there is exposure of the skin, especially fingers, to dry, non-freezing cold. The affected area may itch, appear reddish-blue, be swollen, and painful. Blisters containing clear fluid may form after some time, and the area may become sensitive to cold in the future. Usually there is no permanent damage from chilblains.[8]

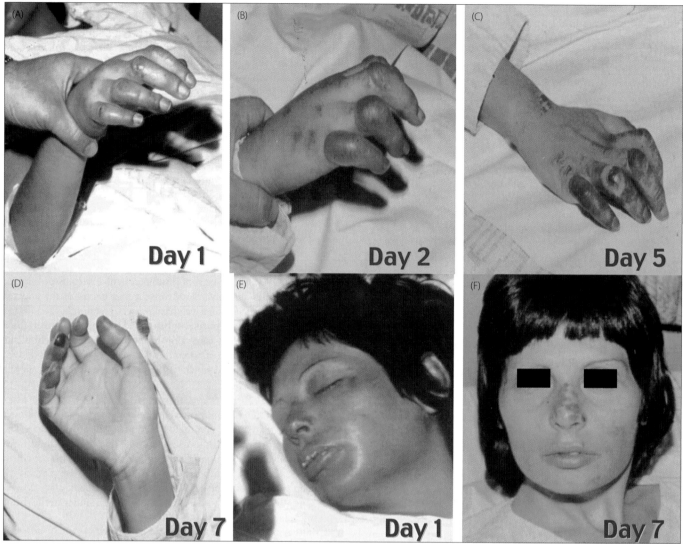

Figure 40.3 Recovery from combined hypothermia and frostbite. An 18-year-old girl was exposed to a snow blizzard for 24 h in a remote rural area. She was not dressed properly and became fatigued and dehydrated after she left her car in an attempt to reach rescue. Two other people who accompanied her died from hypothermia. The girl was rescued with a body-core temperature of 27°C. (A) day 1, 3rd degree frostbite; (B) day 2, seemingly the condition worsens after rewarming in a warm bath of 42°C, three times daily (chlorhexidine gluconate solution added to bath water). Rewarming continued until day 10; (C) day 5; (D) day 7, the proximal flange of the 4th finger is necrotic. This flange was amputated on day 10; (E) the hypothermic, waxy, edematous face of the unconscious patient on admission to the ER. The patient was treated by immersion in a warm bath of 42°C; (F) day 7, post-trauma.

Treatment

Prevention is the best treatment. This includes protecting fingers and toes with dry gloves, dry socks, and boots. Affected areas should be kept warm and dry.

DEHYDRATION AND FLUID CONSUMPTION

Euhydration is represented by a sinusoidal wave indicating the normal, daily body-water content fluctuations that expand and contract within very narrow limits (total body water volume within ± 0.22% of body weight and plasma volume within ± 0.7%). Steady-state conditions of increased and decreased body water content are defined as hyperhydration and hypohydration, respectively. Dehydration refers to the process of losing body water, which leads to hypohydration. Rehydration is the process of adding fluids, leading from a state of hypohydration towards euhydration. Fluid intake exceeding the limits of euhydration leads to hyperhydration, and is referred to as overhydration.

Hypohydration

The adverse effects of hypohydration occur via the impairment of the thermoregulatory and cardiovascular systems, which result in reduced performance and compromised body temperature control. Impairment in physical performance is noticed already at 1% dehydration (600–800 ml water loss), and total collapse is evident when water loss is at around 7% of body weight. The dehydrated subject is described as an apathetic, listless, plodding person straining to finish a given task that he previously performed easily. Cognitive performance is also adversely influenced by body water deficits.[17]

Voluntary dehydration

Thirst is an adequate stimulus for total fluid replacement when at rest. During physical activity or exercise-heat stress, thirst does not appear to be a sufficient stimulus for maintaining body water levels.

Spontaneous drinking occurs only after a considerable amount of water loss (>2% of body weight). In addition, when water is not readily available or if the water is unpalatable, salty, or warm, drinking is also reduced.[14]

The slowdown in voluntary fluid intake, is termed 'voluntary dehydration'. That is, individuals will drink to temporary satiety, but a water deficit remains. Voluntary dehydration is considered the main cause for dehydration during exercise.

Although physical activity accentuates voluntary dehydration, leisure reduces it. Therefore, a water deficit accumulated between meals is usually restored during meals. Awareness of the need for fluid replenishment increases voluntary fluid intake and reduces voluntary dehydration.

Overhydration and hyponatremia

Hyponatremia is commonly defined as sodium plasma concentrations below 135 mEq/L. Clinical symptoms of hyponatremia are not expected to appear unless sodium concentrations are below 130 mEq/L. Whereas subclinical hyponatremia may be common during long (more than 8 hours) exertions in the heat, clinically significant hypontremia is a rare condition.[14, 15]

Theoretically, hyponatremia can result from either excessive loss of sodium in sweat, which is not compensated for by proper salt intake while the extracellular compartment is replenished by adequate water intake, or because of overhydration with hypotonic fluids (e.g., water).

For a healthy individual maintaining a normal diet, to develop a salt deficiency is extremely difficult, perhaps impossible, regardless of the environment and the amount of exercise performed.

The cumulative data suggest that in healthy individuals symptomatic hyponatremia develops mainly because of gross fluid overload. Therefore, electrolyte supplementation may be needed only in rare cases for exercising subjects who: (1) lose more than 8 L of sweat; (2) skip meals; (3) experience a caloric deficit of <1000 kcal/day; or (4) are ill with diarrhea.

Isotonic fluids ('sport drinks')

A debated topic is the 'appropriate' fluid replacement during physical activity, especially in the heat. Some advocate that water is not enough and that it should be enriched with carbohydrates and electrolytes. 'Sport drinks' are commercial or homemade beverages that contain carbohydrates ('to enhance performance') and electrolytes ('to prevent hyponatremia'). In general, the benefit of ingesting sports drinks appears to be their enhanced palatability, which increases fluid consumption.[16, 17]

Physiologically, gastric emptying depends on the osmolality and caloric content of the fluids. Gastric emptying of 'sports drinks' might be slower than that of water. In addition, the rate of intestinal absorption of carbohydrate-electrolyte solutions is slower than the absorption of water.

Therefore, under normal conditions, the use of electrolyte–carbohydrate beverages offers no advantages over water. Consumption of these beverages may be indicated only under conditions of caloric restriction or a state of diarrhea.

Rehydration

At rest and thermal comfort urination is the major cause for loss of body water (around 1.5 L/day). During physical activity or in hot environments, a considerable amount of body water is lost through sweat secretion, enabling evaporative cooling of the body. Sweat secretion can vary considerably, depending on environmental conditions,

work intensity, clothing, gender, age, state of acclimatization, and fitness.

The general concept that prevails is that during prolonged intermittent exercise, the optimal rate of fluid replacement appears to be the rate, which most closely matches the rate of sweating (Fig. 40.4). On average, sweat rates of 1–1.5 L/h during exercise in the heat are common.[14, 17]

To reduce the rate of voluntary dehydration without exposing the individual to the danger involved in dehydration or over-hydration the following should be remembered:

- One should not assume that unlimited quantities of water can be consumed.
- Fluids should be palatable and consumed at regular intervals at a rate sufficient to replace water loss through sweating.
- Fluid intake should be at frequencies and in quantities that will be ingested with ease; volumes of 200–250 mL should be consumed each time.
- Hyponatremia is a potential risk only for activities lasting longer than 8–10 h. There is little physiological basis for the adding of salt to fluid if it is sufficiently available in the diet.

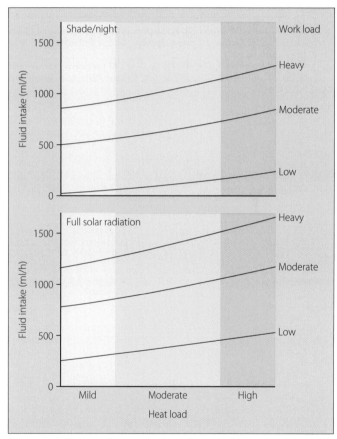

Figure 40.4 Fluid requirements under various conditions of work intensity and heat load. (Levels of heat load are depicted in Fig. 40.1). How to calculate daily fluid requirements. +/−, with and without solar radiation, respectively.

Heat load	Work load	Length	mL/h	Total
Moderate (+)	Moderate	6 h	750	4.5 L
Moderate (−)	Rest	8 h	100	0.8 L
Mild	Moderate	4 h	500	2.0 L
		Total		7.3 L

SUMMARY

Environmental conditions may confine the ability of travelers. Misbehavior and improper preparedness may eventually result in heatstroke and other heat-related injuries when exposed to warm climate. Exposure to cold weather may cause hypothermia and peripheral injuries to the body's extremities. Preventing these devastating conditions, which might also be life-threatening, is possible by the adherence to some simple rules:

- Only fit, healthy, acclimated individuals should conduct physical exercise in adverse climatic conditions.
- Physical exertions should be performed within the physiological limitations; over exertions are life-threatening.
- Work/rest cycles should be planned and adhered to.
- Fluid intake should compensate fluid loss. Euhydration should be attained.
- Clothing should be suitable to the climatic conditions and work intensity.

Casualties of heat or cold weather should be treated vigorously. The sooner body temperature returns to its normal range, the better the prognosis.

REFERENCES

1. Gisolfi CV, Lamb DR, Nadel ER. Perspective in exercise, science and sports medicine. Vol. 6. *Exercise, Heat and Thermoregulation*. Dubuque, IA: Brown & Benchmark; 1993:6.
2. Armstrong LE, Epstein Y, Greenleaf JE, *et al*. ACSM position stand: heat and cold illnesses during distance running. *Med Sci Sports Exerc* 1987; **19**:529–533.
3. Shapiro Y, Seidman DS. Field and clinical observations of exertional heatstroke patients. *Med Sci Sports Exerc* 1990; **22**(1):6–14.
4. Hamlet MP. Prevention and treatment of cold injury. *Int J Circumpolar Health* 2000; **59**:108–113.
5. Mills WJ. and colleagues. Cold injury: a collection of papers. *Alaska Med* 1993; **35**:6–140.
6. Epstein Y, Moran DS, Shapiro Y, Sohar E, Shemer J. Exertional heat stroke: a case series. *Med Sci Sports Exerc* 1999; **31**:224–228.
7. Epstein Y, Sohar E, Shapiro Y. Exertional heatstroke: a preventable condition. *Isr J Med Sci* 1995; **31**:454–462.
8. Burr RE. Medical aspects of cold weather operations: a handbook for medical officers. *USARIEM Report* TN3-4, 1993.
9. Moran DS, Gaffin SL. Clinical management of heat related illnesses. In: Auerbach PS, ed. *Wilderness Medicine*. 4th edn. St. Louis, MO: Mosby; 2001:290–316.
10. Danzl DF, Pozos RS. Accidental hypothermia. *N Eng J Med* 1994; **331**:1756–1760.
11. Giesbrecht GG. Emergency treatment of hypothermia. *Emerg Med* 2001; **13**:9–16.
12. Lloyd EL. ABC of sports medicine. Temperature and performance. I: cold. *BMJ* 1994; 309:531–534.
13. Murphy JV, Banwell PE, Roberts HN. McGrouther DA. Frostbite: pathogenesis and treatment. *J Trauma* 2000; **48**:171–178.
14. Epstein Y, Armstrong LE. Fluid-electrolyte balance during labor and exercise: concepts and misconceptions. *Int J Sport Nutr* 1999; **9**:1–12.
15. Montain SJ, Sawka MN, Wenger LB. Hyponatremia associated with exercise: risk factors and pathogenesis. *Exerc Sports Sci Rev* 2001; **29**:113–117.
16. Gisolfi CV, Lamb DR. Perspective in exercise, science and sports medicine. Vol. 3. *Fluid Homeostasis During Exercise*. Carmel, IN: Benchmark Press, Inc.; 1990:3.
17. Canvertino VA, Armstrong LE, Coyle EF, *et al*. ACSM position stand: Exercise and fluid replacement. *Med Sci Sports Exerc* 1996; **28**:1–5.

CHAPTER 41 Sun-associated Problems

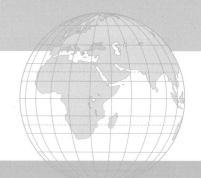

Marilynne McKay

INTRODUCTION

Almost every adult Caucasian has experienced at least one sunburn – it is such a common event that most people do not even think of ultraviolet-induced skin damage as a 'traveler's health problem.' Nothing much can be done for sunburn aside from supportive care until the skin recovers – but fortunately sunscreen agents are widely available and their frequent and appropriate use can prevent painful sunburns entirely. Topical agents that block the sun's harmful rays have decreased the incidence of acute discomfort and disability as well as ameliorated the chronic effects of sun damage, including cutaneous carcinomas. The United Nations Environment Program (UNEP) has estimated that more than 2 million non-melanoma skin cancers and 200 000 malignant melanomas occur globally each year. In the event of a 10% decrease in stratospheric ozone, an additional 300 000 non-melanoma and 4500 melanoma skin cancers could be expected worldwide.[1] Dark-skinned populations have a lower risk of skin cancer than Caucasians because of the protection offered by skin pigmentation. Australia is the most sun-conscious country in the world – its Anti-Cancer Council notes that almost one in two people who live in that country are expected to get skin cancer in their lifetime and every year around 1200 Australians die from this almost totally preventable disease. Sunscreens and protective clothing have made a difference – 20 years after the initiation of the SunSmart Program in Victoria, the number of people under 40 being diagnosed with melanoma in that state fell by 16%.[2]

ULTRAVIOLET RADIATION

The electromagnetic spectrum of ultraviolet (UV) light is made up of visible light, UVC, UVB and UVA. All of these wavelengths can elicit photosensitivity reactions, but UVC, a shorter wavelength, is filtered out by the ozone layer (Fig. 41.1). The others penetrate the ozone layer and reach the earth's surface, although UVB is filtered more by the atmosphere than UVA. UVA and UVB have an additive effect on the skin. UVB, most responsible for sunburning and skin cancer development, is intense during the middle of the day (10 a.m. to 4 p.m.); hence the American Academy of Dermatology advice: 'When your shadow is shorter than you are, look for shade!' UVA is present throughout the day and penetrates more deeply through the skin into subcutaneous fat. UVA ages the skin (produces wrinkles and blotchy pigmentation), contributes to skin cancers, and causes photosensitive rashes (Fig. 41.2). UV protection is good preventive medicine.[3]

The UV Index

The Global Solar UV Index[1] is an estimate of the average maximum solar ultraviolet radiation at the Earth's surface. Recommendations on the calculation, expression and dissemination of the Global Solar UV Index were made in 1995 by the World Health Organization (WHO), the World Meteorological Organization (WMO), United Nations Environment Programme (UNEP) and the International Commission on Non-Ionizing Radiation Protection (ICNIRP). National authorities throughout the world now use the Global Solar

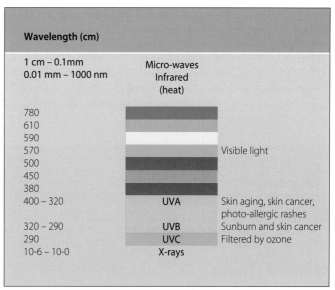

Figure 41.1 Visible and ultraviolet spectrum.

Sun sensitivity	Skin type	Sunburn and tanning history*	Skin colour	Sunburn protection (SPF)
UV Sensitive	I	Always burns easily; never tans	'Celtic'	High 30+
	II	Always burns easily; tans minimally	Fair	High 30+
UV Normal	III	Burns moderately; tans gradually	Average Caucasian	Moderate 12-29
	IV	Burns minimally; always tans well	Olive	Moderate 12-29
UV Insensitive	V	Rarely burns; tans profusely	Brown	Minimal (2-12)
	VI	Never burns; deeply pigmented	Black	Minimal (2-12)

Figure 41.2 Skin types and sun protection. Based on US FDA recommendations. [a]Sunburn and tanning history based on first 30–45 min sun exposure after a winter season of no sun exposure.

UV Index to provide uniform information to the public about daily UV exposure levels so that consistent messages can be provided on what protective measures are necessary with various index values.

The calculation for the UV Index allows for the different skin-damaging effect from each UV wavelength and averages out variations over a 10–30 min timespan. The Index is generally presented as a forecast of the maximum amount of skin-damaging UV expected to reach the Earth's surface at solar noon. (During summer, when daylight saving time is in effect, solar noon in most of Europe is at 14.00 hours (2 p.m.); in the UK and countries with a similar longitude, it is at 13.00 hours (1 p.m.)).

The values of the UV Index range from zero upward – the higher the UV Index number, the greater the likelihood of skin and eye-damaging exposure to UV, and the less time it takes for damage to occur. (Fig. 41.3) Factors affecting the amount of UV radiation entering the atmosphere as well as the UV Index rating include air pollution (which reduces UV radiation), altitude (increases UV intensity), latitude (positioning of the sun in the sky) and distance from the equator. In many countries close to the equator, summertime values can range up to 20. During the European and American summers the Index is generally not more than about eight, but can be higher, especially at beach resorts.

Daily updates of UV levels in the summer are often presented on local television and radio along with weather and environmental information. The UV Index can also be found on a number of websites on the Internet: http://www.srrb.noaa.gov/UV/lindex.html, offers a list of worldwide sites that provide UV index predictions for the next day. Most of these sites also give valuable explanatory information for interpreting the index levels and appropriate steps for avoiding excessive UV.

Heat, humidity and wind can intensify UV effects. In winter, the UV-protective high-level atmospheric ozone layer is typically thinner, and UV damage is also intensified at high elevations and by reflection from snow. UVA damage to eyes can acutely cause snow blindness and long-term exposure can lead to cataracts. UVB and UVA penetrate clouds, so sunburn and snow blindness can occur on cloudy days. Reflection from sand and snow intensifies damaging ultraviolet radiation by 20–30% (and water reflects as much as an additional 100%) (Table 41.1).

SUN PROTECTION FACTOR

The sun protection factor (SPF) value of a sunscreen is defined as the ratio of the energy required to produce a minimal erythema dose (skin reddening or minimal sunburn) through the sunscreen compared with the energy required to produce the same reaction in the absence of the sunscreen. The SPF number gives you some idea how long you can remain in the sun before burning. If, for example, you would normally burn in 10 min without sunscreen, applying a 15 SPF sunscreen may provide you with about 150 min in the sun before burning (15 times the protection). A sunscreen with a SPF of 15 filters out about 92% of UVB rays. An SPF of 30 filters out 97%. SPF applies for UVB rays only – protection against UVA in sunscreens is about 10% of the UVB rating. Similar standards for the determination of SPF have now been established in Australia, the USA, and Europe (Table 41.2).

In 1999, the FDA mandated a new rating scale for sunscreens in the USA to begin in 2001,[4] now delayed to a later date. The new product categories are: minimal sunburn protection (SPF 2 to under 12); moderate sunburn protection (SPF 12 to under 30); high sunburn protection (SPF 30 and above). It should be noted that Australia recently set an upper limit of SPF 30+ based on studies showing that values above 40 offer minimal additional benefit, because even with an SPF of 33, about 97% of the rays that cause erythema are filtered out.[5]

US sunscreen products are also described as providing minimal, moderate, or high protection against tanning. The FDA no longer permits the label 'sunblock' or 'extended wear' claims – i.e., a specific number of hours or an absolute claim such as 'all-day protection.'

	Sun damage			Skin colour		
Global solar UV index	Risk of sun damage	Minutes to sunburn for type I-II skin	Fair, burns (skin type I-II)	Fair, tans (skin type III)	Brown (skin type IV-V)	Black (skin type VI)
1-2	Low	–	Low	Low	Low	Low
3-4	Moderate	20	Medium	Low	Low	Low
5-6	High	15	High-Very high	Medium	Low-Medium	Low
7-8	Very high	10	Very high	High	Medium	Medium
9-10+	Extreme	5	Very high	High	High	Medium

Figure 41.3 The global solar UV index and risk of sun damage by skin color.

Table 41.1 Time required to sunburn fair skin, UV index 6–7

Time	Degree of sunburn
12 min	Perceptible sunburn
30 min	Vivid sunburn
60 min	Painful sunburn
120 min	Blistering sunburn

New labels may say only, 'helps prevent sunburn' and 'higher SPF gives more sunburn protection.'

SPF ratings are established under controlled conditions of humidity, often with artificial UVB exposure – there is no wind, reflection, sweating, or toweling and lotions are typically reapplied hourly. This means that actual use conditions are likely to decrease the SPF value assigned to the product.[6]

Under test conditions, if the SPF of a sunscreen does not change after 20 min of moderate water activity, followed by a 20 min rest period without toweling, followed by 20 additional min of moderate activity in the water, the product can be labeled as 'water resistant,' 'water/sweat resistant', or 'water/perspiration resistant.' 'Very water resistant' sunscreen products have undergone extended water exposure testing to 80 min, while maintaining their labeled SPF values. (This means that a person outside in a pool for 6 h would have to reapply a very water resistant sunscreen at least four times to ensure that the SPF is unchanged.)

The FDA agrees that sunscreen use alone will not prevent all of the possible harmful effects due to the sun. This agency officially states that 'limiting sun exposure, wearing protective clothing, and using sunscreens may reduce the risks of skin aging, skin cancer, and other harmful effects of the sun.' It should be noted that sunscreen chemicals themselves may cause skin reactions; in one randomized clinical trial, one out of five daily sunscreen users had a skin reaction. Review of these cases showed that problems were typically related to irritancy of the product, however – only a small minority showed cell-mediated contact allergy.[7] Fortunately, there are enough different sunscreen ingredients available that it is relatively easy to avoid specific ones – and some of the traditional offenders, such as benzoic acid (formerly PABA) have been modified to be less allergenic. Studies have shown a significant decrease in actinic keratoses appearing on chronically sun-damaged skin when sunscreens are used regularly[8] (Table 41.3).

PROTECTIVE CLOTHING

Light cotton fabrics are not as sun-protective as denim, which is generally considered to be the most effective. Fabric SPF is more a function of the openings in the fabric mesh than the particular fabric type. A cotton/polyester T-shirt has an SPF of around 15, which decreases when the fabric is wet. (An old cotton T-shirt may have a better SPF value when it has been washed a few times due to shrinkage in the hole size of the fabric mesh.) For true lightweight sun-protective clothing (UPF, Ultraviolet Protective Factor of 30+ with UVA and UVB protection), look for Solumbra (Sun Precautions®, 2815 Wetmore Avenue; Everett, WA 98201, www.solumbra.com) or Solarweave® and Solarknit® (Protective Clothing Ltd., 598 Norris Court, Kingston, Ontario K7P 2R9). An Internet search for 'solarweave' will produce other dealers and manufacturers. Sun-protective clothing can be an extremely effective way to prevent long-term UV damage.[9]

Hats should protect the head, ears, neck, and sides of the face, as these areas get almost continual sun exposure, even in winter.

Table 41.2 What most people do not know about sunscreens

Apply sunscreen at least a half-hour before exposure for full skin absorption. For 'water-resistant' protection, benzoic acid-containing sunscreens must be applied at least one hour before immersion. All types of sunscreens must be applied thickly for maximum water-resistance
One application is not enough. Experiments show a time-dependent decrease in SPF within the first few hours after sunscreen application. Swimming and perspiration also reduce the actual SPF value for many sunscreens
Reapply sunscreen after sweating, swimming, toweling and hiking (clothing rubs it off exposed arms and legs). The FDA recommends reapplying sunscreen every 40–80 min – manufacturers can no longer claim 'all-day protection.'
Reapplying sunscreen during the day does NOT extend the period of protection. (SPF 15 means a maximum of SPF 15 protection under ideal conditions and frequent reapplications.)
Multi-day exposure to sunlight increases UV sensitivity on subsequent days of exposure – use higher SPF products then.
One ounce of sunscreen is needed for total body application – less than this lowers the SPF. This means that applied twice a day (as recommended), an 8-ounce bottle of sunscreen should last no more than 4 days per person
The SPF number does not apply to UVA, so an SPF30 product with no UVA screen will be less effective than a product with a lower SPF that contains a UVA screen.
DEET-containing insect repellents may decrease a product's SPF by as much as 30%
Apply sunscreens to all exposed areas of skin including easily overlooked areas such as the rims of the ears, the lips, the back of the neck, and the tops of the feet if in sandals.
Protect eyes with good quality UV-protective sunglasses or goggles in snow or altitude even when cloudy. Always carry a spare pair.
Children receive 50–80% of their lifetime exposure to ultraviolet rays by the time they are 18 years old – start and maintain sunscreen use early. Do not forget a shirt and a hat with a brim!

Table 41.3   Sunscreens

Sunscreen family	Chemical names	Description
para-aminobenzoic Acid (PABA) Derivatives	*Padimate A (amyl dimethyl PABA), and Padimate O (octyl dimethyl PABA).*	Chemicals that block UVB, today's PABAs are mostly PABA esters with fewer problems with stinging, staining, and allergy. They absorb into the top layer of the skin and protect from UVB.
Cinnamates	*2-ethyl-hexyl p-methoxycinnamate (Parsol MCX), octyl methoxycinnamate*	Cinnamates block UVB, rarely cause contact dermatitis and are very insoluble in water.
Salicylates	*Hommenthyl salicylate (homosalate), octyl salicylate and benzyl salicylate*	Weak UVB absorbers but good skin moisturizers, these chemicals are highly water insoluble and tend to be non-irritating.
Phenylbenzimidazole sulfonic acid	*Phenylbenzimidazole sulfonic acid*	A water-soluble UVB blocker that is very lightweight and used frequently in cosmetic moisturizers. No UVA protection.
Benzophenones	*Oxybenzone, dioxybenzone, sulisobenzone*	This group blocks UVA and some UVB. Must be combined with UVB blockers for broad spectrum coverage.
Anthranilates	*Menthyl anthranilate (Maxafil), homomenthyl-N-acetyl anthranilate*	This group absorbs UVB and UVA.
Dibenzoylmethane	*Avobenzone (Parsol 1789)*	Exclusively absorbs in the UVA range and is the top-selling sunscreen agent used in Canada, Australia, and Europe. It was recently re-released in the USA.
Physical Sunscreens	*Titanium dioxide, zinc oxide, Ichthyol, iron pigments, or colored clay*	Opaque substances that block the transmission of visible and ultraviolet radiation to the skin. They are recommended for infants and patients taking photosensitive medications or those with photodermatitis.

Baseball-style caps with transparent mesh backs should be discouraged – the best hats have a wide (at least 2–3 inch) brim that goes all the way around. The Australian 'Slip! Slop! Slap!' campaign says it all: 'Slip on a shirt, slop on the sunscreen, and slap on a hat.'

PHOTOSENSITIVITY

Numerous topical and systemic drugs can interact with ultraviolet radiation to cause photosensitivity, either as a phototoxic or photoallergic reaction.[10] Phototoxic reactions occur minutes to hours after exposure, have a clinical appearance of exaggerated sunburn, and can occur in anyone receiving sufficient exposure to a photosensitizer and light. Photoallergic reactions are the result of cell-mediated immunity and require an initial sensitization period – an acute, subacute, or chronic eczematous rash appears 24 hours or more after exposure. Patients with photoallergic reactions should not take the offending drug again.

Photosensitivity eruptions typically occur in locations with prominent sun exposure such as the face, back of the neck, extensor extremities, and upper chest. Characteristic sites of sparing include the upper eyelids, below the nose and chin, behind the earlobes, and the finger-webs. If a photosensitive drug eruption is suspected, stop the medication if possible – the reaction may persist for weeks (Table 41.4).

Table 41.4   Some medications and additives causing photosensitivity

Anti-infectives	Amantadine, ciprofloxacin, Dapsone, Griseofulvin, Quinolones, Sulfonamides (trimethoprim/sulfisoxazole), Tetracyclines (especially demeclocycline; less frequently doxycycline, oxytetracycline, and tetracycline; minocycline rarely)
Antihistamines	diphenhydramine
Anti-inflammatories	benoxaprofen, ibuprofen, ketoprofen, naproxen, piroxicam
Antimalarials	Fansidar (a sulfa), chloroquine, hydroxychloroquine
Cardiovascular drugs	amiodarone, diltiazem, furosemide, nifedipine, quinidine, thiazide diuretics, triamterene, reserpine
CNS agents	carbamazepine, clomipramine, chlorpromazine, phenothiazines (especially chlorpromazine), tricyclic antidepressants
Miscellaneous	acetazolamide (*Diamox*), oral contraceptives and estrogen, chemotherapy agents, oral diabetes medications (sulfonylureas)
Topical agents	deodorants in soaps, perfumes and citrus herbal products, Coal tar products
Ingestants	*Umbilliferae* (celery), St. John's Wort

Note: This list is not comprehensive. Manufacturer's package inserts should be consulted regarding potential photosensitivity of medications.

SUNBURN

Sunburn develops several hours after exposure, then increases and peaks with the skin's inflammatory response 24 h after exposure, fading in 36–72 h. By the time skin is visibly red (blanches with pressure), it is already burned. If you are responsible for a group of children or adults who will be working or playing in the outdoors, you should make sure they're wearing sunscreen *before* they get outside.

Unfortunately, there is little you can do to reverse skin damage once it is done. Prevent further burning with protective clothing and sunscreens. Analgesics like aspirin or ibuprofen make patients comfortable, but do not decrease the inflammation, which is due to epidermal cell destruction. Topical steroids are of no benefit – a cooling balm of aloe gel, tea, or plain water is as effective (and cheaper).

Systemic steroids such as prednisone may be used for major swelling (sometimes called 'sun poisoning', a non-medical term), but probably will not help most burns. In some cases, narcotic analgesics are needed to treat the pain (Table 41.5).

CONCLUSION

Sun protection should be a priority for all travelers as well as for those who live in areas with a high UV index. All health-care providers should make an effort to educate their patients and raise public awareness about the dangers of overexposure to the sun. Most skin cancers are preventable, and early detection is important. Painful sunburns can be avoided by limiting sun exposure, wearing sun-protective clothing, and the diligent application of protective sunscreen products.

Table 41.5	First aid for sunburn, heat exhaustion and sunstroke	
	Signs and symptoms	**Treatment**
First degree sunburn	Red, painful skin develops within 4 h, peaks at 24 h, lasts 72 h, peels in 4–7 days	1st 48 h: Aspirin or NSAID for pain (no ice), cool wet compresses or baths (with baking soda or pulverized oatmeal), apply soothing water-base gels aloe vera, drink plenty of fluids. After 48 h: continue soaks, add moisturizing lotions
Second degree sunburn	Red, painful skin, blisters, dehydration	As above plus Burow's solution on open blisters; if generalized seek medical attention
Heat exhaustion	Pale, cool, moist skin; sweating, temperature low or normal, weak and rapid pulse, dilated pupils, dry mouth, muscle cramps, headache, nausea, dizziness, fatigue, weakness	Move to cool place indoors or in shade, breeze or fan, lie down, loosen clothing, drink electrolyte solution or cool water with a little salt (1/2 tsp salt/quart of water)
Heat cramps	Muscle cramps, usually in the abdomen and legs; heavy perspiration, lightheadedness, weakness, exhaustion	Follow the same steps as for heat exhaustion, above
Sunstroke	Red, dry, very hot skin (usually no sweating); very high fever, rapid pulse, small pupils, nausea, headache, dehydration, vertigo, disorientation, confusion, combativeness, hypotension, late: loss of consciousness, convulsions	Body temperature is often over 105°, permanent brain or kidney damage or even death can occur. Lower body temperature by immersion in cool water or use cold compresses to head and neck, armpits and groin; loosen or remove clothing, give small sips of fluid

REFERENCES

1. World Health Organization. The Global Solar UV Index. World Health Organization Fact Sheet No 133, revised July. World Health Organization; 1998:available at http://www.who.int/inf-fs/en/fact133.html.
2. Montague M, Borland R, Sinclair C. Slip! Slop! Slap! and SunSmart 1980–2000: Skin cancer control and 20 years of population-based campaigning. *Health Educ Behav* 2001; **28**(3): 290–305. See also http://www.sunsmart.com.au/.
3. Ferrini RL, Perlman M, Hill L. Skin protection from ultraviolet light exposure: American college of preventive medicine practice policy statement. *Am J Prev Med* 1998; **14**:83–86.
4. US Dept of Health & Human Services, Food and Drug Administration. Sunscreen drug products for over-the-counter human use; final monograph. *Federal Register* 64, No. 98, May 21, 1999.
5. AS/NZS 2604:1998 *Sunscreen Products – Evaluation and Classification*. Available from Standards Australia, 1 The Crescent, Homebush NSW 2120, Australia.
6. Patel NP, Highton A, Moy RL. Properties of topical sunscreen formulations. *J Derm Surg Oncol* 1992; **18**:316–20.
7. Foley P, Nixon R, Mario R, Frowen K, et al. The frequency of reactions to sunscreens: results of a longitudinal population-based study on the regular use of sunscreens in Australia. *Br J Derm* 1993; **128**:512–8.
8. Thompson SC, Jolley D, Marks R. Reduction of solar keratoses by regular sunscreen use. *N Engl J Med* 1993; **329**:1147–51.
9. Menter JM, Hollins TD, Sayre RM, et al. Protection against UV photocarcinogenesis by fabric materials. *J Acad Derm* 1994; **31**:711–6.
10. Allen JE. Drug-induced photosensitivity. *Clin Pharm* 1993; **12**:580–587.

CHAPTER 42 Jet Lag

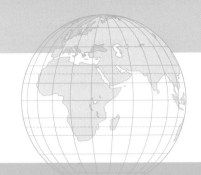

Susan L.F. McLellan

KEYPOINTS

- The suprachiasmatic nuclei act as our internal timekeeper and regulate diurnal variations in body temperature, release of cortisol and growth hormone. Thus, manipulation of the circadian rhythm is complex

- The process of resetting the internal clock is generally agreed to be about 1 day per time zone crossed

- Jet lag tends to increase with age and number of time zones crossed

- Eastward travel is generally more difficult than westward travel with regard to recovery from jet lag

- Light therapy can help speed the resolution of circadian dysynchronism; an eastward traveler should seek light in the morning, and a westward traveler in the afternoon/evening

DEFINITION

'Jet lag' is a condition well known to travelers since the introduction of passenger jet aircraft. The term is commonly used, but the condition manifests itself differently among individuals. Simply defined, it is a combination of malaise, fatigue, derangement of sleep wake cycles, and poor performance, which occurs when travelers cross several time zones rapidly and attempt to follow the time schedule of the new destination.

PHYSIOLOGY

The condition known as jet lag is due primarily to the forced recalibration of the body's natural clock, or circadian rhythms. 'Circadian rhythms' are those innate synchronizations of physiologic processes to natural time cycles, which occur in all animals. These rhythms are present at the cellular level, so that periodicity of firing can be observed in dissected neurons from the suprachiasmatic nuclei of neonatal animals.[1]

In most mammalian species, circadian rhythms are synchronized with the 24 h duration of the earth's rotation and the associated pattern of day and night. The suprachiasmatic nuclei of the hypothalamus act as an internal timekeeper by receiving signals from the environment, including light, food availability, activity, and social cues. Light, specifically outside daylight, is a major cue for the adjustment of the body's 'internal clock' in humans. This clock regulates the release of melatonin, the secretion of which is associated with sleepiness. Daylight levels of light suppress the release of

melatonin from the pineal gland. However, the suppression and release of melatonin is not purely dependent on exposure to light, but is also related to meals and other factors. Furthermore, melatonin also provides feedback to the suprachiasmatic nuclei, therefore controlling its own production and contributing to the modulation of other circadian variables.[2] Other rhythms that appear to be controlled by the suprachiasmatic nuclei are diurnal variations in body temperature and the release of cortisol and growth hormone. A circadian rhythm of cortisol secretion has been identified in infants from the time of birth.[3]

When a traveler crosses several time zones, or meridians, in a short span of time, these circadian rhythms continue to operate on the 'home' schedule for a period of time. The process of resetting the internal clock takes a certain amount of time, generally agreed to be approximately one day per time zone crossed. During this period of time the traveler experiences what is known as jet lag, or circadian dyschronism. Typically after eastward travel it is difficult to fall asleep at the new bedtime, and consequently very difficult to arise in the morning; after westward travel the main complaint is early awakening in the wee hours of the morning. The result is lost total sleep time as well as sleep irregularity.

Contributing to the 'jet lag syndrome' are the conditions that are often associated with preparing for and undertaking long-distance travel. Stress, lack of sleep, culture shock, and the interruption of regular mealtimes and exercise routines may increase the traveler's sense of discomfort and disorientation. There is some disagreement about the extent to which dehydration occurs during a long airplane flight, but certainly reduced mobility and less-than-spacious seating can be a factor. In addition, it is easy for travelers to indulge in excessive alcohol and/or caffeine, both of which may compound the effects of jet lag.

The consequences of the jet lag syndrome extend beyond the loss of vacation time for pleasure-seeking travelers. The decline in cognitive and athletic function has obvious consequences for politicians, diplomats, soldiers, businesspeople, and professional athletes.

EFFECTS

The most obvious evidence of jet lag for most travelers is inability to sleep during destination night and remain alert during destination day. Additional symptoms include headache, gastrointestinal complaints, clumsiness, irritability, difficulty concentrating, and reduction in cognitive and athletic functioning. Individuals vary considerably in their susceptibility to these symptoms. Jet lag tends to be worse for older travelers while infants appear to be less affected. Not surprisingly, the symptoms increase with the number of time zones crossed; eastward travel is usually more difficult to adjust to than westward.

TREATMENTS

A multitude of therapeutic interventions to reduce or eliminate jet lag have been promoted, with varying degrees of scientific evidence to support them. One difficulty in the evaluation of therapies for jet lag is the variability with which the condition presents itself. The best studies use clearly defined measures of cognitive performance and functioning, but the protocols vary among investigators.

Resetting the clock

Pre-travel sleep schedule adjustment

Many travelers find it useful to attempt adjusting their sleep and awakening times by an hour per day for several days before travel in an attempt to coincide with destination time. In addition, immediately resetting one's watch to destination time upon boarding the plane may provide the traveler with an additional mental cue to adjust sleep and eating times (Table 42.1).

Diet

One technique for reducing jet lag is a special diet plan developed at the Argonne National Laboratory of the United States Department of Energy. The 'Argonne diet' has a 'feast then fast' strategy, alternating days of high caloric intake with days of fasting for the 4 days prior to departure. On 'feast' days, the diet therefore calls for high protein breakfasts and high carbohydrate dinners. 'Fast' days allow less than 800 kcal/day, and are supposed to deplete the liver's store of carbohydrates, helping to prepare the internal clock for readjustment. The hypothesis behind this diet plan is that high protein meals increase tyrosine concentrations, promoting an increase in the levels of norepinephrine and dopamine, increasing alertness. High carbohydrate meals elevate tryptophan concentrations, resulting in higher serotonin levels, thought to have a role in sleep regulation and acting as a precursor to melatonin. Although formal studies have not confirmed the efficacy of the diet, it is still frequently cited. A simpler recommendation is simply to follow the recommendation of high protein breakfasts and high carbohydrate dinners upon arrival at the destination.

Light therapy

Exposure to bright light at the appropriate time can help to speed the resolution of circadian dyschronism. The efficacy of this approach depends on timing the light exposure around the nadir of the body temperature, which typically occurs at about 4 a.m. home time. Hence bright light in the internal clock's morning will advance the internal clock, and bright light in the evening will delay it. An eastward traveler should therefore seek light in the morning (05:00–11:00 h), and a westward traveler in the evening (22:00–04:00 h), based on home time. Exposure to bright light should be avoided at times which will produce a phase shift opposite in direction to what is desired.

Even on a cloudy day, daylight is much brighter than most inside lighting. Although early studies indicated that only bright levels of light, similar to daylight, were adequate to affect the internal clock, there is now evidence to suggest that even lower levels of light, such as those in offices and homes, may also play a role in resynchronization.[4] More interestingly, there is evidence that extraocular light exposure may also help adjust the internal clock. Some non-mammalian species of vertebrates are known to have extraocular and extrapineal light sensors. Until recently, no evidence for such a system has been found in mammals. However, a study at Cornell showed that the application of a 3 h pulse of light behind the knee to subjects otherwise kept in low ambient light succeeded in generating a phase response of up to 3 h over a 4 day period compared to controls. One explanatory hypothesis suggests that light falling on a vascular surface acts to increase the serum concentration of neuroactive gases such as nitric oxide and carbon dioxide by dissociating them from heme moieties, and that these gases act on neural pathways in a fashion similar to light. Some degree of evidence to support the steps in such a mechanism, such as the ability of nitric oxide to shift circadian phases, has already been documented.[5]

A number of commercial products are available to help travelers use light exposure to adjust to a new time zone. Computer programs to create the appropriate exposure schedule and caps that shine light on the eyes both have their adherents. A quick Internet search using 'light therapy' or 'phototherapy' will reveal sources for phototherapy aids (Table 42.2). Some hotels are providing 'light boxes' for their patrons' use.[6]

Exercise

For some individuals, vigorous exercise after arrival is helpful in alleviating jet lag. Experiments in hamsters have suggested that exercise can help adjust the internal clock, but its true effect on humans is less clear.[7] Exercise may help by forcing a state of alertness, promoting more restful sleep, or by actually inducing arousal in the central nervous system and affecting the suprachiasmatic nuclei.

Melatonin

Endogenous melatonin is secreted normally in a regular rhythm coinciding with nighttime, from approximately 21:00 h to 08:00 h. The hormone appears to directly affect the internal clock, hence

Table 42.1	Behavioral methods of adjusting circadian rhythm		
Method	Pros	Cons	Efficacy
Sleep schedule adjustment	Inexpensive, easily available	Inconvenient, especially for longer time changes	Good, if able to achieve
Diet	Inexpensive, easily available	Inconvenient, requires careful planning	Recent studies suggest little benefit
Light therapy Sunlight	Inexpensive, easily available	Requires scheduling	Good
Phototherapy devices	Convenient	Relatively expensive, some are bulky	Good
Exercise	Inexpensive, easily available, other health benefits	Requires scheduling, effort	Inconclusive data

Table 42.2	Examples of commercial sources for phototherapy products*
Full Spectrum Light Therapy Products	www.fullspectrumsolutions.com
Apollo Light Therapy Lightboxes	www.apollolight.com
Northern Light Technologies	www.northernlight-tech.com
Light Therapy Centre, The LightMask	www.lightmask.com
ParaLite Brand Full Spectrum Light Therapy	www.paralite.com
True Sun	www.truesun.com
Bio Brite Inc.	www.biobriteinc.com

*Inclusion in this list does not constitute endorsement of any specific product by the author or editors.

altering other circadian rhythms. Among these is the temperature rhythm; melatonin has a temperature lowering effect. The ingestion of exogenous melatonin appears to help induce sleep and to induce a phase shift. The mechanism of the apparent hypnotic effect of melatonin is not completely clear, but may be due to this action in lowering temperature, resetting the internal clock, and/or other mechanisms. Blind persons, who have what is termed 'free-running' circadian rhythms, which tend to oscillate on a schedule slightly longer than 24 h, often have sleep disorders. Melatonin has been found to help 'reset' these rhythms and reduce sleep problems in some blind persons.[8] The drug has been evaluated for the alleviation of symptoms of jet lag, and in most studies appears to show some benefit[9] but not in all.[10] However, in using melatonin to induce a phase shift, the timing of ingestion must be scheduled to advance or delay the internal clock appropriately. Like light exposure, there are situations in which taking melatonin at destination night might cause a phase shift opposite to what is desired, in particular after an eastward journey of greater than nine time zones.[4] The optimal dose amount and dosing regimen have not been determined. One recommendation suggests that the timing of melatonin ingestion for a situation where phase advance is desired would be one hour earlier each day until 15:00 home time is reached, by which time no further adjustment should be necessary. For a phase delay melatonin would be taken, one hour later each day until the dose falls at 06:00 home time. Alternatively, the eastward traveler may take a dose at 18:00–19:00 h home time on the day of departure followed by 4 days of a dose at destination bedtime. The westward traveler needs only take a dose at destination bedtime for the first 5 days after arrival. A dose of 3–5 mg is typically recommended, although much larger doses have been used.

Getting to sleep

Melatonin

The apparent direct hypnotic effect of melatonin has been discussed above. It has been compared in a clinical trial with midazolam for pre-operative premedication and found to confer anxiolysis and sedation without affecting the quality of recovery, whereas the midazolam caused some degree of impairment of cognitive and psychomotor skills.[11] A study on travelers flying from the USA to Switzerland showed that zolpidem was more effective in promoting sleep than melatonin (which was more effective than placebo), but again, more side-effects were noted with the zolpidem and almost none for melatonin.[12] However, at least one study showed adverse effects on vigilance and mental performance after doses of melatonin if the subjects were not allowed to sleep.[13]

Melatonin is sold as an unregulated herbal supplement in the USA and Hong Kong. As such, it has not been formally studied for safety, especially with long-term use, and the standards and quality of available preparations are uncontrolled. In many European countries and Canada, the use of melatonin is strictly regulated or entirely prohibited. In some cases, the importation of even small amounts for personal use may be illegal. Health-care providers and travelers should check local regulations before recommending or transporting melatonin.

Sedatives

Sedatives such as benzodiazepines can be used to help induce sleep at the appropriate hour in the new time zone, but may cause residual drowsiness on awakening. The shorter-acting sedatives, such as zolpidem or temazepam, are less likely to produce such a 'hangover'. Whether the sedatives have any specific effect on the internal clock remains unclear. GABA type A receptors exist in the suprachiasmatic nuclei, so benzodiazepines may have some direct effect, but animal studies are inconclusive and there are no data on humans. Concern has been raised over the use of any sedative while still on a plane, as a sedated sleeper may be less mobile and more prone to deep venous thrombosis (the same, of course, applies to alcohol).

Staying awake

Stimulants

Amphetamines

Amphetamines are effective in promoting alertness, but there remain concerns about their addictive potential and capacity for abuse. There is also some evidence that amphetamines may reduce decision-making ability and psychomotor performance, rather than enhance it.[4] Although they have been studied by the military, they are not currently recommended.

Caffeine

Caffeine clearly has the ability to promote alertness and delay sleep. It does, however, have just as clearly recognized side-effects including tachycardia and the development of a degree of dependence (resulting in the development of the 'caffeine withdrawal headache' upon discontinuation). As caffeine is also a diuretic, there are concerns that over-consumption of the stimulant may promote dehydration, even when taken as a drink. Heart arrhythmias have been reported in some cases. Long acting pharmaceutical preparations of caffeine are available for those who do not enjoy the beverages.

Pemoline

Pemoline is a central nervous system stimulant approved for the treatment of attention deficit disorder in children. It has some potential for abuse, although less than the amphetamines. The exact mechanism of action is unknown but appears to be via dopaminergic pathways. The long half-life, of 12 h, may make this drug less appealing for travelers as it may prevent initiation of sleep when appropriate, however at least one small study by the British military showed improved performance during overnight work with no ill effects on subsequent sleep.[14] The FDA has included a 'black box' warning on its labeling because of several cases of liver failure, but these cases all occurred after long term regular use of the medication.[15]

Modafinil

Modafinil is a non-amphetamine stimulant that has been approved for the treatment of narcolepsy. Its action involves the presynaptic activation of dopamine transmission in promoting wakefulness and the amplification of cortical serotonin release.[16,17] It appears to have minimal side effects, low abuse potential, and does not interfere with normal sleep. Modafinil has been used therapeutically in patients with narcolepsy for several years without the development of tolerance, and is under investigation by the military.[18] The drug has a slow onset of action and a half-life of about 10 h. It also has significant inter-actions with other medications, including anti-seizure medications, some cardiac medications, and oral contraceptives. Although it appears to have potential as a jet lag remedy, modafinil has not been well studied yet for that indication and is available only by prescription.

NADH

Nicotinamide adenine dinucleotide (NADH) is a co-enzyme required for the production of energy in cells. Its effects include the stimula-tion of dopamine, noradrenaline, and serotonin receptors, by which mechanism it is felt to increase mental alertness and clarity and improve concentration. In small studies it has been shown to provide benefit for patients with Alzheimer's, Parkinson's, and chronic fatigue syndrome. A stabilized form for oral consumption is marketed as a nutritional supplement, and therefore, like melatonin, is not under FDA regulation.

The use of NADH in the treatment of jet lag was evaluated with a standardized methodology in a small study. Subjects who received NADH had significantly better cognitive performance and a trend toward reduced sleepiness on the first post-flight day compared with controls and a smaller pilot study showed a similar trends lasting through the second day[19] (Table 42.3).

CONCLUSION

In sum, it appears that some degree of jet lag will remain a compo-nent of trans-meridianal travel for some time to come. The prepared traveler will plan the journey with the expectation of having to make some accommodations for this condition. Most experts recommend

insuring adequate sleep for the several nights prior to travel, given that some sleep deficit is almost sure to occur after arrival. During the flight, moderation is recommended with regard to food, alcohol and caffeine, and of course the respective sedative and stimulating effects of the latter two must be kept in mind when trying to adjust sleep patterns. For many, taking flights that arrive at destination bedtime is a helpful maneuver. Schedules for work or play for the first few days after arrival should be devised taking into account the internal clock's home 'night' and 'day'; important meetings or performances should if possible be scheduled at the time of maximal alertness, or delayed until the traveler has adjusted.

Planning sleep times is also important. As mentioned above, an overall sleep deficit is common. Short naps of 45 min or less may be surprisingly helpful in maintaining alertness,[20] and may be most beneficial at the time which would be the body's temperature nadir (~4 a.m. home time). Longer naps can be beneficial, but should be scheduled so as not to delay the adjustment of the internal clock. If traveling westward, it is preferable to delay sleeping until bedtime at the destination. It is generally felt to be more difficult to advance sleeping time when traveling eastward. In fact, for eastward travel of more than nine time zones, the body response is often to delay the internal clock rather than advance it, as if a longer westward shift had occurred. Travelers may find themselves more easily able to adjust to a new time zone after traveling eastward, for example, ten time zones, if they plan their sleep recalibration to delay the body clock by 14 h rather than try to advance it by 10 h.

Whether or not to use other specific strategies such as those out-lined above will depend on the traveler's needs and itinerary. For very short trips it may be easier to remain on home time rather than attempt to adjust. For longer trips in which no important activities

Table 42.3	Pharmacologic options for jet lag therapy		
Product	**Action**	**Side-effects**	**Availability**
Melatonin	Induce sleep, reset circadian clock	Inappropriate drowsiness may occur	Over the counter in USA, Hong Kong and perhaps elsewhere; restrictions may exist in some countries
Sedatives	Induce sleep	Inappropriate drowsiness, 'hangover', addictive potential	By prescription
Amphetamines	Promote alertness	May reduce decision-making capability; hypertension, tachycardia, addictive potential, may prevent normal sleep	By prescription
Caffeine	Promotes alertness	Jitteryness, hypertension, tachycardia; dependence, may prevent normal sleep	Easily available in various over-the-counter forms
Pemoline	Promotes alertness	Rare liver failure, long half life, mild potential for abuse, may prevent normal sleep	By prescription for attention deficit disorder
Modafinil	Promotes alertness without interfering with sleep	Slow onset of action, many drug interactions	By prescription for narcolepsy
Nicotinamide adenine dinucleotide (NADH)	Promotes alertness, improves mental clarity	Few reported, though limited data	Available over the counter as a nutritional supplement and by mail order

are scheduled for the first several days, a few days of decreased performance may not be an issue. Most travelers will find it useful to consider the possible approaches and select or modify those therapies, that will fit their personal requirements.

REFERENCES

1. Hastings M. The brain, circadian rhythms, and clock genes. *BMJ* 1998; **317**(7174):1704–1707.
2. Arendt J. Melatonin and the mammalian pineal gland. London: Chapman & Hall; 1995.
3. Seron-Ferre M, Riffo R, Valenzuela GJ. Germain AM Twenty-four-hour pattern of cortisol in the human fetus at term. *Am J Obstet Gynecol* 2001; **184**(6):1278–1283.
4. Waterhouse J, Reilly T, Atkinson G. Jet lag. *Lancet* 1997; **350**(9091):1611–1617.
5. Campbell SS, Murphy PJ. Extraocular circadian phototransduction in humans. *Science* 1998; **279**(5349):396–399.
6. Hilton Hotels. Sleep-Tight-Rooms™ available at selected properties – includes a light box 'sunrise clock', and other amenities designed to promote or restore healthy sleep.
7. Reebs S, Mrosovsky N. Effects of induced wheel-running on the circadian activity rhythm of Syrian hamsters: entrainment and phase-response curve. *J Biol Rhythms* 1994; **4**:39–48.
8. Sack RL, Brandes RW, Kendall AR, Lewy AJ. Entrainment of free-running circadian rhythms by melatonin in blind people. *N Engl J Med* 2000; **343**(15):1070–1077.
9. Herxheimer A, Petrie KJ. Melatonin for preventing and treating jet lag. *Cochrane Database Syst Rev* 2001; **1**:CD001520.
10. Brzezinski A. Mechanisms of disease: melatonin in humans. *N Engl J Med* 1997; **336**(3):186–195.
11. Naguib M, Samarkandi AH. The comparative dose-response effects of melatonin and midazolam for premedication of adult patients: a double-blinded, placebo-controlled study. *Anesth Analg* 2000; **91**(2):473–479.
12. Suhner A, Schlagenhauf P, Hofer I, *et al*. Effectiveness and tolerability of melatonin and zolpidem for the alleviation of jet lag. *Aviat Space Environ Med* 2001; **72**:638–646.
13. Zhdanova I, Wurtman R, Lynch H, *et al*. Sleep inducing effects of low doses of melatonin ingested in the evening. *Clin Pharm Ther* 1995; **57**:552–558.
14. Nicholson AN. Turner C Intensive and sustained air operations: potential use of the stimulant. *pemoline Aviat Space Environ Med* 1998; **69**(7):647–655.
15. FDA labeling for Cylert®; 6/17/99.
16. Nishino S, Mao J, Sampathkumaran R, Shelton J. Increased dopaminergic transmissin mediates the wake-promoting effects of CNS stimulants. *Sleep Res Online* 1998; **1**(1):49–61.
17. Ferraro L, Fuxe K, Tnaganelli S, *et al*. Amplification of cortical serotonin release: a further neurochemical action of the vigilance-promoting drug modafinil. *Neuropharmacology* 2000; **39**(11):1974–1983.
18. Lyons TJ, French J. Modafinil: the unique properties of a new stimulant. *Aviat Space Environ Med* 1991; **62**(5):432–435.
19. Viirre ES, Kay GG. *Assessing the efficacy of Pharmaceuticals and Nutraceuticals as countermeasures for jet lag.* Presented at the 7th International Conference of the International Society of Travel Medicine, May 2001.
20. Naitoh P, Kelly TL, Babkoff H. Napping, Stimulant, and Four-Choice Performance. In: Broughton RJ, Ogilvie RD, eds. *Sleep, Arousal, and Performance: Problems and Promises.* Cambridge, MA: Birk Hauser Boston; 1992:198–219.

CHAPTER 43 Motion Sickness

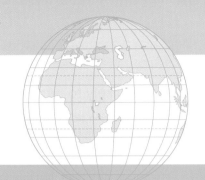

Susan M. Kuhn

KEYPOINTS

- Despite many triggers to motion sickness and the serious difficulties that many have with it, habituation will occur in most people after 3–4 days of sustained motion

- Mal de debarquement syndrome is not well known; it is post-motion vertigo and disequilibrium after disembarking from a ship, even if the traveler is asymptomatic during the journey

- Women are more likely to suffer from motion sickness, particularly around menses and during pregnancy

- Though acupressure is claimed to be effective in the treatment of motion sickness, there are insufficient data supporting any positive impact

- In general, anti-motion sickness medications are more effective if taken prior to the exposure; most induce drowsiness

INTRODUCTION

To travel is to move – so what condition is potentially more relevant to the traveler than motion sickness? In fact, virtually anyone can suffer from this malady, given the right – or more accurately *wrong* – circumstances. The frequency and severity varies, but for some travelers the impact is significant and may ruin a long-awaited and expensive holiday. The secret is to 'be prepared.' The travel health professional must gather sufficient information about an individual's general health, motion susceptibility, and trip itinerary to identify situations in which motion sickness will be a potential risk. For some travelers, counseling on the topic may consist of suggesting the inclusion of an anti-motion sickness medication in a medical kit. For others who will be sailing to the Antarctic, crossing the Sahara desert on camel-back, or for the scuba-diver with severe motion sensitivity, discussing preventive and treatment strategies may be an important component of the pre-travel consultation. Therefore it is essential that the travel health professional have a clear understanding of motion sickness and how it can be prevented or treated.

Triggers of motion sickness

Motion sickness results from exposure to movement or visual suggestion of movement.[1] Traveling through water, on land, and in air may all trigger motion sickness, although seasickness is the most common and notorious form of this condition. Provocative environments include a variety of mechanical vehicles such as ships, planes, cars, buses, trains, carnival rides, and spinning chairs. Riding on the back of an animal can also be a powerful stimulus, particularly those that

cause a lot of swaying or rocking (e.g., camels). Self-propelled motion such as gymnastics or downhill skiing during white-out conditions, or even motion in a state of weightlessness during space flight or floating in water may also be triggers. Scuba-diving or snorkeling in rough water, for example, results in turbulent movement in absence of both the orienting influence of gravity and a visual frame of reference. Luckily, sustained exposure to a constant motion over 3–4 days results in habituation in most individuals.[2] Habituation is thought to be the result of central nervous system compensation, but the exact mechanism has yet to be elucidated. Unfortunately, this tolerance is lost within a similar time period if the motion stops or changes.

Similar symptoms can also result when the movement to which the person has adapted suddenly stops, a kind of 'anti-motion' sickness. The most common example is the transient 'landsickness' sometimes experienced after disembarking from a ship. An unusual and persistent condition known as mal de debarquement syndrome (MDD) is literally an 'illness of disembarkment'. Those who suffer from MDD are usually asymptomatic during the journey, which may include travel by ship, train, or even in space. Symptoms of this form of post-motion vertigo include a sense of disequilibrium along with sensations of swaying or rocking, lasting from a month to years. Explanations are speculative, although it has been suggested that the normal motion compensation during the journey continues when the motion ceases, hence the ongoing perception of movement. MDD does not respond to typical anti-motion sickness medications.[3]

Visual suggestion of movement when the individual is stationary is an equally strong trigger for motion sickness. 'Vection', or illusory self-motion, is created with rotating drums around a stationary patient for laboratory studies.[4] It is also encountered in many real-life situations such as flight simulators, computer games, and movies.

What is motion sickness?

Motion sickness typically consists of a progression of symptoms.[1] The individual initially feels a vague abdominal discomfort sometimes referred to as 'stomach awareness', followed by malaise and nausea which may culminate in vomiting. These gastrointestinal symptoms are associated with measurable changes in gastric muscle activity. Electrogastrography (EGG) in laboratory settings reveals increased and/or uncoordinated muscle activity known as gastric tachyarrhythmia.[4]

In addition to these gastrointestinal effects, other symptoms may include a sense of body warmth, lightheadedness, tachypnea, sighing, yawning, headache, drowsiness, increased salivation, and frequent swallowing. Pallor and sweating is often observed.[1] Lethargy, fatigue and mental slowness that persists after resolution of the gastrointestinal symptoms in some patients has been labeled the 'Sopite syndrome'. Electroencephalography (EEG) monitoring reveals slowing of alpha waves over the frontal areas for about two hours after severe motion sickness, and correlates with this drowsiness and loss in performance.[5]

Who is likely to get motion sickness?

Although motion sickness can occur in virtually anyone, a small proportion of the population is highly resistant while a similar number are very susceptible. The condition is also related to gender and age, and may be influenced by other personal and environmental factors. Women are more likely than men to suffer,[6] particularly near menses and during pregnancy, suggesting a hormonal influence. Symptoms such as nausea and vomiting are uncommon in children under the age of 2, but susceptibility increases thereafter until about 12 to 15 years of age, and then declines steadily and is least common among the elderly.[6] Those who suffer from migraine headaches are more likely to be sensitive to motion. Underlying conditions or medications that cause nausea may mimic or increase the severity of motion sickness as well.

What is the mechanism of motion sickness?

'Motion sickness' is a normal response to an abnormal stimulus, namely conflicting information from the sensory systems that detect and interpret motion with respect to one's surroundings.[7] Contributing input comes from the vestibular, proprioceptive, and visual systems, although past experience or memory of motion sickness may also influence this reaction. Individuals can suffer as a result of a visual perception of movement in absence of a corresponding vestibular sensation, or when there is a sensation of body movement with contradictory visual cues. Processing of this sensory input occurs in the central nervous system, and results in a complex physical response via the autonomic nervous system.

THE VESTIBULAR SYSTEM

Studies comparing persons with normal vestibular systems with those who have bilateral peripheral vestibular deficiencies (e.g., labyrinthectomy) clearly show the inability of the latter to suffer motion sickness.[8] On the other hand, blindness does not confer immunity against the condition. Therefore it appears that a functioning vestibular system is probably essential for the development of motion sickness. Different types of real or perceived movement may trigger motion sickness, including both linear and angular head acceleration. A very powerful stimulus combines these movements, with rotation around a vertical axis and movement in the sagittal plane, known as the Coriolis effect.[1]

The vestibular or balance system works to maintain the physical self in appropriate alignment to the earth (gravity) and to respond to changes in position in space. The semi-circular canals and the vestibule are contiguous and filled with a fluid called endolymph (Fig. 43.1). The three semicircular canals are perpendicular to each other, therefore rotational movement in any direction can be detected as the endolymph shifts and stimulates hair ciliae of the ampulae of the appropriate canal(s) (Fig. 43.2). Hence the semi-circular canals provide information about non-linear acceleration. The vestibule is a fluid-filled space occupied by two membranes perpendicular to each other called the utricle and the saccule. The membrane surfaces are made up of hair cells, which are covered by a gelatinous layer in which microscopic particles (otoliths) are embedded. The mass of the latter can be affected both by linear movements as well as gravity in the absence of motion. Therefore the signals from the utricle and saccule provide information with respect to the head orientation as well as detect linear acceleration in those planes (Fig. 43.3).[1]

The central physiology of motion sickness is less clear, but appears to involve a complex interplay between all levels of the brain and

Figure 43.1 Anatomy of the labyrinth.

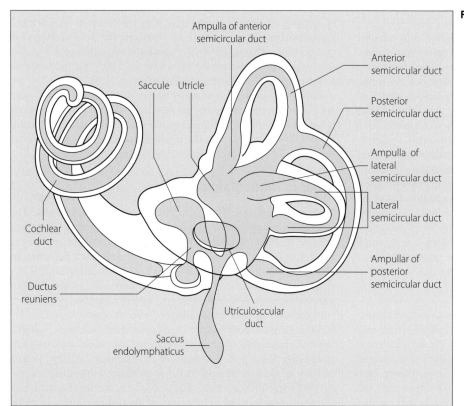

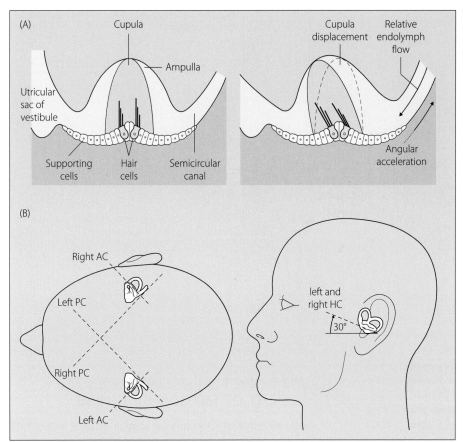

Figure 43.2 The crista. (A) Organ of crista of semicircular canals. (B) Orientation of semicircular canals in skull. HC, horizontal canal; AC, anterior canal; PC, posterior canal.

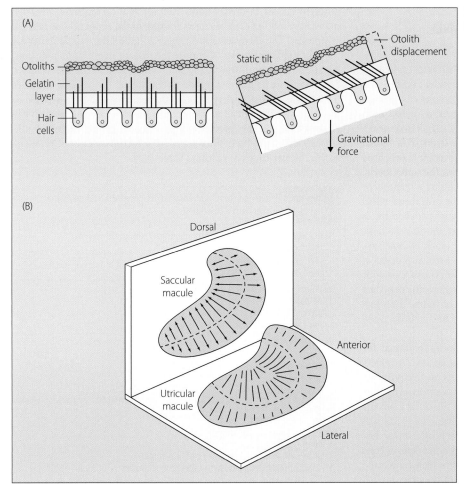

Figure 43.3 (A) Macule within saccule and utricle. (B) Orientation of saccule and utricle in skull.

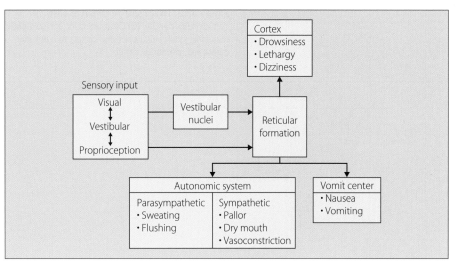

Figure 43.4 Proposed neural pathway resulting in motion sickness.

vestibular, visual, proprioceptive and autonomic centers (Fig. 43.4). This may explain why medications with a variety of mechanisms of action can ameliorate symptoms.[5] Along with the clinical symptoms resembling an adrenalin-like 'fight or flight' response, there is laboratory evidence of sympathetic nervous system and sympathoadrenal-medullary system activation. Both epinephrine and norepinephrine levels rise in subjects reporting motion sickness. Cortisol and beta-endorphin levels do not rise but are elevated at baseline prior to exposure to the stimulus in those who develop motion sickness, possibly suggesting anticipation based on past experience.[4]

NON-MEDICINAL PREVENTION AND TREATMENT OPTIONS

Most environmental preventive approaches have had little evaluation to determine efficacy, particularly in real-life situations. Positioning oneself in the most stable part of the vehicle is commonly recommended, and while it may benefit in some situations, it has been shown to have little impact in severe conditions.[9] Exaggerated movement of the head and upper body appears to be strongly linked to symptoms, possibly greater in certain planes of movement compared with others. If the person is firmly restrained across the upper body, motion sensitivity is reduced or prevented.[10] Assuming a recumbent position presumably has a similar ameliorating or preventive effect and is commonly advised. Minimizing conflicting visual input is another strategy found useful by those who suffer motion sickness, including avoidance of fixation on close objects (such as reading), and instead focusing on a distant point. Although consumption of large meals or certain foods, drinking alcohol, and exposure to poor ventilation or noxious odors have been noted to increase the risk, data to confirm some of these claims is contradictory or sparse. Personal experience with exacerbating factors may prove to be the most useful guide for individual travelers.

Acupressure has been claimed to be an efficacious treatment for motion-sickness and other conditions that induce nausea. A variety of acupressure products are marketed commercially for this purpose. The theory behind wrist bands is that stimulation or pressure at the P6 or Neiguan point (located three finger-widths proximal from the wrist crease between the palmaris longus and flexor carpi radialis tendons) decreases symptoms of nausea. However at least one placebo-controlled study using a commercial band as recommended suggests minimal to no impact on motion sickness, at least in males subjected to very provocative rotational stimuli.[11] Insufficient pressure applied

at this point during stimulation may explain this negative result, but also suggests the potential for incorrect use and at best, variable results. Therefore additional strategies or medications should be offered for situations where motion sickness is very likely or severe (Table 43.1).

MEDICATIONS FOR PREVENTION AND TREATMENT OF MOTION SICKNESS

It is better to anticipate and prevent motion sickness rather than attempt to treat it after it occurs. There are an increasing number of different classes of medications used for motion sickness, although many have similar central effects leading to the reduction or relief of symptoms. The chemoreceptor trigger zone and the emetic center are thought to play key roles, therefore the major categories include anti-histamine (H1), anti-muscarinic, and anti-dopaminergic medications. Stimulants are sometimes added to counteract the adverse effects of the other agents. A variety of other agents have also been studied or used empirically. Not all of the medications discussed are available in all countries, but the travel health practitioner should become familiar with other products since travelers sometimes seek out remedies in the country they are visiting (Table 43.2).

Table 43.1	**Behavioral strategies to prevent or reduce motion sickness**

Select seating in most stable area of vehicle with good visibility
   Mid-ship, near center of vessel
   Over wings of aircraft
   Front seat of car, or front section of train or bus

Minimize upper body and head movement
   Lie recumbent
   Use seat restraint
   Lean against head-rest

Maintain visual orientation
   Fix gaze on distant object or horizon
   Take over driving of car
   Close eyes
   Avoid reading

Personal adjustments
   Eat small, frequent meals
   Avoid alcohol and smoking
   Deep breathing
   Sit in well-ventilated area or open a window
   Avoid or remove odors that exacerbate symptoms

Table 43.2   Medications for the prevention or treatment of motion sickness.

Drug	Oral dose (mg)	First dose (prophylaxis)	Dosing interval (hours)	Route(s) of administration	Comments	Common adverse effects	Availability
Dimenhydrinate (Gravol®, Dramamine®)	Adult: 50–100 Child (years): >12: 50 6–12: 25–50 2–6: 12.5–25	1–2 h prior	>12 years: 4–6 <12 years: 6–8	Oral, i.m., suppository	Not in pregnancy or <2 years	Drowsiness (moderate), vertigo	US, Canada, Europe, Australia, S. Africa
Meclizine (Bonine®, Bonamine®, Antivert®)	Adult: 25–50 Child <12 years: 12.5–25	1–2 h prior	12–24	Oral	Not in pregnancy.	Drowsiness (mild)	US, Canada, Europe
Cinnarizine (Sturgeon®)	Adult: 30 initially, 15 thereafter Child 5–12 years: 15 initially, 7.5 thereafter	1–2 h prior	6–8	Oral	Not in pregnancy. Dose <5 years unknown.	Drowsiness (varies)	Europe, S. Africa
Cyclizine (Marezine®, Marzine®, Valoid®)	Adult: 50 Child: 6–10 years: 25 <6 years: 12.5	1–2 h prior	4–6	Oral or i.m.	Not in pregnancy.	Drowsiness	US (oral), Canada (i.m.)
Buclizine (Buclidin-S Softabs®)	Adult: 50 mg	1 h prior	4–6	Oral	Not in pregnancy or children.	Drowsiness	US, Europe
Promethazine (Phenergan®)	Adult: 25–50 Child: >2 years 0.25–0.5 mg/kg	2 h prior	6–12	Oral, i.m.	May be used in pregnancy. Avoid <2 years.	Severe drowsiness, impaired mental performance	US, Canada, Europe, Australia
Scopolamine hydrochloride (Hyoscine®)	Adult: 0.3–0.6	1 h prior	4–6	Oral or i.m.	Not in pregnancy, childhood, or with glaucoma. Avoid in elderly, with urinary obstruction, or sedatives.	Dry mouth, drowsiness, blurred vision	Europe, Australia
Scopolamine (Transderm-Scop®, Transderm-V®)	Adult: 1.5 in topical form	≥8 h prior	72	Topical patch behind ear (wash hands after applying)			US, Canada, Europe, S. Africa
Dextroamphetamine (Dexedrine®, Dextrostat®)	Adult: 5–10	1–2 h prior	8	Oral	Reserved for extreme conditions, usually in combination with other drugs.	Restlessness, potential for abuse	US, Canada, Europe; illegal to prescribe for motion sickness in some areas
Ephedrine	Adult: 25–50	1–2 h prior	8	Oral	Less effective than dextroamphetamine but not a controlled drug.	Restlessness, tachycardia	US, Canada, Europe, Australia

Antihistamine, anti-muscarinic and anti-dopaminergic medications

There are a large number of potential agents in use around the world. Examples of antihistamines include dimenhydrate, cinnarizine, cyclizine, buclizine and meclizine. The most common phenothiazine used is promethazine, which blocks both dopamine and histamine receptors. Metoclopramide can also be used, and is particularly effective in reducing gastrointestinal symptoms although it is not indicated for motion sickness in some countries. The most common anti-muscarinic medication used is scopolamine. Product presentations for all of these medications vary, in some cases including oral (liquid, tablets, chews), suppositories, topical (skin patches) and injectable formulations.

These drugs have varying degrees of anti-cholinergic effects, most notably with scopolamine. Drowsiness is common with all, but tends to be most pronounced with dimenhydrate, scopolamine, and promethazine. Dry mouth, blurred vision, tachycardia, headache, vertigo, restlessness, euphoria, hallucinations, constipation, urinary retention, and rash may also occur. Scopolamine should be strictly avoided with conditions such as prostatic hypertrophy and glaucoma. Concomitant use of alcohol or other CNS-depressants should be avoided to prevent potentially life-threatening additive effects. These adverse effects may reduce utility of these medications in situations where mental alertness is essential, although they may be partly counteracted by the addition of stimulants. Particular caution should be exercised with the elderly in whom adverse effects such as hallucinations and confusion may be exaggerated, especially since motion sickness is less likely in this age group.

Avoidance of anti-motion sickness medications is usually advised in pregnancy and infancy. For the latter this may not be a frequent issue in view of their relative resistance to the effects of movement. The best option for children under 2 years is probably judicious use of dimenhydrate. On the other hand, pregnant women are at increased risk of motion sickness. If the instigating conditions cannot be avoided or modified, it may become necessary to use medication for prophylaxis or treatment. Most antihistamines including meclizine, cyclizine, and dimenhydrate are considered Category B substances with no evidence of risk in humans. A recent review notes that although promethazine is a category C drug (no adequate studies in humans), it may be the agent of choice.[12] A risk-benefit discussion should be undertaken to plan a course of action for the pregnant individual.

There are a plethora of studies comparing different agents to each other and placebo. While some studies have found certain drugs to be more efficacious than others, a recent study examining seven different products in field conditions found no significant differences in reported symptoms of motion sickness during a sea voyage.[13] Generally, promethazine and scopolamine are considered more effective in extreme conditions than the antihistamines. The side-effect profile is also a useful guide to the selection of one class of agents over another.[5]

It is important to point out that while reduction of the symptoms of motion sickness is appealing, by doing so these medications are interfering with the normal CNS response to conflicting vestibulo-visual input. As a result, adaptation is slowed, and it may actually take the medicated traveler longer to adjust to motion than someone who does not take such drugs.[2]

Treatment of established motion sickness

It is preferable to prevent rather than treat motion sickness, however this may become necessary when the degree of motion is not anticipated, or if the preventive medication proves inadequate. Oral medications are often not tolerated due to established nausea and vomiting, so alternative routes of administration are necessary. Suppositories are one option, and in some circumstances intramuscular injections may be necessary.

Intramuscular (i.m.) dimenhydrate is less effective than i.m. promethazine or scopolamine for treatment of motion sickness. Promethazine has a longer duration of action, but onset is slightly longer than scopolamine by this route. All three can cause marked drowsiness and decreased performance.[14] Benzodiazepines are used in a variety of vertiginous conditions including MDD, and exert their effect by acting on central vestibular pathways.[1] Caution must be exercised if such medications are taken after prophylactic drugs fail given the potentially additive adverse effects.

Adjunctive, New and Experimental Agents

Other categories of medications and foods have been investigated for their utility in the prevention of motion sickness. Stimulants such as caffeine or ephedrine are sometimes combined with other agents to counter side-effects such as drowsiness. Amphetamines such as dextroamphetamine sulfate also have a direct effect on motion sickness[5] via inhibition of vestibular nuclei activity[1], which may be synergistic when used with drugs such as scopolamine or promethazine.[15] Ginger powder has shown variable efficacy, although it may be more useful to counter the gastrointestinal rather than the central effects.[13] Similarity between the EEG activity seen in motion sickness and seizures led to the discovery that the anti-convulsant phenytoin reduces motion-induced nausea.[16] Phenytoin affects a wide variety of sites in the central nervous system, including vestibular nuclei. Blood level monitoring and potentially significant side-effects means it has limited applications for most travelers. Potent anti-emetics such as the 5-HT3 antagonist ondansetron do not appear to have significant benefit in the prevention of motion-induced nausea.[17]

Individualized recommendations for prevention or treatment of motion sickness

Pharmacologic differences between anti-motion sickness drugs result in variable efficacy, onset and duration of activity, as well as adverse effects. Therefore medication selection is based on an assessment of the likelihood and severity of motion sickness, the time before it is expected to occur, the anticipated duration of exposure, as well as the travelers' underlying age and health characteristics. For some occupational travelers, efficacy must be balanced with the impact of adverse effects on job performance. In these cases, combination with sympathomimetic drugs should be considered (Table 43.3)

CONCLUSION

Motion sickness need not be the bane of the traveler's existence. Armed with sufficient knowledge about both the traveler and their itinerary, the travel health professional should be able to offer advice on appropriate behavioral and pharmacologic options that may prevent and treat motion sickness.

Table 43.3 Selection of anti-motion sickness medications

Traveler	Duration of motion	Time prior to departure (for prophylaxis)	Preventive drug options	
			Mild to moderate conditions	Moderate to severe conditions
Healthy adult or teenager	≤6 h	1 h or more	Antihistamines[a]	Promethazine ± amphetamine, dimenhydrinate, scopolamine (oral)
Healthy adult or teenager	>6 h	8 h or more	Antihistamines or scopolamine patch	Scopolamine patch, promethazine ± amphetamine, dimenhydrinate
Elderly	Any	Any	Nil	Consider anti-histamine
Pregnant woman	Any	Any	See text	See text
Child 2–12 years	Any	1 h or more	Meclizine, cyclizine, dimenhydrinate, cinnarizine (>5 years)	Dimenhydrinate, promethazine
Child <2 years	Any	Any	Nil	Dimenhydrinate (0.5 mg/kg) if necessary

[a]meclizine, cyclizine, cinnarizine, buclizine, dimenhydrinate.

REFERENCES

1. Baloh RW. *Dizziness, Hearing Loss, and Tinnitus.* Philadelphia: FA Davis Company; 1998.
2. Wood CD, Stewart JJ, Wood MJ, *et al.* Habituation and motion sickness. *J Clin Pharm* 1994; **34**:628–634.
3. Hain TC, Hanna PA. Rheinberger MA. Mal de Debarquement. *Arch Otolaryngol Head Neck Surg* 1999; **125**:615–620.
4. Koch KL, Stern RM, Vasey MW, *et al.* Neuroendocrine and gastric myoelectrical responses to illusory self-motion in humans. *Am J Physiol* 1990; **258**:E304–E310.
5. Wood CD, Stewart JJ, Wood MJ, Manno BR, Mims ME. Therapeutic effects of antimotion sickness medications on the secondary symptoms of motion sickness. *Aviat Space Environ Med* 1990; **61**:157–161.
6. Mills KL, Griffen MJ. Effect of Seating, vision and direction of horizontal oscillation on motion sickness. *Aviat Space Environ Med* 2000; **71**(10):996–1002.
7. Eyeson-Annan M, Peterkin C, Brown B, Atchinson D. Visual and vestibular components of motion sickness. *Aviat Space Environ Med* 1996; **67**:955–962.
8. Cheung BSK, Howard IP, Money KE. Visually-induced sickness in normal and bilaterally labyrinthine-defective subjects. *Aviat Space Environ Med* 1991; **62**:527–631.
9. Gahlinger PM. Cabin location and the likelihood of motion sickness in cruise ship passengers. *J Travel Med* 2000; **7**:120–124.
10. Mills KL, Griffen MJ. Effect of seating, vision and direction of horizontal oscillation on motion sickness. *Aviat Space Environ Med* 2000; **71**(10):996–1002.
11. Warwick-Evans LA, Masters IJ, Redstone SB. A double-blind placebo controlled evaluation of acupressure in the treatment of motion sickness. *Aviat Space Environ Med* 1991; **62**:776–778.
12. Samuel BU, Barry M. The pregnant traveler. *Infect Dis Clin N Am* 1998; **12**:325–354.
13. Schmid R, Schick T, Steffen R, Tschopp A, Wilk T. Comparison of seven commonly used agents for prophylaxis of seasickness. *J Travel Med* 1994; **1**:203–206.
14. Wood CD, Stewart JJ, Wood MJ, Mims ME. Effectiveness and duration of intramuscular antimotion sickness medications. *J Clin Pharm* 1992; **32**:1008–1012.
15. Dobie TG, May JG. Cognitive-behavioral management of motion sickness. *Aviat Space Environ Med* 1994; **65**:C1–C20.
16. Knox GW, Woodard D, Chelen W, Ferguson R, Johnson L. Phenytoin for motion sickness: clinical evaluation. *Laryngoscope* 1994; **104**:935–939.
17. Levine ME, Chillas MS, Stern RM, Knox G. The effects of serotonin (5-HT3) receptor antagonists on gastric tachyarrhythmia and the symptoms of motion sickness. *Aviat Space Environ Med* 2000; **71**:1111–1114.

CHAPTER 44 # Environmental Issues in Travel Medicine

William B. Bunn and Jessica Herzstein

KEYPOINTS

- Air pollutants such as nitrogen dioxide, sulfur dioxide, carbon monoxide, lead and particulate matter and air toxics can play a major role in traveler's health in certain areas of the world

- Air pollution in urban areas occurs primarily due to motor vehicle emissions, Asia Pacific being one of the most commonly cited examples

- Where coal is a major source of energy, a variety of pollutants are found in the environment as well as indoors that are toxic to humans. Other indoor pollutants include radon, asbestos, formaldehyde and pesticides

- Evaluation of travelers or for placement of expatriates should involve consideration of any underlying cardiopulmonary disease, especially if the destination is an area of high air pollution. Discussion should take place regarding effective ways to reduce or avoid exposure (e.g., best time of day for outdoor exercise)

- There is no globally accepted measurement system for pollution and thus interpretation of reported levels of various pollutants are difficult

INTRODUCTION

Environmental pollution has become a cause of increasing concern for travelers, short-term assignees and expatriates. Reasons for this heightened concern include a significant increase in levels of air pollution, especially in Asia and South America; a better understanding of the health risks of ozone and particulate matter; increased regulatory and medical scrutiny; and growing numbers of adventure, business, and older travelers going to destinations where environmental health is an issue. Water contamination is considered elsewhere so the focus of this chapter will be air pollution.

AIR POLLUTION AS AN INTERNATIONAL ISSUE

Air pollutants are divided into two categories: primary air pollutants and toxic air contaminants. Primary air pollutants commonly listed are carbon monoxide, particulate matter, oxides of nitrogen, lead, ozone and sulfur oxides. Over 250 pollutants are considered toxic air pollutants, e.g., chlorinated hydrocarbons, aldehydes and heavy metals. There is increasing evidence that exposure to both primary air pollutants and toxic air contaminants are associated with adverse health outcomes. Travel to many developing and industrialized countries involves exposure to high levels of some air pollutants, raising issues

about the impact on a traveler's health. A susceptible individual, (e.g. a traveler with pre-existing lung disease), may be at particular risk. In urban areas, air pollution occurs primarily due to motor vehicle emissions (carbon monoxide, carbon dioxide, nitric acid, benzene, particulate materials) and power and heat generation (particulate matter and SO_2 from soft coal combustion and industrial power generation; NO_2 from indoor cooking and heating with gas). Wind-blown dust also is a major contributor to pollution in both urban and rural areas.[1,2]

Internationally, Mexico City is one of the most commonly cited examples of air pollution, with increased levels of all primary pollutants at times during recent years. Indoor air can be a problem due to particulate matter from dust and combustion sources as well as ozone levels in modern buildings which can be one-half to two-thirds those of outdoor levels. Outdoors, increased lead levels related to dust inhalation are a concern. While lead levels in gasoline have been reduced, lead is still used. Thermal inversions occurring in the winter and early spring contribute to particularly high levels of ozone, resulting in eye, mucous membrane, and respiratory irritation in most travelers. Pollution related to thermal inversions, however, is not unique to Mexico City; cities along the entire Pacific coast, from Los Angeles to Lima, experience increased health risks during inversion periods.

Major cities in Asia also have increasing pollution levels. A number of factors combine to increase health risks substantially: traffic congestion; older, poorly maintained vehicles; and industrial pollution sources. Even Katmandu, Nepal, has such high levels of pollution (primarily due to unregulated vehicle emissions) that face masks are commonly worn in downtown areas. Unfortunately, face masks only protect the individual from larger particles and are not effective for most combustion particulate and fine particles from other sources. In China, aside from some cities where natural or liquid petroleum gas is available, coal is the major source of energy, producing high levels of SO_2 and particulate matter indoors. Beijing has a significant particulate problem due to the continued use of brown coal (although its use is declining), and the particulate pollution is dramatically increased by the 'loess' – fine particulate matter blown in by the wind from the Gobi desert. Particulate problems are exacerbated by other phenomena such as forest clearing by burning. In Jakarta, Singapore, and other cities in the region, burning has led to extremely high particulate levels – high enough to necessitate evacuation of multinational expatriates and to restrict visitors with underlying cardio-pulmonary disease. Filtering masks are not useful for smoke and even indoor restriction generally does not reduce exposure to acceptable levels. Therefore, it is best to avoid the region during highly polluted periods if one has underlying pulmonary disease.

Air pollution is not confined to Asia, however; central and eastern European countries have significant levels of all primary pollutants, and particulates, and air toxics are of concern due to limited emissions controls. In Russia, all forms of pollution (air, water, solid and hazardous waste) are a major problem. Mediterranean countries lag behind northern Europe in pollution reduction (for instance, Athens has a significant NO problem), but even northern Europe can experience high particulate levels during the summer months.

In sub-Saharan Africa, the 'harmattan' winds and pollutants blow desert sands from the Sahara over much of Central and Southern Africa. In many major cities (e.g., Accra, Lagos) the particles frequently combine with air pollution from other sources to produce very high exposure levels. Cairo and Alexandria have environmental pollution both from combustion sources and natural sources, such as the above-mentioned harmattan. In the Middle East, sandstorms are common and often necessitate respiratory protection from blown sand; the combination of dust and extreme heat (up to 120–130°F) can lead to significant health risks.

Indoor air pollution is a major issue in a number of countries; pollutants can include radon (Rn), asbestos, lead, formaldehyde, pesticides, respirable particles and environmental tobacco smoke (ETS), biologicals (pollen, fungi, dust mites, etc.), carbon monoxide, nitrogen dioxide, and organic gases (paint, solvents, aerosols, disinfectants, etc.). Radioactive pollutants may be a problem from air, food or water (vegetables are often stored, stored vegetables may be higher risk). Recent increases in trekking and adventure travel have brought the issue of indoor cooking to the attention of travelers. This issue is particularly important in China where indoor air pollution levels are increased greatly during periods of indoor cooking with inadequate ventilation. In addition, air toxins and allergens are more common from indoor air in developing countries. A comprehensive review of pollution including seasonal changes is beyond the scope of this article, but Figures 44.1 and 44.2 present general information on air pollution.[3]

ASSESSING RISK

Although there is growing awareness of the risk from air pollution in many travel destinations, clear guidelines for the prevention of symptoms or disease have not been developed. In order to adequately advise the traveler, travel health providers must assess the potential risk to the traveler based on the extent of air pollution at the planned destination, duration and timing of the trip, underlying health conditions of the traveler, and medical resources available at the destination. The combination of increased risk and inadequate medical facilities in many developing countries is particularly challenging. While anyone can be affected by air pollution, travelers at increased risk of health problems resulting from air pollution or other pollution sources may include those with chronic diseases, the older or very young, and the adventure traveler. In these cases, and particularly for those who suffer from chronic disease, the duration of the trip or expatriation combined with the level of personal exposure will determine what, if any, long-term risks exist. If the combination of increased risk of air pollution and underlying risk of the traveler causes concern, the following actions must be taken.

First, a realistic appraisal of environmental exposure must be made. It is not uncommon to overestimate outdoor air pollution, since cited

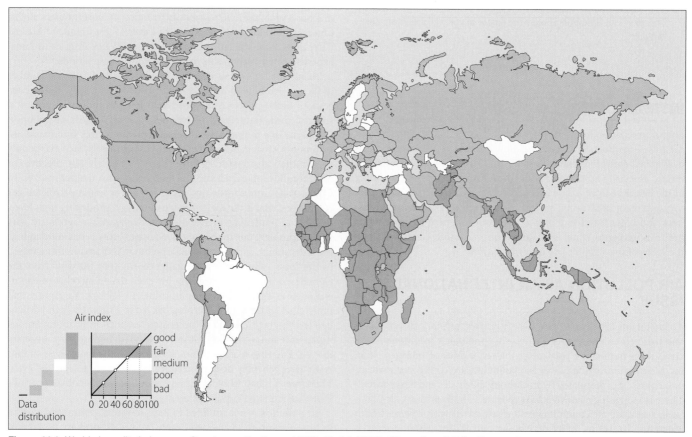

Figure 44.1 World air quality index map. Country results: 0, good (0%); 82, fair (46%); 27, medium (15%); 42, poor (23%); 28, bad (16%); 1, no data (1%).

levels will often be from the period of the greatest pollution levels. Conversely, indoor air pollution is often underestimated, and the traveler must be questioned about combustion sources in the indoor environment. It must be noted, however, that there is no international measurement system, and thus interpretation of reported levels may be difficult (e.g., the levels of particulates reported from Singapore and Jakarta do not directly correspond to µg/m³, the US measurement unit). The underlying risk of disease or disease exacerbation for the traveler or expatriate should be assessed. The exacerbation of pre-existing respiratory or cardiovascular disease (such as congestive heart failure) and the acute health effects from respiratory, mucous membrane, and eye irritation must be considered for all travelers and foreign residents. Adequate oxygenation may be affected by multiple environmental factors including altitude and pollution levels. Asthma, chronic obstructive pulmonary disease, pulmonary fibrosis, and other respiratory diseases and conditions must be assessed. For example, a traveler with sinus drainage or infection who will be flying must be aware of the possibility of barotrauma from air travel. A traveler who usually wears contact lenses should be advised to bring regular eyeglasses along, if she/he will be in an area of heavy dust and ozone.

In order to advise the traveler, the travel health provider must integrate the likelihood and duration of exposure during the trip, possible methods to reduce the levels of exposure, underlying risk of disease or exacerbation of disease, and medical resources available. Therefore, longer term travelers to remote areas may need a full medical evaluation (including vaccines) and travel history similar to an occupational history for workers in high hazard jobs. Physical examination and special testing (e.g., CXR, PFTs) should be performed only as indicated from the travel history.

GENERAL RECOMMENDATIONS AND CONCLUSION

- Discuss with the traveler effective ways to reduce or avoid exposure, such as the best time of day for outdoor exercise, times of the year when outdoor air quality is least affected by pollution, methods of assessing indoor air pollution risks (such as smoke opacity or mucous membrane irritation), the use of face masks, etc. (For example, the air pollution in Mexico City worsens as the day progresses; thus those who exercise outdoors should be advised to do so early in the day.)
- If an underlying health problem exists, ensure that treatment is stabilized before travel commences. Advise that all medications the patient currently takes or has taken in the last 12 months are carried on the trip (such as inhalers for asthmatic travelers) and provide the traveler with the necessary documentation for those medications (e.g., a letter to be used for customs).
- Update all indicated vaccines.
- For each travel destination, try to give the traveler the name and contact information of a physician and/or hospital that can treat the traveler effectively and safely.
- Advise the traveler on the possible need for health and/or evacuation insurance for the trip.
- If the risk is great, advise the traveler to delay travel, to consider another travel destination or to avoid specific areas with potential for high pollutant exposure.

A realistic assessment of health risks – including those due to air pollution, should be conducted for all international travelers, short-term assignees and expatriates for each destination. The travel health provider can ensure that travelers are aware of the risks and are prepared to prevent, minimize, and/or manage these risks.

One guideline for risks due to air quality is the Pollution Standard Index (PSI). The PSI offers general guidance for individuals traveling to polluted areas (see Table 44.1 and Figs 44.1 and 44.2).[4–6] However, a full evaluation of the risk to health for the traveler, particularly if visiting remote areas, should be conducted.

Table 44.1 Pollution Standard Index (PSI) Values and the corresponding descriptors, health effects and suggested actions

Index value	PSI descriptor	General health effects	Suggested actions
0 to 50	Good	None for the general population	None
50 to 100	Moderate	Few for the general population	None
100 to 200	Unhealthful	Mild aggravation of symptoms among susceptible persons; irritation symptoms in the healthy population	Persons with existing heart or respiratory disease should reduce physical exertion and outdoor activity. General population should reduce vigorous outdoor activity.
200 to 300	Very unhealthful	Substantial aggravation of symptoms and reduced exercise tolerance for persons with heart or lung disease; widespread symptoms in the general population.	Elderly and persons with existing heart or respiratory disease should stay indoors and reduce physical activity. General population should avoid vigorous outdoor activity.
over 300	Hazardous	Early onset of certain diseases in addition to substantial aggravation of symptoms and reduced exercise tolerance in healthy persons. At levels over 400, premature death of ill and elderly may result. Healthy persons may experience adverse symptoms that affect normal activity.	Elderly and persons with existing heart or respiratory disease should stay indoors and avoid physical activity. At PSI >400, general population should avoid outdoor activity. All persons should remain indoors with windows and doors closed and should minimize physical exertion.

In addition, nutrition deficiencies of vitamin C, vitamin E, selenium, and riboflavin have been associated with increased susceptibility to ozone and carbon monoxide. PCVs should be encouraged to maintain nutritional diets, and the PCMO should consider multivitamin supplements if a nutritionally sould diet is not possible because of local conditions.

$$PSI = \frac{Days\ pollutant\ level}{National\ Air\ Quality\ Standard\ for\ that\ pollutant.}$$

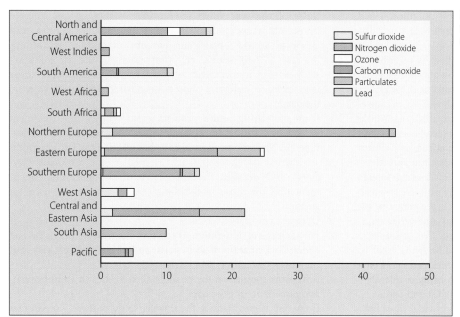

Figure 44.2 Number of cities covered in each region and, the determining pollutant for their air quality scores.

REFERENCES

1. Bunn WB. Environmental Pollution and Travel. *Travel Medicine Monthly* 1999; **3**(10): 1–2.
2. Bunn WB, *et al*. International Environmental Health. In: McCunney RJ, *et al*. A Practical Guide to Occupational and Environmental Medicine, Boston: Little Brown. In press.
3. Maynard RL. *Air Pollution*. In: Herzstein JA, Bunn WB, Fleming LE, Harrington JM, Jeyartnam J, Gardner IR. *International Occupational and Environmental Medicine, 1998*. 35: 569–582.
4. Bergeisen, G. Environmental health: answers to volunteer and staff questions. *Peace Corps/Office of Medical Services, Pollution Standard Index* (PSI), June 1999.
5. Onursal B, Gautam SP. Vehicular air pollution: experiences from seven Latin American urban centers. *World Bank Technical Paper* No. 373; 1997.
6. Prescott-Allen R. The wellbeing of nations: a country-by-country index of quality of life and the environment. *Air* 2001; 80:85.

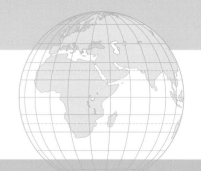

CHAPTER 45 Aircraft Cabin Environment

Michael Bagshaw

KEYPOINTS

■ Though the occupant density, noise and vibration, and relative immobilization may cause physical and/or emotional stresses, the modern commercial aircraft cabin is maintained with adequate environmental control for the comfort of most healthy individuals

■ Cabin air is a combination of both outside air and recirculated air that has gone through HEPA filtration

■ Transmission of illnesses, such as tuberculosis, SARS and other respiratory diseases has been documented aboard aircraft, though transmission of active disease is probably rare. There is no evidence of disease transmission via the environmental control system

■ Automated defibrillators, other sophisticated equipment and telemedicine have saved lives of critically ill passengers. Nonetheless, a passenger's fitness to fly is a responsibility of both the travel health advisor and the traveler

■ Pre-flight notification of special needs and assistance will reduce the stress of a journey and enhance the standard of service delivered by the airlines

INTRODUCTION

The physiology of the human being is optimized for existence at sea level. Most individuals, however, can ascend to around 8000 to 10 000 feet above sea level before lack of oxygen (hypoxia) begins to have ill effects and reduces performance.

With increasing altitude, there is a fall in the atmospheric pressure, together with a decrease in density and temperature. The pressure at sea level in the standard atmosphere is 760 mmHg (29.92 inHg, or 1013.2mb) and this falls to half at 18 000ft, where the ambient temperzature is about –20°C. The composition of the atmosphere remains constant up to the tropopause (36 000 ft), the most abundant gases being nitrogen (78%) and oxygen (21%), with the remaining 1% being argon, carbon dioxide, neon, hydrogen and ozone.

The relationship between the oxygen saturation of hemoglobin and oxygen tension minimizes the effect on the human of the reduction in partial pressure of oxygen. Ascent to an altitude of 10 000 ft produces a fall in the partial pressure of oxygen in the alveoli, but only a slight fall in the percentage saturation of hemoglobin with oxygen. Once altitude exceeds 10 000 ft, however, the percentage saturation of hemoglobin falls quickly, resulting in hypoxia. Indeed, above 8000 ft the effects of lack of oxygen will begin to appear and a decrease in an individual's ability to perform complex tasks and a reduction in night vision can be measured.[1]

Figure 45.1 shows the oxygen dissociation curve of blood. The concentrations of physically dissolved and chemically combined oxygen are shown separately and the curve illustrated is the average for a fit young adult. The actual shape of curve will be influenced by factors such as age, state of health, tobacco use and ambient temperature.

Healthy individuals can tolerate altitudes of up to 8000 to 10 000 ft with no harmful effects. However, in the case of the elderly or of individuals suffering from some diseases of the respiratory or circulatory system, there is less tolerance of the mild hypoxia at even this altitude. In an ideal world, the cabin would be pressurized to simulate sea level conditions. To achieve this would require an extremely strong and heavy aircraft structure with severe implications on load carrying capacity, fuel consumption and resulting effects on the external environment. As a result, a compromise has to be struck, and airworthiness regulations (FAR-JAR 25.841) state that 'pressurized cabins and compartments to be occupied must be equipped to provide a cabin pressure altitude of not more than 8,000 ft at the maximum operating altitude of the aeroplane under normal operating conditions'.

THE PRESSURIZED CABIN

Pressurization is achieved by tapping bleed air from the engine compressors and passing this flow of air through the air-conditioning

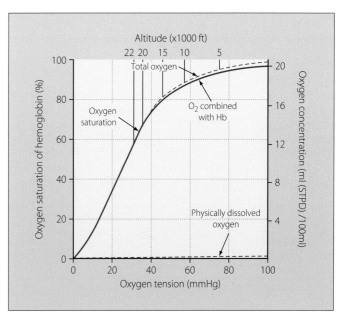

Figure 45.1 The oxygen dissociation curve of blood.

packs into the cabin. The outside air is very dry and cold, and the temperature is also controlled via the air-conditioning packs. The cabin pressure is maintained at the desired level by regulating the flow of air overboard. Figure 45.2 illustrates typical ambient and cabin altitudes for a typical flight.

Figure 45.3 shows how the air circulates in the cabin in the case of single aisle, and while Figure 45.4 shows the airflow patterns in a twin aisle cabin.

As a result of the required cabin pressure change during climb and descent, it is possible for individuals to suffer discomfort as a result of expansion of gas trapped within the body. In particular, gas can be trapped within the gut and within the middle ear and sinuses. Normally this trapped gas is able to escape without any problem, but there may be occasions when this is not so. In particular, the human ear is very sensitive to rates of pressure change, the threshold for detection being 0.132 PSI (0.910 kPa). This is equivalent to a change in cabin altitude of 250 ft (76 m) at sea level. In the human ear the cavity of the middle ear is separated from the outer ear by the tympanic membrane. It communicates with the nasopharynx and in turn the atmosphere by way of the Eustachian tube, the proximal two

thirds of which has soft walls that are normally collapsed. During ascent to altitude, the gas in the middle ear cavity expands and escapes along the Eustachian tube into the nasopharynx, equalizing the pressure across the tympanic membrane. The pharyngeal portion of the Eustachian tube acts as a one-way valve thus allowing expanding air to escape easily to the atmosphere. This can be sometimes felt as a 'popping' sensation as air escapes from the tube during ascent.

During descent, air from the nasopharynx must enter the middle ear to maintain equilibrium. In some individuals, the one-way valve mechanism of the Eustachian tube can prevent passive flow of air back into the middle ear cavity. This causes a relative increase of pressure on the outside of the tympanic membrane pushing it into the middle ear cavity and causing a sensation of fullness, a decrease in hearing acuity and eventually pain. It is possible to perform active maneuvers to open the Eustachian tube, such as swallowing, yawning and jaw movements. In some people these simple maneuvers are not effective and it may be necessary to occlude the nostrils and raise the pressure in the mouth and nose to force air into the middle ear cavities. This increase in pressure can usually simply be achieved by raising the floor of the mouth with the glottis shut, while other individuals raise the pressure in the lungs and the respiratory tract by contracting the expiratory muscles while forcibly exhaling (Valsalva's maneuver).

In addition to regulating the airflow rate required to pressurize the aircraft, the environmental control system controls the flow rate of outside air required to remove contaminants and controls the temperature in the cabin. This requirement is facilitated by the practice of recirculation of approximately 50% of the cabin air. This is achieved by extracting air from the cabin and mixing it with conditioned outside air. Recirculation provides two benefits: one, it allows the total airflow rate to be higher than the flow rate of the outside air, so good circulation in the cabin can be maintained independently of the outside airflow; and two, the conditioned air is mixed with comparatively warm recirculated air before being introduced into the cabin. As a result, the conditioned air is supplied at a much lower tempe-

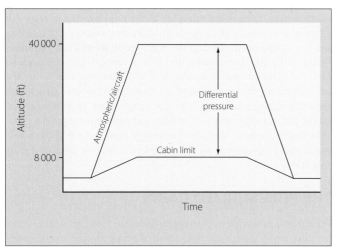

Figure 45.2 Typical cabin pressure flight profile.

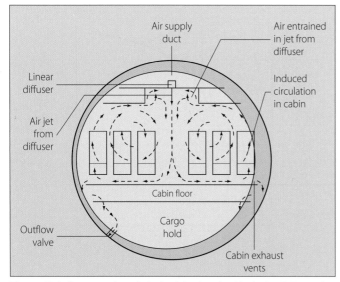

Figure 45.3 Cross-section of single-aisle aircraft with air circulation paths.

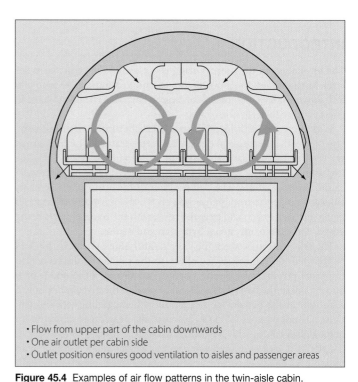

- Flow from upper part of the cabin downwards
- One air outlet per cabin side
- Outlet position ensures good ventilation to aisles and passenger areas

Figure 45.4 Examples of air flow patterns in the twin-aisle cabin.

rature without causing discomfort from cold drafts. The recirculated air will also have picked up moisture from the cabin occupants and the cabin activities, improving the humidity level. In older generation jet aircraft, all the air supplied to the cabin came from outside air, without the benefits of recirculation (improved humidity, reduction in perceived drafts). This practice was inefficient with a substantial energy cost.

In pressurized jet aircraft manufactured since the beginning of the last decade, the recirculated air is passed through filters. These are high efficiency particulate (HEPA) filters, which have an efficiency of 99.97% for 0.3*m particles. They are effective in removing bacteria and viruses from the recirculated air, so preventing their spread through the cabin by this route. Air filters are changed during routine aircraft maintenance, as specified by the manufacturer in the servicing schedule.

Recirculated air is obtained from the area above the cabin or under the floor; air from the cargo bay, lavatories and galleys is not recirculated. The flow rate of outside air per seat ranges from 3.6 to 7.4L/s (7.6–15.6 cubic feet/min) with the percentage of recirculated air distributed to the passenger cabin being of the order 30–55% of the total air supply.[2] The result of filtering the recirculated air is a significant improvement in cabin air quality by the removal of particles and biological microorganisms. It is not technically feasible to pass the compressed air from outside through HEPA filters.

The use of recirculation has been common in the design of building environmental control systems for many years. Building environmental systems are commonly designed and operated with up to 90% of recirculated air, which compares with the maximum recirculated air flow in aircraft of 55%.

The air supply to the flight deck (or cockpit) is derived from the same source, but is delivered at a slightly higher pressure than the air supplied to the cabin. This ensures a positive pressure differential to prevent the ingress of smoke or fumes to the flight deck in the event of a fire or similar in-flight emergency. The flow rate of the flight deck air supply is also slightly higher than that to the cabin because this supply is used for cooling the avionics and other electronic equipment.

HUMIDITY

Humidity is the concentration of water vapor in the air. Relative humidity is the ratio of the actual amount of vapor in the air to the amount that would be present if the air was saturated at the same temperature, expressed as an percentage. Saturated air at high temperatures holds more water vapor than at low temperatures, and if unsaturated air is cooled, it becomes saturated. Humidity in the aircraft cabin is controlled both for human comfort and for aircraft safety. High humidity can lead to passenger and crew discomfort when it is accompanied by high temperature. High humidity can cause condensation, dripping and freezing of moisture on the inside of the aircraft shell, which can lead to a variety of safety problems including corrosion. Condensation can give rise to biological growth so causing adverse effects on cabin air quality.

At a typical aircraft cruising altitude of 30 000ft, the outside air temperature is in the region of –40 °C and is extremely dry, typically containing about 0.15 g/kg of moisture. For pressurized aircraft flying at these levels, the conditioned air entering the cabin has a relative humidity of less than 1%. Exhaled moisture from passengers and crew, together with moisture from galleys and toilet areas, increases the humidity to an average level of 6–10%, which is below the 20% normally accepted as comfort level.[3]

Research has shown that the maximum additional water lost from an individual during an 8-hour period in 0% humidity, compared

with normal day to day loss, is around 100 ml. The sensation of thirst experienced by healthy individuals in the low humidity environment is due to local drying of the pharyngeal membranes, and this itself may lead to the spurious sensation of thirst. There is no evidence that exposure to a low-humidity environment itself leads to dehydration, although local humidity can cause mild subjective symptoms, such as dryness of the eyes and mucous membranes.[4]

No significant effect has been shown on reaction time or other measures of psychomotor performance, although there can be some changes in the fluid regulatory hormones.[4] It is unlikely that low humidity has any long- or short-term ill-effects, provided overall hydration is maintained by drinking adequate amounts of fluid. The body's homeostatic mechanisms ensure that central hydration is maintained, although the peripheral physical effects can lead to discomfort. Dry skin can be alleviated by using moisturizing aqueous creams, particularly just before flight, and dry eye irritation can be alleviated by the use of moisturizing eye drops. Individuals prone to develop dry eyes are advised not to wear contact lenses during long flights in pressurized aircraft.[5] A National Academy of Sciences report identified humidity as one of the areas deserving more attention in future research concerning aircraft cabin environment.[6]

The aircraft cabin is similar to many other indoor environments, such as homes and offices, in that people are exposed to a mixture of external and recirculated air. The cabin environment is different in many respects, (e.g., the high occupant density, the inability of the occupants to leave at will and the need for pressurization). In flight there is a combination of environmental factors including low air pressure and low humidity, as well as low frequency vibration and constant background noise. Although the noise and vibration can contribute to fatigue, the levels are all below those which are accepted as potentially harmful to hearing.[7,8]

OZONE

Ozone is a highly reactive form of oxygen found naturally in the upper atmosphere. It is formed primarily above the tropopause as a result of the action of UV light on oxygen molecules. The amount and distribution of natural ozone in the atmosphere varies with latitude, altitude, season and weather conditions. The highest concentrations in the northern hemisphere are generally found at high altitude over high latitude locations during the winter and spring.

The effects of high-ozone concentration on human beings can include eye irritation, coughing due to irritation of the upper respiratory system, nose irritation and chest pains. As a result of this, the airworthiness regulatory authorities (e.g., US Federal Aviation Authority, European Joint Aviation Authorities) require that transport category aircraft operating above 18 000 ft must show that the concentration of ozone inside the cabin will not exceed 0.25 parts per million by volume (sea level equivalent) at any time, and a time weighted value of 0.1 parts per million by volume (sea level) for scheduled segments of more than 4 h.[9]

For this reason, long haul transport jet aircraft are now equipped with ozone catalytic converters that break down or 'crack' the ozone before it enters the cabin air circulation.

COSMIC RADIATION

Natural radiation consists of cosmic rays from outer space (galactic radiation) and the gamma rays from rocks, earth and building materials. Cosmic radiation is produced when primary photons and alpha particles from outside the solar system interact with components of the earth's atmosphere. A second source of cosmic radiation is the release of charged particles from the sun, which become significant during periods of solar flare ('sun storm'). Cosmic radiation is an ionizing radiation which also includes radiation, such as X-rays and that from radioactive materials. Ionizing radiation is a natural part of the environment in which we live and is present in the earth, buildings, food we eat, and even in the bones of our bodies.

The other type of radiation is known as non-ionizing radiation and this includes ultra violet light, radio waves and microwaves.

Humans, animals and plants have all evolved in an environment with a background of natural radiation and with few exceptions, it is not a significant risk to health.

The amount of cosmic radiation that reaches the earth from the sun and outer space varies and depends on the latitude and height above sea level. The amount of cosmic radiation entering the atmosphere follows an 11–year cycle with the intensity of radiation being lowest when solar activity is at its highest. This is because during high levels of solar activity, the resulting magnetic flux between the sun and the earth deflects much of the galactic cosmic radiation. The most recent solar maximum was in 2001 at which time cosmic radiation levels were at a minimum.

Cosmic radiation is effectively absorbed by the atmosphere and is also affected by the earth's magnetic field. The effect on the body will depend on the latitude and altitude at which the individual is flying and also on the length of time in the air.

Cosmic radiation may be measured directly using sophisticated instruments, as has been done in the Concorde supersonic transport, or can be estimated using a computer software program. These programs look at the route, time at each altitude and the phase of the solar cycle, and calculate the radiation dose received by the aircraft occupant for a particular flight. A number of airlines and research organizations have compared actual measurements taken on board an aircraft with the computer estimations, and the two are very similar.[10]

The effect of ionizing radiation depends not only on the dose absorbed, but also on the type and energy of the radiation and the tissues involved. These factors are taken into account in arriving at the Dose Equivalent measured in Sieverts (Sv). However doses of cosmic radiation are so low that figures are usually quoted in microsieverts (μSv), (millionths of a Sievert) or millisieverts (mSv), (thousandths of a Sievert).

When ionizing radiation passes through the body, energy is transmitted to the tissues which affects the atoms within the individual cells. Very high levels of radiation, such as that from a nuclear explosion, will cause severe cell damage in a human being, particularly to the bone marrow cells and the reproductive cells, which cannot be repaired by the body. Low-level doses of radiation, such as cosmic radiation or medical X-rays, do not cause such severe damage to the cells and in most cases any such damage is repaired satisfactorily by the body's own mechanism. It is not possible to predict a maximum safe threshold of exposure to low levels of radiation, because individuals vary in their biological response.[5,10]

The International Commission for Radiological Protection (ICRP) recommends maximum mean body effective dose limits of 20 milliSieverts per year (mSv/year) (averaged over 5 years) for workers exposed to radiation as part of their occupation (including flight crew), and 1 mSv/year for the general population, with an additional recommendation that the equivalent dose to the fetus should not exceed 1 mSv during the declared term of pregnancy.

For the occupants of the Concorde supersonic transport aircraft, the effective dose rate at cruising altitude has been measured in the range 12–15 microSv/h. On ultra longhaul flights at high latitudes, such as a Boeing 747–400 flying between London and Tokyo, the effective dose rate at cruising altitude is around 5 microSv/h. On shorthaul commercial operations, the effective dose rate in Europe is in the region of 1–3 microSv/hour.

For typical annual flight schedules, crew members accumulate around: 4 or 5 mSv/year on Concorde and longhaul operations, and between 1 or 2mSv/year on European shorthaul operations from cosmic radiation.

For airline passengers, the ICRP recommended limit for the general public of 1 mSv/year equates to about 100 h flying per year on Concorde and about 200 flying hours per year on the trans-equatorial routes. There are essentially two types of airline passenger, the occasional social traveler and the frequent business traveler. The public limit (1 mSv/year) will be of no consequence to the social traveler but could be of significance to the frequent business traveler. The 1 mSv annual limit would be exceeded if the business traveler was flying more than eight trans-atlantic or five antipodean return journeys per year. Business travelers are exposed as an essential part of the occupation, and it is entirely logical to apply the occupational limit of 20 mSv/year to this group.

Cosmic radiation is of no significance at altitudes below about 25 000 ft because of the attenuating properties of the earth's atmosphere. There is no evidence from epidemiological studies of flight crew of any increase in incidence of cancers linked to ionizing radiation exposure, such as leukemia. In general terms, as far as the risk of developing cancer induced by radiation exposure is concerned, it has been calculated that an accumulated dose of 5 mSv/year for 20 years increases the risk of developing cancer (in the general population) from 23–23.4%, i.e. an increase of risk of 0.4% over 20 years. Compared with all the other risks encountered during a working life, this is very low.

Cosmic radiation is both a complex and emotive subject. It cannot be seen, touched, smelled or tasted and yet it is present all around us. While it is known that there is no level of radiation exposure below which effects do not occur, all the evidence indicates that there is an extremely low probability of airline passengers or crew suffering any abnormality or disease as a result of exposure to cosmic radiation.

PESTICIDES IN THE CABIN

The World Health Organization and the International Civil Aviation Organization recommend aircraft arriving through, countries reported with certain indigenous infectious diseases be treated with pesticides.[11] This remains a controversial issue. While it is understandable that countries such as New Zealand would not want to risk the entry of certain vector-borne diseases transmitted by mosquitos, there remains concern about the safety and efficacy of various pesticides used, particularly while passengers are in the cabin (top of descent spraying). There appears to be less concern about using residual pesticides during routine aircraft maintenance. At this time, however, the US Environmental Protection Agency has not promoted the registry of any pesticides in the US for use in aircraft disinsection on American carriers. As vector-borne diseases reemerge, however, these policies may need reevaluation in order to prevent the transmission of disease. Further education of air crew and passengers will be needed, and these issues are being reviewed.

AIRBORNE DISEASE IN THE CABIN

Humans, are the primary source of airborne bacteria and are the most important reservoirs of infectious agents on aircraft. There have been a number of studies carried out and most microorganisms that have been isolated from occupied spaces, including aircraft cabins, are human in source including bacteria which have been shed from exposed skin and scalp and from the nose and mouth.[8] These microorganisms are usually the ones found normally on the human body (normal flora) and very rarely cause infections. The studies have shown no statistically significant differences in concentrations of colonies of bacteria and fungi:

- among different aircraft, airlines or flight durations
- between aircraft cabins and other types of public transport vehicles
- between aircraft cabins and typical indoor and outdoor urban environments.

Because the prime source of infection is person-to-person droplet contact, the risk of exposure to infectious individuals is highest for the passengers seated closest to a source person. Microorganisms suspended in cabin air will be removed by the high efficiency particulate (HEPA) filters during the air recirculation process, but these provide no protection from the cough or sneeze emitted by an infected neighbor. Fortunately, the natural or acquired immunity of most individuals prevents the development of infectious disease. Studies of potential infectious disease transmission on aircraft have considered influenza, legionella, measles and tuberculosis (all of which have been suspected of transmission on board aircraft), meningococcal disease and acute respiratory infections, such as the common cold.[12,13] In fact, the prevalence of transmissible tuberculosis among air travelers is estimated to be 5 to 100 per 100 000 passengers, depending on the route of the plane. Certainly transmission or illness during flight is rarely reported.[14] Available data indicate that infectious agents can be transmitted from person to person aboard aircraft on the ground and during flight, just as they can in any other situation where people find themselves in close proximity. There is no evidence that the pressurized cabin itself makes transmission of disease any more likely. Once the aircraft doors are closed, air conditioning is provided from the auxiliary power unit until it can be supplied from the aircraft engines, so giving the filtration benefits of air recirculation. SARS has been a recent challenge to the airline industry. Limited transmission has probably occurred on board aircraft though the risk is felt to be low. Guidelines are in place for flight crew and management of ill passengers, and can be accessed from www.who.org or www.cdc.gov. In general individuals should not travel on commercial aircraft when they have a febrile illness.

AIRCREW HEALTH

Aircrews, particularly of international fights, are at risk for the same illnesses to which other travelers are exposed. Because of their very short-term stays, and stays that are generally in major cities, they may not be as intensely exposed to some illnesses as others (e.g., malaria). However, their lifestyle may predispose them to other risks. Because of their frequent international travel, flight crews should receive health recommendations that are specifically geared to their travel patterns, itineraries, and lifestyles. For example, an international pilot flying frequently to sub-Saharan Africa would do well not to take routine antimalarial medication, but should take precautions to avoid insect bites and may carry a self-treatment regimen and be instructed to seek medical attention immediately if a fever should occur. The medical department of international carriers should either be able to provide good information and appropriate immunizations to aircrew, or should have an arrangement with a travel clinic for appropriate education of flight crews.

Other than transmission of infectious agents, flight crews have other health concerns that though briefly mentioned here, are best reviewed in an occupational health setting. Issues that have surfaced with regard to pilot health have included the safety of refractive surgery, the use of serotonin reuptake inhibitors, safety of pilots to fly with insulin-dependent diabetes mellitus or even with the human immunodeficiency virus, as well as issues related to pilot fatigue. Flight attendants' concerns have ranged from reproductive health problems, menstrual disorders, chronic back pain, to fears of an increased risk of breast cancer.

PASSENGER HEALTH

Introduction

Flying as a passenger should be no problem for the fit, healthy, and mobile individual. But for the passenger with certain pre-existing conditions, the cabin environment may exacerbate their underlying problems.

Although many problems relate to the physiological effects of hypoxia and expansion of trapped gases, it should be remembered that the complex airport environment can be stressful and challenging to the passenger, leading to problems before even getting airborne.

Although passengers with medical needs require medical clearance from the airline, passengers with disabilities do not. Disabled passengers do need to notify the requirement for special needs, such as wheelchair assistance or assignment of seats with lifting armrests, and this should be done at the time of booking.

An area of little exploration has been air travel stress and anxiety.[15] Whereas typical issues such as fear of flying have been addressed by the airlines in the past, problems that have surfaced related to terrorism and airline security have increased. Passenger lines, terminal crowding, lesser personal services due to cost-cutting, and such have taken a toll on the ease in which air travel is being currently perceived. Addressing these potential problems with the air traveler, particularly with those who have any underlying illness or general anxiety is helpful.

Pre-flight assessment and medical clearance

The objectives of medical clearance are to provide advice to passengers and their medical attendants on fitness to fly, and to prevent delays and diversions of the flight as a result of deterioration in the passenger's well-being. It depends upon self-declaration by the passenger, and upon the attending physician having an awareness of the flight environment and how this might affect the patient's condition.

Most major airlines provide services for those passengers who require extra help, and most have a medical advisor to assess the fitness for travel of those with medical needs. Individual airlines work with their own guidelines, but these are generally based on those published by the Aerospace Medical Association on fitness for travel.[16]

The International Air Transport Association (IATA) publishes a recommended Medical Information Form (MEDIF) for use by member airlines (Fig. 45.5). The MEDIF should be completed by the passenger's medical attendant and passed to the airline, or travel agent, at the time of booking to ensure timely medical clearance.

Medical clearance is required when:

- fitness to travel is in doubt as a result of recent illness, hospitalization, injury, surgery or instability of an acute or chronic medical condition;
- special services are required (e.g. oxygen, stretcher or authority to carry or use accompanying medical equipment such as a ventilator or a nebulizer).

Medical clearance is *not* required for carriage of an invalid passenger outside these categories, although special needs (such as a wheelchair) must be reported to the airline at the time of booking. Cabin crew members are unable to provide individual special assistance to invalid passengers beyond the provision of normal in-flight service. Passengers who are unable to look after their own personal needs during flight (such as toiletting or feeding) will be asked to travel with an accompanying adult who can assist.

It is vital that passengers remember to carry with them any essential medication, and not pack it in their checked baggage.

INCAPACITATED PASSENGERS HANDLING ADVICEŁ
INCAD HANDLING INFORMATION

Answer all questions. Put a (X) in 'Yes' or 'No' boxes.
Use block letters or typewriter when completing this form

Part 1

To be completed by Sales Office/Agent

A Name/Initials/Title

B Proposed itinerary (airline(s), flight number(s) Class(es), date(s), segment(s), reservation status of continuous air journey)

Transfer from one flight to another often requires longer connecting time

C Nature of incapacitation

Medical clearance required? No ☐ Yes ☐

D Is stretcher needed on board? (all stretcher cases must be escorted) No ☐ Yes ☐

Request rate if unknown

E Intended escort (Name, sex, age, professional qualification, segments, if different from passenger). If untrained state 'Travel companion'

For blind and/or deaf state if escorted by trained dog

F Wheelchair needed? No ☐ Yes ☐

Categories are
WCHR - can climb steps/walk cabin
WCHS - unable steps/can walk cabin   WCHC - immobile

Wheelchair category ☐

Own wheelchair?	Collapsible?	Power Driven?	Battery type (Spillable)?
No ☐	No ☐	No ☐	No ☐
Yes ☐	Yes ☐	Yes ☐	Yes ☐

Wheelchairs with spillable batteries are 'restricted articles

G Ambulance needed? No ☐ Yes ☐

To be arranged by airline
No ☐ → specify Ambul Company contact
Yes ☐ → specify destination address

Request rate(s) if unknown

H Other ground arrangements needed? No ☐ Yes ☐

If yes, specify below and indicate for each item, (a) the arranging airline or other organisation, (b) at whose expense, and (c) contact addresses/phones where appropriate, or whenever specific persons are designated to meet/assist the passenger

1 Arrangements for delivery at airport of departure No ☐ Yes ☐ Specify

2 Arrangements for assistance at connecting points No ☐ Yes ☐ Specify

3 Arrangements for meeting at airport of arrival No ☐ Yes ☐ Specify

4 Other requirements or relevant information No ☐ Yes ☐ Specify

K Special in-flight arrangements needed, such as: special meals, special seating, leg rest, extra seat(s), special equipment etc.

(See 'Note(*)' at the end of Part 2 overleaf)

No ☐ Yes ☐

If yes, describe and indicate for each item, (a) segment(s) on which required (b) airline arranged or arranging third party, and (c) at whose expense. provision of special equipment such as oxygen etc. always requires completion of Part 2 overleaf.

L Does passenger hold a 'Frequent traveller's medical card' valid for this trip? (FREMEC) No ☐ Yes ☐

If yes, add below FREMEC data to your reservation requests. If no, (or additional data needed by carrying airline(s)), have physician in attendance complete Part 2 overleaf.

FREMEC
(FREMEC Nr)   (issued by)   (valid until)   (sex)   (age)   (incapacitation)

(incapacit. contd.)   (limitations)

Passengers declaration

I hereby authorize _____

(name of nominated physician)

To complete Part 2 for the purpose as indicated overleaf and in consideration there of I hereby relieve that physician of his/her professional duty of confidentiality in respect of such information, and agree to meet such physician's fees in connection therewith.

Date: _____   Passenger's signature or Agent _____

Figure 45.5 International Air Transport Association (IATA) Medical Information Form (MEDIF).

Part 2	MEDIF Medical information sheet		CONFIDENTIAL

This form is intended to provide confidential information to enable the airlines' medical departments to provide for the passenger's special needs.
To be completed by attending physician
- When fitness to travel is in doubt as evidenced by recent illness, hospitalisation, injury, surgery or instability.
- where special services are required, i.e. oxygen, stretcher, authority to carry accompanying medical equipment.

Completion of the form in block letters or by typewriter will be appreciated.

			Age
Airlines' ref code MEDA01	Patient's name, initial(s), sex		
MEDA02	Attending physician Name and address		
	Telephone contact	Business	Home
MEDA03	Medical data: Diagnosis in details (including vital signs)		
	Day/month/year of first symptoms	Date of diagnosis/injury	Date of operation
MEDA04	Prognosis for the flight		
MEDA05	Contagious communicable disease?	No ☐ Yes ☐ Specify	
MEDA06	Would the physical and/or mental condition of the patient be likely to cause distress or discomfort to other passengers?	No ☐ Yes ☐ Specify	
MEDA07	Would the physical and/or mental condition of the patient be likely to cause distress or discomfort to other passengers?	Yes ☐ No ☐	
MEDA08	Can patient take care of his own needs on board unassisted* (including meals, visit to toilet, etc.)?	Yes ☐ No ☐ If not, type of help needed	
MEDA09	If to be escorted, is the arrangement proposed in part 1/E overleaf satisfactory for you?	Yes ☐ No ☐ If not, type of escort proposed	
MEDA10	Does patient need supplementary oxygen** equipment in flight? (if yes, state rate of flow, 2/41/min). Guidance: supplementary oxygen is not generally required unless dyspnoeic after walking 50 metres. (Charge £100 per journey)	Yes ☐ No ☐ If not, type of escort proposed	Litres per minute ☐ Continuous ☐ Intermittent ☐
MEDA11	Does patient need any medication*, other than self-administered, and/or the use of special apparatus such as a respirator, incubator etc.**	☐ ☐	
MEDA12		☐ ☐	
MEDA13	Does patient need hospitalisation? (If yes, indicate arrangements made or, if none were made indicate 'No action taken)	☐ ☐	
MEDA14		☐ ☐	
MEDA15	Other remarks or information in the interest of your patient's smooth and comfortable transportation:	None ☐ Specify if any**	
MEDA16	Other arrangements made by the attending physician		

Note (*): cabin attendents are not authorized to give special assistance to particular passengers, to the detriment of their service to other passengers. Additionally, they are trained only in first aid and are not permitted to administer any injection, or to give medication.

Important: Fees if any, relevant to the provision of the above information and for carrier - provided special equipment (**) are to be paid by the passenger concerned

Date:	Place:	Attending physician's signature

Figure 45.5 contd.

Deterioration on holiday or on a business trip of a previously stable condition – such as asthma, diabetes, seizure disorder, or accidental trauma – can often give rise to the need for medical clearance for the return journey. A stretcher may be required, together with medical support, and this can incur considerable cost. It is important for all travelers to have adequate travel insurance, which includes provision for the use of a specialist repatriation company to provide the necessary medical support.

Assessment criteria

In determining the passenger's fitness to fly, a basic knowledge of aviation physiology and physics can be applied. Any trapped gas will expand in volume by up to 30% during flight, and consideration must be given to the effects of the relative hypoxia encountered at a cabin altitude of up to 8000 ft above mean sea level. The altitude of the destination airport may also need to be taken into account in deciding the fitness of an individual to undertake a particular journey.

The passenger's exercise tolerance can provide a useful guide on fitness to fly; if unable to walk a distance greater than about 50 m without developing dyspnea, there is a risk that the passenger will be unable to tolerate the relative hypoxia of the pressurized cabin. More specific guidance can be gained from knowledge of the passenger's baseline sea level blood gas levels and hemoglobin value.

Table 45.1 shows the guidelines recommended by one international carrier. This list is not exhaustive, and it should be remembered that individual cases might require individual assessment by the attending physician.

Table 45.1	Guidelines for medical clearance	
Category	**Do not accept**	**Remarks**
Cardiovascular disorders	Uncomplicated myocardial infarction within 7 days Uncontrolled heart failure Open heart surgery within 10 days Angioplasty - No stenting 3 days; With stenting 5 days	Myocardial infarction less than 21 days requires MEDIF assessment. This includes CABG and valve surgery. MEDIF assessment required up to 21 days post-op. Transpositions, ASD/VSD, transplants etc. will require discussion with airline medical advisor
Circulatory disorders	Active thrombophlebitis of lower limbs Bleeding/clotting conditions Blood disorders Hb less than 7.5 g/dL History of sickling crisis within 10 days	Recently commenced anti-coagulation therapy requires assessment MEDIF assessment required for Hb less than 10 g/dL
Respiratory disorders	Pneumothorax which is not fully inflated, or within 14 days after full inflation. Major chest surgery within 10 days. If breathless after walking 50 m on ground or on continuous oxygen therapy on ground	MEDIF assessment required up to 21 days post surgery Consider mobility and all aspects of total journey
Gastrointestinal disorders	General surgery within 10 days G.I. tract bleeding within 24 h	Laparoscopic investigation may travel after 24 h if all gas absorbed. Laparoscopic surgery requires MEDIF up to 10 days. MEDIF required up to 10 days
CNS disorders	Stroke including subarachnoid hemorrhage within 3 days Generalized seizures within 24 h Brain surgery within 10 days	Consider mobility/oxygenation aspects. MEDIF up to 10 days Petit mal or minor twitching – common sense prevails Cranium must be free from air
ENT disorders	Otitis media and sinusitis Middle ear surgery within 10 days Tonsillectomy within 1 week Wired jaw, unless escorted and with wire cutters	If fitted with self quick release wiring may be acceptable without escort
Eye disorders	Penetrating eye injury/intraocular surgery within 1 week	If gas in globe, total absorption necessary – may be up to 6 weeks, specialist check necessary
Acute psychiatric disorders	Unless escorted, with appropriate medication carried by escort, competent to administer such	MEDIF required. Medical, nursing or highly competent companion/relative escort
Pregnancy	After end of 36th week for single uncomplicated After end of 32nd week for multiple uncomplicated	Passenger advised to carry medical certificate.
Neonates	Within 48 h	Accept after 48 h if no complications present
Infectious disease	If in infectious stage	As defined by the American Public Health Association (Benenson)
Terminal Illness	Until individual case assessed by airline medical advisor	Individual case assessment
Decompression	Symptomatic cases (bends, staggers, etc.) within 10 days	May need diving or aviation physician advice
Scuba diving	Within 24 h	
Fractures in plaster	Within 48 h unless splint bi-valved	Extent, site and type of plaster may allow relaxation of guidelines. Exercise caution with fiberglass casts
Burns	Consult airline medical advisor	

The prolonged period of immobility associated with long haul flying can be a risk for those individuals predisposed to develop deep venous thrombosis (DVT). Pre-existing risk factors include:

- blood disorders and clotting factor abnormalities
- cardiovascular disease
- malignancy
- major surgery
- lower limb/abdo trauma
- DVT history
- pregnancy
- estrogen therapy (including oral contraception and hormone replacement therapy)
- older than 40 years of age
- immobilization
- pathological body fluid depletion
- smoking
- obesity
- varicose veins

Although many airlines promote lower limb exercise via the in-flight magazine or videos, and encourage mobility within the cabin, those passengers known to be vulnerable to DVT should seek guidance from their attending physician on the use of compression stockings and/or anti-coagulants. There is currently no evidence that flying, per se, is a risk factor for the development of DVT, but those at high risk should avoid any form of prolonged immobilization. The World Health Organization is currently participating in a comprehensive research program to assess this issue.

CONSIDERATIONS OF PHYSICAL DISABILITY OR IMMOBILITY

In addition to the reduction in ambient pressure and the relative hypoxia, it is important to consider the physical constraints of the passenger cabin. A passenger with a disability must not impede the free egress of the cabin occupants in case of emergency evacuation.

There is limited leg space in an economy class seat and a passenger with an above-knee leg plaster or an ankylosed knee or hip may simply not fit in the available space. The long period of immobility in an uncomfortable position must be taken into account, and it is imperative to ensure adequate pain control for the duration of the journey, particularly following surgery or trauma.

Even in the premier class cabins with more available legroom, there are limits to space. To avoid impeding emergency egress, immobilized or disabled passengers cannot be seated adjacent to emergency exits, despite the availability of increased leg room at many of these positions. Similarly, a plastered leg cannot be stretched into the aisle because of the conflict with safety regulations.

There is limited space in aircraft toilet compartments and if assistance is necessary, a traveling companion is required.

The complexities of the airport environment should not be underestimated, and must be considered during the assessment of fitness to fly. The formalities of check-in and departure procedures are demanding and can be stressful, and this can be compounded by illness and disability, as well as by language difficulties or jet lag.

The operational effect of the use of equipment such as wheelchairs, ambulances and stretchers must be taken into account, and the possibility of aircraft delays or diversion to another airport must be considered. It may be necessary to change aircraft and transit between terminals during the course of a long journey, and landside medical facilities will not be available to a transiting passenger.

There is often a long distance between the check-in desk and the boarding gate. Not all flights depart from or arrive to jetties, and it may be necessary to climb up or down stairs and board transfer coaches. Passengers should specify the level of assistance required when booking facilities such as wheelchairs.

OXYGEN

In addition to the main gaseous system, all commercial aircraft carry an emergency oxygen supply for use in the event of failure of the pressurization system or during emergencies such as fire or smoke in the cabin. The passenger supply is delivered through drop-down masks from chemical generators or an emergency reservoir, and the crew supply is from oxygen bottles strategically located within the cabin. The drop-down masks are automatically released en masse (the so-called 'rubber jungle') in the event of the cabin altitude exceeding a pre-determined level of between 10 000 and 14 000 feet. This passenger emergency supply has a limited duration if provided by chemical generators, usually in the region of 10 minutes. The flow rate is between 4 and 8 L (NTP)/min, and is continuous once the supply is triggered by the passenger pulling on the connecting tube. Oxygen supplied from an emergency reservoir is delivered to the cabin via a 'ring main', and in some aircraft it is possible to plug a mask into this ring main to provide supplementary oxygen for a passenger.

Sufficient first aid oxygen bottles are carried to allow the delivery of oxygen to a passenger in case of a medical emergency in-flight, at a rate of 2 or 4 L (NTP)/min. This cannot be used to provide a premeditated supply for a passenger requiring it continuously throughout a journey, however, since it would then not be available for emergency use.

If a passenger has a condition requiring continuous ('scheduled') oxygen for a journey, this needs prenotification to the airline at the time of booking the ticket. Most airlines make a charge to contribute to the cost of its provision. One major British international airline charges GB£100 per sector, whether the supply is derived from gaseous bottles or via a mask plugged into the ring main.

Normally, it is not possible for a passenger to supply his or her own oxygen. Oxygen bottles, regulators and masks must meet minimum safety standards set by the regulatory authorities, and the oxygen must be of 'aviation' quality, which is a higher specification than 'medical' quality. For further information regarding therapeutic oxygen for airline passengers, see websites: www.medaire.com and www.airsep.com.

IN-FLIGHT MEDICAL EMERGENCIES

An in-flight medical emergency is defined as a medical occurrence requiring the assistance of the cabin crew. It may or may not involve the use of medical equipment or drugs, and may or may not involve a request for assistance from a medical professional traveling as a passenger on the flight. It can be something as simple as a headache, or a vaso-vagal episode, or something major such as a myocardial infarction or impending childbirth.

The incidence is comparatively low, although the media impact of an event can be significant. One major international airline recently reported 3022 incidents occurring in something over 34 million passengers carried in 1 year. The breakdown of these incidents into generalized causes is shown in Table 45.2.[17,18]

The top six in-flight emergency medical conditions reported by the same airline are shown in Table 45.3.[17,18] Any acute medical condition occurring during the course of a flight can be alarming for the passenger and crew because of the remoteness of the environment. The cabin crew receive training in advanced first aid and basic life support and the use of the emergency medical equipment carried on board the aircraft. Many airlines give training in excess of the

Table 45.2	In-flight medical incidents reported in one year by a major airline	
Type of medical incident		(%)
Gastrointestinal system		22.3
Cardiovascular system		21.8
Musculo-skeletal system/skin		13.4
Central nervous system		15.5
Respiratory system		10.2
Uro-genital system		3.3
Metabolic system		2.5
Oto-rhino-laryngology (Ent)		1.4
Miscellaneous		9.6
Total 3022 incidents in 34 million passengers.		

Table 45.3	Six most common in-flight medical incidents reported in one year by a major airline	
Type of medical incident		(%)
Faint		14.9
Diarrhea		11.5
Head injury		6.3
Vomiting		6.1
Collapse		5.4
Asthma		4.9
Total 3022 incidents in 34 million passengers.		

regulatory requirement, particularly when an extended range of medical equipment is carried.

GOOD SAMARITANS

Although the crew are trained to handle common medical emergencies, in serious cases they may request assistance from a medical professional traveling as a passenger. Such assisting professionals are referred to as 'Good Samaritans'. Cabin crew members attempt to establish the *bona fide* of medical professionals offering to assist, but much has to be taken on trust.

The international nature of air travel can lead to complications in terms of professional qualification and certification, specialist knowledge and professional liability. An aircraft in flight is subject to the laws of the state in which it is registered, although when not moving under its own power (i.e., stationary at the airport) it is subject to the local law. In some countries, it is a statutory requirement for a medical professional to offer assistance to a sick or injured person (e.g., France), whereas in other states no such law exists (e.g., UK or USA).

Some countries (e.g., USA) have enacted a Good Samaritan law, whereby an assisting professional delivering emergency medical care within the bounds of his or her competence, is not liable for prosecution for negligence. In the UK, the major medical defense insurance companies provide indemnity for their members acting as Good Samaritans.

Some airlines provide full indemnity for medical professionals assisting in response to a request from the crew, whereas other airlines take the view that a professional relationship is established between the sick passenger and the Good Samaritan and any liability lies within that relationship. At the time of writing, there has been no case of successful action against a Good Samaritan providing assistance on board an aircraft.

Recognition by the airline of the assistance given by the Good Samaritan is complicated by the special nature of the relationship between the professional, the patient and the airline. Indemnity, whether provided by the airline or the professional's defense organization, depends upon the fact that a Good Samaritan act is performed.

If a professional fee is claimed or offered, the relationship moves away from being that of a Good Samaritan act to one of a professional interaction with an acceptance of clinical responsibility. This implies that the professional is suitably trained, qualified and experienced to diagnose, treat and follow up the particular case, and the Good Samaritan indemnity provision no longer applies.

Follow-up of the passenger after disembarkation is frequently difficult, because the sick passenger is no longer in the care of the airline and becomes the responsibility of the receiving hospital or medical practitioner.

AIRCRAFT MEDICAL DIVERSION

Responsibility for the conduct of the flight rests with the aircraft captain who makes the final decision as to whether or not an immediate unscheduled landing or diversion is required for the well being of a sick passenger. The captain has to take into account operational factors as well as the medical condition of the sick passenger.

In practice, it is rarely possible to land immediately because even if a suitable airport is in the immediate vicinity, the aircraft has to descend from cruising altitude, possibly jettison fuel to reduce to landing weight, and then fly the approach procedure to land.

Consideration has to be given to the availability of appropriate medical facilities, and in many cases, it is of greater benefit for the sick passenger to continue to the scheduled destination where the advantage of appropriate facilities will outweigh the risks of continuing the flight.

Operational factors to be considered include the suitability of an airport to receive the particular aircraft type. The runway must be of sufficient length and load bearing capacity, the terminal must be able to accommodate the number of passengers on the flight, and if the crew go out of duty time, there must be sufficient hotel accommodation to allow an overnight stay of crew and passengers.

The cost to the airline may be substantial, including the effects of aircraft and crew unavailability for the next scheduled sector, as well as the direct airport and fuel costs of the diversion. In making the decision whether or not to divert, the captain will take advice from all sources. If a Good Samaritan is assisting, he or she has an important role to play, perhaps in radio consultation with the airline medical advisor.

TELEMEDICINE

Many airlines use an air-to-ground link, which allows the captain and/or the Good Samaritan to confer with the airline medical adviser regarding the diagnosis, treatment and prognosis for the sick passenger. The airline operations department is also involved in the decision-making process. Some airlines maintain a worldwide database of medical facilities available at or near the major airports; others subscribe to a third party provider giving access to immediate medical advice and assistance with arranging emergency medical care for the sick pas-senger at the diversion airport.

The link from the aircraft is made using either radio-telephone voice or data link (VHF or ACARS), high-frequency radio communication (HF) or a satellite communication system (satcom). Satcom is installed in newer, long-range aircraft, and is gradually replacing HF as the industry norm for long-range communication. The advantage is that Satcom is unaffected by terrain, topography or atmospheric conditions, and allows good transmission of voice and data from over any point on the globe. Digitization and telephone transmission of physiological parameters is a well established practice, particularly in remote areas of the world. An aircraft cabin at 37 000 ft can be considered a remote location in terms of availability of medical support, and the digital technology used in Satcom is similar to that used in modern ground-to-ground communication. The advent of Satcom has enabled the development of air-to-ground transmission to assist in diagnosis. Pulse oximetry and ECG are examples of data that can assist the medical advisor to give appropriate advice to the aircraft captain, although the cost/ benefit analysis has to be weighed very carefully.

AIRCRAFT EMERGENCY MEDICAL EQUIPMENT

National regulatory authorities stipulate the minimum scale and standard of all equipment to be carried on aircraft operating under their jurisdiction, which includes emergency medical equipment. These standards stipulate the minimum requirement, although in practice many airlines carry considerably more equipment.

Tables 45.4 and 45.5 give the minimum standard of equipment mandated by the Federal Aviation Administration (FAA) to be carried by aircraft registered in the USA, while Table 45.6 gives the standard determined by the Joint Aviation Authorities (JAA) for aircraft registered in European states.

In determining the type and quantity of equipment and drugs to include in the medical kits, the airline must obviously fulfill the statutory requirements laid down by the regulatory authority. Other factors to be considered are:

- *The route structure and stage lengths flown.* Different countries of the world vary in their regulations on what might be imported and exported, particularly in terms of drugs. For example, it is illegal to import morphine derivatives into the USA, even if securely locked in a medical kit.
- *Passenger expectations.* Premier class business passengers from the developed world expect a higher standard of care and medical provision than passengers traveling on a relatively inexpensive package holiday flight.
- *Training of cabin crew.* The crew must have a knowledge and understanding of the kit contents, for use by themselves or in assisting a Good Samaritan. They must be proficient in first aid, resuscitation and basic life support.
- *Differences in medical cultures.* Ideally, the kit contents should be familiar to any Good Samaritan irrespective of nationality or training. Some authorities require information and drug names to be given in more than one language.

Table 45.4	**Federal aviation regulations part 121: first aid and emergency medical kits**

First-aid kits	Emergency medical kits
Approved first-aid kits required by ß121.309 must meet the following specifications and requirements (1) Each first-aid kit must be dust and moisture proof, and contain only materials that either meet Federal Specification GG-K-291a, as revised, or are approved. (2) Required first-aid kits must be distributed as evenly as practicable throughout the aircraft and be readily accessible to the cabin flight attendants. (3) The minimum number of first-aid kits required is set forth in the following table	The approved emergency medical kit required by ß121.309 for passenger flights must meet the following specifications and requirements: (1) Approved emergency medical equipment shall be stored securely so as to keep it free from dust, moisture, and damaging temperatures. (2) One approved emergency medical kit shall be provided for each aircraft during each passenger flight and shall be located so as to be readily accessible to crew members (3) The approved emergency medical kit must contain, as a minimum, the following appropriately maintained contents in the specified quantities.

No. of passenger seats	No. of first aid kits	Contents	Quantity
0–50	1	Sphygmomanometer	1
51–150	2	Stethoscope	1
151–250	3	Airways, oropharyngeal (3 sizes)	3
More than 250	4	Syringes (sizes necessary to administer required drugs)	4
		Needles (sizes necessary to administer required drugs)	6
(4) Except as provided in paragraph (5), each first-aid kit must contain at least the following or other approved contents:		50% Dextrose injection 50 cc	1
		Epinephrine 1: 1000, single dose ampoule or equivalent	2
Contents	Quantity	Diphenhydramine Hcl injection, single dose ampoule or equivalent	2
Adhesive bandage compresses, 10-inch	16	Nitroglycerin tablets	10
Antiseptic swabs	20	Basic instructions for use of the drugs in the kit	11
Ammonia inhalants	16		
Bandage compresses, 4-inch	8		
Triangular bandage compresses, 10-inch	5		
Burn compound, 1/8-ounce or an equivalent of other burn remedy	6		
Arm splint, non inflatable	1		
Leg splint, non inflatable	1		
Roller bandage, 4-inch	4		
Adhesive tape, 1-inch standard roll	2		
Bandage scissors	1		

(5) Arm and leg splints that do not fit within a first-aid kit may be stowed in a readily accessible location that is as near as practicable to the kit.

Table 45.5	US Aviation Medical Assistance Act (1998)

Rule issued by Federal Aviation Administration (FAA), April 2001
US Aircraft weighing more than 7500 lb and having at least one flight attendant must carry an automated external defibrillator (AED) and enhanced medical kit (EMK) on all domestic and international flights within 3 years

The following items will be added to each EMK
    Oral antihistamine
    Non-narcotic analgesic
    Aspirin
    Atropine
    Bronchodilator inhaler
    Lidocaine and saline
    IV administration kit with connectors
    CPR masks

An EMK is already equipped with
    Sphygmomanometer (measures blood pressure)
    Stethoscope
    Three sizes of oral airways (breathing tubes)
    Syringes
    Needles
    50% dextrose injection (for hypoglycemia or insulin shock)
    Epinephrine (for asthma or acute allergic reactions)
    Diphenhydramine (for allergic reactions)
    Nitroglycerin tablets (for cardiac-related pain)
    Basic instructions on the use of the drugs
    Latex gloves

All crew members will receive initial training on the EMK and on the location, function, and intended operation of an AED. Flight attendants will receive initial and recurrent training in CPR and on the use of AEDs. Medical personnel are frequently onboard and can assist fellow passengers during an in-flight medical event. In addition, a 'Good Samaritan' provision in the aviation medical assistance act of 1998 limits the liability of air carriers and non-employee passengers unless the assistance is grossly negligent or willful misconduct is evident.

- *Equipment and drugs appropriate for likely medical emergencies.* It is important to audit the incidence and outcome of in-flight medical emergencies and maintain a review of the kit content. This review should also take into account changes in medical practice.
- *Space and weight.* The medical equipment must be accessible, but securely stowed. Some airlines divide the equipment and drugs between basic first-aid kits, which are readily accessible on the catering trolleys, and a more comprehensive emergency medical kit that is sealed and stowed with other emergency equipment. Space and weight are always at a premium within the cabin, and the medical kits must be as light and compact as possible.
- *Shelf life and replenishment.* A tracking system for each kit must be in place to ensure that contents have not exceeded their designated shelf life. Similarly, after use of a kit, there has to be a procedure for replenishment. In practice, the aircraft can depart if the kit contents meet the statutory minimum, even though drugs or equipment have been used from the non-statutory part of the kit. Many airlines subcontract the tracking and replenishment to a specialist medical supply company.

RESUSCITATION EQUIPMENT

Although basic cardiopulmonary resuscitation (CPR) techniques are an essential part of cabin crew training, the outcome of an in-flight cardiac event may be improved if appropriate resuscitation equipment is available. This can range from a simple mouth-to-mouth face guard, to a resuscitation bag and mask and airway, to an endotracheal tube and laryngoscope, to an automatic external defibrillator (AED).

The decision on the scale of equipment to be carried has to take account of the same parameters used in determining the content of the emergency medical kits (Table 45.5).

In addition, a cost/benefit analysis has to balance the cost of acquisition, maintenance and training against the probability of need and the expectation of the traveling public.

The European Resuscitation Committee and the American Heart Association endorse the concept of early defibrillation as the standard of care for a cardiac event both in and out of the hospital setting. However, the protocol includes early transfer to an intensive care facility for continuing monitoring and treatment, which is not always possible in the flight environment.

Despite this inability to complete the resuscitation chain, it is becoming increasingly common for commercial aircraft to be equipped with AEDs and for the cabin crew to be trained in their use. This has been mandated in the USA by the FAA (see Table 45.5). Experience of those airlines which carry AEDs indicates that there may be benefits to the airline operation as well as to the passenger. Some types of AED have a cardiac monitoring facility, and this can be of benefit in reaching the decision on whether or not to divert. For example, there is no point in initiating a diversion if the monitor shows asystole, or if it suggests that the chest pain is unlikely to be cardiac in origin.

Lives have been saved by the use of AEDs on aircraft and diversions have been avoided, so it could be argued that the cost/benefit analysis is weighted in favor of carrying AEDs as part of the aircraft medical equipment. Nonetheless, it is important that unrealistic expectations are not raised. An aircraft cabin is not an intensive care unit and the AED forms only a part of the first aid and resuscitation equipment.

Table 45.6	European joint aviation requirements: JAR-OPS 1, sub-part L

First-aid kits

The following should be included in the first-aid kits:
  Bandages (unspecified)
  Burns dressings (unspecified)
  Wound dressings, large and small
  Adhesive tape, safety pins and scissors
  Small adhesive dressings
  Antiseptic wound cleaner
  Adhesive wound closures
  Adhesive tape
  Disposable resuscitation aid
  Simple analgesic (e.g., paracetamol)
  Antiemetic (e.g., cinnarizine)
  Nasal decongestant
  First-aid handbook
  Splints, suitable for upper and lower limbs
  Gastrointestinal antacid +
  Anti-diarrheal medication (e.g., Loperamide +)
  Ground/Air visual signal code for use by survivors
  Disposable gloves

A list of contents in at least two languages (English and one other). This should include information on the effects and side-effects of drugs carried

Note: An eye irrigator, while not required to be carried in the first-aid kit should, where possible, be available for use on the ground

In addition, for aeroplanes with more than nine passenger seats installed, an Emergency medical kit must be carried

The following should be included in the emergency medical kit:
  Sphygmomanometer – non mercury
  Stethoscope
  Syringes and needles
  Oropharyngeal airways (two sizes)
  Tourniquet
  Coronary vasodilator (e.g., nitro-glycerine)
  Anti-spasmodic (e.g., hyoscine)
  Epinephrine 1:1000
  Adrenocortical steroid (e.g., hydrocortisone)
  Major analgesic (e.g., nalbuphine)
  Diuretic (e.g., frusemide)
  Antihistamine (e.g., diphenhydramine hydrochloride)
  Sedative/anticonvulsant (e.g., diazepam)
  Medication for hypoglycemia (e.g. hypertonic glucose)
  Antiemetic (e.g., metoclopramide)
  Atropine
  Digoxin
  Uterine contractant (e.g., Ergometrine/Oxytocin)
  Disposable gloves
  Bronchial dilator, including an injectable form
  Needle disposal box
  Anti-spasmodic drug
  Catheter

A list of contents in at least two languages (English and one other). This should include information on the effects and side-effects of drugs carried

Many airlines have in place a procedure for the follow-up of crew members involved in a distressing event, such as a serious medical emergency. This can be valuable in avoiding long term post-traumatic stress disorder, and also in reinforcing the training that the crew member has already undergone.

CONCLUSION

The pressurized aircraft cabin provides protection against the hostile environment encountered at cruising altitudes.

- Although the partial pressure of oxygen is less than at sea level, it is more than adequate in a pressurized aircraft cabin for normal healthy individuals.

- The cabin air, although dry, does not cause systemic dehydration and harm to health. Dry skin and eyes can lead to discomfort, which can be alleviated by the use of moisturizing creams and eye drops.
- Although up to half of the air in modern pressurized aircraft is recirculated, the amount of fresh air available to each occupant exceeds that available in air conditioned buildings. Recirculating the air has the advantage of reducing cold draughts and increasing the humidity.
- In modern aircraft, all the recirculated air is passed through high efficiency particulate filters which remove more than 99% of particles, including bacteria and viruses.
- There is an extremely low probability of airline passengers or crew suffering any abnormality or disease as a result of exposure to cosmic radiation.

The passenger cabin of a commercial airliner is designed to carry the maximum number of passengers in safety and comfort, within the constraints of cost effectiveness. It is incompatible with providing the facilities of an ambulance, an emergency room, an intensive care unit, a delivery suite, or a mortuary.

The ease and accessibility of air travel to a population of changing demographics inevitably means that there are those who wish to fly who may not cope with the hostile physical environment of the airport, or the hostile physiological environment of the pressurized passenger cabin. It is important for medical professionals to be aware of the relevant factors, and for unrealistic public expectations to be avoided.

Most airlines have a medical advisor who may be consulted before flight to discuss the implications for a particular passenger. Such preflight notification can prevent the development of an in-flight medical emergency that is hazardous to the passenger concerned, inconvenient to fellow passengers, and expensive for the airline.

For those with disability, but not an acute medical problem, preflight notification of special needs and assistance will reduce the stress of the journey and enhance the standard of service delivered by the airline.

The importance of adequate medical insurance coverage for all travelers cannot be over-emphasized. Finally, as is the case in commercial aviation, there is a continuing audit of activity and an on-going risk/benefit analysis. The industry is under constant evolution, and is now truly global in its activity. Application of basic physics and physiology, and an understanding of how this may affect underlying pathology, will minimize the medical risks to the traveling public.[19]

REFERENCES

1. Ernsting J, Nicholson AN, Rainford DJ. *Aviation Medicine*. 3rd edn. Oxford: Butterworth-Heinemann; 1999.
2. Lorengo D, Porter A. *Aircraft Ventilation Systems Study. Final Report*. DTFA-03-84-C-0084. DOT/FAA/CT-TN86/41-I. Washington, DC: Federal Aviation Administration, US Department of Transportation; 1986.
3. de Ree H, Bagshaw M, Simons R, Brown RA. Ozone and relative humidity in airliner cabins on polar routes: measurements and physical symptoms. In: Nagda NL, ed. *Air Quality and Comfort in Airliner Cabins, ASTM STP 1393*. West Conshocken, PA: American Society for Testing and Materials; 2000:243–258.
4. Nicholson AN. Dehydration and long haul flights. *Travel Med Int* 1998; **16**:177–181.
5. Campbell RD, Bagshaw M. *Human Performance and Limitations in Aviation*. 3rd edn. Oxford: Blackwell Science; 1999.
6. Nagda NL, Hudgson M. Low relative humidity and aircraft cabin air quality. *Indoor Air* 2001; **11**:200–214.
7. Bagshaw M, Lower MC. Hearing Loss on the Flight Deck – Origin and Remedy. *Aeronaut J* 2002; **106**(1059):277–289.
8. National Research Council. *The Airliner Cabin Environment and the Health of Passengers and Crew*. Report of the National Research Council. Washington DC: National Academy Press; 2001.
9. US Federal Aviation Regulations FAR25.832 and FAR121.578.
10. Bagshaw M. Cosmic Radiation Measurements in Airline Service. *Radiat Prot Dosim* 1999; **86**:333–4
11. WHO. Recommendations on the disinsecting of aircraft. *Weekly Epidemiological Record* 1985; **60**:45–52.
12. Bruni M, Steffen R. Impact of travel-related health impairments. *J Travel Med* 1997; **4**:61–64.
13. CDC. Exposure to patients with meningococcal disease on aircrafts – United States, 1999–2001. *MMWR* **50**:485–489.
14. Ruder HL. Risk of travel-associated tuberculosis. *Clin Infect Dis* 2001; **33**:1393–1396.
15. McIntosh IB, Swanson V, Power KG. Anxiety and health problems related to air travel. *J Travel Med* 1998; **5**:198–204.
16. Air Transport Medicine Committee, Aerospace medical association. medical guidelines for air travel. *Aviat Space Environ Med* 1996; **67**:B1–B16.
17. Bagshaw M, Byrne NJ. La sante des passagers. *Urgence Prat* 1999; **36**:37–43.
18. Bagshaw M. Telemedicine in British Airways. *J Telemedicine Telecare* 1996; **2**(1):36–38.
19. The Aerospace Medical Association. *Medical Guidelines for Airline Travel*. Copies of this useful material can be obtained from gcarter@asma.org or by telephone: +1 703 739 2240.

CHAPTER 46 Bites, Stings and Envenoming Injuries

Michael V. Callahan

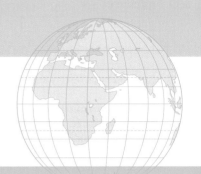

KEYPOINTS

- Pre-travel counseling should include, where applicable, destination specific advice on preventing bites and envenoming injuries, principals of first aid and wound care, and the management of wound infection

- Animal attack injuries can be prevented by recognizing and avoiding predators and by not provoking animals that only attack when threatened. Contaminated wound injuries are common

- Those predisposed to hypersensitivity to hymenoptera (bee) envenomation should be familiar with self-treatment and carry epinephrine auto-injection devices when traveling

- Jellyfish envenomation requires removal of nematocysts from skin with seawater or acetic acid

- Sea urchin, stingray or other spiny wounds should be treated with hot water immersion and removal of foreign bodies

- Snakebite requires basic first aid but rapid removal to the nearest reasonable medical facility is more important than any field treatment

INTRODUCTION

In recent years the growth of the adventure travel market, in particular eco-tourism, extreme dive tours and wilderness safaris, have increased opportunities for travelers to encounter dangerous species. In fact, some tour operators intentionally create encounters between paying clients and dangerous animals (Fig. 46.1). This chapter is divided into three sections: non-venomous injuries resulting from blood-feeding arthropods and animal attack; venomous injuries from arthropods and reptiles; and bite and sting injuries from dangerous marine fauna. Each section includes methods for preventing injuries, principals of first aid and hospital-based wound care, and the management of wound infection.

An attempt should be made to identify those individuals at increased risk and provide destination specific advice. For example, trekkers to Nepal should be advised about the recent increase in rabies in the Himalayas, whereas recreational divers visiting Palau should be discouraged from feeding black-tipped reef sharks, a species that occasionally bites divers who attempt to hand feed them. For travelers to remote destinations pre-travel safety education should be extended to include first aid for bite and sting injuries. A list of credentialed first aid training certification programs is provided in Chapter 32, Table 4.

INSECT BITES

Bites by hematophagous insects, ticks and mites, result from the activities of arthropods seeking a blood meal. As these bites reflect the action of hungry insects, they are more difficult to avoid than are the defensive venomous injuries of scorpions, spiders and bees. Many insect species have specific ranges, ecotones and periods of activity. In turn, the location and timing of human activity influence the likelihood of bites by certain species, and the risk of contracting vector-borne disease. For example, the probability of being bitten by certain species of anopheline mosquitoes is greatest between dusk and dawn.

Treatment

Local reactions to the bite of hematophagous insects vary between species and the sensitivity of the individual. Local reactions include continued bleeding from the bite site due to the continued effects of salivary anticoagulant (e.g., black flies), pruritic lesions (e.g., chiggers), long-lasting granuloma, (e.g., *Ixodid* ticks) and less commonly, hypersensitivity reactions. Bites terminated by the slap of a hand, or other action that tears the insect from its feeding position, may cause mouthparts to be retained in the bite wound. The exoskeleton of many arthropods contain antigenic material leading to chronic inflammation and unsightly lesions. Treatment for these injuries requires close inspection of the wound, a task made easier by using an illuminated magnifying glass, and removal of any foreign body that may

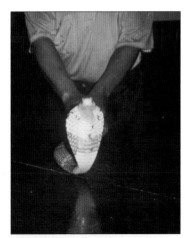

Figure 46.1 Travelers should avoid high-risk wildlife encounters such as workshops that teach tourists how to handle wild cobras.

be present. After inspection, the bite site should be washed with warm water containing dilute antibacterial solution. A list of important hematophagous insects and recommended deterrents is provided in Table 46.1

Several large insects are capable of defending themselves with spines, claws or chelicerae. Species that can cause painful bites or pinches include soldier and leaf-cutter ants, staghorn beetles and praying mantises. While several species are capable of drawing blood, management of injuries requires little more than inspection for retained mouthparts, routine wound care, updating of tetanus prophylaxis and monitoring for secondary bacterial infection.

ANIMAL ATTACK INJURIES

A compilation of annual animal attack fatalities is provided in Table 46.2.[1] Much of the literature on animal bite injuries, in particular factors which influence secondary wound infection, are derived from retrospective series of dog bites.[2,3] However, international travelers may be bitten by a wide variety of exotic, feral and domestic animals, and bite wounds from many of these species are associated with unusual infections.[4]

The wounds caused by animal attack vary with circumstance, and tend to be more significant when caused by large species or carnivores. Injuries resulting from attempted predation, such as the majority of polar bear attacks, tend to be more severe than defensive attack injuries as occur when a sow bear attacks in defense of her cubs. The wounds inflicted are often a combination of punctures; avulsions, abrasions and crush injuries, the last of which may not be apparent until compartment syndrome develops. Injuries caused by horned ungulates such as moose and buffalo, are a combination of massive blunt and penetrating trauma, usually with disastrous amounts of soil contamination (Fig. 46.2).

Prevention of animal attack

Back-country travelers, wildlife photographers, naturalists and others familiar with dangerous species in their home country will still need to learn about native fauna before venturing into foreign ecosystems. Travelers intent on avoiding all dangerous species should be aware that some animals travel beyond the jungle edge and into urban areas, or frequent tourist attractions. For example, tourists are often bitten by monkeys that frequent urban temples in Kampuchea, Thailand and India.

The response to animal attack must change with the situation. The most important determinant is whether the animal is attacking for reasons of self-defense or predation. A large number of unprovoked attacks occur when the predator mistakes the victim, or a part of the victim, for prey. For example, divers may be bitten on the hands by barracuda and sharks that are attracted to shiny rings, watches and bracelets. If attack resulted from an animal's attempts to defend itself, the traveler needs to adopt non-threatening behaviors (backing-away quietly, moving slowly, playing dead). However, if the attacking animal is intent on making the traveler a meal, as is the case with solitary polar bears and lions, the traveler should portray themselves as a large, difficult and unpleasant target. Attack deterrent measures include making loud noises, and trying to appear larger by unzipping coats and flapping them open, holding packs overhead and standing upright. Small children, who are preferentially targeted by hyenas and big cats, should be picked up and carried on the shoulders or back. Running from predators is ill advised as this may trigger a chase reflex, and exposes the unprotected backside to attack. Large predators such as lions, tigers and cougars direct the attack at the head and neck of human victims in a manner similar to the killing bites used on normal prey (Fig. 46.3).

Factors that influence the likelihood of animal attack are listed in Table 46.3.

Table 46.1	Important hematophagous insects and recommended deterrents (see also Chapter 7)	
Mosquito	Mosquitoes are attracted to exhaled CO_2 until they are close enough to rely on thermal and visual senses.	Avoid CO_2 and heat-emitting sources. Maintain air movement to disrupt CO_2 gradients. Wear light-colored clothing. Use repellents (30–45% extended release DEET) or wear permethrin-impregnated clothing.
True Flies	Horseflies and tsetse flies rely on vision whereas sand flies and black flies use CO_2 and thermal detection to locate warm-blooded prey.	Light blue clothing attracts certain species of tsetse flies. Many species preferentially land on dark-colored clothing suggesting lighter shades may serve as a deterrent.
Fleas	Fleabites occur when the preferred host animal is unavailable. Eggs lie in ground cover and may last for weeks so pesticides need to be repeated at 4–6 week intervals.	Long-lasting pesticides help with infestations. Diethyltoluamide (DEET) and permethrin are effective for all but the most voracious species
Lice	Lice are highly specific for certain animal species. Anthrophilic species spend their entire life in human hair. Egg cases ('nits') are resistant to many insecticides; repeated applications are often necessary.	Mild infestations may be treated with lindane. Heavy infestations will likely need topical permethrin.
Chiggers (mite larvae)	*Trombiculid* mites are small arachnid larva (200 µm to 1 mm) that feed on epithelial cells and secrete digestive enzymes, which cause hypersensitivity reactions. Soft tissue edema and severe pruritus are typical findings.	DEET and peremptoriness are both effective. Infestations are treated with benzene hexachloride (Lindane), permethrin or crotamiton
Scabies	*Sarcoptes scabei* are transmitted under crowded conditions. Patients often become sensitized to digested secretions leading to characteristic itching. Infections are identified by distinctive linear tracks, which may be highlighted with dilute povidone-iodine.	Infested areas should be monitored for infection. Scabicidal solution includes benzylbenzoate (20%) or benzene hexachloride. Treatment of close contacts is recommended.

Table 46.2 Annual human deaths from animal attack (1978–1995)

Species	Fatalities	Comments
Venomous snakes	65 000	Annual fatalities are increasing with improved reporting.
Tiger and lion	800	Attacks are decreasing; the majority of attacks are due to individual cats (man-eaters).
Crocodile	600–800	Worldwide, attacks are decreasing, however in Austral-Asian saltwater crocodile attacks are increasing with human encroachment, water activities and protection of species.
Elephant	300	The leading non-predator killer. Attacks by elephants are increasing along game park boundaries. Solitary males are the usual offender.
Hippopotamus	130	Decreasing. There is a high encounter to attack ratio, an indication that attack may occur with little provocation.
Cape buffalo	80	Predominantly game park deaths. Cape buffalo attacks are the leading cause of death among trekkers on Mount Kenya.
Hyena	40	Unattended children are the primary victims.
Feral pig	20	Wounded animals are the primary threat.
Bear	9	Polar bears are the most dangerous species. In the Himalayas, Asiatic black bears are a frequent cause of damage to campsites.
Shark	9	Regional increases in attacks associated with coastal recreation activities.
Alligator	1	Attacks are increasing as protected animals grow to full maturity.
Pythons and boids	<1	Large captive snakes are responsible for rare fatalities
Rhinoceros	<1–4	Decreasing as animals disappear from many areas.

Any activity that place dangerous animals and travelers in close proximity should be avoided. Recent examples from adventure travel advertisements include free-swimming with dangerous species of sharks, caiman wrestling in Brazil, feeding wild monkeys in Africa and free-handling venomous snakes in India. Travelers should also avoid habits that attract foraging animals such as improper storage of food, messy campsites and use of fragrant cosmetics toothpastes and powders. In Asia and South Africa, monkey bite often results from attempts to recover food or possessions from fearless and pugnacious primates.

Treatment of attack injuries

Getting the victim away from the attacking animal, without causing additional injuries, is the first priority. Initial medical care should be basic, easy to improvise, and cause no harm. Medical considerations

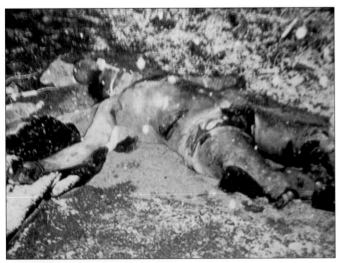

Figure 46.2 Under certain circumstances, horned animals may be easily provoked leading to severe injuries as in this fatality resulting from harassment of a young male buffalo.

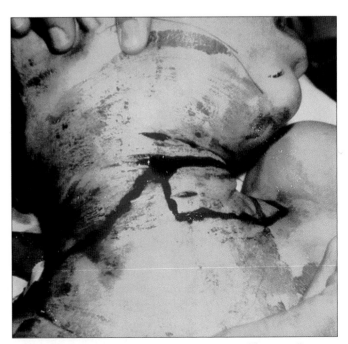

Figure 46.3 Predatory attack from tigers, cougars and lions usually involve bites to the anterior neck as in the case of this 16-year-old woman attacked by a male lion.

Table 46.3 Factors influencing animal attack

Attack unlikely (favorable)	Attack likely (unfavorable)
Omnivore/herbivore	Carnivore
Female	Female with young
Young	Male (breeding season or rut)
	Young adult (recently displaced)
	Territorial species
Plentiful food	Starvation
	Prior human predation (man-eater cats)
Wild (fearful of humans)	Habituated to humans (e.g., temple monkey, camp bear)

for treatment of animal attack victims are shown in Table 46.4.[5–7] A growing number of travelers are using telephone or telemedicine visual links to seek medical advice from physicians back home. Clinicians providing advice to overseas patients should stress the need to follow the procedures in Table 46.4 and not delay cleansing, debridement, imaging or infection prophylaxis while awaiting potential repatriation.

Infection

Animal bite wounds may become infected when microflora from the animal's mouth or from the surrounding environment are inoculated into the wound. Prompt wound decontamination is known to reduce infection and to hasten wound healing.[8] The dentition of the offending species, anatomic location of the wound, and immune status of the victim all influence the likelihood of primary or secondary wound infection. Bites caused by species with filiform dentition, such as mongoose, mustelids (weasel family) and cats, are prone to infection because bacteria are inoculated deep into tissues. Bites to joints may result in tenosynovitis and septic arthritis, whereas bites to bony structures may lead to osteomyelitis. Asplenic patients bitten by certain mammals are at increased risk of severe infection from *Pasteurella* and *Capnocytophaga* bacteria. The bite of several large species of monitor lizards (*Varanus*), which are found throughout tropical Asia and Africa, are prone to mixed infection from oral anaerobes. The septicemia-inducing bite of one species, the komodo dragon (*V. komodoensis*) found on the island of Komodo, Flores and Java, causes fast moving polymicrobial infections leading to septic shock and death in prey animals. Animal hoof, horn and tusk injuries are also likely to be contaminated with environmental microorganisms. Injuries by horned animals such as buffalo and elk may result in large avulsions, which are invariably contaminated with organic matter.

Pigs, both domestic and feral, account for a surprising number of bite and tusk injuries in many developing regions.[9,10] Other animals associated with atypical wound infections include sheep and horses, both of which have been implicated in *Actinobacillus* infections

Table 46.4 Emergency care of animal attack victims

Emergency management
Get victim away from animal.
ABCs: If unconscious, assess airway, breathing, circulation (ABCs) and presence of shock.
Bleeding: Control hemorrhage with direct and indirect pressure and elevation. Traumatic amputations are often ragged, and accompanied by spasm of arterial structures the result of which is less than expected hemorrhage. Bleeding is likely to be adequately controlled using direct pressure rather than tourniquets.
Irrigation: Wounds should be irrigated as soon as possible. In the field, filtered or boil-sterilized water may be used but isotonic fluids produce less tissue damage. Puncture wounds should be irrigated under pressure. Appropriate irrigation pressures may be delivered using an improvised pressure governor made from a 20 cc syringe with 22 g 1.5 inch angiocatheter. When the syringe is emptied over 6 s and using constant pressure, an irrigation force of 3–6 p.s.i. is produced at the catheter tip. Infected wounds should be cultured prior to irrigation.
History: After emergency care is performed, the clinician should obtain an accurate history including the circumstances of the bite, description of the offending animal, documentation of first aid received and changes in wound appearance over time.
Foreign body: Carefully remove any teeth, retained viper fangs, spines and organic mater.
Wound immersion: When resources permit, soak the bite wound in warm water with dilute soap or disinfectant (full strength disinfectant applied to the wound can damage tissue).
Wound dressing: Cover wound with absorbent sterile dressing or clean cloth.
Wound closure: Do not close bite wounds in the field. Wounds may be packed open with sterile dressing.
Immobilize: Bitten extremities should be bandaged, splinted in a functional position and elevated during transport to a local qualified medical facility.
Prophylactic antibiotics: If available antibiotics should be started for all high-risk bites including bites in immunocompromised/asplenic patients, bites to joints, hands, and feet and to extremities with chronic edema. Bites from humans, monkeys, cats, rats and monitor lizards, and those contaminated by organic matter should also receive antibiotics (see Discussion).

Hospital management
Culture: Wounds that present greater than 6 h after attack and those with evidence of infection should be cultured. The laboratory should be instructed to culture for aerobic, anaerobic and fastidious microorganisms.
Radiographs: X-rays should be obtained for all suspicious wounds, and bites to joints.
Debridement: Devitalized tissue should be debrided until a clear base is observed.
Wound approximation: The minority of bite wounds, all low-risk and seen early, may be closed. Select wounds may have edges loosely approximated with sterile closure strips. Skin glue should not be used.
Antibiotics: Treatment should cover anaerobes, such as Provetella, Pasteurella and routine species, such as S. aureus. Oral antibiotics such as amoxicillin-clavulanic acid 875/125 mg b.i.d. (Augmentin) may be used for mild infections. Penicillin-allergic patients will required mixed antibiotic regiments.[5,6] Travelers bitten by old-world monkeys or macaque should be treated with acyclovir (or valacyclovir) to prevent transmission of herpes simiae virus (subtype B virus)[7]
Post-exposure immunization: all patients with severely contaminated wounds receive a tetanus booster. Non-immunized patients should undergo the primary series and be treated with anti-tetanus immunoglobulin. The risk of rabies should be considered using new risk criteria for animal bites and bat contact (see Chapter 10)

following bite injuries.[11] Domestic and feral dogs continue to cause more bite injuries than any other animal – except perhaps for other humans, and many of these are associated with infections by atypical species such as *Capnocytophaga canimoris*,[12] *Staphylococcus intermedius*,[13] and *Neisseria waeveri*.[14] Herpes B virus is enzootic in monkeys and macaques and the majority of species remain asymptomatic. Infection, which can lead to a life-threatening encephalitis, most commonly occurs when humans are bitten or scratched by infected monkeys[15] (Figs 46.4 and 46.5).

Animal wounds associated with increased risk of infection are listed in Table 46.5.

VENOMOUS BITES AND STINGS

The process of delivering venom, known as envenoming, may involve the use of a caudal stinger, as in the case of scorpions and the hymenoptera (bees and wasps); fangs, as in the reptiles, centipedes and spiders; or spines as in certain caterpillars, marine animals and the duck-billed platypus. Venomous injury varies with offending species, with the amount, location and toxicity of venom injected, and the sensitivity of the patient. In the case of envenoming by certain snake, spider and marine species, definitive treatment is only possible using genus, even species-specific antivenin. In the case of the traveler envenomed in foreign countries, antivenin is often difficult to locate, of uncertain activity when available, and prone to side-effects when administered (see treatment).

The physician advising a patient remotely will need to provide comfort while sorting through the patient's description of the offending animal, the progression of symptoms, and then cross-reference this information with medically-significant species native to that region in order to determine whether significant envenoming has occurred. If envenoming is likely, the patient must first access in-country medical services even if international medical evacuation services are immediately available because specific antivenin is more likely to be available in the country where the bite occurred than in the traveler's home country.

Successful triage and clinical decision-making requires that travel medicine clinicians have some familiarity with the range, preferred ecotone, and behavior of venomous animals, and an understanding of how these human–animal encounters occur. An understanding of the description, natural history and initial effects of a given species' venom can play an important role in identifying the offending species

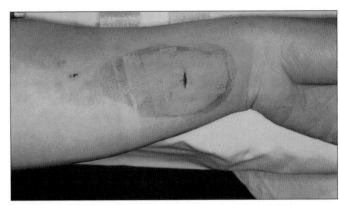

Figure 46.5 Monkey bite to wrist. Monkey bites have a high incidence of bacterial infection and also risk transmission of Herpes B virus, a zoonotic virus associated with fatal cases of encephalitis.

when the animal itself is not available. Examples of this information at work include the clinical diagnosis of scorpion sting, spider bite, and non-envenoming or 'dry' bites by venomous snakes.

Prevention of venomous bites and stings

Methods for preventing encounters with venomous arthropods, reptiles and marine animals are listed in Table 46.6.

Venomous arthropods

Envenoming may occur due to specialized fangs, caudal stingers, dorsal spines or setae. Envenoming result from the defensive actions – usually the final actions – of a spider, wasp, or scorpion that has been swatted or stepped on.

Hymenoptera

The most medically significant venomous arthropods belong to the order hymenoptera, which include bees, wasps, and stinging ants. Together the members of the hymenoptera account for the greatest number of sting injuries, and are responsible for considerable morbidity secondary to hypersensitivity reactions.[16] Hymenoptera venom contains serotonin, histamine and in some tropical hornet

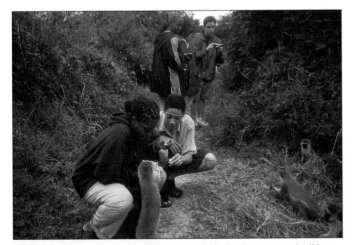

Figure 46.4 Many bites result from attempts to feed or pet semi-wild animals. Monkeys are a frequent and dangerous cause of bites to tourists.

Table 46.5	Animal wounds at high risk of infection
Wounds to joints, hands, feet, tendons and ligaments	
Deep puncture injuries	
Older age	
Certain medical conditions (diabetes, cirrhosis)	
Marine and estuarine injuries	
Contaminated wounds	
Retained teeth, spines, mouthparts	
Carnivores, particularly feline, monkey and monitor lizards	
Delay in wound treatment	
Inappropriate (e.g., early) wound closure	

Table 46.6	Prevention of venomous injuries		
Venomous arthropods	Bees and wasps (Hymenoptera)		Do not wear bright colored clothing, perfumes and aromatic sprays
			Avoid trash cans, flowers and rotting fruit
			Keep wasps away from opened soft drinks
	Centipedes (Scolopendra)		Keep bed sheets off floor
			Wear footwear at night
			Shake out shoes before wearing
Venomous arachnids	Spiders:	Widow spiders (Latrodectus) Banana leaf spiders (Phoneutria) Violin spiders (Loxosceles) Funnel web (Atrax)	Avoid webs
			Keep bed sheets from touching floor
			Use insecticide to reduce prey species
			Inspect privies before sitting (widow spiders)
	Scorpions:	Tityus Buthus Centruroides	Check tub before entering (scorpions)
			Use UV light wands at night (scorpions)
Venomous reptiles	Snakes: Cobras (Naja), mambas, Australian elapids and vipers		Do not attract rodents (which attract snakes that feed on them)
			Do not handle unknown species–even if 'dead'
			Use a flashlight and walking stick after dark.
			Shake out boots and clothing
			Avoid sleeping on the ground
	Lizards		Do not handle Gila monsters or Beaded lizards even if they are 'tame'

species, acetylcholine. The sting injuries cause immediate pain, which tends to decrease over 30 min in the case of honeybees (Apidae) or hours in the case of large hornets (Vespidae). Africanized honeybees, also known as 'killer bees', have venom that is no more toxic than domesticated honeybees. The species is, however, irritable and prone to swarming attacks; victims may be chased considerable distances before the bees give up. Local reactions to hymenoptera stings include a raised papule, often with the stinger-wound in the center, erythema, and edema at the bite site.

Honeybees have a barbed stinger. When the bee attempts to fly away, it is eviscerated, leaving the stinger and the contracting venom gland behind. When present, the stinger-gland complex should be quickly removed to prevent additional venom from being injected into the wound. One effective method of removal makes use of a common fine-toothed comb, which may be used to lift the stinger-gland out of the wound. Additional care of bee stings includes washing with soap and water, verifying tetanus immunization and monitoring for infection. Oral non-steroidal anti-inflammatory agents (NSAIDS) such as ibuprofen are effective in reducing pain, and perhaps swelling, but are of little value after swelling is established. Oral antihistamines are effective at reducing local pruritus, which appears minutes to hours after the sting injury. Cold packs relieve pain associated with hymenoptera sting injuries, but should not be used to treat envenoming injuries caused by other species.

Treatment of hypersensitivity reactions should be initiated as soon as systemic symptoms appear. The most effective therapy is prompt treatment with 1:1000 epinephrine hydrochloride (0.25–0.5 mL subcutaneous). The injection site should be massaged to speed drug absorption. Patients with severe reactions are likely to need a second injection. In recent years, handheld, preloaded epinephrine auto-injectors (e.g., EpiPen™) have become available which facilitate self-treatment by predisposed individuals with minimal training. A small number of sting injuries become infected. Sting injuries that develop

pain, erythema and lymphadenopathy should be treated with antibiotics with activity against gram-positive skin flora.

Spiders and scorpions

Some spider species, such as the hobo spider (*Tageneria*), the violin spider group (recluse spiders; *Loxosceles*) and several types of wolf spiders (*Lycosa*) possess venom capable of causing necrotic skin lesions. In the case of *Loxosceles* spiders the necrosis may be severe. Systemic effects of *Loxosceles* spiders have been reported including renal failure, hepatic insufficiency and hemolysis. No quality antivenin is available for the treatment of *Loxosceles* bite and treatment remains supportive (Fig. 46.6).

Widow spiders (*Latrodectus*) have a worldwide distribution and are responsible for a significant number of neurotoxic envenomings. All widow spiders are a web-dwelling species and it is the female spiders that are responsible for human bites. Widow spiders prefer to build webs near attractants for insects, such as trash dumps, refuse piles and latrines. Bites by widow spiders may initially be mild, however rapid onset of cramping and muscular spasms cause considerable pain. Small children are at increased risk of envenoming and a bad outcome. Antivenins effective against widow spider venom are produced in Australia, South Africa and the United States. The unrelated banana spiders (*Phoneutria*) of South America are another important neurotoxic spider capable of fatal envenoming. Unlike widow spiders, Phoneutria spiders are wandering hunters that often come into contact with humans. An antivenin against *Phoneutria* is produced in Brazil. The most dangerous neurotoxic species are the Australian funnel web spiders (*Atrax*). These large spiders are significantly venomous and unlike the species mentioned above, have a remarkably powerful bite and large fangs, allowing angry specimens to bite through clothing and footwear. An antivenin is made in Australia.

Scorpions are responsible for a significant number of fatalities in Central America, India and North Africa. Most fatalities involve small

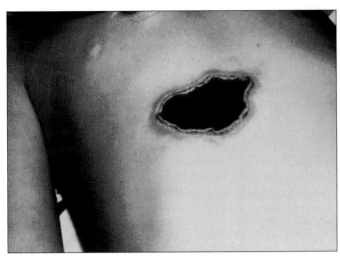

Figure 46.6 Necrotic Loxoscelism from the bite of Loxosceles reclusa, or violin spider in an 8-year-old boy. The child developed acute renal failure, hepatic insufficiency and hemolysis.

Table 46.7	Representative venomous arachnids	
Type/species	**Range**
Spiders	
Widow spiders (*Latrodectus*)	Worldwide
Violin spiders (*Loxosceles*)	Western hemisphere
Banana spiders (*Phoneutria*)	Tropical Americas
Wolf spiders (*Lycosidae*)	Worldwide
Funnel web spiders (*Atrax*)	Australia
Hobo spiders (*Tegeneria*)	Europe, Asia, Northwest USA
Scorpions	
Amazon yellow (*Tityus*)	South America
African scorpions (*Leiurus*)	N. Africa
(*Buthus*)	N. Africa, Spain
Indian scorpions (*Buthotus*)	India, Sri Lanka, Bangladesh
American bark scorpions (*Centruroides*)	S. USA to Colombia

children and debilitated patients. Travelers are likely to be envenomed when they take a shower and step on scorpions that have fallen from the wall into the tub. Many scorpions seek shelter in footwear or between folded clothing, leading to unfortunate encounters. Antivenin is developed against several of the more toxic species such as *Leiurius* and *Centruroides*. In addition to antivenin, neurotoxic bites and stings may be treated with a compression bandage as for neurotoxic snake envenoming (see Snakebite). Medically important spiders and scorpions are provided in Table 46.7.

Venomous reptiles

Snakebite accounts for the majority of severe envenomings in tropical developing countries. Physicians with experience treating snakebite generally agree that while elapids (cobras and kraits) account for the greatest number of deaths, vipers account for the greatest number of bites. Viper venom is rich in enzymes, which cause local pain, swelling, tissue damage, coagulopathy, and for some species, organ damage to the kidneys, adrenals and the pituitary gland.[17] Venom from cobras may be myonecrotic, leading to devastating tissue injury, neurotoxic, leading to respiratory failure, or possess mixed activity. Table 46.8 lists representative species of venomous snakes and their geographic distribution.

If snakebite results in intravenous injection of venom, syncope and death may occur quickly. Deaths occurring within hours usually result from paralysis of respiratory muscles following bites from kraits, mambas, coral snakes and the Philippine cobra (Fig. 46.5). Death after 12 h is likely to be caused by defibrination-related hemorrhage and shock following viper bite. In developing regions, patients may succumb days after the bite, due to complications such as renal failure, secondary wound infection or failure of mechanical ventilation due to power outages.

Table 46.8	Representative venomous snakes by region	
Range	**Species**	
Europe	Vipers	European asp (Vipera berus)
Africa	Elapids	Cobra (Naja, Walterinnesia)
		Mambas (Dendroaspis)
		African Coral snakes (Aspidelaps)
	Vipers	Gaboon viper/puff adder (Bitis)
		Forest vipers (Atheris)
	Ground vipers	Stiletto snakes/burrowing asps (Atractaspis)
	Rear fanged colubrids	Boomslang (Dispholidus)
Americas	Pit vipers	Rattlesnakes (Crotalus)
		Cottonmouth/copperhead (Agkistrodon)
		Central/Southern pit vipers (Bothrops)
	Elapids	Coral snakes (micrurus)
Asia/Australia	Elapids	Asian coral snakes (Maticora/Caliophus)
		Kraits (Bungarus)
		Cobras (Naja)
		Australian elapids (Notechis, Oxyuranus, Pseudechis)
		Sea snakes (Enhydrina)
	Vipers	Daboia (Daboia russelli)
		Saw-scale vipers (Echis)
		Sand vipers (Cerastes)
	Pit vipers	Green tree viper group (Trimeresurus)
		Malayan pit viper (Calloselasma)

A large percentage of cobra and viper bites, between 25 and 40%, are not accompanied by envenoming and may be treated conservatively. The majority of envenoming viper and cobra bites cause local pain, swelling and erythema. Bites from mambas, coral snakes and several Australian species may cause minimal local symptoms suggesting that venom may not have been injected. Indeed, cryptic envenoming by many elapids is often unrecognized until early neurotoxic symptoms such as ptosis or bulbar paralysis appear. Coagulopathy is common for viper bite and is usually first noted at the bite site, where incoagulable blood drains from fang marks. Local necrosis may be significant following bites by most vipers and many species of cobras (Fig. 46.7).

Systemic symptom following snake envenoming include coagulopathy for vipers and neuroparalysis for certain elapids. In the presence of viper hemorrhagins, systemic bleeding may be intense. In southern India and Sri Lanka, envenoming by local daboia (*D. russelli russelli*; previously, *D. r. pulchella* in Sri Lanka) may cause neurotoxic symptoms in addition to DIC-like reactions and myolysis.[18] It should be stressed that the venom of many species varies with region. Such variability influences the effectiveness of antivenin developed using specimens from other regions. An understanding of these limitations is of value for the clinician called upon to evaluate antivenin therapy in a traveler bitten by a dangerous species, and who is being treated with an unfamiliar therapy.

Treatment

Snake envenoming is a medical emergency until proven otherwise. Most snake envenomings are immediately obvious, however, cryptic envenoming, as occurs with several neurotoxic species such as mambas, coral snakes and kraits, cannot be ruled out until the patient has remained symptom-free for at least 18 h. First aid is supportive and is no substitute for antivenin therapy. Definitive treatment of snakebite requires antivenin and skilled medical assessment and care. For this reason, all cases of venomous snakebite should be evaluated as soon as possible at a local medical facility, by a physician with relevant experience.

Pre-hospital care also includes removal of rings, watches and other potentially constrictive items, splinting the bitten limb at or below heart level, and the judicious use of compression dressings (pressure bandages). Compression dressings were originally developed in Australia for use in neurotoxic snakebite[19] and their use in viperidae envenomation is not established. The dressing is wrapped centripetally around the bitten extremity, covering the fang marks. Patients treated with compression wraps require close supervision as increasing pain may prompt the patient to unwrap the dressing, releasing sequestered venom into the systemic circulation. Venom extraction devices, cauterization, and native remedies should be avoided.

On arrival at the medical facility, if coagulopathy is a possibility, blood should be drawn by peripheral venipuncture and left undisturbed in a red top vacutainer or a clean glass test tube. After 20–30 min, the tube should be decanted and the presence of unclotted blood noted. Incoagulable blood indicates envenoming by a viper, or Rhabdophis, a rear-fanged colubrid, which possesses venom with defibrinating activity. Patients who may have been bitten by a neurotoxic species require close monitoring for the development of neurotoxicity. Early symptoms include diplopia, ptosis and bulbar palsy (Fig. 46.8). Evidence of neurologic abnormalities that can not be attributed to other causes (i.e., hyperventilation, narcotic analgesia, etc.) is an indication for immediate treatment with antivenin directed against local neurotoxic species. Polyvalent antivenins, developed to protect against the venom of several species, are commonly used in sub-Saharan Africa, Asia and the tropical Americas. The majority of these antivenins will be unfamiliar to western medical consultants. Antivenin supplies in rural hospitals, where snakebite is likely to be initially treated, is often stored improperly, in short supply and out of date. If the patient is critically envenomed and no alternatives exist, unrefrigerated and expired antivenin should still be used.

Antivenin is stored as either hyperimmune serum or as lyophilized powder, which must be reconstituted prior to intravenous infusion. Attempts to give antivenin by arterial infusion may prove catastrophic in the patient with coagulopathy. Intramuscular injection of antivenin is also not recommended. Although potency varies between manufacturers, antivenin is generally administered in 1–2 vial aliquots over 5–10 min. Pain, paralytic symptoms and blood clotting abnormalities often improve transiently after antivenin however re-treatment is usually necessary (Fig. 46.7). Antivenin therapy may be stopped when no further progression of pain, swelling, or erythema is noted, or when coagulation dyscrasias begin to reverse. If neurotoxicity of bulbar or respiratory muscles is noted, anticholinesterases such as edrophonium may be administered to delay the onset of respiratory failure, and allow time for antivenin to work.

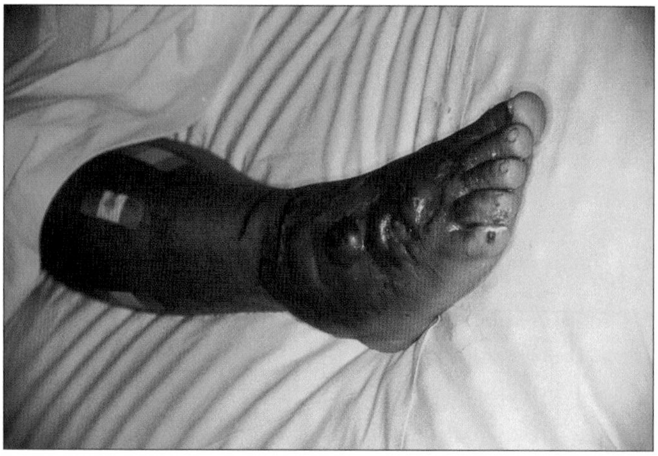

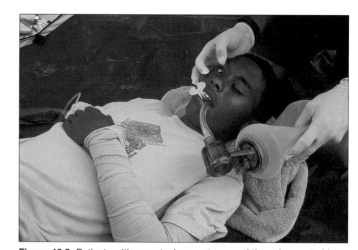

Figure 46.8 Patients with neurotoxic symptoms and those known to bitten by neurotoxic species should be treated with compression dressings and monitored closely. This 8-year-old boy presented 9 h after being bitten by a krait (Bungarus) with diplopia, bulbar palsey and respiratory difficulty. The patient was intubated and treated with compression dressings while waiting for antivenin. Note disconjugate gaze.

Figure 46.7 Bites by vipers and many cobras cause local pain, swelling and ecchymosis as in the case of this Thai woman bitten on the foot by a 1 m long Daboia (Daboia russelli) viper.

Following successful resuscitation and antivenin treatment, patients will need to be monitored for sequelae of envenoming, such as tissue necrosis, renal failure, endocrinopathies and serum sickness reactions from antivenin. Wound care includes debridement of necrotic tissues until clean margins are observed, and daily wound care as for burn injuries. Travelers envenomed by dangerous species should be transported when stable to an appropriate medical center for wound evaluation and initiation of physical therapy. Important points regarding snake envenoming are highlighted in Table 46.9

Several New World lizards, the Gila monster and the Mexican beaded lizard, are venomous. These species possess mandibular venom glands, which secrete moderately toxic venom into the wounds made by the teeth. Deaths from lizard envenoming are rare, however bites occur commonly with pet lizards. No antivenin is available for bites by these lizards.

MARINE ANIMAL BITES, STINGS, AND ATTACKS

Sea urchins, spiney starfish, and fire corals cause many more injuries than do marine predators. Sharks are frequently associated with marine attack injuries on humans, however, less than 100 attacks and fewer than 10 fatalities occur each year. Unprovoked bites from predatory fish such as sharks, often occur when visibility is poor, an observation suggesting that the predator mistook the victim for more typical prey. Other marine species implicated in traumatic marine wounds range from groupers, triggerfish, bluefish, barracuda and moray eels. Wounds caused by shark attack often result in extensive loss of soft tissue, fractures and massive hemorrhage. Bite wounds by other species while less traumatic, may still result in significant blood loss and tissue damage.

Marine envenomings may be caused by vertebrates such as sea snakes and venomous fish or by invertebrates such as anemones, sea plumes, fire corals, and cone shells, which possess a harpoon used to inject venom into the fish that are its primary food source. The diminutive blue ringed octopus, which is found in Indonesian and Australian waters, secretes the potent neurotoxin tetrodotoxin in its saliva. Bites, which may go unnoticed, may cause systemic neurotoxic symptoms including respiratory paralysis and death. As its name suggests, the octopus flashes indigo blue rings along the head and tentacles when disturbed.

Prevention

The majority of invertebrates responsible for human injuries reside in the tropical coastal waters, and within reef systems. Humans who wade, surf, snorkel and scuba dive in these ecosystems should be careful where they sit, step or place their hands. The majority of venomous corals and anemones are distinctive in appearance or color, allowing them to be identified and avoided with relative ease. Many stinging species, such as conus snails, which possess a venomous harpoon, are distinctively patterned.

Stingray injuries, usually the result of waders stepping on camouflaged rays, may be avoided by 'shuffle-footing', whereby the feet slide forward while in continuous contact with the sand. Any stingrays encountered by an advancing human foot, swim off to find a quieter resting site. Protective footwear provides reasonable protection against sharp corals and the smaller venomous creatures. Swimmers, snorkelers and divers should remain vigilant for jellyfish, which often co-exist in large numbers.

Jellyfish, like the anemones and soft corals, deliver venom through a specialized structure known as a nematocyst. Large jellyfish may possess hundreds of thousands, sometimes millions of nematocysts per tentacle, leading to severe envenoming injuries when the victim becomes entangled and struggles to get free. Nematocysts on detached tentacles are capable of delivering venom for many weeks. The box jellyfish (*Chironex fleckeri*), is generally considered to be the most dangerous species. Box jellyfish are a mid-sized species that appear seasonally along Australia's north coast and the tropical Indo-Pacific. The mortality for patients envenomed by box jellyfish ranges from 15–20% and was doubtless higher prior to the advent of antivenin. Envenomed patients may lose consciousness within 2–3 min of being stung, occasionally before they are able to reach the shore. Death is due to hypotension, respiratory paralysis and cardiac arrest. An antivenin is produced from the venom of the box jellyfish. Some marine species such as sea cucumbers secret crinotoxins, that may be absorbed by the unwary handler.

Venomous injuries from marine fish are increasing with the popularity of reef diving and snorkeling. These venoms are usually delivered through specialized caudal or dorsal spines. Several tropical reef fish species such as the stonefish and scorpionfish are particularly toxic; pain associated with envenoming is said to be extreme and intractable. Injuries caused by some species, in particular the stingrays and stonefish are both venomous and traumatic.

Table 46.9 Clinical pearls for snake envenoming
Local pain, swelling, and erythema are the hallmarks of viper and most cobra envenoming bites
Venoms often possess both hemotoxic or neurotoxic activity
The venom of most cobras cause significant tissue injury and not neurotoxicity
The venom of most vipers cause significant tissue injury, and often, systemic coagulopathy
The venom of several colubrids cause minimal local reaction but may cause severe coagulopathy (e.g. *Rhabdophis*, Asian keelback)
Persistent bleeding from the fang marks suggests systemic coagulopathy
Bites from kraits, the Philippines cobra and coral snakes can cause life threatening neuroparalysis with minimal local symptoms
Cryptic envenomation by vipers and the majority of cobras is rare in the absence of local symptoms
Neurotoxic effects of several snake venoms (e.g., kraits) cannot be reversed by antivenin treatment. It is not uncommon for krait paralyzed patients to be artificially ventilated for weeks
Anticholinesterases may delay the onset of paralysis and buy time for antivenin to work.

First aid for severe marine injuries focuses on management of ABCs, control of bleeding, and prompt transport to a hospital. Wound care for marine bites and stings prioritizes irrigation, removal of foreign bodies, use of quality dressings and splinting injured extremities in a functional position. Bite and puncture wounds, and virtually all wounds of hands, feet and other complex structures, should be left open to reduce the likelihood of infection.

Treatment

Treatment of marine envenoming requires identification of the offending species, immediate removal of retained spines or nematocysts, support of ABCs and if indicated and available, administration of antivenin. For jellyfish and soft coral envenoming, attached nematocysts need to be quickly removed before further venom is injected. Adhered tentacles may be removed with an instrument or gloved hand, or by washing with seawater. Under no circumstances should fresh water be used as the hypotonic environment stimulates intact nematocysts to discharge their venom. Nematocysts may also be deactivation by the topical application of alcohol, weak acid solutions and possible weak bases. Although recommendations vary with region, it is generally accepted that the nematocysts of most species (Chironex, Chrysaora and Cyanea) may be inactivated using household vinegar (5% acetic acid) or isopropyl alcohol (50–70%). The value of ethyl alcohol, which is often present on the beaches near where these stings occur, is controversial. Vinegar should not be used to inactivate nematocysts of the unrelated Portuguese Man-o'War jellyfish.[20]

Urchin and starfish spine wounds should initially be treated with hot water immersion (50 °C) for 30–60 min as tolerated or until pain dissipates. In the author's experience, pain invariably returns as the soft tissue around the spine injury cool to body temperature, and so re-treatment will be necessary. Urchin spines should be removed as venom will continue to leach from the spine integument. The first aid provider should be cautioned that the spines are easily broken off with minimal lateral force. During removal of spines, care should be taken to insure that the force is in the reverse direction as the spine's entrance trajectory.

The more severe envenoming injuries of marine fish also show benefit from hot water immersion. The principle difference between these injuries is the amount of corresponding trauma, highest in stingray injuries, or severity of envenoming, highest in the scorpionfish and stonefish stings (Fig. 46.9). Retained spines and spine fragments should be quickly removed and the affected area immersed in hot water as described above. If a skilled medical provider is present and circumstances permit, the wound may be irrigated with sterile hot water. The victim of marine fish envenoming will require follow-up for thorough wound exploration, probable radiographic studies and prophylactic antibiotics. Due to the severity of infections associated with these injuries, travelers should be advised to seek evaluation while overseas, rather then waiting until they return home.

MARINE INFECTIONS

Wound infection is common following traumatic marine injuries, however the range of responsible microorganisms differs from those observed in terrestrial wounds. While staphylococcal and streptococcal wound infections are still common, many marine infections are caused by gram-negative species such as *Vibrio, Aeromonas, Halomonas, Erysipelothrix, Edwardsiella* and *Chromobacterium*.[21,22] Indolent nodular lesions at the site of prior marine injury suggest *Mycobacterium marinum*, a difficult to treat infection that presents weeks after the original wound has healed. Injuries caused by fish spines and broken seashells may result in *Erysipelothrix rhusopathiae* infection, a

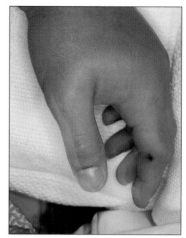

Figure 46.9 Patients envenomed by members of stonefish group, such as this 19-year-old male who received a single spine injury to the hand, experience intense pain.

species that causes a distinctive erythematous cellulitis that spreads quickly from the site of infection. Patients who are immunosuppressed, and those with liver or renal disease are at risk of severe infection from marine vibrios *V.carchariae*,[23] *V. vulnificus* and *V. parahaemolyticus*.[24] In these patients, the appearance of fast moving cellulitis or darkening skin should prompt immediate administration of appropriate intravenous antibiotics and emergency consultation with infectious disease physicians and surgeons (Fig. 46.10).

Infections are not an inevitable consequence of marine wounds. The likelihood of infection is reduced by careful wound inspection, thorough irrigation, and removal of foreign bodies. Injuries from stingrays deserve special mention because the puncture wound often contains remnants of the spine's integument sheath, which if retained increases the likelihood of infection. Culture of marine wounds should be reserved for cases presenting with evidence of infection. Use of antibiotics should be extended beyond treatment to prophylax against high-risk wounds. Antibiotics should be directed against gram-negative microorganisms unless culture and gram stains suggest otherwise.

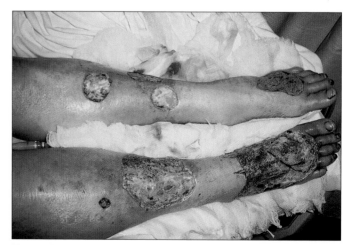

Figure 46.10 Debilitated patients are at increased risk of severe infections by Vibrio vulnificus and related species. This 56-year-old patient with cirrhotic liver disease developed V. vulnificus septicemia and widely scattered hemorrhagic bullae requiring debridement.

Appropriate antibiotics include ciprofloxacin and the extended spectrum fluoroquinolones, trimethoprim-sulfamethoxazole, and third-generation cephalosporins. If *Aeromonas* infections are suspected, aminoglycosides may be added.

REFERENCES

1. Callahan MV. Non-domestic animal attack. In: Keystone, ed. *Wilderness Medicine*. San Diego: University of California; 1998.
2. Goldstein EJC, Citron DM, Fingold SM. Dog bite wounds and infection: a prospective clinical study. *Ann Emerg Med* 1980; **9**:508–513.
3. Talon DA, Citron DM, Abrahamian FM, *et al*. Bacteriologic analysis of infected dog and cat bites. Emergency Medicine Animal Bite Infection Study Group. *N Engl J Med* 1999; **340**:85–92.
4. Goldstein EJ, Citron DM, Merriam CV, *et al*. In vitro activities of the des-fluoro(6) Quinolone BMS-284756 against aerobic and anaerobic pathogens isolated from skin and soft tissue animal and human bite wound infections. *Antimicrob Agents Chemother* 2002; **46**(3):866–870.
5. Vergese A, Hamati F, Berk S, *et al*. Susceptibility of dysgonic fermenter 2 to antimicrobial agents in vitro. *Antimicrob Agents Chemother* 1988; **32**:78–80.
6. Goldstein EJC. Bite wounds and infection. *Clin Infect Dis* 1992; **14**:633–640.
7. Holmes GP, Chapman LE, Stewart J, *et al*. Guidelines for the prevention and treatment of B virus infections in exposed persons. *Clin Infect Dis* 1995; **20**:421–439.
8. Zook EG, Miller M. van Beck *et al*. Successful treatment protocol of canine fang injuries. *J Trauma* 1980; **20**:243–247.
9. Barss P. Ennis S Injuries caused by pigs in Papua New Guinea. *Med J Aust* 1988; **149**(11–12):649–656.
10. Goldstein EJC. Citron Dm, Merkin TE *et al*. Recovery of an unusual Flavobacterium IIb-like isolate from a hand infection following pig bite. *J Clin Microbiol* 1990; **28**:1709–1781.
11. Peel NM, Hornridge KA, Luppino M, *et al*. Actinobacillus spp. And related bacteria in infected wounds of humans bitten by horses and sheep. *J Clin Micrbiol* 1991; **29**:2535–2538.
12. Gallen IW, Ispahani PP. Fulminant Capnocytophaga canimorsus (DF-2) septicaemia. *Lancet* 1991; **337**:308.
13. Talen DA, Goldstein EJC, Staatz D, *et al*. Staphylococcus intermedius: Clinical presentation of a new human dog bite pathogen. *Ann Emerg Med* 1989; **18**:410–413.
14. Anderson BM, Steigerwalt AG, O'Connor SP, *et al*. Neisseria weaveri sp. Nov., formerly CDC group M-5, a gram-negative bacterium associated with dog wounds. *J Clin Microbiol* 1993; **31**:2456–2466.
15. Gp H, Hilliard JK, Klontz KC, *et al*. B virus (herpes virus simiae) infection in humans: Epidemiologic investigations of a cluster. *Ann Intern Med* 1990; **112**:833–839.
16. Nall TM. Analysis of 677 death certificates and 169 autopsies of stinging insect deaths. *J Allergy Clin Immunol* 1990; **75**:185.
17. Tun-Pe, Phillips RE, Warrell DA, *et al*. Acute and chronic pituitary failure resembling Sheehan's syndrome following bites by Russell's viper in Burma. *Lancet* 1987; **ii**:763–767.
18. Jayanthi GP, Gowda TV. Geographic variation in India in the composition and lethal potency of Russell's viper venom. *Toxicon* 1988; **26**:257–264.
19. Sutherland SK, Coulter AR, Harris RD. Rationalization of first-aid measures for elapid snakebite. *Lancet* 1979; **I**:183–186.
20. Fenner PJ, Williamson JA, Burnett JW, *et al*. First aid treatment of jellyfish stings in Australia: response to a newly differentiated species. *Med J Aust* 1993; **158**(498).
21. Graevenitz A von, Bowman J, Notaro C Del, Ritzler M. Human infection with Halomonas venusta following fish bite. *J Clin Microbiol* 2000; **38**(8):3123–3124.
22. Lehane L, Rawlin GT. Topically acquired bacterial zoonoses from fish: a review. *Med J Aust* 2001; **174**(9):480–481.
23. Pavia AT, Bryan JA, Maher KL, *et al*. Vibrio carchariae infection after a shark bite. *Ann Intern Med* 1989; **111**(1):85–86.
24. Howard RJ, Burgess GH. Surgical hazards posed by marine and freshwater animals in Florida. *Am J Surg* 1993; **166**(5):563–567.

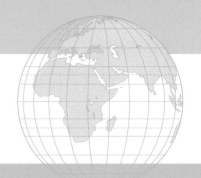

CHAPTER 47 Food-borne Illness

Vernon Ansdell

KEYPOINTS

- Travelers to the Caribbean and Indo-Pacific Ocean regions should be aware of the risk of ciguatera poisoning and avoid consumption of large carnivorous reef fish such as grouper, snapper, amberjack, and barracuda. The toxin survives normal cooking procedures

- Paralytic shellfish poisoning occurs after ingestion of contaminated bivalve mollusks such as clams, mussels, oysters and scallops. The toxin survives normal cooking procedures

- No cases of 'mad-cow' disease due to the agent of Bovine Spongiform Encephalopathy have been reported in travelers and control measures have essentially eliminated current risk in affected countries

- Toxic and unfamiliar mushrooms abound in destination countries. Cooking generally but not always inactivates the toxins

CIGUATERA

It is estimated that there are over 50 000 new cases of ciguatera poisoning worldwide every year making it one of the commonest causes of marine poisoning from a food toxin (Table 47.1). It is widespread in tropical and subtropical waters between the latitudes of 35° North and 35° South and is particularly common in the Pacific and Indian Oceans and the Caribbean Sea.[1,2] Most cases follow ingestion of coral reef fish containing potent toxins such as ciguatoxin or maitotoxin that originate in dinoflagellates found in coral reefs. Average annual incidence rates for ciguatera fish poisoning vary from 5 to 50 per 100 000 in major endemic areas with rates of up to 500 per 100 000 or even higher in some areas of the South Pacific during certain years. Of particular relevance to scuba divers is the fact that many of the symptoms of ciguatera poisoning may closely mimic those of decompression sickness.

The toxins that cause ciguatera poisoning originate from dinoflagellates such as *Gambierdiscus toxicus* that are found on marine algae usually attached to dead coral reefs. Dinoflagellates are ingested by herbivorous fish and the toxins are concentrated as they pass up the food chain to large (usually greater than 6 lb) carnivorous fish and finally to humans.[3] (Fig. 47.1).

Ciguatoxin (CTX) and maitotoxin are among the most lethal natural substances known and may be concentrated up to 50 to 100 times in parts of the fish such as the liver, gastrointestinal tract, roe, and head. The toxins do not affect the appearance, texture, smell, or taste of the affected fish and are not destroyed by gastric acid, cooking or other fish processing methods such as canning, drying, freezing, smoking, salting, or pickling. CTX has recently been completely characterized and synthesized[4] which may lead to advances in the understanding of its mechanism of action and potential therapies. Pacific Ocean, Caribbean and Indian Ocean CTX appear to be structurally different.[5]

Over 400 species of fish have been implicated in ciguatera poisoning. They are mainly carnivorous reef fish such as grouper, snapper, barracuda, jacks, sturgeon, sea bass, and moray eel. Certain herbivorous or omnivorous reef fish such as surgeonfish and parrotfish may also be responsible. Open ocean pelagic fishes such as tuna and mahimahi have not been associated with ciguatera poisoning.

Ciguatera-like illnesses were known in ancient Egypt. Some of the earliest recorded cases in travelers were in the crews sailing with European explorers such as Christopher Columbus and James Cook (Table 47.2). Captain Bligh and his followers apparently developed ciguatera poisoning after the historic mutiny aboard HMS Bounty.

The onset of symptoms is usually within 1–3 h of eating contaminated fish but may occur within 15–30 min or be delayed for up to 30 h. Most symptoms resolve within 1–4 weeks. A wide range of symptoms has been reported, but, typically, there is an acute gastrointestinal illness followed by neurologic symptoms and, rarely, cardiovascular collapse. Gastrointestinal symptoms occur in most cases and include diarrhea, nausea, vomiting, and abdominal pain. They usually occur 1–3 h after eating affected fish and may last for 1–2 days. Neurologic symptoms tend to occur later and may be delayed for up to 72 h. They may last for several months or even years. Neurologic symptoms include paradoxical dysesthesias such as temperature reversal where cold objects feel hot and hot objects feel cold.[6] This is very characteristic of ciguatera poisoning but not pathognonionic since it may also occur in neurotoxic shellfish poisoning. Other neurologic symptoms include paresthesias involving the arms, legs, perioral area, tongue and throat. About one-third of patients report pain in the teeth or a sensation that the teeth are numb or loose. Visual symptoms include blurred vision and transient blindness. Chronic neuropsychiatric symptoms may be very disabling and include malaise, depression, headaches, myalgias, and fatigue.

Cardiac manifestations include bradycardia (possibly due to cholinesterase inhibition), tachycardia, and other arrhythmias. Hypotension in the absence of hypovolemia may be due to the hypotensive properties of maitotoxin. Persistent symptomatic hypotension has been described and is probably due to an increase in parasympathetic tone and impaired sympathetic reflexes. Hypertension has also been described. The cardiac effects of ciguatera poisoning may be serious but usually resolve within 5 days of onset.

General symptoms include profound weakness, chills, sweating, arthralgias, myalgias, and a metallic taste in the mouth. Pruritus, particularly involving the palms and soles, occurs 2–5 days after ingestion of contaminated fish and has been reported in 5 to 89% of cases. It is particularly common in New Caledonia where ciguatera poisoning is

Table 47.1 Summary of seafood toxins

Syndrome	Toxin	Origin of toxin	Seafood vehicle	Geographical distribution	Typical symptoms
Scombroid	Histamine	Histidine converted to histamine by enzyme action	Inadequately refrigerated, histidine rich fish, e.g., mahimahi, tuna, mackerel, skipjack	Worldwide	Flushing, headache, nause, vomiting, diarrhea, urticaria
Ciguatera	Ciguatoxin Maitotoxin	Dinoflagellates. *Gambierdiscus toxicus and others*	Large carnivorous tropical and subtropical reef fish (e.g., barracuda, grouper, moray eel, snapper, jack, seabass)	Tropical and subtropical waters between 35° North and 35° South. Commonest in the Caribbean and South Pacific Islands	Gastroenteritis followed by neurologic symptoms (e.g., dysesthesiae, temperature reversal, pruritus, weakness). Rarely, bradycardia and hypotension
Pufferfish poisoning	Tetrodotoxin		Pufferfish, porcupine fish and rarely ocean sunfish	Worldwide. Commonest in Japan, Indo-Pacific oceans	Perioral parestheriae, nausea, dizziness followed by weakness, numbness, slurred speech, incoordination, respiratory failure
Paralytic shellfish poisoning	Saxitoxin	Dinoflagellates, *Alexandrium species and others*	Bivalve shellfish	Worldwide. Commonest in temperature coastal waters	Paresthesiae of face and limbs, gastroenteritis. Rarely, dysphonia, ataxia, weakness, respiratory failure
Neurotoxic shellfish poisoning	Brevetoxins	Dinoflagellates. *Gymnodinium, breve*	Bivalve shellfish	Rare. Gulf of Mexico and New Zealand	Gastroenteritis and neurologic symptoms (e.g., paresthesiae, temperature reversal, vertigo, ataxia). Respiratory and eye irritation in the presence of aerosol
Diarrhetic shellfish poisoning	Okadaic aad and others	Dinoflagellates. *Dinophysis species*	Bivalve shellfish	Japan, Europe (France), Canada, New Zealand and S. America	Gastroenteritis
Amnesic shellfish poisoning	Domoic acid	Diatoms. *Pseudonitzschia species*	Mussels	Extremely rare, NE Canada only	Gastroenteritis followed by neurologic symptoms (e.g., amnesia, cognitive impairment, headache, seizures)

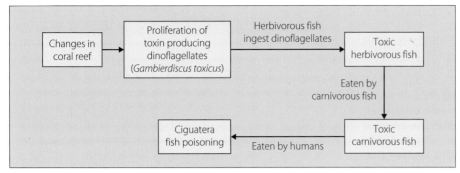

Figure 47.1 Chain of events in ciguatera fish poisoning.

known as 'la gratte' or 'the itch.' It seems to be more common in the Pacific than the Caribbean.

Deaths result from respiratory or cardiac failure and are most common in patients who have eaten parts of the fish known to contain high levels of toxin such as the liver, intestines, or roe. Case fatality rate is usually from 0.1 to 1%, depending on geographic location. A mortality rate of almost 20% was reported in one outbreak in Madagascar when over 500 people became ill after eating a shark.

Disturbances to reef systems and the subsequent proliferation of toxic dinoflagellates have been shown to have an important impact on the incidence of ciguatera poisoning, although there is often a 6- to 24-month time lag. Reef systems may be disrupted by natural disasters such as hurricanes, tidal waves, heavy rains, and earthquakes or manmade activities such as underwater nuclear explosions, coastal construction projects, dredging, shipwrecks, or golf course run-off.

Several factors have been shown to influence the severity of ciguatera poisoning. These include the amount of fish eaten and consumption of parts known to contain high levels of toxin such as the head, liver, intestine, and roe or soup made from those parts. Previous exposure to ciguatera also increases the severity of poisoning, probably as a result of accumulation of toxin or immune sensitization.

Medical management is mainly symptomatic and supportive. If patients are seen within 3 h of ingestion of contaminated fish, emetics such as ipecac or gastric lavage followed by activated charcoal may be indicated. In theory, antiemetics and antidiarrheals should be avoided because they may prolong toxin contact time. Bradycardia responds to atropine. Intravenous fluids are indicated if there is volume depletion and hypotension. Hypotension in the absence of volume depletion is treated with pressors such as dopamine or dobutamine. Intravenous calcium gluconate 10% can be used to treat the inhibited calcium uptake caused by ciguatoxin. Treatment of prolonged ortho-static hypotension may require sodium and fluid replacement, fludrocortisone acetate, and lower extremity support stockings. Lidocaine or mexiletine have been used to treat ventricular arrhythmias. Treatment options for specific symptoms include cyproheptadine or hydroxyzine for pruritus, acetaminophen or nifedipine for headache, and non-steroidal anti-inflammatory agents for musculoskeletal pains. Amitriptyline appears to be effective in treating depression associated with ciguatera poisoning and may also be effective in treating other neuropsychiatric symptoms such as dysesthesias. Chronic fatigue associated with ciguatera poisoning has been treated successfully with fluoxetine (Prozac).

Intravenous mannitol (1 g/kg over 30 min) has been reported to reduce the severity and duration of neurologic symptoms particularly if given within the first 24 h of poisoning.[7] Other studies have not supported this finding.[8] Mannitol should be used with caution, however, and only after ensuring adequate hydration. A potential mechanism of action has not been established. Recent case reports suggest that gabapentin (Neurontin), a drug occasionally used to treat neuropathic pain, may be useful in relieving symptoms late in the illness.

Travelers to endemic areas, particularly the Caribbean and Indo-Pacific regions, should be warned about the risk of ciguatera poisoning and should avoid or limit consumption of reef fish, particularly carnivorous fish weighing over 6 lb. The risk of ciguatera fish poisoning in travelers to an endemic area has been estimated at 300 in 10 000, which is similar to the risk of acquiring hepatitis A. Particularly high-risk fish such as tropical moray eels or barracuda should never be eaten. Travelers should be reminded that it is important to avoid parts of the fish known to contain large amounts of toxin such as the head, liver, intestine, and roe or soup made from these parts and not to consume large reef fish weighing more than 6 lb.

Radioimmune assays or enzyme-linked immunosorbent assays have been developed to investigate ciguatera poisoning and a commercial immunoassay has recently become available for the identification of toxic fish (Cigua-check™, Oceanit Test Systems Inc., Honolulu). The test is easy to perform and very sensitive, but it is relatively expensive (cost approximately US$5 per test). It will probably have limited value for travelers to endemic areas.

Any patient with a history of ciguatera poisoning should avoid consumption of reef fish, fish sauces, shellfish, alcoholic beverages, nuts, and nut oils since they may provoke recurrent symptoms.

Diagnosis of ciguatera poisoning is usually made on clinical grounds. If a portion of the fish is still available, it should be frozen and, if possible, submitted to a laboratory that can test for presence of toxin.

In a survival situation, organ meat should be fed to susceptible animals such as dogs, cats, or mongooses. If the animals show no sign of illness, then the flesh of the fish is probably safe for human consumption.

Table 47.2	Excerpt from the journals of Captain James Cook's voyage in the South Pacific in 1774

The Night before we came out of Port two Red fish about the Size of large Bream and not unlike them were caught with hook and line of which Most of the officers and Some of the Petty officers dined the next day. In the Evening every one who had eat of these fish were seiz'd with Violant pains in the head and Limbs, so as to be unable to stand, together with a kind of Scorching heat all over the Skin, there remained no doubt but that it was occasioned by the fish being of a Poisoness nature and communicated its bad effects to every one who had the ill luck to eat of it even to the Dogs and Hogs, one of the latter died in about Sixteen hours after and a young dog soon after shared the same fate: and it was a week or ten days before all the gentlemen recovered.

SCOMBROID

Scombroid is one of the most common fish poisonings and occurs worldwide in both temperate and tropical waters. The illness often resembles a moderate to severe allergic reaction and occurs after eating improperly refrigerated or preserved fish containing high levels of histamine. Fish that cause scombroid include dark or red muscled fish belonging to the family *Scombridae* such as albacore, bluefin and yellowfin tuna, mackerel, saury, skipjack, and bonito. Various non-scombroid fish may also be responsible including mahimahi (dolphinfish) (Fig. 47.2), sardine, pilchard, anchovy, herring, bluefish, amberjack, and black marlin.[1] Cases of fish poisoning closely resembling scombroid were described by Captain Edmund Fanning while sailing in the North Atlantic in 1797 (Table 47.3).

Fish that cause scombroid have high levels of the amino acid histidine in the flesh. As a result of improper handling and storage after catch, histidine is converted to histamine and other scombrotoxins by bacteria with high histidine decarboxylase activity. These bacteria occur as normal surface flora or secondary contaminants and include *Morganella rnorganii*, *Klebsiella pneumoniae*, *Escherichia coli*, *Aerobacter aerogenes*, and *Plesiomonas shigelloides*.

Conversion of histidine to histamine and other scombrotoxins occurs optimally at 20–30°C, and scombroid typically occurs in fish that have not been promptly refrigerated after capture. Histamine and other scombrotoxins are resistant to freezing, cooking, smoking, or canning.

Symptoms of scombroid poisoning usually appear abruptly 10–60 min after eating contaminated fish, although they may appear within a few min of ingestion or be delayed for several h. Untreated, symptoms typically last for an average of 4 h but may persist for up to 24 h. Symptoms often resemble an acute allergic reaction and are frequently misdiagnosed as an allergy to fish. Affected fish often have a peppery, sharp, metallic. or bitter taste but may be normal in taste and appearance. There are several characteristic symptoms of scombroid poisoning.[1] Flushing of the skin resembling sunburn with a sharply demarcated edge confined to the face and upper body may be present. Pruritus is common, and there may be urticaria or angioneurotic edema. A throbbing headache is often present. Gastrointestinal symptoms include nausea, vomiting, abdominal cramps, and diarrhea. Other clinical features may include perioral paresthesiae, burning of the mouth and gums, conjunctival suffusion, palpitations, blurred vision, and diaphoresis. Scombroid is usually a benign, self-limited illness; rarely, however, it may produce a more serious illness with

Table 47.3	Excerpt from the journals of Captain Edmund Fannings voyage in the North Atlantic 1797

During this period we caught, with hook and grains, as many of the Spanish mackerel, or bonetos, as were wished for; shoals of these fish, as well as the dolphin, being all around us;... On eating of the dolphin and mackerel, almost all on board were affected with a severe pain in the head, which shortly after was much inflamed; the eyes became red, and these distressing symptoms were attended with violent vomiting. Those who were thus affected, were evidently poisoned; the head and some of the limbs began also to swell, which swelling increased, until they had attained a most disagreeable form, having at the same time, a reddish cast over the head and limbs thus swollen... whenever the fish, on being taken out of the water, was immediately cooked, and then eaten, no evil or unpleasant sensation was experienced;...

respiratory compromise, malignant arrhythmias, and hypotension. Serious illness seems to be more likely in the elderly and asthmatics. Patients who are already taking isoniazid may have a severe reaction because the drug inhibits histamine metabolism. Deaths are extremely rare, and none have been reported in recent years. As expected, persons already taking antihistamines tend to have less symptoms.

Diagnosis is usually made on clinical grounds. There may be a clustering of cases, which helps to exclude the possibility of fish allergy. The diagnosis can be confirmed by measuring histamine levels in any leftover fish.

Treatment with histamine-1 antagonists (e.g., diphenhydramine) given orally or parenterally provides symptomatic relief. Newer, second-generation, non-sedating histamine-1 antagonists (e.g., astemizole) have not yet been proved to be as effective. Histamine-2 antagonists (e.g., cimetidine) given orally or parenterally may shorten the course of illness and been particularly useful in controlling headache.[9] A combination of histamine-1 and histamine-2 antagonists may be particularly valuable but rarely may cause hypotension. Steroids have not been shown to be of any benefit. In severe scombroid poisoning intravenous fluids, inhaled bronchodilators, oxygen, and pressor agents may be indicated. Gastric lavage or catharsis may be worthwhile if large quantities of contaminated fish have been consumed within the previous few h.

The most important preventive measure is to chill the fish promptly after capture and maintain adequate refrigeration until the fish is prepared for consumption. Fish kept at 15–20°C or less prior to cooking should be safe for consumption.

PUFFERFISH (FUGU) POISONING

Pufferfish or fugu poisoning occurs after ingestion of fish containing tetrodotoxin, a potent neurotoxin. Potentially toxic fish are distributed widely throughout the world and include pufferfish, porcupine fish, and ocean sunfish.[1] The toxin is usually concentrated in the ovaries, liver, intestines, and skin of the fish. Pufferfish poisoning has been recognized since ancient Egyptian times. One of the earliest recorded outbreaks of pufferfish poisoning in travelers may have involved Captain Cook and members of his crew who became ill after eating pufferfish liver while sailing in the South Pacific during their second voyage around the world in 1774 (Table 47.4).

Most cases of pufferfish poisoning occur in Japan where pufferfish or fugu is eaten as a very expensive and prized delicacy. The fugu is filleted, thinly sliced, and then arranged in traditional patterns such as a crane. The fugu experience is characterized by tingling of the lips and tongue, a sensation of generalized warmth and flushing, and a feeling of euphoria and exhilaration. Over the 78-year period from 1886 to 1963 there were 6386 cases of fugu poisoning in Japan with

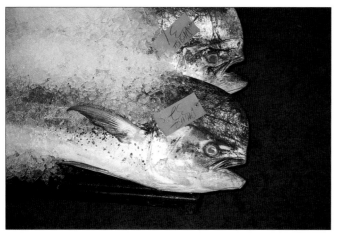

Figure 47.2 Mahimahi (dolphin fish) a common cause of scombroid poisoning. Prompt refrigeration, using ice as shown here, will prevent poisoning (Photo by David Ansdell).

Table 47.4	Excerpt from the journals of Captain James Cooks voyage in the South Pacific in 1774

This afternoon a fish being struck by one of the natives near the watering place, the Captain's clerk purchased it, and sent it to him after his return on board. It was of a new species, something like a sun-fish, with a large, long, ugly head. Having no suspicion of its being of a poisonous nature, they ordered it to be dressed for supper; but, very luckily, the operation of drawing and describing took up so much time that it was too late, so that only the liver and roe were dressed, of which the two Mr. Fortsters and the Captain did but taste. About three o'clock in the morning they all found themselves seized with an extraordinary weakness and numbness all over their limbs. The Captain had almost lost the sense of feeling; nor could he distinguish between light and heavy bodies, of such as he had strength to move; a quart pot full of water and a feather being the same in his hand. They each took an emetic, and after that a sweet, which gave them much relief. In the morning, one of the pigs which had eaten the entrails was found dead.

approximately 59% mortality. Increased awareness of fugu poisoning and strict regulation and training of licensed fugu chefs has resulted in far fewer cases and lower mortality in recent years. For example, in the 10-year period from 1967 to 1976, there were 1105 cases and 372 deaths (34% mortality), and from 1983 to 1992 there were only 449 cases and 49 deaths (1% mortality). Nowadays, all cooks and restaurants handling fugu must be licensed, and most cases of pufferfish poisoning occur in inexperienced fishermen who prepare their own food. In 1996, three cases of fugu poisoning occurred in San Diego in chefs who ate prepackaged, ready-to-eat fugu illegally imported from Japan.

Tetrodotoxin is a heat-stable, water-soluble, non-protein toxin that is 50 times more potent than strychnine. It acts by binding to sodium channels and blocking axonal nerve transmission and results in ascending paralysis and respiratory failure. In addition to pufferfish, porcupine fish and ocean sunfish, tetrodotoxin has been found in other marine animals such as the blue-ringed octopus, starfishes, flatworms, various crabs, and mollusks.

Levels of toxin are usually highest in the ovaries, liver, intestine, and skin. The toxin does not alter the taste or appearance of the fish, and it is not destroyed or inactivated by cooking, canning, freezing, or smoking.

The onset of symptoms of pufferfish poisoning may occur within ten min of ingestion of toxic fish or be delayed for up to 4 h or longer. Severe cases are usually associated with ingestion of large amounts of toxin and early onset of symptoms. Initial symptoms include perioral paresthesiae and numbness, nausea, and dizziness. Later on there may be more generalized paraesthesia and numbness, dysarthria, ataxia, ascending paralysis, and a variety of other symptoms such as headache, hypersalivation, diaphoresis, vomiting, abdominal pain, and diarrhea. In the most severe cases, there is widespread paralysis, respiratory failure, bradycardia and other arrhythmias and hypotension. Most deaths are due to respiratory failure and occur within the first 6 h. The prognosis is usually excellent in patients who survive the first 24 h.

Diagnosis is made on clinical grounds. There is no specific antidote for tetrodotoxin and treatment is aimed at limiting absorption of toxin and treating the adverse effects. Absorption of toxin can be limited by gastric lavage, which is indicated if patients are seen within 3 h of ingestion of toxic fish. Emetic agents such as ipecac should probably be avoided because of the risk of aspiration. In severe cases, intravenous fluids, vasopressors, endotracheal intubation, and ventilatory support may be indicated. Bradycardia may respond to atropine.

It is impossible to guarantee that fish are free from toxin, and travelers should be advised to avoid any potentially toxic fish even when prepared by trained chefs in licensed restaurants. In life-threatening (survival) situations, travelers should take advantage of the water-soluble properties of the toxin. Viscera and skin must not be eaten under any circumstances, but the muscle of the fish can be shredded into small pieces, kneaded, and soaked in water for at least 4 h in an attempt to remove toxin prior to consumption.

PARALYTIC SHELLFISH POISONING

Paralytic shellfish poisoning (PSP) has been recognized for over 200 years. The first recognized outbreak in travelers was in 1793 and was reported in Captain George Vancouver's A Voyage of Discovery to the North Pacific Ocean and Round the World. PSP is the most common and most serious form of shellfish poisoning and occurs after eating contaminated bivalve mollusks (clams, cockles, mussels, oysters, and scallops) containing saxitoxin and other potent neurotoxins produced by dinoflagellates (e.g., *Alexandrium* species). Saxitoxin, like ciguatoxin and tetrodotoxin, causes paralysis by blocking sodium channels in nerve cell membranes. It is 50 times more potent than curare. Saxitoxin and other toxins that cause PSP are heat stable and survive normal cooking procedures.

As in other forms of shellfish poisoning, outbreaks of PSP often follow dinoflagellate blooms. In the past, most cases of PSP occurred in cold, temperate waters above latitude 30° North and below latitude 30° South. Recently, outbreaks in tropical and subtropical waters have become more frequent, with cases reported from countries such as Guatemala, El Salvador, Mexico. Thailand, Singapore, Malaysia, Papua New Guinea, India, and the Solomon Islands.

Symptoms of PSP usually occur within 30 to 60 min of eating toxic shellfish but can be delayed for 3 h or longer. Early symptoms include paresthesiae of the face, lips and tongue, and later the arms and legs. Affected persons may complain of lightheadedness or a floating sensation. Other symptoms may include headache, increased salivation, nausea, vomiting, and diarrhea. Hypertension may be an important finding. Severe cases are usually associated with ingestion of large doses of toxin and clinical features such as ataxia, dysphagia, and mental status changes. Flaccid paralysis occurs in the most severe cases with respiratory insufficiency as a result of paralysis of the diaphragm and chest wall muscles. Deaths are typically caused by respiratory failure and tend to occur within 12 h of eating toxic shellfish. Prognosis is good for patients who survive past 12 h. Recovery usually occurs within a week but may occasionally be prolonged for several weeks.[10]

Case fatality rate averages 6% but may be as high a 44%. Mortality is higher in children, who seem to be particularly sensitive to the effects of the toxin. Travelers to developing countries who are tempted to eat shellfish should be reminded that the highest mortality from PSP occur in areas with poor access to good quality medical care.

Diagnosis is usually made on clinical grounds although in special circumstances, it can be confirmed by a standard mouse bioassay method.

There are no antidotes for PSP, but saxitoxin and other toxins that cause PSP bind well to charcoal and, if safe, oral charcoal should be given. Victims should be observed for at least 24 h for respiratory insufficiency. Mechanical ventilation may be necessary. Atropine should be avoided since saxitoxin and its derivatives may be anticholinergic.

PSP can be prevented by avoiding potentially contaminated shellfish. This is particularly important in children who are at greater risk of fatal illness. It is important to emphasize that cooking will not destroy the toxin. Because of the lack of sophisticated medical facilities for resuscitation and mechanical ventilation, it is prudent for all travelers to developing countries to always avoid potentially toxic shellfish.

NEUROTOXIC SHELLFISH POISONING

Neurotoxic shellfish poisoning (NSP) occurs after eating bivalve mollusks (e.g., oysters, clams, scallops, and mussels) contaminated by heat-stable brevetoxins produced by the marine dinoflagellate Gymnodinium breve. G. breve is an important cause of red tides and has been responsible for the deaths of large numbers of fish, sea birds, and even marine mammals such as manatees.

NSP usually presents as a gastroenteritis accompanied by neurologic symptoms and often resembles mild paralytic shellfish poisoning or ciguatera poisoning. No deaths have been reported in humans. Inhalation of aerosolized brevetoxins from the seaspray associated with a red tide may cause an acute respiratory illness often referred to as aerosolized red tide respiratory irritation (ARTRI).

NSP was first described on the west coast of Florida in 1844. Since then, it has been reported from the Gulf of Mexico, the east coast of Florida, the North Carolina coast, and New Zealand. It is expected to be reported from other areas of the world in the future.

Symptoms of NSP may develop within 15 min of ingestion of contaminated shellfish or be delayed for up to 18 h. Gastrointestinal symptoms include abdominal pain, nausea, vomiting, and diarrhea. There may be myalgias and dizziness. Neurologic symptoms include circumoral paresthesias, paresthesias of the arms and legs, temperature reversal, vertigo, and ataxia. Symptoms may last for several h or a few days. Symptoms of ARTRI occur almost immediately after exposure and include a non-productive cough, wheezing, conjunctivitis, and rhinorrhea. Asthmatics are particularly susceptible, and there is some anecdotal evidence of long-term pulmonary symptoms following ARTRI in the elderly or those with pre-existing lung disease.

Treatment of NSP and ARTRI is symptomatic and supportive. Preventive measures include avoiding shellfish associated with red tides and limiting coastline exposure to red tides and aerosolized brevetoxins. Particle masks can be used to prevent inhalation of aerosolized toxins.

DIARRHEIC SHELLFISH POISONING

Diarrheic shellfish poisoning (DSP) results from ingestion of contaminated bivalve mollusks (clams, mussels, and scallops) containing okadaic acid and other toxins produced by various marine dinoflagellates.

Historically, DSP was reported predominantly from Japan and European countries such as the Netherlands, Italy, and Spain. As a result of increased global spread of toxic dinoflagellates, however, outbreaks have recently been reported from Canada, South America, Australia, New Zealand. and Indonesia. As in other shellfish poisonings, outbreaks tend to follow red tides or dinoflagellate blooms. Okadaic acid triggers sodium release by intestinal cells and produces diarrhea. Symptoms usually appear 30 min to 6 h after ingestion of contaminated shellfish, although onset may be delayed for up to 12 h. Typically, symptoms last for up to 4 days and include diarrhea, abdominal cramps, nausea, vomiting, weakness, and chills. The severity of symptoms is usually related to the amount of toxin ingested. No fatalities have been reported. Diagnosis is usually made on clinical grounds and treatment is symptomatic and supportive.

AMNESIC SHELLFISH POISONING

Amnesic shellfish poisoning (ASP) is a recently described toxic encephalopathy. It was first identified in 1987 after an outbreak involving over 100 Canadians who had eaten mussels contaminated by domoic acid harvested off Prince Edward Island. Domoic acid is a heat-stable toxin produced by diatoms such as Nitzschia pungens.

High levels of toxin have been demonstrated in shellfish in areas such as the Pacific Northwest, the Gulf of Mexico, and off the west coast of Scotland, although no clinical cases have been reported from those areas.

In the Prince Edward Island outbreak, symptoms of ASP developed within 15 min to 38 h (median 6 h) of ingestion of contaminated mussels. Acute gastrointestinal symptoms were very common and included nausea, vomiting, abdominal cramps, and diarrhea. Neurologic features occurred in over one-third of patients and included headaches, short-term memory loss, confusion, disorientation, dizziness, seizures, and comas. Several patients developed long-term cognitive dysfunction. There were four deaths, all in patients over 70 years of age.

Treatment for ASP is symptomatic and supportive. Potentially contaminated shellfish, particularly those associated with red tides, should never be eaten.

BOVINE SPONGIFORM ENCEPHALOPATHY AND NEW VARIANT CREUTZFELDT-JAKOB DISEASE

First recognized in the UK in 1996, new variant Creutzfeldt-Jakob Disease (vCJD) is an invariably fatal, rapidly progressive dementia that occurs in humans. It is suspected to be one of the transmissible spongiform encephalopathies linked to an outbreak of bovine spongiform encephalopathy (BSE) or 'mad cow disease 'that began in the UK in 1986 and has affected almost 200 000 cattle worldwide.[11,12] The vast majority of cases have been reported from the UK. The disease causing agent is thought to be a self replicating protein known as a prion and the human form (vCJD) probably occurs mainly as a result of ingestion of beef on the bone and ground beef products such as beef burgers and sausages contaminated by central nervous system tissue such as brain, spinal cord and retina from infected cattle. Prions are resistant to common treatments such as heat and are not destroyed by usual forms of cooking.

Since BSE was first discovered, large numbers of cases have been diagnosed in native cattle mainly in the UK but also in various other European countries, Japan and Israel. A small number of cases have also been identified in Canada, the Falkland Islands and Oman but only in animals imported from the UK (Fig. 47.3). Intense public health measures to control BSE in cattle have been successful, particularly in the UK, in reducing the number of new cases reported (Fig. 47.4).

To date (July 2003), there have been 147 definite and probable cases of vCJD (137 in the UK, 6 in France, 1 in Ireland, and 1 in Italy, together with 1 case diagnosed in the USA and 1 case diagnosed in Canada, both believed to have been contracted in the UK). In contrast to the traditional forms of CJD, vCJD seems to affect younger patients (average age 29 years, compared with 65 years) and has a longer duration of illness (average of 14 months as opposed to 4.5 months). Clinically, patients with vCJD experience psychiatric symptoms such as depression, anxiety, apathy, withdrawal, or a schizophrenia-like psychosis early in the illness. In about half of the patients, unusual sensory symptoms such as unpleasant dysesthesia, 'stickiness' of the skin or frank pain may also occur in the early stages. As the disease progresses, there is ataxia, involuntary movements and progressive dementia. In the end stages, patients are usually completely immobile and mute.[13]

Although the number of reported cases of BSE has fallen considerably, cases of vCJD continue to be reported. It is important to emphasize, however, that because of the very long incubation period, any cases of vCJD that are being diagnosed now were probably contracted 10 or more years previously.

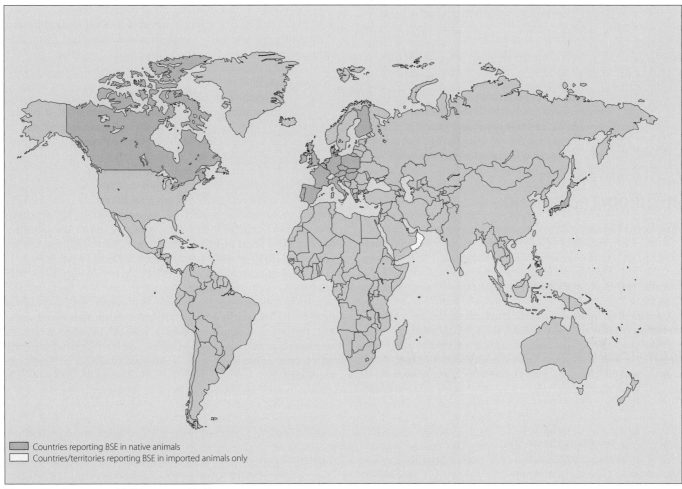

Figure 47.3 Documented BSE cases worldwide.

To date, no cases of vCJD have been reported in travelers and the risk of vCJD for current travelers is considered to be extremely small. The UK and Ireland have apparently eradicated BSE in cattle less than 30 months of age and production of beef from older cattle is illegal. As a result, one estimate from the Centers for Disease Control suggests that the current risk in travelers to the UK may be as low as one case per billion servings of beef. The risk for the rest of Europe may be even lower although there is a concern that in some countries such as Portugal, the risk may be somewhat higher because of inexperience in implementing relevant public health measures. The very small risk of infection for travelers can be reduced even further by avoiding those beef and beef products that are more likely to have been contaminated with cattle nerve tissue than muscle meat. Examples include beef on the bone and ground beef products, such as beef burgers and sausages. Milk and milk products such as cheese and butter do not present any risk of vCJD. Currently, cattle are the only known food animal species with disease caused by the BSE agent. Experiments have shown, however, that sheep are susceptible to infection with the BSE agent and there is a theoretical concern that vCJD may also occur as a result of eating sheep or goat. In addition, concerns have been raised recently about the risks of eating chicken breasts that may have become contaminated by beef protein powder.

Since large numbers of apparently healthy people may be incubating vCJD, there is a theoretical concern about iatrogenic transmission as a result of blood transfusion or organ transplantation in

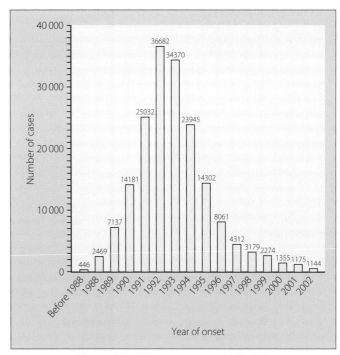

Figure 47.4 BSE cases per year in the UK.

countries where the illness occurs. In addition, since the BSE agent is resistant to autoclaving and other sterilization techniques, there is a concern about infection from surgical instruments during neurosurgery, eye surgery or ear, nose and throat surgery. Further concerns include the possibility that transmission of BSE agent could occur via bovine derived vaccines. Fortunately, travelers to areas where vCJD or BSE have been reported can be reassured that most experts feel that the risk of transmission via these situations is thought to be extremely small. In addition, in many countries a variety of measures have been implemented, to limit the risk even further. For example, in the UK, blood for transfusion is filtered to remove white blood cells and plasma is imported.

MUSHROOM POISONING

Mushroom poisoning is a rare but potentially very serious hazard for travelers. Since facilities for the diagnosis and treatment of mushroom poisoning may be unavailable or inadequate in many foreign, particularly developing, countries or in wilderness regions, there is an increased risk of a complicated or even fatal outcome in travelers in those areas.

A variety of toxins have been extracted from mushrooms. Most are heat labile, but may not be completely destroyed by cooking.

Toxins in mushrooms cause a variety of clinical syndromes (Table 47.5) and a history of recent mushroom ingestion should always be sought in travelers who present with suspicious symptoms.

Onset of illness is usually within a few hours of ingestion of toxic mushrooms and cases in returned travelers are most likely to be seen if they have brought back mushrooms and consumed them after returning. Since some of the non-gastrointestinal symptoms may last for several days, however, certain travelers may not present until after returning home.

Most toxic mushrooms cause gastrointestinal symptoms – nausea, vomiting, abdominal pain and diarrhea – beginning 1–2 h after ingestion and resolving in 6–12 h. Occasionally, symptoms may be severe enough to require fluid and electrolyte replacement. In general, if gastrointestinal symptoms are delayed for 4 h or more after ingestion, there is an increased chance that one of the highly toxic mushrooms such as *Amanita phalloides* or death cap mushroom is responsible and a complicated or even fatal outcome is more likely. General symptoms of mushroom poisoning often include chills, myalgias and headache. Mushroom toxins may also produce a variety of neurologic, renal or hepatic syndromes (Table 47.5) that can be difficult to diagnose unless there is a high index of suspicion.[14]

Unless very experienced, travelers should not attempt to identify mushrooms that are considered safe to eat. Not uncommonly, non-toxic mushrooms in Europe and North America closely resemble highly toxic mushrooms found in other parts of the world and vice versa. There have been a number of tragic deaths in immigrants from SE Asia as a result of misidentifying and ingesting highly toxic mushrooms such as *Amanita phalloides* or death cap mushroom.

Table 47.5	Mushroom poisoning			
Syndrome	Incubation	Clinical Features	Mushrooms involved	Treatment
Gastrointestinal (multiple)	Usually 1-2h Rarely >4h	Nausea, vomiting, abdominal pain, diarrhea	Multiple	Symptomatic and supportive. Fluid and electrolytes. Gastric lavage, catharsis.
Hallucinations (psilocybin, psilocin)	15–30mins (30-60mins)	Hallucinations, euphoria, loss of time, sensation, tachycardia, hypertention	Psilocybe, Panaeolus, Gymnopilus species	Symptomatic and supportive.
Anticholinergic (muscarine)	15–30mins	Salivation, sweating, lacrimation, urination, GI symptoms. Bradycardia, hypotension, constricted pupils	Amanita, Inocybe, Clitocybe species	Symptomatic and supportive. Fluid and electrolytes, atropine for bradycardia or to control secretions.
Delirium (ibotenic acid, muscimol)	<30 mins (20–90mins)	Delirium, hyperactivity, alteration in visual perception, ataxia, seizures, muscle twitching	Amanita and other species	Symptomatic and supportive. Antiseizure medications
Disulfiramlike (coprine)	2–6h, symptoms 15–30 mins after alcohol	Nausea, vomiting, headache, flushing, palpitations	Coprinus species	Symptomatic and supportive fluid and electrolytes. Avoid alcohol.
Renal	2–20 days	Thirst, nausea, paresthesias, taste impairment, renal failure	Cortinarius species	Symptomatic and supportive. Fluid and electrolytes. Dialysis and renal transplantation
Hepatorenal (Amatoxins, phallotoxins)	4–16h	Nausea, vomiting, abdominal pain, diarrhea. Hepatic and renal failure	Amanita phalloides and other species	Symptomatic and supportive. Fluid and electrolytes. Thioctic acid. Dialysis, renal/liver transplantation

REFERENCES

1. Van Hoesen KB, Clark RF. Seafood Toxidromes. In: Auerbach PS, ed. *Wilderness Medicine.* 4th edn. St. Louis, MO: Mosby; 2001:1285–1326.

2. Lewis RJ. The changing face of ciguatera. *Toxicon* 2001; **39**(1):97–106.

3. Legrand P. AM. The epidemiology of ciguatera fish poisoning. *Toxicon* 1994; **32**(863).

4. Hirama M, Oishi T, Uehara H, *et al.* Total synthesis of ciguatoxin CTX3C. *Science* 2001; **294**(5548):1904–1907.

5. Hamilton B, Hurbungs M, Vernoux JP, Jones A, Lewis RJ. Isolation and characterisation of Indian Ocean ciguatoxin. *Toxicon* 2002; **40**(6):685–693.

6. Bagnis R, Kuberski T, Langier S. Clinical observations on 3009 cases of ciguatera fish poisoning in the South Pacific. *Am J Trop Med Hyg* 1979; **28**:1067.

7. Palafox NA, Buenconsejo-Lum L, Riklon S, *et al.* Successful treatment of ciguatera fish poisoning with intravenous mannitol. *JAMA* 1988; **259**:2740.

8. Schnorf H, Taurarii M, Cundy T. Ciguatera fish poisoning: a double-blind randomized trial of mannitol therapy. *Neurology* 2002; **58**(6):873–880.

9. Blakesley ML. Scombroid poisoning; prompt resolution of symptoms with cimetidine. *Ann Emerg Med* 1983; **12**:104

10. Gessner BD, Middaugh JP. Paralytic shellfish poisoning in Alaska: a 20-year retrospective analysis. *Am J Epidemiol* 1995; **141**:766.

11. Will RG, Ironside JW, Zeidler M, *et al.* A new variant of Creutzfeldt-Jakob disease in the UK. *Lancet* 1996; **347**:921–925.

12. Andrews NJ, Farrington CP, Cousens SN, *et al.* Incidence of variant Creutzfeldt-Jakob disease in the UK. *Lancet* 2000; **356**:481–482.

13. Spencer MD, Knight RSG, Will RG. First hundred cases of variant Creutzfeldt-Jakob disease: retrospective review of early psychiatric and neurological features. *BMJ* 2002; **324**:1479–1482.

14. Schneider S, Donnelly M. Mushroom Toxicity. In: Auerbach PS, ed. *Wilderness Medicine.* 4th edn. St. Louis, MO: Mosby; 2001:1141–1160.

CHAPTER 48   # Injuries and Injury Prevention

Jeffrey Wilks

KEYPOINTS

- Injuries are the leading cause of travel-related mortality with motor vehicle trauma and drowning being the most important

- Fractures, lacerations, dislocations and sprains are the most common injuries experienced by tourists

- When driving in a foreign country travelers should avoid alcohol, fatigue, jet-lag, all night-driving and familiarize themselves with local driving customs

- Never drive or ride on a moped or motorbike in a foreign country

- Avoid overcrowded public transport

- Never swim at an unmarked or unguarded beach

INTRODUCTION

According to the *Concise Oxford Dictionary*, an accident is 'an event that is without apparent cause, or is unexpected; an unfortunate event, especially one causing physical harm or damage'.[1] While it is true that most accidents involving tourists are unexpected, at least for the person injured, the causes and consequences of many accidents are now reasonably well understood by many health and tourism authorities. The current challenge is to use available information effectively in the design and implementation of risk management and injury prevention programs.[2]

Injuries are the leading cause of travel-related mortality worldwide,[3] accounting for up to 25 times more deaths than infectious disease. Injuries to tourists are also a significant burden to hospitals and health care systems, both at the tourist destination[4,5] and in terms of continuing care when the patient returns home.[6]

Hargarten and Güler Gürsu[3] emphasize the fact that injuries are not accidents or random events, though common usage favors the term 'accident' to describe many injuries and unexpected outcomes.

As injuries among tourists are 'caused' by identifiable factors, and can therefore be prevented in many cases, this chapter reviews the types of injuries experienced by tourists, their etiology and treatment, and various prevention initiatives. The text uses both terms 'accident' and 'injury' to convey the fact that most injuries occur in the context of tourists being in unfamiliar environments and participating in unfamiliar activities.[7]

SNAPSHOTS OF INJURIES AMONG TOURISTS

Tourist accidents and injuries can be identified and monitored at several levels, providing snapshots at a particular time and for a particular destination. Wilks and Grenfell[8] identify four major levels for these snapshots.

Fatalities

As noted above, injuries are the leading cause of travel-related mortality worldwide, accounting for up to 25% of all deaths among travelers (Table 48.1). At the level of serious injury causing death, reviews of the travel medicine and tourism literature show tourists are most often killed in motor vehicle crashes and by drowning.[9–12] Other causes of travel-related injury death, though less common, include homicides, suicides, airplane crashes, and animal and marine bites/stings.[3]

Information about deaths of travelers is very useful to travel medicine practitioners as it provides a general foundation for pre-travel advice based on the geographical location of accidents. Unfortunately, the collection of information on travelers' deaths relies heavily on local police and coroners' reports, and cooperation by consular authorities, so fatality studies are expensive, time consuming and difficult to conduct. In addition, because of the way information is collected, fatality studies are often limited in what they can say about the external factors or causes of death. For this level of detail, the more controlled environment of a hospital setting provides the greatest insights into tourist accidents and injuries.

Table 48.1   Travel-related injury deaths

Year	Author(s)	Sample population	Injury deaths (%)
1991	Hargarten et al.[9]	2463 deaths of American travelers in 1975 and 1984	25
1991	Paixao et al.[10]	952 deaths of Scottish travelers between 1973 and 1988	21
1995	Prociv[11]	421 deaths of Australian travelers during 1992/93	18
2000	MacPherson et al.[12]	309 deaths of Canadian travelers in 1995	25

Hospital inpatient admissions

The second level is that of serious injury requiring admission to hospital. Reviews of the travel medicine and tourism literature again identify motor vehicle accidents and near-drowning/non-fatal submersion as leading causes of hospital admission.[5,7] Other injuries that result in tourists being admitted to hospital include fractures, lacerations and soft tissue injuries. Hospital admissions are a very rich and important source of information for travel medicine practitioners, as most hospitals routinely collect data on external causes of injuries. This can provide greater insight into the mechanisms of injury. For example, many of the presenting fractures, lacerations, sprains and dislocations are the result of falls by tourists.[5] This knowledge can be used to design and implement appropriate injury prevention initiatives, such as the use of personal protective clothing and footwear, safety harnesses and helmets, depending on the particular activity being undertaken.

Published studies also identify some variation in the relative frequency of presenting injuries according to destination. For example, in a study of seven coastal hospitals in Queensland, Australia, Nicol et al.[5] found decompression illness associated with scuba diving to be the second most frequent reason for overseas visitor hospital admissions. In contrast, reviewing visitor hospital admissions in New Zealand, Bentley et al.[13] found that tourist injuries were most frequently associated with skiing, mountaineering and trekking.

Analysis of hospital admissions can also identify useful variations between local residents and tourists, pointing to areas where injury prevention initiatives should be focused. For example, Table 48.2 shows that in one study the proportion of overseas visitors admitted to hospital for fractures, contusions, dislocations, sprains and burns, was very similar to that of local residents[5] and other Australians from inter-state. However, overseas visitor injuries are clearly much higher for water-related activities, especially decompression illness associated with scuba diving.

Overall, hospital inpatient admissions are a very good general monitoring tool for all tourist destinations, since most hospitals worldwide routinely collect patient information in a standard format (International Classification of Diseases, either ICD-9-CM or ICD-10). The World Tourism Organization currently recommends hospital monitoring as part of each destination's visitor safety and security program.[2]

Outpatient treatments and general medical practice

Tourist injuries not requiring inpatient admission to hospital are often treated at outpatient clinics and in general medical practices. While relatively few studies tend to be reported at this level, those that are available are rich in practical information. For example, Hartung et al.[14] investigated 276 ocean sports-related injuries in Hawaii using information obtained by emergency room personnel at hospitals and acute-care clinics. They found swimming, board surfing and scuba diving were the main activities associated with injury, while lacerations, stings and decompression illness were the primary diagnoses for treatment. Based on their identification of groups at risk for injury, Hartung et al.[14] were able to recommend specific injury prevention initiatives, including improved warning signs on beaches and targeted education for both tourists and local residents.

In a more recent study, Wilks et al.[15] reported on 1183 outpatient clinic visits by tourists on three tropical island resorts off the coast of Queensland, Australia. Injuries accounted for 38% of clinic visits, with lacerations, fractures, bites/stings and sprains being the main types of injury treated. Again, the advantage of using trained health

Table 48.2　Injury admissions for seven coastal hospitals in Queensland, Australia

Type of Injury	Overseas visitors			Interstate visitors			Queensland residents		
	Frequency	(%)	Rank	Frequency	(%)	Rank	Frequency	(%)	Rank
Fractures	107	41.0	1	214	40.0	1	421	42.2	1
Decompression illness	35	13.4	2	11	2.1	10	23	2.3	9
Open wounds	21	8.0	3	70	13.1	2	150	15.1	2
Intracranial injury – no fracture	18	6.9	4	54	10.1	3	125	12.5	3
Drowning/non-fatal submersions	9	3.5	5	7	1.3	12	5	0.5	13
Internal injury to chest, abdomen and pelvis	9	3.5	5	12	2.2	8	25	2.5	8
Poisoning and toxic effects	9	3.5	5	44	8.2	4	60	6.0	5
Complications of medical/surgical care	9	3.5	5	32	6.0	5	61	6.1	4
Contusions	8	3.1	9	18	3.4	6	30	3.0	7
Dislocations	8	3.1	9	15	2.8	7	31	3.1	6
Sprains	6	2.3	11	11	2.1	10	13	1.3	10
Burns	4	1.5	12	6	1.1	13	8	0.8	11
Effect of foreign body	2	0.8	13	12	2.2	8	7	0.7	12
Other	16	6.1	–	29	5.4	–	38	3.8	–
Total	261			535			997		

With permission of the Australian Healthcare Association,[5] and unpublished data.

personnel and a standard international reporting system (in this case the ICD-9-CM) is that the causes of injuries could be identified (Table 48.3) and prevention initiatives developed based on specific injury findings.

For example, Table 48.3 shows that coral cuts were the main source of lacerations for island resort guests. Following this study, island management purchased additional sandshoes and made them available to guests for both guided and unaccompanied reef walks. Similarly, the study findings on bites and stings led to several large wasp nests being removed from the resort golf course, while information on marine stingers was specifically included in guest orientation briefings.

Wilks and Grenfell[8] note that studies conducted by medical practitioners at this level tend to concentrate on outbound patients, while monitoring of inbound visitors is most often undertaken by social scientists and allied health professionals. With the growing interest in tourist health and safety worldwide,[2] there is now a reasonably large tourism literature focusing on travel-related injury and prevention. Much of this literature is useful and relevant for medicine practitioners preparing their patients for overseas travel.

Other health areas

The final level of information can generally be described as other health areas, including treatment, support and advice provided for tourists by paramedic and emergency services, the Coast Guard, pharmacists, lifeguards and local citizens. In Australia, Surf Life Saving Queensland (Fig. 48.1) is an excellent example of a community-based organization playing a major role in tourism and injury prevention. During the 2000–2001 season, Surf Life Saving Queensland members performed 3370 rescues and 42 resuscitations, provided 14 964 first aid and 9176 marine stinger treatments, and initiated 15 2578 preventative actions.[16] These services were acknowledged with 2001 state and national tourism industry awards.

In a recent study of 431 international backpackers in North Queensland, Peach and Bath[17] reported that 62% experienced a health and safety problem, commonly, insect bites, sunburn, headaches, lacerations, coral cuts, ear infections and diarrhea. While the injuries experienced by this group are generally the same as those reported from Queensland hospital[5] and outpatient clinic studies,[15] the finding that only 54% of the backpackers had been offered health and safety information prior to departure on their travels is alarming. Where information was offered to these backpackers it was mainly vaccination advice.

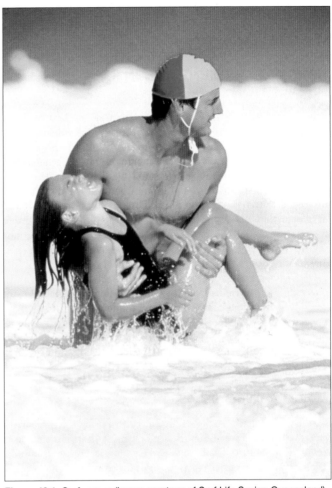

Figure 48.1 Surf rescue (Image courtesy of Surf Life Saving Queensland).

The point to be highlighted here is that travel health and safety advice must be specific and relevant for a particular destination. As noted by Behrens *et al.*[18]

'*A crucial pre-requisite for giving balanced advice and assessing health risks is accurate epidemiological data on travel morbidity and mortality, preferably related to geographical risk*'

Table 48.3	Main causes of injuries (E-codes) for island resort guests
Injury	**Causes (number)**
Lacerations	Coral cuts (29); striking against objects or other people (14); cutlery, knives, broken glass (14); boating or water sports (9); falls (7); over-exertion (3).
Fractures	Falls (6); boating or water sports (3).
Bites/stings	Sandflies and insects (51); marine stingers (29); wasps and bees (7); other animals (5).
Sprains	Falls (10); boating or water sports (4).
Ear problems	Air pressure (33) – mainly from scuba diving.
Sun/heat	Exposure (29).
Other injuries	Other – burns, chemicals, horse-riding, machinery (17); exposure (13); poisonings (10); boating or water sports (7); falls (5); striking against objects or other people (5); over-exertion (3).

With permission of the Australian Healthcare Association.[15]

If injuries are the main form of harm travelers are likely to experience at a particular destination, then pre-travel advice and preparation should adequately address the potential injury risks.

RISK MANAGEMENT AND INJURY PREVENTION

Risk management is now an accepted part of modern business. Standard steps in the risk management process include identification, analysis and evaluation, as well as treatment of risk. This is not a new approach. In Australia and New Zealand, for example, a general standard for risk management has been available since 1995 (Fig. 48.2).[19] Applied to tourist accidents and injuries, most of the discussion in this chapter has so far concerned identification of risk based on sources of information. Across the four levels where snap-shots are available, fractures, lacerations, dislocations and sprains are the most common injuries experienced by tourists. The main external causes of these injuries include motor vehicle crashes, falls, and water-related accidents.

Having identified motor vehicle and water-related accidents as the most common concerns for most tourist destinations, the following sections focus on these two main areas of injury, using the risk management framework to analyze and evaluate the issues. The risk management framework is also useful for describing prevention and education initiatives in terms of treatment, review and communication of identified risks.

Motor vehicle crashes

Motor vehicle crashes consistently emerge from the travel medicine literature as the most common cause of injury death for tourists.[20] Yet, worldwide there has been very little empirical research into the factors contributing to such crashes. Prior to the Sydney 2000 Olympic Games, Australian tourism and transport authorities began to focus on international visitor safety, and to seek ways of preventing road crashes involving tourists. In the risk analysis phase it was revealed that the rate of tourist deaths on Australian roads was double that for all Australians.[21] Detailed analysis at a state level showed that road crash fatalities were only one very general measure of the problem. When research was extended to include tourists admitted to hospital, those receiving outpatient and first aid treatments, and crashes involv-

ing property damage only, the social costs in the State of Queensland were conservatively estimated to be ~A$19 million in 1 year.[21]

Further analysis and evaluation of tourist road crash factors revealed the following:[20–23]

- International visitor crashes were *less likely* to involve high risk driving behaviors such as alcohol use or speeding;
- International visitor crashes were *more likely* to involve disorientation, particularly driver fatigue, failure to keep to the left (correct) side of the road, head-on crashes and overturning their vehicle;
- International visitors who drive on the right side of the road at home were *more likely* than left side of the road visitor drivers to be involved in a head-on crash;
- German, English, American and Japanese tourists were identified as possible 'at risk' groups on Australian roads.

The Australian research program concluded that tourist road crashes appear to be largely the product of unfamiliarity with local driving conditions and disorientation (Fig. 48.3). Key recommendations on risk treatment from a parliamentary symposium[21] convened to discuss tourist road safety included educational initiatives encouraging international drivers to:

- be mindful of the effects of medication, alcohol and jet-lag when they reach their destination
- take a rest after a long distance flight, especially before taking charge of a motor vehicle
- familiarize themselves with Australian road rules and traffic signs
- request a full familiarization of their rental vehicles (particularly if it is a type of vehicle they have not driven before, such as a 4-wheel drive or campervan) and a briefing on their travel route from staff of the hire company before leaving the airport or car depot
- always wear a seat belt (and use child restraints) both to comply with Australian law and as a safety measure
- drive a rental vehicle around the car park before heading onto a public road for the first time;
- plan to drive only in daylight hours
- build in rest stops every 2 h to counter driver fatigue.

Most of these messages are applicable to other destinations worldwide. They can be reinforced or brought to the attention of travelers via brochures, websites and in-flight videos in the language of the target audience. However, as noted by the tourism and transport experts attending the parliamentary symposium,[21] the best results will be obtained if these messages are communicated to tourists before they leave home. For this reason, travel medicine practitioners have been urged to include road safety information in their pre-travel advice.

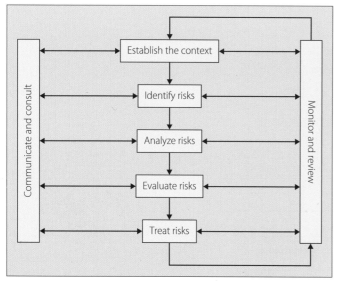

Figure 48.2 Risk management overview.[19]

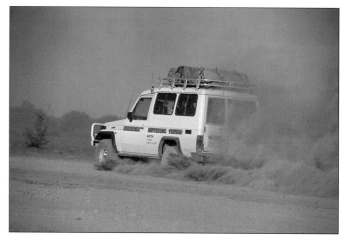

Figure 48.3 Accidents are often associated with unfamiliar vehicles and driving environments (Image courtesy of Tourism Queensland)

The advantage of road travel in Australia, and in other developed countries, is that rental vehicles and public roads are generally maintained at a reasonable safety standard according to government regulations. To some extent the visitor has some control over driving in an unfamiliar environment. In developing nations, however, the visitor is more likely to be a passenger in a car, bus, minivan or local transport variation (for example, Jeepneys in the Philippines, Tuk-Tuks or motorized rickshaws in Thailand, or in the back of a truck in parts of Africa). In most cases, hiring a vehicle with a driver is recommended as a less expensive and safer way to travel than driving yourself. For example, the injury rate for visitors hiring mopeds or small motorbikes in tourist destinations is very high.[24,25]

While some of the following points may seem to be common sense, experience shows that safety on the roads in developing countries can be markedly enhanced by:

- avoiding night travel in countries with poor road conditions
- when hiring a vehicle (with or without a driver) take time to inspect the tires, brakes, lights and seatbelts
- if the driver of the vehicle is reckless, then stop and get out
- avoid overcrowded public transport, both for road safety reasons and because pickpockets often target visitors in crowded public areas
- if possible, carry a mobile phone in case of vehicle breakdown or other emergency. Mobile phones for rent or sale are widely available at many destinations, though having your own GSM phone should ensure more reliable communications, and lastly,
- inform friends and local authorities about your movements on a regular basis, including anticipated time of arrival at each destination. In the case of an accident, wherever possible stay with your vehicle and wait for help to arrive.

A final recommendation concerns seatbelts and child restraints in vehicles. In many countries seatbelts are not required to be fitted in motor vehicles, or may only be required in the front seats.[26] Hargarten[27] reports that seatbelts are frequently not available in hire cars in developing countries. Ideally, child seats or baby capsules should be taken on each journey, since there is really no other safe way to restrain a young child in a motor vehicle except with the appropriate age-related equipment.

Water-related injuries

Many of the water sports and water-related activities offered to tourists (e.g., surfing, scuba diving, snorkeling, water-skiing) are both novel and unfamiliar. Even swimming can present difficulties for tourists who have no background, skills or ability in the water. Drowning is consistently reported as a leading cause of injury death among tourists,[9–12] while near-drowning or non-fatal submersion also appears in hospital[4,5,28] and general accident reports.[7,29] As an island holiday destination, with an emphasis on beaches, water sports and the Great Barrier Reef, Australia has recognized water-related injuries as a significant risk area for international visitors.[30]

There are several specific water-related activities that can be identified as problematic for tourists, depending on geographical location. Snorkelling[31] and scuba diving[32] are two areas where tourists appear to experience more problems than local residents. Analysis and evaluation of the risks associated with snorkeling and scuba diving reveal the following:

- the main causes of death are drowning and cardiac events
- pre-existing medical conditions, inexperience, failure to dive according to a set plan, and panic, are the major contributing factors to scuba fatalities
- pre-existing medical conditions, notably epilepsy, and cardiac disease, as well as fatigue, and panic, are the main contributing factors to snorkeling fatalities

- the main non-fatal injuries associated with scuba diving are decompression illness and barotrauma.

In response to the worldwide media publicity surrounding the disappearance of American scuba divers Thomas and Eileen Lonergan on the Great Barrier Reef,[32] the Queensland government extensively reviewed its workplace health and safety standards relating to recreational scuba diving and snorkeling. The resulting industry standards are a benchmark in terms of risk management, and have been adopted by several other countries. Risk treatment and prevention measures include:[33]

- health screening for participants in scuba diving and snorkeling
- mandatory supervision of dive and snorkeling sites by designated lookouts
- counting and recording passengers back on board vessels to ensure no persons are left behind
- ensuring that suitable and well maintained diving and snorkeling equipment is available
- having in place an emergency plan, trained rescue staff, first aid equipment and oxygen
- provision of detailed instructions/briefing on the site and the requirements for conducting the dive or snorkel activity (Fig. 48.4)
- an emphasis on diving and/or snorkeling in 'buddy pairs'. That is, with a partner (Fig. 48.5).

Between 1992 and 1998, there were 119 tourist deaths due to drowning in Australia, an average of 17/year.[29] Alcohol and drug use clearly play a role in some water-related injuries, but overall accidents in this area mainly appear to be the result of an unfamiliar environment and participation in unfamiliar activities. For example, many tourists have a serious lack of appreciation of the potential dangers associated with swimming at unpatrolled beaches. Pictorial signs are now used widely throughout the world to warn of local dangers, including rip currents, marine stingers, sharks and restricted access zones. However, these aids will only be effective if their messages are reinforced by education campaigns and targeted tourist information initiatives before travelers leave home.

A general reminder must also be made about supervising small children around any body of water. In many parts of the world, especially developing nations, swimming pools are often not situated in fenced areas so it is essential to survey water recreation facilities when staying at hotels and resorts abroad. In their *Health and Safety Handbook*, the Federation of Tour Operators[34] provides very detailed information on swimming pool safety, including the following points to remember – points that are relevant for both children and adults on holidays:

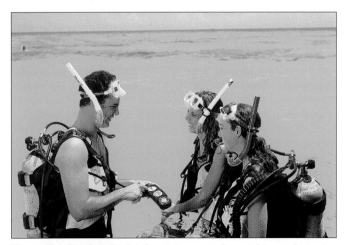

Figure 48.4 Detailed dive briefings are a compulsory safety requirement (Image courtesy of Tourism Queensland).

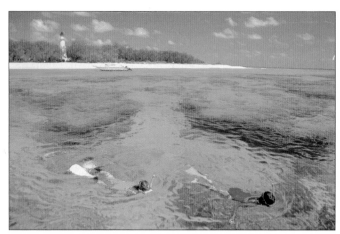

Figure 48.5 Safety can be enhanced by snorkeling and diving in 'buddy pairs' (Image courtesy of Tourism Queensland).

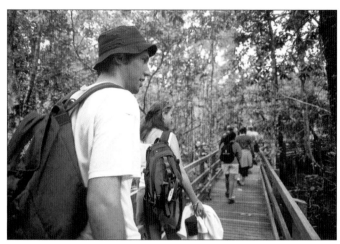

Figure 48.6 Tourists must be adequately prepared for outback and remote travel (Image courtesy of Tourism Queensland).

- Please familiarize yourself with the depth of your pool, the deep and shallow areas, and the steepness of slopes in the pool.
- Please ensure children are supervised at all times.
- Avoid using the pool when alone.
- Do not swim at night.
- Eat after swimming, not before.
- Only fools mix alcohol and swimming.
- Avoid using drinking glasses and glass bottles around the pool area, and
- Do not dive from the poolside into water less that 1.5 m deep. Never bring furniture, household items etc. directly onto the poolside, as this can cause accidents and tempt members of your party to dive from them.

The last point about diving into potentially shallow water is equally pertinent at other aquatic locations. Each year a number of tourists suffer severe spinal and other impact injuries from diving or jumping into shallow water. While it may seem less adventurous, the safe approach is to wade into the water first, check for rocks or other obstacles under the surface, before considering entering the water from any height.

Outdoor and wilderness-based injuries

The United Nations has designated 2002 as the International Year of Eco-tourism, http://www.un.org/documents/ecosoc/res/1998/eres1998-40.htm. This endorsement, coupled with the growing popularity of adventure tourism and outdoor activities, will see more tourists traveling to remote locations. Unless tourists are adequately prepared for the great outdoors (Fig. 48.6), it is also likely that there will be more wilderness-based injuries and the need for medical evacuations. Already there are signs of an increase in Queensland hospital admissions of bites by venomous spiders, snakes and marine animals.[35] In both New Zealand[13] and Queensland[35] the number of overseas visitor hospital admissions due to horse-riding injuries also appears to be increasing.

Based on existing research,[15,17] lacerations, fractures, bites/stings, sunburn and sprains are the main types of injury likely to be experienced in outback and remote areas. However, as noted by Wilks *et al.*[15] some medical evacuations are also likely. From three island tourist resorts there were 14 medical evacuations over a 6 month period. The reasons for evacuation and subsequent hospital admission were angina, deep vein thrombosis, asthma, fractured ankle, dislocated shoulder, wound to fingers, bite or sting, barotrauma, broken tooth, contusion, back injury, abdominal pain, vestibular neuronitis, and readmission for a patient recently discharged from hospital.

Detailed preparation must be undertaken before participating in outdoor activities. At a minimum, this should include trip planning, advising friends or authorities of trip details and expected time of arrival at designated locations, appropriate clothing and footwear, a first aid kit, adequate food and water, and reliable communication facilities. A basic understanding of local flora and fauna, and current skills and knowledge in first aid are also essential for tourists venturing off the beaten track.[36]

CONCLUSION

The World Tourism Organization[2] recommends that 'every state should develop a national policy on tourism safety commensurate with the prevention of tourist risk'. All destinations have a major responsibility to protect their visitors and, in turn, their reputation. Similarly, travel medicine practitioners need to monitor the risk of injury according to geographical location in order to provide balanced and accurate pre-travel advice. In this chapter, a risk management framework was suggested as a way of identifying tourist accidents and injuries across four levels: fatalities, hospital inpatient admissions, outpatient treatments/general medical practice, and other health areas. Motor vehicle accidents and water-related injuries were then examined in detail, highlighting current research findings and prevention initiatives. A brief mention was made of outdoor and wilderness injuries, since the popularity of eco-tourism and adventure travel is likely to increase the number and diversity of accidents in remote locations. Detailed preparation for outdoor activities was highlighted as central to accident and injury prevention.

REFERENCES

1. Thompson D, ed. *The Concise Oxford Dictionary of Current English*, 9th edn. Oxford: Clarendon Press; 1995.
2. World Tourism Organization. *Safety and Security in Tourism: Partnerships and Practical Guidelines for Destinations*. Madrid: World Tourism Organization; 2003.
3. Hargarten SW, Güler Gürsu K. Travel-related injuries, epidemiology, and prevention. In: DuPont HL, Steffen R, eds. *Textbook of Travel Medicine and Health*. Hamilton, Ontario: BC Decker; 1997:258–261.
4. Walters J, Fraser HS, Alleyne GAO. Use by visitors of the services of the Queen Elizabeth Hospital, Barbados, WI. *WI Med J* 1993; **42**:13–17.
5. Nicol J, Wilks J, Wood M. Tourists as inpatients in Queensland regional hospitals. *Aust Health Rev* 1996; **19**:55–72.

6. Cossar JH. Travelers' health: a medical perspective. In: Clift S, Page SJ, eds. *Health and the International Tourist.* London: Routledge; 1996:23–43.

7. Page SJ, Meyer D. Injuries and accidents among international tourists in Australasia: scale, causes and solutions. In: Clift S, Grabowski P, eds. *Tourism and Health: Risks, Research and Responses.* London: Pinter; 1997:61–79.

8. Wilks J, Grenfell R. Travel and health research in Australia. *J Travel Med* 1997; 4:83–89.

9. Hargarten S, Baker T, Guptill K. Overseas fatalities of United States citizen travelers: an analysis of deaths related to international travel. *Ann Emerg Med* 1991; **20**:622–626.

10. Paixao ML, Dewar RD, Cossar JH, et al. What do Scots die of when abroad? *Scott Med J* 1991; **36**:114–116.

11. Prociv P. Deaths of Australian travelers overseas. *Med J Aust* 1995; **163**:27–30.

12. MacPherson DW, Guérillot F, Streiner DL, et al. Death and dying abroad: the Canadian experience. *J Travel Med* 2000; 7:227–233.

13. Bentley T, Meyer D, Page S, Chalmers D. Recreational tourism injuries among visitors to New Zealand: an exploratory analysis using hospital discharge data. *Tourism Manage* 2001; **22**:373–381.

14. Hartung G, Goebert D, Taniguchi R, Okamoto G. Epidemiology of ocean sports-related injuries in Hawaii: Akahele O Ke Kai. *Hawaii Med J* 1990; **49**:52–56.

15. Wilks J, Walker S, Wood M, et al. Tourist health services at tropical island resorts. *Aust Health Rev* 1995; **18**:45–62.

16. Surf Life Saving Queensland. *The Life of the Beach: Annual Report 2000–2001.* Brisbane: Surf Life Saving Queensland; 2001.

17. Peach HG, Bath NE. Health and safety problems and lack of information among international visitors backpacking through North Queensland. *J Travel Med* 2000; 7:234–238.

18. Behrens RH, Steffen R, Looke DFM. Travel medicine: 1. Before departure. *Med J Aust* 1994; **160**:143–147.

19. Standards Australia and Standards New Zealand. *Risk Management. Australian/New Zealand Standard AS/NZS 4360.* Strathfield: Standards Association of Australia; 1999.

20. Wilks J. International tourists, motor vehicles and road safety: a review of the literature leading up to the Sydney 2000 Olympics. *J Travel Med* 1999; **6**:115–121.

21. Wilks J, Watson B, Hansen R, eds. *International Visitors and Road Safety in Australia: A Status Report.* Canberra: Australian Transport Safety Bureau; 1999.

22. Wilks J, Watson B, Hansen J. International drivers and road safety in Queensland, Australia. *J Tourism Stud* 2000; **11**:36–43.

23. Wilks J, Watson B. Assisting 'at risk' tourist road users in Australia. *Travel Med Int* 2000; **18**:88–92.

24. Purkiss SF. Motorcycle injuries in Bermuda. *Injury* 1990; **21**:228–230.

25. Carey MJ, Aitken ME. Motorbike injuries in Bermuda: a risk for tourists. *Ann Emerg Med* 1996; **28**(4):424–429.

26. Wilks J, Watson B, Faulks IJ. International tourists and road safety in Australia: developing a national research and management programme. *Tourism Manage* 1999; **20**:645–654.

27. Hargarten SW. Availability of safety devices in rental cars: an international survey. *Travel Med Int* 1992; **10**:109–110.

28. Wilks J, Coory M. Overseas visitors admitted to Queensland hospitals for water-related injuries. *Med J Aust* 2000; **173**:244–246.

29. New South Wales Injury Risk Management Research Centre. *Analysis of Drowning in Australia and Pilot Analysis of Near-drowning in New South Wales.* Sydney: Australian Water Safety Council; 2000.

30. Australian Water Safety Council. *National Water Safety Plan.* Sydney: Australian Water Safety Council; 1998.

31. Edmonds CW, Walker DG. Snorkeling deaths in Australia, 1987–1996. *Med J Aust* 1999; **171**:591–594.

32. Wilks J. Scuba diving and snorkeling safety on Australia's Great Barrier Reef. *J Travel Med* 2000; 7:283–289.

33. Division of Workplace Health and Safety. *Industry Code of Practice: Compressed Air Recreational Diving and Recreational Snorkeling.* Brisbane, Australia: Division of Workplace Health and Safety; 1999.

34. Federation of Tour Operators. *Health and Safety Handbook.* Lewes, England: Federation of Tour Operators; 1999.

35. Wilks J, Coory M. Overseas visitor injuries in Queensland hospitals: 1996–2000. *J Tourism Stud* 2002; **13**:2–8.

36. Wilks J. *Risk management in tourism and hospitality.* Paper presented at the Parks Victoria Risk Management Seminar, Victoria University, Melbourne, 5 November 2001.

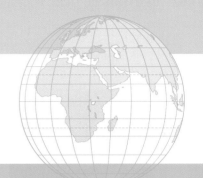

CHAPTER 49 Healthcare Abroad

John W. Aldis

KEYPOINTS

- Life-threatening conditions are often managed surprisingly well in even rather under-developed medical systems

- Except in the most acute of emergencies, most travelers end up in the hands of treating physicians who can speak English

- The desire of the traveler to await evacuation from a place where adequate care is already available should consider the consequences the delay in operating or initiating therapy would have on outcome

- A number of vendors allow a patient to store personal medical records on a website in order to allow worldwide access

- List of physicians at a destination is available from embassies and from ISTM, www.istm.org and IAMAT www.iamat.org

- The financing of medical care at a remote location is often very problematic

- Travelers need to be familiar with the difference between air evacuation companies, insurance companies, and medical assistance companies

INTRODUCTION

An unexpected illness or medical emergency can be extremely frightening for the traveler in a strange place where they do not know the country and do not speak the language. Preparation and anticipation of medical problems should start at the time of the first pre-travel medical consultation in order to prevent even a minor illness abroad from turning into an anxiety-provoking crisis. It is both inaccurate and potentially harmful to our patients to make a blanket assumption that every ill traveler (or long-term expatriate) must return home to receive any adequate medical care. Even in many developing countries there are wealthy elites that can support a limited number of private medical facilities with state-of-the art technology and well-trained (often abroad) professionals (Fig. 49.1). Even in acute life threatening situations, an accurate picture of at least three parameters are necessary: (1) the patient's medical condition, (2) the availability and quality of medical care at the remote location, and (3) the availability and feasibility of emergency medical evacuation. Delaying appropriate care that is readily available in order to effect an evacuation may in fact be detrimental to the patient and can be exceptionally expensive.

Assessing a patient's condition and needs, the capability of the local health-care system to meet those needs and how medical evacuation can best be accomplished is often difficult even when a physician is located in the same city as the patient. Except in the most acute of emergencies, most travelers land in the hands of treating physicians who can speak English. If the traveling patient always has his regular physician's office telephone numbers, a fax number, a pager number and an e-mail address, the treating physician overseas will be able to discuss the patient's problems with a physician who knows that patient best (Table 49.1). A number of vendors allow a patient to store personal medical records on a website in order to allow worldwide access. This needs to be set-up pre-travel.

ASSESSMENT OF AVAILABILITY OF CARE OVERSEAS

Travelers can and should begin to organize the sources of medical care prior to departure. The US State Department's site for its embassies' American Citizens' Services offices (www.travel.state.gov/acs.htm) is useful, although many areas are not included.[1] Other governments have similar information on their websites.[2, 3] Commercial services such as International SOS Assistance and *Travax EnCompass* from Shoreland, Inc., provide corporate and private travel physicians (for a fee) with a list of worldwide medical facilities and contact information. For non-urgent care the International Society of Travel Medicine's website (www.istm.org) provides a list of its members from about 60 countries with contact information for each physician. The International Association for Medical Assistance to Travellers (IAMAT, www.iamat.org) is a good resource for both travelers and travel medicine physicians to find physicians and facilities in 125 countries. Finally, 'premium' credit card companies, health insurance firms, and, of course, medical evacuation and medical assistance companies all provide lists of doctors and medical facilities at overseas locations. If traveling with a tour group, policies and procedures may be in place for referrals to medical care overseas. Enquiries should be made in advance.

Of course there is a wide range of travelers with differing needs: newborns, young children, teenagers, single (unaccompanied) adults, couples, elderly people, and people with medical problems of various degrees of seriousness. Then there are the different circumstances of the patients' travel: long-term versus tourists (solo or part of a group tour), government- or company-sponsored travelers, students, missionaries, etc. Each of these factors affect a patient's ability to access local health-care facilities, pay for local medical care, or take advantage of emergency medical evacuation if that is deemed necessary. It is impractical to treat the overseas traveler with a one-size-fits-all approach, as one must look for the optimal 'fit' between the patient's illness, the availability of local medical care, and the patient's financial situation.

Patients/travelers with established medical problems should plan even before they depart. Long-stay travelers moving overseas with a

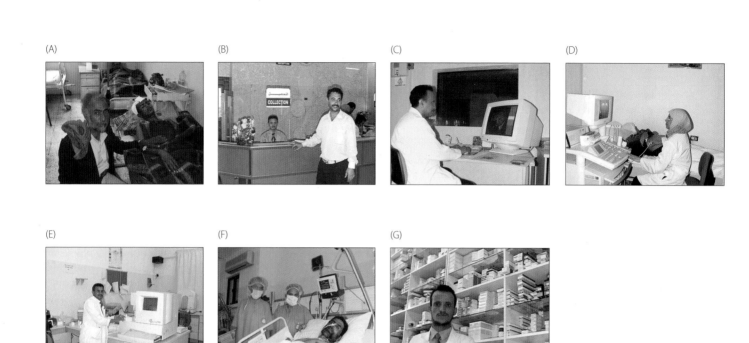

Figure 49.1 Even in the poorest developing countries such as Yemen, where only limited medical care is available to most local people (A), there is often a wealthy elite in the main cities that can support state-of-the-art medical facilities (B). Shown to illustrate this situation is the Yemen German Hospital where all expected technology and services such as (C) MRI; (D) obstetrical ultrasound; (E) automated laboratory; (F) ICU, and (G) a well stocked pharmacy, is available.

company or organization can often read available country reports prepared by the organizational medical department and communicate ahead of time with fellow expatriates already in or previously posted to that location. They should also be very clear in advance what their own organization's policies toward in-country care versus medical evacuation is. Hospitals in some developing countries are often much more specialized than one might expect. There are 'orthopedic hospitals,' 'obstetric/pediatric hospitals,' 'cancer hospitals,' and 'infectious disease hospitals' each of which may be preferable to a general hospital in a limited area. Large cities in developing countries that are not among the most medically austere can often support a number of generally high-quality private general hospitals. Nevertheless, each one often excels in certain specialty areas and can be relatively deficient in others. Local knowledge from colleagues, other expatriates, or an embassy is crucial.

PAYMENT FOR MEDICAL CARE OVERSEAS

The financing of medical care at a remote location is often very problematic. Local hospitals rarely accept insurance, but some major multinational insurers have been moving aggressively to improve this

Table 49.1	Travelers should always have on their person contact information for a personal physician
Office and home phone numbers	
Fax number	
E-mail address	
Mailing address	
Website	
Pager number	

situation mainly in frequent travel destinations.[3] Personal checks, travelers' checks, credit cards, or personal promises from the patient or his family are usually equally useless and cash payment in local currency is often demanded. For those who have contracted with medical evacuation and assistance companies, they will often step in to 'front' the money to pay the hospital bill. The patient's embassy may also assist in helping the patient transfer funds from his/her bank account into the local currency. Travelers with health insurance at home should enquire prior to departure regarding documentation requirements and pre-authorization for possible reimbursement for costs incurred overseas. Although there are a number of strategies, adequate cover for both medical expenses and evacuation (these two do not always go hand in hand) is advisable for all travelers who can afford it. Less affluent travelers often cannot afford to pay for their care, and they are less likely to be covered by medical evacuation insurance so an acute problem often represents more of a crisis for them.

POTENTIALLY LIFE-THREATENING EMERGENCIES

The management of major trauma at a remote location is very similar to anywhere else. Ideally, the patient will be taken to the best hospital in the area, and the early medical management is left in the hands of the physicians there. If applicable, early contact with a medical assistance service for consideration of subsequent medical evacuation or possibly transfer to a higher level of care should it be needed should be effected.

Acute and serious medical problems are, perhaps, somewhat different from trauma because (a) they are often related to chronic, ongoing medical problems familiar to the patient and the hometown physician and (b) the nature of the problem may allow more time to adjust the management than is the case with acute trauma. Angina, GI bleeding, and cerebrovascular stroke are all good examples of serious medical problems that may strike travelers. In many developing countries, thrombolytic therapy or coronary angiography and angioplasty are unavailable or unreliable. While medically evacuating the patient to another country might be possible, the inevitable delay, the risks because of the patient's unstable condition, and the considerable cost of moving an unstable patient must all be considered before a decision is made to move a seriously ill patient. Again, early discussion with a medical assistance company as well as the patient's regular hometown physician is vital (Fig. 49.2). In any case, it is important to have someone accompany the patient to the local medical facility to help with the local language, to call others for more assistance, to notify family, to help in acquiring adequate funds, and for other support. This person might come from the hotel where the patient was staying, from the patient's business office, or perhaps a friend or even a neighbor.

Fortunately, life-threatening conditions are often managed surprisingly well in even rather under-developed medical systems. Even when the care is less than 'state of the art,' it often reflects 'standard' medical care more than is the case for many less serious problems. One should never delay seeking medical care for obviously life-threatening situations for fear of the local medical care system.

SOURCES OF MEDICAL CARE AND ASSISTANCE IN AN EMERGENCY

In medical emergencies, finding the right doctor or medical facility is only part of the problem. Making airline bookings, finding cash to pay the often very large medical bills, assuring a smooth interface between connections on international emergency medical travel, and coordinating the medical care between different local medical facilities are daunting tasks. There are no easy answers, but without good management and coordination of all of the aspects of the crisis, even the best medical care will not assure a good outcome.

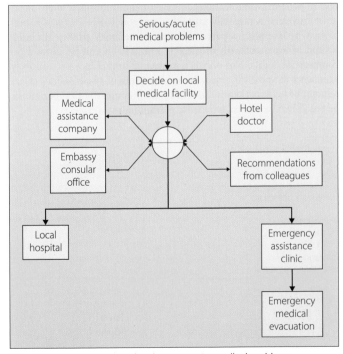

Figure 49.2 Management of serious or acute medical problems.

International medical assistance company clinics

These medical facilities, which are owned by international assistance companies, are found only in larger cities in areas that are otherwise severely medically underserved and that have a large number of tourists and businesses. While the clinics are usually staffed with local physicians, there are almost always some foreign medical staff as well. Sometimes the foreign physicians are prohibited from seeing patients directly as they may be only licensed to serve as 'medical coordinators' by the local government. Nevertheless, when the medical situation is particularly serious, the local and expatriate clinicians usually work hand-in-hand. The clinics usually resemble most closely what patients are familiar with in their home countries, and they are often able to obtain imported medicines and equipment more easily than local clinics. In most cases they *are* the local experts regarding the best local in-patient facilities and the best local clinicians for their patients. These clinics are usually closely tied to medical evacuation systems, and they are usually the best choice for seriously ill patients who need to be stabilized before they can be medically evacuated. They are also often the best clinics for short-term visitors or for expatriate patients who are particularly anxious about using local medical care for even minor problems.

Foreigners' clinics and international clinics

In recent years, physicians and hospitals in many countries have set up 'Foreigners' Clinics' or a dedicated office within their facility to cater to the needs of visitors and long-term expatriates who are guests in their countries. These clinics are usually found only in larger cities, and they often serve as the best 'front door' for foreign patients to the local health-care system. While many of the physicians speak English these services will often provide translators to accompany patients as they move from department to department within the facility.

In countries with more 'socialized' health-care systems such as many countries in Asia, these clinics are often designated as the clinic where all foreign patients are expected to go for care. In fact, such rules are commonly ignored and patients may usually go to whichever clinic they prefer. Many long-term expatriates prefer to choose their own clinics, but newcomers will first try out the Foreigners' Clinic. Since these clinics are usually staffed by local physicians with few ties with medical evacuation facilities, their emphasis is often to encourage local management of the medical problems. While in most cases this is to the patients' advantage, there is sometimes a 'resistance' to getting second opinions or to medically evacuating patients that might (under other circumstances) be transported outside of the country for more advanced levels of care.

Embassies and embassy clinics

In some particularly underdeveloped countries, the most reliable level of medical care is found in the embassy medical clinics. The USA, Germany, and France often have local medical staff (usually at least a nurse, sometimes a physician), and their clinics are stocked with imported medicines and equipment. Unfortunately, these clinics must usually restrict their services to their own embassy community, and 'outsiders' can rarely obtain direct health care through them. The local governments limit their services strictly to the diplomatic personnel, and it is usually not legal for the clinics to charge fees for any services to cover the costs of non-official care.

The embassy health units do provide valuable information about local health risks and available health-care resources for foreigners. In particular, the American Citizens' Services in the Consular Section of each American Embassy keeps an updated list of local medical facilities and clinicians deemed to be reliable, which is available to any American upon request. Usually the complete list is provided with no designation as to the best physician or the best medical facility. The embassy can help in contacting medical assistance and evacuation companies, help organize transfer of funds from home, notify family and friends at home, and assist in arrangements for repatriation of remains. They cannot pay upfront cash for medical expenses, medical evacuation, or repatriation of remains.

Foreign missionary clinics

These are only found in underdeveloped countries and of potential use to travelers in very medically austere areas where they may be the best medical resource in the area. The foreign staff members in the clinics are generally dedicated, well trained, and acutely aware of the local health-care problems. However, these clinics usually do not like to be perceived as being there for the affluent travelers, they do not operate on a fee-for-service basis, so it is often difficult for travelers to obtain care in the clinics.

Local clinics

These clinics are most attractive to budget travelers and some familiarity with the local language is necessary. Physicians will usually do their best to meet the foreign patient's needs and expectations. The care is often quite adequate for many problems but the quality is less predictable in these settings.

Hotel doctors

Often the hotels will insist that their guest consult their own physician when one of the guests falls ill, even when a local clinic might well be able to provide a higher level of medical care. Although the hotel doctors often speak reasonable English, their stature in the local medical care system is sometimes not high. In serious medical situations, they may provide useful contacts with the local health-care system, but too often their main qualification for their job is their political or family connections.

A final point: 'ask for the professor'

The first clinicians to greet the patients at a facility in an emergency situation are usually not the health-care system's most experienced ones. It is sometimes helpful to request the assistance of one of the 'professors' (or teachers) if at a teaching facility or to insist on the appropriate certified specialist if at a private facility. These senior physicians often speak better English and usually have more experience and training in Western-style medicine.

EMERGENCY MEDICAL EVACUATION

Most medical evacuations are most quickly and economically accomplished using regularly scheduled commercial airline flights and not a Lear Jet packed with equipment and highly trained personnel sweeping out of the sky to rescue the unfortunate traveler. Medical evacuation or medical assistance companies can arrange the travel with the airline, outfit the necessary medical equipment, and provide the medical personnel. Medical evacuation companies can choose to use a dedicated plane to transport the patient but this depends on availability of the aircraft, the availability of funding, and the nature of the medical problem (Table 49.2).[4, 5]

Often, the decision to medically evacuate a patient is based as much on the wishes of the patient and the availability of funds to pay for the transportation as on the nature of the medical problem or the local availability of medical care. One good example of this scenario would be a young patient with symptoms and signs of acute appendicitis. The local medical care may be such that a simple appendectomy done in a timely manner would be the best course of action, whereas organizing a medical evacuation might seriously delay the surgical procedure and result in a much more complicated outcome.

Another scenario involves the decision to medically evacuate a patient, when in fact, it is the X-ray or lab result which is in question. Assuming the patient is stable, it is often faster, easier, and much less expensive to send a questionable X-ray to a consultant in another city with higher level medical care available than it is to send the patient. A 'positive malaria smear' or 'an X-ray showing tuberculosis' simply do not necessarily mean the same thing as when they come from laboratories in more developed medical systems. If these can be hand-carried to the consultant at a relatively nearby medical facility, it is even better. While such an approach will not necessarily obviate the need for emergency medical travel, it often does and it almost always adds clarity to the diagnosis and the clinical management decisions.

Some commercial airlines have strict guidelines regarding the transport of patients with infectious illnesses or conditions that might affect other travelers. A mentally unstable (and potentially uncontrollable) patient or one with a particularly offensive smell from a draining wound or a patient with meningitis would likely not be allowed on commercial flights. Not only is a private air ambulance prohibitively expensive in some circumstances, even some of these operators are reluctant to risk contamination of their equipment with tuberculosis or possible resistant bacteria from a draining wound.

Table 49.2	Factors supporting emergency medical evacuation
Medical evacuation is medically required (based on the opinion of the local and/or the remote physician) and the patient agrees with the decision:	
The medical situation is serious enough to justify the expense of emergency medical travel	
The patient's condition is such that delaying the travel (i.e., delaying the patient's medical evacuation) would appreciably worsen the condition	
The patient's medical condition is such that the medical benefits of the travel outweigh the risks	
Medical services at the medical evacuation destination point are appreciably better than where the patient is presently located	
The medical services at the destination point are capable of either dealing with the patient's medical problem(s) or stabilizing the patient for onward travel	
The patient can afford the emergency medical travel	
The medical evacuation system available in that region is capable of providing the support necessary	

Three different kinds of companies may play a role in covering the costs for the medical evacuation. The planes that actually accomplish the medical evacuation are either owned or leased by air evacuation companies that, in turn, provide the services to individual patients or to insurance companies who cover individual or corporate travelers. Medical assistance companies may provide emergency medical evacuation in addition to their wider range of services that they provide to their individual or corporate clients, but these companies are usually backed by an insurance company that covers the costs of the medical travel. Finally, there are the insurance companies themselves, which may provide medical evacuation insurance directly to individual travelers or to the assistance companies to cover their risk (Table 49.3).

Travelers should be counseled on the differences between these types of companies and on what coverage is provided by an individual or corporate policy the traveler is depending on for the stay abroad. Many policies have a number of exclusions including coverage for traveling family members, some psychiatric conditions, pre-existing medical conditions, pregnancy complications and travelers over the age of 75. An assistance company providing support for an overseas corporate site may not be in a position to evacuate the patient unless the insurance company backing them covers the travel or some other funding can be arranged. Since medical evacuations may cost US$100 000 or more and a guarantee of payment is needed by the medical evacuation company before they can act, this sort of 'misunderstanding' can have tragic consequences.

How does one choose a medical evacuation service? Of course, if the patient is already covered by an insurance policy (either through a medical assistance service or independently), that decision is already made. In most emergencies when the patient does not already have medical evacuation insurance, it is usually prudent to rely on the advice of the medical assistance company on site who is probably already caring for the patient. Alternatively, one can request the advice of the local hospital's medical staff but those physicians may resist any effort to move the patient away from their care. Finally, calling a large internationally reputable medical evacuation and assistance company rather than a local operator can often start things moving in the right direction with the minimum of delay. The best advice is to use a company who knows the local health-care system and which can deal with the bureaucratic hurdles of the country where the patient is located.

URGENT AND ROUTINE CARE ISSUES FOR SHORT-STAY TRAVELERS

When travelers who are in transit or on a short visit in a foreign country become seriously ill or injured, it is sometimes easier to deal with their repatriation, should that become necessary. They already have tickets for their onward travel, and these can usually be used for their travel to their home or a location where the level of medical care is adequate. However, without any familiarity with the local situation, they may find it more difficult to access the health-care system or to have on hand sufficient local currency to deal with medical costs. In emergency situations, someone (traveling companion, business colleague, relative) should accompany the victim to the most appropriate medical facility that can be rapidly ascertained in an ambulance (if available) or less desirably a taxi. Once emergency care has been accessed the companion can help contact the embassy, the assistance company or relatives for further advice or help.

For non-urgent problems like diarrhea, urinary or respiratory infections, the traveler may be able to self-treat if accompanied by a properly stocked personal medical kit (see Chapters 8, 14 and 19). An appropriate physician may be found from the embassy list, the assistance company, local colleagues, or as a last resort the hotel desk. In most developing countries all drugs except for narcotics are available without prescription so that a traveler in many situations may do well to contact his/her personal physician at home for advice and the generic names of any drugs that may be indicated.

ON-GOING ROUTINE CARE FOR EXPATRIATES

Many expatriates and their families get annual home leave, and if in good health, continue to use their hometown physicians for routine care and the occasional phone call for minor ailments.

It is therefore useful for the hometown physicians to discuss with their patients what medical interventions might best be done 'at post' (at the remote location), and which can more easily (and safely) be accomplished during the families' periodic trips back home. Table 49.4 lists some types of care that the physician may address during a discussion with the families as they prepare to embark on a long-term assignment to a medically austere location.

Choosing a local physician and medical facility is even more of a challenge than is the case back home but needs to be done soon after arrival before any medical problems arise.[6] The list (Table 49.5) puts English competency at the top, and that is probably the single most important factor. While some expatriates speak the local languages fluently, most people have trouble with a second language when in the midst of a medical crisis. The finer points of communication are lost, and the patient too often over- or under-interprets what it is the doctor is trying to say. The medical office should be visited and questions asked.

After deciding on a source of healthcare, post the name, address and phone number to the preferred doctor and the hospital in the house. Every person in the family as well as the domestic staff should be familiar with these as well as road directions to get there as emergency vehicles may or may not be an option. The 911 number or other familiar emergency numbers may not work in the new country, so if there are emergency phone numbers they should be posted and familiar to all.

Table 49.3	The different roles of companies with whom travelers may contract

Air evacuation companies – provide air evacuation services on a fee-for-service basis to individual clients, corporate clients, or insurance companies

Assistance companies – provide a wider range of services (medical, technical, security, medical evacuation, and other travel-related support) usually to insurance companies or directly to corporate or individual clients.

Insurance companies – provide various forms of risk cover for travelers or assistance companies but generally contract for the air evacuation service.

Table 49.4	Distribution of medical care for the expatriate family
Care obtained locally	**Care by home-town physician**
Acute medical problems	Initial assessment and treatment schedules to address chronic medical problems
Regular assessments of chronic medical problems	Periodic health screening with special attention to chronic problems
Ongoing psychiatric care	Periodic update assessments of psychiatric conditions
Acute dental problems	Regular dental checks and attention problems before they become serious later
Antibiotics and OTC medications which are urgently needed	Prescription and OTC refills and delivery of medications to the remote site
Identification of learning issues of school children	Formal assessment of learning issues, recommendations for treatment, and periodic follow-up
Administer immunizations only under unusual circumstances	All routine (and location-specific) pediatric and adult immunizations[4]
Only emergency hospitalizations or surgical procedures	Surgical procedures, major diagnostic work-ups, inpatient care which can be delayed until return home
Good coordination of care with the patient's hometown health-care provider	Careful coordination of care with the physician(s) providing care at the remote site.

MANAGEMENT OF CHRONIC MEDICAL PROBLEMS

For long-term 'expatriate' patients, the most important aspect of the management of chronic, ongoing medical problems in expatriates is continuity of the clinical management. This becomes more complicated when the patients are living in medically austere environments or when they are traveling from one country to another every few months or years. Through careful and coordinated sharing of the clinical responsibilities, the expatriate patients can receive both close monitoring of their medical conditions and long-range continuity of their clinical care.

Ideally, the hometown physician will be aware of the patient's medical conditions, and the patient will be well advised as to the frequency and type of follow-up care, that is expected. This may involve a wide variety of procedures such as BP measurements, periodic lab testing, etc. The particular tests, which will be done locally, will depend on what local testing is available and reliable. This is usually coordinated by clinicians at the remote location, and the results can then be screened locally and then forwarded on to the hometown physician if necessary. Normally the patient will serve to transmit the test results to his physician. That not only allows the patient to convey his own concerns to his physician, but in most cases, it is easier for the patient to contact his own physician. This process allows the patient's personal physician to monitor progress of the medical condition and to make appropriate and timely adjustments in management.

One area that is particularly difficult to manage overseas is that of children's special learning problems and other childhood developmental or psychiatric conditions. Parents are often willing to 'risk it' and try to manage the problems themselves, but this is often extremely difficult or impossible in many overseas settings. The simple matter of getting a supply of methylphenidate for children with ADHD becomes unimaginably complicated since the drug is a Schedule-II

Table 49.5	Factors in choosing a local physician
Competency in English (or patient's native language)
Recommendations by a fellow foreigner in the community
Prominence in medical community
Medical specialty
Ability to refer to specialists when necessary
Hospital affiliations
Availability of appointments
Availability of off-hours care
Availability of emergency care in tandem with the office practice
Costs and methods of payment

drug and many overseas medical systems do not recognize its value; the government simply will not allow it to be imported into the country.

RETURNING REMAINS HOME

Many travel insurance policies cover the costs of returning the remains of a deceased person to their home country. Even with this financial assistance (usually in the form of reimbursement after the fact) the process is often complicated and expensive. In most cases, the Consular Officer from the deceased person's embassy, should act as the family's representative with the local authorities. The Consular Officer will assist in shipping or arranging for burial of remains and prepare necessary documents including a Consular report of death based on the local country's death certificate.

REFERENCES

1. A Safe Trip Abroad. US State Department Publication 10942. Washington, DC. 2002.
2. International Association for Medical Assistance to Travelers Directory of Physicians. Guelph, Canada. 2003.
3. Leggat PA, Carne J, Kedjarune U. Travel insurance and health. *J Travel Med* 1999; **6**(4):243-8.
4. Hargarten SW, Bouc GT. Emergency air medical transport of U.S.-citizen tourists: 1988 to 1990. *Air Med J* 1993; **12**(10):398-402.
5. Kramer W, Domres B, Durner P, Stockert K. Evaluation of repatriation parameters: an analysis of patient data of the German Air Rescue. *Aviat Space Environ Med* 1996; **67**(9):885-9.
6. De Jongh R and Rey-Herme P. Travel and Expatriate Medicine. In: International Occupational and Environmental Medicine. Herzstein J, *et al* Eds. Mosby, St. Louis. 1998. pp 211-22.

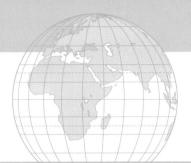

CHAPTER 50 Personal Security and Crime Avoidance

David O. Freedman

INTRODUCTION

Crimes and violent acts against persons occur with some regularity while traveling. Because tourists and business travelers are perceived to be both wealthy and possibly carrying large sums of money and valuables, they are often the specific targets of criminals. Despite this, little formal research has been done to prioritize or rank personal protection measures or even to define which of a long list of frequently given recommendations have any real benefit at all. Nevertheless, security experts agree that a large proportion of criminal occurrences are avoidable if travelers adhere to a number of these common sense guidelines. The 'key points' (see above) should be reviewed during the pre-travel consultation and the rest given in an easy to follow written format for the traveler to carry with them.

The cornerstone of personal safety is situational awareness. Every city, no matter whether in a rich or in a poor country has unsafe zones of varying size where personal risk is high. Most individuals know where these zones are in their own home city; the same level of knowledge should be obtained by all travelers prior to or as soon as possible after arrival at any destination. Once the high-risk zones and high-risk activities are identified – avoid them.

Travelers must not only be constantly aware of the general environment in the destination city or town but also stay constantly alert to the ongoing minute-by-minute situation in the traveler's immediate personal proximity as he/she moves through the day. Travelers should know the country's history, its culture, and follow current events for the destination in the media prior to departure and during the stay. This can be accomplished by use of Consular Information Sheets (Table 50.1), corporate or organizational security reports, and reports from threat assessment consultancies (Table 50.2). However, good statistical data on crime and violent events is often not kept in many countries. In those places where data is kept, for political and economic reasons it is often not easily available to foreign consulates, consultants, or international authorities. Thus in many cases, the most accurate and timely advice on districts, regions or situations to avoid may be from friends, colleagues, clients, tour operators, or the hotel concierge. Such advice is usually based on recent real experiences of other travelers and should be sought immediately on arrival. In addition, embassies usually monitor incidents involving their own citizens and can provide some guidance when asked.

Table 50.1	Consular websites with comprehensive security and risk information
Website for:	**Website address**
US Department of State Travel Warnings and Consular Information	www.travel.state.gov/travel_warnings.html
UK Foreign and Commonwealth Office Country Advice	www.fco.gov.uk/travel (Select Country Advice)
Canada Department of Foreign Affairs & International Trade Travel Reports	www.voyage.gc.ca/dest/intro-en.asp
Australia Department of Foreign Affairs and Trade Travel Advice by Country	www.dfat.gov.au/consular/advice/advices_mnu.html
US Department of State Overseas Security Advisory Council (OSAC), Daily Global News Bulletins	www.ds-osac.org

Table 50.2	Major consultancies specializing in risk management and security
Kroll Inc. Risk Consulting www.krollworldwide.com New York, NY, USA +1 212 593 1000 (tel) +1 212 593 2631 (fax)	
Control Risks Group Risk Consultancy www.crg.com London, UK + 44 20 7222 1552 (tel) + 44 20 7222 2296 (fax)	
Global Business Access, Ltd. Consulting www.globalltd.com Bethesda, MD, USA +1 301-767-9570 (tel) +1 301-767-1935 (fax)	
iJet Travel Intelligence Travel Risk Management www.ijet.com Annapolis, MD, USA 410-573-3860 (tel) 410-573-3869 (fax)	
International SOS Assistance www.intsos.com Singapore +65 6338 2311 (tel)	

The second over-riding crime avoidance principle is to not be a creature of habit. This applies equally to the short stay hotel guest as to the higher profile corporate expatriate. Jogging at the same time each early morning and following the same route from a well known business hotel identifies a potential target just as easily as for the expatriate who leaves the house vacant each Saturday morning to go grocery shopping.

Complex security issues that are beyond the scope of the typical travel clinic patient interaction are not covered here. These include hostile surveillance, kidnapping and hostage situations, hijackings, surviving in hostile situations during armed conflict, and recognition of land mine risks. A number of highly experienced risk consultancies, usually staffed by former law enforcement, espionage, and military personnel are available to provide appropriate risk management, threat assessment, and training packages to organizations and corporations (see Table 50.2). The basics of many of these issues are covered elsewhere.[1-3]

Larger organizations and corporations that may contract out their travel medicine needs to outside clinics often have corporate security departments which will have already provided destination specific risk ratings and written security reports to employees and expatriates on an ongoing basis. This will include very specific information on safe and unsafe districts within a destination city and lists of hotels and residential areas considered to be the most desirable and safe. Country and city specific security reports are available from most of the risk consultancies (Table 50.2).

Personal safety as pertains to injury prevention, motor vehicle crash protection, and prevention of drowning is covered in Chapter 48.

BEFORE DEPARTURE

Before departing, or sometimes before booking, travelers should seek advice from their own country's consular website regarding local safety and political stability. The most comprehensive English language Consular websites are shown in Table 50.2. These countries all have consular personnel on the ground in most destinations so can provide detailed situational information. These consular reports contain much street and district specific information so are best printed and carried during travel. More than one national website should be checked when assessing a destination, as language used in reports from one country may reflect political influences or threat situations targeted only at the citizens of that particular reporting country. In recent years, the trend for consular reports has been away from blanket 'go' or 'no-go' labels for entire destination countries and more towards an enumeration of risk in specific parts of those countries. In addition, risk levels have been introduced into the reports so that leisure travelers may be advised to avoid travel but essential travel may be sanctioned within certain geographic limits. In addition, for specific situations or enhanced information, citizens can usually telephone their own embassy at the destination and obtain details from the security attaché that may be too sensitive or complex to post on the public consular reports.

PRIORITIES UPON ARRIVAL

Unfortunately, the initial airport arrival constitutes one of the highest threat situations of the entire trip. Travelers are tired from the journey, unfamiliar with the surroundings, the arrivals lobby is usually crowded and noisy, and directions and signs may be in a foreign language. This is a natural magnet for criminals in any country. An advance plan needs to be in place. Travelers who are to be met at the airport in a high-risk destination by an individual, tour company representative, or driver not personally known to them should be instructed not to leave the arrivals lobby with anyone who does not know a pre-arranged verbal recognition code. Company signboards as well as a travelers name are easily copied by anyone in the arrivals area. Missed pick-ups often occur, no matter how meticulous the arrangements were. Travelers should always know the address of exactly where they are supposed to get to on arrival and also have phone numbers for appropriate local contact people.

Many airports have kiosks in the terminal rented to reputable taxi concessionaires where pre-paid taxi rides can be purchased and where travelers will be then led to a waiting car. Next best is to look for an organized taxi rank with cars lined up, accepting passengers in sequence, and that is located within the airport perimeter. Avoid at all costs, individuals on foot soliciting for passengers solo in the airport arrivals area. In any country, many criminals purport to be taxi drivers or taxi operators.

Travelers should put a system into place to always ensure that someone knows where they are and what the expected schedule is at all times. If staying for any length of time, travelers should register with their country's embassy and be familiar with appropriate modes of contact should emergency situations arise.

Unless otherwise mandated by law (uncommon), passports should be locked in a safe at home or in the hotel and a photocopy of the face page carried at all times on the travelers person. The photocopy should include any necessary visa as well as the legal entry stamp to the country, as authorities are usually on the lookout for individuals who entered illegally. Additional photocopies or at least passport number and issue details should be kept in a separate place.

Travelers should learn telephone-dialing sequences even for short stays immediately on arrival and certainly before an emergency situation arises. Travelers should be aware of the dial sequence necessary to access both local and long-distance circuits from their hotel room, residence, place of business, and/or locally on leased or personal mobile phone. They should ascertain all emergency phone numbers, including police, fire, ambulance, as well as neighbors, key business colleagues, and the hotel if applicable. These should be posted prominently in the home, if applicable, and carried on the person at all times. Organizations with local operations often have laminated wallet cards with key contact points regularly made up and these can be delivered to all arriving employees or visitors right at the airport.

The hotel desk or colleagues should be questioned upon arrival about common local scams and distraction techniques used by pickpockets and thieves. Thieves often work in groups of two, one to distract and the other to take.

MOBILE PHONES

Even the poorest countries generally have high quality mobile phone service. Efficient and rapid communication with sources of potential help when a traveler finds him/her self in a high-risk situation can provide solutions to that particular situation or can help to minimize the time the traveler is exposed to that threat.

A locally purchased or leased mobile phone is best, because of ease of dialing local numbers and the ease with which local people can dial the traveler. Organizations or companies that have short-term visitors or staff coming in from other countries can consider providing a local mobile phone upon arrival. Alternatively, frequent travelers should carry their own GSM band phone so that they can roam on the local network. GSM band service is the most prevalent in the world and is available in almost every country, although it is only a minor player in the USA and Canada. GSM coverage maps for any country can be checked at www.gsmworld.com/roaming/gsminfo/index.shtml. GSM frequencies in the Americas differ from other parts of the world, but tri-band GSM handsets that automatically detect the ambient GSM signal are available from all GSM operators worldwide. In the USA, many mobile phone operators that on a day-to-day basis use non-GSM technical standards have, combination handsets available for sale or temporary rental to travelers.

IN THE HOTEL

In high threat countries, hotel locations should be carefully selected using advance knowledge and are ideally located in proximity to planned activities. Rooms on floors three to six are generally regarded as optimal for safety and security. They are harder to break into from the outside of the hotel but are accessible to firefighting equipment. Travelers should look for fire safety instructions in the room upon arrival and also familiarize themselves with escape routes. Travelers may consider counting doors in the corridor in order to find exits in case of poor visibility due to dark or smoke.

The hotel room door should be locked at all times. For those anticipating stays in budget accommodations, compact locking and door opening blocking devices are cheap and readily available. Doors should not be opened to strangers and a call to the front desk can be made to confirm the identity of someone knocking at the door. Room safes are less secure than individual safe deposit boxes at the front desk but may be preferable, depending on model type, to a large hotel safe readily accessible to many hotel employees.

Room numbers should not be disclosed to any but the closest personal friends and colleagues. Meet visitors in the lobby. Room keys that identify the room number together with the hotel should be left with the concierge upon leaving the building. Hotel business cards with address and phone number in the local language should be carried on the person at all times.

Disagreement exists about the wisdom of informing the hotel desk about expected time of return to the hotel. This is probably unwise in general, but may be considered if a traveler is to be returning late at night and no-one else is aware of the anticipated destination and schedule.

OUT AND ABOUT

Travelers should radiate confidence and know exactly where they are going. Situational awareness requires planning ahead before venturing out. If the terrain and routes are already familiar, little planning time will be required. However, all travelers need to have good knowledge of high-risk areas and potentially high-risk situations. Methods for ascertaining these have been described above, but it is important to remember that high-risk areas can change with time so even frequent travelers need to do an assessment on each visit. Consult local media regularly to keep up with current events and potentially volatile situations. Routes should be decided either mentally or using a map before setting out. Maps should not be studied in the street as this broadcasts vulnerability.

Travelers should not wear expensive clothing or jewelry or carry expensive cameras or electronics. They should dress to blend in as much as possible and definitely avoid clothing that declares their nationality or any indication of local or global political beliefs. Travelers should always carry either a mobile phone or whatever phone cards or coins are needed to operate a public telephone.

Travelers should be constantly attentive to surroundings and be wary of any stranger who engages them in any form of conversation or touches their person in any way no matter how accidental the contact may appear to be. Travelers should never accept any sort of food or drink from strangers on the street, in bars, or from taxi drivers; drugging is common in many places. One's drink should never be left unattended at the bar. While out on foot, travelers should always have one hand free to protect themselves and their valuables. Specific targets for thieves are shoulder bags, outside pouches of backpacks, and cameras that hang from straps. Valuables should be slung across the chest and preferably under a jacket or shirt so that they are less accessible to thieves. Luggage or personal belongings should never be given to anyone who cannot be directly supervised or observed.

Even if the area is familiar, travelers need always use extra caution in tourist sites, market places, elevators, crowded subways, train stations and at festivals. Isolated beaches should always be avoided and even popular and safe beaches should be avoided after dark and in the early morning hours. Joggers are at risk of losing even shoes and clothing whose name brands may have high value in many countries. Curiosity is dangerous and political gatherings and any sort of crowd should always be avoided but particularly in potentially unstable civil environments. Travelers should be aware of special dates and anniversaries on which any public place is best avoided.

Travelers should never withdraw money from ATMs or change money at a money-changing establishment after dark. Darkness makes it simple for potential assailants to observe discreetly from a relatively short distance. After obtaining cash, travelers should verify carefully that they are not being followed.

In any country many criminals pose as willing sex partners. The set-up may entail a sex-for-hire scenario or may appear as a casual or accidental meeting in a hotel, bar, restaurant or even on the street. Whether the liaison moves on to the traveler's hotel/apartment or a location of the criminal's choice carries equal risk of a poor outcome. Potentially intimate encounters with host-country nationals should be avoided at all times. Travelers should avoid being intoxicated at night on the street and taxis should be used even for short distances in this situation.

Long-stay travelers should be constantly alert to their immediate environment and make mental notes of the usual neighborhood and work environments. This makes anomalies, out of place persons, and suspicious situations more instantly obvious.

TAXIS AND PUBLIC TRANSPORT

The taxi situation varies greatly by country and the guidelines here will often need to be adapted to local conditions. In general, travelers should use only 'registered' taxis, but the guidelines for identifying these require local knowledge that must be ascertained upon arrival.

For day-to-day use, radio taxis are always the safest, although in many countries with a well-enforced system of registration, taxis found in marked ranks may be equally safe. Local colleagues can usually inform as to the phone numbers of reputable radio taxi operators. If it is possible to adequately communicate with the radio dispatcher when ordering the taxi, travelers should obtain the car number or license plate number of the taxi that has been dispatched. If the situation requires the taxi driver to ring up over an apartment block intercom, a pre-arranged recognition signal should be requested from the telephone dispatcher.

The fare should always be fixed before entering any taxi, even if sign language must be used. Travelers anticipating taxi travel should always have local money in small denominations, as change for large bills is never available even if it is on board. Taxis should never be shared with unknown passengers.

Hotels often have their own vehicles and drivers for hire. These are usually very over-priced but generally safe and reliable. However, travelers need to beware of hotel doormen who when asked for a taxi will put the traveler into a taxi operated by an accomplice who will at best just overcharge and at worst rob the traveler. Warning signs would include a taxi parked to a side away from a marked taxi line or rank or a taxi apparently taken out of turn.

Public transportation, particularly if overcrowded, presents many safety risks that are detailed in Chapter 48. In addition, public vehicles present a situation where foreigners will both stand out and will be relatively stationary targets for a fixed period of time. Travelers should ride public transportation in pairs if possible. Thieves often work in pairs, so travelers should avoid continuing to move in the direction of anyone that suddenly appears and is positioned in a way to be blocking the path forward. Public transportation should be avoided at night at all costs. Travelers should never sit in a train car that is otherwise empty of other passengers.

CAR TRAVEL

Travelers should never drive themselves or travel by private car at night in a foreign country particularly in rural areas. Of all the recommendations in this chapter, this is the one that has the strongest support from the literature and by consensus of security experts. This has to do equally with crime avoidance as well as the injury prevention issues covered elsewhere in this book. Local travel at night in the company of trusted and close colleagues may be unavoidable and is perhaps somewhat safer, but out of town travel even under these circumstances is still usually extremely dangerous. After an appropriate period of acclimatization, driving in a personal automobile at night to familiar local venues in non high-risk neighborhoods can be

considered but this still represents some increase in the chance of being a victim of a crime.

Whether traveling locally or between cities by car in a destination country efficient communications can greatly reduce exposure time and risk of attack in case of getting lost or breakdowns. Even if not carried on a day-to-day basis, a mobile telephone should be borrowed or leased for out of town travel.

Where appropriate, travelers should consider hiring a local driver who is familiar with the terrain, the road rules, driving customs and has been personally recommended. This is especially important for remote areas and where language is an issue. The sobriety of the driver should be verified each time the car is entered. Because of prevailing wages in poorer countries, the cost of a car and driver is usually similar to the cost of renting the car itself. When renting a car or car and driver, travelers should avoid those with any sort of rental markings.

En route, car doors should be kept locked at all times and the windows should be kept closed as much as is feasible. In hot climates air conditioned cars should be sought for this reason. As at home, travelers should not pick up hitchhikers. Travelers need to be alert at all times even as a passenger. Carjacking and grab and run thefts happen when stopped at gas stations, parking lots, or in slow city traffic.

LEARN LOCAL REGULATIONS EARLY

Travelers should make efforts to learn in advance the rules and regulations of the destination country. Procedures to follow when involved in a motor vehicle incident need to be known. Penalties for breaking the law can be surprisingly severe. An embassy can help ensure legal representation but cannot over-rule local laws. Some countries have a 'zero tolerance' policy with severe penalties for those driving under the influence of alcohol or other drugs. Drug violations, firearms possession, photography of government or military installations, and antiques purchases are frequent cause of detention by local authorities.

CONCLUSION

All experts agree that travelers should give up valuables without struggle once confronted. Money and passports can be replaced; human lives cannot.

REFERENCES

1. Rogers C, Sytsma B. *World Vision Security Manual. Safety Awareness for Aid Workers*. Geneva: World Vision; 1999, www.marcpublications.com.
2. Pelton RY. *Come Back Alive: The Ultimate Guide to Surviving Disasters, Kidnapping, Animal Attacks and Other Nasty Perils of Modern Travel*. Garden City, NY: Doubleday; 1999.
3. Pelton RY. *The World's Most Dangerous Places* 4th edn. London: Harper Collins; 2000.

CHAPTER 51 Post-travel screening

Jan C. Clerinx and Alfons Van Gompel

KEYPOINTS

- The medical history is the cornerstone of post-travel screening

- Asymptomatic short-term travelers rarely need a medical posttravel examination

- The long-term traveler or expatriate needs a more thorough medical interview to assess potential exposure to a variety of infections

- Adventurous travelers frequently adopt lifestyles which put them at greater risk for unusual infections

- Minimal laboratory tests include a complete blood count, a WBC differential count, liver transaminases and creatinine levels, as well as serological tests according to risk of infection

INTRODUCTION

Many travel clinics provide both pre-travel counseling as well as post-travel screening and care. Pre-travel counseling focuses on the patient's ability to travel or to live in a different physical environment, and on preventing common infectious diseases by means of vaccination, chemoprophylaxis, and behavioral counseling. During the post-travel screening of asymptomatic travelers, the physician estimates the risk of occult travel-related infections and their potential impact on the traveler's health. In a travel clinic, the investigation of a pre-existing illness is not part of the post-travel health screening, but in many hospitals both travel and non-travel-related health services are often managed by the same medical staff. Integration of preventative and curative travel medicine services leads to a better knowledge of travel related infections and helps to improve the quality of both pre-travel counseling and post-travel screening.[1]

Far more useful than any other test, the medical history is the cornerstone of the post-travel screening process, focusing on infectious diseases transmitted by various routes.[2] Additionally, older, long-term travelers and expatriates may benefit most from an assessment of common non-infectious conditions such as cardiovascular disease, neoplasia and the impact of trauma. For those intending to travel again, it offers an ideal opportunity for counseling on travel-related behaviour and preventative measures, and for reviewing the immunization status and chemoprophylaxis.

Laboratory tests are often insensitive (resulting in false negative results), non-specific (resulting in false positive results) and may not be available for the diagnosis of, subclinical disease or infections during their incubation period as is the case for malaria. Qualitative diagnostic tests are useful to detect infection, but (semi) quantitative tests are often essential to determine the 'parasite load'. This may be of importance for malaria, schistosomiasis and some filarial infections.

A cost/benefit analysis of post-travel screening of asymptomatic travelers has not received much attention. Post-travel screening of itself will in most cases not have an impact on patient morbidity and mortality. When broadening its mandate towards medical counseling (i.e., pre-and post-exposure disease prevention), its impact on individual health status may be equivalent to that of health check-ups for cardiovascular and neoplastic diseases, and to the periodic medical examinations in occupational medicine.[3] Relying too heavily on laboratory results alone often leads to repeated follow-up visits to test the validity of the test results, rather than focusing on the potential morbidity of the infection. One might reasonably question the cost-effectiveness of investigating too thoroughly, especially for infections that have minimal morbidity.[4,5]

WHO AND WHEN TO SCREEN?

According to WHO guidelines, a medical examination is advisable after a long stay in the tropics, but is deemed unnecessary for asymptomatic short-term travelers who did not experience any health problems or only trivial self-limited ailments such as diarrhea, or a febrile episode of short duration.[6] Symptomatic travelers will benefit from a post-travel examination by an experienced health professional.

To be useful to the asymptomatic traveler, and to alleviate his/her fears of having acquired some 'exotic' disease, a post-travel examination has to be able to rule out the presence of subclinical disease. This requires knowledge of the pre-patent period (time from infection until a laboratory diagnosis can be made) of the targeted infectious diseases, as well as of the shortcomings of laboratory procedures to detect subclinical infection. Screening for sexually transmissable diseases deserves special consideration and speedy intervention.[1]

There is still some uncertainty about the ideal timing to conduct a post-travel medical examination. Infections with a long pre-patent period (eg., intestinal helminth infections) may be overlooked if infection has occurred immediately before the screening process. The traveler needs to be informed about potential disease manifestations that might occur in the future depending on exposure, and a second medical evaluation at a later date might be considered. Also, patients should be offered access to urgent consultation (by travel clinic personnel and/or a tropical disease expert), especially when fever may herald potentially serious diseases such as malaria, amebic liver abscess, and acute schistosomiasis (Katayama fever).

Targeted population

Those who might benefit most from a post-travel medical examination, may be determined according to potential risk of exposure to infectious disease, demographic factors (age, gender, socio-economic status) and travel characteristics (duration, destination, exposure). Immigrants, refugees and adopted children from tropical countries constitute a specific subgroup that is not specifically dealt with in this chapter. Moreover, these travelers often visit relatives and friends in their country of origin, but only rarely do they consult for post-travel screening when they are asymptomatic.

The asymptomatic short-term traveler or expatriate

Asymptomatic short-term travelers, whether tourists or professionals, rarely need medical post-travel screening, if they have been aware of potential health risks and if they do not report exposure to a particular infection. This implies that travelers have been correctly instructed before traveling, which of course, is often not the case. A review of imported malaria cases has shown that many travelers to popular tourist destinations such as the Gambia and Senegal did not even seek advice on malaria prevention and yellow fever vaccination.

Routine post-travel screening is probably unnecessary in short-term travelers who have experienced a self-limited illness, as these symptoms rarely herald the onset of a chronic or recurring illness associated with significant morbidity.

For some professional corporate travelers, a post-travel screening procedure constitutes an integral (often compulsory) part of the periodic medical evaluation in occupational medicine.

Conducting a history of exposure to infection should include specific types of food and water ingestion, arthropod exposure, fresh water contact, sexual contacts, blood exposure (injections) and animal bites/contact. Thus, post-travel screening in short-term travelers without a particular health risk could be restricted to individuals with a chronic underlying health condition whose symptoms can be con-founded by those of a newly acquired infectious disease.

The asymptomatic long-term traveler or expatriate

This group is subjected to a more thorough medical interview to assess potential exposure to a wide variety of infections.

This includes exposure to air-borne diseases (tuberculosis, SARS), arthropod-borne diseases (malaria, filariasis, trypanosomiasis), water-borne infections (schistosomiasis), soil transmitted helminth infections (strongyloidiasis, hookworm, intestinal helminths), food-borne parasites (amoebiasis, giardiasis, intestinal helminths) and STDs. If a specific exposure has been identified, one has to estimate the magnitude of the risk incurred. Systematic questioning often brings to the surface a potential medical problem that can be resolved early in its course.

Expatriates and long-term travelers may expect a general health assessment for more mundane cosmopolitan disorders, as these services are often lacking in the country of residence. This includes cardiovascular disorders, and preventive screening for malignancies, including prostate, breast and colonic cancer, according to the national guidelines or practices.

The asymptomatic adventurous traveler

Adventurous travelers frequently adopt lifestyles similar to those of the indigenous population of the countries visited, and present a greatly increased risk for unusual infections. Here, the physician needs to question in detail local eating habits and the consumption of exotic foods. Eating raw meat and fish, undercooked food, unusual ingredients such as reptiles, drinking unpurified water and unpasteurised dairy products all constitute a risk for unusual infections such as anisakiasis, gnathostomiasis, trichinosis, sarcocystosis, brucellosis, and porocephalosis.

Exposure to specific environments may lead to specific infections: fresh water contact while bathing or swimming in lakes, ponds or rivers, or when wading through flooded areas (schistosomiasis, frequent; leptospirosis), bat-infested caves (histoplasmosis, rabies: rare, but specific high risk environment), game parks infested with tse-tse flies (East African trypanosomiasis: rare, but serious mortality risk), walking safaris (tick bite fever, frequent), equatorial forests (loiasis and onchocerciasis in West and Central Africa: occasional, only long-stay travelers), and marine environment (stings of fish and coelenterates, coral reefs).

Travelers presenting with self-identified risk factors and/or disease symptoms during travel

Travelers who have experienced a particular health problem are more readily inclined to consult for a variety of reasons. They may be worried about the possible long-term consequences, or they are looking for confirmation of a diagnosis established elsewhere. Although answers to the travelers concerns are not always possible, the physician may wish to seize the opportunity (especially in case of the frequent traveler) to provide counseling on important disease manifestations and presumptive treatment strategies, and advice on specific diseases associated with that particular exposure. Some travelers are mistakenly convinced that exposure to certain diseases makes them more susceptible to complications during future travel, e.g., after malaria or amebiasis; however, this may be the case for Dengue fever.

Fear of infecting others is another incentive to consult. This issue applies to well-defined professional positions where air-borne or (indirect) fecal-oral transmission may affect vulnerable groups of people (elderly, institutions for mentally retarded, immunocompromised patients, food industry etc.).

GENERAL SCREENING

Medical interview

More important than any set of laboratory tests, the medical interview is the cornerstone of the post-travel screening process. It is the basic tool for assessing exposure to specific infections and for estimating the magnitude of risk. It needs to be stressed that risk perception of the traveler often differs widely from the objective risks incurred. Therefore, a versatile and flexible history by an experienced physician remains the essential component of post-travel medical screening.

For an appropriate travel risk assessment in asymptomatic travelers, the questions are listed in Tables 51.1, 51.2 and 51.3. Using a concise printed questionnaire will often speed up a general risk assessment. These items provide an adequate picture of the existing health risks to steer clinical examination, laboratory investigations and counseling.

Table 51.1	Self administered questionnaire in post-travel screening
Demographic factors	Age, gender
Travel characteristics	Destination, duration of stay and date of return
Vaccinations Including year of last dose	Polio, diphtheria, tetanus Hepatitis A and B Yellow fever Typhoid fever Meningococcal meningitis type A and C Japanese encephalitis Other (rabies, Tick-borne encephalitis)
Malaria chemoprophylaxis	Drug regimen used, adherence and duration of intake

Table 51.2	Post-travel screening questionnaire
Basic medical information	Weight change, tobacco, alcohol and psychotropic drug use, concomitant medication
Purpose of travel	Holiday, professional travel, visiting relatives and friends (VFR), adventure sports etc.
Physical environment	Destination, duration, transport means, travel route, type of accommodation, altitude
Specific environment	Freshwater contact (rivers, lakes, flooded areas), caves, marine environment, forests, game parks, etc.
Food intake habits	Exposure to raw meat and fish, undercooked food, unusual ingredients, unpurified water, unpasteurized dairy products
Previous disease history	Chronic diseases and allergic conditions (asthma, eczema, urticaria)
Malaria protection	Physical protection, type of antimalarial drugs, dosage, and duration of intake
STD Risk	Protective measures, contact with risk groups
Blood-borne risks	IVDU, needle prick accidents, trauma, blood transfusion
Diseases during travel	Fever, intestinal and skin diseases, STDs

Physical examination

In asymptomatic travelers, physical examination is of limited value. However, unsuspecting individuals may present with lymphadenopathy, splenomegaly, hypertension, cardiac or pulmonary dysfunction or a skin disorder that may require attention. If the medical history reveals a specific complaint, carrying out a physical examination may yield useful information, and helps to reassure patient and physician alike. The extent of the examination is guided by the nature of the ailment.

General Screening Test

General laboratory tests

A minimal set of tests comprises a complete blood count, WBC diffential count, and determination of liver transaminase and creatinine levels. This may provide important information on possible infection, and on liver and kidney function.

Table 51.3	Specific exposure risks for tropical infectious diseases
Physical environment (exposure)	**Disease risk**
Urban environment	Dengue[bc]
Fresh water contact (swimming, wading, rafting)	Schistosomiasis Leptospirosis
Estuaries, rivers (borders)	Soil transmitted helminths Onchocerciasis Leptospirosis Cutaneous larva migrans West-African sleeping sickness[a]
Tropical forests	Filariasis (blood) Viral hemorrhagic fevers
Caves	Histoplasmosis, rabies
African game parks (tse-tse infested)	East-African sleeping sickness[a]
Tropical grass land (walking safaris)	Tick bite fever[a] Tsutsugamushi fever[c]

[a]Africa
[b]Central and South-America
[c]S.E. Asia

Urinalysis, including urine microscopy, heme dipstick, and proteinuria is essential when urinary schistosomiasis is suspected, but will usually fail to detect light infections, as is often the case in travelers. It does not necessarily yield reliable information on renal disease, bladder cancer or urinary tract infection in asymptomatic persons.[4]

Determining fasting blood glucose levels and blood lipids as a marker for diabetes and cardiovascular disease risk is optional but certainly recommended as part of a general health screening in long-term expatriates.

Blood eosinophil count

This screening test has generally been accepted in clinical practice as a useful method to indicate possible helminth infection (worms), especially with nematodes or trematodes, but not with non-invasive cestodes.[7] Eosinophilia is more marked when blood or tissue migration occurs, as in strongyloidiasis, schistosomiasis, blood filariasis and intestinal helminths (ascaris, hookworm), but less so in lymphatic filariasis.

However, in many individuals harboring subclinical helminth infections, the eosinophil count is normal. When using a low cut-off level of 450 eosinophils/mm3 (0.45 bil/L) as a screening marker for helminth infection, the test lacks specificity as well. Since the prevalence of helminth infections is usually low in asymptomatic travelers, relying only on eosinophilia to diagnose parastic infections leads to unnecessarily high costs in terms of follow-up visits and additional laboratory examinations.[7]

Consequently, the eosinophil count does not add substantial value to stool examination and serological tests for the detection of parasitic infections (see below). It can be assumed, however, that the yield would be higher in travelers with high eosinophil counts (absolute count >1000/mm3 or >1.0 bil/L), and that further diagnostic workup would be better restricted to this subpopulation.

Likewise, extremely high levels of IgE in long-term travelers or expatriates are indicative of past or present helminth infection as well, and do not merely reflect an allergic condition.

Abdominal ultrasound

At present ultrasound may only be considered as a secondary diagnostic procedure in asymptomatic travelers presenting with abnormal liver and urinary tract function tests, or as part of a screening strategy for prostate disorders in the elderly. The latter applies specifically to long-term expatriates and missionaries without access to quality healthcare in the country of residence.

Resting ECG

A resting ECG has had its indication when prescribing halofantrine as a standby emergency antimalarial treatment. It might identify persons presenting with the 'long Q-T' syndrome who are vulnerable for a specific malignant ventricular tachycardia ('*torsade de pointes*') when treated with drugs that promote Q-T prolongation. Halofantrine is no longer considered a first choice in the treatment of malaria.

SPECIFIC SCREENING ITEMS

The main objective of these tests is to provide information on occult infection with tuberculosis, STDs, hepatitis and on intestinal and extraintestinal parasitic diseases. See also Table 51.4.

Screening for tuberculosis (TB)

The probability of becoming infected in areas highly endemic for TB depends on the specific environment in which the density of infected droplets and the duration of inhalation determine its likelihood. Basically, this happens only in a confined space protected from sunlight and air flow, and contaminated with droplets from an index case with active pulmonary tuberculosis. In contrast, the risk of infection outdoors is comparatively negligible. Consequently, the risk of TB will be minimal in short-term travelers.

However, infection risk increases substantially in long-term travelers and expatriates. Incidence rates of TB infection in long-term, low budget travelers are comparable to those of the indigenous population of these areas, and is estimated in a recent Dutch study at 2.8/1000 person-months, a >100-fold increase of risk. However, disease risk estimated at 0.6/1000 person-months remains relatively modest in absolute terms.[8]

Table 51.4	Diagnosis of exposure to common travel-related infections			
	Incubation period	Diagnostic procedure	Use of test	Time elapsed after which an acute symptomatic infection becomes very unlikely
Amebiasis	1 d – >6 m	Stool microscopy Stool antigen test[a] Serum antibody test[a]	Infection E.h./E.d. Infection (E.histolytica) Tissue invasion E.h	6 m [b] – but may be longer
Malaria (P. falciparum)	9 d – 35 d	Thick film, antigen test Serum antibody test[a]	Active infection/disease Postinfection confirmation Chronic suppressed infection	Nonimmunes : 3 m Semi-immunes : 4 y
Malaria (benign tertian-quartan)	10 d – >1 year	Thick film, (antigen test) Serum antibody test[a]	Active infection/disease Postinfection confirmation	Benign tertian : 2-4 y Quartan : > 10 y
Typhoid	7 d – 45 d[a]	Blood culture Stool, urine culture[a] Serum antibody test (Widal)	Active disease Convalescent carrier state Postinfection (controversial, not reliable)	2 m
Tuberculosis	>30 d	Tuberculin skin test[a]	Latent infection Active infection/disease	2 to 4 m Reactivation lifelong
Schistosomiasis	21 d – >60 d	Serum antibody tests[a] Microscopy stools, urine[a] Microscopy rectal snips[a] Antigen in stool, urine[a]	Latent infection/Katayama syndrome Active infection/disease Active infection/disease Active infection/disease	3 to 6 m– exceptionally longer
Intestinal helminths	3 d – >60 d	Stool microscopy[a]	Active infection	2 m
Filariasis (bancroftian)	? – >1year	Serum antibody tests[a] Serum antigen test[a] (nocturnal) microfilaremia	Exposure Active infection. Active infection	Up to 2 y
Filariasis (onchocercosis)	3 m – >15 m	Serum antibody tests[a] Cutaneous, ocular microfilaria[a]	Exposure (low sensitivity) Active infection	Up to 2 y
Filariasis (loiasis)	? – >12 m	Serum antibody tests[a] Microfilaremia[a]	Exposure Active infection	Up to 2 y
Strongyloidoiasis	7 d – >21 d	Serum antibody tests[a] Stool microscopy (concentration)[a]	Exposure, active infection Active infection	1 m (reactivation lifelong)
HIV	14 d – >90 d	Serum antibody test (HIV-elisa)[a] HIV-wb[a]	Active infection: screening Active infection: confirmation	3 – 6 m
Syphilis	9 d – >90 d	RPR and vdrl[a] TPHA, FTA[a]	Active infection Confirmation postexposure, posttreatment	3 m

[a]Useful in asymptomatic travelers.
[b] d, days; m, months; Y: years

Health-care workers, on the other hand, are are at significant risk (7.9/1000 person-months), some of them to MDR tuberculosis. For this high-risk category, strict follow-up by tuberculin skin testing before and after exposure is highly recommended.

Chest X-ray

Routine chest X-ray is an often performed, but nonspecific and insensitive screening test for latent pulmonary tuberculosis infection. In industrialized countries with low levels of endemic TB, mass chest X-ray as a means of controlling TB has long been abandoned. Consequently a chest X-ray cannot be recommended as a routine screening procedure for TB in asymptomatic travelers.

If considered, it should be restricted to expatriates or adventurous travelers with a positive tuberculin skin test reaction, the more so if there has been exposure to a known or strongly suspected pulmonary TB case in the household or at the workplace, or when BCG vaccination has been given in the past.

Tuberculin skin testing

Tuberculin skin testing (skin reaction after intradermal injection of 1 to 5 IU PPD) is by far more sensitive and specific than a chest X-ray to identify TB exposure. A change from a negative skin reaction before travel to a positive one on return indicates exposure to TB, i.e., latent tuberculosis infection. Typically, the tuberculin reaction turns positive 6 weeks after TB exposure, but conversion can take longer, sometimes up to 2–4 months.

As a diagnostic test, it is fraught with problems in its practical application (two visits) and interpretation. To be reliable, the response must be read at 72 h, and the technique of intradermal injection as well as the reading of the result must be performed correctly by experienced personnel. False negative reactions are frequent when these are not correctly performed.9 Tuberculin reaction is less reliable during pregnancy, old age, diabetes, corticosteroid treatment, and is unreliable in immunodeficient individuals. BCG vaccination during childhood may result in a positive skin test for many years thereafter. Some authors recommend a second pre-travel tuberculin skin test within a short interval (1-3 weeks) to detect a booster effect as a means to increase specificity, but patients are not very compliant with this cumbersome procedure.

Whether tuberculin skin testing should be performed in all long-term travelers and residents in the tropics is yet subject to debate. The American Thoracic Society advocates tuberculin testing only for persons likely to be recently infected, particularly those who have been in close contact with a known infectious case. Although post-exposure prophylactic treatment averts progression to active disease in most cases, limiting oneself to the detection and treatment of clinically apparent tuberculosis remains at present the most cost-effective strategy.[10]

Sexually transmitted diseases

Studies conducted among travelers from various countries on their attitude towards STDs indicate a high rate of unprotected sexual contacts with new partners, primarily with persons from the countries visited.[11] STDs have become a pivotal part of a post-travel screening, largely due to the HIV pandemic. Thus there is a great need to include STD risk prevention strategies in the pre-travel counseling sessions, and to have them reinforced during a post-travel screening.

Screening STDs in asymptomatic travelers returning home serves a two fold goal: limiting secondary transmission through prevention and treatment, and reassuring the traveler.

Screening for STD should involve detection of HIV, syphilis, gonorrhea and chlamydia, genital herpes and condylomata.

HIV and syphilis are conveniently detected by serological techniques. On the other hand, screening for gonorrhea and chlamydia involves sampling of the urethra and/or cervix directly, either by means of bacterial culture, antigen tests or PCR, or indirectly from the detection of an abnormal number of white blood cells in a first pass of urine. Direct sampling may be unacceptable to asymptomatic patients, particularly women. Studies on chlamydia prevalence suggest that direct sampling be reserved for a subgroup of patients engaging in sexually high risk behavior, i.e., frequent unprotected sex with multiple partners.[11,12]

Screening for HIV has by far become the most compelling issue in post-exposure STD screening. It may prevent transmission and may improve personal infection management. Though the potential benefit of antiretroviral treatment soon after HIV seroconversion remains undetermined, early detection and treatment will offer the infected patient the option to preserve the full potential of the immune system. Since serological screening for HIV has become very reliable in terms of specificity and sensitivity, it should not be restricted to high risk travelers only.[13]

Some STDs have a long incubation period. For HIV testing it is accepted practice to conduct a second antibody test three months after exposure, although some individuals take longer to seroconvert. In the case of syphilis it can take some time after the disappearance of the primary chancre, which may go totally unnoticed, before the basic screening tests (VDRL or RPR) become positive. Therefore it is mandatory to conduct a second examination for STDs at least 3 months after exposure. To prevent transmission during the period before seroconversion, safe sexual practices, foremost through condom use, need to be emphasized.

Recipients of blood transfusions in developing countries where blood screening procedures are often less complete and reliable, are candidates for repeated screening for HIV and syphilis. In such a context there is a potential risk for acquiring hepatitis B and C, or for trypanosomiasis as well. During the incubation period, blood recipients need to adopt safe sexual practices.

Viral hepatitis

As hepatitis B may be considered as a STD and/or as an infection highly endemic in the tropics, it has its place in the post-travel screening procedure. Vaccination offers satisfactory protection in most people. In unvaccinated travelers who have been recently exposed to unprotected sex with a partner likely to be chronically infected with hepatitis B, or who received injections or tattoos etc., testing for hepatitis B surface antigen will detect recent infection or the carrier state. Testing for both hepatitis B surface and core antibody will provide information on past exposure and seroconversion, or on previous vaccination in unsuspecting travelers.

Screening for hepatitis A may be indicated for unvaccinated, frequent or long-stay travelers who may have had a subclinical infection and wish is to know whether they require the vaccine for future travel. Hepatitis A antibody prevalence among unvaccinated people from industrialized countries born after World War II is low, and morbidity increases with age.

Although the prevalence of hepatitis C is relatively high in some developing countries, sexual practices do not play an important role in transmission. Systematic screening of asymptomatic low/medium risk travelers has not been proven to be cost-effective.[14] Apart from persons with a history of intravenous drug use, screening for hepatitis C should be restricted to travelers who have received a blood transfusion in a developing country where blood screening may be substandard.

Parasitic diseases

Although parasitic infections in travelers are not rare, only a handful of these organisms potentially cause serious morbidity: schistosomiasis, strongyloidiasis, and invasive amebiasis.[15]

Schistosomiasis

Infection with *Schistosoma spp.* should be be suspected in any traveler who has been in contact with potentially infested fresh water in endemic areas. This includes swimming or bathing in rivers, lakes, ponds, and irrigated wet rice fields, and also wading through seasonally flooded areas with runoffs from contaminated fresh water sources. Even when the parasite burden is light, infection may sometimes cause severe neurological impairment, most notably transverse myelitis following embolization of schistosome eggs, or adult worms in the spinal cord.[16]

The first stage of infection usually passes unnoticed, although a pruritic, papular rash ('swimmers' itch) may sometimes appear soon after exposure. Primary infection with *Schistosoma mansoni* may cause an hypersensitivity reaction with fever and cough when adult worms begin producing eggs, the so called 'Katayama syndrome'. Marked hypereosinophilia is frequent. As the incubation period of this syndrome ranges from three weeks to three months, any possible risk should lead the practitioner to warn travelers of potential future symptoms: fever, persistent cough and/or dyspnea. Schistosome antibodies and schistosome eggs in stools or in rectal biopsies do not appear until at least 4–8 weeks after inoculation, and it may take weeks after the onset of the febrile episode that the final diagnosis can be established.[17] A follow-up examination is advisable after at least three months in asymptomatic individuals. Longterm residents or travelers in endemic regions rarely incur heavy parasite loads. Therefore, late stage latent disease manifestations such as periportal liver fibrosis by *Schistosoma mansoni* are hardly ever seen in this risk group.

Infection with *S. hematobium* causes non-specific urinary tract inflammation, involving the ureter and bladder wall, sometimes associated with pseudopolyps and obstruction. These changes result in microscopic hematuria in the unsuspecting traveler when the parasite load is moderate to high, often leading to cystoscopy for suspicion of bladder malignancy.[17] Stool or urine microscopy is a rather insensitive method to diagnose active intestinal or urinary schistosomiasis. The 'rectal snip' technique is at least ten times more sensitive and requires 4–6 superficial rectal biopsies, squeezed between microscopy slides, to observe the characteristic eggs containing a viable miracidium, embedded in the mucosa.

Detection of schistosome antibodies is currently the preferred routine screening test for infection. Seroconversion usually occurs within three months, but occasionally takes up to one year. Antibody detection is both sensitive and specific, but does not provide information about the worm load. A positive test does not necessarily mean that infection is still active, as antibody titers remain detectable many years after successful treatment.

Schistosome antigen tests are currently being developed and might replace egg detection in the future as a probe for active infection.

Strongyloidiasis

Strongyloidiasis may persist lifelong through its endogenous re-infection cycle and may produce a potentially lethal disseminated hyperinfection in patients put on high dose steroids or immunosuppressants, or in immunocompromised persons. Eosinophilia is often absent (20–60%) or eosinophils may only be mildly elevated. Suspicion of infection is high in patients with a history of intermittent pruritis, serpiginous urticaria, hypereosinophilia, and/or a positive serology. Stool microscopy for the detection of rhabditiform larvae should be the next diagnostic procedure. Although the sensitivity of a single stool examination is too low to be reliable, it may be markedly increased by repeating stool examinations (20–30% for a single exam, up to 100% after seven stool exams), or by performing specific concentration methods like the 'Baermann' concentration or the agar culture test.[18] Though the latter techniques are not complicated, they are time-consuming and thus not cost-effective as a screening test in asymptomatic travelers. It is yet unclear how serology and stool concentration tests for *S. stercoralis* compare, but combining both in suspected cases probably produces the best results, with a sensitivity of 97% in some series.

Detecting *S. stercoralis* antigen in stool using an ELISA technique is a useful alternative to detect infection, is relatively specific and sensitive, but is currently only available in specialized centers.

Invasive amebiasis

Detection of amebic infection is still problematic. Amebic colitis and liver abscess are by far the most important clinical manifestations of invasive amebiasis However, the patient may remain asymptomatic with a latent infection for many months or even years.

Stool microscopy is not a reliable test for *E. histolytica* infection. It is important to remember that the vast majority of asymptomatic amebic cyst passers harbor the non-pathogenic *E. dispar* species (>90%), indistinguishable microscopically from the potentially invasive *E. histolytica* species. While only *E. histolytica* deserves treatment, one has to rely on techniques that identify the pathogenic species.[19]

For the diagnosis of the asymptomatic *E. histolytica* carrier state, the current gold standard diagnostic test relies on a DNA amplification procedure, through PCR, from fecal material containing cysts. Unfortunately, the process is tricky and cumbersome, and therefore still out of reach of a clinical laboratory. Recently, *E. histolytica* copro-antigen tests have been developed and their performance seems adequate.

Serum antibody tests for *Entamoeba histolytica* have proven their value in active invasive disease, and data are encouraging on their use in asymptomatic cyst carriers. It would be tempting, as some authors report, to use the antibody test as a marker for microinvasive infection in asymptomatic cyst carriers; however, antibodies persist for many months after successful treatment. More comparative studies among diagnostic tests are needed to define the best strategy.

It is as yet unclear whether treatment with non-absorbed 'contact' amebicides will suffice in the management of asymptomatic *E. histolytica* carriers. A positive serum antibody test in an asymptomatic individual probably indicates subclinical invasion and might warrant combination treatment with 'tissue' amebicides such as metronidazole, although this approach is controversial.

Other intestinal parasites

Other intestinal nematode infections (*Ascaris lumbricoides*, *Trichuris trichiura*, hookworm) rarely achieve parasite burdens that lead to significant symptoms in adult travelers and expatriates, with the exception of the rare aberrant migration of an adult ascaris into the bile duct.[20] Occasionally, peptic-ulcer like symptoms may appear, even in light hookworm infections.

In asymptomatic travelers, direct microscopy (with and without use of a concentration method) of a single stool sample is usually sufficiently sensitive to detect the majority of clinically significant nematode infections (*A. lumbricoides*, *T. trichiura*, *A. duodenale*, *N. americanus*) and pathogenic intestinal protozoa; however, it is notable that *S. stercoralis* is often not found by these methods (see above).

Among the intestinal protozoa seen in asymptomatic travelers, *Giardia lamblia* is the most common. It can be detected by means of microscopy of a single, concentrated stool sample stained with Lugol, but in some cases multiple samples may be required. Cross infection between close partners and family members, particularly young children, is not unusual, and, although controversial, treatment of asymptomatic infections might be warranted in high risk situations.[21] Occasionally, *Isospora belli* and *Cyclospora cayetanensis* are found by simple microscopy in stools of asymptomatic travelers. Detection of *Cryptosporidium spp.* however, requires specific staining methods. Treatment is not warranted in asymptomatic or convalescing persons, as these infections are self-limited (except in the immunocompromised) and rarely transmitted by direct contact.

An ever expanding array of copro-antigen tests have been introduced in the previous decade, and will continue to increase in the near future. Currently available antigen tests for *Giardia lamblia* and *Cryptosporidium spp.* perform as well as microscopy, and are less time-consuming. As a consequence, there is a tendency for antigen tests to supplant microscopy that requires more skilled technical expertise. However, since a large number of copro-antigen kits must be used simultaneously to screen for potentially pathogenic intestinal parasites this might push up the screening price tag to unacceptable levels. In the asymptomatic traveler it would probably be advisable to restrict copro-antigen screening to the 'big three' of intestinal parasites (*E. histolytica*, *Strongyloides stercoralis*, and *Schistosoma spp.*), once these tests have proven their diagnostic value.

Other parasitic infections

For many parasitic diseases, serum antibody tests still provide the main diagnostic screening tool to detect exposure or latent infection in asymptomatic travelers. Most techniques currently used are based on an ELISA or on an immunofluorescent antibody assay.

The tests are relatively easy to standardize and to perform, and therefore quite convenient, however, sensitivity or specificity is often uncertain in asymptomatic or light infections. Antibody tests do not provide information on parasite viability nor on parasite burden, (e.g.,schistosomiasis) and the antibody response may persist many years after exposure and curative treatment.

Malaria

Many travelers who have been treated for malaria during travel are anxious to have the diagnosis confirmed. The malaria antibody response persists for at least 2 months after treatment. Therefore, antibody detection may be used in the retrospective diagnosis of malaria in non-immune travelers.[22]

Recurrent infection with benign tertian malaria (*P. vivax*, *P. ovale*) is prevented by treating the latent liver stage. Malaria antibody testing enables the clinician to differentiate between a past *P. falciparum* and a benign tertian malaria infection. Malaria antibody assays cross-react with each other but can be semi-quantified. To interpret correctly the results, the incriminating species produces the highest antibody titer. This does not apply so much to quartan malaria with *P. malariae*. Retrospective malaria antibody testing is not frequently utilized in North America.

Filariasis

In asymptomatic travelers, antibody testing is the usual procedure to detect filarial infection, although the serological response does not identify a particular species. In fact, the test is highly non-specific because of significant cross-reactivity with other helminths.

Blood microfilaria may sometimes be found in a 'thick film' from unsuspecting long-term travelers infected with *Mansonella perstans*, and occasionally in those with Loa loa. Case reports of lymphatic filariasis in asymptomatic travelers are scarce.

However, focused detection requires either microfilaria concentration techniques, or provocation tests (DEC-test). Night-time sampling for microfilaria in bancroftian filariasis (*Wuchereria bancrofti*) has been largely supplanted by filarial antigen detection. These tests may take up to one year to turn positive. after exposure.

Diagnosis of cutaneous filariasis with *Onchocerca volvulus* requires detection of microfilaria in skin snips or in exudate from superficial scarifications of the affected skin. Ophthalmologic examination of the cornea and the anterior chamber may reveal microfilaria, or characteristic corneal lesions (punctate keratitis).

Occasionally, relatively mild symptoms may occur periodically in loiasis (Calabar swellings, superficial ocular migration) and in onchocerciasis (pruritis) some time after exposure.

Trypanosomiasis

Serological screening for American trypanosomiasis (*T. cruzi*) should be restricted to adventurous travelers who have been exposed to triatomid bugs in poor housing facilities in endemic areas in South America. Screening for West African trypanosomiasis (*T. gambiense*) should be restricted to the occasional long-term resident and missionary who reports exposure to tse-tse flies in areas in Africa known for intense transmission. East African trypanosomiasis does not require screening since it has a short incubation period and always produces an acute febrile disease.

Expert advice should be sought in case serology is found to be positive.

REFERENCES

1. McLean JD, Libman M. Screening the returning travelers. *Inf Dis Clin Trav Med* 1998; **12**(2):431–443.
2. Whitty CJ, Carroll B, Armstrong M, *et al*. Utility of history, examination and laboratory tests in screening those returning to Europe from the tropics for parasitic infection. *Trop Med Int Health* 2000; **5**(11):818–823.
3. Carroll B, Dow C, Snashall D, Marshall T, Chiodini PL. Post-tropical screening: how useful is it? *BMJ* 1993; **307**(6903):541.
4. The Canadian Task Force on the Periodic Health Examination. *The Canadian Guide to Clinical Preventive Health Care*. Ottawa: Canada Communication Group-Publishing; 1994.
5. Wintour K, Jones ME. *Routine Medical Evaluation of Expatriate Volunteers - Retrospective Analysis of 613 Patients*. 7th Conference of the International Society of Travel Medicine (CISTM7), Innsbruck, 27–31 May 2001: Abstract FC09.03
6. WHO. *Vaccination Requirements and Health Advice*. Geneva: International Travel and Health; 2001. Yearly update see : www.who.int/ith.
7. Weller PF. Eosinophilia in travelers. *Med Clin North Am* 1992; **76**:1413–1432.
8. Cobelens FG, Deutekom H van, Draayer-Jansen IW, *et al*. Risk of infection with Mycobacterium tuberculosis in travelers to areas of high tuberculosis endemicity. *Lancet* 2000; **356**(9228):461–465.
9. Lifson AR. Mycobacterium tuberculosis infection in travelers: tuberculosis comes home (commentary). *Lancet* 2000; **356**(4423)
10. Rieder HL. Risk of travel-associated tuberculosis. *Clin Infect Dis* 2001; **33**(8):1393–1396.
11. Matteelli A, Carosi G. Sexually transmitted diseases in travelers. *Clin Infect Dis* 2001; **32**(7):1063–1067.
12. Wang CC, Celum CL. Global risk of sexually transmitted diseases. *Med Clin North Am* 1999; **83**(4):975–995.
13. Bos JM, Fennema JS, Postma MJ. Cost-effectiveness of HIV screening of patients attending clinics for sexually transmitted diseases in Amsterdam. *AIDS* 2001; **15**(15):2031–2036.
14. Singer ME, Younoussi ZM. Cost-effectiveness of screening for hepatitis C virus in asymptomatic average risk adults. *Am J Med* 2001; **111**(8):667–668.
15. Libman MD, MacLean D, Gyorkos TW. Screening for schistosomiasis, filariasis, and strongyloidiasis among expatriates returning from the tropics. *Clin Infect Dis* 1993; **17**:353–359.
16. CDC. Acute schistosomiasis with transverse myelitis in American students returning from Kenya. *MMWR* 1984; **33**:445–447.
17. Harries AD, Fryatt R, Walker J, Chiodini PL, Bryceson ADM. Schistosomiasis in expatriates returning to Britain from the tropics: a controlled study. *Lancet* 1986; **86**(i):86.
18. Mahmoud A. Strongyloidiasis. *Clin Infect Dis* 1996; **23**(5):949–952.

19. Ravdin JI, Petri WA. Entamoeba histolytica (Amoebiasis). In: Mandell GL, Bennett JE, Dolin R, eds. *Principles and practice of infectious diseases. 4th edn.* New York: Churchill Livingstone; 1995:2395–2408.

20. Gilles HM. Soil-transmitted helminths. In: Cook GC, ed. *Manson's Tropical Diseases.* 20th edn. London: Saunders; 1996:1369–1412.

21. Farthing MJ, Cevallos AM, Kelly P. Intestinal protozoa. In: Cook GC, ed. *Manson's Tropical Diseases.* 20th edn. London: Saunders; 1996:1255–1298.

22. Jelinek T, Sonnenburg F von, Kumlien S, Loscher T, Nothdurft HD. Retrospective immunodiagnosis of malaria in nonimmune travelers returning from the tropics. *J Travel Med* 1995; **2**(4):225–228.

CHAPTER 52 Fever

Mary E. Wilson and Eli Schwartz

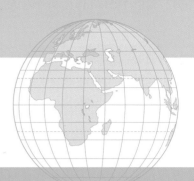

KEYPOINTS

- A total of 2–3% of returned travelers present with fever

- Infections with a worldwide distribution account for 50% of the fevers

- The approach to feverish patient has to consider travel and exposure history, incubation period, mode of exposure and impact of pre-travel vaccination

- Many febrile infections are associated with focal signs and symptoms that can limit the differential diagnosis

- Routine laboratory results may provide clues to the final diagnosis

INTRODUCTION

Fever in a returned traveler demands prompt attention. While fever may be the manifestation of a self-limited, trivial infection, it can also presage an infection that could be rapidly progressive and lethal. International travel expands the list of infections that must be considered but does not eliminate common, cosmopolitan infections. Initial attention should focus most urgently on infections that are treatable, transmissible, and that cause serious sequelae or death.[1] The characteristics of the places visited and recency of travel will affect the urgency and extent of the initial work up. This chapter will focus on identifying the cause of fever in a returned traveler. The reader should refer to other sources for the specifics of therapy.

EPIDEMIOLOGY OF FEVER IN TRAVELERS

How common is fever in returning travelers?

Fever in the absence of other prominent findings has been reported in 2–3% of European and American travelers to developing countries. Among 784 American travelers who traveled three months or less to developing countries, 3% reported fever unassociated with other illness.[2] These results are similar to those reported in classic studies by Steffen *et al.*[3] in which 152 of 7886 (almost 2%) of Swiss travelers with short-term travel to developing countries reported 'high fevers over several days' on questionnaires completed several months after return. Of those with fever, 39% reported fever only while abroad, 37% had fevers while abroad and at home and 24% had fevers at home only.

Another source of information about illness in travelers is GeoSentinel, a global network of 27 travel and tropical medicine clinics, doing systematic surveillance on travelers since 1996. Analysis of the database available as of late 2001 showed that 22.6% (4063 of 17 993) of ill-returned travelers (including outpatients and hospitalized patients) had fever as a chief complaint (Leisa Weld, unpublished data, 2002).

Causes of fever in returned travelers

Published series that examine the causes of fever after travel yield relevant data. Findings from three studies (one each in Canada,[4] the UK,[5] and Australia[6]) that examined causes of fever after tropical travel are shown in Table 52.1. Malaria was the most common diagnosis among those requiring hospitalization for fever, accounting for 27–42% of admissions in two recently published series.[4,6] Among 336 travelers and migrants in Switzerland who presented to an outpatient clinic with a history of fever or malaise and who had blood tests for malaria, 29% had laboratory confirmation of malaria.[7] Infections, such as respiratory tract infections, hepatitis, diarrheal illness, urinary tract infections and pharyngitis, with a broad or worldwide distribution, accounted for more than half of fevers in some series[4,5] and the cause of fever remained undefined in about one-quarter of cases. Specific agents most often identified, in addition to malaria, include dengue fever, hepatitis A, rickettsial infections, streptococcal pharyngitis, typhoid fever, gastrointestinal infections (caused by campylobacter, salmonella, shigella) and amebic liver abscess. In the GeoSentinel database among travelers with a confirmed diagnosis, malaria was the most common specific agent identified in travelers with fever (Leisa Weld, unpublished data, 2002).

Differences between travelers and local residents

Important differences exist between short-term travelers to developing countries and residents or long term visitors in types of infections commonly seen and in clinical manifestations. These differences reflect differences in likelihood of exposure to infections and age and intensity of exposure. For example, melioidosis (caused by the gram-negative soil- and water-associated bacterium *Burkholderia pseudomallei*) is a common cause of community-acquired sepsis in northern Thailand, yet is rarely seen in short-term travelers. In many developing countries hepatitis A is not viewed as an important problem. Clinical disease is largely unknown because most children are infected at a young age when infection is mild and often unrecognized. Older children and adults are immune, but the virus regularly contaminates food and water and poses a threat to non-immune travelers who enter the area. Katayama syndrome, an immune-complex mediated disease, is seen in travelers and persons newly infected with schistosomiasis but not in residents of endemic areas who have been repeatedly exposed to the parasite.[8]

Table 52.1	Causes of fever from published series (UK, Canada, Australia)		
	Doherty (195) (%) of total	MacLean (587) (%)	O'Brien (232) (%)
Malaria	42	32	27
Respiratory tract infection[a]	2.6	11	24
Diarrhea/dysentery	6.7	4.5	14
Dengue	6.2	2	8
Hepatitis	3 (hepatitis A only)	6	3 (hepatitis A only)
Enteric fever	1.5	2	3
UTI/pyelo	2.6	4	2
Rickettsial	0.5	1	2
Tuberculosis	1.6	1	0.4
Amebiasis/liver abscess	0	1	1
No diagnosis	24.6	25	9

[a]Respiratory tract infection: includes URI, pneumonia, and bronchitis

APPROACH TO THE PATIENT WITH FEVER

The travel and exposure history

The fever pattern and clinical findings for many infections are similar. A detailed history of where a person has lived and traveled (including intermediate stops and modes of travel), dates of travel and time since return, as well as activities during travel (such as types of accommodations, food habits, exposures including sexual exposures, needle and blood exposures, animal and arthropod bites, water exposures) and vaccinations and other preparation before travel and prophylaxis or treatment during or after travel are essential in developing a list of what infections are possible based on potential exposures and usual incubation periods.

During the work up the clinician should keep in mind that fever after exotic travel may reflect infection with a common, cosmopolitan pathogen acquired during travel or after return home. At the same time, it should be noted that unfamiliar infections can be acquired in industrialized countries (such as plague, Rocky Mountain spotted fever, tularemia, Lyme disease, hantavirus pulmonary syndrome in North America and visceral leishmaniasis, hemorrhagic fever with renal syndrome and other hantaviral infections, and tick-borne encephalitis in Europe).

A detailed review of the clinical course, supplemented by the physical examination and laboratory data will help to determine more likely causes and also to identify any infections that might require urgent interventions, hence expedited diagnostic studies. The process involved in the evaluation can be summarized in these questions:

- What diagnoses are possible based on the geographic areas visited?
- What diagnoses are possible based on the time of travel, taking into account incubation periods?
- What diagnoses are more likely based on activities, exposures, host factors, and clinical and laboratory findings?
- Among the possible diagnoses, what is treatable, transmissible or both?

Incubation period

Incubation time is a valuable tool in evaluating a febrile patient. Knowledge of the incubation periods can allow one to exclude infec-

tions that are not biologically plausible. For example, dengue fever typically has an incubation of 3–14 days. Thus fever that begins more than two weeks after return from Thailand is not likely to be related to dengue fever. Remote travel is sometimes relevant but most severe, acute life-threatening infections result from exposures that have occurred within the past 3 months. Important treatable infections that may occur more than 3 months after return include malaria, amebic liver abscess and visceral leishmaniasis. In the study by O'Brien et al.[6] that analyzed hospitalized patients with fever after travel, 96% were seen within 6 months of return from travel. Although the initial focus should be on travel within the past 3–6 months, the history should extend to include exposures a year or more earlier, if the initial investigation is unrevealing. Approximately 30% of patients with vivax malaria in the USA had onset of symptoms more than 6 months after return. In 2–4% of cases of malaria symptoms may begin a year or more after return.[9,10] Table 52.2 lists many of the infections seen in travelers by time of onset of symptoms relative to the exposure and the initial clinical presentation. In assessing potential incubation period one must take into account the duration of the trip (and points of potential exposure during travel) and time since return.

Mode of exposure

Infections that can be acquired by a single bite of an infective arthropod, ingestion of contaminated food or beverages, swimming in contaminated water, or from direct contact with an infected person or animal are most often seen in short-term travelers. Casual sexual contact with new partners is common in travelers (5–50% among short-term travelers) and inquiry about sexual exposures should be included as part of the history of an ill traveler. A recent study found that 15% of Canadians reported sex with a new partner or potential exposure to blood and body fluids through injections, dental work, tattoos, or other skin perforating procedures during international travel.[11] This history is important to review even in returned travelers who are not acutely ill. Examples of specific exposures associated with infections are listed in Table 52.3. In many instances, travelers will be unaware of exposures. For example, patients with mosquito and tick-borne infections may not recall any bites. In contrast, patients who have had freshwater exposure (such as swimming, wading, bathing, or rafting) that places them at risk for schistosomiasis will typically

Table 52.2   Causes of fever by usual incubation periods and geographic distribution

Disease/organism	Distribution
Incubation <2 weeks	
Undifferentiated fever	
Malaria	Tropics, subtropics, especially Africa
Dengue	Topics, subtropics, especially Asia
Rickettsial infections	
Spotted fever rickettsiae	Widespread; species vary by region
Typhus group rickettsiae	All continents
Scrub typhus	Especially Asia
Leptospirosis	Global; more common in tropics
Typhoid and paratyphoid	Global; high risk in Indian subcontinent
Brucellosis	Widespread; more common in developing areas
Acute HIV	Global
Tularemia	Especially N America and Europe
Relapsing fever	
(tick-borne)	Widespread
(louse-borne)	Limited foci
Fever and hemorrhage	
Meningococcemia, leptospirosis, and other acute bacterial infections	
Dengue (see above)	
Lassa fever	Africa, especially western, sub-Saharan
Yellow fever	Sub-Saharan Africa and tropical Latin America
Hemorrhagic fever with renal syndrome	Primarily Asia and Europe
Crimean-Congo hemorrhagic fever	Africa, eastern Europe and western Asia
Other hemorrhagic fevers in Africa:	
Ebola, Marburg, Rift Valley fever	
Hemorrhagic fevers from South America caused by Junin, Machupo, Sabia, Guanarito viruses	
Fever and CNS findings	
Meningococcal meningitis and many bacteria, viruses, and fungi with wide distribution	
African trypanosomiasis (sleeping sickness)	Focal areas of sub-Saharan Africa
Japanese encephalitis	Primarily Asia
Tick-borne encephalitis	Central and eastern Asia; far eastern Russia, Asia
Polio	Primarily Africa, parts of Asia
West Nile encephalitis	Widespread in Africa, Europe, Asia, Americas
Rabies	Most common in parts of Africa, Asia, Latin America
Angiostrongylus cantonensis	Most common in East, SE Asia, scattered cases elsewhere
Fever and pulmonary findings	
Influenza and other respiratory viruses, pneumococcal pneumonia, mycoplasma, Chlamydia, coronavirus	
Legionnaires'	Widespread; outbreaks in hotels, in cruise ships
Acute histoplasmosis	Especially in the Americas
Acute coccidioidomycosis	Americas
Hantavirus pulmonary syndrome	Widespread, especially in the Americas
Q fever (see below)	
Melioidosis	Especially SE Asia
Incubation 2 weeks to 2 months	
Malaria, typhoid fever, leptospirosis, brucellosis, African trypanosomiasis, melioidosis, and many of the hemorrhagic fevers and fungal infections can have incubation periods that exceed 2 weeks.	
Amebic liver abscess	Most common in developing regions
Toxoplasmosis, acute	Worldwide
Hepatitis A	Most common in developing areas
Hepatitis E	Widespread; outbreaks in Asia, Africa, Latin America
Schistosomiasis (acute)	Mainly in Africa; also in Asia, Latin America
Q fever	Widespread
Bartonellosis (*B. bacilliformis*)	Especially mountain areas of South America
Incubation >2 months	
Many of these infections can have incubation period shorter than 2 months	
Malaria, amebic liver abscess, melioidosis, and rabies, listed above, can have incubation >2 months.	
Hepatitis B	Worldwide
Leishmaniasis, visceral	Areas of risk in Africa, Asia, South America, southern Europe
Tuberculosis	Worldwide with wide range in incidence rates
Filariasis, lymphatic	Tropical regions
Fascioliasis	Sheep and cattle raising areas

Table 52.3	Examples of specific exposures leading to infections causing fever
Exposure	**Infections**
Sex, blood and body fluid exposures (includes injections, tattoos, medical procedures)	Hepatitis A, hepatitis B, hepatitis C, hepatitis D (coninfection with hepatitis B), CMV, HIV, syphilis
Freshwater (occupational or recreational contact)	Schistosomiasis, leptospirosis
Rodents (and their excreta)	Hantaviruses, Lassa fever and other hemorrhagic fevers, plague, rat-bite fever
Dogs, bats, other animals (bites and saliva exposure)	Rabies, herpes B virus (monkeys), mouth bacteria
Soil	Several fungi (e.g., histoplasmosis, coccidioidomycosis)
Ingestions	Raw vegetables, water plants: fascioliasis Unpasteurized milk and milk products: brucellosis, salmonellosis, tuberculosis Raw or undercooked shellfish: clonorchiasis, paragonimiasis, vibrios, hepatitis A Raw or undercooked animal flesh: trichinosis, salmonella, E. coli O157: H7, campylobacter, toxoplasmosis
Animal and animal products	Q fever, brucellosis, tularemia, anthrax, plague, toxoplasmosis, psittacosis

recall the exposure with focused questioning, though they may have been unaware that the exposure carried any risk for infection.

Impact of pre-travel vaccination

The history should include a review of pre-travel vaccines, including dates of vaccination, types of vaccines received, and number of doses for multidose vaccines. Vaccines vary greatly in efficacy, and knowledge of vaccine status can influence the probability that certain infections will be present. For example, hepatitis A and yellow fever vaccines have high efficacy and only rare instances of infection have been reported in vaccinated travelers. In contrast, the typhoid fever vaccines (oral and parenteral) give incomplete protection and do not protect against *Salmonella paratyphi*.[12] The protective efficacy with the available typhoid vaccines was estimated to be 60–72% in field trials in endemic regions.[13]

CLINICAL PRESENTATIONS

Many febrile infections are associated with focal signs or symptoms, which may help to limit the differential diagnosis. Undifferentiated fever can be more challenging. The following sections discuss common clinical presentations with focus on more common diseases causing each. Other chapters provide more detailed discussions of diarrhea, skin diseases, and respiratory diseases.

Undifferentiated fever

Always look for malaria

Malaria remains the most important infection to consider in anyone with fever after visiting or living in malarious areas. In non-immune travelers falciparum malaria can be fatal if not diagnosed and treated urgently. Although most patients with malaria will report fever, as many as 40% or more may not have fever at the time of initial medical evaluation.[14] Risk of malaria varies greatly from one endemic region to another, but in general risk is highest in parts of sub-

Saharan Africa; most severe and fatal cases in travelers follow exposure in this region. Tests to look for malaria should be done urgently (same day) and repeated in 8–24 h if the initial blood smears are negative. Infected erythrocytes may be sequestered in deep vasculature in patients with falciparum malaria so few parasites may be seen on a blood smear even in a severely ill patient.

Prompt evaluation is most critical in persons who have visited areas with falciparum malaria in recent weeks. In the USA, almost 90% of reported patients with acute falciparum malaria had onset of symptoms within a month of return to the USA.[9] Use of chemoprophylaxis may ameliorate symptoms or delay onset. No chemoprophylactic agent is 100% effective, so malaria tests should be done even in persons who report taking chemoprophylaxis. Many antimicrobials (e.g., TMP-SMX, azithromycin, doxycycline, clindamycin) have some activity against plasmodia. Taking these drugs for reasons unrelated to malaria may delay onset of symptoms of malaria or modify the clinical course.

Although fever and headache are commonly reported in malaria, gastrointestinal and pulmonary symptoms may be prominent and may misdirect the initial attention toward other infections. Thrombocytopenia and absence of leukocytosis are common laboratory findings.

Dengue

Dengue, a mosquito-transmitted flavivirus that exists in four serotypes, is the most common arbovirus in the world. It is increasing in incidence in endemic areas and is an increasingly common cause of fever in returned travelers.[15–17] Dengue is found in tropical and subtropical regions throughout the world. Among travelers dengue is seen most often in visitors to Southeast Asia and Latin America (including the Caribbean) and infrequently in travelers to Africa. Because humans are the main reservoir for the dengue virus, which is transmitted primarily by the *Aedes aegypti* mosquito that inhabits urban areas and lives in close association with humans, travelers visiting only urban areas can become infected. Symptoms of dengue, also known as breakbone fever, typically begin 4–7 days (range 3–14 days) after exposure. Common findings are fever, frontal headache, and myalgia. Approximately 50% of patients have skin findings, which can be a diffuse erythema or a maculopapular or petechial eruption. Intense itching may be present toward the end of the febrile period. Leukopenia, thrombocytopenia, and elevated transaminases are common laboratory findings. The most serious forms of infection, dengue hemorrhagic fever (DHF) and dengue shock syndrome (DSS) occur primarily in persons who have a second dengue infection with a different serotype. This helps explain why these complications are rare among travelers. In a well-characterized outbreak in Cuba, 98.5% of DHF/DSS cases were in persons with a prior dengue infection. The attack rate of DHF/DSS was 4.2% in persons with prior dengue infection who became infected with a new serotype.[18]

Supportive care, including i.v. fluids, can be lifesaving in DHF/DSS. Diagnosis is usually confirmed by serologic tests; viral isolation or detection of viral RNA by PCR is available in some laboratories. Because specific IgM antibodies take several days to develop (usually present by day 5 of illness), serologic diagnosis may not be possible in the early febrile period. IgG antibody response can be difficult to interpret because of extensive cross reactions with other flaviviruses (e.g., yellow fever, Japanese encephalitis).[19]

It is likely that only a minority of cases that occur in travelers are documented. Two Israeli studies try to estimate the attack rate in travelers. Among 104 young Israeli adults who had spent at least 3 months in tropical areas, four (3.8%) had dengue-specific IgM antibodies, suggesting recent dengue infection.[20] In another study, the attack rate was 3.4/1000 travelers to Thailand in 1998.[21] In 1998, the 90 laboratory diagnosed infections reported to the US Centers for Disease Control reflected a 70% increase from 1997.[15]

Rickettsial infections

Rickettsial infections are widely distributed in developed and developing countries and often named for a geographic region where they are found, though names can mislead. *Rickettsia rickettsii*, the cause of Rocky Mountain spotted fever in the USA is found throughout the Americas from Canada to Brazil. Rickettsial infections, such as South African tick-bite fever (*R. africae*), Mediterranean tick typhus (*R. conorii*), and murine or endemic typhus (*R. typhi*), are important treatable infections in travelers.[22] They are being increasingly recognized in travelers, probably reflecting increased travel to high risk areas, such as southern Africa, and increased awareness among clinicians.[23] Diagnosis is usually made with serologic tests.

Clinical presentations of the rickettsial infections are varied, depending on the species. Most rickettsial infections are transmitted by arthropods, such as ticks and mites, and an eschar may mark the inoculation site. Eschars are often small (<1 cm in diameter), asymptomatic, and may be overlooked. In South African tick bite fever, eschars are often multiple (>50% of cases). Among 78 cases of tick typhus in German travelers, 87.2% had an eschar at the time of evaluation, but only 17.9% recalled having a tick bite at that site.[22] More than 70% had acquired their infections in southern Africa. Rashes may be present but many rickettsial infections (even among the spotted fever group rickettsia) are spotless. *R. australis*, *R. africae*, and rickettsialpox can cause a vesicular rash that may be mistaken for varicella, monkeypox, or even smallpox. High fever, headache, and normal or low white blood cell count and thrombocytopenia are characteristic. Lymphadenopathy may be present. Infections may be confused with dengue fever. Rickettsiae multiply in and damage endothelial cells and cause disseminated vascular lesions. Without treatment, the illness may persist for 2–3 weeks. Response to tetracyclines is generally prompt.

Other tick-borne infections, human monocytic ehrlichiosis and human granulocytic ehrlichiosis,[24] are most commonly diagnosed in the USA but are also found in Europe, Africa, and probably Asia.

Clinical findings include prominent fever and headache. These infections may also be associated with leukopenia, thrombocytopenia and they respond to treatment with tetracyclines.

Enteric fever

Enteric fever (typhoid and paratyphoid fever) is another infection that causes fever and headache and can be associated with an unremarkable physical examination, though a faint rash (rose spots) may appear at the end of the first week of illness. Laboratory findings include a normal or low white blood cell count, thrombocytopenia, and elevation (usually modest) of liver enzymes. Gastrointestinal symptoms, such as diarrhea, constipation and vague abdominal discomfort may be present, as well as dry cough. In contrast to the abrupt onset of fevers in dengue and rickettsial infections, the onset of typhoid fever may be insidious. Leukocytosis in a patient with typhoid fever should raise suspicion of intestinal perforation or other complication. Diagnosis should be confirmed by recovery of *Salmonella typhi* (or *S. paratyphi*) from blood or stool.[25] Culture of bone marrow aspirate may have higher yield than blood or feces but is generally not favored by clinicians and patients. Serologic tests lack sensitivity and specificity. Increasing resistance of *S. typhi* to many antimicrobials makes it important to isolate the organism and to do sensitivity testing. Resistance to ampicillin, TMP-SMZ, and chloramphenicol is now common, and resistance has also been reported to quinolones.

The efficacy of typhoid vaccines in published studies varies widely depending on the type of vaccine, number of doses, and population studied. As noted above, the efficacy of commonly used vaccines may be 60–70%.[13] The important observation for clinicians evaluating returned travelers is that typhoid fever remains a concern (albeit lower) in persons who have received a typhoid vaccine. Infections with *S. paratyphi* may be relatively more common as a cause of typhoid fever in vaccinated populations because vaccine protects mainly against *S. typhi*.[12,25]

Leptospirosis

Although leptospirosis has a broad geographic distribution, infections in humans are more common in tropical and subtropical regions. Recreational activities of travelers, including white water rafting in Costa Rica and other sports involving water exposures, have been associated with sporadic cases and large outbreaks.[26] Among 158 competitive swimmers in the Eco-Challenge in Malaysia in 2000, 44% met the case definition for acute leptospirosis.[27] Although clinical manifestations may be protean, common findings include fever, myalgia, and headache. Among 353 cases reported from Hawaii, 39% had jaundice and 28% conjunctival suffusion.[28] Other findings such as meningitis, rash, hemorrhage, and uveitis may be present. Multiple different serovars exist, and clinical presentation and severity vary with infecting serovar. In a large Brazilian urban outbreak in 1996, 43% of cases of leptospirosis were initially misdiagnosed as dengue fever.[29] It is important to recognize leptospirosis because antibiotic treatment significantly shortens duration of illness.[28]

Acute schistosomiasis

Acute schistosomaisis (Katayama fever) follows exposure to freshwater infested with cercariae that penetrate intact skin. The disease, seen primarily in non-immunes, manifests 3–8 weeks after exposure. Clinical manifestations include high fever, myalgia, lethargy, and intermittent urticaria.[30] Dry cough, dyspnea, sometimes with pulmonary infiltrates are noted in the majority of patients.[31] Eosinophilia, often high grade, is usually present. In one outbreak involving 12 travelers the median duration of fever was 12 days (range of 4–46 days) and 10 of 12 had eosinophilia during the first 10 weeks of infection.[30]

Amebic liver abscess

An amebic abscess can cause fever and chills that develop over days to weeks. Although focal findings may not be prominent, 85–90% of patients will report abdominal discomfort and about 70–80% will have right upper quadrant tenderness on examination.[32] Extension of infection to the diaphragmatic surface of the liver may lead to cough, pleuritic or shoulder pain, and right basilar abnormalities on chest X-ray, which may initially suggest a pulmonary process. The abscess can be seen by ultrasound and serology for *Entamoeba histolytica* is usually positive.

Hemorrhagic fevers

Several infections, in addition to exotic infections, such as Ebola and Marburg, can cause fever and hemorrhage in travelers and many are treatable. Leptospirosis, meningococcemia, and other bacterial infections can cause hemorrhage. Rickettsial infections can produce a petechial rash or purpura, and severe malaria may be associated with disseminated intravascular coagulation. Many viral infections, in addition to dengue, can cause hemorrhage. Most are arthropod-borne (especially mosquito or tick) or have rodent reservoir hosts. Among those reported in travelers are dengue fever (DHF), yellow fever, Lassa fever, Crimean Congo hemorrhagic fever, Rift Valley fever, hemorrhagic fever with renal syndrome (and other hantavirus-associated infections), Kyasanur Forest disease, Omsk hemorrhagic fever, and several viruses in South America (Junin, Machupo, Guanarito, Sabia). Other geographically focal infections can cause hemorrhagic fever and would be expected primarily in travelers who visit rural or remote areas. Lassa fever responds to ribavirin therapy if started early. Several of the viruses can be transmitted during medical care, so it is important to institute barrier isolation in a private room pending a specific diagnosis. Identification of viral agents causing hemorrhage may require the assistance from staff working in special laboratories, such as one available at CDC. (Assistance is available through the Special Pathogens Branch, Division of Viral and Rickettsial Diseases, CDC, Atlanta, GA 404 639 1511). Even when specific treatment is not available, good supportive care can save lives.

Fever and CNS changes

Neurological findings in the febrile patient indicate the need for prompt workup. High fever alone or in combination with metabolic alternations precipitated by systemic infections can cause changes in the mental status in the absence of CNS invasion. One must consider common, cosmopolitan bacterial, viral, and fungal infections that cause fever and CNS changes. Additional considerations in travelers include Japanese encephalitis, rabies, West Nile, polio, tick-borne encephalitis, and a number of other geographically focal viral infections, such as Nipah virus.

Outbreaks of meningococcal infections (meningococcemia and meningitis) have been associated with the annual pilgrimage to Mecca in Saudi Arabia for the Hajj. Beginning in 2000, for the first time ever, infection with *Neisseria meningitidis* serogroup W-135 caused outbreaks of meningococcal disease in pilgrims and subsequently in their contacts in multiple countries. Pilgrims vaccinated with the quadrivalent meningococcal vaccine (serogroups A, C, W-135 and Y) can still carry *N. meningitidis*. Dengue fever can cause neurological findings that mimic Japanese encephalitis. In a study in Vietnam, dengue-associated encephalopathy was found in 0.5% of 5400 children admitted with DHF.[33] Meningitis may be present in leptospirosis. The parasite *Angiostrongylus cantonensis* causes sporadic infection in many countries and was responsible for an outbreak of eosinophilic meningoencephalitis in travelers to Jamaica in 2000.[34] African trypanoso-

miasis (sleeping sickness), transmitted by an infective tsetse fly, initially causes a non-specific febrile illness. A chancre marks the site of the bite. If untreated, trypanosomes can infect the CNS and cause lethargy. A recent increase in cases has been noted in travelers to Tanzania and Kenya. Patients with malaria, typhoid fever, and rickettsial infections often have severe headache, but CSF is typically unremarkable in these infections. Cerebral malaria causes altered mental status and can progress to seizures and coma. Mefloquine taken for malaria chemoprophylaxis has rarely been associated with seizures and other neuropsychiatric side-effects but fever typically is absent. Neuroschistosomiasis can be seen in travelers, but fever usually is not present at the time of the focal neurological changes, caused by ectopic egg deposition.

Sexually transmitted infections, such as HIV and syphilis, whether acquired at home or during travel can involve the CNS. Lyme and ehrlichiosis are other treatable infections that can cause prominent neurological findings. Other treatable infections that are unfamiliar to clinicians in many geographic areas include Q fever, relapsing fever, brucellosis, bartonellosis, anthrax, and plague.

Fever and pulmonary findings

Prominent respiratory symptoms in a febrile recently returned traveler (including cruise ship traveler) should suggest common respiratory pathogens, such as *Streptococcus pneumoniae*, influenza, other respiratory viruses, mycoplasma, as well as Legionnaires disease and severe acute respiratory syndrome (SARS). The recent global epidemic of SARS has put health-care workers at significant risk of infection. Although fever, chills, headache, myalgia and dry cough are the common presenting features, the syndrome cannot be differentiated clinically or radiologically from other causes of atypical pneumonia. Therefore, health-care providers managing such patients who have recently returned from a SARS-endemic area, must institute both air-borne and contact precautions.[35,36–38] The fungal infections, histoplasmosis and coccidioidomycosis, have caused recent outbreaks in travelers.[39,40] Risk factors for inhalation of air-borne spores and subsequent infection have included exploration of caves and proximity to excavation or construction sites. Fever, headache, myalgia, and cough have been common. Q fever is a prominent cause of fever and pneumonia in some areas, e.g. Spain. Tuberculosis is a risk, especially for persons who spend months or longer in areas with high rates of tuberculosis. Symptoms may begin months or years after return.

Pulmonary infiltrates and respiratory symptoms may be present during the pulmonary migration phase of many parasites, including hookworm, ascaris, and strongyloidiasis. Schistosomiasis may cause fever and pulmonary infiltrates in its early stage (Katayama syndrome) due to immunological reaction to antigen release outside the pulmonary bed.[8,31] Respiratory failure occurs in hantavirus pulmonary syndrome and adult respiratory distress syndrome (ARDS) may complicate severe malaria. Hemorrhagic pneumonia is sometimes reported with leptospirosis. Other treatable infections with pulmonary findings are anthrax, plague, and tularemia.

The possibility of pulmonary emboli should also be kept in mind in travelers who have recently experienced long intercontinental flights. Low grade fever and pulmonary findings may initially suggest an infectious disease.

Persistent and relapsing fevers

Diagnoses to be considered in patients with persistent or relapsing fevers include malaria, typhoid fever, tuberculosis, brucellosis, CMV, toxoplasmosis, relapsing fever, melioidosis, Q fever, visceral leishmaniasis, histoplasmosis (and other fungal infections), West African trypanosomiasis, and infections that may be unrelated to exposures during travel, such as endocarditis.

LABORATORY CLUES

Routine laboratory studies

Results of routine laboratory findings may provide clues to the diagnosis in the febrile traveler. An elevated white blood cell count may suggest a bacterial infection, but a number of bacterial infections, such as uncomplicated typhoid fever, brucellosis, and rickettsial infections are associated with a normal or low white blood cell count. Table 52.4 provides a summary of findings on routine laboratory studies for infections commonly seen in febrile travelers.

Elevated liver enzymes

In the past hepatitis A virus was the most common cause of hepatitis after travel to developing regions. With the increasing awareness of this risk and the use of the hepatitis A vaccine, acute hepatitis A now is seen primarily in persons who failed to receive vaccine (or immune globulin) before travel. Hepatitis B remains a risk for unvaccinated persons. Hepatitis E, transmitted via fecally contaminated water or food, clinically resembles acute hepatitis A. Cases have been reported in travelers.[41] Mortality may be 20% or higher in women infected during the third trimester of pregnancy.

Many common as well as unusual systemic infections cause fever and elevation of liver enzymes. Among those that may be a concern, depending on geographic exposures, are yellow fever, dengue and other hemorrhagic fevers, typhoid fever, leptospirosis, rickettsial infections, toxoplasmosis, Q fever, syphilis, psittacosis, and brucellosis. Transaminases are often elevated in these infections. Parasites that directly invade the liver and bile ducts (e.g., amebic liver abscess and liver flukes) often cause right upper quadrant pain, tender liver and elevated alkaline phosphatase. Drugs and toxins can damage the liver so a careful review of these agents should be part of the history.

Fever and eosinophilia

Eosinophilia is sometimes an incidental finding on laboratory testing. When it is found in a person who has visited or lived in tropical, developing countries, it is a clue that should suggest several specific parasitic infections.[42] Before beginning an extensive work up to look for parasites, however, it is important to review carefully the general medical history for other processes that may be associated with eosinophilia and to review drug history (including drugs received during travel, over the counter drugs and drugs that may have been given by injection during travel). Many parasitic infections are not associated with eosinophilia or may be associated with eosinophilia only during one stage of development. Infections that can cause both eosinophilia and fever include acute schistosomiasis (Katayama syndrome), trichinosis, fascioliasis, gnathostomiasis, lymphatic filariasis, tropical pulmonary eosinophilia, toxocariasis, and loiasis. Many of these helminthic infections are seen primarily in persons with prior residence or prolonged stays in tropical developing countries. Acute coccidioidomycosis, resolving scarlet fever, and a few other non-helminthic infections may also be associated with eosinophilia, but in these infections eosinophilia usually is not high grade or persistent. The protozoan infections, malaria, amebiasis, giardiasis, and leishmaniasis, are not associated with eosinophilia.

Initial diagnostic workup

A careful, complete physical examination should be carried out, looking with special care for rashes or skin lesions, lymphadenopathy, retinal or conjunctival changes, enlargement of liver or spleen, genital lesions, and neurological findings. The initial laboratory evaluation in a febrile patient with a history of tropical exposures should generally include all or most of the following:

- complete blood count with a differential and estimate of platelets
- liver enzymes
- blood cultures
- blood smears for malaria
- urinalysis
- chest radiograph

Table 52.4 Usual laboratory findings and diagnostic tests for infections common in febrile travelers

	WBC-total	Eosinophils	Platelets	Liver enzymes	Diagnostic tests
Viral infections					
Dengue fever	Very low	Normal/low	Very low	Mild elevation	Serology; isolate virus; pcr
Viral hepatitis (A, B, E)	Normal/low	Normal/low	Normal/low	Very high	Serology
Bacterial infections					
Typhoid fever	Normal/low	Very low	Normal/low	Mild elevation	Isolate bacteria (blood, feces)
Rickettsial infections	Normal/low	Normal/low	Normal/low	Mild elevation	Serology; pcr; immunohistochemistry
Leptospirosis	Normal/high	Normal/low	Normal/low	Mild to very high	Serology; isolate (special media required)
Brucellosis	Normal/low	Normal/low	Normal/low	Mild elevation	Isolate bacteria; serology
Protozoa					
Malaria	Normal/low	Normal/low	Low	Mild elevation	Identify parasites on blood smear; detect antigen in blood
Visceral leishmaniasis	Low	Normal/low	Low	Normal or elevated	Identify parasite in tissue; culture; pcr
Amebic liver abscess	Normal/high	Normal/low	Normal	Normal or elevated	Serology; identify trophozoites in tissue/aspirate
Helminth					
Acute schistosomiasis (Katayama fever)	Normal/high	Very high	Normal	Mild elevation	Serology; identify eggs may be absent (at time of symptom onset)

If malaria is suspected, it is essential not only to request the appropriate tests for malaria, but also to make certain that tests are done expeditiously and by knowledgeable persons. In a patient with persisting fever, a repeat physical examination will sometimes identify new findings (e.g., new rash, splenomegaly) that can provide useful clues to the diagnosis. Table 52.4 lists tests used to diagnose common infections in febrile returned travelers.

The process of travel may lead to medical problems. The immobility associated with travel may predispose to deep vein thrombosis; sinusitis may flare up during or after travel, related to changes in pressure during ascent and descent. Non-infectious disease causes of fever, such as drug fever, and pulmonary emboli, should also be considered if initial studies do not confirm the presence of an infection.

Management

Prompt diagnosis and urgent treatment may be necessary to save the patient's life. During the evaluation and treatment, the clinician should also keep in mind the public health impact. Outside resources, such as CDC or other reference laboratories with special expertise may be needed to provide diagnostic studies or other support. Familiar infections (e.g., salmonella, campylobacter, gonorrhea) may be caused by multi-drug resistant organisms. It is especially important to recognize the potential for multidrug resistance in infections, such as typhoid fever, that can be lethal. Absence of response to what should be appropriate treatment should lead the clinician to consider drug resistance, the possibility of the wrong diagnosis, or presence of two infections. A number of case reports document the simultaneous presence of malaria and typhoid fever, amebic liver abscess and hepatitis A, and other dual infections (see Fig. 52.1).[43,44]

SOURCES OF CURRENT INFORMATION AND ASSISTANCE

Knowledge of the epidemiology of infections in a given geographic area is valuable but detailed, up-to-date information about a specific location may be unavailable. Electronic databases are a useful source of current information about disease outbreaks and alerts about antimicrobial resistance patterns. A review by Keystone *et al.* lists useful websites, including some with country or region-specific information.[45]

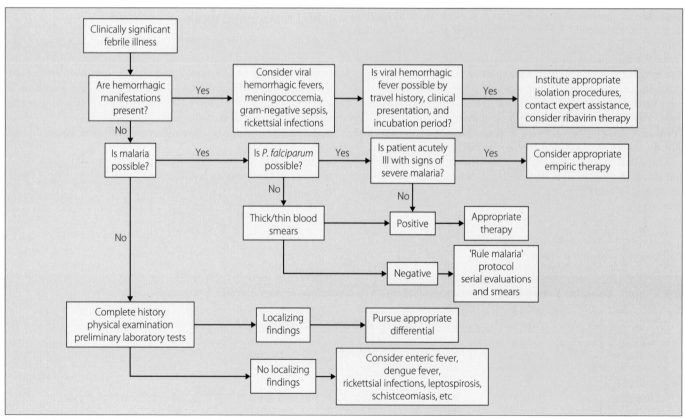

Figure 52.1 Flowchart for the management of a febrile patient.

REFERENCES

1. Wilson ME, Pearson R. Fever and systemic symptoms. In: Guerrant RL, Walker DH, Weller PF, eds. Tropical infectious diseases. *Principles, Pathogens, and Practice*. Philadelphia: Churchill Livingstone; 1999:1381–1399.
2. Hill D. Health problems in a large cohort of Americans traveling to developing countries. *J Travel Med* 2000; 7:259–266.
3. Steffen R, Rickenbach M, Willhelm U, *et al*. Health problems after travel to developing countries. *J Infect Dis* 1987; 156:84–91.
4. Doherty JF, Grant AD, Bryceson AD. Fever as the presenting complaint of travelers returning from the tropics. *Quart J Med* 1995; 88:277–281.
5. MacLean J, Lalonde R, Ward B. Fever from the tropics. *Travel Medicine Advisor* 1994; 5:27.2–27.14.
6. O'Brien D, Tobin S, Brown GV, Torresi J. Fever in returned travelers: review of hospital admissions for a 3-year period. *Clin Infect Dis* 2001; 33:603–609.
7. D'Acremont V, Landry P, Mueller I, Pecoud A, Genton B. Clinical and laboratory predictors of imported malaria in an outpatient setting: an aid to

the medial decision making in returning travelers with fever. *Am J Trop Med Hyg* 2002: **66**:481–486.

8. Ribeiro de Jesus A, Silva A, Santana LB, *et al.* Clinical and immunologic evaluation of 31 patients with acute Schistosomiasis mansoni. *J Infect Dis* 2001; **185**:98–105.

9. Centers for Disease Control and Prevention. CDC Surveillance summaries. Malaria Surveillance: United States, 1997. *MMWR* 2001; 50(SS-1):25–44.

10. Centers for Disease Control and Prevention. CDC Surveillance Summaries. Malaria Surveillance – United States, 1998. *MMWR* 2001; 7:1–18.

11. Correia JD, Shafer RT, Patel V, *et al.* Blood and body fluid exposure as a health risk for international travelers. *J Travel Med* 2001; **8**:263–266.

12. Schwartz E, Shlim DR, Eaton M, *et al.* The effect of oral and parenteral typhoid vaccination on the rate of infection with Salmonella typhi and Salmonella paratyphi among foreigners in Nepal. *Arch Intern Med* 1990; **150**:349–351.

13. Levine MM, Ferreccio C, Cryz S, *et al.* Comparison of enteric coated capsules and liquid formulation of Ty21a typhoid vaccine: a randomized controlled field trial. *Lancet* 1990; **336**:891–896.

14. Dorsey G, Gandhi M, Oyugi JH, Rosenthal PJ. Difficulties in the prevention, diagnosis, and treatment of imported malaria. *Arch Intern Med* 2000; **160**:2505–2510.

15. Centers for Disease Control and Prevention. Imported dengue – United States, 1997 and 1998. *MMWR* 2000; **49**:248–253.

16. Jelinek T. Dengue fever in international travelers. *Clin Infect Dis* 2000; **31**:144–147.

17. Schwartz E, Mendelson E, Sidi Y. Dengue fever among travelers. *Am J Med* 1996; **101**:516–520.

18. Guzman MG, Kouri G, Valdes L, *et al.* Epidemiologic studies on dengue in Santiago de Cuba, 1997. *Am J Epidemiol* 2000; **152**:793–799.

19. Schwartz E, Mileguir F, Grossman Z, Mendelson E. Evaluation of serological-based diagnosis of dengue fever among travelers. *J Clin Virology* 2000; **19**:169–173.

20. Postasman I, Srugo I, Schwartz E. Dengue seroconversion among Israeli travelers to tropical countries. *Emerg Infect Dis* 1999; **5**:824–827.

21. Schwartz E, Moskovitz A, Pstasman I, Peri G, Grossman Z, Alkan ML. The changing epidemiology of dengue fever in travelers to Thailand. *Eur J Clin Microbiol Infect Dis* 2000; **19**:784–786.

22. Jelinek T, Loscher T. Clinical features and epidemiology of tick typhus in travelers. *J Travel Med* 2001; **8**:57–59.

23. Raoult D, Rournier PE, Fenollar F, *et al.* Rickettsia africae, a tick-borne pathogen in travelers to sub-Saharan Africa. *N Engl J Med* 2001; **344**:1504–1510.

24. Olano JP, Walker DH. Human ehrlichiosis. *Med Clin N Amer* 2002; **86**(2): 375–392.

25. Shlim DR, Schwartz E, Eaton M. Clinical importance of Salmonella paratyphi A infection to enteric fever in Nepal. *J Travel Med* 1996; **2**:165–168.

26. Centers for Disease Control and Prevention. Outbreak of leptospirosis among white-water rafters – Costa Rica, 1996. *MMWR* 1997; **46**:577–579.

27. Centers for Disease Control and Prevention. Update: outbreak of acute febrile illness among athletes participating in Eco-Challenge-Sabah 2000 – Borneo, Malaysia, 2000. *MMWR* 2001; **50**:21–24.

28. Katz AR, Ansdell VE, Effler PV, Middleton CR, Sasaki DM. Assessment of the clinical presentation and treatment of 353 cases of laboratory-confirmed leptospirosis in Hawaii, 1974–1988. *Clin Infect Dis* 2001; **33**:1834–1841.

29. Ko AI, Reis MG, Dourado CMR, *et al.* Urban epidemic of severe leptospirosis in Brazil. *Lancet* 1999; **354**(4 Sept):820–825.

30. Visser LG, Polderman AM, Stuuiver PC. Outbreak of schistosomiasis among travelers returning from Mali, West Africa. *Clin Infect Dis* 1995; **20**:280–285.

31. Schwartz E, Rozenman J, Perelman N. Pulmonary manifestations of early Schistosoma infection among nonimmune travelers. *Am J Med* 2000; **109**:718–722.

32. Hughes MA, Petri WA, Jr. Amebic liver abscess. *Infect Dis Clin North Am* 2000; **14**:565–582.

33. Cam BV, Fonsmark L, Hue NB, *et al.* Prospective case-control study of encephalopathy in children with dengue hemorrhagic fever. *Am J Trop Med Hyg* 2001; **65**:848–851.

34. Slom TJ, Cortese MM, Gerger SI, *et al.* An outbreak of eosinophilic meningitis caused by Angiostrongylus cantonensis in travelers returning from the Caribbean. *N Engl J Med* 2002; **346**:668–675.

35. Miller JM, Tam TWS, Maloney S, *et al.* Cruise ships: high-risk passengers and the global spread of new influenza viruses. *Clin Infect Dis* 2000; **31**:433–438.

36. Lee N, Hui D, Wu A, *et al.* A major outbreak of severe acute respiratory syndrome. *N Engl J Med* 2003; **348**;1986–94.

37. Booth CM, Matukas LM, Tomlinson GA, *et al.* Clinical Features and short-term outcomes of 144 patients with SARS in the Greater Toronto Area. *JAMA* 2003:**289**:1–9.

38. Centers for Disease Control & Prevention. Updated interim domestic infection control guidance in the health care and community setting for patients with suspected SARS. Available at: http://www.cdc.gov/ncidod/sars/ic.html.

39. Centers for Disease Control and Prevention. Update: outbreak of acute febrile respiratory illness among college students – Acapulco, Mexico, March 2001. *MMWR* 2001; **50**:359–360.

40. Cairns L, Blythe D, Kao A, *et al.* Outbreak of coccidioidomycosis in Washington State residents returning from Mexico. *Clin Infect Dis* 2000; **30**:61–64.

41. Piper-Jenks N, Horowitz HW, Schwartz E. Risk of hepatitis E to travelers. *J Travel Med* 2000; **7**:194–199.

42. Schulte C, Krebs B, Jelinek T, *et al.* Diagnostic significance of blood eosinophilia in returning travelers. *Clin Infect Dis* 2002; **34**:407–411.

43. Gopinath R, Keystone JS, Kain KC. Concurrent falciparum malaria and salmonella bacteremia in travelers: report of two cases. *Clin Infect Dis* 1995; **20**:706–708.

44. Schwartz E, Piper-Jenks. Simultaneous amebic liver abscess and hepatitis A infection. *J Trav Med* 1998; **5**:95–96.

45. Keystone JS, Kozarsky PE, Freedman DO. Internet and computer-based resources for travel medicine practitioners. *Clin Infect Dis* 2001; **32**:757–765.

CHAPTER 53 Skin Diseases

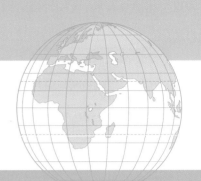

Eric Caumes

KEYPOINTS

- Dermatoses are the third most common health problem in travelers

- Skin problems occurring while abroad are cosmopolitan; most of these dermatoses are related to infectious origin, insect bites, envenomization or solar allergy

- The dermatoses occurring after return are usually of infectious origin, and about 50% are tropical diseases

EPIDEMIOLOGICAL DATA

In the 1980s, dermatoses were considered the fifth most common cause of health problems related to travel, being reported by 1.2% of 7886 short-term Swiss visitors to developing countries.[1] In the same period another study showed that sunburns and insect stings were reported by 10% and 3%, respectively, of 2665 Finnish travelers worldwide.[2]

Today dermatoses are considered as the third most common cause of health problems in travelers (after diarrhea and respiratory tract infection). Indeed it has been reported during travel by 8% of 784 American travelers worldwide.[3] Of the 63 dermatoses observed in this cohort, 14 were related to insect's bites or stings, 10 to sun expo-sure, seven to dermatophytes, seven to contact allergy and five to infectious cellulitis.

Dermatoses diagnosed abroad

Similarly, on-site studies of health impairment during travel showed that dermatoses were one of the three main reasons for consultation in travelers abroad. In Nepal, two studies showed that dermatoses were the third most frequent presenting illness among tourists: skin diseases accounted for 12% of 860 health impairments among 838 French tourists[4] and in another report for 10% of 19 616 presentations of patients of all nationalities at a private clinic.[5] Bacterial and fungal skin infections as well as scabies infestation were the most common travel-associated dermatoses in Nepal, accounting for 4.35%, 1.86% and 2%, respectively, of 860 health impairments in French tourists.[4]

Moreover, in the Maldives and Fiji, dermatoses were the most frequent presenting illnesses in tourists, with sunburns and superficial injuries documented most often.[6,7] Similarly, dermatoses were the most frequent reason for consultation in USA military troops in Thailand, accounting for 19% of 1299 patient visits to three military clinics, during a 33-day exercise.[8] In Fiji, injuries (including those due to contact with marine creatures) and skin rash (frequently related to sunburn) each accounted for 10% of clinic visits by tourists, while skin infections accounted for 13%.[6] In the Maldives, superficial injuries (usually caused by contact with coral and shells) and 'sun allergies' accounted for 14% and 13%, respectively, of health impairments among tourists.[7]

Dermatoses diagnosed upon return

Results of studies of travelers returning from tropical countries show that dermatoses are the third cause of health impairment in this setting, after fever and diarrhea. A prospective study has helped to more specifically identify the spectrum of travel-associated dermatoses observed after return. A total of 269 patients who presented to a tropical disease clinic in Paris with a travel-associated dermatosis were evaluated.[9] Skin lesions appeared while the patient was still abroad in 61% of cases and within 2 months after return in 39%. Among the latter group of patients, the median time of onset after departure from the tropics was 7 days (0–52 days). A firm diagnosis was made in 260 (97%) of the 269 cases (Table 53.1).[8] Of these, 260 firm diagnoses, 137 (53%) involved an imported tropical disease.

In summary, the spectrum of travel-related dermatoses seems to be closely related to the geographic location visited and the onset of signs and symptoms relative to the date of return. Sunburns, arthropod-related reactions and superficial injuries are most often seen during the patient's stay abroad and are prominent in hot seaside areas. Skin infections, most particularly pyoderma, are ubiquitous and are a common cause of dermatoses abroad and after return. Infectious cellulitis is certainly the most severe dermatoses to be encountered by travelers. Tropical dermatoses are usually seen after the traveler returns, given the prolonged incubation period of these diseases.

TROPICAL DERMATOSES IN THE TRAVELER

Limited knowledge of tropical dermatoses among Western physicians can delay the diagnosis and effective treatment. This is well illustrated by a study of cutaneous leishmaniasis where the median time interval from when the lesions were first noticed to when treatment was instituted was 112 days (range, 0–1032 days).[10] Similarly 55%, of 64 patients with cutaneous larva migrans had already consulted a general practitioner or a dermatologist (mean number of consultations: two; range: 1–6) before the correct diagnosis was made.[11] Therefore it is reasonable to bear in mind that about 50% of the dermatoses seen in travelers after their return are of tropical origin.[9]

Hookworm-related cutaneous larva migrans

Cutaneous larva migrans (CLM) (also called creeping eruption, creeping verminous dermatitis, clam digger's itch, sand worm eruption, plumber's itch) is the most frequent travel-associated skin disease of

Table 53.1	Travel associated dermatoses diagnosed in 269 French travelers presenting to a tropical disease unit in Paris in 1991–1993	
Diagnosis	**Number of cases (%)**	
Cutaneous larva migrans	65 (24.9)	
Pyodermas	48 (17.8)	
Arthropod-related pruritic dermatitis	26 (9.7)	
Myiasis	25 (9.3)	
Tungiasis	17 (6.3)	
Urticaria	16 (5.9)	
Rash with fever	11 (4.1)	
Cutaneous leishmaniasis	8 (3.0)	
Scabies	6 (2.2)	
Injuries*	5 (1.9)	
Cutaneous fungal infections	5 (1.9)	
Exacerbation of preexisting illness	5 (1.9)	
Sexually transmitted disease	4 (1.5)	
Cutaneous herpes simplex	3 (1.1)	
Septicemia	3 (1.1)	
Acute venous thrombosis	2 (0.7)	
Pityriasis rosea	2 (0.7)	
Mycobacterium marinum infection	2 (0.7)	
Acute lymphatic filariasis	1 (0.4)	
Traumatic abrasion	1 (0.4)	
Miscellaneous**	3 (1.1)	
Undetermined	9 (3.3)	
Total	269 (100)	

*Injuries included local envenomation (one case), superficial injuries caused by contact with marine creatures (two cases) and cellulitis-like reactions presumably caused by arthropods (two cases).
**Miscellaneous diagnoses were lichen planus, erythema nodosum (manifesting infection with *Salmonella enteritidis*) and Reiter's syndrome (of unknown etiology).

(5–34 days) in one study[12] and the median incubation period was 10 days (4–38 days) in the other.[13] The eruption usually lasts between 2 and 8 weeks but has been reported to last up to 2 years. For instance, in a series of 44 British patients, the median duration of symptoms was 8 weeks (range, 1–104 weeks).[15] The itchiness has been shown to disappear much sooner than the eruption (on average 7.2 days earlier).[12]

Apart from pruritus, the most frequent clinical sign of CLM is an erythematous, linear or serpiginous lesion that is approximately 3 mm wide and may be up to 15–20 mm in length (Fig. 53.1). The mean number of lesions per patient varies from one[9,14] to three.[11] The most frequent anatomic locations of CLM lesions are the feet, followed by the buttocks and trunk.[9,11,12,14,15] The larva advances a few millimeters to a few centimeters daily. Vesiculobullous lesions (Fig. 53.2) and at a lesser extent impetiginization (Fig. 53.3) are common. Super infection has been estimated at 8% in one study.[11] Edema and vesiculobullous lesions were observed in 6% and 9% of 67 French patients[9] as opposed to 17% and 10% of 60 Canadian patients.[14] In the Canadian outbreak all the lesions were located on the feet and a more significant number (40%) of patients reported bullous lesions.[12] Systemic signs and symptoms such as erythema multiforme, dry cough, wheezing and eosinophilic pneumonitis have been rarely reported.

Blood eosinophilia varied from 0–37% (mean 5%) among forty German patients with CLM.[16] Nonetheless, blood tests are not necessary to assess the diagnosis which is usually based on the characteristic clinical findings and a history of possible exposure. The differential diagnoses include the other dermatoses that give rise to serpiginous or linear migrating cutaneous lesions (see, creeping eruptions).

There is a particular form of hookworm-related cutaneous larva migrans, known as hookworm folliculitis, which usually occurs on the buttocks (Fig. 53.4). The largest series include seven patients.[17] The diagnosis is made clinically when the serpiginous tracks are seen among the lesions of folliculitis or relies on histopathological grounds when the hookworm larva is found in the sebaceous follicular canal.

The treatment of choice for CLM is the topical application of a 15% liquid suspension (or ointment) of thiabendazole applied three times per day for at least 5 days.[18] Topical thiabendazole may be difficult to use in cases of multiple lesions or lesions located on the soles. Of all the efficient oral antihelminthic agents, ivermectin has the advantage of being well tolerated with high efficacy when taken in a single dose, the cure rate varying from 77%[11] to more than 94%.[9,19] Oral thiabendazole (50 mg/kg per day) for two to three consecutive days is effective but its use is limited by the occurrence of adverse events such as

tropical origin. CLM is caused most often by the larvae of hookworms (*Ancylostoma braziliense*), of dogs, cats or other mammals. It is widely distributed in tropical and subtropical countries worldwide. CLM is acquired by skin contact with infective larvae in the soil, usually while landing or walking on the beaches in hot seaside areas.

Two outbreaks have been observed in travelers. In a group of 32 Canadian who acquired CLM (25% of exposed persons) in Barbados, risk factors for developing the illness were younger age (39 versus 41 years, *P* = 0.014) and less frequent use of protective footwear while walking on the beach (risk ratio of four for people who never wear sandals to and on the beach).[12] Interestingly, 90% of travelers reported seeing cats whereas only 5% of the group noticed dogs on the beach and around the hotel area. The other outbreak involved a group of 13 (87% of exposed persons) British military personnel who acquired CLM during a training exercise in Belize.[13]

The incubation period of CLM is usually a few days and rarely goes beyond one month. Among three large series of 64 French travelers, 67 French travelers and 60 Canadian travelers, the cutaneous lesions appeared after return in 55%,[11] 51%,[9] and 55%,[14] respectively, with the median time of onset being 16 days (1–120 days),[11] 8 days (range, 0–28 days)[9] and 5 days (range, 0–30 days)[14] after return. Similarly, in the two above mentioned outbreaks of CLM, the median time from the start of the trip to the development of the eruption was 15 days

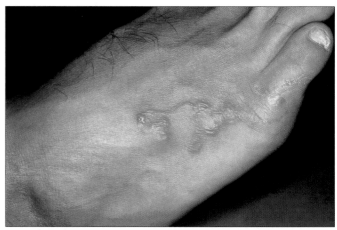

Figure 53.1 Serpiginous track of cutaneous larva migrans (CLM) (French West Indies).

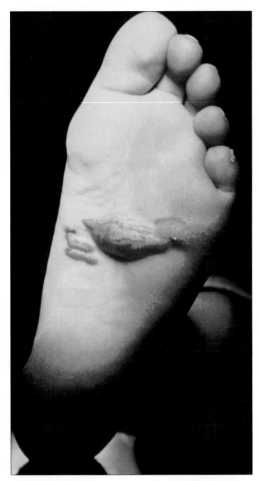

Figure 53.2 Vesiculobullous lesion over CLM track (Brazil).

dizziness, nausea, vomiting, and headaches. Oral albendazole (400 to 800 mg/day) for three consecutive days is also effective and well tolerated. A single 12 mg oral dose of ivermectin was significantly more efficacious in a prospective comparative study than a single 400 mg oral dose of albendazole (100% versus 46%; $P = 0.017$).[20] To avoid CLM on tropical beaches frequented by dogs and cats, it is best to wear shoes, to use a mattress, or to lie on the sand washed by the tide.

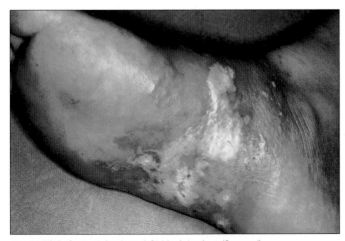

Figure 53.3 Super infection of CLM of the foot (Senegal).

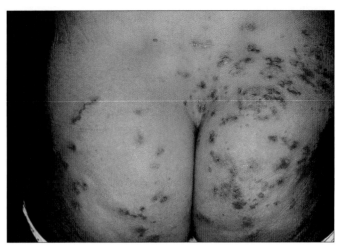

Figure 53.4 Hookworm folliculitis (Senegal).

Localized cutaneous leishmaniasis

Localized cutaneous leishmaniasis (LCL) occurs in tropical and warm temperate countries and is transmitted by sandflies. Old World LCL (caused primarily by *L. major and L. tropica*) mainly occurs in travelers to the sub-Saharan and North Africa, the Mediterranean basin, and the Middle East. The Indian subcontinent and China seem to be less at-risk destinations. New World LCL (caused primarily by the species of *L. braziliensis* and *L. mexicana* complexes) mainly occurs in travelers to the forested parts of Latin America. Workers in the Amazon forest are particularly at risk.

Of all the clinical forms of cutaneous leishmaniasis, LCL occurs more often in travelers as compared to immigrants. Of the 59 cases of cutaneous leishmaniasis reported to the National Institutes of Health from 1973 to 1991, there were 42 cases of LCL (23 Old World, 19 New World), four cases of recurrent cutaneous leishmaniasis (RCL), 2 cases of mucosal leishmaniasis (ML) and 10 cases of diffuse cutaneous leish-maniasis (DCL).[21] LCL was essentially observed in American travelers whereas RCL, ML and DCL occurred mainly in immigrants to the USA.

Between 1985 and 1990, the CDC provided a pentavalent derivative of antimony for 59 American travelers with New World LCL. A total of 26 (46%) of those treated were expatriates and 23 (39%) were tourists.[10] Of the 15 (26%) patients who had stayed in a forest region for a week or less, at least six were exposed for no more than two days. LCL has been shown to be more frequent among people traveling for professional reasons than among tourists and among men than women.[9,10] Small outbreaks are observed among travelers, with attack rates of 17–42% in a group of students in Guatemala and Belize and 15–23% in a group of tourists in Peru.[10] These attack rates may go up to 100% for workers in the Amazon forest.[9] The incidence of LCL has been estimated at 1 per thousand travelers to Surinam and 1 per million travelers to Mexico.[10]

The incubation period varies from a few days to a few months. The median time interval between return from the tropics and the onset of cutaneous lesions has been estimated to be 15 days (range, 7–30 days) in one study,[21] 52 days (7–104 days) in another study[9] whereas the median maximum possible incubation period was 30 days (range, 1 day to 5 months) in another report.[10]

The clinical forms of LCL include papule (Fig. 53.5), nodule (Fig. 53.6), plaque (Fig. 53.7) , ulcer (Fig. 53.8) or nodular lymphangitis (Fig. 53.9). Cutaneous ulcer is the most frequent clinical presentation (at least in the New World) and is commonly characterized by a well-circumscribed border, a crusted base and the absence of pain.

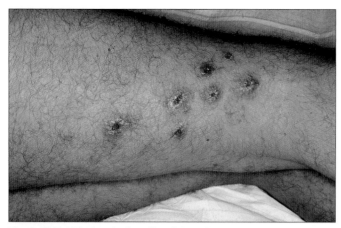

Figure 53.5 LCL, papular form (Saudi Arabia).

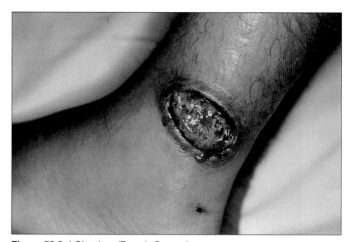

Figure 53.8 LCL, ulcer (French Guyana).

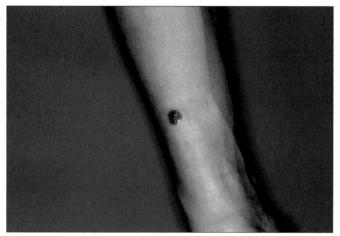

Figure 53.6 LCL, nodular form (Ethiopia).

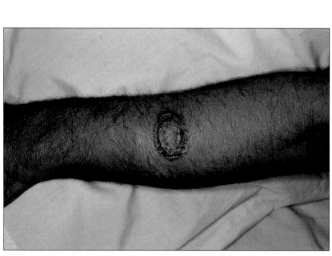

Figure 53.7 LCL , erythematosquamous plaque (Algeria).

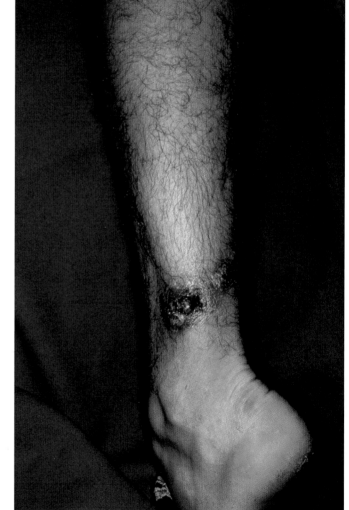

Figure 53.9 LCL, nodular lymphangitis (French Guyana).

The average number of cutaneous lesions varies from one to three and rarely exceeds 10/patient. Usual features of LCL include the anatomic location on exposed skin (face, arms, legs), absence of pain, chronicity (more than 15 days duration), and failure of antibiotics (which are often prescribed, given that it often looks like pyoderma).

Late destructive ML is rather more frequently observed in immigrants than in travelers.[21] Nonetheless, it has been described in immunocompromised persons who have traveled in the past to endemic areas, and have been infected with a *Leishmania* species (e.g., *L. braziliensis*) that have the potential for mucous involvement. The differential diagnosis of LCL includes pyoderma, anthrax, myiasis, arthropod bite or sting, tick eschar and sporotrichosis mostly in case of nodular lymphangitis (see, nodular lymphangitis).

Diagnosis is usually made by evaluating a slit skin smear of the cutaneous lesion stained with Giemsa under light microscopy.[22] Skin biopsy from the edge of the ulcer may reveal the characteristic amastigotes within macrophages but is less sensitive than culture. *Leishmania* species may be cultured on various media (e.g., Novy-MacNeal-Nicolle). DNA and monoclonal antibodies may also be used for *Leishmania* antibody analyses and species identification.

Only four drugs have showed significant efficacy in the treatment of LCL in placebo controlled trials (most of them coming from the New World). The mainstay of treatment is pentavalent antimonial agents given intramuscularly in New World LCL and intralesionally in Old World LCL. Other treatments include pentamidine salts, fluconazole and ketoconazole, which have been evaluated in a few species only. In some instances, mainly cases originating from the Old World, absence of treatment may be considered, given that the cutaneous lesions heal spontaneously in nearly all the patients within one year.

Myiasis

Cutaneous myiasis is the infestation of human tissues by *Diptera* fly larvae. According to the results of three series of imported cases in Western countries, various forms of cutaneous myiasis are observed in travelers. In a series of 25 cases imported in France, 20 were due to *Cordylobia anthropophaga* (the tumbu fly), four to *Dermatobia hominis* (the human botfly), and one to *Cochliomyia hominivorax*.[9] In a series of 19 cases imported in England, nine were due to *C. anthropophaga*, four to *D hominis*, one to *C hominivorax* and one to *Oestrus ovis*.[23] In a series of 13 cases imported in Germany, six were infected with *C. anthropophaga*, six with *Dermatobia hominis* and one with *Hypoderma lineatum*.[24]

Furuncular myiasis is caused primarily by *C. anthropophaga* in sub-Saharan Africa and *D. hominis* in Central and South America. Depending on which fly is involved (the tumbu fly or the botfly), the presentation of myiasis differs by the place of acquisition, duration of maturation, number and anatomic location of cutaneous lesions, and the ability to manually extract the larvae (Table 53.2). *C. anthropophaga* larvae penetrate the skin after hatching from eggs deposited on clothing and bed linens hung to dry outdoors and which have not been ironed. The infestation by *D. hominis* larvae develop from fly eggs carried to the human by a biting mosquito. In both cases, the larvae develop by successive molts. The incubation period varies from days to weeks (7–10 days for the tumbu fly and 15–45 days for the botfly).

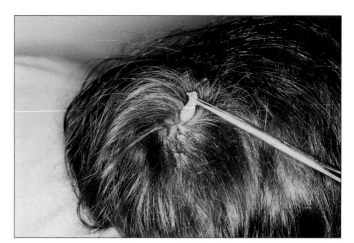

Figure 53.10 Cutaneous myiasis due to *D. hominis* (French Guyana).

The cutaneous lesion is a one to two centimeter furuncle-like lesion with a central punctum through which serosanguineous or purulent fluid discharges (Figs 53.10 and 53.11). Importantly, the patient complains of a crawling sensation within the lesion and movements of the larvae may be seen within the central punctum. *C. anthropophaga* lesions are more commonly multiple whereas *D. hominis* lesions usually number from one to three. Indeed, the number of maggots removed from the skin was markedly higher in six patients infected with the Tumbu fly (average of five) compared with the six with botfly (average of 1.7).[24] *C. anthropophaga* lesions are usually located on areas of the body covered by clothing (such as the trunk) whereas *D. hominis* lesions are commonly located on exposed areas of the body (such as the scalp, face, forearms, and legs). The largest number of lesions ever reported was 94 in a child from Ghana infected by *C. anthropophaga*.[25]

The diagnosis of myiasis is made by the identification of the larva from the lesion. The differential diagnosis primarily includes pyoderma, LCL and tungiasis. The treatment is the removal of the larvae. It is important to avoid breaking the larvae in that incomplete removal may result in a hypersensitivity or foreign body reaction to the larvae. In the case of *C. anthropophaga*, manual pressure to the lateral aspects of the lesion easily allow the expression of the maggot. With *D. hominis*, extraction is facilitated by placing an occlusive agent (e.g., paraffin, petrolatum, pork fat, toothpaste cap) onto the lesion may cause the larva to migrate to the skin surface.[26]

Table 53.2	Furuncular myiasis	
Diptera (fly)	***Cordylobia anthropophaga (Tumbu fly)***	***Dermatobia hominis (Human bot fly)***
Distribution	sub-Saharan Africa	Latin America
Duration	9 days	6–12 weeks
Localization	Covered areas	Uncovered areas
Number of lesions	1–94[25]	1–3
Removal	Local pressure	Extraction

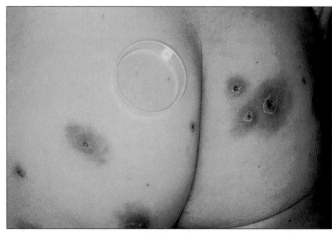

Figure 53.11 Cutaneous myiasis due to *C. anthropophaga* (Senegal).

Tungiasis

Tungiasis is the infestation by the female sand flea, *Tunga penetrans* (also called chigoe flea, jigger flea). It is widely distributed throughout Latin America, the Caribbean, Africa and Asia up to the west coast of India.[27] The sand flea penetrates human skin, feeds on blood, and produces eggs within its abdomen. In the largest study of 17 imported cases, the median lag time between return and onset was 5 days (range, 2–10 days) and the median lag time between return and presentation was 12 days (range, 5–40 days).[9] This confirms that the time of exposure to the onset of cutaneous lesions is short and that the flea may survive more than one month. The cutaneous lesion is a black papule (at the site of penetration) that develops into a nodule through which the eggs of the flea are expelled (Fig. 53.12). There is a limited number of nodules (most commonly one) which are usually located on the feet (subungual, sole, toe) and lower extremities. The diagnosis relies on clinical findings and is confirmed by the morphology of the flea. The differential diagnosis includes myiasis, pyoderma and foreign body reaction. The treatment is the removal of the flea by excision and curettage.

Ciguatera

Ciguatera is a significant cause of pruritus which may last months after the initial event.[28] This is a fish poisoning which is acquired by the consumption of certain tropical marine reef fish in tropical and subtropical regions (also see Chapter 47). The diagnosis relies on history of fish consumption, other cases in travelers sharing the same food habit, a short incubation period (2–30 h), and the association to gastrointestinal signs and symptoms, fatigue, myalgias (particularly of the lower extremities), pruritus, and neurosensory manifestations (perioral and distal extremity paresthesias and altered temperature sensation). The reversal of the temperature sensation (i.e., cold beverages and objects are described as feeling hot) is unique to ciguatera. There may be cardiovascular impairment. Whereas gastrointestinal symptoms resolve in a few hours, myalgias, pruritus and neurosensory symptoms last longer. Treatment is essentially supportive.

Other tropical dermatoses of interest for travelers

Many other tropical dermatoses (i.e., acute filariasis, loiasis, onchocerciasis, cutaneous gnathostomiasis, west and east African trypanosomiasis, mucosal leishmaniasis, genital amebiasis, Buruli's ulcer, cutaneous anthrax) have been observed in travelers. East African trypanosomiasis, which is on the rise, may be revealed by trypanosomal

chancre (Fig. 53.13). Nonetheless, only a few cases have been reported. In contrast, a series of five cases of acute onchocerciasis acquired in west or central Africa and responsible for limb lymphoedema (Fig. 53.14) have been reported.[29]

Numerous cases (including clusters) of tropical diseases which cause febrile rash (e.g., rickettsial diseases, dengue fever, acute schistosomiasis) have been reported in travelers (see febrile rash).

COSMOPOLITAN DERMATOSES

Pyodermas

Pyodermas are one of the most common dermatoses in travelers. The lesions usually appear while the patient is still abroad. The clinical spectrum ranges from impetigo (Fig. 53.15) and ecthyma to erysipelas and necrotizing cellulites.[9] The most common bacterial species involved are *Staphylococcus aureus* and *Streptococcus pyogenes*. Cutaneous lesions may act as a portal of entry for septicemia. In a series of 19 cases of impetigo in travelers, 63% were secondary to an insect bite.[9] This points towards the importance of insect protection in the prevention of pyodermas. In addition, travel first aid kits should include antibiotics effective against bacterial infections, at least in susceptible persons (history of erysipelas or infectious cellulites, pres-ence of venous or lymphatic insufficiency).

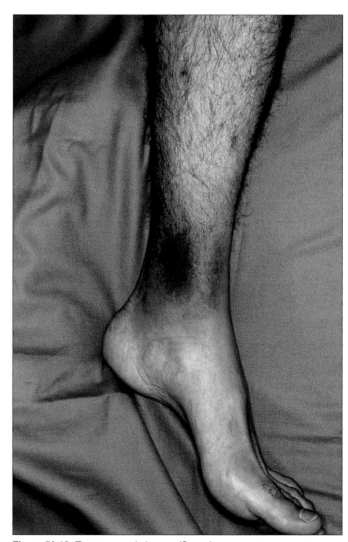

Figure 53.13 Trypanosomal chancre (Congo).

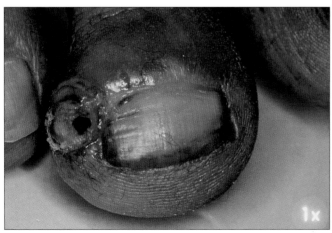

Figure 53.12 Tungiasis of the toe (Ivory Coast).

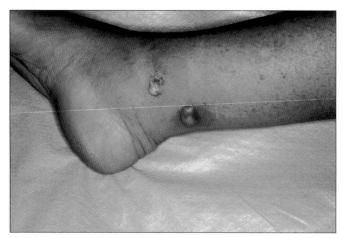

Figure 53.15 Impetigo complicating arthropod bites (French West Indies).

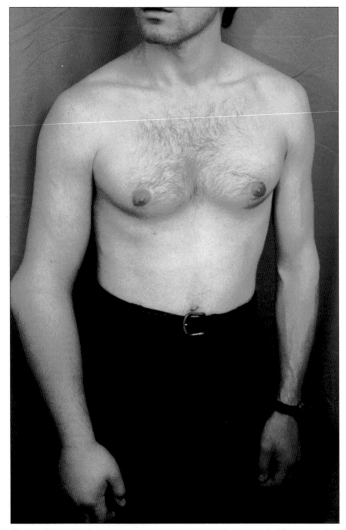

Figure 53.14 Limb lymphoedema related to onchocerciasis (Cameroon).

Dermatophytosis

Dermatophytosis, or tinea, is a worldwide cutaneous infection but its incidence is higher in the tropics and subtropics. Tinea infections rank among the most common skin diseases observed during travel abroad.[3,4]

Tinea corporis is a fungous infection of the glabrous skin located on the non-hairy parts of the face, neck, trunk, and limbs with the exception of the axillae, groins, hands and feet. *T. soudanensis* appears to be a common cause of infection in Africa whereas *T. rubrum* is more common in Asia and Latin America, and *T. mentagrophytes* in South-east Asia. The characteristic lesion is a well-defined round or oval erythematous plaque with a vesicular border and central clearing.

Tinea barbae is a fungous infection of the hairy parts of the face as beard and moustache. It could be observed in travelers returning from rural areas who were in close contact with cattle, horses and other animals.

Tinea cruris and *axillaris* may be common in travelers due to the excessive perspiration and friction of the major intertriginous areas, such as groins, axillae and submammary folds. *T. rubrum*, *E. floccosum* and *T. soudanense* are the main agents of tinea cruris. Tinea of the intertriginous areas are often asymmetrical, located around the folds and form erythematous, scaly patches that progress to polycyclic borders.

Tinea of the feet is probably the most common dermatophytic infection to be encountered in travelers who are not going barefoot or wearing sandals. The predominant agent of *Tinea pedis* is *T. rubrum*, and to a lesser extent *T. mentagrophytes*, *T. soudanense* and *E. floccosum*. Three clinical varieties may be described: the intertriginous type, the vesicular, bullous or vesiculobullous type, and the squamous or hyperkeratotic type.

Tinea unguium, the dermatophytic infection of nails, is responsible for whitish, yellow or brownish discoloration which extends from the free border or sides towards the base of the nails. It is more often located on the feet.

Scalp ringworm is a common variety of dermatophytosis in children coming back from visiting friends and relatives in Africa.

Tinea versicolor is a chronic, superficial yeast infection of the epidermal stratum corneum. It is worldwide but extremely common in the tropics and subtropics. Tinea versicolor is caused by the hyphal form of *Malassezia furfur*. The characteristic clinical lesion is a well-defined round or oval macule covered with adherent fine scales. The macules may remain isolated, but have a tendency to coalesce, and cover large areas of the body on the chest, shoulders, back and neck. Usually asymptomatic, the eruption may become pruritic in hot climates. The diagnosis is evoked on the distribution, shape and appearance of the patches and the fingernail test, which demonstrates the fine scales, limited to affected spots. The final diagnosis relies on the microscopic examination of a scotch tape.

Arthropod-related dermatoses

Exposure to an arthropod (see Chapter 46) is a common cause of skin lesions in travelers.[9] Attempts to identify the implicated arthropod are often difficult in that arthropods of different species may give rise to similar dermatologic manifestations. Nonetheless, epidemiological exposures suggested by history are useful.

The clinical picture varies according to the nature of skin injury (e.g., traumatic injury, local envenomation, hypersensitivity reaction). The predominant feature of the arthropod reaction is prurigo, an eruption of intensely pruritic erythematous and excoriated papules (Fig. 53.16). This reaction is considered to be an evolutive stage of papular urticaria related to a hypersensitivity reaction to the bites of insects such as fleas, bedbugs, and less commonly mosquitoes, chiggers, and mites. Arthropod bites may also result in vesiculobullous lesions and papular urticaria. Cutaneous lesions are self-limited.

Oral antihistamines and topical corticosteroids may improve the symptoms.

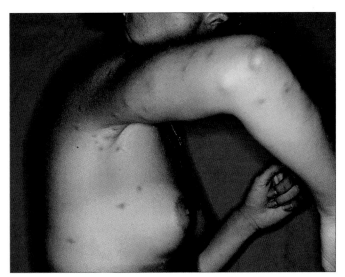

Figure 53.16 Prurigo after exposure to thrombiculidae ((Brazil).

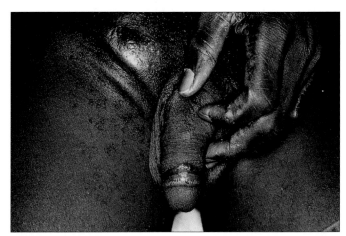

Figure 53.17 Genital ulcer associated with inguinal bubo, chancroid (Mali).

Scabies

Scabies is the most common cause of generalized pruritus in travelers.[9] Scabies is acquired by skin-to-skin contact. Clinically, the patient complains of pruritus within 4 weeks of contact in case of primary exposure. In patients with a history of previous scabies exposure, pruritus may occur within a few days. The more specific skin findings include burrows, papulonodular genital lesions, and pustules on the hands. Other skin changes are secondary to pruritus and include excoriation, lichenification and impetiginization.

The diagnosis is made by the microscopic identification of the *S. scabiei* var. *hominis* mite, eggs or feces on skin scrapings of a cutaneous lesion. Treatment includes permethrin cream 5%, lindane 1% (*gamma-benzene hexachloride*), benzyl benzoate (in Europe) and ivermectin. Bedding and clothing must be laundered or removed from contact for at least 3 days. Personal and household contacts must also be treated.

Sexually transmitted infections

Sexually transmitted diseases (STD) are particularly frequent in travelers. Genital discharge and genital ulcerations were respectively the 7th and 8th causes of health problems in Swiss travelers.[1] In Finnish travelers, 39% of round the world travelers and 30% of tourists to Thailand reported having had 'high risk' behavior.[2] Gonococcal infection is the most frequent cause of STDs in travelers.[1]

STDs contracted in tropical areas may be unusual (donovanosis, lymphogranuloma venerum) or have a different antibiotic susceptibility profile to that seen in Western countries. Genital ulceration suggests primary syphilis, herpes and chancroid, possibly donovanosis and rarely lymphogranuloma venerum. A genital discharge points to gonococcal, *Chlamydia trachomatis* or *Mycoplasma spp.* infections. Inguinal suppurative bubo suggests chancroid when it is close to a genital ulcer (Fig. 53.17) and lymphogranuloma venerum when it proceeds to a self-healing genital lesion. When these pathogens are acquired abroad it is preferable to test for antimicrobial susceptibility as most strains are resistant to common antibiotics.

Cercarial dermatitis

Cercarial dermatitis (also called clam digger's dermatitis, schistosome dermatitis, sedge pool itch, swimmer's itch) is caused by the infes-

tation of the skin by cercariae (larvae) of non-human schistosomes whose usual hosts are birds and small mammals.[30] Cercarial dermatitis is acquired by skin exposure to fresh and at lesser extent salt water. The cercariae penetrate intact human skin within a few minutes. Cercarial dermatitis occurs in swimmers and those with occupations that include water exposure. There are sporadic reports and few outbreaks reported from all continents.

The time from exposure to onset of symptoms varies from a few minutes to a maximum of 24 h after exposure. A prickling sensation during or shortly after exposure to infested water may be reported. Typically, and approximately one hour later, the cutaneous lesions begin as a pruritic macular erythematous eruption that progresses to a papular, papulovesicular and urticarial eruption. The eruption typically covers skin surfaces that are exposed to water but the skin surfaces that are covered by swimwear are not spared. The eruption peaks in 1–3 days and lasts 1–3 weeks. In case of previous contact, the clinical findings may begin sooner, with increased severity and a prolonged course.

The diagnosis is made by history of exposure and the characteristic clinical findings. The differential diagnosis includes seabather's eruption, contact dermatitis (secondary to marine plants, hydroids and corals), and insect bites. Cercarial dermatitis is self-limited. Oral antihistamines and topical steroids reduce the symptoms.

Seabather's eruption

Seabather's eruption (also called sea lice) is acquired by skin exposure to salt water inhabited by larvae of sea anemone and jelly fish.[31] Seabather's eruption is caused by the larvae discharging toxin from nematocysts into human skin. Seabather's eruption has been reported on the Atlantic coast of the USA, the Caribbean, Central and South America, and in South-east Asia. It probably exists worldwide in tropical and subtropical marine environments.

The time from exposure to onset of symptoms is usually a few minutes to 24 h. Individuals with a history of previous exposures may develop a prickling or stinging sensation or urticarial lesions while in the water. The clinical features include pruritic, erythematous macules, that progresses to papules, vesicles, and urticarial lesions. The anatomic distribution typically includes skin surfaces covered by swimwear and uncovered skin surfaces where there is friction (e.g., axillae, medial thighs, surfer's chest). The eruption is more pronounced in areas that are more confined (e.g., waistband). The eruption can last from 3 days to 3 weeks.

The diagnosis is made by the characteristic clinical findings and history of exposure. The differential diagnosis include cercarial dermatitis, contact dermatitis (secondary to marine life inhabitants) and insect bites. Seabather's eruption is self-limited. Oral antihistamines and topical steroids may reduce the symptoms.

Marine life dermatitis

Dermatoses associated with contact with a marine creature (see Chapter 46) are one of the most frequent causes of disease in travelers to tropical islands.[6,7]

The most dangerous creatures are the coelenterate, which are found worldwide in tropical and subtropical waters.[32] Contact with Portuguese man-of-war, fire coral, jelly fish, and sea anemone immediately produces a stinging sensation that varies from a slight burning sensation to excruciating pain. The cutaneous lesions appear at the site of exposition within a few minutes, begin as macules and papules, and may progress to vesicles, bulles and ulceration (Fig. 53.18). Contact with a jelly fish may result in systemic symptoms such as hypotension, muscle spasm and respiratory paralysis and may be fatal.[33] Sea urchins and other echinoderms may produce similar cutaneous and systemic symptoms as observed with coelenterake.

The other dangers of marine environment include shark and Moray eel bites, stone and fire fish stings, sea leech burns, and coral cuts and scratches.

Photosensitivity and photo-induced disorders

Ultraviolet irradiation have both acute and chronic effects on the skin (Chapter 41). In the traveler, skin changes due to acute sun exposure are common, including sunburn, phototoxic reactions, both drug-induced and plant-induced (phytophotodermatitis), photoallergic reactions, solar urticaria, polymorphic light eruption, actinic prurigo and hydroa vacciniforme.

Chronic sun exposure over the years result in dermatoheliosis, including chronic actinic dermatitis, lentigines, actinic keratoses, and skin cancer.

Other cosmopolitan infections of interest for travelers

Hypersensitivity reaction to drugs, not only daily medications but prophylaxis, must always be considered in the differential diagnosis of urticaria and exanthema in travelers.

Exacerbation of chronic diseases such as acne, atopic dermatitis, lupus erythematosus, dermatomyositis, pemphigus foliaceus, and several of the porphyries may occur and some of them result from sun exposure.

Other dermatoses of interest include miliaria rubra, frost bite, plant-related dermatoses, and contact dermatitis.

DIAGNOSIS OF A SKIN LESION IN THE TRAVELER

The evaluation of a traveler with skin lesions first include an extensive patient history with a focus on possible epidemiologic exposures.[34] The differential diagnosis is broadened. It depends on factors such as geographic location visited, length of stay as well as many other entities (Table 53.3).

Complete physical examination will focus on the appearance of cutaneous lesions because dermatological diseases are classified according to their morphologic characteristics such as: type (e.g., macule, papule, nodule, vesicle, ulcer), color (e.g., skin colored, red, brown, blue, black, hyperpigmented, hypopigmented, depigmented), shape or configuration (e.g., round, oval, annular, serpiginous, linear, zosteriform, reticulated) and distribution (e.g., localized, generalized, limited to a specific anatomic location).

Further diagnostic studies such as blood tests and serologies, skin biopsy and cultures, and imaging techniques may be warranted according to the results of clinical examination.

Diseases with dermatological manifestations that are encountered by travelers are listed according to the type of cutaneous lesion and history in Table 53.4. In addition some symptoms, signs or syndromes warrant further consideration given their frequency in travelers.

Pruritus

The diagnosis of a pruritic dermatosis mainly relies on the location of the symptoms and the presence of more specific cutaneous signs (Table 53.5). Generalized pruritus usually orients towards scabies, one of the most common causes of skin disease in travelers. Another significant cause of pruritus is ciguatera fish poisoning.

Table 53.3	Relevant historical data in the evaluation of skin lesions in the traveler

Travel history
    Duration of travel
    Duration of time since return
    Geographic locations visited
    Recent outbreaks of disease in locations visited
    Fellow travelers with similar signs and symptoms
    Means of transportation
    Housing and lifestyle, dietary habits
    Clothing and shoes worn
    Exposures: beach, fresh or salt water, rural, plants, insects, animals, sexual contacts
    Medications: therapeutic and prophylactic
    Use of personal preventive measures: insect repellent, mosquito net
    Previous medical care
    Immunization against tetanus

Dermatologic history
    Underlying skin diseases
    Alteration of skin integrity during travel
    Time of onset relative to potential exposures
    Time of onset relative to return
    Description of initial presentation and anatomic distribution of lesion(s)
    Description of progression of lesion(s)

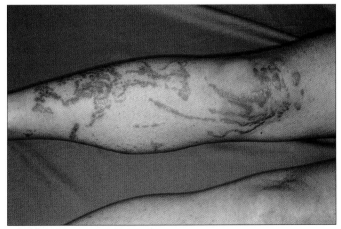

Figure 53.18 Erythematous flagellations after contact with jelly fish (Thailand).

Table 53.4   **Dermatoses encountered by travelers according to the type of cutaneous lesion and nature of exposure**

Clinical presentation	Short-term traveler	Long-term traveler and immigrant
Papules and nodules	Adverse drug reaction, acne exacerbation, milaria rubra, sea urchin granuloma Arthropod bites, tungiasis, myiasis, tick granuloma, lice Pyodermas, mycobacterial infection Leishmaniasis, scabies, cercarial dermatitis, gnathostomiasis, seabather's eruption Sporotrichosis	Leprosy, tuberculosis, mycetoma, pinta, bartonellosis, glanders, yaws Orf, milker's nodules Onchocerciasis, cysticercosis, schistosomiasis, dirofilariasis, sparganosis, trypanosomiasis Paracoccidioidomycosis, paragonimiasis, chromomycosis, West African histoplasmosis, lobomycosis
Erythematous plaque	Bacterial cellulitis, pyoderma, Lyme disease Leishmaniasis Dermatophytosis (tinea)	African trypanosomiasis
Vesicles and bullae	Sunburn, blister beetle dermatitis, contact dermatitis, irritant dermatitis, phytophotodermatitis, milaria rubra, fixed drug eruption Arthropod bites, Bullous impetigo Herpes simplex infection Cutaneous larva migrans, cercarial dermatitis, seabather's eruption	Varicella infection Dracunculiasis
Ulcers	Spider bite Ecthyma, pyodermas, tache noire (tick eschar) Herpes simplex infection Leishmaniasis Sporotrichosis	Cupping Mycetomas, anthrax, tuberculosis, mycobacterial infection, cutaneous diphtheria, glanders, melioidosis, plague[a], yaws[a], tularemia[a] Cutaneous amebiasis, dracunculiasis West African histoplasmosis, North American blastomycosis, paracoccidioidomycosis, chromomycosis

Any of the diseases listed above that may affect the short-term traveler may also affect the long-term traveler and immigrant and vice versa
[a]Primary inoculation site

Table 53.5   **Causes of pruritus in travelers**

Localized pruritus	Contact dermatitis, irritant dermatitis, phytophotodermatitis, arthropod bite, lice, seabather's eruption Cercarial dermatitis, cutaneous larva migrans, enterobiasis (perianal), gnathostomiasis, loiasis, strongyloidiasis (larva currens)
Generalized pruritus	Adverse drug reactions, ciguatera fish poisoning, atopic dermatitis exacerbation Varicella (in adult) Scabies Loiasis, onchocerciasis, African trypanosomiasis Schistosomiasis, ascariasis, hookworm, trichinellosis and strongyloidiasis (in association with urticarial rash during invasive phase)

Table 53.6   **Causes of creeping eruption**

Nematode's larva	Strongyloidiasis (larva currens) Cutaneous larva migrans Gnathostomiasis Hookworm ('ground itch')
Nematode' adult	Loiasis Dracunculiasis
Maggot	Myiasis (due to *Gasterophilus* and *Hypoderma* spp.)

Self-limited and localized pruritus orients towards an allergic reaction to insect bites or stings.

Creeping eruption

Creeping eruption is defined by a linear or serpiginous cutaneous track, slightly elevated, erythematous, and mobile. This eruption has to be distinguished from other non-creeping dermatoses which give rise to serpiginous or linear cutaneous lesions.

The numerous causes of creeping eruption have been reviewed recently.[35] All of them are of parasitic origin (Table 53.6). Some diseases are related to the subcutaneous migration of various helminthic larvae (i.e., cutaneous larva migrans related to hookworms or other nematodes, larva currens, gnathostomiasis). Others are the consequence of the subcutaneous migration of a fly's maggot (migratory myiasis), or adult nematode (*Loa loa*, *Dracunculus medinensis*).

Urticaria

Acute urticaria is a common reason for consultation. The causes of urticaria are numerous (Table 53.7). The travel history may provide epidemiologic clues such as exposure to fresh water (Katayama fever associated with acute schistosomiasis), ingestion of fish (anisakiasis), undercooked meats (trichinellosis), and raw vegetables (ascariasis), or walking barefoot (hookworm, strongyloïdiasis). Adverse drug reactions must also be considered in the differential diagnosis of urticaria.

Febrile rash

The occurrence of febrile maculopapular rash warrants immediate attention. It primarily points to adverse drug reaction or viral infection (Table 53.8). The most frequent cause of febrile rash in travelers

Table 53.7	Causes of urticaria in travelers or expatriates
Adverse drug reaction	
Hepatitis A infection	
Invasive phase of schistosomiasis, ascariasis, hookworm, trichinellosis, strongyloidiasis, and fascioliasis	
Rupture of cyst during hydatidosis	

Table 53.8	Causes of fever and maculopapular rash in travelers
Adverse drug reaction	
Meningococcemia (purpura), typhoid fever, syphilis, rat-bite fever, leptospirosis, trench fever, rickettsial infections, brucellosis	
Measles, rubella, Epstein Barr Virus, HIV and cytomegalovirus primary infection, dengue, other arboviral infections, viral hemorrhagic fever.	
African trypanosomiasis, trichinellosis, toxoplasmosis	

is dengue (Fig. 53.19) with a frequency estimated at 30%. The development of a rash within 10 days after return is suggestive of arboviral infection, mostly in case of mucous membrane involvement. Moreover, the association of rash and fever may herald a life-threatening infectious disease such as hemorrhagic viral fever, meningococcemia, rickettsial infections (Fig. 53.20), or typhoid fever.

Edema

Localized edematous plaque anywhere on the body surface is always suggestive of infectious cellulitis when inflammatory and of a reaction to arthropod (cellulitis like reaction) when pruritic. When localized to a limb, it points to acute lymphatic filariasis, lymphoedema of onchocerciasis, or Calabar swelling of loiasis. It may also suggest gnathostomiasis when located on the trunk and American trypanosomiasis or trichinellosis when located on the face.

Nodular lymphangitis

Nodular lymphangitis is defined by an eruption of nodules located along the lymphatic vessels of a limb, usually the arm or forearm, thus

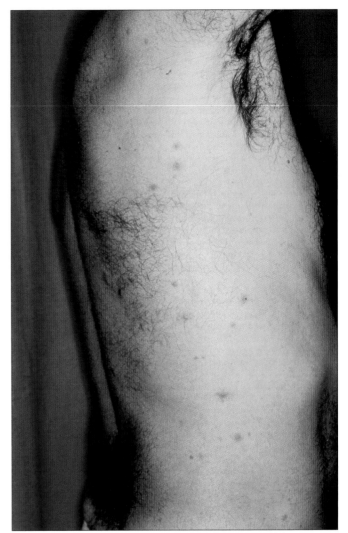

Figure 53.20 Febrile rash in African tick bite fever (South Africa).

conferring the so-called sporotrichoid pattern.[36] This condition primarily suggests cutaneous leishmaniasis and sporotrichosis. However, this sign has been linked to many other causes such as tularemia, cat-scratch disease, pyogenic or mycobacterial infection.

Travelers abroad must be instructed to take precautions to prevent the most common skin diseases during travel. They must be appropriately vaccinated against tetanus before departure and specifically instructed to avoid arthropods bites and sun overexposure. They should be informed of the risk of acquiring localized cutaneous leishmaniasis, cutaneous larva migrans, tungiasis and pyoderma. Travel first aid kits should include antibiotics effective against bacterial skin infection, oral antihistamines and corticosteroid ointments.

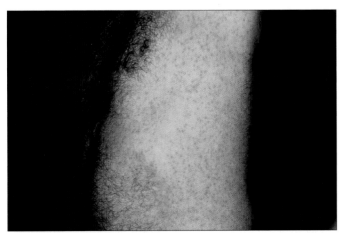

Figure 53.19 Febrile rash in dengue fever (Thailand).

REFERENCES

1. Steffen R, Rickenbach M, Wilhelm U, Helminger A, Schar M. Health problems after travel to developing countries. *J Infect Dis* 1987; **156**:84–91.
2. Peltola H, Kironseppa H, Holsa P. Trips to the south; a health hazard. Morbidity of Finnish travelers. *Scand J Infect Dis* 1983; **15**:375–381.
3. Hill DR. Health problems in a large cohort of Americans traveling to developing countries. *J Travel Med* 2000; **7**:259–266.
4. Caumes E, Brücker G, Brousse G, *et al*. Travel associated illness in 838 French tourists in Nepal in 1984. *Travel Med Int* 1991; **9**:72–76.
5. Shlim DR. *Learning from experience: travel medicine in Kathmandu.* Travel medicine 2. Proceedings of the Second Conference on International Travel Medicine, Atlanta: International Society of Travel Medicine, 1992.

6. Raju R, Smal N, Sorokin M. *Incidence of minor and major disorders among visitors to Fiji.* Travel medicine 2. Proceedings of the Second Conference on International Travel Medicine, Atlanta: International Society of Travel Medicine, 1992.

7. Plentz K. *Nontropical and noninfectious diseases among travelers in a tropical area during five year period (1986–1990).* Travel medicine 2. Proceedings of the Second Conference on International Travel Medicine, Atlanta: International Society of Travel Medicine, 1992.

8. Sanchez JL, Gelnett J, Petruccelli BP, Fraites RF De, Taylor DN. Diarrheal disease incidence and morbidity among United States military personnel during short-term missions overseas. *Am J Trop Med Hyg* 1998; **58**:299–304.

9. Caumes E, Carrière J, Guermonprez G, *et al.* Dermatoses associated with travel to tropical countries: a prospective study of the diagnosis and management of 269 patients presenting to a tropical disease unit. *Clin Infect Dis* 1995; **20**:542–548.

10. Herwaldt BL, Stokes SL, Juranek DD. American cutaneous leishmaniasis in US travelers. *Ann Intern Med* 1993; **118**:779–784.

11. Bouchaud O, Houzé S, Schiemann R, *et al.* Cutaneous larva migrans in travelers: a prospective study, with assessment of therapy with Ivermectin. *Clin Infect Dis* 2000; **31**:493–498.

12. Tremblay A, MacLean JD, Gyorkos T, Mac Phersen DW. Outbreak of cutaneous larva migrans in a group of travelers. *Trop Med Intern Health* 2000; **5**:330–334.

13. Green AD, Mason C, Spragg PM. Outbreak of cutaneous larva migrans among British Military Personnel in Belize. *J Travel Med* 2001; **8**:267–269.

14. Davies HD, Sakuls P, Keystone JS. Creeping eruption. A review of clinical presentation and management of 60 cases presenting to a tropical disease unit. *Arch Derm* 1993; **129**:588–591.

15. Blackwell V, Vega-Lopez F. Cutaneous larva migrans: clinical features and management of 44 cases presenting in the returning travelers. *Br J Derm* 2001; **145**:434–437.

16. Jelinek T, Maiwald H, Nothdurft HD, Loscher T. Cutaneous larva migrans in travelers: synopsis of histories, symptoms and treatment of 98 patients. *Clin Infect Dis* 1994; **19**:1062–1066.

17. Caumes E, Ly F, Bricaire F. Cutaneous larva migrans with folliculitis: report of seven cases and review of the literature. *Br J Derm* 2002; **146**:1–3.

18. Caumes E. Treatment of cutaneous larva migrans. *Clin Infect Dis* 2000; **30**:811–814.

19. Enden E Van Den, Stevens A, Gompel AV. Treatment of cutaneous larva migrans. *N Engl J Med* 1998; **339**:1246–1247.

20. Caumes E, Carrière J, Datry A, Danis M, Gentilini M. A randomized trial of ivermectin versus albendazole for the treatment of cutaneous larva migrans. *Am J Trop Med Hyg* 1993; **49**:641–644.

21. Melby PC, Kreutzer RD, Mc Mahon-Pratt D, Gam AA, Neva FA. Cutaneous leishmaniasis: review of 59 cases seen at the National Institutes of Health. *Clin Infect Dis* 1992; **15**:924–937.

22. Herwaldt BL. Leishmaniasis. *Lancet* 1999; **354**:1191–1199.

23. McGarry JW, McCall PJ, Welby S. Arthropod dermatoses acquired in the UK and overseas. *Lancet* 2001; **357**:2105–2106.

24. Jelinek T, Nothdurft HD, Rieder N, Loscher T. Cutaneous myiasis: review of 13 cases in travelers returning from tropical countries. *Int J Derm* 1995; **34**:624–626.

25. Biggar RJ, Morrow H, Morrow RH. Extensive myiasis from tumbu fly larvae in Ghana, West Africa. *Clin Pediatr* 1980; **19**:231–232.

26. Brewer TF, Wilson ME, Gonzalez E, Felsenstein D. Bacon therapy and furuncular myiasis. *JAMA* 1993; **270**:2087–2088.

27. Sanusi ID, Brown EB, Shepard TG, Grafton WD. Tungiasis; report of one case and review of the 14 reported cases in the United States. *J Am Acad Derm* 1989; **20**:941–944.

28. Bavastrelli M, Bertucci P, Midula M, Giardini O, Sanguigni S. Ciguareta fish poisoning: an emerging syndrome in Italian travelers. *J Travel Med* 2000; **8**:139–142.

29. Nozais JP, Caumes E, Datry A, *et al.* A propos de cinq nouveaux cas d'oedème onchocerquien. *Bull Soc Path Ex* 1997; **90**:335–338.

30. Gonzalez E. Schistosomiasis, cercarial dermatitis and marine dermatitis. *Derm Clin* 1989; **7**:291–300.

31. Freudenthal AR, Joseph PR. Seabather's eruption. *N Engl J Med* 1993; **329**:542–544.

32. Auerbach PS. Marine envenomations. *N Engl J Med* 1991; **325**:486–495.

33. Suntrarachun S, Roselieb M, Wilde H, Sitprija V. A fatal jellyfish encounter in the gulf of Siam. *J Travel Med* 2001; **8**:150–151.

34. Lucchina LC, Wilson ME, Drake LA. Dermatology and the recently returned traveler: infectious diseases with dermatologic manifestations. *Int J Derm* 1997; **36**:167–181.

35. Elgarth ML. Creeping eruption. *Arch Derm* 1998; **134**:619–620.

36. Kostman JR, DiNubile MJ. Nodular lymphangitis: a distinctive but often unrecognized syndrome. *Ann Intern Med* 1993; **118**:883–888.

CHAPTER 54　Persistent Travelers' Diarrhea

Bradley A. Connor and Brian R. Landzberg

KEYPOINTS

- Although most cases of travelers' diarrhea are acute and self-limited, it is important for physicians who treat returning travelers to be aware of a significant percentage of patients who develop persistent gastrointestinal symptoms

- The pathogenesis of persistent travelers' diarrhea generally falls into one of three broad categories: persistent infections, post-infectious processes or chronic gastrointestinal illnesses unmasked by an enteric infection

- Giardiasis is, by far, the most likely persistent infection to be encountered in these patients, making empiric therapy for it a reasonable option

- Many patients with persistent travelers' diarrhea exhibiting typically lower gastrointestinal symptoms, no constitutional symptoms and normal stool and blood evaluation suffer from a post-infectious irritable bowel syndrome

- Patients with post-infectious irritable bowel syndrome will benefit greatly from reassurance from the physician and symptomatic therapy

INTRODUCTION

Fortunately, acute and self-limited illnesses comprise the preponderance of cases of travelers' diarrhea. However, an important minority of patients will develop a more protracted course, lasting weeks, months or even years. Persistent travelers' diarrhea (PTD) is a syndrome frequently encountered by clinicians but poorly studied and characterized. After a review of the various pathogenetic mechanisms underlying the syndrome, we will address the usual concerns shared by both physician and patient in ruling out a persistent infection or infestation, as well as to focus attention on other common and probably underappreciated etiologies of this syndrome. Many of these patients will have long cleared the offending pathogen, and are presenting with post-infectious sequelae, be they inflammatory, malabsorptive, or functional. Others may be suffering from a chronic non-infectious gastrointestinal disease, such as idiopathic inflammatory bowel disease, colorectal carcinoma or celiac sprue which has been unmasked and brought to medical attention by a superimposed enteric infection. When initial stool studies reveal the presence of a persistent pathogen, the management is generally quite straightforward. When this is not the case, however, effective management requires the understanding and application of sound principles of gastroenterology, infectious disease and travel medicine.

DEFINITIONS AND EPIDEMIOLOGY

Travelers' diarrhea (TD) may be defined as diarrhea which develops while abroad in or shortly upon return from a developing country. The dividing line between *acute* and *chronic diarrhea* has generally been accepted to occur at a symptom duration of four weeks.[1] The term *persistent diarrhea* is often used to describe a syndrome of inter-mediate duration, lasting more than 14 days, particularly in children.[2] In this chapter, the terms chronic and persistent travelers' diarrhea will be used interchangeably to describe a syndrome of at least three weeks duration, although the authors prefer the latter term, *persistent*, as it is appropriately less precise and implies a process which began acutely but lingered unexpectedly. In addition, many patients with PTD have the diarrhea itself as a relative minor complaint, over-shadowed by associated cramping pain, bloating, excessive flatulence or tenesmus, and even constipation, all of which we will include here under the rubric of PTD.

Acute travelers' diarrhea visits 20–50% of travelers to tropical and semitropical areas, including Latin America, parts of the Caribbean, southern Asia and Africa, is usually self-limited to a duration of less than one week and is the most common malady encountered by that group.[3,4] An overview of several studies, however, found that between 3 and 10% of travelers may have diarrhea lasting more than two weeks and that 0.8–3% of travelers will have symptoms lasting more than a month.[5–8] A Peace Corps study involving 4607 American volunteers spending 2 years in 21 endemic countries found a prevalence of PTD of 1.7%. A study of 7886 Swiss travelers remaining outside their country for less than 3 months, found PTD to occur in 0.9%. The third study, of students traveling to several Latin American cities, found PTD to occur in 2.9%. The risk of PTD in these studies appeared greatest in travelers to West Africa, Nepal and the Far East. PTD also poses a large problem for the military, with, for example, 16% of 1163 returned Gulf War veterans reporting chronic diarrhea (as defined as three or more loose stools in 24 h lasting more than 6 months) compared with 3% of 2538 non-deployed military personnel.[9] Interestingly, no infectious cause was found in the vast majority of these patients.

PATHOGENETIC MECHANISMS

One can broadly subdivide the syndrome of PTD into several pathogenetic subsets: persistent infection or infestation, post-infectious processes and chronic gastrointestinal illnesses unmasked by an infection (Table 54.1).

Persistent infection or infestation

The infections acquired by travelers often recapitulate those acquired by the indigenous children of the developing world, the two groups

Table 54.1 **Differential diagnosis of chronic travelers' diarrhea**

Persistent infections or infestations
  Protozoans
    Mastigophora: Giardia lamblia
    Coccidia: Cryptosporidium parvum, Isospora belli
    Ciliophora: Balantidium coli
    Microspora: Enterocytozoon bieneusi, Septata intestinalis
    Eimeriidae: Cyclospora cayetanensis
    Rhizopoda: Entamoeba histolytica
    Histomonads and trichomonads: Dientamoeba fragilis
  Helminths
    Strongyloides stercoralis
    Schistosoma spp.
    Ascaris lumbricoides
    Capillaria philippinensis
  Bacteria
    Enterobacteriaceae: Escherichia coli (especially *enteroadherent),
      Shigella spp, non-typhoidal Salmonella,
      Campylobacter spp., Yersinia enterocolitica,
      Vibrionaceae: Aeromonas spp, Plesiomonas spp.
      Clostridium difficile*
  Viruses
  Unknown pathogen
    Brainerd diarrhea
    Tropical sprue

Post-infectious processes
  Post infectious malabsorptive states
    Disaccharide intolerance
    Bacterial overgrowth
  Post-infectious irritable bowel syndrome

Chronic gastrointestinal diseases unmasked by an enteric infection
  Idiopathic inflammatory bowel disease
    Ulcerative colitis
    Crohn's disease
    Microscopic colitis
  Celiac sprue
  Colorectal adenocarcinoma
  Acquired immunodeficiency syndrome

sharing in common a naïveté to the pathogens of the environment.[10] Attention will be focussed here on some of the most commonly encountered persistent pathogens in PTD as well as some unusual and interesting infections with which most clinicians may not be familiar. A more complete list of the relevant pathogens can be found in Table 54.1.

Parasites

Parasites, as a group, are the pathogens most likely to be isolated from patients with PTD, with their probability relative to bacterial infections, increasing with increasing duration of symptoms. In a study of travelers to Nepal, protozoans were detected in 10% of travelers with gastrointestinal symptoms lasting less than 14 days and in 27% of patients with symptoms lasting more than 14 days.[11,12] After passing the three to 4-month mark of symptom duration, however, it becomes decreasingly likely that one will encounter a persistent parasite and more likely that one is dealing with a post-infectious phenomenon. Parasites of the proximal small bowel are an especial concern when malabsorption is present in the presenting clinical syndrome. The parasites most likely to be encountered in PTD are discussed in brief below.

Giardia lamblia

Giardia lamblia, a flagellated protozoan of the class Mastigophora, is, by far the most commonly encountered pathogen in patients with PTD (Fig. 54.1). Suspicion for giardiasis should be particularly high when upper gastrointestinal symptoms predominate[13] (see Clinical approach section). Untreated, symptoms may last for months, even in the immunocompetent host. The diagnosis can often be made through stool microscopy, however as the parasite infests the very proximal small bowel, it is often too degraded prior to defecation to be recognized at microscopy. It is unclear if specific *Giardia* antigen testing by enzyme linked immunosorbent assay significantly enhances sensitivity over multiple careful examinations of stool.[14]

Sampling of the duodenum for *Giardia* may be accomplished through several means. A string test, in which a long string is swallowed, carried by peristalsis into the duodenum and extracted per os has fallen out of favor due to some unreliability.[15] Upper gastrointestinal endoscopy with aspiration of duodenal juice and duodenal biopsy is probably the most sensitive means of making the diagnosis. Biopsy specimens generally show the typical trophozoites appearing as small wavy lines inhabiting the intestinal brush border but not invading the epithelium.

Giardia is usually cured with therapy consisting of metronidazole 250 mg thrice daily for 7 days or tinidazole as a single 2 g dose or 2 g/day for 2 days. Occasionally, a repeat course may be required. Recently metronidazole and tinidazole resistance has been reported. Albendazole 400 mg daily for 7 days, which has cured 100% of children tested, found more mixed success in travelers.[16,17] Quinacrine 100 mg t.i.d. and other alternatives have been listed in Table 54.2. Given the very high prevalence of *Giardia* in PTD, empiric therapy is reasonable in the appropriate clinical setting, after negative stool microscopy and in lieu of duodenal sampling.

Entamoeba histolytica

Entamoeba histolytica has the versatile capacity to produce acute or chronic symptoms which may vary from mild diarrhea to severe, even fatal, colitis, or dysentery. Its prevalence, however, has probably historically been overestimated as a cause of TD and PTD. Only relatively recently have we become aware of *E. dispar*, a morphologically indistinguishable and non-pathogenic protozoan, which seems to vastly outnumber its pathogenic cousin in stool isolate prevalence, by a factor of 10:1.[18,19] Diagnosis is typically made by finding cysts or trophozoites in stool microscopy specimens or by blood serology. Illness with amebiasis usually takes one of three forms. The first is asymptomatic cyst passage, detected in screening stool specimens. Non-dysenteric amebiasis, the second form, often presents with cyclical alternations of diarrhea and constipation with fatigue.

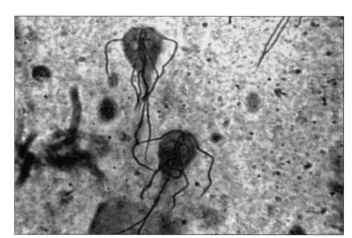

Figure 54.1 *Giardia lamblia* trophozoites, classically described as reminiscent of a face, are seen in this wet prep of stool. (Courtesy of Murray Wittner, MD, Albert Einstein College of Medicine, Bronx, New York).

Table 54.2	Treatment options for giardiasis
Drug	**Regimen**
Metronidazole	250 mg t.i.d. x 5 d
Quinacrine	100 mg t.i.d. x 5 d
Furazolidone	100 mg q.i.d. x 7–10 d
Paromomycin	25–30 mg/kg per d in 3 doses x 7 d
Albendazole	400 mg q.d. x 5 d
Tinidazole	2 g (single dose or x 2 daily doses)

Amebic colitis, manifested by bloody diarrhea with cramping pain and tenesmus, is the third and most severe form of illness and is relatively uncommon in travelers. Stool specimens from patients falling into the first two categories should be carefully analyzed to ensure that the protozoan found is not *E. dispar*, an isolate which should simply be ignored. Patients in the first category with documented *E. histolytica* should be treated a luminal cysticidal agent alone, such as paromomycin 500 mg t.i.d. for 10 days, iodoquinol 650 mg t.i.d. for 20 days (may not be available at standard pharmacies), or diloxanide furoate.[20–22] For patients in the second and third categories, therapy consists of metronidazole 750 mg t.i.d. for 10 days or tinidazole 2 g daily, followed by a luminal cysticidal agent.

Dientamoeba fragilis

A relatively rare cause of PTD, is generally diagnosed by stool microscopy and effectively treated by iodoquinol 650 mg t.i.d. for 20 days or tetracycline 500 mg q.i.d. for 10 days.[23]

Microsporidia

Microsporidia including *Enterocytozoon bieneusi* and *Encephalitozoon intestinalis* have been identified in patients with PTD.[24,25]

Cyclospora cayetanensis

Cyclospora cayetanensis is a relatively recently recognized pathogen which is of particular concern in the patient with PTD acquired in the late spring and early summer months[26] (Fig. 54.2). Although its greatest media attention arose in the setting of outbreaks in North America traced to Guatemalan raspberries, it is a prevalent cause of diarrhea in travelers and expatriates.[27,28] In data from Nepal and Peru before effective therapy was known, cases of diarrhea typically lasted 6 or more weeks. Symptoms are usually upper gastrointestinal and associated with profound fatigue, anorexia, weight loss and malabsorption.[29] Although it is twice as large as *Cryptosporidium*, detection of the 8–10 micron protozoan often requires obtaining a modified acid fast stain of the stool. While often mimicking bacterial gastroenteritis at its onset and giardiasis, unlike the others, *Cyclospora* will not respond to empiric quinolones or metronidazole, respectively. The effective therapy, trimethoprim-sulfamethoxazole, (given as one double strength tablet b.i.d. for 7–10 days) is now relatively seldom used for treating diarrhea, thus such patients are likely to seek care after having failed multiple empiric therapy regimens.[30] Alternative therapies for those allergic or refractory to trimethoprim-sulfamethoxazole are sorely lacking.

Cryptosporidium parvum

Although originally described as an opportunistic pathogen causing diarrhea in AIDS patients, a 1993 water-borne outbreak of *C. parvum* affecting 400 000 Milwaukee residents demonstrated that the immunocompetent were also at significant risk.[31] *C. parvum* has been reported

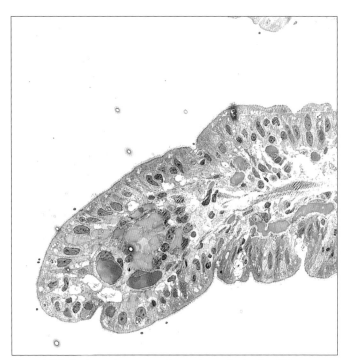

Figure 54.2 Electron microscopy of an endoscopic duodenal biopsy specimen (× 1.1 K) revealing multiple *Cyclospora cayetanensis* organisms identified with dots around villus.

as a cause of PTD in travelers from Egypt, Mauritius and elsewhere.[32] The largest travel-related outbreak occurred when 7 out of 34 Finnish students traveling to Leningrad became ill with profuse diarrhea.[33] Like *Cyclospora*, *C. parvum* is more easily found upon acid-fast staining of stool specimens. In the immunocompetent, a self-limited illness usually lasting less than one month is observed. Though no consistently effective therapy exists for this illness, paromomycin has been met with some success in AIDS patients and immunocompetent travelers.[34]

Isospora belli

Isospora belli has been reported as a cause of diarrhea in travelers returning to the USA from the Caribbean, India and West Africa.[35] Like the previous two protozoans, acid-fast staining of the stool is helpful. Successful therapy generally includes a 10-day course of trimethoprim-sulfamethoxazole double-strength qid or pyrimethamine-sulfadiazine.

Bacteria

Enterobacteriaceae

Enterobacteriaceae, such as enterotoxigenic *Escherichia coli*, *Campylobacter* and *Salmonella*, which play the major role in acute travelers' diarrhea,[36] are probably a relatively uncommon cause of PTD as a persistent or recurrent infection. *Salmonella* and *Shigella*, however have both been reported to result in a carrier state; a recrudescence of symptoms days to weeks later is theoretically possible.

Enteroadherent *E. coli* (EAEC) have been implicated as an important cause of chronic diarrhea in children, AIDS patients and travelers.[37–39] Despite the non-invasive implication of its name, evidence of enterocolonic inflammation from EAEC is often evinced by the presence of fecal leukocytes and occult blood. Quinolones have been used safely and effectively to treat EAEC in affected travelers.[40,41] *Aeromonas*, *Plesiomonas* and *Yersinia enterocolitica* are other pathogens to consider in their ability to cause subacute symptoms and have all been reported in patients with PTD.[42,43]

C. difficile

C. difficile is an extremely relevant pathogen to consider in the patient with PTD. Its clinical presentation may vary from acute to chronic and from mildly increased stool frequency to bloody diarrhea to toxic megacolon. Consequently, the initial workup of PTD should always include a *C. difficile* stool toxin assay. Many PTD patients have taken malaria prophylaxis including mefloquine, chloroquine or doxycycline, or antibiotics for acute travelers' diarrhea which place them at risk for this opportunist.[44] It is an especial consideration in the patient with continuing PTD which seems refractory to multiple courses of empiric antibiotic therapy. Therapy with metronidazole or oral vancomycin is generally successful, although recurrence may occur in upwards of 10% of patients.

Unknown pathogens

There exist many patients with a syndrome of PTD which bears the clinical and epidemiological characteristics of a persistent infectious disease, yet in which extensive microbiological analysis to date has failed to find a responsible pathogen. One has only to look back in recent history to predict that this is a category which will shrink in the future as diagnostic techniques, such as new stains, polymerase chain reaction, and enzyme-linked immunosorbent assay (ELISA) techniques improve and our knowledge of emerging pathogens increases. Cases of travelers' diarrhea due to *Campylobacter jejuni*, *Cryptosporidium parvum*, Enteroadherent *E. coli* and *Cyclospora cayetanensis* were deemed idiopathic infectious disease until the recent recognition of these organisms as common human pathogens in 1977, 1982, 1985 and 1991, respectively.[45–48]

Tropical sprue

Tropical sprue identifies a syndrome of persistent travelers' diarrhea associated with malabsorption, steatorrhea, fatigue and deficiencies of vitamins absorbed in both the proximal and distal small bowel (folate and B_{12}, respectively).[49] It most commonly affects longer-term travelers and expatriates in certain areas of endemicity in the tropics, although short-term travelers are still at risk for it[50] (Fig. 54.3). It occurs more commonly in travelers with close contact with the indigenous population, often follows an acute infectious diarrhea and is seen in household and seasonal epidemics. It has been included in the section of persistent infections causing PTD as it has long been known to reflect an infectious process. However, while modern microbiology and epidemiology provides evidence to support this statement, the past century has accomplished little in identifying a particular responsible pathogen. Competing theories implicate an overgrowth of mixed fecal flora versus various protozoan species including *Cryptosporidium*, *Isospora* and *Cyclospora*.[51] Endoscopic and histopathological changes resemble those of celiac sprue including fissuring and scalloping of mucosal folds and villous atrophy with crypt hyperplasia (Fig. 54.4).[49]

The incidence of tropical sprue has declined dramatically over the years. Less than 1% of the returned travelers we see in a referral center for PTD have tropical sprue. And in an active clinic in Nepal geared

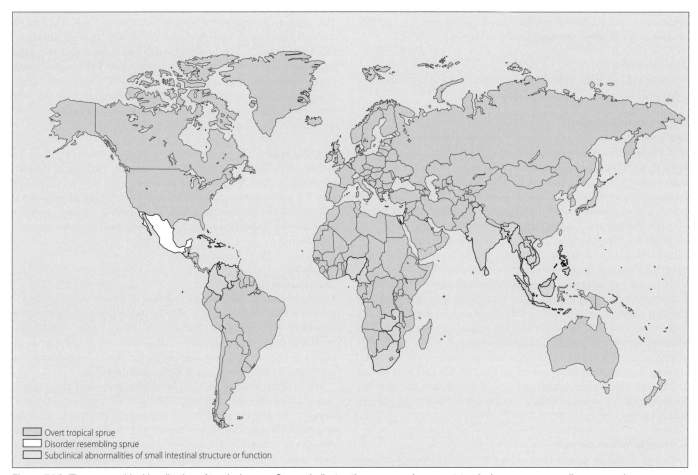

☐ Overt tropical sprue
☐ Disorder resembling sprue
☐ Subclinical abnormalities of small intestinal structure or function

Figure 54.3 The geographical localization of tropical sprue. Orange indicates those areas where overt tropical sprue occurs; yellow areas where a disorder resembling sprue occurs; and green areas where only subclinical abnormalities of small intestinal structure or function have been observed.

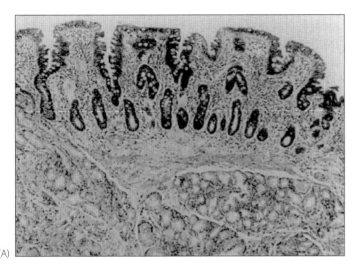

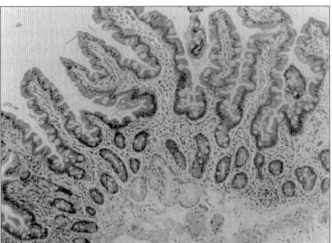

Figure 54.4 Jejunal morphology in a traveler from the UK with tropical sprue. (A) before and (B) after treatment with tetracycline and folic acid.[49]

toward the care of travelers and expatriates, the diagnosis is made only 5–6 times among approximately 1500 patients presenting with diarrhea per year.[52] Whether this reflects that tropical sojourns tend to be shorter with the present ease of transcontinental flight, or the present recommendations to start quinolone antibiosis with the onset of acute diarrhea is unknown.

Treatment has generally consisted of tetracycline 250 mg q.i.d. for at least 6 weeks with folate supplements, though shorter courses, bid dosing and substitution with doxycycline have been tried successfully. Because the diagnosis is presently so rarely made, and the course of treatment is so prolonged, empiric therapy for this should be discouraged.

Brainerd diarrhea

Brainerd diarrhea was first described in 1983 when an epidemic of chronic diarrhea occurred in Brainerd, Minnesota, in which the unpasteurized milk of a local dairy was epidemiologically identified as the source.[53] Although presumably infectious, extensive microbiological analysis has failed to identify a responsible pathogen and no antimicrobial agents have been found to be effective. Seven subsequent Brainerd epidemics have been reported since its initial description, including six in the USA, and one on a cruise ship in the Galapagos Islands of Ecuador.[54,55] The watery diarrhea, associated with urgency, frequency (10–20 stools/day), cramping, weight loss and a waxing and waning pattern, lasts from 2–42 months. At one

year follow-up of the initial outbreak, 12% of patients were subjectively normal, 40% were improved and 48% had unrelenting diarrhea. Biopsy specimens of the colon revealed a prominence of intra-epithelial lymphocytes without markers consistent with lymphocytic or collagenous colitis. It is unknown whether this entity reflects a frequent cause of sporadic PTD.

Post-infectious processes

Post-infectious malabsorptive states

Malabsorption due to persistent infection or infestation of the proximal small bowel, such as giardiasis or tropical sprue, is readily recognized and understood by most clinicians. Less attention, however, has been paid to the issue of malabsorption which persists after an acute infection, such as a bacterial or viral gastroenteritis, has cleared. Disaccharidases, such as the enzymes used to digest lactose and sucrose, normally reside in the brush border overlying the intestinal epithelium. Any acute inflammatory process will readily disrupt the fragile brush border, leaving the patient with transient lactose and sucrose intolerance, which may take several weeks to resolve.[56,57] In some patients with underlying subclinical disaccharidase deficiency, a more permanent lactose intolerance may be seen following gastroenteritis. Exacerbation of symptoms with dairy products and concentrated sweets may not be elicited unless specifically queried and may not even be apparent to the patient. Malabsorption of xylose, folate and B_{12} has been well documented to occur in the setting of acute gastroenteritis.[58] In most of the patients in this report malabsorption was quite transient, however a handful showed continued malabsorption lasting weeks to months after the acute gastroenteritis had resolved.

Occasionally, the changes in bowel motility following acute TD can result in stasis and secondary bacterial overgrowth, ultimately leading to a combined osmotic and secretory diarrhea. This diagnosis should be entertained in the setting of positive fecal fat analysis and D-xylose testing in which both non-invasive and endoscopic duodenal sampling have failed to find a persistent pathogen. The diagnosis is confirmed by lactulose hydrogen breath testing and usually responds to antibiotic therapy, including tetracyclines, amoxicillin-clavulanate and quinolones.[59] The prevalence of bacterial overgrowth in the PTD setting is unknown and many of these patients may be cured by tetracycline empirically administered for tropical sprue. Some authors have suggested that it has been widely underdiagnosed in the setting of chronic gastrointestinal symptoms in general, though rigorous studies on the subject are lacking.[60]

Post-infectious irritable bowel syndrome

The concept of a short, self-limited enteric infection resulting in long-standing neurogastroenterological and motility sequelae is not novel, but appears to be underappreciated. For example, it has long been known that post-viral gastroparesis is an important subset of symptomatic delayed gastric emptying, though it generally quite under-diagnosed except in the hands of gastrointestinal motility subspecialists. So it seems that an enteric infection of the type acquired in travel may leave the host with an altered neurogastroenterological milieu and altered gastrointestinal motility. *Campylobacter*, perhaps the most common cause of bacterial gastroenteritis, has long been known to result in a syndrome of chronic gastrointestinal symptoms meeting the criteria for irritable bowel syndrome (IBS)[61] (Table 54.3). An important study of 38 patients followed in two out-breaks of *Salmonella enteritides* phage Type 4 found approximately one third to develop a chronic IBS.[62] In this study, patients who developed IBS were more likely to have had a severe initial infective illness, but whether this reflects an increased dose of organism or host factors was

Table 54.3	Criteria for the diagnosis of irritable bowel syndrome

Manning criteria	Rome II criteria
Abdominal pain eased with defecation Pain associated with change in frequency of defecation Pain associated with change in consistency of stool Abdominal distention Feeling of incomplete evacuation after defecation Mucus in the stool.	Greater than or equal to 12 weeks (need not be consecutive) in the preceding 12 months of abdominal discomfort or pain with 2 or 3 of the following features: • Relieved by defecation • Onset associated with change in frequency of stool • Onset associated with change in form (appearance) of stool

unclear. The study also demonstrated abnormally increased rectal sensitivity and decreased rectal compliance in a manner similar to what has been seen in 58% of IBS patients in general, suggesting they may constitute a pathophysiologically distinct subset of the IBS population.[63] The symptoms seen in the post-Salmonella patients exclusively localized to colon, consisting of small volume, cramping diarrhea and urgency with no reports of nausea, vomiting or other upper tract symptoms. The authors posit that these patients probably had an enterocolitis rather than a gastroenteritis, however neither imaging nor endoscopy were performed and this remains speculative.

Is post-infectious irritable bowel syndrome (PIBS) different from IBS? Clinically the syndromes are similar, both defined by the absence of constitutional symptoms or weight loss and the presence of abdominal pain which is both associated with an alteration of bowel habits and relieved by defecation.[64,65] Both IBS and PIBS can be subcategorized into syndromes of diarrhea predominance, constipation predominance and pain–gas–bloat predominance, with patients in the latter two groups often not suffering from diarrhea at all. Divergently however, our unpublished clinical experience with this syndrome suggests men and women to be equally likely to develop PIBS, whereas IBS which presents to the physician is much more prevalent in women, demonstrating a ratio of at least 2:1. PIBS has also been known on occasion to respond to antibiotics. While there exist virtually no published data on antibiotic treatment in this group of patients, our own experience as well as that shared with us by colleagues seeing a large volume of such patients, include many anecdotes of such patients responding to transient antibiotic therapy, often intended for another purpose such as an intercurrent urinary tract or upper respiratory infection.

Like IBS, psychological factors play a contributory role in those patients seeking medical care.[66,67] A review of 75 patients with acute gastroenteritis, found that the 22 patients which went on to develop PIBS had higher baseline and follow-up scores for anxiety, depression, somatization and neurotic trait than did those who promptly returned to normal bowel function.[68] In this study, lactose maldigestion was interestingly not an important factor. In animal models, enteric infection has been shown to lead to persistent dysfunction of neuromuscular tissue.[69] Unlike IBS, rigorous human data on natural history, visceral hyperalgesia, neurogastroenterological changes and motility changes as well as the success of various therapies of PIBS simply do not yet exist.

Why is it important to give this entity a name and definition? From the physician's standpoint, once a diagnosis has been made, attention can be appropriately focused away from diagnostic efforts and onto symptomatic therapy and reassurance, the importance of which can-

not be overstated. And psychologically, patients need to have a diagnosis and find comfort in one. Many sufferers are consumed with the concern of harboring a parasite, or worse, an intestinal cancer. All too often we have seen such patients, desperate to have an explanation for their symptoms, fall prey to practitioners who may provide false diagnoses of parasites from in-office stool microscopy and dispense potentially harmful and unnecessary drug therapy. Finally, from a more global perspective, giving this syndrome a name may help facilitate research in the area, which is sorely lacking.

The key concepts here are to consider the diagnosis of PIBS in the young PTD patient with a typically lower gastrointestinal symptom complex and without constitutional symptoms, rule out a structural cause or persistent pathogen with reasonable certainty, reassure the patient and offer symptomatic relief.

Chronic gastrointestinal diseases unmasked by an enteric infection

Travelers' diarrhea has an important potential to uncover latent non-infectious gastrointestinal disease. In the case of celiac sprue (gluten-sensitive enteropathy) and colonic adenocarcinoma, it seems clear that the acute infection acquired in travel is not causative, but merely superimposed on diseased bowel with impaired reserve function or friability, leading to persistent diarrhea or bleeding and bringing the patient to medical attention. In the case of inflammatory bowel disease, it remains somewhat unclear if the travelers' diarrhea is only unmasking the chronic disease or actually initiating it.

Idiopathic inflammatory bowel disease

Idiopathic inflammatory bowel disease (IBD) was diagnosed in 25% of patients in a retrospective British review of 129 cases of bloody diarrhea acquired in or within two weeks upon return from a tropical sojourn.[70] These patients denied gastrointestinal complaints predating travel, begging the question if the infection acquired in travel was actually responsible for the initiation of the autoimmune cascade of IBD. As many of the prevailing hypotheses of the pathogenesis of IBD begin with an initiating antigenic pathogen in the setting of an alteration in intestinal permeability and a genetically determined imbalance of pro- and anti-inflammatory responses, such a scenario would seem quite plausible. The most common form of IBD uncovered in this setting is ulcerative colitis, however Crohn's Disease[71] and microscopic colitides, including collagenous and lymphocytic colitis, have also been seen. The latter group demonstrates a normal gross colonoscopic examination, however random biopsy specimens will evince the underlying inflammatory process.

Celiac sprue

Celiac sprue is a disease of the small bowel in which genetically susceptible individuals sustain villous atrophy and crypt hyperplasia in response to exposure to antigens found in many grains, leading to malabsorption. From studies of healthy blood donors, we know that clinically apparent disease with malabsorptive diarrhea accounts for only the tip of the celiac sprue iceberg, with the majority of cases being subclinical or presenting with associated symptoms of osteoporosis, anemia and the like.[72] As 1:250 healthy Americans seem to harbor latent celiac disease, based on the screening of blood bank donations, it is important to consider the unmasking of this entity by an enteric superinfection in patients with PTD. The disease is diagnosed by compatible gross and microscopic duodenal examination and by the presence of anti-endomysial, anti-gliadin, anti-tissue trans glutaminase and anti-reticulin antibodies[73] and is treated by a very effective, if difficult to maintain, gluten free diet (Fig. 54.5).

Colorectal cancer

Colorectal cancer must be a consideration in patients with PTD, particularly those passing blood per rectum or found to have fecal occult blood or new iron deficiency anemia.[74] This is especially true if hematochezia persists after the diarrhea has resolved. In any such patient over the age of 50 years old, a full colonoscopy should be performed, even if the symptoms seem consistent with infectious colitis. Colorectal cancer is too prevalent in the USA, with the average lifetime risk of the individual approaching 6%, and the consequences of missing an early diagnosis too great not to request a complete colonic luminal evaluation in the older patient. In the patient younger than 40 years old, the prevalence of cancer is substantially lower and flexible sigmoidoscopy or expectant management may be reasonable options.

CLINICAL APPROACH

History and physical examination

As with any other medical complaint, the most important diagnostic tools in PTD remain the complete history and physical examination. A detailed history of present illness is particularly essential. It is first necessary to establish the diagnosis of a chronic or persistent diarrhea. For example, a complaint of PTD of 8 weeks of diarrhea may, upon further questioning, turn out to be three separate episodes of acute diarrhea, the most recent of which brings the patient to the office, changing the differential diagnosis considerably. In eliciting the history of present illness therefore it is critical to listen for gaps in wellness; a hiatus of 5–7 days without diarrhea suggests that an infection may have cleared and a new one begun.[75] In addition, vomiting and fever usually occur at the onset of enteric infections, so that if a patient reports weeks of diarrhea followed by the initiation of vomiting and fever, the likelihood is that the patient suffers from a new superimposed acute infection, rather than a chronic one. Travelers may develop multiple enteric infections, as suggested in a study of travelers to Nepal, in which 17% were diagnosed with more than one stool pathogen.[76]

The history should be used to anatomically localize the pathology to either small or large bowel. Diarrhea which is large volume, but relatively infrequent should suggest a small bowel process, testament to the bulk of fluid absorption normally occurring in the small bowel, as well as the capacitance of the non-inflamed colon as a reservoir for stool. Other symptoms localizing to the upper gastrointestinal tract include nausea, vomiting, eructation and pyrosis. Symptoms such as copious flatus or stools which are foul-smelling, floating or associated with oil droplets suggest a small bowel process associated with malab-

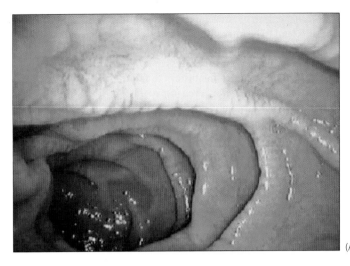

(A)

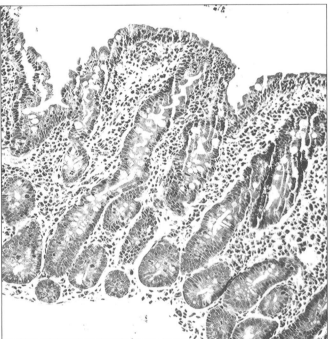

(B)

Figure 54.5 (A) Endoscopic photograph of a patient with PTD due to unmasked celiac sprue showing classic mucosal fissuring and scalloping of folds. (B) Low power light photomicrograph of a duodenal biopsy specimen revealing marked villous blunting and crypt hyperplasia, consistent with sprue. Laboratory values in this patient were notable for iron and folate deficiency with a normal B_{12} level consistent with a duodenal process and positive antigliadin and anti-tissue transglutaminase antibodies. A gluten free diet was recommended.

sorption. The frequent, relatively small volume diarrhea associated with infraumbilical cramping, implies a colonic process (like Brainerd diarrhea), in which additional symptoms of tenesmus, bloody mucus or frank hematochezia would herald a colitis or dysentery. Fever, sweats or chills would favor the presence of a continued invasive pathogen, but may also be seen in unmasked idiopathic inflammatory bowel disease or cancer.

Weight loss raises a concern for an ongoing infectious, malabsorptive, inflammatory or malignant process and should be seen as inconsistent with merely functional syndromes such as PIBS, as would symptoms which awaken the patient from sleep. Bacterial infections will generally be abrupt and severe in onset with a steady daily pattern. The symptoms of protozoan illnesses tend to be milder at onset, beginning with the passage of a few loose movements per day. They will also tend to be intermittent, with a few days on and few days off, as is typically seen with Entameba and Cyclospora. Giardiasis tends to behave more like a bacterial process in its consistency of symptoms.

It is also important in the history to inquire about any preceding gastrointestinal symptoms, even if patients are slow to offer them. These are often found in patients with unmasked idiopathic inflammatory bowel disease or PIBS. Family history of gastrointestinal ailments and personal history of non-steroidal anti-inflammatory drug use or smoking patterns may influence the likelihood of IBD. If, and only if, no evidence of malabsorption or constitutional symptoms exists, then the diagnosis of post-infectious irritable bowel syndrome should be considered.

Oftentimes, you will be the second or third physician encountering the patient, and it important to be aware of all preceding diagnostic and therapeutic management, including pre-, intra- and post-travel care. Many of these patients have taken antibacterial agents, malarial prophylaxis and the like, predisposing them to antibiotic associated diarrhea and *C. difficile* in addition to gastrointestinal side-effects of the medications apart from changes in bowel flora. The particular antibiotics given are important. Did they include broad gram negative coverage, like a quinolone? Did the patient take trimethoprim-sulfamethoxazole which would have covered *Cyclospora*?

In addition to the careful gastrointestinal history, a detailed travel history is important. In which season did the patient travel, Cyclospora being most prevalent in the spring and early summer months? Was the patient in rural or urban areas? Did the symptoms worsen on the airplane ride home? (Air pressure changes in flight may cause inflamed bowel to distend, creating more discomfort.)

Physical examination, though less helpful than history in these patients, remains important. Observed weights (especially serial) and assessments of temporal wasting and skin turgor provide useful insights into the nutritional and volume status of the patient. Marked lower abdominal tenderness should raise concern for the presence of a colitis, be it infectious, ischemic or idiopathic inflammatory bowel disease. Mild tenderness in the left lower quadrant may be seen in PIBS, as it is with IBS, relating to spasm of the sigmoid colon. Epigastric and right upper quadrant tenderness may be seen in giardial infections but is neither specific nor sensitive. Edema may be seen in the presence of either malabsorption or protein-losing enteropathy. Any positive physical examination findings listed above, other than mild left lower quadrant tenderness, probably preclude the diagnosis of PIBS. Fecal occult blood testing and testing for fecal leukocytes are also useful, and if positive, suggest the presence of an invasive or inflammatory, typically colonic, pathogen or process. Occult fecal blood should, in an older patient, alert the clinician to the alternative possibility of an unmasked gastrointestinal malignancy and lead to colonoscopic evaluation. Testing for fecal leukocytes is unnecessary when gross or occult blood is present in the stool as it will always be positive in that setting, regardless of the presence of an inflammatory process.

Non-invasive laboratory workup

Stool studies

Stool studies should be the first diagnostic step in the evaluation of PTD, after the history and physical examination. These may be very helpful when positive, but are notoriously insensitive. Upper gastrointestinal parasites are often missed and pathogenic bacteria are often misclassified as normal flora unless examined in specialized laboratories. We generally recommend at least three ova and parasite examinations with wet prep, trichrome stain and modified acid-fast stain, in addition to culture and C. difficile toxin assay. A large retro-

spective review of stool microscopy specimens submitted to the Kaiser Permanente system in California found that sending three specimens rather than one increased the yield for *E. histolytica*, *G. lamblia*, and *D. fragilis* by 22.7%, 11.3% and 31.1%, respectively.[77] Acid-fast staining is very helpful in the detection of *Cyclospora*, *Cryptosporidia* and *Isospora* spp and is not performed unless specifically requested in most laboratories. Concentration of the stool will also increase the yield of finding these protozoans. Antigen assays, such as the one which exists for *G. lamblia* appear to only minimally heighten sensitivity.

The accuracy of fecal light microscopy is exquisitely dependent on the skill, experience and integrity of the technician reading the slides. It is therefore important for clinicians to develop a relationship and a level of confidence with a particular laboratory. The authors have had personal experience both with laboratories which are very insensitive in finding parasites as well as those which are notorious for over-diagnosing infestation when it does not exist.

Another important caveat in obtaining stool microscopy of which to be aware, is the potential detection of non-pathogenic protozoans, often identified in avid travelers to developing countries. Many of these have been listed in Table 54.4. Unnecessary attention, patient angst and drug therapy have been lavished on these organisms which are essentially clinically irrelevant and are harmful only in distracting the clinician from further workup and iatrogenic complications of unneeded therapy.

When edema is present, and when the serum albumin appears to be disproportionately reduced compared with other markers of malnutrition or malabsorption, the diagnosis of a protein-losing enteropathy may be addressed by obtaining a 24–72 h stool collection and blood sample for alpha-1-antitrypsin clearance.

Blood testing

As in the workup of any chronic diarrheal illness, reasonable laboratory evaluation for PTD would begin with a complete blood count with differential. Eosinophilia would suggest the presence of a lingering parasitic infestation, recalling that this is seen with invasive helminths and not protozoans. Leukocytosis with neutrophilia favors a bacterial process, and when marked (greater than 20 000 cells/dL) suggests *C. difficile* infection. Lymphocytosis may be seen in viral processes. An elevated erythrocyte sedimentation rate or C-reactive protein, although neither sensitive nor specific, may be seen in either an infectious or inflammatory process and should steer the differential diagnosis away from PIBS. Abnormalities in albumin or prothrombin time may be seen in malabsorption or malnutrition. Abnormally low values for iron or folate suggest a process in the proximal small bowel, whereas deficiency in vitamin B_{12} generally

Table 54.4	Non pathogenic protozoans

Entamoeba spp. (non-*histolytica*)
    E. hartmanni
    E. moshkovskii
    E. coli
    E. dispar (distinguished from *histolytica* only with specialized analysis)	

Blastocystis hominis	
Endolimax nana	
Iodamoeba butschlii	
Chilomastix mesnili	
Enteromonas hominis	

stems from ileal disease, relating to the area or normal absorption. The presence of both B$_{12}$ and folate deficiency should raise suspicion for tropical sprue in its typical ability to involve wide-reaching segments of the alimentary canal.

With or without the benefit of a positive fecal fat assessment, D-xylose testing is indicated as a confirmatory, non-invasive test for small bowel malabsorption. The absorption of this pentose monosaccharide occurs by passive diffusion through the gut, neither dependent on pancreaticobiliary secretion (like triglycerides) nor brush border digestion (like lactose), nor a sodium hexose co-transporter (like most other monosaccharides). It therefore may be taken as a pure marker of small bowel mucosal permeability and surface area. After drinking a 25 g bolus of D-xylose, the patient may either submit a 5 h urine collection, or have a venous sample drawn. A normal result is excretion of greater than 20% of the xylose load into the urine. Markedly positive results, i.e. those less than 15% are typically seen in tropical sprue.

Other reasonable bloodwork might include an electrolyte panel, thyroid function tests, amebic, HIV and celiac serologies.

Endoscopic evaluation

The authors believe that most patients with PTD who have had unrevealing non-invasive evaluation (Table 54.5) as elaborated above should be considered for an endoscopic evaluation, although empiric therapy is an equally acceptable first-line approach, such as for parasitic illness like *Giardia* or bacterial illness. There are advantages and disadvantages to both strategies. There are no randomized data on the subject of empiric therapy versus endoscopic evaluation for PTD and generally recommendations have come from infectious disease subspecialists rather than gastroenterologists, the former who do not have endoscopy as a tool immediately at hand. However, the argument for empiric therapy is the avoidance of procedures which carry some cost and some minimal risk. The use of antimicrobials or antiparasitic agents when no pathogen has been documented may confuse rather than clarify the issue. These medications, in addition to the risk of allergic reaction and other side effects particular to the individual drugs, alter bowel flora and may muddle the picture by introducing antibiotic-associated diarrhea, with or without pseudomembranous colitis. In addition, a lack of response to an empiric course of therapy may simply reflect antibiotic resistance rather than an incorrect diagnosis. While empiric therapy remains an important tool in our armamentarium, and an acceptable first line approach, there exist selected groups of patients, in whom an endoscopic evaluation should be performed, including: (1) patients failing one or two unsuccessful empiric courses, (2) all patients older than 50 with occult or gross fecal blood and (3) the setting of malabsorptive symptoms or signs. Endoscopy provides a sensitive means of identifying a lingering parasitic infestation or tropical sprue as well as identifying underlying structural gastrointestinal processes including idiopathic inflammatory bowel disease, celiac sprue and colorectal carcinoma. It also provides an objective marker to follow in patients with persistent symptoms. From an evidence-based medicine standpoint, it demonstrates a useful diagnostic yield in the workup of chronic diarrhea in general,[78] however the yield in PTD remains poorly studied.

The choice of upper gastrointestinal endoscopy versus colonoscopy (or sigmoidoscopy) returns us to the importance of the medical history, using the clues as described above for localizing a process to the small or large bowel. Of key importance is that the endoscopist should take biopsies and aspirates of the duodenum at EGD and the colon (and possibly terminal ileum) at lower endoscopy, regardless of the presence of gross mucosal disease, as the changes may be only visible at the microscopic level. The role for evaluation of these specimens by transmission electron microscopy (EM) remains unclear.

Presently it is to be considered an investigational tool to be used by those with research interests in the area.

Outlined in Figure 54.6 are management algorithms for the various clinical syndromes grouped under PTD. There is certainly room for debate in many of the steps of these algorithms and prospective clinical trials are essentially non-existent. And, of course, all diagnostic and therapeutic interventions must be tailored to the unique aspects of each individual patient (Table 54.6). Consequently, these should not be regarded as a standard of care in treating such patients, but rather as a reasonable clinical approach based upon extensive personal experience and review of existing data.

Therapy

Empiric anti-infective therapy is both a useful diagnostic and therapeutic tool. A response to a quinolone or macrolide would simultaneously support the diagnosis of and treat bacterial disease. A response to a nitroimidazole might be similarly useful in clinically suspected giardiasis or amebiasis as would trimethoprim-sulfamethoxazole for suspected cyclosporiasis. Many authors have recommended empiric courses of therapy for tropical sprue in the patient with PTD and malabsorption.[79] As mentioned previously, we no longer recommend this particular approach for several reasons including the dramatically diminishing incidence of tropical sprue, the lengthy courses of therapy required and the increasing awareness of other etiologies including unmasked celiac disease. In the patient with PTD and upper symptoms and without malabsorption, we would still more strongly advise against empiric tropical sprue therapy as this entity was found quite rarely in this setting, based on the Nepalese and other data. In the patient with diarrhea associated with upper gastrointestinal symptoms and without malabsorption, an empiric course of metronidazole to cover giardiasis would be an appropriate intervention (see Fig. 54.6).

Symptomatic therapy is another important aspect of the clinical management of PTD, particularly in PIBS, and begins with diet modifications. Due to the compromise of the brush border with a transient enteric infection, a trial should be undertaken of sequential avoidance of dairy products, sorbitol containing products, fruit juices, concentrated sweets and high fat items, in that order. In patients with colitis, a low residue, low fiber diet should be advised.

Table 54.5	Non-invasive evaluation
Blood	**Stool**
All patients	**All patients**
Complete blood count with differential	Culture and sensitivity
Electrolytes	Ova and parasites (three specimens)
Albumin	Giardia antigen ELISA
Prothrombin time	C. difficile toxin assay
Folate	Fecal occult blood
Iron studies	Fecal fat (qualitative)
Vitamin B$_{12}$	Fecal leukocytes
TSH	
Erythrocyte sedimentation rate or c-reactive protein	**Selected patients**
	Fecal alpha-1 antitrypsin clearance
Selected patients	
Celiac serologies	
TSH	
Amebic serology	
D-xylose (after 25 g load, urine level also acceptable)	
HIV ELISA	

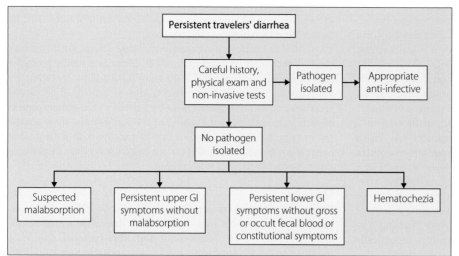

Figure 54.6A

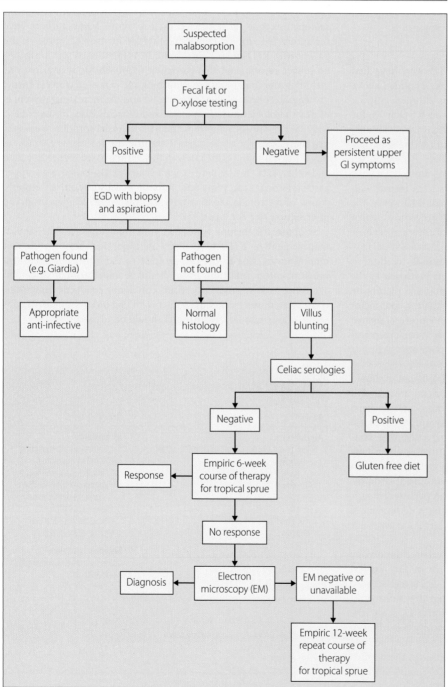

Figure 54.6B

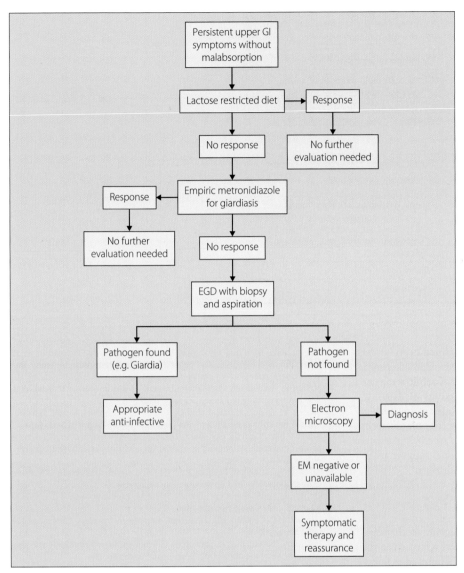

Figure 54.6C

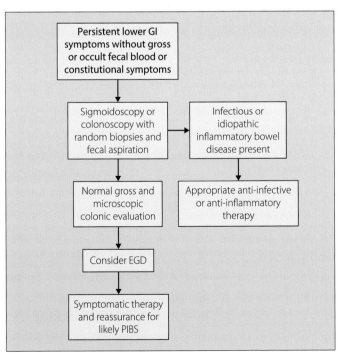

Figure 54.6D

Figure 54.6E

Figure 54.6 Clinical management algorithms (A–E) for persistent travelers' diarrhea.

Table 54.6 Selected clinical patterns of persistent travelers' diarrhea and likely etiologies

Clinical pattern	Common diagnoses
Large gaps in symptoms with long periods of wellness or onset of fever and emesis more than one week into illness	Consider multiple episodes of acute travelers' diarrhea rather than PTD.
Predominantly upper gastrointestinal symptoms, including eructation, nausea and epigastric discomfort, and small volume, infrequent diarrhea	*Giardiasis, Cyclosporiasis,* celiac sprue.
Predominantly lower gastrointestinal symptoms without blood per rectum or constitutional symptoms.	Post-infectious irritable bowel syndrome
Blood or bloody mucus per rectum, or frequent, small-volume diarrhea, tenesmus, lower abdominal cramping	Colonic processes including: *Amoebiasis, C. difficile,* bacillary dysentery (C. jejunae, shigellosis, salmonellosis), unmasked colonic adenocarcinoma, unmasked idiopathic IBD.
Weight loss without malabsorption	Malignancy or AIDS
B_{12} and folate deficiency	Tropical sprue

Based upon the nature of the symptoms, antispasmodics and other drugs useful in IBS, such as hyoscyamine, chlordiazepoxide, clinidium, Limbitrol and fiber in the form of psyllium or methylcellulose may be helpful. For the patient with predominant symptoms of diarrhea, loperamide, diphenoxylate, and tincture of opium are invaluable. Probiotics such as Lactobacillus and Saccharomyces boulardii seem to improve symptoms in some of these patients as well.[80] In patients with PIBS, remember that reassurance and emotional support are as important as dietary recommendations and drug therapy.

CONCLUSION

This chapter has reviewed the various pathogenetic mechanisms underlying PTD as well as outlined a logical clinical approach to the patient suffering from it. Particularly when initial stool studies fail to reveal a persistent pathogen, considerable clinical acumen is required to appropriately direct diagnostic and therapeutic efforts to pursue diagnoses either not addressed or missed by the initial evaluation. Of course, every effort should be made to identify a persistent infection or infestation, and we should remain ever vigilant for emerging pathogens. It is equally essential, however, for the clinician to develop a level of comfort in the absence of a specific microbiological or histopathological diagnosis, as the majority of patients with PTD will not have one. In such cases, one must implement the tools of a thorough history and physical examination, blood and stool evaluations, empiric therapy and endoscopy to localize the problem to the small or large bowel, to characterize the problem as a persistent infection, post-infectious syndrome, or the unmasking of a chronic gastrointestinal disease, and to treat the patient accordingly. In the patient with lower abdominal symptoms without constitutional symptoms, and in whom persistent infection and structural gastrointestinal disease have been reasonably ruled out, that is PIBS, offering a diagnosis, reassurance and symptom-based therapy will prove extremely beneficial.

REFERENCES

1. American Gastroenterological Association Medical Position Statement. Guidelines for the evaluation and management of chronic diarrhea. *Gastroenterol* 1999; **116**:1461–1463.

2. International Working Group on Persistent Diarrhoea. Evaluation of an algorithm for the treatment of persistent diarrhea: A multicenter study. *Bull WHO* 1996; **74**:478.

3. Steffen R, Rickenbach M, Wilhelm U, *et al.* Health problems after travel to developing countries. *J Infect Dis* 1987; **156**:84–91.

4. Steffen R. Epidemiological studies of travelers' diarrhea, severe gastrointestinal infections and cholera. *Rev Infect Dis* 1986; **8**(suppl 2):S122–S130.

5. Merson MH, Morris GK, Sack DA. Travelers' Diarrhea in Mexico: A prospective study of physicians and family members attending a congress. *N Engl J Med* 1976; **294**:1299.

6. Addis DG, Tauxe RV, Bernard KW. Chronic diarrheal illness in U.S. Peace Corps volunteers. *Int J Epidemiol* 1990; **19**:217–218.

7. Steffen R, Linde F van der, Gyr K, Schar M. Epidemiology of diarrhea in travelers. *JAMA* 1983; **249**:1176–1180.

8. Dupont HL, Capsuto EG. Persistent diarrhea in travelers. *Clin Infect Dis* 1996; **22**:124–128.

9. Fukuda K, Nisenbaum R, Stewart G. Chronic multi-system illness affecting Air Force veterans of the Gulf War. *JAMA* 1998; **280**:981.

10. Shlim DR, Hoge CW, Rajah R, *et al.* Persistent high risk of diarrhea among foreigners in Nepal during the first 2 years of residence. *Clin Infect Dis* 1999; **29**:613–616.

11. Hoge CW, Shlim DR, Echevarria P. Epidemiology of diarrhea among expatriate residents living in a highly endemic environment. *JAMA* 1996; **275**:533–538.

12. Taylor DN, Houston R, Shlim DR. Etiology of diarrhea among travelers and foreign residents in Nepal. *JAMA* 1988; **260**:1245–1248.

13. Ortega YR. Adam R. Giardia: Overview and Update. *Clin Infect Dis* 1997; **25**:545–550.

14. Addis DG, Mathews HM, Stewart JM. Evaluation of a commercially available enzyme-linked immunosorbent assay for Giardia lamblia testing in stool. *J Clin Microbiol* 1991; **29**:1137.

15. Goka AK, Rolston DD. MAthan VI. The relative merits of faecal and duodenal juice microscopy in the diagnosis of giardiasis. *Trans R Soc Trop Med Hyg* 1990; **84**:66.

16. Kollaritsch H, Jeschko E, Wiedermann G. Albendazole is highly effective against cutaneous larva migrans but not against Giardia infection: Results of an open pilot trial in travelers returning from the tropics. *Trans R Soc Trop Med Hyg* 1993; **87**:689.

17. Dutta AK, Phadke MA, Bagade AC. A randomized multicentre study to compare the safety and efficacy of albendazole and metronidazole in the treatment of giardiasis in children. *Indian J Pediatr* 1994; **61**:689.

18. Jackson TF. Entamoeba histolytica and Entamoeba dispar are distinct species; clinical, epidemiological and serological evidence. *Int J Parasitol* 1998; **28**:181.

19. Reed SL. Amebiasis: an update. *Clin Infect Dis* 1992; **14**:385–391.

20. Anand AC, Reddy PS, Saiprasad GS, Kher SK. Does non-dysenteric intestinal amoebiasis exist? *Lancet* 1997; **349**:89–92.

21. Nanda R, Baveja U, Anand BS. Entamoeba histolytica cyst passers: clinical features and outcome in untreated subjects. *Lancet* 1984; **1**:301–303.

22. Petri WA, Singh U. Diagnosis and Management of Amebiasis. *Clin Infect Dis* 1999; **29**:1117–1125.
23. Cuffari C, Oligny L, Seidmen EG. Dientamoeba fragilis masquerading as allergic colitis. *J Pediatr Gastroenterol Nutr* 1998; **26**:16.
24. Raynaud L, Delbac F, Broussolle V. Identification of Encephalitozoon intestinalis in travelers with chronic diarrhea by specific PCR amplification. *J Clin Microbiol* 1998; **36**:37.
25. Wanke CA, DeGirolami P, Federman M. Enterocytozooan bieneusi infection and diarrheal disease in patients who were not infected with human immunodeficiency virus: Case report and review. *Clin Infect Dis* 1996; **23**:816.
26. Connor BA. Cyclospora. In: Blaser MJ, *et al.*, eds. *Infections of the Gastrointestinal Tract 2e*. Maryland: Lippincott, Williams and Wilkins; 2002:1029–1038.
27. Herwaldt BL, Ackers ML. An outbreak in 1996 of cyclosporiasis associated with imported raspberries. Cyclospora Work Group. *N Engl J Med* 1997; **336**:1548.
28. Hoge CW, Shlim DR, Echeverria P, *et al.* Epidemiology of diarrhea among expatriate residents living in a highly endemic environment. *JAMA* 1996; **275**:533–538.
29. Connor BA, Shlim DR, Scholes JV, *et al.* Pathologic changes in the small bowel in nine patients with diarrhea associated with a coccidian-like body. *Int Med* 1993; **119**:377–382.
30. Hoge CW, Shlim DR, Ghimire M, *et al.* Placebo-controlled trial of co-trimoxazole for Cyclospora infections among travelers and foreign residents in Nepal. *Lancet* 1995; **345**:691–693.
31. MacKenzie WR, Hoxie NJ, Proctor ME, *et al.* A massive outbreak in Milwaukee of Cryptosporidium infection transmitted through the public water supply. *N Engl J Med* 1994; **331**:161.
32. Gatti S, Cevini C, Bruno A, *et al.* Cryptosporidiosis in tourists returning from Egypt and the island of Mauritius. *Clin Infect Dis* 1993; **16**:344–345.
33. Jokipii AMM, Hemila M, Jokipii L. Prospective study of acquisition of Cryptosporidium, Giardia lamblia, and gastrointestinal disease. *Lancet* 1985; **1**:487–489.
34. Bissuel F, Cotte L, Rabodonirina M, *et al.* Paramomycin: an effective treatment for cryptosporidiosis in patients with AIDS. *Clin Infect Dis* 1994; **18**:447.
35. Shaffer N, Moore L. Correspondence – chronic travelers' diarrhea in a normal host due to Isospora belli. *J Infect Dis* 1989; **159**:596–597.
36. Steffen R, Linde F van der, Gyr K, Schar M. Epidemiology of diarrhea in travelers. *JAMA* 1983; **249**:1176–1180.
37. Bhan MK, Raj P, Levine MM. Enteroaggregative Escherichia coli associated with persistent diarrhea in a cohort of rural children in India. *J Infect Dis* 1989; **159**:1061–1064.
38. Matthewson JJ, Jiang ZD, Zumla A. Hep 2 cell adherent Escherichia coli in patients with human immunodeficiency virus-associated diarrhea. *J Infect Dis* 1995; **171**:1636.
39. Gascôn J, Vargas M, Quinté L. Enteroaggregative Escherichia coli strains as a cause of travelers' diarrhea: a case control study. *J Infect Dis* 1998; **177**:1409–1412.
40. Glandt M, Adachi JA, Mathewson JJ, *et al.* Enteroaggregative Escherichia coli as a cause of travelers' diarrhea: clinical response to ciprofloxacin. *Clin Infect Dis* 1998; **29**:335–338.
41. Boockenooghe AR, DuPont HL, Jiang ZD, *et al.* Markers of enteric inflammation in enteroaggregative Escherichia coli diarrhea in travelers. *Am J Trop Med Hyg* 2000; **62**:711–713.
42. Rautelin H, Hanninen ML, Sivonen A. Chronic diarrhea due to a single strain of Aeromonas caviae. *Eur J Clin Microbiol Infect Dis* 1995; **14**:51.
43. Rautelin H, Sivonen A, Kuikka A. Enteric Plesiomonas shigelloides infections in Finnish patients. *Scand J Infect Dis* 1995; **27**:495.
44. Golledge CL, Riley TV. Clostridium difficile-associated diarrhea after doxycycline malaria prophylaxis. *Lancet* 1995; **345**:1377–1378.
45. Skirrow MB. Campylobacter enteritis: a 'new' disease. *BMJ* 1977; **2**:9–11.
46. Centers for Disease Control. Cryptosporidiosis: an assessment of chemotherapy of males with acquired immunodeficiency syndrome (AIDS). *MMWR Morb Mortal Wkly Rep* 1982; **31**:589–592.
47. Mathewson JJ, Johnson PC, DuPont HL, *et al.* A newly recognized cause of travelers' diarrhea: Enteroadherent Escherichia coli. *J Infect Dis* 1985; 1985; **151**:471–475.
48. Hoge CW, Shlim DR, Rajah R, *et al.* Epidemiology of diarrheal illness associated with coccidian-like organism among travelers and foreign residents in Nepal. *Lancet* 1993; **341**:1175–1178.
49. Farthing MJG. Tropical Malabsorption and Tropical Diarrhea. In: Feldman M, Scharschmidt BF, Sleisenger MH, ed. *Sleisenger & Fordtran's Gastrointestinal and Liver Disease*, 6th edn. Philadelphia, PA: WB Saunders; 1998:1574–1584.
50. Klipstein FA. Tropical sprue in travelers and expatriates living abroad. *Gastroenterology* 1981; **80**:590–600.
51. Cook GC. Aetiology and pathogenesis of postinfective tropical malabsorption (tropical sprue). *Lancet* 1984; **i**:721–723.
52. Shlim DR. Response to Letter to the Editor: Tropical sprue as a cause of traveler's diarrhea. *Wilderness Environ Med* 2000; **11**:140–141.
53. Osterholm MT, MacDonald KL, White KE. An outbreak of a newly recognized chronic diarrhea syndrome associated with raw milk consumption. *JAMA* 1986; **256**:484–490.
54. Mintz ED, Weber JT, Guris D. An outbreak of Brainerd diarrhea among travelers to the Galapagos Islands. *J Infect Dis* 1998; **177**:1041.
55. Parsonnet J, Wanke CA, Hack H. Idiopathic chronic diarrhea. In: Blaser MJ, Smith PD, Ravidin JI, eds. *Infections of the Gastrointestinal Tract*. New York, NY: Raven Press; 1995:311–323.
56. Montgomery RD, Beale DJ, Sammons HG, Schneider R. Postinfective malabsorption: a sprue syndrome. *BMJ* 1973; **2**:265–268.
57. Greene HL, McCabe DR, Merenstein GB. Protracted diarrhea and malnutrition in infancy: changes in intestinal morphology and disaccharidase activities during treatment with total intravenous nutrition or elemental diets. *J Pediatr* 1975; **87**:695.
58. Lindenbaum J. Malabsorption during and after recovery from acute intestinal infection. *BMJ* 1965; **2**:326–329.
59. Attar A, Flourie B, Rambaud JC, *et al.* Antibiotic efficacy in small intestinal bacterial overgrowth-related chronic diarrhea: A crossover, randomized trial. *Gastroenterol* 1999; **117**:794–720.
60. Pimentel M, Chow EJ, Lin HC. Eradication of small intestinal bacterial overgrowth reduces symptoms of irritable bowel syndrome. *Am J Gastroenterol* 2000; **95**:3503–3506.
61. Neal KR, Hebden J, Spiller R. Prevalence of gastrointestinal symptoms six months after bacterial gastroenteritis and risk factors for development of the irritable bowel syndrome: postal survey of patients. *BMJ* 1997; **314**:719–782.
62. McKendrick MW, Read NW. Irritable bowel syndrome-post salmonella infection. *J Infect* 1994; **29**:1–3.
63. Bewrgin AJ, Donnelly TC, McKendrick MW, Read NW. Changes in anorectal function in persistent bowel disturbance following salmonella gastroenteritis. *Gui J Gastroenterol Hepatol* 1993; **5**:617–620.
64. Vanner SJ. Predictive value of the Rome criteria for diagnosing the irritable bowel syndrome. *Am J Gastroenterol* 1999; **94**:2912–2917.
65. Drossman DA, Whitehead WE, Camilleri M. Irritable bowel syndrome: a technical review for practice guideline development. *Gastroenterol* 1997; **112**:2120–2137.
66. Esler MD, Goulston KJ. Levels of anxiety in colonic disorders. *N Engl J Med* 1973; **288**:16–20.
67. Drossman DA, McKee DC, Sandler RS. Psychological factors in the irritable bowel syndrome. A multivariate analysis of patients and non-patients with irritable bowel syndrome. *Gastroenterol* 1988; **95**:701–708.
68. Gwee KA, Graham JC, McKendrick MW, *et al.* Psychometric scores and persistence of irritable bowel after infectious diarrhea. *Lancet* 1996; **347**:150–153.
69. Collins SM, Hurst SM, Main C. Effect of inflammation on enteric nerves. Cytokine induced changes in neurotransmitter content and release. *Ann NY Acad Sci* 1992; **664**:415–424.
70. Harries AD, Myers B, Cook GC. Inflammatory Bowel Disease: a common cause of bloody diarrhea in visitors to the tropics. *BMJ* 1985; **291**:1686–1687.
71. Case Records of the Massachusetts General Hospital. Case 29–1992. *New Engl J Med* 1992; **91**(327):182–191.
72. Trevisiol C, Not T, Berti I, *et al.* Screening for celiac disease in healthy blood donors at two immuno-transfusion centres in northeast Italy. *Ital J Gastroenterol Hepatol* 1999; **31**:584–586.
73. Ladinser B, Rossipal E, Pittschieler K. Endomysium antibodies in celiac disease: an improved method. *Gut* 1994; **35**:776–778.
74. Case records of the Massachusetts General Hospital. Case 33-1993. *N Engl J Med* 1993; **329**:561–568.
75. Taylor DN, Connor BA, Shlim DR. Chronic diarrhea in the returned traveler. *Med Clin N Am* 1999; **83**:1033–1052.
76. Taylor DN, Houston R, Shlim DR. Etiology of diarrhea among travelers and foreign residents in Nepal. *JAMA* 1988; **260**:1245.
77. Hiatt RA, Markell EK, Ng E. How many stool examinations are necessary to detect pathogenic intestinal protozoa? *Am J Trop Med Hyg* 1995; **53**:36–39.
78. Shah RJ, Fenoglio-Preiser C, Bleau BL, Gianella RA. Usefulness of colonoscopy with biopsy in the evaluation of patients with chronic diarrhea. *Am J Gastroenterol* 2001; **96**:1091–1095.
79. Taylor DN, Connor BA, Shlim DR. Chronic diarrhea in the returned traveler. *Med Clin N Am* 1999; **83**:1033–1052.
80. Kirchhelle A, Fruhwein N, Toburen D. Treatment of persistent diarrhea with S. boulardii in returning travelers: results of a prospective study. *Fortschr Med* 1996; **114**:136.

CHAPTER 55 Eosinophilia

Amy D. Klion

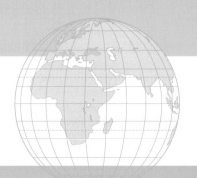

INTRODUCTION

Eosinophilia, as defined by ≥450 eosinophils/μL in the peripheral blood, occurs in up to 10% of travelers[1] and may be caused by a variety of conditions, including allergies and asthma, drug hypersensitivity, infection, neoplasm and other miscellaneous disorders (Table 55.1). Although the utility of screening for eosinophilia in returned travelers remains controversial, eosinophilia may be the first (or only) indication of a condition associated with potentially serious sequelae, such as schistosomiasis or strongyloidiasis, and is often useful in guiding the diagnostic evaluation in symptomatic patients. In this chapter, the causes of eosinophilia in travelers will be reviewed and a systematic approach to patients with eosinophilia in the presence and absence of symptoms will be presented.

EOSINOPHIL BIOLOGY

Eosinophils are bone marrow-derived leukocytes that are predominantly found in peripheral tissues that interface with the environment, such as the lungs, skin and gastrointestinal tract.[2] Whereas eosinophil levels in the peripheral blood are normally ≤450/mm³, eosinophil numbers can increase dramatically in certain disease states, including acute helminth infection and hypereosinophilic syndrome, reaching levels of greater than 20 000/mm³. In these situations, blood eosinophils may undergo characteristic morphologic and functional changes that have been associated with 'cellular activation' and eosinophil-induced tissue damage, including endomyocardial fibrosis and peripheral neuropathy.

Peripheral blood eosinophil levels exhibit diurnal variation, with the highest levels occurring in the early morning when endogenous corticosteroid levels are low. Levels may be decreased (eosinopenia) in acute bacterial and viral infections, acute malaria, pregnancy and in response to certain medications, including corticosteroids, epinephrine and estrogens. In contrast, the use of β-adrenergic blockers can result in a mild increase in eosinophil counts.

The development of eosinophilia in response to a particular stimulus (ex. helminth infection, allergen exposure) is dependent not

Table 55.1 Conditions associated with eosinophilia[a]

Allergic disorders
Asthma
Atopic dermatitis
Allergic rhinitis

Drug hypersensitivity (see Table 55.2)

Infection
Parasitic
Helminth
Ectoparasite (scabies, myiasis)
Protozoan (*Isospora belli*, sarcocystis)
Bacterial (resolving scarlet fever, chronic tuberculosis)
Fungal (coccidiomycosis, allergic bronchopulmonary aspergillosis)
Viral (human immunodeficiency virus)

Neoplasm
Eosinophilic leukemia (rare)
Myelogenous leukemia
Lymphoma, especially Hodgkin's
Adenocarcinoma of the bowel, lung, ovary or other solid organs

Connective tissue disorders
Churg-Strauss vasculitis
Systemic lupus erythematosus
Rheumatoid arthritis

Primary eosinophilic disorders
Idiopathic hypereosinophilic syndrome
Eosinophilic gastroenteritis
Chronic eosinophilic pneumonia
Familial hypereosinophilia
Episodic angioedema and eosinophilia
Kimura's disease

Other
Hypoadrenalism
Sarcoid
Ulcerative colitis
Radiation
Cholesterol embolization

[a]Lists are not exhaustive.

only on the nature of the offending agent but on the host immune response to that agent. In the case of helminth infection, the stage of parasite development, the location of the helminth within the host and the parasite burden are important determinants of the host immune response, and consequently of the degree of eosinophilia. Although tissue invasion by the parasite tends to be associated with a pronounced peripheral blood eosinophilia, the eosinophil response may be restricted to the involved tissues. Finally, eosinophilia is more pronounced in travelers to endemic areas (i.e., individuals not previously exposed to helminth infections) than in residents of helminth-endemic areas who have had exposure to parasite antigens.[3,4]

CAUSES OF EOSINOPHILIA

Overview

Although the list of potential etiologies of eosinophilia is overwhelming, the most commonly identified cause of eosinophilia in returned travelers is unquestionably helminth infection. It should be noted, however, that the absence of eosinophilia does not exclude the presence of a parasitic disease. Allergic diseases, including drug hypersensitivity, account for the second largest group of travelers with eosinophilia in most studies. Consequently, although the initial evaluation of travelers with eosinophilia should include screening for the most common helminth infections, non-infectious causes of eosinophilia should be considered before an extensive evaluation for unusual parasitic causes of eosinophilia is undertaken.

A definitive diagnosis is found in 16–45% of travelers with eosinophilia,[1] and the likelihood of a definitive diagnosis increases with the length of travel and the degree of the eosinophilia (>60% in patients with ≥16% eosinophils[1]). Surprisingly, the presence or absence of symptoms does not appear to influence the diagnostic yield.[5]

Allergic disorders/asthma

Allergic disorders, including allergic rhinitis, atopic disease, and asthma, are extremely common in the general population and are a common cause of mild eosinophilia. Changes in the external environment associated with travel can lead to an exacerbation (or improvement) in allergic disease; however, marked eosinophilia (≥3000 eosinophils/mm³) is rare in the absence of another cause (ex. helminth infection, drug hypersensitivity).

Drug hypersensitivity

Among the non-infectious causes of eosinophilia in travelers, drug-related hypersensitivity reactions are among the most common, accounting for up to 20% of cases of eosinophilia in some studies.[6] Although any drug has the potential to cause eosinophilia, some are more likely to do so, including many of the agents used to prevent or treat malaria and travelers' diarrhea (i.e., quinine, quinolones, tetracyclines, and sulfonamides). Prescription and non-prescription drugs, as well as dietary supplements and herbal medications, have been implicated (Table 55.2).

In most instances, drug-induced eosinophilia is entirely asymptomatic. End organ involvement, such as pulmonary infiltrates, interstitial nephritis, hepatitis or rash, can occur, however, and may be suggestive of hypersensitivity to a particular agent. In addition, some drugs are associated with specific syndromes, such as tryptophan-induced eosinophilia myalgia syndrome or the aspirin triad (asthma, nasal polyps and aspirin hypersensitivity).

Infection

Helminths

Helminth infections are the most commonly identified cause of eosinophilia in travelers, accounting for 30–60% of patients depending on the study.[6,7] Although intestinal nematode infection, filariasis, strongyloidiasis and schistosomiasis comprise the majority of cases in most studies, the precise causes depend on the particular population studied, and the location and duration of travel. It is important to remember that although helminth infection is a common cause of eosinophilia, not all patients with documented helminth infection have eosinophilia. In one study of 1107 travelers with schistosomiasis, only 44% had eosinophilia.[8] Similar findings have been reported in other helminth infections, including strongyloidiasis and hookworm infection.[9] In addition, helminths that do not invade tissues at all during their life-cycle, such as *Trichuris* and *Enterobius*, rarely cause eosinophilia.

Whereas eosinophilia is common in a wide variety of helminth infections, marked eosinophilia tends to be associated with tissue invasion and is seen in a relatively limited number of infections (Table 55.3). In some infections, including ascariasis and hookworm

Table 55.2	Common drugs associated with eosinophilia in travelers
Clinical manifestation	Drug(s)[a]
Asymptomatic or skin rash	Antibiotics, including penicillins, cephalosporins, quinolones, quinine and quinine derivatives, macrolides
Pulmonary infiltrates	Nonsteroidal anti-inflammatory agents; Sulfa-containing drugs
Hepatitis	Tetracyclines; Semisynthetic penicillins
Interstitial nephritis	Cephalosporins; Semisynthetic penicillins
Asthma, nasal polyps	Aspirin

[a]Note: this list is limited to common drugs that may be used in the treatment and prevention of travel-related illnesses, such as malaria, traveler's diarrhea, skin and upper respiratory infections.

Table 55.3	Helminth infections associated with eosinophilia

Mild to moderate eosinophilia (≤3000/mm³)

Anisakiasis[a]	Echinostomiasis
Capillariasis[a]	Enterobiasis
Coenurosis	Heterophyiasis
Cysticercosis	Hymenolepsiasis
Dicrocoeliasis	Metagonimiasis
Dirofilariasis	Sparganosis
Dracunculiasis	Trichuriasis
Echinococcosis	

Marked eosinophilia (>3000/mm³)

Angiostrongyliasis[a]	Mansonellosis
Ascariasis[a]	Onchocerciasis
Clonorchiasis[a]	Opisthorchiasis[a]
Fascioliasis[a]	Paragonimiasis[a]
Fasciolopsiasis	Schistosomiasis[a]
Gnathostomiasis	Strongyloidiasis[a]
Hookworm infection[a]	Trichinosis[a]
Loiasis	Visceral larva migrans
Lymphatic filariasis	

[a]Eosinophilia predominantly during acute phase of infection

infection, marked eosinophilia is seen only in the early phase of infection when developing larvae migrate through the lungs or other tissues and come into contact with the cells of the host immune system. In most instances, eosinophilia gradually resolves over time with or without anthelmintic treatment. However, chronic eosinophilia does occur in some infections (Table 55.4).

Ectoparasites

Scabies infestation occurs worldwide and is an unusual, but treatable, cause of eosinophilia in travelers.[10] Sensitization to the mites and their eggs typically produces intense itching, rash and erythema, which is accompanied by mild to moderate eosinophilia in up to 10% of cases. Although data regarding eosinophilia and other common ectoparasite infestations are lacking, hypersensitivity reactions can occur in response to flea, bedbug and tick bites. Rare cases of hyper-eosinophilic syndrome secondary to myiasis (infestation by fly larvae) have been reported with complete resolution following removal of the larvae.[11]

Protozoa

Protozoan infections, including giardiasis and amebiasis, are not associated with eosinophilia. Consequently, the identification of protozoa in the stool should prompt further search for an underlying cause. Infection with the intestinal coccidian parasite, *Isospora belli*, which causes diarrhea and malabsorption, is a rare exception to this rule and has been associated with eosinophilia in a minority of cases.[12] The parasite may be detected in the stool by modified acid-fast stain, or in intestinal biopsies. *Sarcocystis* has also been associated with acute symptomatic eosinophilic myositis in a few case reports.[13]

Other

Bacterial, fungal and viral infections typically cause eosinopenia and may suppress eosinophilia from other causes. An important exception is HIV infection. Numerous studies have demonstrated an increased risk of sexually transmitted diseases, including HIV, in travelers. Increased eosinophil counts in HIV infected individuals may be the direct result of immune dysregulation produced by the HIV infection itself or may occur secondary to drug hypersensitivity or hypoadrenalism.[14] Peripheral blood eosinophilia may also accompany eosinophilic pustular folliculitis, a chronic pruritic dermatosis seen in advanced HIV disease.[15] Other notable exceptions include coccidioidomycosis[16] and chronic tuberculosis,[17] which can be acquired during travel and are associated with eosinophilia in a minority of cases.

Other causes

Eosinophilia can be seen in a variety of common disorders associated with dysregulation of the immune response, including neoplasms, connective tissue diseases, sarcoidosis,[18] and ulcerative colitis.[19] Less frequent etiologies include hypoadrenalism, irradiation and a variety of primary eosinophilic disorders (see Table 55.2). Although these disorders are unlikely to be caused by travel, eosinophilia arising from any of these conditions may first be detected during a post-travel evaluation.

CLINICAL SYNDROMES

Skin/soft tissue involvement

Dermatologic problems (Table 55.5) are among the most frequent complaints in returning travelers and are commonly associated with eosinophilia.[20,21] In a prospective study of returning French travelers,

Table 55.4	Helminthic causes of eosinophilia of >2 years' duration
Cysticercosis[a]	Mansonellosis
Clonorchiasis	Onchocerciasis
Echinococcosis[a]	Opisthorchiasis
Fascioliasis	Paragonimiasis
Gnathostomiasis	Schistosomiasis
Hookworm infection	Strongyloidiasis
Loiasis	Visceral larva migrans
Lymphatic filariasis	

[a]Intermittent eosinophilia due to cyst leakage

Table 55.5	Evaluation of eosinophilia with dermatologic manifestations	
Clinical manifestation	Most common etiologies	Diagnostic tests
Urticaria	Helminth infection	Stool for ova and parasites, serology
	Drug hypersensitivity	
	Idiopathic	
Chronic pruritic dermatitis	Onchocerciasis	Skin snips, serology
	Scabies	Skin scraping
	Drug hypersensitivity	
Subcutaneous nodules	Onchocerciasis	Skin snips, excisional biopsy, serology
	Myiasis	Visual inspection
Migratory angioedema	Loiasis	Serology, midday blood filtration for microfilariae
	Gnathostomiasis	Serology, excision of parasite
Serpiginous lesions	Cutaneous larva migrans	Visual inspection
	Strongyloidiasis	Serology, stool for larvae

*Helminth infections that commonly cause urticaria include ascariasis, fascioliasis, gnathostomiasis, hookworm infection, filariasis, paragonimiasis, schistosomiasis, strongyloidiasis, trichinosis, and visceral larva migrans

cutaneous larva migrans, arthropod-related pruritic dermatitis, myiasis, urticaria and scabies, all of which can be associated with eosinophilia, were among the ten most frequent dermatologic diagnoses.[20] Of note, exacerbations of pre-existing skin conditions, such as atopic dermatitis, eczema and psoriasis, can be precipitated by tropical climates and should be included in the differential diagnosis of travel-related dermatologic disorders.[21] Although skin biopsy (or skin snips in suspected onchocerciasis) may be necessary in some cases, many dermatologic causes of eosinophilia can be identified by observation alone.

Urticaria is a frequent symptom in the general population and may be idiopathic or related to a variety of allergies. In travelers with eosinophilia, urticaria may signal the presence of a drug allergy or a helminth infection. Transient pruritic skin rashes also occur in response to a variety of stimuli, including but not limited to the penetration of the skin by a variety of helminth larvae, such as hookworm species, *Strongyloides* and schistosomes. The differential diagnosis of persistent or recurrent dermatitis and eosinophilia is more restrictive with onchocerciasis, scabies, and hypersensitivity reactions among the most common causes in travelers.

Subcutaneous nodules may be present in a number of infections also associated with eosinophilia, including onchocerciasis, dirofilariasis, paragonimiasis, fascioliasis, echinococcosis, cysticercosis, coenurosis, sparganosis, and myiasis. In many of these infections, including onchocerciasis and cysticercosis, subcutaneous nodules are painless and easily overlooked. Since excisional biopsy of such nodules can be diagnostic, a careful skin and soft tissue examination should be undertaken if one of these infections is suspected. Over time, with death of the parasite, nodules may calcify and become detectable in soft tissue films.

Invasion of the skin by larval maggots of the *Diptera* species (myiasis) typically produces painful nodules that may be confused with a furuncle. Visible movement of the maggot within the characteristic central punctum is common, however, and generally leads to the correct diagnosis. Painful subcutaneous nodules that migrate are the hallmark of sparganosis, a disease caused by migration of tapeworm larvae of *Spirometra* species through the subcutaneous tissues of humans or other paratenic hosts.[22]

Localized, intermittent, migratory angioedema is characteristic of loiasis, a filarial infection that is endemic in Central and West Africa. Infective *Loa loa* larvae are transmitted through the bite of infected *Chrysops* flies and develop into adult worms that migrate through the subcutaneous tissues provoking a hypersensitivity reaction (Calabar swelling).[3] Swellings are most common on the extremities and face and typically resolve within a few days, only to recur weeks to months later. Eyeworm (migration of the adult worm across the subconjunctiva) occurs in up to 20% of infected patients and, when present, is diagnostic of loiasis. Peripheral eosinophilia is present with rare exception and is frequently marked (>3000 eosinophils/mm³). Complications, including endomyocardial fibrosis and encephalitis, are uncommon and are thought to be due to the host immune response to the parasite. In the absence of demonstrable parasites in the peripheral blood or subcutaneous tissues, a presumptive diagnosis can be made in the setting of eosinophilia, positive serology and an appropriate exposure history.

Migrating *Gnathostoma* larvae can cause migratory angioedema indistinguishable from that of loiasis, although localized pain, pruritus and erythema are more frequent and the swellings tend to last longer (1–2 weeks).[23] Migration of larvae to deeper tissues and organs (visceral gnathostomiasis) can occur producing a wide variety of symptoms. Endemic in parts of Southeast Asia, Central and South America, gnathostomiasis is usually acquired by ingestion of the parasite in inadequately cooked freshwater fish or other intermediate hosts. As in loiasis, symptoms may appear months to years after infection, and eosinophilia is often striking. Whereas recovery of the parasite is necessary for a definitive diagnosis of gnathostomiasis, positive serology in a traveler with migratory subcutaneous swellings, eosinophilia and an appropriate exposure history is highly suggestive of the diagnosis.

Cutaneous larva migrans, or creeping eruption, results when the larval stages of animal hookworms inadvertently penetrate human skin. The appearance of the intensely pruritic, reddened serpiginous track, found most commonly on the feet or buttocks, is diagnostic.[24] *Larva currens*, the serpiginous skin lesions seen in chronic strongyloidiasis, can be easily distinguished from creeping eruption by the evanescent nature of the lesions and the speed with which they migrate (5–10 cm/h).[25] Whereas eosinophilia is present in a minority of patients with creeping eruption, it is common in patients with strongyloidiasis and may be the first clue to the diagnosis.

Pulmonary manifestations

Migration of helminth larvae through the lung can cause eosinophilia and migratory pulmonary infiltrates, or Loeffler's syndrome (Table 55.6).[26] The most common cause of Loeffler's syndrome is infection with *Ascaris lumbricoides*, an intestinal nematode that is worldwide in distribution. Patients typically present with nonproductive cough and substernal burning occurring 1–2 weeks after ingestion of embryonated eggs on contaminated foodstuffs. The symptoms resolve once larval migration is finished (within 5–10 days), but chest X-ray abnor-

Table 55.6	Causes of eosinophilia with pulmonary manifestations

Transient infiltrates
Ascariasis, hookworm infection, strongyloidiasis, drug hypersensitivity, acute eosinophilic pneumonia

Chronic infiltrates
Tropical pulmonary eosinophilia, strongyloidiasis, drug hypersensitivity reactions, hypereosinophilic syndrome, chronic eosinophilic pneumonia, Churg-Strauss vasculitis

Eosinophilic pleural effusion
Helminths (toxocariasis, filariasis, paragonimiasis, anisakiasis, echinococcosis, strongyloidiasis)
Other infections (coccidiomycosis, Tb)
Other causes (malignancy, hemothorax, drug reactions, pulmonary infarct, rheumatologic disease, pneumothorax)

Parenchymal invasion with or without cavitation
Paragonimiasis, tuberculosis, allergic bronchopulmonary aspergillosis, echinococcosis (rare)

malities and eosinophilia may persist for weeks. Diagnosis is complicated by the fact that eggs may not be apparent in the stool for months, at which time the eosinophilia has generally resolved. Consequently, the detection of *Ascaris* eggs in the stool of a traveler with marked eosinophilia should prompt a search for another cause of the eosinophilia. Symptoms are few during the intestinal stage of infection, except in extremely heavy infections, where intestinal obstruction may occur.

Acute schistosomiasis may present with eosinophilia, cough and transient pulmonary infiltrates; however, the presence of concomitant gastrointestinal and constitutional symptoms helps distinguish this from Loeffler's syndrome.[27] Although hookworm and *Strongyloides* larvae also pass through the lungs early in infection, this is rarely associated with pulmonary symptoms.

Unlike the transient migratory infiltrates of Loeffler's syndrome, the pulmonary infiltrates of tropical pulmonary eosinophilia, a hyperreactive form of lymphatic filariasis, persist in the absence of anthelmintic therapy.[28] Nocturnal cough or wheezing is characteristic and the eosinophilia is accompanied by extremely high levels of serum IgE and antifilarial antibodies. A similar syndrome can be seen in strongyloides infection.[29] Other causes of pulmonary infiltrates recurring over a period of weeks to months include drug reactions, and several rare idiopathic disorders (e.g., hypereosinophilic syndrome, chronic eosinophilic pneumonia, and Churg Strauss vasculitis).

Eosinophilic pleural effusions have been described in the setting of numerous helminth infections, including echinococcosis, paragonimiasis and disseminated strongyloides infection. Fungal and mycobacterial infections, hypersensitivity reactions, malignancy, pulmonary infarct and hemothorax have also been implicated.[30]

Relatively few infections give rise to eosinophilia and lesions of the pulmonary parenchyma. Although tuberculosis should be considered in any traveler with a cavitary lesion, eosinophilia in tuberculosis is exceedingly uncommon. Other infections to consider in the appropriate epidemiologic setting include paragonimiasis, which can present with cavitary infiltrates and hilar adenopathy, and pulmonary echinococcosis, which typically presents as a solitary cystic lesion.

Gastrointestinal symptoms

Gastrointestinal symptoms are the most frequent complaint in returned travelers presenting to travel clinics.[31] When accompanied by peripheral blood eosinophilia, they are most often indicative of a helminth infection, although the onset of a non-infectious gastrointestinal disorder associated with eosinophilia, such as inflammatory bowel disease or eosinophilic gastroenteritis may coincide with travel.

Transient gastrointestinal symptoms, including nausea, diarrhea, vomiting and abdominal pain, occur in the early stages of a number of helminth infections, including trichinosis, schistosomiasis, paragonimiasis, and hookworm infection. These symptoms may precede the characteristic clinical manifestations of the infection, as in trichinosis, where abdominal pain and diarrhea, if present, develop in the first week after ingestion of contaminated pork (or other meats) as the larvae migrate to the intestine. The well-recognized syndrome of eosinophilia, myalgia, fever and periorbital edema, typically does not appear until 1–2 weeks later as new larvae migrate through the tissues and encyst in the muscle.[32] Diagnosis in these early stage infections can be difficult as serologic tests are often negative and production of larvae and/or eggs may not have been initiated.

Although liver fluke infections are uncommon in travelers, they do occur and need to be considered in the differential diagnosis of recurrent cholangitis and eosinophilia in travelers. Obstruction of the biliary system by an echinococcal cyst or aberrant migration of an adult Ascaris worm has also been reported. In *Fasciola* infection, migration of the fluke larvae through the liver parenchyma causes an acute syndrome of eosinophilia, abdominal pain, fever, and variable hepatomegaly that can last for up to 4 months.[33] Multiple small tunnel-like hypodense lesions can be seen in CT scans of the liver, and represent microabscesses. Other helminth infections, including toxocariasis,[34] can produce a similar clinical syndrome.

Neurologic disease

Neurologic syndromes (Table 55.7) associated with eosinophilia are relatively infrequent in travelers, but include eosinophilic meningitis,

Table 55.7	Evaluation of eosinophilia with neurologic manifestations	
Clinical manifestation	Most common etiologies	Diagnostic tests
Headache and meningeal signs	Angiostrongylus Gnathostomiasis Coccidioidomycosis Drug hypersensitivity Neoplasm, esp. Hodgkin's lymphoma	Lumbar puncture[a], serology
Headache and/or seizures	Cysticercosis Echinococcosis Schistosomiasis Paragonimiasis Fascioliasis Trichinosis Toxocariasis Sparganosis	CT, MRI, serology
Transverse myelitis	Schistosomiasis	Spine MRI, serology (serum and CSF), stool or urine exam for ova, rectal snip
Peripheral neuropathy	Loiasis	Serology, midday blood filtration for microfilariae

[a]Larvae of Angiostrongylus may be detected in the CSF

seizures, focal neurologic deficits, peripheral neuropathy, transverse myelitis and eosinophilic myeloencephalitis.

The most common cause of eosinophilic meningitis in travelers is infection with the rat lungworm, *Angiostrongylus cantonensis*, although infection with other helminths, fungal infections, drug hypersensitivity and other non-infectious causes may also be implicated. Angiostrongylus infection is most prevalent in Southeast Asia and the Pacific, but is present in other tropical areas worldwide, including the Caribbean.[35] Infection occurs following ingestion of an infected mollusk, vegetables or other uncooked foods contaminated with mollusk slime. Although gastrointestinal symptoms may occur soon after ingestion of the larvae, the most common presenting complaint is an intermittent excruciating headache occurring after an incubation period of 2–30 days. Cranial nerve palsies may also be present. Lumbar puncture reveals an elevated opening pressure, pleocytosis with ≥10% eosinophils, elevated protein and normal glucose. Infection is self-limited as larvae do not reach maturity in the human host, and treatment is supportive. Peripheral eosinophilia is marked early in infection but decreases as the infection resolves.

Headache and/or seizures in a patient with eosinophilia may be the presenting symptom of a number of helminth infections that affect the central nervous system, including cysticercosis, schistosomiasis, and echinococcosis. Focal neurologic findings may also be present. Many of these infections have a characteristic appearance on imaging studies that may facilitate diagnosis. For example, the presence of both cystic lesions with surrounding edema and calcifications in the brain parenchyma is highly suggestive of cysticercosis; whereas soap bubble cystic lesions in a grape-like cluster with calcification are characteristic of *Paragonimus* infection and septate lesions with daughter cysts are typical of echinococcal disease. In contrast, the mass lesions with surrounding edema that can occur in the brain and spinal cord in schistosomiasis are indistinguishable from the mass lesions of other causes.

Other neurologic syndromes that occur in association with eosinophilia include peripheral neuropathy secondary to nerve compression by angioedema in loiasis, transverse myelitis in schistosomiasis, and potentially fatal eosinophilic myeloencephalitis due to gnathostomiasis.

Fever

Since fever can suppress eosinophilia, it is not surprising that the potential etiologies of fever and eosinophilia are few. Drug hypersensitivity should be excluded in all patients. The possibility of a parasitic infection, such as acute schistosomiasis, visceral larva migrans, trichinellosis, fascioliasis, or gnathostomiasis, should also be considered depending on the exposure history.

Asymptomatic eosinophilia

As many as one-third of returned travelers with eosinophilia are asymptomatic at the time of presentation with helminth infection, notably schistosomiasis, filariasis, strongyloidiasis, and hookworm infection, listed as the most frequently identified treatable cause in most studies.[1,7]

Schistosomiasis

Endemic in 74 countries in Africa, Asia, Central and South America, schistosomiasis is acquired when infective larvae (cercariae) swimming in fresh water penetrate the skin. A mild dermatitis at the site of penetration is sometimes seen within a few hours to 1 week after exposure. Acute schistosomiasis (Katayama fever) may occur 2–12 weeks after exposure and is characterized by fever, headache,

myalgias, right upper quadrant pain, bloody diarrhea, and pulmonary symptoms.[27] Eosinophilia is usually present in acute infection and may be marked. Although the acute symptoms resolve without treatment within 3–4 months after exposure, the eosinophilia may persist for many years. Central nervous system involvement is uncommon in travelers, but can lead to permanent deficits,[36] underlining the importance of early diagnosis and treatment.

The gold standard for the diagnosis of schistosomiasis remains the detection of viable parasite eggs in the stool, urine or a tissue biopsy. However, as many as 50% of patients with chronic schistosomiasis[37] and most patients with acute schistosomiasis,[27] will not have eggs detected in stool or urine examinations. Serologic tests are more sensitive and can detect infection prior to the appearance of eggs in the stool or urine, but do not distinguish between active and past infection,[38] limiting their utility in the detection of infection in long-term residents of endemic countries and travelers with a history of prior infection.

Filarial infection

The most frequently identified cause of eosinophilia in travelers returning from Africa is *Loa loa* infection. Although symptoms, including urticaria, myalgias, arthralgias, migratory angioedema (Calabar swellings) and eyeworm, are common, some travelers and most residents of endemic areas remain asymptomatic despite microfilariae detectable in the peripheral blood.[39] Whereas the clinical manifestations of *Mansonella perstans* infection, which is endemic in tropical Africa, the Caribbean and northeastern South America, can mimic those of loiasis; most infected travelers are asymptomatic.[40]

Endemic in parts of Africa and Central and South America, onchocerciasis ranks second among the filarial infections that afflict travelers. Infection typically presents with a pruritic papular dermatitis and eosinophilia, although asymptomatic infection does occur.[4] Palpable subcutaneous nodules, when present, are useful from a diagnostic standpoint, but are uncommon in travelers, who generally have light infections. The keratitis and blindness that characterize onchocerciasis in some regions of Africa are rarely, if ever, seen in temporary residents of these areas.

Lymphatic filariasis is estimated to affect 120 million people worldwide, but is a relatively uncommon cause of eosinophilia in travelers. Although acute clinical manifestations, including adenolymphangitis, fever, and recurrent swelling of the extremities or genitalia, may be seen in travelers, progression to chronic lymphedema or elephantiasis is rare.[41] Other filariae that occasionally infect travelers include *Mansonella streptocerca,* which is endemic in western and central Africa, and *Mansonella ozzardi,* which is found in Central and South America and on some Caribbean islands.[42]

A definitive diagnosis of filarial infection can be made by the detection of microfilariae or their DNA in the blood or skin, identification of an adult worm, or, in the case of lymphatic filariasis due to *Wuchereria bancrofti,* by the demonstration of circulating antigen in the peripheral blood.[43] Serology may be useful in making a presumptive diagnosis in visitors to endemic areas who have suggestive clinical symptoms or unexplained eosinophilia.

Strongyloidiasis

In most series, *Strongyloides* infection accounts for a high percentage (up to 38%) of unexplained eosinophilia in travelers and immigrants.[9,44] Worldwide in distribution, *Strongyloides* infection is acquired by penetration of exposed skin by infective stage larvae. Early in infection, the developing larvae migrate through the lungs and pulmonary symptoms may predominate. Later, infection may be associated with intermittent creeping eruption (*larva currens*), urticaria, or gastrointestinal symptoms, but is often asymptomatic. Because of the capacity of the third stage larvae to reinvade the intestinal mucosa or skin of the infected host, untreated strongyloidiasis can persist for decades.[45] More importantly, life-threatening dissemination may occur in the setting of immunosuppression.[46]

Stool examination is an insensitive means of diagnosis in strongyloidiasis, as larvae are often shed sporadically and in very low numbers. In a study of strongyloidiasis in Brazilian patients with hematologic malignancies, the probability of finding larvae in the stool was only 47% when four samples were examined.[47] Eosinophilia is present in 40–80% of immunocompetent patients with strongyloidiasis and may be the only clue to the diagnosis. However, the eosinophilia generally decreases over time and may or may not be present during hyperinfection syndromes.[46] Serologic tests remain the most sensitive and specific method of diagnosis in travelers.[9,48] Although antibody levels decrease following treatment and may be a useful marker of response to therapy, levels remain positive for long periods of time after treatment limiting their use as a screening tool in previously infected populations.

Hookworm infection

Although some patients with chronic hookworm infection complain of vague abdominal pain or nausea, most are asymptomatic. Eosinophilia is usually mild, but may exceed 3000/mm³ in some cases.[49] Since hookworm infection is self-limited in the absence of treatment, eosinophilia rarely persists for longer than 3 years.

EVALUATION OF PATIENTS WITH EOSINOPHILIA

Eosinophilia (Fig. 55.1) should always be confirmed with an absolute eosinophil count (eosinophils/μL blood), since an increased percentage of eosinophils may reflect a decrease in the number of non-eosinophil leucocytes (ex. neutropenia) rather than a true increase in eosinophils. Once eosinophilia has been established, the next problem is to establish the etiology. Since the numbers of potential causes of eosinophilia are many, and the diagnostic tests required to distinguish between them are extensive, a careful history and a physical examination is an essential first step in directing the evaluation. Pre-travel eosinophil counts, if available, are useful in determining whether the eosinophilia is travel-related. Similarly, pre-existent medical problems (ex. asthma, atopic disease) associated with eosinophilia should be excluded. A detailed drug history, including over the counter medications, vitamins and dietary supplements, should be obtained, and drugs or other agents associated with eosinophilia should be discontinued if possible.

An accurate exposure history is crucial to the evaluation of eosinophilia. Since many infectious agents have restricted geographic distribution, or a limited life span, a detailed review of recent and past travel can narrow the differential diagnosis significantly. For example, eosinophilia and migratory angioedema in a patient who has traveled only to Southeast Asia would suggest gnathostomiasis, whereas identical symptoms in a patient from West Africa would likely be due to loiasis. Similarly, abdominal symptoms and eosinophilia occurring in a traveler whose last potential exposure was 3 years prior to evaluation is not likely to be due to ascariasis (life span 1–2 years), but could be indicative of hookworm (life span ≤6 years) or *Strongyloides* infection (life span in decades). The duration of exposure is also helpful, as some parasite infections, such as filariasis, paragonimiasis and cysticercosis, are uncommon in short term travelers; whereas others, such as schistosomiasis or trichinosis,[32] can occur after a single exposure.

It is often more difficult to obtain a reliable dietary and behavioral history. Although most studies have demonstrated an increased incidence of certain infections, including schistosomiasis and HIV, in travelers who report risk-taking behavior, the absence of such a history did not exclude infection.[5] Nevertheless, significant exposures, such as a history of swimming in Lake Malawi or ingestion of raw pork, may prompt a more thorough search for a particular etiologic agent.

Up-to-date information with respect to recent outbreaks or epidemics in the regions visited should be sought, since unusual causes of eosinophilia may be more likely in these settings (ex. the recent outbreak of eosinophilic meningitis caused by *Angiostrongylus* in a group of students visiting the Caribbean[35]). A history of illness in travel companions can be extremely helpful, since some infections may occur in clusters as a result of exposure to a common contaminated source (ex. schistosomiasis in a group of rafters on the Omo River in Ethiopia[50] or trichinosis diagnosed in 13 travelers on a cruise to Alaska[51]).

A detailed symptom history should be elicited, including symptoms that occurred during or soon after travel but have since resolved, as they may provide important clues to the underlying diagnosis. Similarly, a careful physical examination should be performed, with particular attention paid to the dermatologic examination, since skin and soft tissue findings, such as *larva currens* (the fleeting serpiginous rash of strongyloidiasis) and the mild unilateral limb swelling due to early lymphatic filariasis, are easily missed.

Although the exposure history, symptoms and signs may help to narrow down the possible etiologies of eosinophilia in travelers and guide the diagnostic evaluation, specific features of the eosinophilia can also be useful in this regard. For example, intermittent eosinophilia is characteristic of echinococcosis and cysticercosis, and reflects the inflammatory response to leakage of cyst contents. Marked eosinophilia (≥3000/mm³) is most commonly associated with tissue invasive helminth infections and drug hypersensitivity reactions.

If the history and physical examination do not point to a specific diagnosis, three stool specimens collected 48 h apart should be obtained to look for ova and parasites. Specimens should be examined by direct smear and using a concentration technique. In patients with potential exposure to *Schistosoma haematobium*, urinalysis and examination of three midday urine specimens for ova and parasites should also be performed.

Whereas routine stool examination will detect most helminths with an intestinal phase in their life-cycle, their sensitivity is poor in the detection of strongyloidiasis and schistosomiasis, two common infections that may be asymptomatic, prolonged (up to several decades) and associated with potentially life-threatening complications (hyperinfection syndrome and central nervous system involvement, respectively). Tissue parasites, including filariae, *Trichinella* and agents of visceral larva migrans, will also be missed. Consequently, serologic assessment for the most common helminth infections (schistosomiasis, strongyloidiasis, filariasis, and toxocariasis (in children)) is recommended as suggested by the exposure history.

The utility of additional screening tests, including liver function tests, IgE levels and chest radiography, remains controversial in asymptomatic returned travelers. These tests, as well as other diagnostic procedures, including biopsies, radiologic studies and specific serologic tests, should be guided by the patient's symptoms and exposure history. For example, the initial evaluation of a returned traveler with jaundice and eosinophilia following a trip to rural China should include stool examination for ova and parasites, liver function studies and abdominal imaging, as well as serologies for schistosomiasis, toxocariasis and the liver flukes. In contrast, evaluation of the same traveler complaining of dyspnea and cough should include a chest X-ray, sputum for larvae, eggs and acid-fast bacilli, and serologic studies for schistosomiasis, strongyloidiasis, and filariasis.

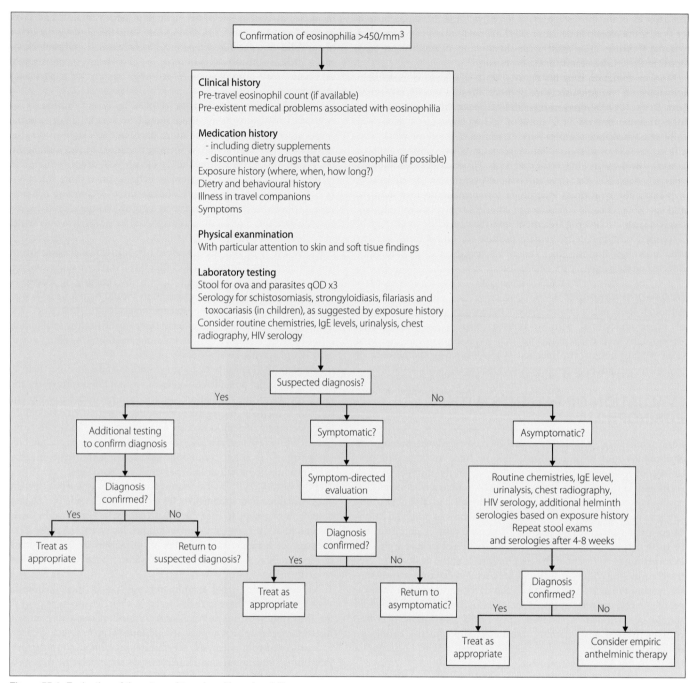

Figure 55.1 Evaluation of the returned traveler with eosinophilia.

Because of the long prepatent period characteristic of some helminth infections, eosinophilia may occur at a time that parasitologic diagnosis is not possible, ex. prior to egg secretion or antibody positivity. The clinical manifestations of early infection may be markedly different from those occurring later further obscuring the diagnosis (ex. acute schistosomiasis). Repeat stool examinations and/or serology should be considered in 4–8 weeks.

APPROACH TO THE PATIENT WITH UNDIAGNOSED EOSINOPHILIA

Despite extensive evaluation, up to 50% of cases of eosinophilia remain undiagnosed.[7,9] In such cases, the role of empiric therapy with alben-

dazole or ivermectin remains controversial since most studies have demonstrated resolution of the eosinophilia in 3–6 months with or without the administration of anthelmintics.[7] In patients with eosinophil counts ≥1500/mm3, evaluation for eosinophil-related end organ damage is warranted, as well as a comprehensive evaluation for non-infectious etiologies of eosinophilia, including myeloproliferative disorders.

CONCLUSION

Although screening for eosinophilia may not be appropriate in all cases, it can be a useful tool in the evaluation of returned travelers, particularly those with potential exposure to helminth infections.

Because of the wide spectrum of causes of eosinophilia, a careful exposure and symptom history is crucial to narrow down the diagnostic possibilities. The initial evaluation of all travelers with eosinophilia should include screening for the most common helminth infections to which they may have been exposed, since several of these, including strongyloidiasis, schistosomiasis and filariasis, are associated with potentially serious long-term sequelae. Non-infectious causes should be considered however, before an extensive evaluation for unusual parasitic causes of eosinophilia is undertaken.

REFERENCES

1. Schulte C, Krebs B, Jelinek T, *et al.* Diagnostic significance of blood eosinophilia in returned travelers. *Clin Infect Dis* 2002; **34**:407–411.
2. Weller PF. The immunobiology of eosinophils. *N Engl J Med* 1991; **324**:1110–1118.
3. Klion AD, Massougbodji M, Sadeler B-C, Ottesen EA, Nutman TB. Loiasis in endemic and non-endemic populations: immunologically mediated differences in clinical presentation. *J Infect Dis* 1991; **163**:1318–1325.
4. McCarthy JS, Ottesen EA, Nutman TB. Onchocerciasis in endemic and nonendemic populations: differences in clinical presentation and immunologic findings. *J Infect Dis* 1994; **170**:736–741.
5. Whitty CJM, Carroll B, Armstrong M, *et al.* Utility of history, examination and laboratory tests in screening those returning to Europe from the tropics for parasitic infection. *Trop Med Int Health* 2000; **5**(11):818–823.
6. Van den Ende J, van Gompel A, van den Enden E, de Meulenaere T, Vervoort T. Hypereosinophilia after a stay in tropical countries. *Trop Geogr Med* 1994; **46**:191.
7. Harries AD, Myers B, Bhattacharrya D. Eosinophilia in Caucasians returning from the tropics. *Trans R Soc Trop Med* 1986; **80**:327–328.
8. Whitty CJ, Mabey DC, Armstron M, Wright SG, Chiodini PL. Presentation and outcome of 1107 cases of schistosomiasis from Africa diagnosed in a non-endemic country. *Trans R Soc Trop Med Hyg* 2000; **94**(5):531–534.
9. Libman MD, MacLean JD, Gyorkos TW. Screening for schistosomiasis, filariasis, and strongyloidiasis among expatriates returning from the tropics. *Clin Infect Dis* 1993; **17**:353–359.
10. Deshpande AD. Eosinophilia associated with scabies. *Practitioner* 1987; **231**:455.
11. Starr J, Pruett JH, Yunginger JW, Gleich GJ. Myiasis due to *Hypoderma lineatum* infection mimicking the hypereosinophilic syndrome. *Mayo Clin Proc* 2000; **75**:755–759.
12. Junod C. *Isospora belli* coccidiosis in immunocompetent subjects (a study of 40 cases seen in Paris). *Bull Soc Pathol Exot* 1988; **81**:317–325.
13. Arness MK, Brown JD, Dubey JP, Neafie RC, Granstrom DE. An outbreak of acute eosinophilic myositis attributed to human *Sarcocystis* parasitism. *Am J Trop Med Hyg* 1999; **61**:548–553.
14. Skiest DJ, Keiser P. Clinical significance of eosinophilia in HIV-infected individuals. *Am J Med* 1997; **102**(5):449–453.
15. Rosenthal D, LeBoit PE, Klumpp L, Berger TG. Human immunodeficiency virus-associated eosinophilic folliculitis. A unique dermatosis associated with advanced human immunodeficiency virus infection. *Arch Dermatol* 1991; **127**:206–209.
16. Harley WB, Blaser MJ. Disseminated coccidioidomycosis associated with extreme eosinophilia. *Clin Infect Dis* 1994; **18**:627–629.
17. Flores M, Merino Angulo J, Tanago JG, Aquirre C. Late generalized tuberculosis and eosinophilia. *Arch Intern Med* 1983; **143**:182.
18. Renston JP, Goldman ES, Hsu RM, Tomasheski JF. Peripheral blood eosinophilia in association with sarcoidosis. *Mayo Clin Proc* 2000; **75**:586–590.
19. Keene WR. Uncommon abnormalities of blood associated with ulcerative colitis. *Med Clin North Am* 1966; **50**:535–541.
20. Caumes E, Carriere J, Guermonprez G, Bricaire F, Danis M, Gentilini M. Dermatoses associated with travel to tropical countries: a prospective study of the diagnosis and management of 269 patients presenting to a tropical disease unit. *Clin Infect Dis* 1995; **20**:542–548.
21. Kain K. Skin lesions in returned travelers. *Med Clin N Am* 1999; **83**:1077–1102.
22. Sarma DP, Weilbaecher TG. Human sparganosis. *J Am Acad Dermatol* 1986; **15**:1145–1148.
23. Rusnak JM, Lucey DR. Clinical gnathostomiasis: case report and review of the English-language literature. *Clin Infect Dis* 1993; **16**:33–50.
24. Jelinek T, Maiwald H, Nothdurft HD, Loscher T. Cutaneous larva migrans in travelers: synopsis of histories, symptoms, and treatment of 98 patients. *Clin Infect Dis* 1994; **19**:1062–1066.
25. von Kuster LC, Genta RM. Cutaneous manifestations of strongyloidiasis. *Arch Dermatol* 1988; **124**:1826–1830.
26. Loeffler W. Transient lung infiltrations with blood eosinophilia. *Int Arch Allergy Appl Immunol* 1956; **8**:54.
27. Hiatt RA, Sotomayor ZR, Sanchez G, Zambrana M, Knight WB. Factors in the pathogenesis of acute schistosomiasis mansoni. *J Infect Dis* 1979; **139**(6):659–666.
28. Ottesen EA, Nutman TB. Tropical pulmonary eosinophilia. *Annu Rev Med* 1992; **43**:417–424.
29. Rocha A, Dreyer G, Poindexter RW, Ottesen EA. Syndrome resembling tropical pulmonary eosinophilia but of non-filarial aetiology: serological findings with filarial antigens. *Trans R Soc Trop Med Hyg* 1995; **89**:573–575.
30. Rubins JB, Rubins HB. Etiology and prognostic significance of eosinophilic pleural effusions. *Chest* 1996; **110**:1271–1274.
31. Ryan ET, Wilson ME, Kain KC. Illness after international travel. *N Engl J Med* 2002; **347**:505–516.
32. McAuley JB, Michelson MK, Schantz PM. *Trichinella* in travelers. *J Infect Dis* 1991; **164**:1013–1016.
33. Arjona R, Riancho JA, Aguado JM, Salesa R, Gonzalez-Macias J. Fascioliasis in developed countries: A review of classic and aberrant forms of the disease. *Medicine* (Baltimore) 1995; **74**:13–23.
34. Schantz PM, Glickman LT. Toxocaral visceral larva migrans. *N Engl J Med* 1978; **298**:436–439.
35. Slom TJ, Cortese MM, Gerber SI, *et al.* An outbreak of eosinophilic meningitis caused by *Angiostrongylus cantonensis* in travelers returning from the Caribbean. *N Engl J Med* 2002 **346**:668–675.
36. Scrimgeour EM, Gadjusek DC. Involvement of the central nervous system in *Schistosoma mansoni* and *S haematobium* infection: review. *Brain* 1985; **108**:1023–1038.
37. Harries AD, Fryatt R, Walker J, Chiodini PL, Bryceson ADM. Schistosomiasis in expatriates returning to Britain from the tropics: a controlled study. *Lancet* 1986; **1**:86–88.
38. Tsang VCW, Wilkins PP. Immunodiagnosis of schistosomiasis. *Immunol Investigat* 1997; **26**:175–188.
39. Nutman TB, Miller KD, Mulligan M, Ottesen EA. *Loa loa* infection in temporary residents of endemic regions: recognition of a hyperresponsive syndrome with characteristic clinical manifestations. *J Infect Dis* 1986; **154**(1):10–18.
40. Adolph PE, Kagan IG, McQuay RM. Diagnosis and treatment of *Acanthocheilonema perstans* filariasis. *Am J Trop Med Hyg* 1962; **11**:76.
41. Wartman WB. Filariasis in American armed forces in World War II. *Medicine* 1947; **26**:332–392.
42. Klion AD, Nutman TB. Loiasis and Mansonella infections. In: Guerrant RL, Walker DH, Weller PF, eds. *Tropical Infectious Diseases. Principles, Pathogens & Practice.* Philadelphia: Churchill Livingstone; 1999: 861–872.
43. Harnett W, Bradley JE, Garate T. Molecular and immunodiagnosis of human filarial nematode infections. *Parasitology* 1998; **117**(**suppl**):S59–71.
44. Nutman TB, Ottesen EA, Ieng S, *et al.* Eosinophilia in Southeast Asian Refugees: Evaluation at a Referral Center. *J Infect Dis* 1987; **155**(2):309–313.
45. Pelletier LL. Chronic strongyloidiasis in World War II Far East ex-prisoners of war. *Am J Trop Med Hyg* 1984; **33**:55.
46. Longworth DL, Weller PF. Hyperinfection syndrome with strongyloidiasis. *Curr Clin Top Infect Dis* 1986; **7**:1.
47. Nucci M, Portugal R, Pulcheri W, *et al.* Strongyloidiasis in patients with hematologic malignancies. *Clin Infect Dis* 1995; **21**:675–677.
48. Loutfy MR, Wilson M, Keystone JS, Kain KC. Serology and eosinophil count in the diagnosis and management of strongyloidiasis in a non-endemic area. *Am J Trop Med Hyg* 2002; **66**:749–752.
49. Maxwell C, Hussain R, Nutman TB, *et al.* The clinical and immunologic responses of normal volunteers to low dose hookworm (*Necator americanus*) infection. *Am J Trop Med Hyg* 1987; **37**:126–134.
50. Istre GR, Fontaine RE, Tarr J, Hopkins RS. Acute schistosomiasis among Americans rafting the Omo River, Ethiopia. *JAMA* 1984; **251**:508–510.
51. Singal M, Schantz PM, Werner SB. Trichinosis acquired at sea-report of an outbreak. *Am J Trop Med Hyg* 1974; **25**:675–681.

CHAPTER 56 Respiratory Diseases

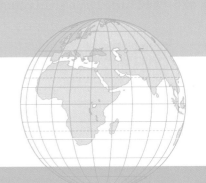

Alberto Matteelli and Nuccia Saleri

KEYPOINTS

- The estimated monthly incidence of acute febrile respiratory tract infections is 1261/100 000 travelers

- Lower tract respiratory infections account for 50% of all RTI in travelers

- There are no definitive factors associated to an increased risk of acquiring respiratory infections

- High-risk groups such as infants, small children, the elderly and subjects with chronic tracheobronchial or pulmonary disease are at increased risk of developing severe clinical consequences should infection occur

- Prevention of RTI in the traveler usually relies on vaccines

- There is mounting evidence on the association between travel and increased risk for infection with *M. tuberculosis*

INTRODUCTION

Respiratory diseases represent a frequent,[1] potentially life-threatening[2] health problem in travelers, and a reason for concern due to the possibility of importation of infections such as influenza, diphtheria, or tuberculosis.[3–5]

This chapter gives a general overview of the pathogens causing respiratory tract infections (RTI), their clinical presentation and standard management procedures. Some details are given for the etiological agents responsible for outbreaks in travelers. A few diseases with limited tropical distribution which may represent a specific hazard for travelers to these destinations are also shortly discussed. Tuberculosis is presented in a separate paragraph.

CAUSATIVE AGENTS AND CLINICAL PRESENTATION

It is generally assumed that travelers are infected by the same sort of organisms of the respiratory tract regardless the destination of travel. The resulting clinical picture is determined by the combined effect of the type of causative agent and the site of the inflammatory response. Multiple signs are usually combined in a given patient but it is often possible to distinguish upper from lower tract infections.

Usual causative agents of acute upper respiratory tract infections are listed in Table 56.1. Most of the cases are due to viruses and evolve as uncomplicated disease resolving without specific treatment. The infection of the nasal airways determines an acute coryzal illness, traditionally referred to as a common cold, presenting with nasal discharge and obstruction, sneezing and sore throat. It is caused by a group of infections, all of viral nature, for the most part belonging to five families: rhinovirus, parainfluenza virus, respiratory syncytial virus, enterovirus (especially coxsackievirus A21), and coronaviruses. Acute laryngitis is characterized by hoarseness of voice with a deepened pitch with possible episodes of aphonia. Often these signs are associated to those of coryza and pharyngitis. The large majority of episodes are due to viral agents, including parainfluenza virus, rhinovirus, influenza virus, and adenovirus. Bacteria, represented by *C. diphteriae*, *Branhamella catarrhalis* and *Haemophilus influenzae*, may rarely play a role in this condition, and are almost invariably associated to pharyngitis. The acute inflammation of the pharynx causes the pharyngitis syndrome, which presents with soreness, scratchiness and irritation. Most cases are of viral etiology, and appear in the contest of the coryzal syndrome or influenza, rather than as an isolated entity. Rhinovirus and coronavirus are the most common causative agents, but adenovirus and herpes simplex virus may also be implicated, usually in more severe clinical cases. Other viral causes of pharyngitis in the context of a generalized infection are Epstein-Barr virus (EBV) and the Human Immunodeficiency Virus (HIV). The pharyngitis/tonsillitis syndrome is caused by bacteria in up to 15% of the cases, the most important agent being represented by *Streptococcus pyogenes* (Group A β-hemolytic streptococcus) and, more rarely, *Corynebacterium diphtheriae*.

Lower respiratory infections are characterized by bronchial and pulmonary parenchyma involvement. The most common etiologic agents of pneumonia are listed in Table 56.2. Viruses commonly occur, but bacteria are responsible for a significant proportion of community acquired cases. *S. pneumoniae* and *H. influenzae*, as well as *M. pneumoniae* and *C. pneumoniae* are most frequent but pneumonia may also be caused by mycobacterial, fungal, and parasitic agents. Young children may sometimes be affected by severe forms of tracheobronchitis, characterized by dyspnea accompanied on inspiration by characteristic stridulous notes caused by inflammation in the subglottic area. The large majority of cases are due to viruses with a few being due to diphtheria, *H. influenzae*, or *M. pneumoniae* infection.

A list of common complications of RTI is presented in Table 56.3. Otitis media is the most common, especially among young children. *Streptococcus pneumoniae* is responsible for most such cases.

EPIDEMIOLOGY

Steffen estimated the monthly incidence of acute febrile respiratory tract infections to be 1261/100 000 travellers.[1] In that analysis RTI ranked third after travelers' diarrhea and malaria among all infectious problems of the travelers. However, that rate, which is equivalent to 0.2 episodes per person per year, is much lower than the incidence of common respiratory diseases among adults in the USA, which is

Table 56.1	Most common etiologic agents of upper respiratory tract infections	
	Viral	Bacterial
Coryzal syndrome	Rhinovirus Parainfluenza virus Respiratory syncytial virus Enterovirus Coronavirus	
Laryngitis	Influenza virus A and B Parainfluenza virus Rhinovirus Adenovirus	Corynebacterium diphtheriae Haemophilus influenzae Branhamella catarrhalis
Pharyngitis	Rhinovirus Adenovirus Coronavirus Enterovirus Influenza virus Parainfluenza virus Respiratory syncytial virus Epstein-Barr virus Herpes Simplex Virus Human Immunodeficiency Virus type 1	Streptococcus pyogenes Group C β-hemolytic Streptococci Corynebacterium diphtheriae Mycoplasma pneumoniae Chlamydia pneumoniae

Table 56.2	Most common etiologic agents of pneumonia		
Bacterial	Fungal	Viral	Other
Streptococcus pneumoniae	Histoplasma capsulatum	Influenza A	Coxiella burnetii
Staphylococcus aureus	Coccidioides immitis	Influenza B	Mycobacterium tuberculosis
Haemophilus influenzae	Aspergillus spp	Adenovirus type 4 and 7	Ascaris lumbricoides
Mixed anaerobic bacteria		Hantanvirus	Strongyloides stercoralis
Escherichia coli		Corona virus	Paragonimus westermani
Klebsiella pneumonia			
Pseudomonas aeruginosa			
Legionella spp			
Mycoplasma pneumoniae			
Chlamydia pneumoniae			
Chlamydia psittaci			

Table 56.3	Common complications of respiratory tract infections and common etiologic agents of otitis media	
Complications	Agents of otitis media	
Otitis media	Streptococcus pneumoniae	
Sinusitis	Streptococcus Group A	
Epiglottitis	Staphylococcus aureus	
Mastoiditis	Haemophilus influenzae	
Periorbital cellulitis	Branhamella catarrhalis	
Peritonsillar abscess		
Retropharyngeal abscess		
Adenitis		

around four episodes per person per year.[6] The difference is likely to be attributable to underreporting among travelers, because a large proportion of RTI are mild, not incapacitating, and do not require hospital care.

The incidence of RTI is similar in developing and developed nations. In a classic study comparing incidence rates in travelers to different areas RTI occurred in 3.7/1000 travel days to Latin America, 3.5/1000 to Oceania, and 3.1/1000 to the Caribbean.[7]

In the literature there are large variations in the proportion of respiratory infections among all causes of illness in returning travelers. Comparison among studies, however, is difficult and differences are likely to reflect diverse diagnostic procedures and definition of syndromes rather than true epidemiological differences. Still, RTI consistently rank in the highest belt of most frequently diagnosed conditions. Incidence rates have been recently reviewed by Denny and Kallings, ranging from 4–42%.[8] As they correctly point out, proportions made on a population group should be differentiated from those made on an ill group. A few additional reports have become available since the above review has been published. Among 1469 British package holiday tourists 7.6% had respiratory infection, and this condition was over-ranked by travelers' diarrhea only.[9] Respiratory illness occurred in 26% of 748 travelers from the USA, second only to diarrhea.[10] O'Brien studied a group of 232 sick travelers at a tertiary hospital in Australia mainly returned from Asian destinations: RTI were second after malaria accounting for 24% of the cases.[11] In that series lower tract infections accounted for 50% of all RTI, and were almost equally distributed between bacterial pneumonia and influenza.[11] Bacterial pneumonia was significantly more common in patients aged >40 years with an OR of 5.5. One fourth of upper tract infections were due to group A streptococcus. Our own data of an unpublished multicenter hospital study in Italy including 541 travelers with fever showed that 8.1% had a respiratory syndrome, one third of whom had pneumonia. TB was responsible for 29% of pneumonia cases. Among cases with RTI and no signs of pneumonia, malaria was the underlying disease in 11 of 27, despite the fact that malaria is reportedly not associated to respiratory symptoms.

RISK FACTORS

There are no definitive factors associated to an increased risk of acquisition of respiratory infections. However, some persons are at increased risk of developing severe clinical consequences should infection occur. High-risk groups include people at the extreme of the ages, infants, small children and the elderly, and subjects with chronic tracheobronchial or pulmonary disease. There is convincing evidence that chilling is not an important risk factor for these diseases. The reduced pressure of inspired oxygen found on airline flight or high altitude destinations may adversely affect infants breathing patterns.[12] It has been suggested that if a concomitant respiratory tract infection is present hypoxia can reach levels to be a significant risk for sudden infant death.

Respiratory infections are the most common diagnosis for passengers and crew seeking medical care on board ships.[13] In addition, cruise travelers are at increased risk for legionellosis, influenza or pneumococcal disease.[2] Reasons for increased susceptibility of cruise ship travelers to respiratory infections include passengers factors, such as age, underlying illnesses and physical conditions, as well as environmental factors, like the heavy use of secretional spas (increasing difficulties to maintain safe water systems) and the confinement in relatively close quarters.[14]

TRANSMISSION

The spread of agents such as streptococci or meningococci is by direct, person to person, contacts transmitted by large droplets. Common occurrence is as sporadic and isolated cases, because droplets are too large to contaminate the air environment, and fall quickly to the ground unless they come in contact with mucous membranes in the very close proximity of the source case.

Other pathogens are transmitted by tiny droplet nuclei (less than 10 µm in diameter), that are dispersed widely and randomly, remain viable in the air for hours, may be inhaled and pass easily through the narrow bronchioles. These agents lead to infection in a large number of people, presenting as clusters of disease among those exposed. *Influenza* virus and *M.tuberculosis* disseminate in this way.

Legionella is an air-borne disease with a unique chain of transmission. It is a free living bacteria which multiplicates in the water systems forming biofilms in cooling towers, waterpipe fittings, and showers. From the domestic water systems legionella spreads to the human host in the aerosols generated by showerheads, whirlpools, or cooling systems. This transmission chain justify the existence of outbreaks in hotels and cruise ships.

MANAGEMENT OF THE RESPIRATORY SYNDROME

An example of decision algorithm for respiratory tract infections in travelers is presented in Figures 56.1 and 56.2. A syndromic management algorithm should effectively differentiate upper from lower respiratory tract infections to anticipate causative agents and guide treatment decisions. It should also identify complications requiring specific treatment. There is no generally accepted definition for the respiratory syndrome: cough with runny nose, or either of this with any one of headache, fever or shortness of breath are widely used for study purposes.

Among upper respiratory tract infections (Fig 56.1) the isolated coryzal syndrome is rarely cause of medical consultation. It is easily identified through the patient history and typical manifestations, no additional diagnostic procedures are required and symptomatic treatment provides quick relief. The diagnosis of laryngitis is clinical, and antibiotic treatment is not routinely envisaged. The diagnosis of pharyngitis is also clinical. It is important to differentiate group A streptococcal infections in this group of patients because this condition may determine late complications which are readily preventable by antibiotic treatment. Reportedly, bacterial pharyngitis is associated with more severe pharyngeal pain, odynophagia and higher fever, with grayish-yellow exudate on the tonsils and enlarged cervical lymphatic glands. However, clinical criteria are unreliable to identify bacterial pharyngitis/tonsillitis, because a typical presentation occurs in less than a half of the cases. Rapid antigen detection tests are available with reported specificity of over 90% and sensitivity of 60–95%, and should be performed on initial evaluation on specimens collected by throat swab. The need to perform a bacterial culture if a rapid test is negative is still debated. Supportive care is the only therapy for the majority of cases which are due to viruses. Antibiotic treatment is warranted if the rapid test demonstrates streptococcal infection. Presumptive antibiotic treatment may be prescribed to cases when clinical suspicion of streptococcal infection is high and the clinical manifestations are severe, to be discontinued if the culture result is negative. A treatment course with penicillin for 10 days is appropriate to treat pharyngitis due to *S.pyogenes*. Diphtheria is a rare cause of pharyngitis with potentially fatal outcome. It is characterized by thick and gray pharyngeal and tracheal membranes, bleeding upon attempted removal. Microscopic examination of direct stained pharyngeal smear is unreliable, and clinical suspicion of diphtheria must be confirmed by culture isolation of a toxigenic strain of *Corynebacterium diphtheriae*. The mainstay of therapy is diphtheria antitoxin, associated with antibiotic treatment with penicillin or macrolides.

Complications of upper RTI include focal inflammation and toxin-mediated toxicity. The most frequent form of focal inflammation are otitis and sinusitis (Table 56.3), usually sustained by bacterial infections. *Streptococcus pneumoniae* is responsible for most cases, and initial treatment should be effective against this agent. Pharyngo-tonsillitis may be complicated by pharyngeal abscess which also requires prompt and appropriate antibacterial therapy. The selected treatment regimen should be effective not only against Group A streptococcus, but also against *S. pneumoniae*, *H. influenzae*, *B. catarrhalis* and *S.aureus* which are more troublesome agents. Protected penicillins and third generation cephalosporins may be the treatment of choice. Toxin mediated toxicity is basically observed in the case of diphtheria.

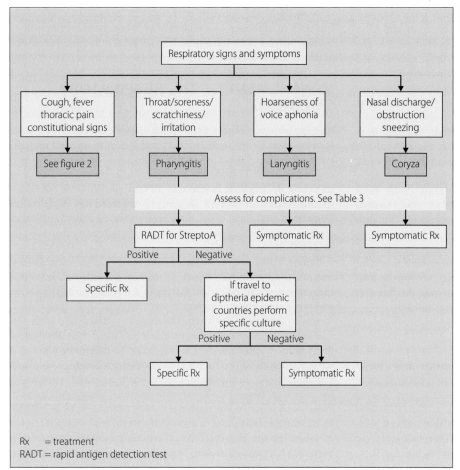

Figure 56.1 Decision algorithm for acute upper respiratory tract infections.

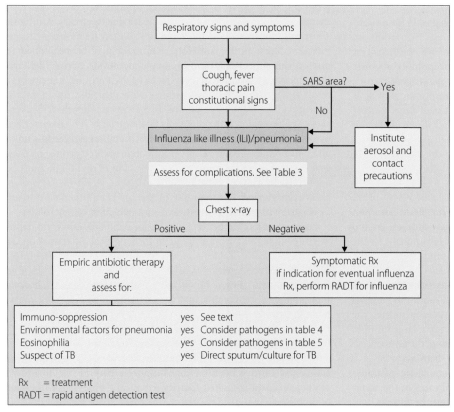

Figure 56.2 Decision algorithm for acute lower respiratory tract infections.

Clinical signs suggestive of pneumonia include productive cough, thoracic pain, and shortness of breath. A chest X-ray should be routinely performed, because the demonstration of an abnormal chest radiograph consistent with pneumonia differentiates a patient population that may benefit from antibiotic therapy from patient populations that will not (Fig. 56.2). Although the majority of cases with radiological evidence of pneumonia may still have a viral infection, the proportion of cases due to bacteria is high enough to warrant systematic antibacterial treatment. The chest film is not helpful in making a specific etiologic diagnosis, however, lobar consolidation, cavitation and large pleural effusions support a bacterial cause. Pneumococcal disease is often characterized by abrupt onset of fever, cough, rapid respiration, and lobar consolidation on chest film. Atypical pneumonia caused by *M. pneumoniae* and *C. pneumoniae* are characterized by gradual onset of symptoms, cough progressive from dry to productive, chest film worse than symptoms, and normal peripheral white blood cell counts. Overall, however, clinical presentation is not specific enough to make etiologic diagnosis, and effective methods to recognize the causative agent of pneumonia are not available. The sputum Gram stain is a simple, quick and inexpensive procedure but its helpfulness for aiding in the etiologic diagnosis is unclear. The main advantages are the identification of *P. carinii* in patients with AIDS or acid-fast bacilli in patients with tuberculosis. The utility of the sputum culture is also unclear, since the procedure is insensitive, only half of the patients with pneumonia may produce sputum and contamination occurs in one third of the patients. An advantage of routine sputum Gram stain and culture is that these procedures would capture rare causes of pneumonia like melioidosis. Because the cause of pneumonia cannot be determined on the basis of any specific clinical, radiographic, or laboratory parameter, antibiotic therapy is usually begun empirically. Treatment should be effective on *S. pneumoniae*, the most frequently responsible agent, and on agents of atypical pneumonia: *M. pneumoniae*, *C. pneumoniae*, and legionella infections. Amoxicillin and amoxicillin-clavulanic acid should be associated with a macrolide. Alternatively, the new respiratory tract quinolones can be used alone. Presumptive treatment should be replaced by more specific treatment when a high degree of suspicion of the etiology of diagnosis is reached.

Immunocompromised patients are susceptible to diseases which are very rarely observed in the immunocompetent host, such as *P. carinii*, cytomegalovirus or *Cryptococcus neoformans* pneumonia. Determining the presence of malignancy, neutropenia, chronic use of steroids or myelosuppressive agents, or the presence of HIV infection is therefore an important component of the patient history. Environmental factors may be risk markers for some specific causes of pneumonia and pharyngitis, as summarized in Table 56.4. Information on the type of recent travel is important as a history of ship cruise should alert for the possibility of legionella of influenza infections. Tropical destinations are a prerequisite to suspect exotic infections like melioidosis, paragonimiasis or fungal infections. Behavioral parameters, like possible contact with rats or bats are necessary to suspect plague/hantavirus or histoplasmosis respectively. Pneumonia with eosinophilia in a traveler is often suggestive of specific infections, a list of which is presented in Table 56.5. Treatment of tuberculosis should be started only following a positive sputum smear or culture have been obtained.

Influenza is often included among the causes of lower tract respiratory infection. The definition of influenza like illness (ILI) requires the presence of fever or feverishness with cough or sore throat. Quick laboratory evidence of influenza infection can be obtained by detection of viral antigens in nasopharyngeal aspirates. This may be important for groups of patients at increased risk of influenza morbidity and mortality. Antiviral treatment may be considered for patients with ILI aged greater than 65 years or who have certain underlying chronic conditions like pulmonary or cardiac disease. Amantadine and rimantadine are effective against type A virus, which is responsible for the totality of influenza cases among travelers.

PREVENTION IN TRAVELERS

Prevention of RTI in the traveler usually relies on vaccines, and, in a few specific conditions such as influenza in the elderly, by self-administered treatment to ameliorate the course of the resulting disease (Table 56.6). Public health interventions are important to minimize the risk of acquiring a new RTI, or limit the scale of epidemic outbreaks, while behavioral interventions and chemoprophylaxis play a little role.

Diphtheria is one of the major vaccine preventable diseases, which can be virtually eliminated by effective immunization programs, using diphtheria toxoid. The primary vaccination schedule consists of four doses of the toxoid before two years of age. Boosters every 10 years are required to sustain a protective immunological response, especially in areas of low transmission of the bacteria. Sporadic cases of diphtheria have been reported in adult travelers who had received full childhood vaccination including diphtheria toxoid.[15] A booster

Table 56.4	Important environmental factors in respiratory tract infections
Pneumonia	
Anthrax	Biological war; exposure to cattle
Melioidosis	Travel to endemic areas
Brucellosis	Exposure to cattle
Plague	Travel to endemic areas and contact with rats
Tularemia	Hunting or otherwise exposure to wild animals
Psittacosis	Exposure to birds
Leptospirosis	Adventurous travel
Coccidioidomycosis	Travel to endemic areas
Histoplasmosis	Exposure to bat droppings
Q fever	Exposure to infected animals
Legionnaires' disease	Ship trip or enclosure in epidemic foci
Hantavirus	Exposure to rodents
Pharyngitis	
Diphtheria	Travel to epidemic countries

Table 56.5	Causative causes of pneumonia and eosinophilia
Ascaris lumbricoides	
Strongyloides stercoralis	
Mycobacterium tuberculosis	
Chlamydia psittaci	
Coccidioides immitis	
Histoplasma capsulatum	
Paragonimus spp	
Echinococcus granulosus	
Visceral larva migrans	
Schistosoma spp	
Dirofilaria immitis	
Ancylostoma spp	

Table 56.6	Prevention of respiratory tract infections in travelers
Prevention strategy	**Preventable condition**
Vaccine	Primary vaccination
	Haemophilus influenzae
	Diphtheria
	Influenza
	Streptococcus pneumoniae
	Booster
	Diphtheria
Early presumptive treatment	Influenza
Public health interventions	Influenza
	Guidelines for international response
	Legionellosis
	Alert networks (EWGLI)
	Guidelines for safe water systems
Behavioural interventions	Paragonimiasis
	Avoid eating raw crabs or crayfish
	Histoplasmosis
	Avoid bat caves
	Leptospirosis
	Avoid adventurous travel
	Plague
	Avoid contacts with rodents
	Anthrax / Q fever
	Avoid contact with cattle and sheep

dose of combined diphtheria-tetanus toxoid (Td) is an acceptable option to protect travelers to countries with epidemics of the disease. Influenza virus vaccine are available against current epidemic types. Vaccination is a cost-saving intervention among the elderly and subjects with chronic cardiac and pulmonary diseases under influenza epidemic conditions, as it effectively reduces influenza-related morbidity and mortality.[16] Special groups may be considered for influenza vaccination for reasons of convenience, such as athletes participating at the Olympic games. As a consequence of the 1998 epidemic of influenza in Alaska and the Yukon Territory, The National Advisory Committee on Immunization of Canada recommended influenza vaccination for people at high risk of influenza complications before embarking on travel to destinations where influenza was likely to be circulating.[17] At the same time some cruise lines initiated policies to vaccinate crew members to decrease the risk for influenza transmission to travellers.[18] Subjects who have received the influenza vaccine in the previous 6 months do not deserve to be re-vaccinated because specific antibody titers remain high for at least 6 months.[19] Vaccination against *H. influenzae* (type B only) is now part of the childhood immunization program in many industrialized countries; its possible role in adult unimmunized travelers is unclear. The capsular polysaccharide vaccine against *S. pneumoniae* is of questionable efficacy in the elderly[20] and it is not recommended in children below 2 years of age. An effective vaccine against group A streptococcus is currently under development but will not be available for many years.

Persons at high risk for complications of influenza infection who have no access to vaccination because of shortage in vaccine supplies might receive a prescription for self-administered amantadine or rimantadine.[18] Both drugs can reduce the duration of influenza A illness and viral shedding if administered within the first 24–48 h of onset of influenza-like illness

The response to emerging influenza pandemics is an important task for public health interventions. International guidelines were established after the identification in Hong Kong of the first known human outbreak of infection by the influenza A (H5N1) virus, previously known to infect only birds.[21] Massive efforts were put in place by international organizations for the identification and containment of the outbreak, including the slaughtering of 1.6 million chickens, the putative source of the infection.[22] Control measures of legionellosis are based on the application of guidelines for maintaining safe water systems in international tourist locations and cruise ships.[23] These include proper disinfection, filtration and storage of source water, avoidance of dead ends in pipes, proper cleaning and maintenance of spas, and periodic replacement of devices likely to amplify or disseminate the organism.

The early recognition of outbreaks is exceedingly important in the management of individual cases of diseases like legionellosis. The European Working Group for Legionella Infections (EWGLI) is a network created to report legionella cases diagnosed in patients who have been traveling within the likely incubation period of two weeks, together with geographical location of suspected source of transmission. Members of the group report cases of Legionnaires' disease to the coordinating center, which then notifies all EWGLI members of any disease cluster. Other international global and regional surveillance networks, including GeoSentinel and TropNetEurop, play a pivotal role in early detection and public warning of travel related epidemics.[24,25]

INFECTIONS OF THE RESPIRATORY TRACT ASSOCIATED TO EPIDEMICS

Influenza

Influenza is the most important of the viral respiratory infections, sustained by the influenza viruses type A and B. The virus is responsible for recurrent epidemics due to the emergence and spread of a novel type of virus. World-wide pandemics resulting in a high number of illnesses and millions of deaths occurred in 1918, 1957, and 1968, each one lasting for approximately 2–3 years. While large epidemics are due to human viral strains, small outbreaks have been associated to avian and swine viruses. The last such outbreak has been described in Hong Kong in 1997, where an avian influenza virus resulted in 18 proven human cases, of which five were fatal, with a case-fatality rate of 18% in children and 57% in adults older than 17 years.[21] Transmission was direct from chicken to humans rather than from person to person and the outbreak remained an isolated accident.

Travelers acquire influenza both as sporadic cases and as clusters from a common source aboard ships, airplanes, or in tour groups. All described outbreaks are caused by the type A virus, and are characterized by the involvement of a large proportion of the population at risk, and the explosive nature of the epidemic. In 1998, approximately 40 000 tourists and tourism workers were affected by an influenza outbreak in Alaska and the Yukon Territory.[26]

Influenza is a self-limiting disease, which produces high morbidity and is responsible for lethal cases among the youngest and the eldest. The hallmark of the clinical presentation of influenza is a febrile illness with cough, resulting from involvement of trachea and bronchi. Fever characteristically lasts 3–5 days, but dry cough may persist for much longer. Pneumonia is the most frequent complication. Part of the cases are due to direct involvement of the lungs by the influenza virus, the remainder being attributable to bacterial superinfections mainly from *S. pneumoniae*, *H. influenzae*, and group A *Streptococcus*. Otitis media and sinusitis are other serious complications. Complications are more frequent and severe among patients with chronic diseases of the lung or the heart. Early diagnosis of influenza can be based on rapid antigen detection tests. Viral isolation is the method of reference but it is seldom used in clinical care. Antibody determination is also rarely used for diagnosis in clinical settings. Treatment is symptomatic in most cases. For severe cases in debilitated subjects the neuraminidase inhibitor antivirals amantadine and rimantadine are effective on type A virus, and reduce the duration of the illness and viral shedding if administered within 48 h of symptom onset.

Legionellosis

Legionella infections occur world-wide as sporadic cases. Endemic legionellosis is responsible for approximately 2% of community acquired pneumonia, the highest incidence is in people aged over 40 years, but only a fraction of these cases are recognized. Legionellosis also presents as clusters in large, common-source, outbreaks. A number of such outbreaks have been described among travelers. A European Working Group on Legionella Infection involving 29 countries was started in 1987. In 1997 the network identified 1360 cases of legionellosis, 22% of whom were related to travel, mostly within Europe.[27] In Sweden 15–30% of all legionella infections are related to travel, either international or domestic.[28] In the UK this proportion presents an increasing trend since the 1970s, with a pick at 46%.[29] Countries whose tourist industries are expanding appear to have higher rates of infection. The Mediterranean region in Europe has been the origin of most reported outbreaks, but no area is immune from the risk, as exemplified by the recent identification of the first cluster of cases associated with a hotel in Bangkok.[30]

Transmission is air-borne, but the source of infection is the environment rather than other persons.

The incubation period is classically considered as 2–10 days, although 16% of 188 cases described in a recent large outbreak in the Netherlands reported incubation periods exceeding 10 days.[31] The clinical spectrum is wide, ranging from subclinical to lethal manifestations. The overt picture of legionellosis is that of a lobar pneumonia with abrupt onset characterized by high fever, severe headache and confusion.[28] Patchy infiltrates are often present bilaterally. Mortality may be as high as 20% if diagnosis and antibiotic treatment is delayed. Diagnosis is challenging because sensitive and friendly diagnostic tests are not widely available. Urine antigen tests are very helpful for rapid diagnosis, but they are not widely used as legionellosis is considered a rare disease. Serological diagnosis requires a fourfold or higher rise in antibody titers in paired acute and convalescent phase sera, and its usefulness is very limited in clinical terms. Isolation of the bacteria from respiratory secretions is possible but cumbersome; however, this is essential to apply molecular techniques to match patients' isolates with those of the environment, in order to provide evidence for clusters and the common source of the infection. Macrolides are the treatment of choice, clarithromycin and erythromycin should be administered for 3 weeks to avoid relapses. Co-trimoxazole and fluoroquinolones are also effective.

Diphtheria

Diphtheria is considered eliminated in the immunized population of industrialized countries, with toxigenic strains no longer circulating among the native population. However, importation of the organism from developing countries where diphtheria remains endemic poses a constant threat, particularly among subgroups of travelers with low vaccination levels. Eastern Europe has been the theatre of a large-scale resurgence of diphtheria during the 1990s, due to the collapse of the health systems and consequent disruption of the vaccination programs. Almost 20 000 cases of diphtheria were reported in 1993 mainly in the former Russia Federation and Ukraine, with cases identified in neighboring countries including Poland, Norway, Finland and Germany.[32] Re-emergence of diphtheria has been described in susceptible trav-

elers to these areas.[33] Travelers to endemic areas may act as asymptomatic carriers of the bacterium, and determine secondary cases in unimmunized children in non-endemic areas.[4]

Diphtheria presents as a respiratory disease with cough and fever, characterized by pseudomembranous pharyngitis with membrane formation and cervical lymphadenitis, sometimes evolving to cervical edema (bull-neck). Pharyngeal and tracheal membranes are described as thick and gray, bleeding upon attempted removal. A chest X-ray may show subglottic narrowing and bilateral lung hyperinflation. Lethal complications are due to airway mechanical obstruction at laryngeal level and to myocarditis and neuritis resulting from acute systemic toxicity caused by a toxin. Cardiac toxicity consist of both cardiac heart failure and potentially fatal arrhythmia. Clinical suspicion of diphtheria must be confirmed by culture isolation of the bacteria, which demonstrates the presence of a toxigenic strain of *Corynebacterium diphtheriae*. Microscopic examination of direct stained pharyngeal smear is unreliable. The mainstay of therapy is diphtheria antitoxin, which must be administered as early as possible to neutralize circulating, unbounded toxin. Antibiotic treatment with penicillin or macrolides is indicated to eradicate the organism and terminate toxin production. The notification of a diphtheria case must prompt the implementation of control measures to prevent the spread of toxigenic *C. diphtheriae*, including taking nose and throat swabs from close contacts, antibiotic prophylaxis, and full immunization or booster doses depending on contacts' immunization history.

TROPICAL RESPIRATORY INFECTIONS

This term identifies infectious diseases that are particularly or uniquely prevalent in tropical countries. The climate in this region offers an ideal environment for pathogenic organisms, their vectors, or their intermediate hosts.

Melioidosis

The most common clinical manifestations of melioidosis is a localized infection with regional lymphadenitis, but community acquired septicemia and pneumonia are also common. The disease is caused by *Burkholderia pseudomallei (Pseudomonas pseudomallei)*, an aerobic gram negative bipolar staining bacillus which is free living in earth and water in many tropical and subtropical countries. Melioidosis is rare outside the main endemic regions, namely Southeast Asia and Northern Australia. Reactivation melioidosis has been reported among tourists, immigrants and Vietnam veterans decades after leaving endemic regions. The infection is acquired by inhalation, ingestion or from contaminated injuries. Many big mammals (cows, horses, pigs) are the reservoir. Human to human transmission is extremely rare.[34]

Lung involvement consists of acute necrotizing pneumonia or chronic granulomatous or fibrosing lung disease mimicking tuberculosis. The diagnosis of pulmonary melioidosis is difficult. It might be suspected in travelers from endemic areas, though cases have reported from areas considered to be non-endemic.[35] The diagnosis can be confirmed by gram stain (gram negative bipolar stained safety-pin appearance) and culture of respiratory specimens. The presumptive diagnosis of melioidosis may be based on a positive IHA or ELISA serology.[36,37] IHA titers above 1:80 are suggestive of active infection but can also be seen in asymptomatic subjects in endemic regions.[37] Current therapy recommendations are ceftazidime or imipenem plus trimethoprim-sulfamethoxazole, doxycycline or amoxicillin-clavulanic acid, for a period of 2–6 weeks. Maintenance therapy for 3–6 months using either trimethoprim-sulfamethoxazole, doxycycline or amoxicillin clavulanic acid is also necessary. A vaccine against mehoidosis is not available, and there is no role for chemoprophylaxis. Low risk behaviors, like avoiding bathing or walking in rice paddies and still water should be recommended for short-term travelers.

Leptospirosis

Pulmonary involvement in leptospirosis is not rare, usually manifested by a dry cough, occasionally with blood stained sputum. Although being a zoonosis of world-wide dimension the infection has significantly higher diffusion in the tropical belt.

Leptospirosis is due to several serovars of a spirochetal bacteria, *Leptospira interrrogans*. Transmission occurs by accidental contact with urine, contaminated water, and soil. Clinical manifestation of leptospirosis may vary from asymptomatic infection to fulminant disease. Severe cases are characterized by liver and renal failure with mortality as high as 30% in untreated cases. Pulmonary complication often contribute to the fatal outcome: they include extensive edema and alveolar hemorrhages in the contest of an ARDS episode. The radiological findings are those of ARDS. The diagnosis requires the isolation of the bacteria from blood or urine samples. As an alternative, a microhemagglutination serological test provides evidence of the disease in coupled sera of acute and convalescent phases. Penicillin and tetracycline's are effective for the treatment of the disease.

Prevention of leptospirosis is difficult, especially in tropical areas where the disease is not limited to high-risk groups. Prevention of rodent–human contacts is important. A human vaccine and the use of tetracycline chemoprophylaxis (200 mg/week) are available but are indicated for well defined high-risk populations only.

Anthrax

Pulmonary anthrax is caused by the inhalation of spores produced by the bacteria *Bacillus anthracis*. Cutaneous disease is the commonly observed form in natural infection. The pulmonary form is of concern for the use of anthrax aerosols as a biological weapon against a civilian population, due to the possibility of rapid dissemination and rapidly fatal outcome.[38] Naturally acquired anthrax may occur in developing countries where the risk is still significant in rural parts of Asia, Africa, Eastern Europe, South and Central America as a result of contaminated soil and a few cases have been described in travelers who import souvenirs.

Inhalation anthrax results in an extremely severe mediastinitis due to the penetration of the pathogen from the pulmonary alveoli and its spread to hilar lymph nodes. The incubation period is 2–5 days, but the spores can germinate up to 60 days after exposure. Pathogenesis is mediated by a toxin responsible for hemorrhagia, edema, and necrosis. The presenting symptoms are nonspecific, with mild fever, malaise, and a nonproductive cough. After a period of a few days in which the patient's condition apparently improves, a second phase begins with high fever, respiratory distress, cyanosis, and subcutaneous edema of the neck and thorax. Crepitant rales are evident on auscultation. The chest film reveals mediastinal widening and frequently a pleural effusion. Inhalation anthrax is almost invariably fatal with a very short time between the onset of the second phase, mediastinal signs, and death. The diagnosis of inhalation anthrax is extremely difficult outside epidemic conditions. PCR and ELISA tests for a protective antigen are available at specialized centers. The most useful bacteriologic test in case of suspicion, however, is blood culture of *B. anthracis*. Direct examination and Gram stain of the sputum specimen are unlikely to be diagnostic. A serologic ELISA test is available, although a significant increase in titer is usually obtained only in convalescent subjects who survive. Treatment of inhalation anthrax should be as early as possible to provide chances of success. *B. anthracis* is sensitive to penicillin and penicillin 1.2 million units (or intra-venously 18 to 24 million units daily in severe cases) or doxycycline for 7–10 days are the drug of choice for the naturally acquired disease. In the contest of biological war, because of the high likelihood that *B. anthracis* strains are engineered to be resistant to these two classes of antibiotics, the treatment of choice is ciprofloxacin 400 mg intra-venously every 12 h. Ancillary treatment to sustain vascular volume, cardiac, pulmonary, and renal functions is essential in severe cases. A human inactivated cell free vaccine is available in case of biological attack. Post-exposure prophylaxis following exposure to an anthrax aerosol would require the use of ciprofloxacin for a period of 60 days.

Plague

Plague usually presents as lymphadenitis and septicemia. Pulmonary forms are rarely observed, secondary to inhalation of the causative agent, *Yersinia pestis*, from coughing patients affected by the disease. Plague is considered a re-emerging disease because of the increase of the worldwide number of reported cases, the occurrence of epidemics (such as the one in India in 1994), and the gradual expansion in areas of low endemicity (including the USA). Over 85% of the cases of 1996 were reported from Africa where, more then 85% of the cases occurred in just two countries, Madagascar and United Republic of Tanzania.[39] The major recent world-wide plague epidemic occurred in India, where a total of 5150 suspected pneumonic or bubonic cases occurred from August to October 1994, causing travel and trade disruption and resulting in severe economic repercussions.[40] Travelers are rarely affected by plague while visiting endemic areas, for example no visitors were affected during the 1994 epidemic in India. Campers or visitors staying in rodent infested lodges are exposed to the highest risk of infection.

In humans, pneumonia may follow septicemia or may be a primary event in the case of airborne transmission. Plague should be suspected in febrile patients who have been exposed to rodents or other mammals in the known endemic areas of the world. The presence of buboes in this setting is highly suspicious. The bacterium may be isolated on standard bacteriologic media from culture samples of blood and bubo aspirate. The Gram stain may reveal Gram negative coccobacilli with polymorphonuclear leukocytes. Rapid diagnostic tests like the direct immunofluorescence test for the presumptive identification of *Y. pestis* F1 antigen are of interest for the quick management of patients with the suspect of the disease.[41] Serologic tests to detect antibodies to the F1 antigen by passive hemoagglutination assay or enzyme-linked immunosorbent assay methods are available. A fourfold increase in titer (or a single titer of 1:16 or more) may provide presumptive evidence of plague in culture negative cases. Antibiotic treatment should be started on the basis of clinical suspicion. Streptomycin 30 mg/kg per day intramuscularly in two divided doses for 10 days is the drug of choice. Whenever streptomycin is contraindicated due to allergy, tetracycline's or chloramphenicol should be administered.

A formalin-killed whole cell vaccine is licensed and available for subjects at specific risk for plague, but its efficacy is questionable. Those who may have contact with rodents in endemic areas are candidates for vaccination. Personal hygiene (avoidance of lice by using insect repellents) and safe behaviors (avoidance of contacts with rodents) represent the most important preventive measures for travelers. Plague is an internationally quarantinable disease. Pulmonary infections present a particular risk for human epidemics due to the contagiousness of the organism. Doxycycline (100 mg twice daily for 7 days) prophylaxis of family members of index cases is indicated within the standard 7-day maximum plague incubation period.

Paragonimiasis

Lung involvement is constant in paragonimiasis because the adult stage of the causative agent live in the pulmonary district, and may survive up to 20 years in the human host. Paragonimiasis is an helmintic disease caused by trematodes of the genus *Paragonimus*: *P. westermani* is the most diffuse species. The infection is endemic in South East Asia (including Thailand, the Philippines, Vietnam, China and Taiwan), South America and Africa. The distribution is determined by the presence of the intermediate host and human habits to eat them raw. The disease is well described, though rare, in travelers to endemic regions.[42] The incubation period may vary from one to several months after exposure.

Symptoms are characterized by a chronic bronchopneumonic process with productive cough, thoracic pain and low grade fever, sometimes hemoptysis. The chest X-ray is not characteristic, and may present with single or bilateral infiltrates and cavity formation. The main differential diagnosis is with tuberculosis: in paragonimiasis there are no constitutional signs and general conditions may remain good for several years despite persistent respiratory signs. The diagnosis requires the identification of the eggs in the sputum or in feces by the use of concentration methods. The treatment of choice is praziquantel 25 mg/kg three times a day for two consecutive days. Prevention is based on avoidance of eating raw crayfish and crabs.

Coccidioidomycosis and histoplasmosis

Coccidioidomycosis and histoplasmosis are two fungal infections acquired by the respiratory route and therefore primarily involving the respiratory system. Coccidioidomycosis is caused by inhalation of *Coccidioides immitis*, a dimorphic fungus found in the dust and soil. The pathogen is present only in semiarid regions of the Americas. Symptomatic disease develop in approximately 40% of individuals infected by *C. immitis*, presenting as a flu-like syndrome. The radiological finding is often that of hilar pneumonia with lymphadenitis and pleural involvement. In a recently described outbreak of coccidioidomycosis in a 126-member church group traveling to Mexico the average incubation period was 12 days (range 7–20 days), and chest pain was present in 76% and cough in 66% of the affected travelers.[43] The diagnosis is serological, antibodies appear 1–3 weeks after the onset of symptoms.

Histoplasmosis is caused by the infection with a soil-inhabiting dimorphic fungus, *Histoplasma capsulatum*. The agent is ubiquitous, but diffusion is higher in the tropical belt and the USA. The disease may evolve as a mild, spontaneously resolving condition, but severe and systemic disease may develop in immunocompromised patients. In an outbreak of histoplasmosis among college students from the USA to Acapulco 229 persons developed an acute febrile respiratory illness with cough, shortness of breath, chest pain, or headache.[44] The chest X-ray may show both patchy infiltrates or interstitial pneumonia. Diagnosis may be extremely difficult unless the disease is considered in the differential diagnosis, and most cases are unrecognized and considered as bacterial bronchitis or flu. Confirmation of the disease requires testing of acute- and convalescent-phase serum specimens. A urine antigen test for histoplasmosis is not sensitive, but it is highly specific for diagnosis of acute pulmonary disease.

Both fungal infections are sensitive to the azoles (fluconazole and itraconazole) and amphotericin B.

Tuberculosis

Tuberculosis (TB) is a widely distributed infection and a leading cause of human morbidity and mortality. Travel interacts with TB increasing the risk of reactivated TB among immigrants and the risk of infection among travelers. The problem of TB among immigrants is beyond the scope of this chapter. We discuss here the risk of TB among travelers from low to high endemicity countries and that associated to air flights.

TB among travelers from low to high endemicity areas

There is mounting evidence on the association between travel and increased risk for infection with *M. tuberculosis*. Lobato first demonstrated that US children who had traveled abroad had a significantly higher probability to have a positive tuberculin skin test compared to children without a history of travel.[45] More recently Cobelens has measured the risk of acquiring *M. tuberculosis* infection among long term (3 months or more) Dutch travelers to Africa, Asia, and Latin America at 3.3% per year. This rate is very similar to that of native populations in the visited countries, and much higher than the 0.01% yearly risk in the Netherlands.[5] Other identified factors for increased TB risk among travelers were being a health care worker, a longer cumulative duration of travel, and a loger total time spent in TB endemic countries.[46] Thus, this demonstrates a previously unrecognized high risk for TB infection among travelers, limited to travels with a duration of 3 months or more.

The evidence of association between travel and TB disease is on the contrary elusive. In the most well-known report describing health associated diseases, TB was not mentioned[1] and TB was not present in a list of causes of mortality among American missionaries in Africa.[47] We have recently actively searched for TB diagnosis among travelers in the data generated by GeoSentinel, a surveillance network of travel/tropical medicine clinics, designed to monitor global trends and disease occurrence among travelers. From January 1997 to November 2000, the system registered seven TB cases among travelers/ expatriates which were likely to be associated to travel.[48] It is likely that TB cases associated to travel do occur, but they go unrecognized.

Prevention of tuberculosis in the traveler

Three possible preventive strategies against TB may be envisaged: vaccination, chemoprophylaxis, and detection and treatment of travel-acquired latent tuberculosis infection.

A vaccine against *M. tuberculosis* is available since 1921, consisting in an attenuated strain of *M. bovis*. The protective efficacy from this vaccine ranged from 0–80%, in a series of prospective studies. The general understanding of its action is that the vaccine protects against disseminated disease but does not prevent infection and, possibly, focal disease. The consequence, confirmed by clinical trials, is that BCG effectively protects against a potentially fatal form of tuberculosis in infant and child populations only.[49] Based on this knowledge, the vaccine cannot be recommended to adult travelers because of its unproven efficacy, but it might be administered to children below 5 years of age who travel to TB endemic areas for periods of 6 months or longer.

Chemoprophylaxis with isoniazid during travel is usually not indicated, independently from the estimate of the risk of infection, because of inconclusive evidence of the capacity of chemoprophylaxis to reduce the risk of acquisition of infection with *M. tuberculosis*.

The rational for tuberculin skin testing and preventive therapy of latent tuberculosis infections acquired during travel is that the risk of disease following infection is highest in the first 1–2 years, and that preventive therapy is effective in eradicating dormant tubercle bacilli. Travelers acquiring the infection during the travel may be identified by skin conversion in pre- and post-travel tests (Fig. 56.3). However,

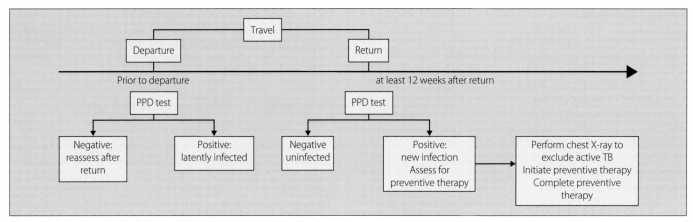

Figure 56.3 Prevention of TB disease in long-term travelers: identification and treatment of new infections.

tuberculin skin testing and preventive therapy have several drawbacks of operational feasibility, lack of sensitivity/specificity, and poor adherence that will be discussed shortly. At present, the detection of tuberculosis infection is based on the skin reaction to the intradermal injection of *M. tuberculosis* antigens and detection of an area of induration (conventionally 10 mm or more) at 72 h. Skin testing of travelers is useful only if the pre-travel test is negative and a post-travel test is conducted 3 months after returning home, to allow for the time of the immune system to mount a significant skin reaction in case of infection. This therefore requires at least two encounters with the traveler before and two after the travel. The possible interference of the booster effect on the significance of a positive tuberculin test might even require two tests (four encounters) before the travel,[5] though this is considered unnecessary by most. Sensitivity and specificity of tuberculin skin test are far from optimal. Rieder estimated that the positive predictive value of a positive tuberculin test with a basic prevalence of 2% is 16%, and is increased only marginally even by a 1% risk of infection during a travel.[50] Preventive therapy carries additional operational problems. Clinical trials have consistently demonstrated that a standard course of 6–12 months of daily isoniazid is over 90% effective in preventing reactivated TB.[51] However, under field conditions adherence is less than optimal and efficacy is significantly reduced. Finally, the isoniazid chemoprophylaxis regimen is not effective against isoniazid-resistant strains, which now may represent from 5–10% of all strains in resource poor countries. Because of all these drawbacks, Rieder has estimated that 14 travelers should be exposed to isoniazid treatment in order to eradicate a single case of latent infection.[50] In summary, a universal strategy of tuberculin testing and preventive therapy for travelers cannot be advocated, at this moment, for both economic and epidemiologic reasons.

TB and air travel

In the past few years several episodes of potential transmission of TB infection during air travel have been reported, raising anxiety in both the general population and health authorities. As a consequence of this, WHO has produced a summary report on this issue, the main conclusion of which is that tuberculosis acquired during air travel is of little epidemiological importance.[52] This statement is based on the review of seven investigations of 2600 persons exposed to one infectious crew member and six passengers over a total of 191 flights.[52] No active TB cases occurred, and possible transmission of infection occurred in only two instances. The risk was limited to flights of over

8 h duration, and for the seats in close proximity to the index case. In fact, airplane-cabin air is exchanged every 3–4 min in contrast to the air in offices and homes, which is exchanged every 5, and 12 min, respectively. A laminar flow ventilation system is in place on airplanes, and despite modern airplanes use to re-circulate up to 50% of the cabin air, this seems not to be a way of dissemination of small droplet nuclei. On these basis, medical screening of the almost 2 billion air passengers over 1 year is impossible and unnecessary. Prevention guidelines are that persons with infectious TB should postpone air travel. Epidemiological investigation for contacts of infectious passengers are indicated only within 3 months from exposure for passengers of travels of more than 8 h duration.[52]

The risk of TB transmission on ship[53] or train[54] has been described as well, but, similarly, it is of little epidemiological importance.

SARS

In November 2002, reports from Guangdong Province in Southern China suggested that more than 300 cases of a mysterious, highly contagious pneumonia had occurred. This severe atypical pneumonia appeared to be particularly prevalent among health care workers and their families. As the condition began to spread from China, on March 13, 2003, the World Health Organization issued a global alert about the outbreak and subsequently named this condition Severe Acute Respiratory Syndrome (SARS). By May 21, 2003 7,956 cases and 666 deaths had been reported from 28 countries.[55]

A novel coronavirus distinct from those previously reported in animals and humans causes SARS; the parent virus has not yet been discovered.[56,57] The virus is transmitted person-to-person by inhalation of droplets, but aerosol transmission may occur in "super spreaders," patients who are severely ill and excreting large viral loads. Since the virus can remain viable on surfaces for several days, mucous membrane contamination (i.e. conjunctiva) or ingestion have not been ruled out as possible modes of transmission. Sixty percent of SARS cases have occurred among health care workers who have not been adequately protected.[58] The incubation period of SARS is 3 to 11 days with a median of 5 days. The syndrome often begins with a prodrome of headache, myalgia and fatigue, progressing a day later to fever above 38°C and subsequently to a non-productive cough and/or shortness of breath. Patients may present with fever and non-specific symptoms 1-3 days before respiratory symptoms begin. Gastrointestinal symptoms (nausea, vomiting and diarrhea) occur in approximately 20% of patients.[59,60] In the series of 144 patients seen in Toronto hospitals, the chest x-ray was normal in 25% of individuals on admission.[61] Unilateral and bilateral infiltrates were observed in 46% and 29% of the patients respectively. Most patients eventually developed multifocal opacities. Laboratory investigations typically show lymphopenia and to a lesser extent thrombocytopenia; during hospitalization many patients develop hypocalcemia, hypo-magnesemia, hypokalemia and hypophosphatemia.

The diagnosis of SARS until recently has been on the basis of a case definition which included a possible contact history, fever and respiratory symptoms. Although not available for use by routine laboratories, serology and PCR used for viral RNA detection will be standard diagnostic tests in the very near future. The treatment of SARS has not yet been determined. Corticosteriod therapy and the antiviral drug ribavirin have been used most frequently with little certainly of their efficacy. Recent reports suggest that most patients recover in spite of not receiving these drugs.[62] The mortality rate from SARS ranges from 3-10% with a median of 5%. Those with the highest mortality rate are the elderly (>60 yrs) and those with underlying co-morbid conditions such as diabetes and chronic lung disease.

Since health-care providers are at the greatest risk or acquiring SARS, a high index of suspicion, based on the travel history and knowledge of current epidemics, is needed so that aerosol and contact prevention measures can be initiated even before direct contact with the patient occurs. A face shield, N-95 masks, gown, gloves and booties are recommended. All surfaces must be carefully wiped down with a disinfectant after the patient has left the room.[63]

Prevention of SARS among travelers will be remarkably difficult during epidemic periods. The only sure way to prevent infection is to avoid locations where outbreaks have occurred. Air travel appears to be relatively safe since only 14 cases have been reported from 35 flights carrying infected passengers. Twelve occurred among passengers seated within 4 rows of the index case and two were flight attendants.

As of this writing, SARS remains a global problem with no end in sight. The infection has strained public health systems to the breaking point and has led to millions of dollars lost in tourism and productivity in affected counties. The new reality of SARS is that intercontinental travel and the dramatically increased mobility of people will make outbreak containment of this infectious disease on a global scale a serious, if not impossible challenge.

CONCLUSION

Respiratory infections represent the third most frequent health problem for international travelers. Incidence is underestimated, mainly because the majority of infections are mild and not incapacitating. Most are due to cosmopolitan agents and 'tropical' infections are rare.

Travel facilitates the spread of cluster epidemics such as influenza and legionellosis, and is associated with an increased risk of infection with *M.tuberculosis*. The route of acquisition for most respiratory infection is by direct contact, which makes prevention through behavioral interventions very difficult. Preventative therapy mainly relies on vaccines.

The threat of spreading infections transmitted through the respiratory route is exemplified by the epidemic of Severe Acute Respiratory Syndrome (SARS). Rapidly spread all over the world by air travel and with a fatality rate of up 10% it has caused travel and trade disruption, with an economic loss of several billions. The clinical management of respiratory infections would greatly be enhanced by the use of standardized management algorithms, based on a better understanding of disease epidemiology. International health polices and regional and global networking can also play a pivotal role in the control of these infections.

REFERENCES

1. Steffen R. *Health risk for short term travelers.* Steffen R, Lobel HO, Haworth J, Bradley DJ eds. Travel Medicine: Proceedings of the First Conference on International Travel Medicine, 1989.
2. Jernigan DB, Hofmann J, Cetron MS, *et al.* Outbreak of Legionnaires' disease among cruise ship passengers exposed to a contaminated whirlpool spa. *Lancet* 1996; **275:**545–547.
3. Sato K, Morishita T, Nobusawa E, *et al.* Surveillance of influenza viruses isolated from travelers at Nagoya International Airport. *Epidemiol Infect* 2000; **124:**507–514.
4. Farizo KM, Strebel PM, Cen RT, *et al.* Fatal respiratory disease due to Corynebacterium diptheriae: case report and review of guidelines for management, investigation, and control. *Clin Infect Dis* 1993; **16:**59–68.
5. Cobelens FGJ, Deutekom H van, Draayer-Jansen IWE, *et al.* Risk of infection with mycobacterium tuberculosis in travelers to areas of high tuberculosis endemicity. *Lancet* 2000; **356:**461–65.
6. Dingle JH, Badger GF, Jordan WS Jr, *et al.* Illness in the Home: Study of 25,000 Illnesses in a Group of Cleveland Families. Cleveland: The Press of the Western Reserve University; 1969.
7. Kendrick MA. Study of illness among Americans returning from international travel; July. *J Infect Dis* 1972; **126:**684–685.
8. Denny FW Jr, Kallings I. Respiratory tract infections. In: DuPont H, Steffen R, eds. *Textbook of Travel Medicine and Health, second edition.* Hamilton/London: BC Decker; 2001:269–279.
9. Evans MR, Shickle D, Morgan MS. Travel illness in British package holiday tourists: prospective cohort study. *J Infect* 2001; **43:**140–147.
10. Hill DR. Health problems in a large cohort of Americans traveling to Developing Countries. *J Travel Med* 2000; **7:**259–266.
11. O'Brien D, Tobin S, Brown GV, Torresi J. Fever in returned travelers: review of hospital admissions for a 3-year period. *Clin Infect Dis* 2001; **33:**603–609.
12. Parkins KJ, Poets CF, O'Brien LM, Stebbens VA, Southall DP. Effect of exposure to 15% oxygen on breathing patterns and oxygen saturation in infants: interventional study. *BMJ* 1998; **316:**887–894.
13. Dreake DE, Gray CL, Ludwig MR, Hill CD. Descriptive epidemiology of injury and illness among cruise ship passengers. *Ann Emerg Med* 1999; **33:**67–72.
14. Edelstein P, Cetron MS. Sea, wind, and pneumonia. *Clin Infect Dis* 1999; **29:**39–41.
15. Hart PE, Lee PYC, Macallan DC, Wansbrough-Jones MH. Cutaneous and pharyngeal diphtheria imported from the Indian subcontinent. *Postgrad Med J* 1996; **72:**619–620.
16. Gross PA, Hermogenes AW; Sacks HS, *et al.* The efficacy of influenza vaccine in elderly persons: a meta analysis and review of the literature. *Ann Intern Med* 1995; 123:518–527.
17. National Advisory Committee on Immunization (NACI). Statement on influenza vaccination for the 1998-1999 season: an Advisory Committee Statement (ACS). *Can Commun Dis Rep* 1998; 24: 1–12.
18. Centres for Diseases Control and Prevention. Outbreak of influenza A infection – Alaska and the Yukon territory. *Morb Mortal Wkly Rep* 1999; 48: 545–546.
19. Buxton JA, Skowronski DM, Ng H, *et al.* Influenza revaccination of elderly travelers: antibody response to single influenza vaccination and revaccination at 12 weeks. *J Infect Dis* 2001; 184: 188–191.
20. Ortquist A, Hedlund J, Burman LA, Elbel A, Hofer M, Leinonten M, *et al.* Randomised trial of a 23-valent pneumococcal capsular polysaccharide vaccine in the prevention of pneumonia in middle-aged and elderly people. *Lancet* 1998; 351: 399–403.
21. Snaken R, Kendal AP, Haaheim LR, Wood JM. The next influenza pandemic: lessons from Hong Kong, 1997. *Emerg Infect Dis* 1999:5 Available at: http://www.cdc.gov/ncidod/EID/vol5no2/snaken.html
22. World Health Organization. Influenza pandemic preparedness plan. Responding to an influenza pandemic or its treat: the role of WO and guidelines for national and regional planning. Geneva: The Geneva World Health Organization; 1999.
23. Health and Safety Executive. *The control of Legionellosis including Legionnaires' disease.* London: Health and Safety Executive; 1991:1–19.
24. Freedman DO, Kozarsky PE, Weld LH. Cetron MS. GeoSentinel: the global emerging infections sentinel network of the international society of travel medicine. *J Travel Med* 1999; **6:**94–98.
25. Jelinek T, Corachan M, Grobush M, *et al.* Falciparum malaria in European tourists to the Dominican Republic. *Emerg Infect Dis* 2000; **6:**537–8.
26. Zane S, Uyeki T, Bodnar U, *et al.* Influenza in travelers, tourism workers, and residents in Alaska and the Yukon Territory. Presented at the 6th Conference of the International Society for Travel Medicine, Montreal, Canada, 1998.

27. Freedman DO, Woodlall J. Emerging infectious diseases and risk to the traveler. *Med Clin North Am* 1999; **83**:865–883.

28. World Health Organization. Epidemiology, prevention and control of legionellosis: memorandum of a WHO meeting. *Bull World Health Organ* 1990; **68**:155–164.

29. Joseph CA, Harrison TG. Ilijiac-car D, Bartlett C. Legionnaires' disease in residents of England and Wales: 1997. *Commun Dis Public Hlth* 1998; **1**:252–257.

30. Anonymous. Cluster of cases of Legionnaire's disease associated with a Bangkok hotel. *Commun Dis Rep CDR Wkly* 1999; **9**:147.

31. Boer JW Den, Yzerman EPF, Schellekens J, et al. A large outbreak of Legionnaires' disease at a flower show, the Netherlands, 1999. *Emerg Infect Dis* 2002; **8**:37–43.

32. World Health Organization. *Plan of action for the prevention and control of diphtheria in the European Region (1994-1995)*. WHO Document ICP/EPI 038, Copenhagen. Geneva: World Health Organization; 1994.

33. Anonymous. Diphtheria acquired during a cruise in the Baltic Sea. *Commun Dis Rev* 1997; **7**:210.

34. Chaowagul W, White NJ, Dance DAB, et al. Melioidosis: a major cause of community acquired septicemia in northeastern Thailand. *J Infect Dis* 1989; **159**:890–899.

35. Peetermans WE, Wijngaerden EV, Eldere JV, Verhaejen J. Melioidosis brain and lung abscess after travel to Sri Lanka. *Clin Infect Dis* 1999; **28**:921–922.

36. Dharakul T, Anuntagool SS, Chaowagul N, et al. Diagnostic value of an antibody enzyme-linked immunosorbent assay using affinity-purified antigen in an area endemic for melioidosis. *Am J Trop Med Hyg* 1997; **56**:418–423.

37. Appassakij H, Silpojakul KR, Wansit R, et al. Diagnostic value of indirect hemoagglutination test for melioidosis in an endemic area. *Am J Trop Med Hyg* 1990; **42**:248–253.

38. Inglesby TV, Henderson DA, Bartlett JG, et al. Anthrax as a biological weapon. Medical and public health management. *JAMA* 1999; **281**:1735–1745.

39. Perry RD, Fetherston RD. Yersinia pestis – aetiologic agent of plague. *Clin Microbiol Rev* 1997; **10**:35–66.

40. World Health Organization. Human plague in 1996. *Wkly Epidemiol Rec* 1998; **47**:366–369.

41. Chanteau S, Rabarijaona L, O'Brien T, et al. F1 antigenaemia in bubonic plague patients, a marker of gravity and efficacy of therapy. *Trans R Soc Trop Med Hyg* 1998; **92**:572–573.

42. Guiard-Schmid JB, Lacombe K, Osman D, et al. La paragonimose: une affection rare à ne pas méconnaitre. *Presse Med* 1998; **27**:1835–1837.

43. Cairns L, Blythe D, Kao A, et al. Outbreak of coccidioidomycosis in Washington State residents returning from Mexico. *Clin Infect Dis* 2000; **30**:61–64.

44. Centres for Diseases Control and Prevention. Outbreak of acute febrile respiratory illness among college students – Acapulco, Mexico, March 2001. *Morb Mortal Wkly Rep* 2001; **50**:359–360.

45. Lobato MN, Hopewell PC. Mycobacterium tuberculosis infection from countries with a high prevalence of tuberculosis. *Am J Respir Crit Care Med* 1998; **158**:1871–75.

46. Cobelens FGJ, Deutekom H van, Draayer-Jansen IWE, et al. Association of tuberculin sensitivity in Dutch adults with history of travel to areas with a high incidence of tuberculosis. *Clin Infect Dis* 2001; **33**:300–4.

47. Frame JD, Lange DR, Frankenfield DL. Mortality trends of American missionaries in Africa, 1945–1985. *Am J Trop Med Hyg* 1992; **46**:686–90.

48. Matteelli A, Gurtman A, Torresi J, Weld L. Tuberculosis in travelers and long term immigrants, Abs. FC05.05. Presented at the 7th conference of the International Society of Travel Medicine, Innsbruck, Austria, 27–31 May 2001.

49. Smith PG, Fine PEM. BCG vaccination. In: Davies PDO, ed. *Clinical tuberculosis*. London: Chapman and Hall; 1998:417–431.

50. Rieder HL. Risk of travel-associated tuberculosis. *Clin Infect Dis* 2001; **33**:1393–1396.

51. International Union against Tuberculosis Committee on Prophylaxis. Efficacy of various durations of isoniazid preventive therapy for tuberculosis: five years of follow-up in the IUAT trial. *Bull World Health Organ* 1982; **60**:555–564.

52. World Health Organization. Tuberculosis and air travel: guidelines for prevention and control. WHO/TB/98.256. Geneva: World Health Organization.

53. Houk VN, Baker JH, Sorensen K, et al. The epidemiology of tuberculosis infection in a close environment. *Arch Environ Health* 1968; **16**:26–50.

54. Moore M, Valvay SE, Ihle W, et al. A train passenger with pulmonary tuberculosis: evidence of limited transmission during travel. *Clin Infect Dis* 1999; **28**:52–56.

55. WHO, Cumulative number of reported probable cases of Severe Acute Respiratory Syndrome. *www.who.int/crs/sars/country/2003_05_21/en/*, accessed May 21, 2003.

56. Drosten C, Gurther S, Preiser W, et al. Identification of a novel coronavirus in patients with Severe Acute Respiratory Syndrome. *N Engl J Med* 2003; **348**:1967–76.

57. Ksiazek TG, Edman D, Goldsmith CS, et al. A novel coronavirus associated with Severe Acute Respiratory Syndrome. *N Engl J Med* 2003; **348**:1953–66.

58. Lee N, Hui D, Wu A, et al A major outbreak of Severe Acute Respiratory Syndrome. *N Engl J Med* 2003; **348**:1986–94.

59. Poutamen SM, Low DE, Henrey B, et al. Identification of Severe Acute Respiratory Syndrome in Canada. *N Engl J Med* 2003; **348**:1995–2005.

60. Booth CM, Matukas LM, Tomlinson GA, et al. Clinical features and short-term outcomes of 144 patients with SARS in the Greater Toronto Area. *JAMA* 2003; **289**:1–9.

61. Centers for Disease Control and Prevention. Severe Acute Respiratory Syndrome and Coronavirus testing. – United States 2003. Available at: www.cdc.gov/mmwr/preview/mmwrhtml/mm5214al.html.

CHAPTER 57 Emerging Problems in Travel Medicine

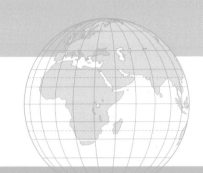

Michelle Weinberg and Martin Cetron

KEYPOINTS

- As international travel grows and diversifies, the risk of emerging infectious diseases among travelers will increase

- The emergence of infectious diseases among travelers involves a constant interaction between the pathogen, host immunity, vectors and zoonotic hosts and behaviors and exposures during travel

- Travel medicine clinicians play a crucial role and should work closely with public health officials and laboratory scientists to monitor the resurgence of known pathogens and the emergence of new diseases among travelers

- The participation of travel medicine providers in global surveillance activities, such as GeoSentinel, will greatly enhance the detection and prevention of emerging infectious diseases among travelers

INTRODUCTION

According to the World Health Organization, in the last three decades a new pathogen has been identified at a rate of approximately one per year.[1] (Fig. 57.1) With the growth of international travel, travelers have a special role in the detection and potential transmission of these diseases. In 1950, there were 50 million international tourist arrivals. By 2001, this figure had increased to over 693 million international tourist arrivals. The World Tourism Organization predicts the number of arrivals will increase to more than 1 billion by 2010.[2] Emerging infectious diseases may also have a unique impact on travelers. Despite a lower pathogen burden, non-immune travelers may develop severe acute clinical manifestations of infectious diseases compared with the local population that may have full or partial immunity due to chronic exposure. Travel medicine specialists have an important, and probably, underestimated role in surveillance for emerging infectious diseases. Clinicians should become familiar with the concept of emerging infectious diseases, be knowledgeable of recent examples of emerging infectious diseases, and develop a framework from which to approach diagnostic challenges in patients with possible travel-related emerging infectious diseases.

Emerging infectious diseases encompass two groups of pathogens: newly-discovered organisms, and known organisms with characteristics that have changed, for example, acquired antibiotic resistance. A pathogen may also be considered an emerging infectious disease because the population affected has changed, for example, by engaging in activities that increase the risk of exposure or because of altered host susceptibility.

In 1992, the Institute of Medicine issued a report, *Emerging Infections: Microbial Threats to Health in the United States* identifying six factors that contribute to disease emergence and re-emergence: (1) changes in human demographics and behavior, (2) advances in technology and changes in industrial practices, (3) economic development and changes in land usage, (4) dramatic deterioration of the public health infrastructure required to address infectious diseases, (5) microbial adaptation and change and (6) expanding international travel and commerce.[3]

Emerging infectious diseases have become a 'hot topic' in public health. They are the focus of special public health programs, meeting sessions at numerous international conferences, and countless articles in the lay press that have captured the public's attention. In conducting a literature search for 'emerging infectious diseases', more than 300 articles were published between 1993–mid 2002, compared with none prior to 1993.

Yet, the concept of emerging infectious diseases should not be new for most travel medicine clinicians. Travel medicine specialists must routinely consider diseases that do not usually affect the local population or occur in the geographic area where they practice medicine. Clinicians caring for travelers have an important role in the detection of emerging infectious diseases. Yet they are also faced with an incredible challenge; how does the clinician know when the fever in the traveler is caused by malaria or an unusual pathogen? Surveillance for emerging infectious diseases relies on astute clinicians with a high index of suspicion, laboratorians who perform diagnostic testing, and public health officials who identify potential sources and risk factors for infection among travelers with diverse exposures and who may present for medical care in disparate locations. Regardless of the current level of interest, the emerging infectious disease concept is useful for travel medicine clinicians. In particular, it is helpful to have a framework from which to approach the evaluation of a patient. Six key elements in clinical practice can assist with the detection of emerging infectious diseases among travelers (Table 57.1).

Historically, improvements in transportation technology have been a driving force in the spread of infectious diseases. In the 1880s, the development of the steamboat had a major role in the spread of plague throughout Asia and the Americas.[4] Air travel has dramatically enhanced the potential transmission of emerging infectious diseases. The speed of international travel now enables a person to travel around the world in 36 h, which is less than the incubation period of many infectious diseases. Increased access to international travel with low cost airfares and the diversity of flights has further contributed to the growth of international travel. Economic recession and the terrorist events of September 11th 2001 led to a temporary decrease in international tourism arrivals by 0.6%, compared with 2000[5]; however, tourism industries are predicting tremendous growth for the future. By 2020, global receipts from tourism are expected to double to 2 trillion dollars.[2]

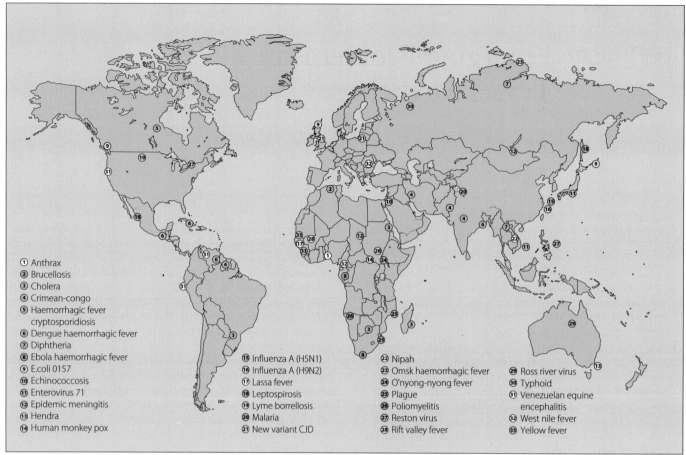

Figure 57.1 Unexpected outbreaks: examples of emerging and re-emerging infectious diseases 1994–1999. *Source*: World Health Organization. Removing Obstacles to Healthy Development, 1999.

① Anthrax
② Brucellosis
③ Cholera
④ Crimean-congo
⑤ Haemorrhagic fever cryptosporidiosis
⑥ Dengue haemorrhagic fever
⑦ Diphtheria
⑧ Ebola haemorrhagic fever
⑨ E.coli 0157
⑩ Echinococcosis
⑪ Enterovirus 71
⑫ Epidemic meningitis
⑬ Hendra
⑭ Human monkey pox
⑮ Influenza A (H5N1)
⑯ Influenza A (H9N2)
⑰ Lassa fever
⑱ Leptospirosis
⑲ Lyme borrellosis
⑳ Malaria
㉑ New variant CJD
㉒ Nipah
㉓ Omsk haemorrhagic fever
㉔ O'nyong-nyong fever
㉕ Plague
㉖ Poliomyelitis
㉗ Reston virus
㉘ Rift valley fever
㉙ Ross river virus
㉚ Typhoid
㉛ Venezuelan equine encephalitis
㉜ West nile fever
㉝ Yellow fever

Table 57.1	Six key elements in clinical practice to assist in the detection of emerging infectious diseases among travelers
Type	**Description**
Emerging infectious disease framework	Evaluate the patient in light of the framework of four factors influencing the emergence of infectious diseases among travelers: pathogen, host immunity, vectors and zoonotic hosts, and risk behaviors and exposures during travel.
Clinical features	Document clinical features of the illness at presentation and during evolution. This can help identify new clinical syndromes associated with a known pathogen and characterize the clinical features associated with a new pathogen. Avoid limiting the differential diagnosis of an unusual clinical picture to a poorly matched diagnosis; it is better to label the condition as 'unknown' and accurately describe the features.
Diagnostic testing	Obtain clinical specimens for diagnostic testing, and communicate with laboratory scientists and pathologists about the clinical features and travel history so that they can consider performing additional diagnostic tests.
Therapy	Monitor progress during therapy. Failure to respond to therapy may represent the first clue that you are dealing with an emerging infectious disease.
Epidemiological data collection	Collect detailed epidemiological information that is essential to investigating an outbreak or identifying common sources, including travel itinerary, activities and exposures during travel, lodging arrangements, sources of food and water, and information about other travelers on the trip.
Reporting to public health authorities	Report unusual cases or clusters to public health authorities and look for recent information about diseases that may be occurring in areas where the patient traveled. Public health officials may be notified of sporadic cases of persons with similar clinical findings or exposures from several clinicians who might not otherwise have communication, and thus, can assist in identification of clusters or outbreaks of emerging infectious diseases. Obtain current information about global disease occurrences and emerging infectious diseases.

The public health impact of emerging infectious diseases among travelers depends on the potential for transmission beyond the traveler and the sustainability of this infection in another geographic region. (Fig. 57.2) While the magnitude of travel-related emerging infectious diseases has not been systematically evaluated, the burden of emerging infectious diseases among travelers is greatly affected by whether the occurrence is an individual case or an outbreak. The persons at risk for infection may be limited to only the traveler or the local population may also be affected. Illnesses among travelers can represent sentinel indicators for undetected diseases that affect the local population, especially in developing countries where diagnostic options are limited. These diseases may be identified first among travelers, who may have greater access to diagnostic testing upon return. Non-immune travelers who cross the 'prevalence gap' from a non-endemic to endemic area may acquire diseases or present with severe clinical manifestations that are not seen in the local, immune population. The traveler may carry a pathogen from one geographic region to another, infecting other persons either along the route of travel or in the traveler's final destination.

Emerging infectious diseases may require the use of additional resources for diagnosis and treatment, and to address potential media and public concerns that occur. The economic cost of outbreaks associated with certain emerging infectious diseases has been documented. In 1991, cholera was re-introduced into Peru via contaminated ship ballast water and subsequently spread throughout most of Latin America during 1992–1993. The re-introduction of cholera into Peru was estimated to cost Peru US$770 million in 1991. The plague epidemic in India in 1995 cost US$1.7 billion. Other outbreaks have been associated with substantial costs, for example the influenza A (H5N1) outbreak in Hong Kong led to the destruction of all poultry in the territory and the 1999 Nipah outbreak in Malaysia resulted in widespread pig destruction.[6] Travel-related emerging infections may also have political and economic consequences, as both perceived and real risks may impact tourism. International tourism is one of the major sources of foreign-currency earnings for many countries. In 1999, total international tourism receipts were an estimated US$555 billion, greater than all other international trade categories, including automotive products, chemicals, food and fuels.[2]

The relationship between travelers and emerging infectious diseases can be represented as a framework with four major axes: pathogen, host immunity, vectors and zoonotic hosts, and risk behaviors and exposures during travel. Each of these major axes is affected by other factors. (Fig. 57.2) It would be impossible to review every possible emerging infectious disease among travelers in this chapter, in part, because of the rapidly changing nature of infectious diseases. However, examples of emerging infectious diseases among travelers will be described within the context of one of the four major axes of the framework. When appropriate, the impact of the emerging infectious diseases among affected populations will also be discussed.

THE PATHOGEN

Pathogens can evolve over time and the alteration of characteristics, such as virulence factors, may cause a known pathogen to become an emerging infectious disease. Examples include the development of drug resistance in a variety of organisms, such as multi-drug resistance tuberculosis, and malaria.

ENTERIC ORGANISMS

The evolution of antibiotic resistance among enteric pathogens, particularly in Southeast Asia, highlights the practical importance of emerging infectious diseases for clinicians and its impact on the management of ill travelers with diarrhea. The development of antibiotic resistance is often multifactorial, involving genetic mutation in response to environmental pressures; for example, fluoroquinolone resistance has been correlated with use of these antibiotics in veterinary and human medicine.[7,8] In Thailand, the nalidixic acid

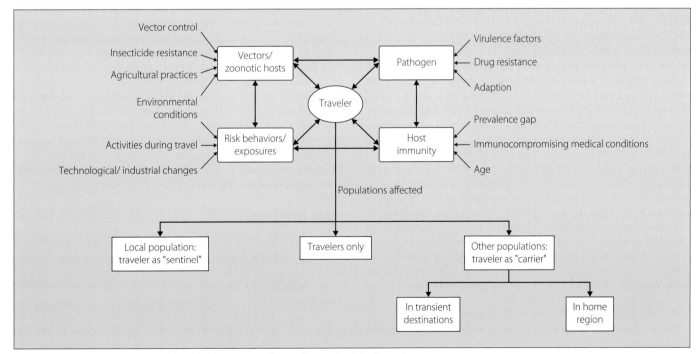

Figure 57.2 Framework for the relationship between travelers and emerging infectious diseases.

and fluoroquinolone resistance was first identified in the 1990s and now occurs among 1–2% of isolates of ETEC and non-S. dysenteriae type 1 Shigella. Campylobacter is one of the most important diarrheal pathogens for travelers to Thailand and is the leading cause of diarrhea among US military personnel deployed in Thailand. In a study of campylobacter antibiotic resistance trends in Thailand, campylobacter isolates collected in 1987 and 1990 were susceptible to ciprofloxacin. However, by 1993, 40% of the isolates were resistant to ciprofloxacin. In 1995, 84% of the isolates were resistant to fluoroquinolones and 7–15% were resistant to azithromycin.[9,10] These changes in antimicrobial susceptibility have led some clinicians to recommend the use of azithromycin, rather than ciprofloxacin, for empiric treatment for travelers' diarrhea acquired in Thailand, and have also raised a warning about the possible emergence of azithromycin-resistant organisms.[8]

Studies of travelers returning from Southeast Asia have demonstrated the emergence of Salmonella isolates with reduced susceptibility to fluoroquinolones. Among Finnish travelers returning from Southeast Asia, the annual percent of reduced ciprofloxacin susceptibility isolates increased from 3.9% in 1995, to 23.5% in 1999. In the travelers returning from Thailand, the percentage of reduced ciprofloxacin susceptibility increased from 5.6–50.0%. The reduced susceptibility was also associated with multidrug resistance.[11] Similar findings have been reported among travelers from the United Kingdom.[12] In the USA, a study of persons with typhoid fever between 1996–1997 identified antibiotic resistant Salmonella isolates among travelers. A total of 74 isolates (25%) were resistant to one or more antibiotics and 17% were multi-drug resistant to five or more antibiotics. A total of 81% of the patients had traveled internationally in the six weeks prior to illness onset. Patients with multidrug resistant Salmonella were more likely to report travel to the Indian subcontinent.[13] With the evolution of environmental pressures and antibiotic use among humans and animals, enteric organisms and their antibiotic resistance trends will remain important emerging infectious disease problems among travelers.

Cyclospora cayetanensis, a coccidian parasite that causes gastrointestinal illness, is an excellent example of a newly emerging organism that was detected among travelers. Cyclospora infection was first identified in three persons by Ashford in Papua New Guinea in 1977.[14] Sporadic cases were reported among 11 travelers to Latin American, the Caribbean, Southeast Asia or India.[15,16] However, cyclospora became more widely recognized when it was associated with outbreaks of gastrointestinal illness among travelers and expatriates in Nepal.[17] Between June–November 1989, 55 persons with prolonged watery diarrhea were found to have an alga-like organism with characteristics of coccidian and cyanobacteria species. In subsequent studies, the organism was detected in 108 (11%) of 964 persons with gastrointestinal illness. Outbreaks occurred seasonally during the warm monsoon season of May–August. In 1992, an estimated 7% of the US Embassy population and 4% of the other 2000 expatriates seen at the Katmandu clinic were infected.[18,19] Studies of Peruvian children demonstrated that the pathogen was associated with 11 episodes of diarrhea in 51 children (ages 1 month–2 years) from whom weekly fecal specimens were collected. These researchers demonstrated the sporulation and excystation of the organism, resulting in its confirmation as cyclospora, the same pathogen originally identified by Ashford.[17,20] The cyclospora example highlights how the reemergence of an organism among travelers can be associated with delayed recognition of the pathogen, especially when various investigators use different nomenclature to describe their observations.

Other studies have confirmed the greater importance of cyclospora infection among travelers compared to the local population. During the wet season, cyclospora was the main cause of gastrointestinal

illness among expatriates living in West Java, Indonesia, and was detected in 11.5% of persons with gastrointestinal illness. In contrast, the organism rarely occurred among the local population. During a 1-year study of gastrointestinal illness among 263 Indonesians, no cyclospora infections were detected. In a study of 348 Indonesian schoolchildren, only two children were infected and both were asymptomatic.[21]

Influenza

Influenza is the classic example of an organism that has undergone mutation and reemerges cyclically over time. Alterations in viral surface glycoproteins, neuraminidase and hemagglutinin, of 'influenza A' virus have led to antigenic shifts and large epidemics. An influenza pandemic, with more than 20 million deaths occurred in 1918–1919 following the emergence of H1N1 strain from swine. The emergence of H2N2 and H3N2 was associated with antigenic shifts in 1957 and 1968, respectively. In 1997, the H5N1 strain emerged in Hong Kong, and was responsible for illness in 18 persons and six deaths.[22,23] Studies have shown that the probable source of this new strain was poultry and strongly suggest that the virus was spread directly from poultry to humans, rather than passing through an intermediate, 'mixing' host such as swine.[24] Before the human cases, large-scale outbreaks of avian influenza with H5N1 occurred in parts of Hong Kong. Molecular studies showed greater than 99% sequence homology between the human and avian isolates. Additional studies are being conducted to determine the source of the H5N1 strain; current evidence suggests that the strains may have been reassortants from multiple co-circulating avian influenza virus strains, possibly involving geese or teal. In response to the outbreak, the Hong Kong government mandated the slaughter of all poultry, more than 1.5 million chickens, in farms and markets. The poultry slaughter and the inefficient human-to-human transmission were important factors that may have prevented more widespread infection with this strain. In 1999 and 2001, H5N1 strains were identified in poultry but no human cases were detected. In May 2001, H5N1 caused a cluster of poultry deaths and the government ordered another territory-wide poultry slaughter.[22] In March 1999, the government detected another avian influenza virus H9N2, which caused mild infection in two children.[25] While these new strains have not been detected among travelers, the potential for exposure and subsequent spread via travelers exists.

Recent outbreaks of influenza among cruise ship passengers highlight how unique circumstances of travel can lead to the emergence of known pathogens. Travelers may carry influenza when traveling from their country of origin to the opposite hemisphere during non-influenza season of the destination country, for example, persons who travel to the Southern from the Northern Hemisphere during April through September. Outbreaks of influenza have also occurred among persons traveling in large groups regardless of the season.[26–31] Since influenza vaccine is not usually available during off-season months, these outbreaks can be especially difficult to control and prevent.

Host immunity

Host immunity is an important risk factor for the emergence of infectious diseases among travelers. Even 'healthy', non-immune travelers may be at greater risk for selected infectious diseases if they cross the prevalence gap from a non-endemic to an endemic area. Examples include endemic mycoses, which will be discussed later in this chapter. International travel has become more accessible to populations with decreased immunity. Improvements in medical care, longer life expectancy and a highly functional lifestyle have led to increased international travel among the elderly and immunocompromised persons, including persons with cancer or human immunodeficiency virus (HIV) infection.

While several articles providing medical advice for HIV-infected travelers have been published,[32,33] data on the numbers of travelers with HIV infection or other immunocompromising conditions is limited and additional research in this area is greatly needed. Studies among HIV-infected persons have shown that rather than discouraging persons from traveling, some persons decide to travel when they learn that they have HIV infection or more severe disease. In a study among 41 HIV infected persons who had traveled during the preceding 2 years, 20% of the travelers visited foreign countries for an average of 3 weeks. Of the 25 foreign countries visited, 60% were developing countries. Among the travelers, 26–30% stated that the reason for travel was progression of disease and anticipation of a final opportunity to travel. The majority of travelers were severely immunocompromised with a median CD4+ count for all travelers of 120/mm³.[34]

Persons with HIV infection may be at higher risk for acquiring a variety of pathogens and may also acquire more severe disease, including tropical diseases such as measles, visceral leishmaniasis, microsporidiosis, and fungal infections such as cryptococcus, histoplasmosis, coccidioidomycosis, penicilliosis. HIV-infected persons with higher degrees of immunosuppression may be at greater risk for some vaccine-preventable diseases because they may be less likely to respond to certain vaccines or because some vaccines may be contraindicated.[33,34]

Similar to the lack of data about immunocompromised travelers, there are little data about the number of travelers who are young children, elderly or have chronic medical conditions. However, perhaps the best indication has been the growth of travel industry with special services targeted to some of these populations. The travel industry has developed tours to exotic destinations for elderly travelers and international travel packages targeted to persons who require dialysis or supplemental oxygen for chronic medical conditions. Escort services are also available for travelers with complex medical conditions.

The example of influenza outbreaks associated with cruise ships demonstrates the critical relationship between the pathogen and host immunity. Persons who are older than 50 years of age, immunocompromised conditions and persons with underlying medical conditions such as chronic pulmonary or cardiac disease are at greater risk for complications of influenza, including pneumonia. Outbreaks of influenza have occurred among cruise ship travelers in the United States, Alaska and Northern Europe during summer months. Infection has been associated with crew members and passengers. As high-risk travelers, elderly cruise ship passengers have been greatly affected by influenza outbreaks. One of the first documented out-breaks of influenza among cruise ship passengers occurred in August 1997 when international tourists traveling on a cruise along the United States eastern coastline became ill.[26,28] In July 1998 and June 1999, outbreaks of influenza A occurred among land and sea travelers to Alaska and the Yukon Territory; surveillance identified 898 persons with influenza-like illness (cough or sore throat and fever or feverishness). Elderly passengers were heavily impacted by the outbreak and 3.2% of the ill passengers developed pneumonia; in 1998, the median age of persons with influenza-like illness was 72 years.[29–31] In the summer of 2001, an outbreak of influenza B occurred on a cruise ship in Northern Europe and 70 persons developed influenza-like illness. Similar to prior outbreaks, the median age of ill passengers was 68 years. The spread of this outbreak was likely limited by early implementation of surveillance and control measures.[27] Whether the pathogen affects other high-risk travelers or undergoes an antigenic shift, influenza warrants close surveillance and collaboration among clinicians, public health authorities and laboratory scientists.

VECTORS AND ZOONOTIC HOSTS

The emergence of vector-borne diseases involves the dynamic interaction among some or all of the components of the framework: the pathogen, host immunity, risk behaviors and exposures and changes in the vectors. For example, the malaria parasite has developed resistance to many antimicrobials used for prophylaxis and treatment. The growth of adventure travel has led to increased exposure to African trypanosomiasis among persons participating in safaris.[35–37] Host immunity has important implications for the emergence of dengue shock syndrome (DSS) and dengue hemorrhagic fever (DHF) among travelers. The risk of developing DHF is greater for previously infected persons who are reinfected with a different serotype. The pathogenesis is thought to be due to antibody-dependent immune enhancement. The current widespread distribution of all four dengue viral serotypes increases the risk for DHF/DSS. Since primary infection may be mild or asymptomatic, many travelers may not know whether they have been previously infected. Studies of travelers with febrile illness after returning from endemic areas have shown dengue seroprevalence ranging from 7–45%.[38–43] Travelers originally from endemic areas who are visiting friends and relatives may be at greatest risk for DSS/DHF.[38]

The impact of these types of factors on vector-borne diseases is addressed in the chapters dedicated to the specific organisms; this section will focus on vector-related aspects of emergence. Vector populations are affected by environmental conditions such as changes in climate, rainfall, agricultural practices, and deforestation. The deterioration of vector control programs, the re-infestation of areas where vectors had been eliminated, the expansion of vectors to previously uninhabited areas and the development of insecticide resistance have contributed to the emergence of vector-borne infectious diseases.[44] As vector-borne diseases reemerge locally, the risk to travelers will increase. In addition to malaria and dengue, other vector-borne diseases that may become important for travelers include Japanese encephalitis, yellow fever, African trypanosomiasis and West Nile virus.

Malaria

Malaria infects over 300–500 million people globally and thousands of travelers, and is responsible for more than 1 million deaths annually.[45,46] Anopheles mosquitoes have been able to adapt to a variety of local conditions; the vectors have altered biting habits depending on geographic distribution and developed resistance to insecticides such as DDT. The use of bednets impregnated with pyrethroids has reduced the risk of acquiring malaria. However, resistance is emerging to pyrethroids and few alternatives are being developed.[44,47]

Local changes in vector distribution and population migration can affect the risk of malaria for tourists. In 1999–2000, 13 cases of *P. falciparium* malaria were first identified among European tourists to a resort area of the Dominican Republic that had previously been considered low risk for malaria. An outbreak of malaria occurred among the local residents and was traced back to importation from Haitian migrant construction workers. Hurricane George changed environmental conditions, increasing vector breeding sites and the vector population.[48] Dominican health authorities were able to intervene and eliminate risk of malaria transmission in this area; however, the outbreak demonstrates the complex dynamics of vector-borne diseases, the sentinel role and potential impact of mobile populations and how this may alter the risk for travelers, even for a limited period of time.

Malaria is also an excellent example of how travelers may be carriers of infections that impact communities upon return. In the USA, malaria was eliminated during the mid-twentieth century and, in 1970, the USA received certification of malaria eradication.[49] However, the importation of malaria by mobile populations in the USA has led to outbreaks of locally acquired mosquito-borne malaria. Several requirements must be met to have malaria transmission: the presence of anopheline larvae or infective adults, weather conditions that permit the completion of the sporogonic cycle in the mosquito gut and persons with gametocytes.[49,50] Between 1957 through 1994, 74 persons with probable locally acquired mosquito-borne malaria transmission were identified from 21 US states. Some of the outbreaks were linked to malaria importation by migrant workers, or have occurred in areas with large immigrant communities or near international airports. Many of these outbreaks occurred during seasons with unusually hot or humid climate.[50] Between 1992 and 2002, ten outbreaks involving 17 cases of probable locally acquired mosquito-borne malaria were reported to CDC. In 2002, two cases of locally acquired, Plasmodium vivax were reported in Virginia and, for the first time, pools of Plasmodium vivax-infected Anopheles mosquitoes were identified in the area.[49] While most of these outbreaks have not been sufficient to sustain long-term transmission, the risk of locally acquired malaria will continue to emerge as environmental conditions enhance vector populations and international travel among tourists, immigrants and other mobile populations increases.

Dengue

Dengue represents a significant emerging infectious disease among travelers and is currently causing pandemic activity in Latin America, Asia and Africa. Factors influencing the resurgence include population growth and urbanization, vector expansion, and the widespread use of non-degradable containers where Aedes breed.[3,51] More than 100 countries are affected by dengue and 2.5 billion people in the tropics and subtropics are at-risk. Before 1970, only nine countries in the world had DHF epidemics; the number had increased more than four-fold by 1995. In the 1950s, an average of 908 cases per year of DHF were reported to WHO; in 1998, a total of 1.2 million cases of dengue and DHF, including 3442 deaths were reported to WHO. Since diagnostic capacity and surveillance systems are variable, the number of reported cases is likely to be an underestimate of the true incidence. Based on statistical modeling, there are an estimated 51 million infections per year.[52] The situation of dengue in Latin America is an excellent example of emergence over time. In the 1940–1960s, the Aedes aegypti mosquito was eradicated in Central America, South America and Mexico as part of a program to eliminate the risk of urban yellow fever. However, parts of the Caribbean, the United States and Venezuela remained infected and the vector re-infested most of Latin America when the program ended in the 1970s.[53] The potential spread of dengue in the Western hemisphere increased after the identification of Aedes albopictus in Texas in 1985. The vector was imported into the USA in used tires from Asia and subsequent spread to 25 US states and areas in Latin America.[54] Outbreaks of dengue have occurred in Texas along the US-Mexico border.[55–57] In 2002, major epidemics of dengue and DHF occurred throughout Latin America.[58] Several countries in Latin America declared national emergencies in response to the outbreaks.

Yellow fever

Yellow fever has the potential for resurgence among travelers. Between 1990 and 1998, yellow fever increased worldwide and WHO received reports of 13 236 cases and 3589 deaths.[59] However, an estimated 200 000 cases of yellow fever are thought to occur annually.[60] Between 1996 and mid-2002, six travelers from the USA and Europe died of imported yellow fever. All of these travelers were visiting areas of high risk but were unvaccinated.[59,61] The decline of vector control programs and the potential spread of sylvatic yellow fever to urban areas have contributed to the possible resurgence of yellow fever, especially in Latin America.[60]

Japanese encephalitis

Even Japanese encephalitis (JE), which rarely occurs in travelers, may become a significant infectious disease problem. An estimated 10 000 deaths due to JE occur annually.[62] JE is an emerging infectious disease in Asia, and has been associated with rural coastal areas and areas with pig farming. In the late 1980s, JE spread across Western Papua New Guinea, probably through travel by the mosquito vector and, by 1995 and 1998, reached Torres Strait and northern mainland in Australia, respectively. The virus was isolated from Culex gelidus, a major vector of JE in Southeast Asia; this vector had not previously been identified in Australia, but has now become well established.[63,64] As more persons travel to Asia for exotic trips to rural areas and participate in non-tourist activities, the risk of exposure to JE may increase. Although JE is vaccine-preventable, the traveler must start vaccination at least one month before departure and return for multiple vaccinations; these factors may prevent travelers from being vaccinated.

West Nile virus

West Nile virus, a mosquito-borne flavivirus, was first identified in the USA in 1999; the first cases occurred in New York City in a geographic area near an international airport and a large, diverse immigrant community. Infected mosquitoes and birds were detected in many areas. Although the mechanism of importation has not been determined, genetic studies have shown that the West Nile virus strain circulating in New York was most closely related to a strain circulating in Israel from 1997 to 2000 and suggest that the virus was imported into the USA from the Middle East.[65] West Nile spread rapidly and more than 39 states have reported human cases; as of mid-November 2002, 3,605 persons with West Nile infection and 212 deaths had been reported.[66] The virus had also spread to Canada.[67]

African trypanosomiasis

African trypanosomiasis, caused by infection with Trypanosoma brucei complex and transmitted by the bite of a tsetse fly, is an emerging disease among travelers. An estimated 300 000 persons are currently infected with trypanosomiasis and an estimated >60 million persons live in high-risk areas.[68] Prior to 2001, less than 15 cases had been reported among travelers.[37] Several countries in Central Africa have experienced a dramatic increase in trypanosomiasis. The increase in trypanosomiasis in this area has been primarily attributed to West African trypanosomiasis, T.b. gambiense, for which humans are the most important reservoir. The expansion has occurred in Western and Central African countries affected by population movements, disruptions in health services, poor vector control, and political unrest in countries such as Central Africa Republic, Côte d'Ivoire, Guinea, Angola, Sudan and Democratic Republic of Congo where the number of cases increased from 7700 in 1990 to 27 044 in 1998.[36,44,68–70] While travelers are considered to be at low risk for West African trypanosomiasis, cases of East African trypanosomiasis have recently been reported among travelers to games parks in Tanzania and other countries. East African trypanosomiasis, which is caused by T.b. rhodesiense, is maintained through a reservoir of domestic and wild game animals. In January–March 2001, a cluster of nine patients (five

European travelers and one South African tourist) were infected during visits to game parks in Tanzania, Kenya and Zanzibar; one case was fatal.[37,38] During a 2-week period in 2002, two travelers from England were infected, one traveled to the same game parks in Tanzania and Kenya, and the other visited game parks in Zambia; only six cases of trypanosomiasis had been reported in the previous 14 years in England.[36]

Schistosomiasis

Schistosomiasis is an excellent example of how alterations in vector populations can lead to changes in the distribution of disease and increase the risk for travelers. It demonstrates the role of travelers as sentinel indicators for undetected foci of infection that may affect the local population. The risk of infection of Schistosoma mansoni associated with bathing in a fresh water basin under Hassan Gari Bira Falls was first detected in Djibouti when French and Djiboutian tourists became infected after visiting the area. Seventeen cases were diagnosed in tourists. Among 35 local village inhabitants who were subsequently tested for schistosomiasis, 80% were infected.[71] Schistosomiasis associated with exposure to Lake Malawi was also first identified among travelers. In 1991, members of a scientific team conducting research on the biology of fishes around the Lake contracted schistosomiasis. In 1992, two US Peace Corps volunteers developed central nervous system schistosomiasis after exposure to freshwater at Cape Maclear of Lake Malawi. Prior to the detection of these infections, this area had been considered to be free of schistosomiasis. In a study of 440 expatriates whose freshwater exposure was limited to Lake Malawi, 32% tested positive for antibodies to schistosomiasis.[72] Schistosome-infected snail vectors were also found at several locations along the lake. Further studies indicated that the snail vectors had dramatically increased after the reduction of its natural predator, the placodon fish. Following the implementation of a bednet project for malaria prevention, the local population used the bednets for fishing and consequently depleted the population of this molluscivore fish.[73]

RISK BEHAVIORS AND EXPOSURES DURING TRAVEL

Risk behaviors, activities and exposures during travel are critical risk factors for emerging infectious diseases among travelers. The purpose of travel may increase the risk of emerging infectious disease. According to the World Tourism Organization, leisure, recreation and holidays represent the main purpose of visit for 62% of international tourists worldwide. Business accounts for 18%; persons traveling to visit family and friends, participate in religious activities, receive health treatment or other reasons has grown in the last 10 years to 20% of the market share. Eighty-two percent of the travelers to South Asia are traveling for leisure, recreation and holiday purposes compared to the Americas (66%) and Africa (65%).[2]

The diversification of international travel, in both destination and activities, has changed the spectrum of infectious diseases risks associated with international travel. Ecotourism has become a new part of the travel package and has been promoted by the tourism industry. The United Nations declared 2002 as the International Year of Ecotourism; a journal dedicated to ecotourism exists. Sports vacations, nature activities and cultural and rural tourism in Africa and Asia are among the highest growth areas for travel.[74] Travelers can live with indigenous tribes in the Amazon or hunt with tribesmen in Africa. As travelers search for exotic activities, travel destinations have shifted to different, and more distant regions. In 1999–2000, tourist arrivals to South Africa increased by 19.3%, Brazil by 17.2%,

and Costa Rica by 9.6%. By 2020, the World Tourism Organization predicts that China will surpass France as the world's top destination with 186.6 million visitors annually. Although Europe will continue to receive the largest number of international arrivals with 717 million tourists, the East Asia/Pacific region is growing at the fastest rate and the number of tourist arrivals is predicted to increase to 397 million in 2020. Between 1995 and 2020, the highest average annual increases in visitor arrivals is predicted to shift to the East Asia/Pacific (6.5%), South Asia (6.2%), Africa (5.5%) from the traditional destinations of the Americas (3.9%) and Europe (3.0%). Most travel continues to be intra-regional, however, intra-continental travel is growing at a faster annual rate of 5.4% compared with a 3.8% annual growth for intraregional travel. By 2020, an estimated 377 million persons will be intra-continental travelers.[2,74]

Cutaneous leishmaniasis

The growth of exotic travel to remote areas has led to the emergence of several infectious diseases not commonly seen among tourists visiting usual destinations. American cutaneous leishmaniasis, a parasitic infection transmitted by the bite of a sandfly, has been detected among persons participating in educational and research activities in rural areas of Latin America. The yearly number of cases of American cutaneous leishmaniasis is estimated to be at least 59 300 and the population at risk is estimated to be 39 million persons. Between January 1985 and April 1990, 59 civilian US travelers with American cutaneous leishmaniasis were identified. Of the 58 travelers interviewed, 46% were conducting field studies or school projects, such as studying birds, and nocturnal animals and 32% were tourists or visitors, 7% were tour guides, and 7% were missionaries, 5% were nature photographers and 3% were landowners. Diagnostic delays occurred in many cases because some clinicians were unfamiliar with cutaneous leishmaniasis. The median time from noticing lesions to the release of drug was 112 days (range 13–1022 days).[75] As travel to remote tropical areas becomes more common and the tourism industry encroaches into undeveloped forest areas, travelers will be at greater risk.

Leptospirosis

Leptospirosis is another infectious disease that has emerged among travelers as a result of exotic exposures and adventure travel activities. In August–September 2000, athletes from 29 US states and 26 countries participated in the Eco-Challenge-Sabah 2000 multisport expedition race in Borneo, Malaysia, and likely acquired leptospirosis from water from the Segama River. The outbreak was rapidly detected by GeoSentinel, a global network of travel medicine providers. While leptospira was known to be endemic in Malaysian Borneo, it was not recognized to cause a large burden of disease in the local population. Of the 158 athletes contacted, 109 reported illness and 68 (44%) had illness that met the case definition. Twenty-five (34%) of the case-patients required hospitalization. Leptospirosis has also been reported among white-water rafters to Costa Rica.[76,77]

Endemic mycoses

Endemic mycoses, such as coccidioidomycosis and histoplasmosis have been reported among adventure travelers and persons participating in community service work in endemic areas.[78] The risk of endemic mycoses highlights the relationship between host immunity, the pathogen and type of exposures during travel. Histoplasmosis can be asymptomatic, but can also present as a spectrum of illness, ranging from mild flu-like illness to acute pulmonary infection and disseminated extrapulmonary disease. Persons with immunocompromising conditions are at higher risk for severe disease. *Histoplasma capsulatum* exists throughout the world; however, non-immune travelers from low prevalence areas who engage in high-risk activities, such as entering caves with bats, are at greater risk of acquiring symptomatic fungal infection. The detection of histoplasmosis, especially among travelers to Latin America has increased. Histoplasmosis has been reported among groups of travelers who entered caves in Costa Rica, Ecuador, Peru, Nicaragua and Belize. Many of these reported have two similar features: involvement in high-risk activities, such as visiting a cave with bats, and a high attack rate among exposed persons, including young, non-immunocompromised individuals.[78–82]

In addition to adventure travelers exposed to bat-infested caves, histoplasmosis has been reported among tourists vacationing in endemic areas. In March 2001, a large outbreak of acute pulmonary histoplasmosis occurred among healthy college students who visited Acapulco, Mexico during their spring break. In the USA, 44 colleges in 22 states reported 229 students with acute febrile pulmonary illness. The infection was associated with staying at a luxury hotel where construction was occurring; the students were likely exposed to dust from the construction work.[83,84]

Outbreaks of coccidioidomycosis have occurred among two groups of US travelers who were participating in construction work in endemic areas of Mexico. In 2000, an outbreak of coccidioidomycosis occurred among US travelers to Hermosillo, Mexico who were involved in church reconstruction. Among the travelers, eight (23%) had serologically confirmed coccidioidomycosis and seven travelers developed symptomatic infection.[85] A similar outbreak of coccidioidomycosis was reported among Washington state residents who traveled to another area of Mexico to assist with construction work at an orphanage. Twenty-one (17%) of the 126 travelers had serologically confirmed infection; of these persons, 95% developed symptomatic infection.[86] Fungal infections have important implications for travelers who are immune suppressed or have other high-risk characteristics. Risk factors for disseminated coccidioidomycosis include African American or Asian race, immunocompromising conditions and pregnancy. Persons with immunocompromising conditions, such as acquired immunodeficiency syndrome, are also at greater risk for disseminated histoplasmosis.[78] As more immunocompromised persons travel, endemic mycoses among travelers may increase.

Sexually transmitted diseases

Sexually transmitted diseases, in particular drug-resistant organisms, are emerging infectious diseases in sexually active travelers. Several studies have demonstrated that even travelers who are not considered 'sex tourists' may engage in more frequent sexual activity while traveling and that condom use is variable.[87,88] In an anonymous survey of 213 persons seeking pre-travel advice at private clinics in Australia prior to travel to Thailand, 17% of travelers planned or hoped to have sexual contact while in Thailand and 39.4% stated they would have sexual contact depending on whom they met.[87] In a postal survey of adults residing in a semi-rural general medical practice area in the UK, 5% of 354 persons who had traveled abroad had sexual intercourse with a new partner during their last trip. Factors associated with having sexual intercourse with a new partner included getting drunk, being single, young and traveling alone. Twelve of 17 (71%) persons reporting carrying condoms and 53% reported using condoms. However, 12 of the 17 also reported having intercourse at least one time without using a condom.[89] In another survey of persons aged 18–34 years in the UK, one in ten persons who traveled abroad without a partner in the previous two years reported sexual intercourse with a new partner during their trip.[90]

Sexual activity among travelers has been associated with the transmission and emergence of *Neisseria gonorrhoeae* with fluoroquinolone resistance (ciprofloxacin MIC $\geq$ 1.0 µg/mL) or intermediate resistance (ciprofloxacin MIC = 0.125–0.5 µg/mL) in the USA. In the USA, fluoroquinolones have been among the recommended regimens for treatment of uncomplicated gonococcal infections. In parts of Asia and the Pacific, up to 50% of *N. gonorrhoeae* strains have decreased susceptibility to fluoroquinolones and, in the Philippines and Hong Kong, up to 10% of isolates tested have been resistant.[91] In 1995, a US traveler from Colorado acquired fluoroquinolone resistant *N. gonorrhoeae* while on a 'dating tour' in the Philippines. He reported having sex with seven or eight female commercial sex workers during his trip.[92] Travelers with fluoroquinolone-resistant *N. gonorrhoeae* who imported infection into the US, have led to sustained local transmission.[93] In 1993–1994, three persons with fluoroquinolone-resistant *N. gonorrhoeae* were identified in Hawaii; all three persons had traveled to or had sex partners who had recently traveled to Southeast Asia.[94] In 1997, 1.4% of gonococcal isolates from Hawaii that were tested as part of CDCs Gonococcal Isolate Surveillance Project (GISP) were fluoroquinolone-resistant. In 1999, the percentage had increased to 9.5% and, by 2000, 14.3% of the Hawaiian isolates were resistant to fluoroquinolones, compared with 0.2% of the isolates from the 25 other cities that participate in GISP.[95] Among 62 persons from Hawaii who were interviewed, 52% reported international travel during the 30 days before diagnosis or having a sex partner with a history of recent international travel.[96] In 2002, CDC altered the treatment guidelines and consequently, the use of fluoroquinolones for the treatment of *N. gonorrhoeae* in Hawaii or infection acquired in Asia or the Pacific is no longer recommended.[95]

Meningococcal disease

As previously described, adventure travel, sexual behavior and other environmental exposures are associated with emerging infectious diseases among travelers. However, the exposures may be as simple as the convergence of large numbers of travelers, such as the Hajj pilgrimage. The emergence and continuing evolution of meningococcal infection in conjunction with the Hajj highlights the critical role of travelers in the transmission of the organism to other populations. Travelers who have participated in the Hajj pilgrimage have carried meningococcal infection to Saudi Arabia and other parts of the world. During the Hajj, approximately 2 million people from more than 140 countries visit Mecca and Medina in Saudia Arabia.[97] In 1987, a large outbreak of meningococcal disease occurred among Hajj participants and the Saudi population. The outbreak was caused by a single group A *N. meningitidis* clonal complex, designated III–1. Molecular studies suggested that the strain originated in Nepal and was probably brought to the Middle East by Hajj pilgrims. Outbreaks in Qatar and other Persian Gulf states were associated with travelers who carried the Hajj strain back to their countries of origin. Pilgrims also carried the clone, which was not previously found in isolate surveys from Africa, back to sub-Saharan Africa. In spring 1988, 7500 cases of group A *N. meningitidis* occurred in Chad; electrophoretic enzyme typing indicated that this clone was the same as the Hajj strain.[98] In response to the outbreaks, the Saudi government required vaccination with A/C bivalent vaccine, annual vaccination campaigns for local population and compulsory administration of oral ciprofloxacin for persons coming from sub-Saharan Africa to reduce carriage rate.[97]

Despite these control measures, the Hajj pilgrims became associated with the emergence of W135 strain of *N. meningitidis*. In 2000, a large outbreak of W135 occurred among more than 400 Hajj pilgrims and their contacts in Saudi Arabia and 16 countries (UK, Belgium,

USA, France, Morocco, Kuwait, Saudi Arabia, Oman, Indonesia, Singapore, Denmark, Finland, Sweden, Norway, Germany and the Netherlands).[97,99,100] Twenty-six of the outbreak-associated isolates were compared to 50 W135 isolates that were collected from around the world from 1970 through 2000. The study demonstrated that the outbreak isolates were members of a single clone of the hypervirulent electrophoretic type (ET)-37 complex. Rather than representing the emergence of a new strain, this outbreak was caused by the expansion of this clone that had been circulating since the 1970s and had actually been associated with the Hajj as early as 1996 when it was isolated from a patient in Indonesia who had just returned from the Hajj. The strains were also closely related to isolates that later caused large outbreaks in the Gambia in the 1990s and in Algeria and Mali in 2000.[100]

While meningococcal vaccine can prevent illness, it does not prevent carriage; cases of meningococcal infection have occurred in contacts of Hajj pilgrims. Among 90 cases of W135 meningococcal infection that were identified in nine European countries from March–July 2000, 13% of cases were in pilgrims (all vaccinated against A/C), 34% were household contacts of pilgrims and 23% were contacts outside the household and 29% had no known contact with pilgrims. Among the European cases, 14 deaths occurred.[101]

In 2000, Taha and colleagues predicted the impact of Hajj travelers on the spread of W135 to Africa. The authors warned that quadrivalent vaccine containing a W135 component, rather than the bivalent A/C vaccine which has been used in public health activities in Africa, could be required in Africa as a result of spread of Hajj-associated strains.[102] In 2002, large outbreaks of W135 occurred in Africa. In Burkina Faso, more than 12 000 persons developed W135 infection and at least 1500 died.[103] However, quadrivalent vaccine supplies were insufficient to be used as part of the public health response to the outbreaks.[104] In 2002, the Saudi Government changed the vaccination requirement for Hajj pilgrims to the quadrivalent vaccine.[97]

CONCLUSION

The framework for the emergence of infectious diseases among travelers involves a constantly evolving interaction between the pathogen, host immunity, vectors and zoonotic hosts and behaviors and exposures during travel. As international travel grows and diversifies, the risk of emerging infectious diseases among travelers will increase. Travel medicine clinicians will continue to play a crucial role and should work in close collaboration with public health officials and laboratory scientists to monitor the resurgence of known pathogens and the emergence of new diseases among travelers (Table 57.2). The participation of travel medicine providers in global surveillance activities, such as GeoSentinel, will greatly enhance the detection and prevention of emerging infectious diseases among travelers.

Table 57.2	Internet resources for information about emerging infectious diseases
Organization	**Internet site**
US Centers for Disease Control and Prevention	
Travelers' Health	http://www.cdc.gov/travel/
Morbidity Mortality Weekly Report	http://www.cdc.gov/mmwr
Emerging Infectious Disease Journal	http://www.cdc.gov/ncidod/EID/index.htm
European surveillance	http://www.eurosurv.org
Geosentinel	http://www.istm.org/geosentinel/geosentinel_main.html
Infectious Disease Society of America Emerging Infections Network	http://www.idsociety.org/EIN/TOC.htm
Health Canada	http://www.TravelHealth.gc.ca
ProMed	http://www.promedmail.org
World Health Organization	
Outbreaks	http://www.who.int/disease-outbreak_news
Surveillance and Response	http://www.who.int/emc
Weekly Epidemiological Report	http://www.who.int/wer/
International Travel and Health	http://www.who.int/ith/

REFERENCES

1. Heymann DL, Rodier GR, and the WHO Operational Support Team to the Global Outbreak Alert and Response Network. Hot spots in a wired world: WHO surveillance of emerging and re-emerging infectious diseases. *Lancet Infect Dis* 2001; 1:345–353.
2. World Tourism Organization. *Tourism Market Trends 2000.* Madrid: World Tourism Organization; 2002. Available at: http://www.worldtourism.org/market_research/facts&figures/menu.htm.
3. Lederberg J, Shope RE, Oaks SC, eds. Institute of Medicine. *Microbial Threats to Health in the United States.* Washington, DC: National Academy Press, 1992.
4. Hays JN. *The Burdens of Disease.* New Brunswick: Rutgers University Press; 1998: 183.
5. World Tourism Organization. *Tourism Proves as a Resilient and Stable Economic Sector.* Madrid: World Tourism Organization; 2002. Available: http://www.world-tourism.org.
6. World Health Organization. *WHO Global Epidemic Detection and Response 2000.* Geneva: World Health Organization; 2000. Available at: http://www.who.int/emc/surveill/index.html.

7. Engberg J, Aarestrup FM, Taylor DE, *et al.* Quinolone and macrolide resistance in Campylobacter jejuni and *C. coli:* resistance mechanisms and trends in human isolates. *Emerg Infect Dis* 2001; 7:24–34.
8. Kuschner RA, Trofa AF, Thomas RI, *et al.* Use of azithromycin for the treatment of Campylobacter enteritis in travelers to Thailand, an area where ciprofloxacin resistance is prevalent. *Clin Infect Dis* 1995; 21:536–541.
9. Hoge CW, Gambel JM, Srijan A, *et al.* Trends in antibiotic resistance among diarrheal pathogens isolated in Thailand over 15 years. *Clin Infect Dis* 1998; 26:341–345.
10. Isenbarger DW, Hoge CW, Srijan A, *et al.* Comparative antibiotic resistance of diarrheal pathogens from Vietnam and Thailand, 1996–1999. *Emerg Infect Dis* 2002; 8:175–180.
11. Hakanen A, Kotilainen P, Huovinen P, *et al.* Reduced fluoroquinolone susceptibility in Salmonella enterica serotypes in travelers returning from Southeast Asia. *Emerg Infect Dis* 2001; 7: 996–1003.
12. Threlfall EJ, Ward LR. Decreased susceptibility to ciprofloxacin in Salmonella enterica serotype Typhi, United Kingdom. *Emerg Infect Dis* 2001; 7:448–450.

13. Ackers ML, Puhr ND, Tauxe RV, *et al.* Laboratory-based surveillance of Salmonella serotype Typhi infections in the United States: antimicrobial resistance on the rise. *JAMA* 2000; **283**(20):2668–2673.

14. Ashford RW. Occurrence of an undescribed coccidian in man in Papua New Guinea. *Ann Trop Med Parasitol* 1979; **73**:497–500.

15. Soave R, Dubey JP, Ramos LJ, *et al.* An intestinal pathogen? (abstract). *Clin Res* 1986; **34**:533A.

16. Long EG, Ebrahimzadeh A, White EB, *et al.* Alga associated with diarrhea in patients with acquired immunodeficiency syndrome and in travelers. *J Clin Micro* 1990; **28**(6):1101–1104.

17. Herwaldt B. Cyclospora cayetanensis: a review, focusing on the outbreaks of Cyclosporiasis in the 1990s. *Clin Infect Dis* 2000; **31**:1040–1057.

18. Shlim DR, Cohen MT, Eaton M, *et al.* An alga-like organism associated with an outbreak of prolonged diarrhea among foreigners in Nepal. *Am J Trop Med Hyg* 1991; **45**:383–389.

19. Hoge CW, Shlim DR, Rajah R, *et al.* Epidemiology of diarrhoeal illness associated with coccidian-like organism among travelers and foreign residents in Nepal. *Lancet* 1993; **341**:1175–1179.

20. Ortega YR, Sterling CR, Gilman RH, *et al.* Cyclospora species: a new protozoan pathogen of humans. *N Engl J Med* 1993; **328**:1308–1312.

21. Fryauff DJ, Krippner R, Prodjodipuro P, *et al.* Cyclospora cayetanensis among expatriate and indigenous populations of West Java, Indonesia. *Emerg Infect Dis* 1999; **5**:585–588.

22. Chan PKS. Outbreak of avian influenza A(H5N1) virus infection in Hong Kong in 1997. *Clin Infect Dis* 2002; **34**(suppl 2):S58–S64.

23. Centers for Disease Control and Prevention. Isolation of avian influenza A(H5N1) viruses from humans - Hong Kong, May-December 1997. *MMWR* 1997; **46**:1204–1207.

24. Class ECJ, Osterhaus ADME, Beek R van, *et al.* Human influenza A H5N1 virus related to a highly pathogenic avian influenza virus. *Lancet* 1998; **351**:472–477.

25. Peiris M, Yuen KY, Leung CW, *et al.* Human infection with influenza H9N2. *Lancet* 1999; **354**(9182):916.

26. Miller JM, Tam TWS, Maloney S, *et al.* Cruise ships: high-risk passengers and the global spread of new influenza viruses. *Clin Infect Dis* 2000; **31**:433–438.

27. Centers for Disease Control and Prevention. Influenza B virus outbreak on a cruise ship - Northern Europe, 2000. *MMWR Morb Mortal Wkly Rep* 2001; **50**:137–140.

28. Centers for Disease Control and Prevention. Outbreak of influenza-like illness in a tour group - Alaska. *MMWR* 1987; **36**:697–699, 704.

29. Centers for Disease Control and Prevention. Outbreak of influenza A infection - Alaska and the Yukon Territory, June-July 1998. *MMWR* 1998; **47**(638)

30. Centers for Disease Control and Prevention. Update: outbreak of influenza A infection – Alaska and the Yukon Territory, July-August 1998. *MMWR* 1998; **47**:687–688.

31. Centers for Disease Control and Prevention. Outbreak of Influenza A infection among travelers – Alaska and the Yukon Territory, May-June 1999. *MMWR* 1999; **48**:545–546, 555.

32. Karp CL. Preparation of the HIV-infected traveler to the tropics. *Curr Infect Dis Rep* 2001; **3**:50–58.

33. Gompel A Van, Kozarsky P, Colebunders R. Adult travelers with HIV infection. *J Travel Med* 1997; **4**(3):136–143.

34. Kemper C, Linett A, Kane C, *et al.* Travels with HIV: the compliance and health of HIV-infected adults who travel. *Int J STD AIDS* 1997; **8**:44–49.

35. Jelinek T, Bisoffi Z, Bonazzi L, *et al.* Cluster of African Trypanosomiasis in travelers to Tanzanian national parks. *Emerg Infect Dis* 2002; **8**(6):634–635.

36. Moore DAJ, Edwards M, Escombe R, *et al.* African trypanosomiasis in travelers returning to the United Kingdom. *Emerg Infect Dis* 2002; **8**(1):74–76.

37. Ripamonti D, Massari M, Arici C, *et al.* African sleeping sickness in tourists returning from Tanzania: the first 2 Italian cases from a small outbreak among European travelers. *Clin Infect Dis* 2002; **34**:e18–e22.

38. Jelinek T. Dengue fever in international travelers. *Clin Infect Dis* 2000; **31**:144–147.

39. Jelinek T, Dobler G, Holscher M, *et al.* Prevalence of infection with dengue virus among international travelers. *Arch Intern Med* 1997; **157**:2367–2370.

40. Lopez-Velez R. Perez-Casas, Vorndam AV, *et al.* Dengue in Spanish travelers returning from the tropics. *Eur J Clin Microbiol Infect Dis* 1996; **15**:823–826.

41. Lyerla R, Rigau-Perez JG, Vorndam AV, *et al.* A dengue outbreak among camp participants in a Caribbean island, 1995. *J Travel Med* 2000; **7**:59–63.

42. Schwartz E, Moskovitz A, Potasman I, *et al.* Changing epidemiology of dengue fever in travelers to Thailand. *Eur J Clin Microbiol Infect Dis* 2000; **19**:784–786.

43. Postasman I, Srugo I, Schwartz E. Dengue seroconversion among Israeli travelers to tropical countries. *Emerg Infect Dis* 1999; **5**:824–827.

44. Molyneux DH. Vector-borne infections in the tropics and health policy issues in the twenty-first century. *Trans R Soc Trop Med Hyg* 2001; **95**:1–6.

45. World Health Organization. Malaria. Geneva, Switzerland: World Health Organization; 2002:Online. Available:http://www/who/int/inf-fs/en/InformationSheet01.pdf.

46. World Health Organization. Malaria. In: Martinez L., ed. *International Travel and Health,* 2002 edn. Geneva, Switzerland: World Health Organization; 2002:130–148: Online. Available:http://www/who/int/ith/chapter07_01.html

47. Molyneux DH, Looreesuwan S, Liese B, *et al.* Global campaign to eradicate malaria: malaria is paradigm of an emergent disease (letter). *BMJ* 2001; **323**(571)

48. Jelinek T, Corachan M, Grobusch M, *et al.* Falciparum malaria in European tourists to the Dominican Republic. *Emerg Infect Dis* 2000; **6**:537–538.

49. Centers for Disease Control and Prevention. Local transmission of Plasmodium vivax Malaria - Virginia, 2002. *MMWR* 2002; **51**:921–923.

50. Zucker JR. Changing patterns of autochthonous malaria transmission in the United States: a review of recent outbreaks. *Emerg Infect Dis* 1996; **2**(1):37–43.

51. Rigau-Perez JG, Gubler DJ, Vorndam AV, *et al.* Dengue: a literature review and case study of travelers from the United States, 1986–1994. *J Travel Med* 1997; **4**:65–71.

52. World Health Organization. Strengthening Implementation of the global strategy for dengue fever/dengue haemorrhagic fever prevention and control. Geneva: World Health Organization; 1999.

53. Isturiz RE, Gubler DJ, del Castillo JB. Dengue and dengue hemorrhagic fever in Latin America and the Caribbean. *Infect Dis Clin North Am* 2000; **14**:121–140.

54. Moore CH, Mitchell CJ. Aedes albopictus in the United States: ten-year presence and public health implications. *Emerg Infect Dis* 1997; **3**:329–334.

55. Centers for Disease Control and Prevention. Dengue – Texas. *MMWR* 1980; **29**:451.

56. Centers for Disease Control and Prevention. Dengue fever at the U.S.-Mexico border, 1995–1996. *MMWR* 1996; **45**:841–844.

57. Centers for Disease Control and Prevention. Underdiagnosis of dengue – Laredo, Texas, 1999. *MMWR* 2001; **50**:57–59.

58. Pan American Health Organization. Dengue in the Americas: number of reported cases of dengue and dengue hemorrhagic fever in the Americas by country, 2002. Available at http://www.paho.org/English/HCP/HCT/VBD/dengue-cases-2002.htm.

59. Monath TP, Cetron MS. Prevention of yellow fever in persons traveling to the tropics. *Clin Infect Dis* 2002; **34**:1369–1378.

60. Monath TP. Yellow fever: an update. *Lancet Infect Dis* 2001; **1**:11–20.

61. CDC. Fatal yellow fever in a traveler returning from Amazonas, Brazil, 2002. *MMWR* 2002; **51**:324–325.

62. World Health Organization. Japanese encephalitis: public health status and recommended interventions. Geneva, Switzerland: World Health Organization; 2002:Online. Available:http://www.who.int/vaccines/en/japanenceph.shtml#strategies.

63. MacKenzie JS, Chua KB, Daniels PW, *et al.* Emerging viral diseases of Southeast Asia and the Western Pacific. *Emerg Infect Dis* 2001; **7**(suppl):497–504.

64. Johansen CA, Hurk AF van den, Ritchie SA, *et al.* Isolation of Japanese encephalitis virus from mosquitoes (Diptera: Cullicidae) collected in the Western Province of Papua New Guinea, 1997-1998. *Am J Trop Med Hyg* 2000; **62**:631–638.

65. Petersen LR. Roehrig JT. West Nile Virus: a reemerging global pathogen. *Emerg Infect Dis* 2001; **7**:611–614.

66. Centers for Disease Control and Prevention. Weekly update: West Nile virus activity - United States, November 14, 2002. Atlanta: Centers for Disease Control and Prevention; 2002:Online. Available:http://www.cdc.gov/od/oc/media/wncount.htm.

67. World Health Organization. West Nile virus, Canada - update. *Wkly Epidemiol Rec* 2002; **45**:374.

68. World Health Organization. African trypanosomiasis fact sheet. Geneva, Switzerland: World Health Organization; 2001:Online. Available:http://www.who.int/inf-fs/en/fact259.html.

69. Nieuwenhove S Van. Gambiense sleeping sickness: reemerging and soon untreatable? *Bull WHO* 2000; **78**:1283.

70. World Health Organization. WHO report on global surveillance of epidemic-prone infectious diseases. Geneva, Switzerland: World Health Organization; 2000:Online. Available: http://www.who.int/emc-documents/surveillance/docs/whocdscsrisr2001.html/African_Trypanosomiasis/African_Trypanosomiais.html.

71. Koeck JL, Modica C, Tual F, *et al.* Discovery of a focus of intestinal schistosomiasis in the Republic of Djibouti. *Med Trop* 1999; **59**(1):35–38.

72. Cetron MS, Chitsulo L, Sullivan JJ, *et al.* Schistosomiasis in Lake Malawi. *Lancet* 1996; **348**:1274–1278.

73. Stauffer JR, Arnegard ME, Cetron M, *et al.* Controlling vectors and hosts of parasitic diseases using fishes. *BioScience* 1997; **47**:41–49.

74. Foroohar R. Getting off the beaten track. *Newsweek* 2002; **July 22**:30D–30H.

75. Herwaldt BL, Stokes SL, Juranek DD. American cutaneous leishmaniasis in U.S. travelers. *Ann Intern Med* 1993; **118**:779–784.

76. Centers for Disease Control and Prevention. Public health dispatch; outbreak of acute febrile illness among participants in EcoChallenge Sabah 2000, Malaysia, 2000. *MMWR* 2000; **49**(36):816–817.

77. Centers for Disease Control and Prevention. Update: outbreak of acute febrile illness among athletes participating in Eco-Challenge-Sabah 2000; Borneo, Malaysia, 2000. *MMWR* 2001; **50**:21–24.

78. Panackal A, Hajjeh RA, Cetron MS, *et al.* Fungal infections among returning travelers. *Clin Infect Dis* 2002; **35**:1088–1095.

79. Centers for Disease Control and Prevention. Cave-associated histoplasmosis – Costa Rica. *MMWR Morb Mortal Wkly Rep* 1988; **37**(20):312–313.

80. Valdez H, Salata RA. Bat-associated histoplasmosis in returning travelers: case presentation and description of a cluster. *J Travel Med* 1999; **6**:258–260.

81. Nasta P, Donisi A, Cattane A, *et al.* Acute histoplasmosis in spelunkers returning from Mato Grosso, Peru. *J Travel Med* 1997; **4**:176–178.

82. Buxton JA, Dawar M, Wheat LJ, *et al.* Outbreak of histoplasmosis in a school party that visited a cave in Belize: role of antigen testing in diagnosis. *J Travel Med* 2002; **9**(1):48–50.

83. Centers for Disease Control and Prevention. Outbreak of acute respiratory febrile illness among college students - Acapulco, Mexico, March 2001. *MMWR* 2001; **50**(14):261–262.

84. Centers for Disease Control and Prevention. Update: outbreak of acute febrile respiratory illness among college students - Acapulco, Mexico, March 2001. *MMWR* 2001; **50**(18):359–360.

85. Centers for Disease Control and Prevention. Coccidioidomycosis in travelers returning from Mexico - Pennsylvania, 2000. *MMWR* 2000; **49**:1004–1006.

86. Cairns L, Blythe D, Kao A, *et al.* Outbreak of coccidioidomycosis in Washington state residents returning from Mexico. *Clin Infect Dis* 2000; **30**:61–64.

87. Mulhall BP, Hu M, Thompson M, *et al.* Planned sexual behaviour of young Australian visitors to Thailand. *Med J Aust* 1993; **158**:530–535.

88. Mulhall B. Sex and travel: studies of sexual behaviour, disease and health promotion in international travellers - a global review. *Int J STD AIDS* 1996; **7**:455–465.

89. Gillies P, Slack R, Stoddart N, *et al.* HIV-related risk behaviour in UK holiday makers. *AIDS* 1992; **6**:339–341.

90. Bloor M, Thomas M, Hood K, *et al.* Differences in sexual risk behaviour between young men and women traveling abroad from the UK. *Lancet* 1998; **352**:1664–1668.

91. Knapp JS, Fox KK, Trees DL, *et al.* Fluoroquinolone resistance in Neisseria gonorrhoeae. *Emerg Infect Dis* 1997; **3**:584.

92. Centers for Disease Control and Prevention. Fluoroquinolone-resistant Neisseria gonorrhoeae – Colorado and Washington, 1995. *MMWR* 1995; **44**:761–764.

93. Trees DL, Sandul AL, Neal SW, *et al.* Molecular epidemiology of Neisseria gonorrhoeae exhibiting decreased susceptibility and resistance to ciprofloxacin in Hawaii, 1991–1999. *Sex Trans Dis* 2001; **28**(6):309–314.

94. Centers for Disease Control and Prevention. Decreased susceptibility of Neisseria gonorrhoeae to fluoroquinolones – Ohio and Hawaii, 1992–1994. *MMWR* 1994; **43**:325–327.

95. Centers for Disease Control and Prevention. 2002 Sexually transmitted diseases treatment guidelines. *MMWR* 2002; **51**(RR-6):36–37.

96. Centers for Disease Control and Prevention. Fluoroquinolone-resistant Neisseria gonorrhoeae – Hawaii, 1999, and decreased susceptibility to azithromycin in N.gonorrhoeae, Missouri, 1999. *MMWR* 2000; **49**:833–837.

97. Memish ZA. Meningococcal disease and travel. *Clin Infect Dis* 2002; **34**:84–90.

98. Moore PS, Reeves MW, Schwartz B, *et al.* Intercontinental spread of an epidemic group A Neisseria meningitides strain. *Lancet* 1989; **2**(8657):260–263.

99. Popovic T, Sacchi CT, Reeves MW, *et al.* Neisseria meningitides serogroup W135 isolates associated with ET-37 complex (letter). *Emerg Infect Dis* 2000; **6**:428–429.

100. Mayer LW, Reeves MW, Al-Hamdan N, *et al.* Outbreak of W135 meningococcal disease in 2000: not emergence of a new W135 strain but clonal expansion within the electrophoretic type-37 complex. *J Infect Dis* 2002; **185**:1596–1605.

101. Aguilera JF, Perrocheau A, Meffre C, *et al.* Outbreak of serogroup W135 meningococcal disease after the Hajj pilgrimage, Europe, 2000. *Emerg Infect Dis* 2002; **8**:761–767.

102. Taha MK, Achtman M, Alonso JM, *et al.* Serogroup W135 meningococcal disease in Hajj pilgrims. *Lancet* 2000; **356**:2159.

103. World Health Organization. Meningococcal disease, serogroup W135, Burkina Faso. *Wkly Epidemiol Rec* 2002; **18**:152–155.

104. World Health Organization. Urgent call for action on meningitis in Africa – vaccine price and shortage are major obstacles. *Wkly Epidemiol Rec* 2002; **40**:330–331.

Glossary of Tropical Diseases for the Travel Medicine Practitioner

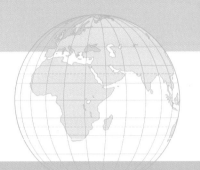

AFRICAN TRYPANOSOMIASIS (SLEEPING SICKNESS)

Epidemiology:

African trypanosomiasis or sleeping sickness, a disease that occurs only in rural foci in Africa between 15° North and 20° South latitude, is caused by two protozoan parasites: *Trypanosoma brucei gambiense* in West and Central Africa and *T.b. rhodesiense* in East Africa. Tsetse flies transmit Gambian trypanosomiasis in forested areas along rivers and streams and Rhodesian trypanosomiasis in the Savannah where game animals are abundant. African trypanosomiasis occurs rarely among travelers, most often among persons visiting game parks in East Africa. Recently, there was as increase in numbers of cases of Rhodesian trypanosomiasis among North American and European travelers, particularly those who visited game parks in Tanzania.

Clinical:

An inflamed nodule (inoculation chancre) may develop at the site of the tsetse fly bite, which is usually quite painful. Fever, chills, headache, rash, lymphadenopathy, and anemia occur in the first weeks to months after infection. Trypanosomes later invade the central nervous system, producing progressive neurological deterioration, coma, and death. Rhodesian sleeping sickness runs a rapid course with myocarditis, early invasion of the central nervous system, and death within months of onset. In Gambian sleeping sickness, the initial illness is more indolent, and nervous system involvement and death may not occur for several years, often after a long period of time in which there are no symptoms.

Diagnosis:

Microscopic demonstration of parasites in blood, lymph node aspirates, and cerebrospinal fluid. Screening serologic tests are available mostly in endemic countries.

Treatment:

Early infection with no central nervous system involvement: pentamidine (Gambian only), suramin. Central nervous system involvement: melarsoprol eflornithine (Gambian only).

Prevention:

Avoid tsetse-infested areas. Note that tsetse flies can bite through light clothing, and repellents do not prevent bites.

AMEBIASIS

Epidemiology:

Amebiasis is caused by the protozoan parasite *Entamoeba histolytica*, which is spread by the fecal-oral route either by direct person-to-person contact or by ingestion of amebic cysts in contaminated food and water. The infection occurs worldwide but is most frequent in areas with poor sanitation such as Mexico and other parts of Latin America, India, and Southern and West Africa.

Clinical:

Most infections with *E. histolytica* are asymptomatic, and many persons who shed amebas in their stool are in fact infected with the morphologically identical but nonpathogenic *E. dispar*. Symptomatic persons may complain of mild abdominal pain and loose stools, but in more severe cases, bloody diarrhea (dysentery), generalized abdominal pain, and sometimes fever and toxicity occur. Less commonly, amebic liver abscesses develop and produce fever, right upper quadrant pain, and enlargement of the liver.

Diagnosis:

Microscopic examination of stool; stool antigen test; PCR-based assay of stool; serology. *E. histolytica* can be differentiated from *E. dispar* with stool antigen tests, PCR or serology.

Treatment:

Invasive disease: metronidazole or tinidazole and luminal amebacide (iodoquinol, diloxanide furoate, or paromomycin); *asymptomatic infection:* luminal amebicide.

Prevention:

Avoid potentially contaminated food and water; hand washing before meals; good personal hygiene.

AMERICAN TRYPANOSOMIASIS (CHAGAS' DISEASE)

Epidemiology:

The protozoan parasite *Trypanosoma cruzi*, which causes American trypanosomiasis or Chagas' disease in Mexico, Central and South America, is transmitted in the faeces of its night-biting insect vector, the triatomine bug (kissing bug, reduviid bug), which infests poorly constructed houses in rural areas. Infection can also results from blood transfusions and organ transplants from infected donors or from transplacental transmission of parasites from an infected mother. Successful control programs in parts of South America have nearly eliminated both insect-borne and transfusion-associated transmission to human beings, but transmission continues in other parts of Latin America, and there are still approximately 16–18 million infected persons throughout the Americas. The parasite will never be eradicated because it infects over 100 species of wild and domestic animals as well as human beings. Chagas disease is exceptionally rare among travelers.

Clinical:

Most infections are asymptomatic. A small percentage of persons with acute Chagas' disease present with a self-limiting mononucleosis-like illness, which in <10% of cases is complicated by myocarditis or meningoencephalitis. All infected persons remain infected for life, and after several months, enter a chronic asymptomatic phase. Most persons never develop symptoms of chronic Chagas' disease, but 20–30% of persons within 1–4 decades develop a progressive cardiomyopathy that causes congestive heart failure, sudden cardiac death, arrhythmias, and heart block), or denervation of the esophagus or colon that leads to megaesophagus or megacolon and difficulty swallowing or defecating, respectively.

Diagnosis:

Acute stage: microscopic identification of parasites in blood. *Chronic stage:* serology (blood culture, xenodiagnosis, and PCR-based assays less sensitive).

Treatment:

Nifurtimox; benzimidazole in early infections; supportive measures or cardiac transplant for cardiomyopathy, surgery for megaesophagus or megacolon.

Prevention:

Avoid contact with triatomine bugs by not sleeping in poorly constructed houses or camping in rural areas where Chagas' disease is endemic. If such exposure is unavoidable, search bedding for bugs before sleeping and use a bed net. Avoid blood transfusions in endemic areas, especially where blood donors are not screened.

ASCARIASIS

Epidemiology:

The roundworm *Ascaris lumbricoides* infects more than a billion persons in warm climates where sanitation in inadequate. Infection results from ingestion of microscopic eggs shed in the faeces of persons infected with adult worms that live in the lumen of the small bowel for about one year. Eggs become infectious several weeks after being shed in the faeces onto soil, and readily contaminate uncooked vegetables and drinking water.

Clinical:

Most infections are asymptomatic. Occasionally, a reaction to migrating larvae produces cough, wheezing, pulmonary infiltrates, and eosinophilia during the first weeks of infection. In children, moderate to heavy infection with adult worms causes malnutrition, and large numbers of worms can become entangled and obstruct the small bowel. Adult worms that may reach 8–10 inches in length are occasionally passed through the rectum, mouth, or nose. Even a single wandering adult can cause biliary or pancreatic obstruction.

Diagnosis:

Microscopic identification of eggs in stool; identification of adult worms passed in faeces.

Treatment:

Albendazole, mebendazole, pyrantel pamoate.

Prevention:

Avoiding uncooked vegetables; hand washing before meals; drinking clean water.

CHOLERA

Epidemiology:

The diarrheal disease cholera, is transmitted by ingestion of food or water contaminated with the bacterium *Vibrio cholerae,* which is shed in the faeces and vomitus of infected persons. Cholera occurs sporadically and in epidemics in over 60 countries in Asia, Africa, and South America where there is inadequate sanitation and a lack of clean water. Most travelers are at minimal risk, even when cholera is endemic or epidemic.

Clinical:

Most infections are subclinical or consist of a mild, self-limiting diarrhea. In severe cases the abrupt onset of nausea, vomiting, and diarrhea leads to massive fluid loss and dehydration. Without treatment, shock and death can occur within hours.

Diagnosis:

Culture of stool or rectal swab; rapid tests for antigen in stool.

Treatment:

Ciprofloxacin, ofloxacin, levofloxacin, tetracycline, doxycycline, azithromycin, trimethoprim-sulfamethoxazole, furazolidone; oral rehydration solution.

Prevention:

Single dose of an oral vaccine available in some countries (rarely recommended for travelers other than those working in high risk areas without adequate sanitation for long periods of time). Proof of vaccination periodically required for entry to some countries. Avoid potentially contaminated water and food, especially fish and shellfish.

CIGUATERA POISONING

Epidemiology:

Ciguatera poisoning results from ingestion of fish containing toxins produced by dinoflagellates. Barracuda, snapper, jack, sea bass and other tropical reef fish that acquire the toxin from herbivorous fish are most commonly implicated. The ciguatoxic fish cannot be recognized by appearance, taste, or smell, and cooking does not destroy the toxin.

Clinical:

Symptoms appear 4–30 h after ingestion and include nausea, vomiting, diarrhea, abdominal pain, pruritus, myalgia, paresthesias around the mouth and in the extremities, hot sensation on exposure to cold, and a sensation of loosening of the teeth. Death may occur in up to 10% of persons from shock or respiratory failure. Certain symptoms may persist for months.

Diagnosis:

Clinical. Fish can be tested by an assay for toxin.

Treatment:

Intravenous mannitol. Supportive and symptomatic treatment.

Prevention:

Avoiding ingestion of potentially ciguatoxic fish and their viscera: in particular, all moray eels, reef fish in regions where ciguatera is endemic, oversized reef fish (e.g., >6 lb). The assay for toxin is expensive and not likely to be useful to most travelers.

DENGUE

Epidemiology:

Dengue is a viral infection transmitted primarily by daytime-biting *Aedes aegypti* mosquitoes that breed in stagnant water, in vases, buckets, tires and other containers around houses in urban and periurban areas. The four different serotypes of dengue cause more than 100 million infections a year in the Caribbean, Latin America, sub-Saharan Africa, tropical Asia, and the Pacific islands, and its incidence is rising throughout the world. The risk to travelers to endemic areas is low, except during epidemics.

Clinical:

Infections in non-immune adults are frequently symptomatic, while infections in non-immune young children are asymptomatic or extremely mild. Classic dengue fever begins after an incubation period of 3–8 days with the abrupt onset of fever, chills, headache, myalgia, arthralgia, rash, generalized lymphadenopathy, neutropenia, and often thrombocytopenia. Because of the phenomenon of immune enhancement, persons infected for a second time (with a different serotype) are at risk for life-threatening dengue hemorrhagic fever and dengue shock syndrome, characterized by plasma leakage, hemoconcentration, and bleeding and/or shock. The great majority of travelers from nonendemic areas have not experienced previous infection and are not at risk for dengue hemorrhagic fever and shock syndrome.

Diagnosis:

Serology, isolation of virus from serum.

Treatment:

No specific treatment available. Supportive care, including vigorous fluid replacement for dengue hemorrhagic fever and shock syndromes.

Prevention:

No vaccine available as of this writing. Protective clothing, repellents, and other measures to prevent mosquito bites, especially early morning and late afternoon.

FILARIASIS

Epidemiology:

There are three important diseases caused by filarial worms: lymphatic filariasis due mainly to *Wuchereria bancrofti* and *Brugia malayi;* onchocerciasis or river blindness caused by *Onchocerca volvulus;* and loiasis caused by the 'eye worm' *Loa loa.* Lymphatic filariasis is transmitted by evening and night-biting mosquitoes in rural and urban foci in the tropics, including in Haiti, Dominican Republic, northeastern coast of South America, sub-Saharan Africa, Egypt, South and Southeast Asia, China, and the Western Pacific islands. Day-biting black flies that breed in rapidly flowing rivers and streams transmit onchocerciasis in Mexico, Guatemala, northern South America, and sub-Saharan Africa. Loiasis is limited to the rain forests of West and Central Africa, where it is transmitted by day-biting deer flies. Infections with these parasites occur primarily in persons living in endemic areas for long periods of time.

Clinical:

Most infections with all three filarial worms are asymptomatic and frequently elicit eosinophilia. Clinical manifestations of lymphatic filariasis include intermittent episodes of lymphangitis and lymphadenitis, lymphedema that can progress to elephantiasis, hydrocele, and tropical pulmonary eosinophilia. Onchocerciasis is manifested by pruritus, rashes, damaged skin, subcutaneous nodules, progressive visual impairment, and blindness. Persons with loiasis may experience migratory pruritic swellings in the skin and subcutaneous tissues or an adult worm migrating under the conjunctiva.

Diagnosis:

Lymphatic filariasis: microscopic examination of blood for microfilariae (for most parts of the world done best around midnight), card test for antigen in blood. Onchocerciasis: skin snips for microfilariae. Loiasis: microscopic examination of blood for microfilariae (during the day). Serology sensitive, but not species specific.

Treatment:

Lymphatic filariasis: diethylcarbamazine (DEC) (note that albendazole and ivermectin are used only in endemic areas for transmission control). Onchocerciasis: ivermectin. Loaiasis: DEC. Chemoprophylaxis: DEC for loiasis.

Prevention:

Prevention of insect bites by use of repellents, protective clothing, bed-nets (latter only for some areas where lymphatic filariasis is transmitted by mosquitoes that bite indoors at night).

GIARDIASIS

Epidemiology:

Giardia lamblia is a single-celled protozoan of the small bowel. Giardiasis occurs worldwide, especially in developing countries where sanitation and public water treatment systems are poor. The infection is transmitted most often by drinking contaminated water and by person-to-person transmission by the fecal-oral route.

Clinical:

Symptoms of giardiasis include nausea, bloating, diarrhea, flatulence weight loss, rotten egg burps, and fatigue. Symptoms may persist for weeks or months. Many infected persons are asymptomatic.

Diagnosis:

Microscopic examination of the stool, stool antigen test, or PCR.

Treatment:

Metronidazole, tinidazole, albendazole, quinacrine, paromomycin.

Prevention:

Drinking purified water, hand washing before meals; good personal hygiene.

HEPATITIS A

Epidemiology:

Hepatitis A, the most common vaccine-preventable infection among travelers, is a viral infection transmitted worldwide by the fecal-oral route, usually via contaminated food and water or close personal or sexual contact. High risk of infection is associated with travel to countries with poor sanitation, where transmission is intense and most people become infected during childhood. In remote areas of these countries, the risk may be as high as 5 cases per 1000 persons per week. Levels of transmission are lower in industrialized countries with adequate sanitation, but outbreaks (often due to an infected food handler) also occur.

Clinical:

Infections in children are usually asymptomatic or mild, but severity increases with increasing age. In symptomatic cases, after an incubation period of 2–6 weeks, typical manifestations include fever, nausea, anorexia, fatigue, jaundice, tender hepatomegaly, dark urine and light stools. Symptoms usually resolve in several weeks to months, but mortality from acute hepatic failure is as high as 3% in persons over the age of 50 years. Reinfections and chronic infections do not occur.

Diagnosis:

Serology distinguishes acute or recent infection from previous infection.

Treatment:

No effective drug available. Supportive care; avoidance of alcohol and other hepatic toxins.

Prevention:

Two doses of hepatitis A vaccine 6–12 months apart prevent infection for at least 10–20 years and probably for life. A single dose of vaccine elicits an antibody response within two weeks and complete protection within 4 weeks. Intramuscular immune globulin (0.02 mg/kg and 0.06 mg/kg for travel up to 3 and 6 months, respectively) provides immediate protection. Although immune globulin alone or administered with the first dose of hepatitis A vaccine has been recommended for unvaccinated travelers with immediate departures, many travel medicine clinicians give the vaccine alone to such travelers. Avoidance of potentially contaminated food and water.

HEPATITIS B

Epidemiology:

Hepatitis B virus is transmitted from person to person via infected blood and other body fluids. Important exposures include unprotected sexual contact; transfusion of unscreened blood products; exposure to unsterilized syringes, needles or other sharp instruments (e.g., during dental or medical procedures, injecting drug use, body piercing, tattooing, acupuncture); and contact with blood or open wounds (e.g., by health-care workers or household members). Chronic hepatitis B infection occurs worldwide. The prevalence is <2% in North America, Western and northern Europe, Australia, and New Zealand. Rates are higher elsewhere and exceed 7% in the Amazon basin, Haiti, Dominican Republic, Africa, Pacific Islands, the Middle East, Southeast Asia, China, Korea, Indonesia, and the Philippines.

Clinical:

Most cases are asymptomatic or mild. After an incubation period of 6 weeks to 6 months, persons with acute hepatitis B experience the gradual onset of fatigue, anorexia, nausea, abdominal pain, and occasionally rash, arthralgia or jaundice. Death due to acute hepatic necrosis occurs in about 1% of infected persons. Approximately 5% of adults become chronic carriers of the virus, and are at risk of developing chronic hepatitis, cirrhosis, or liver cancer.

Diagnosis:

Serology to detect hepatitis B antigens or anti-hepatitis B antibodies.

Treatment:

Supportive care and avoidance of alcohol and other hepatic toxins. Interferon alpha, lamivudine for chronic infection.

Prevention:

Hepatitis B vaccine for travelers with potential exposures in moderate to high prevalence areas, stays >3 months, or chronic liver disease. Standard schedule of vaccination is three doses at 0, 1 and 6 months. Accelerated schedules (0, 1, 2 months or 0, 7, 21 days with a booster at 1 year) recommended for imminent travel, confers protection of 80% of vacinees at 1 month. Hepatitis B immune globulin following exposure for unvaccinated persons. Avoidance of unsafe sexual practices, potentially contaminated needles, blood transfusions in areas where donors are not screened, and other risky exposures.

HEPATITIS C

Epidemiology:

Hepatitis C virus is transmitted by exposure to blood (transfusions, contaminated needles, syringes and sharp instruments) and less commonly by unsafe sexual contact or perinatally. Hepatitis C occurs throughout the world. The prevalence is <3% in North America and Europe and higher in Africa, South America, and parts of Asia. The risk of transmission from transfusion is increased in areas where blood donors are not screened.

Clinical:

Most infections are asymptomatic. Symptomatic acute hepatitis, which occurs in <10% of infected persons, is manifested by anorexia, nausea, abdominal pain, and in some cases jaundice. Up to 80% of infected persons develop chronic infection and are at risk for developing cirrhosis or liver cancer.

Diagnosis:

Serology.

Treatment:

Interferon alpha, ribavirin.

Prevention:

No vaccine available. Avoidance of blood transfusions in areas where donors are not screened, avoidance of contact with blood or potentially contaminated needles or sharp instruments, safe sexual practices.

HEPATITIS D

Epidemiology:

Hepatitis D virus (delta virus) only infects persons who are already infected with hepatitis B or who become infected with hepatitis B and D at the same time. Like hepatitis B, hepatitis D is transmitted through contact with contaminated blood, sexual contact, and close household contact. Sporadic cases and epidemics have occurred among intravenous drug users. Non-parenterally spread hepatitis D is endemic in Italy, other Mediterranean countries, and the Middle East, while it is both endemic and epidemic in remote areas of the Amazon, where household contact is largely responsible for its spread.

Clinical:

Hepatitis D superinfection in persons with chronic hepatitis B often causes a severe acute hepatitis with high mortality, and survivors are at extremely high risk of chronic hepatitis and cirrhosis. When hepatitis B and D viruses are acquired at the same time, the infection is less severe and often self-limiting.

Diagnosis:

Serology to detect hepatitis D antigens or anti-hepatitis D antibodies.

Treatment:

Supportive measures, avoidance of alcohol and other hepato-toxins.

Prevention:

No vaccine for hepatitis D available, but prevention of hepatitis B by vaccination prevents hepatitis D. Avoidance of contact with blood or potentially contaminated needles or sharp instruments, safe sexual practices.

HEPATITIS E

Epidemiology:

Hepatitis E is transmitted by the fecal-oral route, largely via contaminated water and occasionally by direct person-to-person contact. It is endemic in tropical and subtropical areas, particularly in Asia, Mexico, and North Africa and has produced outbreaks in India, Nepal, Pakistan, China and Southeast Asia.

Clinical:

Similar to hepatitis A, hepatitis E is often subclinical but can also cause a self-limiting illness with fatigue, anorexia, nausea, abdominal pain, fever and jaundice. Unlike hepatitis A, it causes fulminant hepatitis with 20% mortality in women during the third month of pregnancy.

Diagnosis:

Serology.

Treatment:

Supportive care, avoidance of alcohol and other hepatotoxins.

Prevention:

No vaccine available. Avoidance of potentially contaminated food and water.

HOOKWORM INFECTION

Epidemiology:

The human hookworms (*Necator americanus, Ancylostoma duodenale*) infect nearly as many people as Ascaris worldwide and like Ascaris, thrive in warm areas with poor sanitation. Transmission results from contact of bare skin with fecally contaminated soil containing tiny larvae that hatch from eggs shed in the faeces of an infected person.

Clinical:

Most infections are asymptomatic. Pulmonary symptoms and infiltrates on chest x-ray may occur during the first weeks of infection. Adult worms feed on blood, and heavy, chronic infections can result in iron-deficiency anemia. Eosinophilia may be present in chronic infections, but is most intense during the first months of infection. Infection with dog or cat hookworms leads to a migrating, pruritic, serpingous rash called cutaneous larva migrans or 'creeping eruption'.

Diagnosis:

Microscopic examination of stool for eggs.

Treatment:

Albendazole, mebendazole, pyrantel pamoate.

Prevention:

Shoes and other methods of preventing direct contact of bare skin with potentially infected soil.

JAPANESE ENCEPHALITIS

Epidemiology:

Japanese encephalitis is a common viral disease transmitted by *Culex* mosquitoes to birds, domestic animals, and people in Asia and the Western Pacific. The risk is greatest for short-term travelers and expatriates living in rural agricultural areas, especially where rice is produced and pigs are raised. Transmission occurs from late spring to early fall in temperate areas, such as Japan, Korea, People's Republic of China, and eastern Russia, from July to December in northern India and Nepal, and at other times of the year or year round in other endemic areas that extend from India through Southeast Asia to the Philippines, Indonesia, Malaysia, Taiwan, Papua New Guinea and the Western Pacific.

Clinical:

Only one in several hundred infections are symptomatic. For those who become ill, after an incubation period of 4–14 days, fever, headache, myalgia, nausea, and vomiting are followed by confusion, motor abnormalities, seizures, and often coma. In symptomatic cases, mortality can reach 30% in children and the elderly, and up to 25% of survivors have permanent neurological damage.

Diagnosis:

Serologic tests of cerebrospinal fluid, serum; viral isolation from blood, CSF.

Treatment:

Supportive measures; no specific treatment available.

Prevention:

All travelers to endemic areas: measures to prevent mosquito bites. Persons planning long (e.g., >30 days) stays in rural farming areas during transmission season or persons anticipating extensive outdoor exposure in these areas: consider Japanese encephalitis vaccine (three doses at least 10 days before travel).

LEPTOSPIROSIS

Epidemiology:

Leptospirosis is caused by the spirochete *Leptospira interrogans*. It is a common zoonosis with a worldwide distribution and is acquired by skin contact with fresh water (floods, swamps, and moist soil) contaminated with the urine of infected animals such as rats or mice. Contact with excreta directly may result in infection. The organism enters the body through cuts or abrasions of skin or through mucous membranes. Recent outbreaks have occurred among ecotourists (hiking, swimming, rafting, kayaking).

Clinical:

Many cases are mild or asymptomatic. Typically, clinical disease manifests in two phases with fever, headache, conjunctival suffusion, myalgia, jaundice, renal insufficiency, and aseptic meningitis.

Diagnosis:

Dark field examination of urine and serological tests.

Treatment:

Doxycycline, penicillin.

Prevention:

Avoiding fresh water and animal contact, especially during periods of flooding. Chemoprophylaxis with doxycycline 200 mg/week or using the drug in the same regimen as for malaria chemoprophylaxis.

MALARIA

Epidemiology:

Malaria is a blood-borne protozoan disease transmitted by female *Anopheles* mosquitoes to an estimated 300–500 million persons in tropical and subtropical areas in Africa, Asia, and the Americas. The risk of infection varies according to season, altitude, and geographic area, with the highest risk to persons traveling to certain parts of Papua New Guinea, Solomon Islands, Vanuatu and sub-Saharan Africa (including in urban areas). In general, the risk to travelers is lower in the Indian subcontinent and lowest in Latin America and Southeast Asia. *Plasmodium falciparum* is the species of malaria parasite that causes severe complications and death, while *P. vivax, malariae,* and *ovale,* are rarely fatal. Chloroquine-resistant *P. falciparum* has spread to most malarious areas, and chloroquine resistance in *P. vivax* is spreading as well.

Clinical:

Features common to all species include fever (may be irregular or occur every other day or every three days depending on species), rigors, headache, nausea, vomiting, myalgia, anemia, and thrombocytopenia. Falciparum malaria may be complicated by coma and other evidence of insult to the central nervous system, respiratory or renal failure, shock, and death. *Vivax* and *ovale* malarias relapse if treatment does not include primaquine.

Diagnosis:

Microscopic examination of thick and thin blood smears; tests for detecting antigen in blood.

Treatment:

Chloroquine for infections with all four species except those acquired in areas with known chloroquine resistance; otherwise, quinine or quinidine, doxycycline, pyrimethamine and sulfadoxine (Fansidar'), mefloquine, atovaquone and proguanil (Malarone'), artemisin and its derivatives. Primaquine is added to prevent relapses of *P. vivax* or *ovale*.

Prevention:

Avoidance of mosquito bites with repellant, protective clothing, bed nets (preferably insecticide-impregnated), remaining in screened areas. Prophylaxis with chloroquine for travel to areas without chloroquine resistance; otherwise mefloquine, doxycycline, atovaquone/proguanil; addition of primaquine for *P. vivax* or *ovale* infections.

MENINGOCOCCAL MENINGITIS

Epidemiology:

Meningococcal meningitis is a highly lethal infection of the central nervous system caused by the bacterium *Neisseria meningitidis.*

Infection is spread by direct person-to-person contact, and aerosols and respiratory droplets from patients and asymptomatic persons carrying the organism in their nose. Cases occur worldwide. In temperate zones, sporadic cases and outbreaks occur most often during the winter. The risk to travelers is low, but in the 'meningitis belt' of sub-Saharan Africa, which extends from Senegal to Ethiopia, outbreaks occur during the dry months (November to June). Outbreaks have been associated with population movements and pilgrimages.

Clinical:

Most infections are asymptomatic and lead to asymptomatic carriage that can be a source of infection for others. Meningococcal meningitis is characterized by fever, headache, nausea, vomiting, stiff neck, hemorrhagic rashes, and circulatory collapse (which can also result from bacteremia without meningitis). With treatment the case fatality rate is 5–15%, and 20% of survivors are left with permanent neurological damage.

Diagnosis:

Smears and cultures of blood and cerebrospinal fluid. Tests for antigen in cerebrospinal fluid may yield falsely negative results.

Treatment:

Ceftriaxone or cefotaxime, chloramphenicol. Some strains are relatively resistant to penicillin.

Prevention:

Single dose of quadrivalent vaccine for: travelers to the meningitis belt in Africa in the dry season who will have close contact with local populations; pilgrims to Mecca for the Hajj (required by Saudi Arabia for entry). Avoid crowded confined spaces. Prophylactic antibiotics (ciprofloxacin, rifampin, ceftriaxone) after close contact with a person with meningococcal disease.

PLAGUE

Epidemiology:

Plague is a zoonotic disease of rodents caused by the bacterium *Yersinia pestis.* It is transmitted from rodents by fleas or directly by respiratory droplets from persons with pneumonic plague. Plague in wild rodents occurs in areas of western North America, South America, sub-Saharan Africa, Asia, and Russian Federation.

Clinical:

Initially, symptoms include fever, chills, headache, myalgia, and malaise. Lymph nodes that drain the site of the fleabite become greatly enlarged and painful. Infection can spread to (or originate in) the lungs, and disseminate through the bloodstream to cause shock and meningitis. Without treatment, mortality is about 60% for bubonic plague and 100% for pneumonia and septicemia.

Diagnosis:

Examination of lymph node aspirate, blood, sputum, or cerebrospinal fluid by microscopy, direct immunofluorescence, and culture; serology.

Treatment:

Streptomycin, gentamicin, tetracycline, doxycycline, chloramphenicol.

Prevention:

For persons who will have exposure to rodents and fleas in epizootic areas: three doses of plague vaccine at 0, 3, 8–9 months. Prophylaxis with tetracycline, doxycycline, trimethoprim-sulfamethoxazole for unavoidable exposures.

RABIES

Epidemiology:

Rabies is a fatal viral disease transmitted from rabid animals by bites and less commonly scratches or contact of animal saliva with mucous membranes or breaks in the skin. In developing countries, transmission is largely from dogs, but rabies can be contracted by exposure to a broad range of domestic and wild animals, including cats, monkeys, and bats. Canine rabies is highly endemic in parts of Mexico, El Salvador, Guatemala, Peru, Colombia, Ecuador, the Indian subcontinent, Thailand, Vietnam, and the Philippines. Of the remaining countries, approximately 50 are currently rabies-free, including many Caribbean islands, Japan, Taiwan, Australia, New Zealand and countries in Scandinavia, parts of Europe, and Oceania.

Clinical:

The incubation period depends on severity of the wound and its distance from the central nervous system and can be as short 9 days and as long as a year or more. Initially, there are fever, headache, sensory changes at the site of the bite, apprehension, and soon after, excitability, hallucinations, spasms of swallowing muscles leading to fear or swallowing, seizures, and delirium. Death occurs within a few days of onset.

Diagnosis:

Direct immunofluorescence of skin or brain tissue obtained by biopsy; isolation of virus from brain, saliva, and cerebrospinal fluid; PCR.

Treatment:

Supportive and palliative care.

Prevention:

For travel to remote endemic areas, prolonged stays in endemic areas, and activities that may lead to exposure: *predeparture vaccination* (with HCDV, PCEC, or RVA vaccines) on days 0, 7, 21 or 28. Avoidance of wild and stray animals. *Post exposure:* vigorous cleaning of bite wound and other potentially contaminated areas with soap and water, prompt medical attention, two doses of rabies vaccine and, depending on exposure and vaccination status, rabies immune globulin.

SEVERE ACUTE RESPIRATORY SYNDROME (SARS)

Epidemiology:

SARS is new clinical syndrome which was first reported from China in November, 2002. It is caused by a novel Coronavirus which is transmitted person-to-person by inhalation of droplets and, in unusual cases, by aerosol transmission. It may also be transmitted by mucous membranes contamination and possibly by ingestion of stool. The virus has been documented in 28 countries, with large outbreaks, mostly affecting health-care workers and their families, occurring in mainland China, Hong Kong, Singapore, Taiwan, and Toronto, Canada.

Clinical:

The incubation period of SARS is 3–11 days. The syndrome often begins with a prodrome of headache, myalgia, and fatigue, progressing over several days to fever, cough, and shortness of breath. Gastrointestinal symptoms occur less often. Although the mortality rate is approximately five percent, it appears to be considerably higher in older individuals. The chest X-ray may be normal early on and progress quickly to show unilateral and bilateral infiltrates. Many patients develop lymphopenia, thrombocytopenia, and hypocalcemia.

Diagnosis:

The diagnosis of SARS has, until recently, been based on a case definition which included a possible contact history, fever and respiratory symptoms. The most reliable diagnostic test is serology which is positive within 28 days of symptom onset. PCR is less reliable but may be positive in tissue samples, BAL secretions and naso-pharangeal swabs.

Treatment:

The treatment of SARS has not yet been determined.

Prevention:

Avoid areas in which SARS is known to be active in the community. Stringent handwashing may be helpful. Barrier techniques, including the use of an N-95 mask, are mandatory in the management of an acute case.

SCHISTOSOMIASIS

Epidemiology:

Schistosomiasis (also known as bilharzia) is caused by infection with schistosomes, flatworms (trematodes or flukes) that live in the lumen of veins that drain the intestines or lower urinary tract. Infection is acquired during fresh water contact when bare skin is penetrated by cercariae (larval parasites) that are shed from certain species of freshwater snails. Snails become infected with a different type of larva that hatches from eggs excreted in human faeces or urine into fresh water. Approximately 200 million persons in South America, the Caribbean, Africa, the Middle East, People's Republic of China, Southeast Asia, and the Philippines suffer from schistosomiasis. Certain rivers (e.g., the Nile River, the Omo River in Ethiopia) and lakes (e.g., Lake Victoria, Lake Malawi) are notorious sources of infection for travelers from nonendemic areas.

Clinical:

Infections in travelers are usually light and asymptomatic. Previously uninfected persons may present with manifestations of acute schistosomiasis (Katayama fever) 3–6 weeks after exposure, including fever, headache, myalgia, cough, abdominal pain, urticarial rash, hepatosplenomegaly, and eosinophilia. Aberrant deposition of eggs in the brain or spinal cord can lead to cerebral mass lesions, seizures, focal neurological signs, and transverse myelitis. Chronic schistosomiasis usually lasts about 3–5 years but can persist for as long as 30 years. Eosinophilia is present in less than half of chronically infected persons. Heavy infections are rare in travelers with short exposures, but can cause chronic diarrhea, hepatic fibrosis, and portal hypertension with splenomegaly and esophageal varices (*Schistosoma mansoni, japonicum*), or hematuria, bladder polyps, urinary tract infections, obstructive uropathy and bladder cancer (*S. hematobium*).

Diagnosis:

Serology, microscopic identification of eggs in stool, urine, rectal or bladder biopsy in selected cases. Diagnostic tests may be negative during the first 6 weeks of infection.

Treatment:

Praziquantel.

Prevention:

Avoidance of contact with bodies of fresh water in endemic areas (note that salt water, very rapidly flowing water, chlorinated water, water heated to 50 °C for at least 5 min, and snail-free water that has been held for ≥36 h are safe). Vigorous toweling of rubbing skin with alcohol immediately after accidental exposure may prevent infection.

STRONGYLOIDIASIS

Epidemiology:

Strongyloidiasis, infection with the intestinal roundworm *Strongyloides stercoralis,* occurs worldwide, but most commonly in developing areas with poor sanitation where infection results from contact of bare skin with larvae on fecally contaminated soil. Unlike most other worms that infect human beings, *Strongyloides* can complete its life cycle within the same host, and therefore infections persist for years, decades, or a lifetime. Because infective larvae are shed intermittently in the faeces, the parasite can also be spread by direct person-to-person contact, even in temperate and cold climates.

Clinical:

Asymptomatic infections are common. During the early stage of infection, patients may complain of cough and wheezing. Gastrointestinal complaints (abdominal pain and diarrhea) and pruritic rashes (urticaria and a migrating rash called *larva currens*) occur during chronic infection. Immunosuppressed persons, especially those receiving corticosteroids, may develop highly lethal hyperinfection with dissemination of larvae throughout the body. Many, but not all patients have eosinophilia, which usually disappears in patients taking corticosteroids or experiencing hyperinfection.

Diagnosis:

Microscopic examination of stool, small bowel aspirates or biopsy samples (for larvae); serology.

Treatment:

Ivermectin, albendazole, thiabendazole.

Prevention:

Shoes and other methods of preventing direct contact of bare skin with potentially infected soil.

TAPEWORM INFECTION

Epidemiology:

The beef tape worm *(Taenia saginata)*, pork tapeworm *(Taenia solium)*, and fish tapeworm *(Diphyllobothrium latum)*, are long flatworms that live in the intestinal tract of human beings and produce eggs that are shed in the faeces. After cattle and swine ingest the eggs, larvae emerge that are carried by the bloodstream to muscle and other tissues where they develop into cysticerci (cystic larval parasites). Freshwater fish become infected with a larval parasite (without a cyst wall) in a similar but more complex way. After humans ingest uncooked or poorly cooked infected meat or fish, the larval parasite emerges and develops into an adult tapeworm that lives in the intestines for years. In the case of the pork tapeworm, persons can also become infected with cysticerci by ingesting eggs shed in his or her own stool or in the stool of

another person harboring an adult tapeworm. The fish tapeworm is endemic in cool lake regions, while the beef and pork tapeworms are transmitted in developing areas with poor sanitation and inadequate inspection of meat.

Clinical:

Most persons harboring an adult tapeworm have no symptoms other than passing egg-laden tapeworm segments per rectum. About 1% of persons with a fish tapeworm develop macrocytic anemia because the worm is able to deprive its host of vitamin B_{12}. Cysticercosis, human infection with *T. solium* cysticerci, is often asymptomatic, especially when the cysts are located in subcutaneous tissue or muscle. Cysts in the central nervous system can cause seizures and other neurological symptoms, typically when they begin to degenerate several years after infection.

Diagnosis:

Microscopic examination of stool for eggs; identification of passed segments; serology (for *T. solium* infection and cysticercosis); stool antigen test (for *T. solium*).

Treatment:

Adult tapeworms: praziquantel; niclosamide; cysticercosis: praziquantel, albendazole.

Prevention:

For prevention of tapeworm infection: avoiding poorly cooked or uncooked beef, pork, or fish that may be infected with the larval tapeworm. For prevention of cysticercosis: handwashing; personal hygiene; avoiding food or water potentially contaminated with *T. solium* eggs; treatment of persons harboring an adult tapeworm.

TICK-BORNE ENCEPHALITIS

Epidemiology:

Tick-borne encephalitis is a viral infection of the central nervous system that is transmitted between March and October by ticks (principally *Ixodes ricinus*) in Scandinavia, Western and Central Europe, and countries of the former Soviet Union. Persons who spend time in forests, meadows, or pastures are at risk, as are persons who drink unpasteurized dairy products from infected cows, sheep or goats.

Clinical:

Infection is usually subclinical. Initial symptoms include an influenza-like illness in <1% of persons, which in an even smaller percentage of infected persons, leads to encephalitis that can be fatal or produce paralysis and other permanent neurological damage. The disease is more severe in older persons.

Diagnosis:

Isolation of virus from blood, tissue, cerebrospinal fluid (rare); serologic testing of cerebrospinal fluid and serum.

Treatment:

Supportive care including anticonvulsants, ventilatory support.

Prevention:

For extended intense exposures only: three doses of tick-borne encephalitis vaccine over 6–12 months. Protective clothing, use of repellents, prompt removal of ticks, avoidance of unpasteurized dairy products.

TYPHOID

Epidemiology:

Typhoid fever (enteric fever) is transmitted by ingestion of the bacterium *Salmonella typhi* in food or water contaminated by faeces of infected persons. Typhoid occurs primarily in areas without adequate sanitation and clean drinking water. The risk is especially high for travelers to the Indian subcontinent, Southeast Asia, Indonesia, Peru, and Haiti.

Clinical:

Typhoid begins gradually with fever, chills, headache, anorexia, and malaise, which are followed by sustained high fevers, toxic appearance, abdominal pain, and hepatosplenomegaly. Patients are often constipated, although diarrhea occurs in about 50% of infected persons. Without treatment, illness lasts two to 6 weeks and may be complicated by gastrointestinal bleeding, bowel perforation, shock, and death in as many as 30% of untreated patients. Up to 5% of persons become chronic typhoid carriers.

Diagnosis:

Culture of blood, bone marrow, stool, and urine; serology (Widal reaction of variable sensitivity and specificity).

Treatment:

Ciprofloxacin, ofloxacin, levofloxacin, ceftriaxone, cefotaxime effective against most isolates. Resistance to trimethoprim-sulfamethoxazole, ampicillin, amoxicillin, chloramphenicol frequent in some areas; increasing quinolone resistance in South Asia.

Prevention:

Vaccination for travelers with anticipated prolonged exposure to potentially contaminated food and drink, especially in remote rural areas. Available vaccines about 70% efficacious: single dose of bacterial polysaccharide (Vi); multiple doses of oral attenuated live Ty21a vaccine. Avoidance of potentially contaminated food and water.

TYPHUS (SCRUB, TICK)

Epidemiology:

Scrub typhus (tsutsugamushi fever) is caused by the rickettsia *Orienta tsutsugamushi*, which is transmitted by the bite of larval mites (chiggers). The term tick typhus encompasses a number of tick-borne infections caused by various rickettsias in different parts of the world (e.g., *Rickettsia conorii* in southern Europe, Africa, and Asia, and *R. africae* in East and Southern Africa). The reservoir of infection includes domestic dogs, rodents, and livestock. People become infected in grassy or shrub-covered areas while on safari, treks, or camping trips.

Clinical:

An erythematous skin lesion with a black necrotic center develops at the site of the tick bite, and the patient develops fever, headache, rash (often absent in *R. africae* infection), myalgia, regional lymphadenopathy, leukopenia, and thrombocytopenia.

Diagnosis:

Serology.

Treatment:

Doxycycline, ciprofloxacin, chloramphenicol.

Prevention:

Avoidance of tick- and mite-infested areas; use of protective clothing, repellents, prompt removal of ticks. For unavoidable exposures to scrub typhus only: weekly doxycycline.

VIRAL HEMORRHAGIC FEVERS (LASSA, EBOLA, MARBURG)

Epidemiology:

The viral hemorrhagic fevers include infections caused by a variety of organisms with different geographic distribution. Of these, Lassa fever, Ebola hemorrhagic fever, and Marburg hemorrhagic fever are well known for their high mortality and ready ability to infect healthcare workers and household members who come in contact with body fluids and secretions of infected persons. Lassa fever virus is found in West Africa, where it also is spread from infected rodents and their excreta. Marburg and Ebola viruses are found most often in Central and East Africa, respectively. The risk of infection to travelers other than clinicians and laboratory workers assisting with an outbreak is very low.

Clinical:

Initial manifestations include fever, headache, sore throat, myalgia and fatigue, which are followed in severe cases by coagulopathy, spontaneous hemorrhage into skin, mucous membranes and gastrointestinal tract, and shock. Mortality is highest for Ebola infection and can exceed 90%.

Diagnosis:

Viral isolation from blood, tissue; serology; antigen detection, PCR.

Treatment:

Ribavirin (Lassa only). Supportive care.

Prevention:

No vaccine available. Avoid contact with rodents and rodent excreta. Barrier isolation of infected persons; disinfection of blood, body fluids and tissue, and contaminated materials; strict precautions in laboratories; level 4 biosafety laboratory for viral isolation.

WHIPWORM INFECTION

Epidemiology:

The whipworm, *Trichuris trichiura*, an extremely common intestinal parasite, occurs in warm climates where sanitation is inadequate. Infection results from ingestion of microscopic eggs shed in the faeces of persons infected with the adult worms that live for up to seven years in the colon. Eggs become infectious after several weeks in the environment and readily contaminate uncooked vegetables and drinking water.

Clinical:

Most infections are asymptomatic, and eosinophilia is mild or absent. Heavy infections cause chronic diarrhea, abdominal pain, dysentery and rectal prolapse, while even moderate infections in children can impair growth and cognitive development.

Diagnosis:

Microscopic examination of stool for eggs.

Treatment:

Albendazole, mebendazole.

Prevention:

Avoiding uncooked vegetables; hand washing before meals; drinking clean water.

YELLOW FEVER

Epidemiology:

Yellow fever is a mosquito-borne viral disease found only in parts of tropical South America and Africa. Exposure to the sylvatic cycle of transmission among mosquitoes and monkeys occurs in South American rain forests and in jungles and moist savannah in Africa. Occasional outbreaks of urban yellow fever in African cities are the result of viral transmission from person to person by peridomestic Aedes aegypti mosquitoes. Although yellow fever is a rare cause of illness in travelers, recently there have been cases among North American travelers to the Amazon region.

Clinical:

Most cases are mild or subclinical. Severe cases begin abruptly within a week of exposure with fever, headache, myalgia, nausea, vomiting, and back pain, followed several days later by jaundice, hematemesis, melena, purpura, renal failure, coma, and death in up to 50% of cases.

Diagnosis:

Viral isolation (tissue culture, mouse or mosquito inoculation), detection of viral antigens or genome in blood or post-mortem tissue, serology.

Treatment:

No specific treatment available. Supportive care with strict adherence to blood and body fluid precautions.

Prevention:

Immunization with single dose of live, attenuated vaccine (17D) within 10 days of travel to countries reporting yellow fever, rural areas within endemic zones of countries not reporting yellow fever, and countries requiring a valid International Vaccination Certificate from an approved Yellow Fever Vaccination Center. Revaccination every 10 years. Insect repellent, protective clothing, and other measures to prevent mosquito bites, especially during early morning and late afternoon.

The Body of Knowledge for the Practice of Travel Medicine

Jay S. Keystone

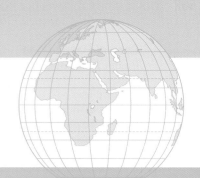

INTRODUCTION

The field of travel medicine has grown dramatically as greater numbers of people travel to exotic and remote destinations. Approximately 600 million travelers cross international borders annually. However, studies suggest that only about 8% seek pre-travel health advice, many of whom receive information from practitioners who are ill equipped to provide current and accurate information. Travel medicine has become increasingly complex due to dynamic changes in global infectious disease epidemiology, changing patterns of drug resistance, and a rise in the number of travelers with chronic health conditions.

WHY DO WE NEED A BODY OF KNOWLEDGE?

This 'Body of Knowledge' was created to guide the professional development of individuals practicing travel medicine and to shape curricula and training programs in travel medicine. It is also expected to serve as a vehicle for establishing the content validity of a credentialing process.

WHAT IS A BODY OF KNOWLEDGE?

It is the scope and extent of knowledge required for professionals working in the field of travel medicine. Major content areas include the global epidemiology of health risks to the traveler, vaccinology, malaria prevention, and pre-travel counseling designed to maintain the health of the traveling public.

HOW WAS THE BODY OF KNOWLEDGE DEVELOPED?

In September 1999, the International Society of Travel Medicine Executive Board established a group of travel medicine experts from (ISTM) its membership to define the scope of knowledge in the field of travel medicine worldwide. The final draft of their report was converted to survey format and mailed to 110 ISTM members worldwide, who were representative of the diversity within the profession. The respondents provided further input into the relative importance of each of the content areas. The results of their efforts contributed significantly to the 'Body of Knowledge' presented as follows.

I. EPIDEMIOLOGY

    A.   Basic concepts (e.g. morbidity, mortality, incidence, prevalence)

    B.   Geographic specificity/global distribution of diseases and potential health hazards

II. IMMUNOLOGY/VACCINOLOGY

    A.   Basic concepts and principles (e.g., live vs. inactivated vaccine, measurement of immune response)

    B.   Handling, storage, and disposal of vaccines and related supplies

Types of Vaccines/Immunizations

Indications/contraindications, routes of administration, dosing regimens duration of protection, immunogenicity, efficacy, potential adverse reactions and medical management of adverse reactions associated with the following vaccinations:

    C.   Bacille Calmette-Guerin
    D.   Cholera
    E.   Diphtheria
    F.   Encephalitis, Japanese
    G.   Encephalitis, tick-borne
    H.   Hepatitis A
    I.   Hepatitis B
    J.   Hepatitis A and B combined
    K.   Immune globulin
    L.   Influenza
    M.   Lyme
    N.   Measles
    O.   Meningococcal
    P.   Mumps
    Q.   Plague
    R.   Pneumococcal
    S.   Poliomyelitis
    T.   Rabies
    U.   Rubella
    V.   Tetanus
    W.   Typhoid
    X.   Varicella
    Y.   Yellow fever

III. PRETRAVEL CONSULTATION/MANAGEMENT

Patient Evaluation

    A.   Relevant medical history (e.g. previous vaccinations, allergies, chronic illness)

    B.   Evaluation of ravel itineraries/risk assessment (e.g. pre-existing activities, travel to rural vs. urban areas)

    C.   Assessment of fitness/contraindications to travel (e.g. pre-existing illness, fitness to fly)

Special Populations

Unique management issues pertaining to the following populations:

D. Athletes
E. Corporate travelers
F. Elderly travelers
G. Infants and children
H. Immigrants/expatriates
I. Pregnant travelers
J. Travelers with chronic diseases (diabetes, chronic obstructive pulmonary disease, cardiovascular disease)
K. Travelers with disabilities
L. Travelers who are immunocompromised, including HIV and AIDS

Special Itineraries

Unique management issues associated with the following activities/itineraries:

M. Cruise ship travel
N. Diving
O. Extended stay travel
P. Extreme travel
Q. Mass gatherings (e.g. the Hajj)
R. Wilderness/remote regions travel

Prevention and Self Treatment

S. Travel health kits
T. Chemoprophylaxis (e.g. malaria, traveler's diarrhea, filariasis)
U. Self treatment (e.g. diarrhea, malaria)
V. Personal protective measures (e.g. restriction of outdoor activity at dawn and dusk and barrier protection (e.g., bed nets, insect repellents)

Precautions (and Reasons for Precautions) Regarding:

W. Food consumption
X. Water consumption and purification
Y. Contact with fresh and salt water
Z. Walking barefoot
AA. Animal contact
BB. Close interpersonal contact (e.g. sexually transmitted diseases)
CC. Safety and security

IV. DISEASES CONTRACTED DURING TRAVEL

Geographic risk, prevention, transmission, possible symptoms and appropriate referral/triage of:

Diseases Associated with Vectors

A. Dengue
B Encephalitis, Japanese
C. Encephalitis, tick-borne
D. Filariasis (e.g. Loa loa, bancroftian, onchocerciasis)
E. Hemorrhagic fevers
F. Leishmaniasis
G. Lyme
H. Malaria
I. Plague
J. Rift Valley fever
K. Trypanosomiasis, American

M. Typhus fever
N. Yellow fever
O. Other

Diseases Associated with Person-to-Person Contact

P. Diphtheria
Q. Hepatitis B
R. Hepatitis C
S. Influenza
T. Measles
U. Meningococcal disease
V. Mumps
W. Pertussis
X. Pneumococcal disease
Y. Rubella
Z. Sexually transmitted diseases
AA. Tuberculosis
BB. Varicella
CC. Other

Diseases Associated with Ingestion of Food and Water

DD. Amebiasis
EE. Cholera
FF. Cryptosporidiosis
GG. Cyclosporiasis
HH. Giardiasis
II. Hepatitis A
JJ. Hepatitis E
KK. Poilomyelitis
LL. Seafood poisoning/toxins
MM. Transmissable spongiform encephalopathy
NN. Travelers' diarrhea
OO. Typhoid fever
PP. Other

Diseases Associated with Bites Stings

QQ. Envenomation (e.g. jelly fish, sea urchin, scorpion, snake)
RR. Rabies

Diseases Associated with Water/Environmental Contact

SS. Cutaneous larva migrans
TT. Legionella
UU. Schistosomiasis
VV. Tetanus

V OTHER CONDITIONS ASSOCIATED WITH TRAVEL

Conditions Occurring During or Immediately Following Travel

Symptoms, prevention, and treatment of:

A. Motion sickness
B. Barotrauma
C. Thrombosis/embolism
D. Jet lag

Conditions Associated with Environmental Factors

Symptoms, prevention and treatment of:

E. Sunburn, heat exhaustion and sun stroke
F. Frostbite and hypothermia

G. Respiratory distress/failure (associated with humidity, pollution, etc.)

H. Altitude sickness

Threats to Personal Security

Precautions regarding:

I. Transportation/motor vehicle accidents

J. Violence-related injuries

Psychocultural Issues

Unique management issues associated with:

K. Culture shock/adaptation

L. Repatriation

VI. POST-TRAVEL MANAGEMENT

A. Screening/assessment of returned travelers

B. Emergencies and triage

C. Conditions requiring referral to a specialist

Diagnostic and Management Implications of the Following Symptoms:

D. Diarrhea

E. Eosinophilia

F. Fever

G. Nausea and/or vomiting

H. Skin problems

I. Other

VII. GENERAL TRAVEL MEDICINE ISSUES

Medical Care Abroad

A. Procedures for locating medical care abroad

B. Blood transfusion guidelines for international travelers

C. Limitations of standard medical coverage during international travel and alternative medical insurance for international travelers

D. Aeromedical evacuation

Travel Clinic Management

E. Equipment

F. Supplies and disposables

G. Resources for laboratory testing

H. Documentation and record keeping (e.g vaccination certificate requirements, reporting of adverse events)

I. Infection control procedures

J. Management of medical emergencies

Travel Medicine Information/Resources

K. International health recommendations/advisories (e.g. World Health Organization and national pulbic health organizations)

L. International Health Regulations

M. National/regional recommendations, including national/regional differences

N. Information for travelers

CONCLUSION

The field of travel medicine encompasses a wide variety of disciplines including epidemiology, infectious disease, public health, tropical medicine, and occupational health. As a unique and growing specialty, it has become necessary to establish standards of practice in the field

itself. These standards have been established to identify the scope of competencies expected of travel medicine practitioners, guide their professional training and development, and ensure an acceptable level of patient care.

This Body of Knowledge will serve as the basis for an examination being developed for all travel health professionals. This exam was administered prior to the opening of the CISTM 8 in New York in May 2003. Practitioners who successfully complete this examination will be awarded a Certificate of Knowledge in Travel Medicine by the ISTM. Information about the Certificate of Knowledge examination will be available at www.istm.org.

Copyright ISTM.

FURTHER READING

1. World Health Organization. *Intestional Parasites. Basic Laboratory Methods in Medical Parasitology.* Geneva: World Health Organization; 1991:67–79.
2. Crook P, Mayon-White R, Reacher M. Enhancing, surveillance of cryptosporidiosis; test all faecal specimens from, children. *Commun. Dis. Pub. Health* 2002; **5**:112–113.
3. Chiodini PL. A 'new' parasite human infection with *Cyclospora cayetanensis*. *Trans R Soc Trop Med Hyg* 1994; **88**:369–371.
4. Eberhard ML, Pieniazek NJ, Arrowood MJ. Laboratory diagnosis of *Cyclospora* infections. *Arch Pathol Lab Med* 1997; **121**:792–797.
5. Van Gool T, Snidjers F. Reiss P. *et al.* Diagnosis of intestinal and disseminated microsporidial infections in patients with HIV by a new rapid fluorescence technique. *J Clin Pathol* 1993; **46**: 694–699.
6. Weber R. Bryan DT, Owen RL, Wilcox CM, Gorelkin L, Visvesvara GS. Improved light microscopical detection of microsporidial spores in stool and duodenal aspirates. *N Engl J Med* 1992; **326**:161–166.
7. Sestak K, Ward LA, Sheoran A, Feng X, Akiyoshi, DE, Ward HD, Tzipori, S. Variability among *Cryptosporidium parvum* and genotype 1 and 2 immunodominant, surface glycoproteins. *Parasit Immunol* 2002; **24**:213–219.
8. Garcia LS., Laboratory identification of the microsporidia. *J Clin Microbiol* 2002; **40**:1892–1901.
9. Sloan LM, Rosenblatt JE. Evaluation of enzyme-linked immunosorbent assay for detection of *Cryptosporidium* spp. in stool specimens. *J Clin Microbiol* 1993; **31**: 1468–1471.
10. Limor JF, Lal AA, Xiao L. Detection and differentiation of Cryptosporidium parasites that are pathogenic for humans by real-time PCR. *J Clin Microbiol* 2002; **40**:2335–2338.
11. Quintero-Betancourt W, Peele PR, Rose JB. *Cryptosporidium parvum* and *Cyclospora cayetanensis*: a review of laboratory methods for detection of these waterborne parasites. *J Microbiol Meth* 2002; **49**:209–224.
12. Rosoff JD, Sanders CA, Sonnad SS *et al.* Stool diagnosis of giardiasis using a commercially available enzyme immunoassay to detect *Giardia*-specific antigen 65 (GSA 65). *J Clin Microbiol* 1989; **23**:1997–2002.
13. Jackson TF. *Entamoeba histrolytica* and *Entamoeba dispar* are distinct species; clinical, epidemiological and serological evidence. *Int J Parasitol* 1998; **28**:181–186.
14. Haque RK, Kress S, Wood T, et al. Diagnosis of pathogenic *Entamoeba histolytica* infection using a stool ELISA based on monoclonal antibodies to the galactose-specific adhesin *J Infect Dis* 1993; **167**:247–249.
15. Aguirre A, Warhurst DC, Guhl F, Frame 1. Polymerase chain reaction-solution hybridization enzyme-linked immunoassay (PCR-SHELA) for the differential diagnosis of pathogenic and non-pathogenic *Entamoeba histolytica*. *Trans R Soc Trop Med Hyg* 1995; **89**:187–188.
16. Britten D, Wilson SM, McNerney R, Moody AH, Chiodini PL, Ackers JP. An improved colorometric PCR-based method for detection and differentiation of *Entamoeba histolytica* and *Entamoeba dispar* in faeces. *J Clin Microbiol* 1997; **35**:1108–1011.
17. Lujan HD, Conrad JT, Clark CG, et al. Detection of microsporidia spore-specific antigens by monoclonal antibodies. *Hybridoma* 1998; **17**:237–243.
18. Cisse OA, Ouattara A, Thellier M *et al.* Evaluation of an immunofluorescent-antibody test using monoclonal, antibodies against *Enterocytozoon bieneusi* and *Encephalitozoon intestinalis* for diagnosis of intestinal microsporidiosis in Bamako (Mali). *J Clin Microbiol* 2002; **40**:1715–1718.
19. Franzen C, Muller A, Hartmann P, *et al.* Polymerase chain reaction for diagnosis and species differentiation of microsporidia. *Folia Parasitol (Praha)* 1998; **45**:140–148.
20. Rinder H, Janitschke K, Aspock H, *et al.* Blinded, externally controlled multicenter evaluation of light microscopy and PCR for detection of microsporidia in stool specimens. The Diagnostic Multicenter Study Group on Microsporidia. *J Clin Microbiol* 1998; **36**:1814–1818.

Index

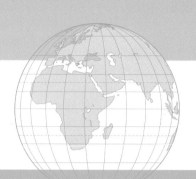

Note: Page references in **bold** refer to Figures and Tables

ELSEVIER CD-ROM LICENCE AGREEMENT

YOU UNDERSTAND THAT, EXCEPT FOR THE LIMITED WARRANTY RECITED ABOVE, ELSEVIER, ITS AFFILIATES, LICENSORS, THIRD PARTY SUPPLIERS AND AGENTS (TOGETHER 'THE SUPPLIERS') MAKE NO REPRESENTATIONS OR WARRANTIES, WITH RESPECT TO THE PRODUCT, INCLUDING, WITHOUT LIMITATION THE PROPRIETARY MATERIAL. ALL OTHER REPRESENTATIONS, WARRANTIES, CONDITIONS OR OTHER TERMS, WHETHER EXPRESS OR IMPLIED BY STATUTE OR COMMON LAW, ARE HEREBY EXCLUDED TO THE FULLEST EXTENT PERMITTED BY LAW.

IN PARTICULAR BUT WITHOUT LIMITATION TO THE FOREGOING NONE OF THE SUPPLIERS MAKE ANY REPRESENTATIONS OR WARRANTIES (WHETHER EXPRESS OR IMPLIED) REGARDING THE PERFORMANCE OF YOUR PAD, NETWORK OR COMPUTER SYSTEM WHEN USED IN CONJUNCTION WITH THE PRODUCT, NOR THAT THE PRODUCT WILL MEET YOUR REQUIREMENTS OR THAT ITS OPERATION WILL BE UNINTERRUPTED OR ERROR-FREE.

EXCEPT IN RESPECT OF DEATH OR PERSONAL INJURY CAUSED BY THE SUPPLIERS' NEGLIGENCE AND TO THE FULLEST EXTENT PERMITTED BY LAW, IN NO EVENT (AND REGARDLESS OF WHETHER SUCH DAMAGES ARE FORESEEABLE AND OF WHETHER SUCH LIABILITY IS BASED IN TORT, CONTRACT OR OTHERWISE) WILL ANY OF THE SUPPLIERS BE LIABLE TO YOU FOR ANY DAMAGES (INCLUDING, WITHOUT LIMITATION, ANY LOST PROFITS, LOST SAVINGS OR OTHER SPECIAL, INDIRECT, INCIDENTAL OR CONSEQUENTIAL DAMAGES ARISING OUT OF OR RESULTING FROM: (I) YOUR USE OF, OR INABILITY TO USE, THE PRODUCT; (II) DATA LOSS OR CORRUPTION; AND/OR (III) ERRORS OR OMISSIONS IN THE PROPRIETARY MATERIAL.

IF THE FOREGOING LIMITATION IS HELD TO BE UNENFORCEABLE, OUR MAXIMUM LIABILITY TO YOU IN RESPECT THEREOF SHALL NOT EXCEED THE AMOUNT OF THE LICENCE FEE PAID BY YOU FOR THE PRODUCT. THE REMEDIES AVAILABLE TO YOU AGAINST ELSEVIER AND THE LICENSORS OF MATERIALS INCLUDED IN THE PRODUCT ARE EXCLUSIVE.

If the information provided in the Product contains medical or health sciences information, it is intended for professional use within the medical field. Information about medical treatment or drug dosages is intended strictly for professional use, and because of rapid advances in the medical sciences, independent verification of diagnosis and drug dosages should be made.

The provisions of this Agreement shall be severable, and in the event that any provision of this Agreement is found to be legally unenforceable, such unenforceability shall not prevent the enforcement or any other provision of this Agreement.

GOVERNING LAW This Agreement shall be governed by the laws of England and Wales. In any dispute arising out of this Agreement, you and Elsevier each consent to the exclusive personal jurisdiction and venue in the courts of England and Wales.